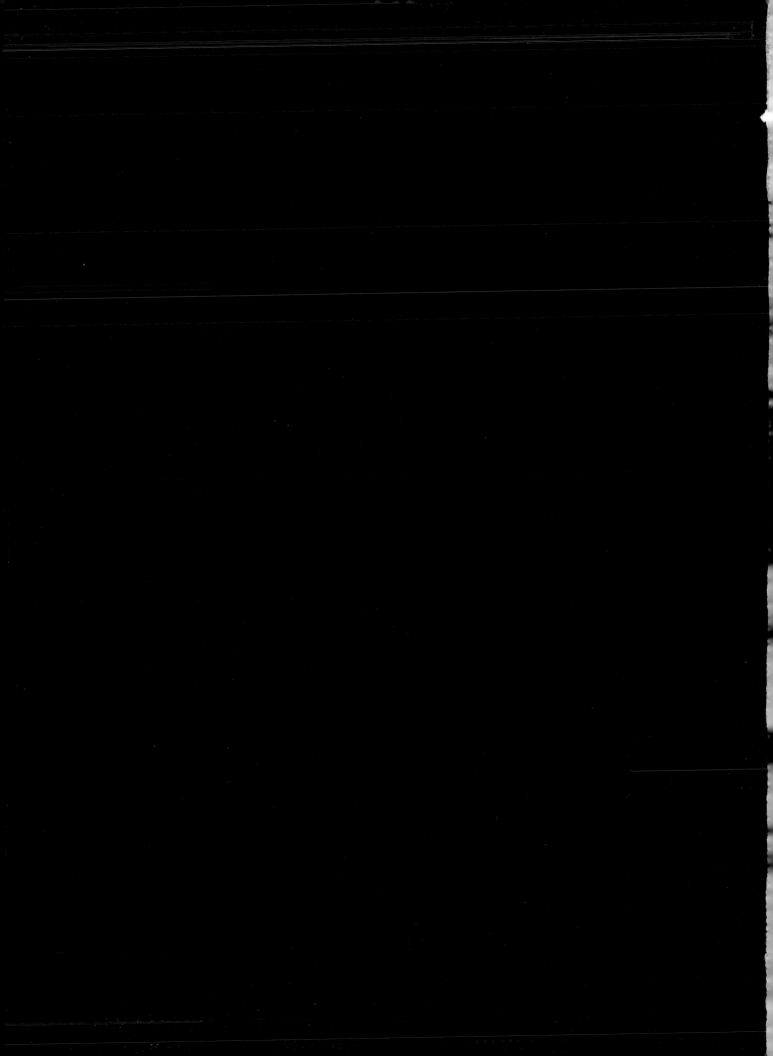

CONTEMPORARY
ORTHODONTICS

CONTEMPORARY ORTHODONTICS

WILLIAM R. PROFFIT, D.D.S., Ph.D.
Kenan Professor and Chairman, Department of Orthodontics,
School of Dentistry, University of North Carolina,
Chapel Hill, North Carolina

with

Henry W. Fields, Jr., D.D.S., M.S., M.S.D.
Professor, Orthodontics,
Dean, College of Dentistry, The Ohio State University,
Columbus, Ohio

and

James L. Ackerman
L'Tanya J. Bailey
J.F. Camilla Tulloch

THIRD EDITION

With 1939 Illustrations

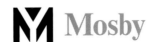 Mosby

An Imprint of Elsevier Science

St. Louis   London   Philadelphia   Sydney   Toronto

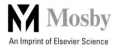

Editor: Penny Rudolph
Developmental Editor: Kimberly Frare
Project Manager: Dana Peick
Production Editor: Jodi Everding
Designer: Judi Lang

THIRD EDITION

Mosby, Inc.
An Imprint of Elsevier Science
11830 Westline Industrial Drive
St. Louis, Missouri 63146

Printed in United States

Library of Congress Cataloging-in-Publication Data

Proffit, William R.
    Contemporary orthodontics / William R. Proffit with Henry W.
  Fields ... [et al.]. — 3rd ed.
       p.   cm.
  Includes bibliographical references and index.
    ISBN 1-55664-553-8 (alk. paper)
    1. Orthodontics.   I. Fields, Henry W.   II. Title.
RK521.P76   1999
617.6'43—dc21   99-24758

02 03 04 / 9 8 7 6 5 4 3

Contributors

James L. Ackerman, D.D.S.
Private Practice, Bryn Mawr, Pennsylvania;
Formerly Professor and Chairman, Department of Orthodontics,
University of Pennsylvania, School of Dental Medicine,
Philadelphia, Pennsylvania

L'Tanya J. Bailey, D.D.S., M.S.D.
Associate Professor and Graduate Program Director,
Department of Orthodontics,
School of Dentistry, University of North Carolina,
Chapel Hill, North Carolina

J.F. Camilla Tulloch, B.D.S., D. Orth.
G. Fred Hale Professor,
Department of Orthodontics,
School of Dentistry, University of North Carolina,
Chapel Hill, North Carolina

Preface

As in previous editions, the objective of *Contemporary Orthodontics* is to provide a comprehensive overview of this subject that is accessible to students, useful for residents, and a valuable reference for practitioners. Our goal has been to put information into a perspective that facilitates clinical use in a rational way.

This third edition follows the basic outline of previous editions, incorporating much new information without changing the overall approach and organization. There is an increased emphasis on the use of computer database applications and computer simulations in diagnosis and treatment planning, a particular focus on clinical decisions based on data instead of on anecdote and opinion, and additional material on clinical biomechanics that reflects the continued rapid progress in this area.

For use in the dental curriculum and residency programs, the book now is supplemented with extensive audiovisual and computer-based teaching materials. The slide-tape sequences that supplemented basic and applied growth and development sections have been replaced with computer teaching programs (available in both Windows and Macintosh versions), and several new video cassettes incorporate computer graphics. The most impressive advance in these supplemental teaching materials, however, is the availability of computer self-tests (for instruction, not evaluation), which not only tell students if they have correctly answered questions about the material they just studied but also they tell them why answers are correct or incorrect and display appropriate graphics (graphs, clinical photos, etc.) to reinforce the message. These tests now accompany both the video and computer programs for basic and applied growth and development. The result has been a further increase in the number of students who really master the material, beyond the improvements produced by self-instruction without this reinforcement.

Further information about supplemental teaching materials, including video cassettes, computer teaching programs, and computer self-tests, can be obtained by contacting the Department of Orthodontics, University of North Carolina School of Dentistry, Chapel Hill, NC 27599-7450, or by visiting the department's home page on the Internet at http://ortho.dent.unc.edu.

We thank Marion Blackburn for new and revised artwork for this edition, Ramona Hutton-Howe for photographic support, and Faith Patterson for careful organization and management of the revision. Particular thanks also go to Drs. Kelly Mitchell, Andy Hass, Bo-Hoon Joo, and Mr. Will Harvey for their assistance in obtaining new illustrations and background material. A number of individuals have reviewed areas of the manuscript and kindly contributed illustrations; specific acknowledgement is provided at appropriate points throughout the book.

William R. Proffit
Henry W. Fields, Jr.

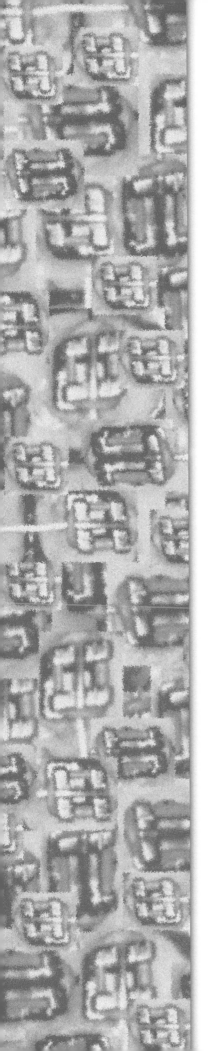

Contents

CONTEMPORARY
ORTHODONTICS

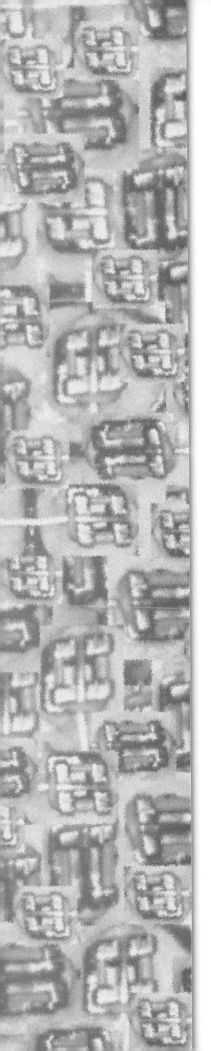

SECTION

I

THE ORTHODONTIC PROBLEM

CHAPTER 1

Malocclusion and Dentofacial Deformity in Contemporary Society

The changing goals of orthodontic treatment
    Orthodontics (dentofacial orthopedics)
The usual orthodontic problems: epidemiology of
    malocclusion
Why is malocclusion so prevalent?
Need and demand for orthodontic treatment
    Need for orthodontic treatment
    Demand for orthodontic treatment

THE CHANGING GOALS OF ORTHODONTIC TREATMENT

Crowded, irregular, and protruding teeth have been a problem for some individuals since antiquity, and attempts to correct this disorder go back at least to 1000 BC. Primitive (and surprisingly well designed) orthodontic appliances have been found in both Greek and Etruscan materials.[1] As dentistry developed in the eighteenth and nineteenth centuries, a number of devices for the "regulation" of the teeth were described by various authors and apparently used sporadically by the dentists of that era.

After 1850, the first texts that systematically described orthodontics appeared, the most notable being Norman Kingsley's *Oral Deformities*.[2] Kingsley (Figure 1-1), who had a tremendous influence on American dentistry in the latter half of the nineteenth century, was among the first to use extraoral force to correct protruding teeth. He was also a pioneer in the treatment of cleft palate and related problems.

Despite the contributions of Kingsley and his contemporaries, their emphasis in orthodontics remained the alignment of the teeth and the correction of facial proportions. Little attention was paid to the dental occlusion, and since it was common practice to remove teeth for many dental problems, extractions for crowding or malalignment were frequent. In an era when an intact dentition was a rarity, the details of occlusal relationships were considered unimportant.

In order to make good prosthetic replacement teeth, it was necessary to develop a concept of occlusion, and this occurred in the late 1800s. As the concepts of prosthetic occlusion developed and were refined, it was natural to extend this to the natural dentition. Edward H. Angle (Figure 1-2), whose influence began to be felt about 1890, can be credited with much of the development of a concept of occlusion in the natural dentition. Angle's original interest was in prosthodontics, and he taught in that department in the dental schools at Pennsylvania and Minnesota in the 1880s. His increasing interest in dental occlusion and in the treatment necessary to obtain normal occlusion led directly to his development of orthodontics as a specialty, with himself as the "father of modern orthodontics."

The publication of Angle's classification of malocclusion in the 1890s[3] was an important step in the development of orthodontics because it not only subdivided major types of malocclusion but also included the first clear and simple definition of normal occlusion in the natural dentition. Angle's postulate was that the upper first molars were the key to occlusion and that the upper and lower molars should be related so that the mesiobuccal cusp of the upper molar occludes in the buccal groove of the lower molar. If this molar relationship existed and the teeth were arranged on a smoothly curving line of occlusion (Figure 1-3), then normal occlusion would result. This statement, which 100 years of experience has proved to be correct—except when there are aberrations in the size of teeth, brilliantly simplified normal occlusion.

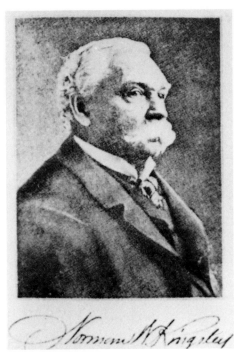

FIGURE 1-1 Norman Kingsley's self-portrait. Kingsley, who was a noted sculptor and artist as well as an influential dentist, also served as Dean of the School of Dentistry at New York University.

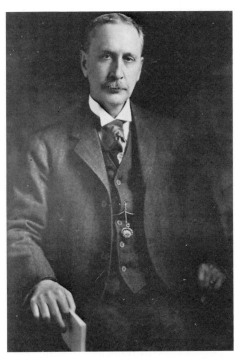

FIGURE 1-2 Edward H. Angle in his early forties, near the time that he established himself as the first dental specialist. From 1905 to 1928, Angle operated proprietary orthodontic schools in St. Louis; New London, Connecticut; and Pasadena, California, in which many of the pioneer American orthodontists were trained.

Angle then described three classes of malocclusion, based on the occlusal relationships of the first molars:

Class I   Normal relationship of the molars, but line of occlusion incorrect because of malposed teeth, rotations, or other causes

Class II   Lower molar distally positioned relative to upper molar, line of occlusion not specified

Class III   Lower molar mesially positioned relative to upper molar, line of occlusion not specified

Note that the Angle classification has four classes: normal occlusion, Class I malocclusion, Class II malocclusion, and Class III malocclusion (Figure 1-4). Normal occlusion and Class I malocclusion share the same molar relationship but differ in the arrangement of the teeth relative to the line of occlusion. The line of occlusion may or may not be correct in Class II and Class III.

With the establishment of a concept of normal occlusion and a classification scheme that incorporated the line of occlusion, by the early 1900s orthodontics was no longer just the alignment of irregular teeth. Instead, it had evolved into the treatment of malocclusion, defined as any deviation from the ideal occlusal scheme described by Angle. Since precisely defined relationships required a full complement of teeth in both arches, maintaining an intact dentition became an important goal of orthodontic treatment. Angle and his followers strongly opposed extraction for orthodontic purposes. With the emphasis on dental occlusion that followed, however, less attention came to be paid to

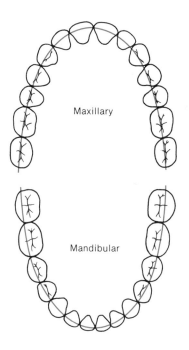

FIGURE 1-3 The line of occlusion is a smooth (catenary) curve passing through the central fossa of each upper molar and across the cingulum of the upper canine and incisor teeth. The same line runs along the buccal cusps and incisal edges of the lower teeth, thus specifying the occlusal as well as interarch relationships once the molar position is established.

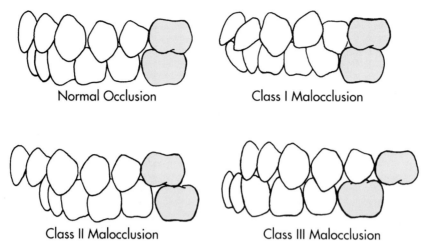

FIGURE 1-4   Normal occlusion and malocclusion classes as specified by Angle. This classification was quickly and widely adopted early in the twentieth century. It is incorporated within all contemporary descriptive and classification schemes.

facial proportions and esthetics. Angle abandoned extra-oral force because he decided this was not necessary to achieve proper occlusal relationships.

As time passed, it became clear that even an excellent occlusion was unsatisfactory if it was achieved at the expense of proper facial proportions. Not only were there esthetic problems, it often proved impossible to maintain an occlusal relationship achieved by prolonged use of heavy elastics to pull the teeth together as Angle and his followers had suggested. Extraction of teeth was reintroduced into orthodontics in the 1930s to enhance facial esthetics and achieve better stability of the occlusal relationships.

Cephalometric radiography, which enabled orthodontists to measure the changes in tooth and jaw positions produced by growth and treatment, came into widespread use after World War II. These radiographs made it clear that many Class II and Class III malocclusions resulted from faulty jaw relationships, not just malposed teeth. By use of cephalometrics, it also was possible to see that jaw growth could be altered by orthodontic treatment. In Europe, the method of "functional jaw orthopedics" was developed to enhance growth changes, while in the United States, extraoral force came to be used for this purpose. At present, both functional and extraoral appliances are used internationally to control and modify growth and form.

As the 21st century begins, orthodontics differs from what was done previously in three important ways: (1) there is more emphasis now on dental and facial esthetics, and less on details of dental occlusion. This has resulted from the advent of orthognathic surgery, which makes it possible to correct facial disproportions that previously were not treatable, and the development of computer imaging methods that allow the orthodontist to share facial concerns with patients in a way that was not possible until recently; (2) patients now expect and are granted a greater degree of involvement in planning treatment. No longer is it appro-

priate for the paternalistic doctor to simply tell patients what treatment they should have. Now patients are given the opportunity to participate in selecting among treatment options—which the computer imaging methods also facilitate. The recent text by Sarver[4] illustrates both these developments very nicely; and (3) orthodontics now is offered much more frequently to older patients as part of a multidisciplinary treatment plan involving other dental and medical specialties. The goal is not necessarily the best possible dental occlusion or facial esthetics but the best chance for long-term maintenance of the dentition. This increased emphasis on treatment coordinated with other dentists has the effect of integrating orthodontics back into the mainstream of dentistry, from which Angle's teachings had tended to separate it. All three of these recent developments are reflected in the later chapters of this book.

The goal of modern orthodontics can be summed up as the creation of the best balance among occlusal relationships, dental and facial esthetics, stability of the result and long-term maintenance, and restoration of the dentition. The two cases shown in Figures 1-5 through 1-10 demonstrate the excellent results that can be attained through orthodontics. The current definition of orthodontics indicates the change in focus.

Orthodontics (Dentofacial Orthopedics)

Orthodontics now is formally defined (by the American Association of Orthodontists) as: the area of dentistry concerned with the supervision, guidance and correction of the growing and mature dentofacial structures, including those conditions that require movement of teeth or correction of malrelationships and malformations of related structures by the adjustment of relationships between and among teeth and facial bones by the application of forces and/or the stimulation and redirection of the functional forces within the craniofacial complex.

Text continued on p. 9

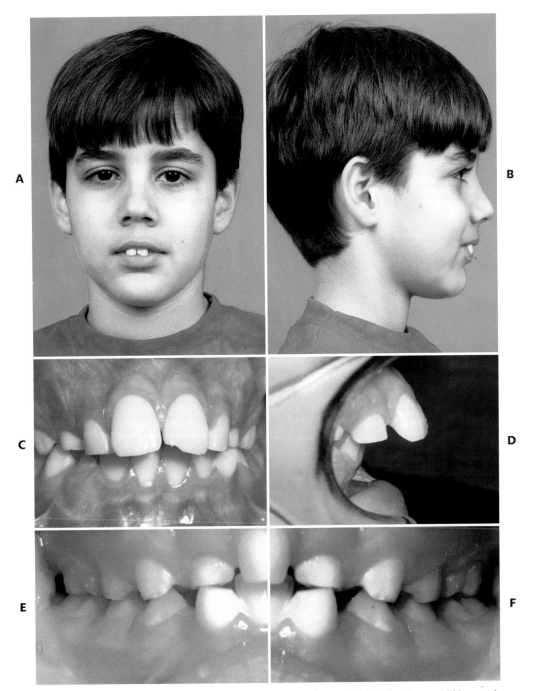

FIGURE 1-5   Pre-treatment facial (**A,B**) and intra-oral views (**C-F**) of a 12-year-old boy with Class II division 1 malocclusion. His chief complaint was the protruding upper incisors, which created both esthetic and functional problems. Examination of the facial profile shows that, as usually is the case with Class II problems, the major problem is an underdeveloped lower jaw. Note also the deep bite anteriorly, because the lower incisors have erupted up against the palate.

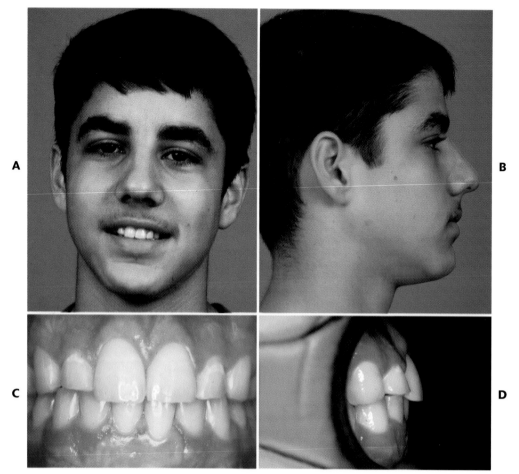

FIGURE 1-6 Post-treatment (age 14) facial (**A,B**) and intra-oral views (**C,D**) of the boy in Figure 1-5. He wore a headgear to the upper molars and had a complete fixed appliance in place for 26 months of active treatment. Note the improved facial appearance and resolution of both overjet and overbite.

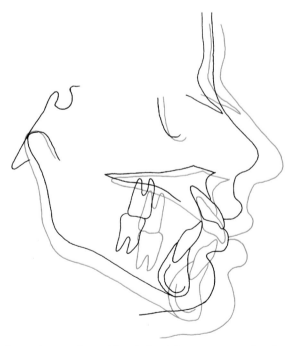

FIGURE 1-7 Cephalometric superimposition before/after treatment for the patient in Figure 1-5. Note the favorable downward-forward growth of the mandible and minimal forward growth of the maxilla, along with retraction of the maxillary incisors, some forward movement of the lower teeth, and differential eruption of the lower posterior teeth. The improvement during treatment occurred because of a combination of growth modification and tooth movement.

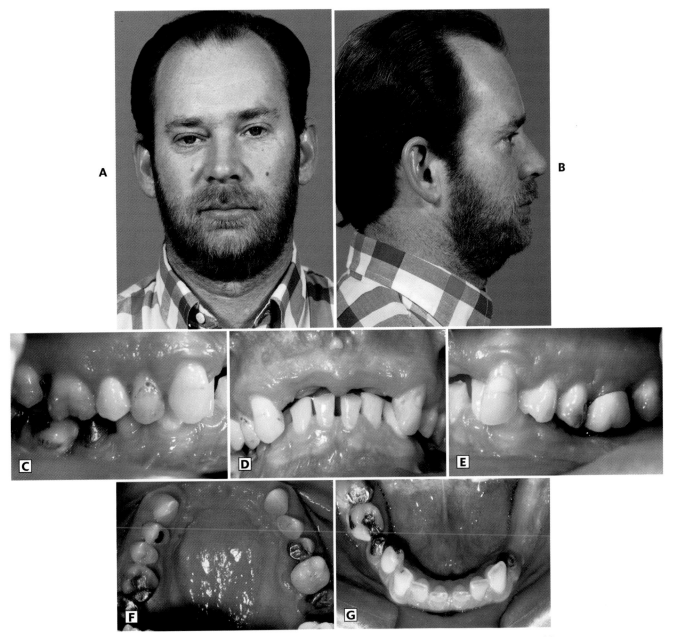

FIGURE 1-8 Pre-treatment facial (**A,B**) and intra-oral (**C-G**) views of a 42-year-old man with severe Class II malocclusion and loss of multiple teeth due to trauma to palatal tissues from his impinging overbite, caries, and periodontal disease. His primary motivation was satisfactory replacement of his upper incisors and preventing loss of all his teeth, but he also hoped for improved function and esthetics. He was willing to accept periodontal, orthodontic, surgical, and prosthodontic treatment.

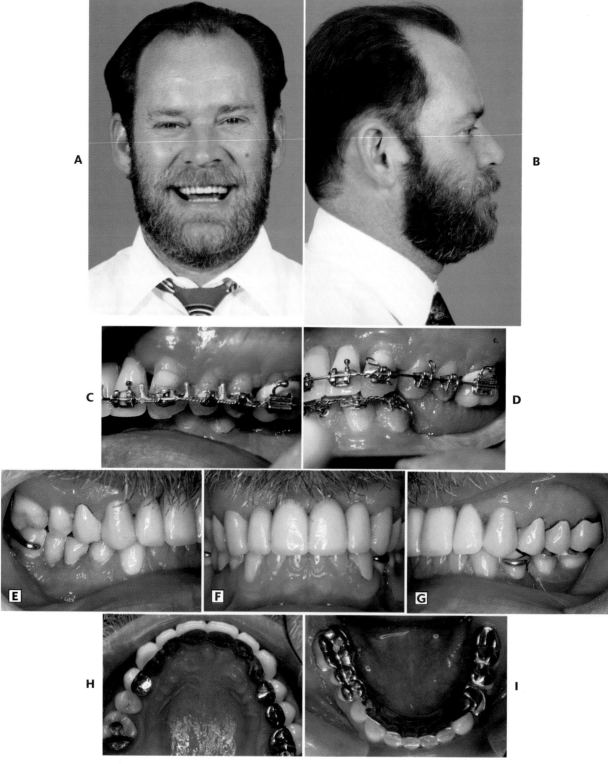

FIGURE 1-9   For the patient in Figure 1-8, post-treatment (age 44) facial (**A,B**) views; dental relationships immediately before (**C**) and after (**D**) orthognathic surgery to bring the lower jaw forward; and dental relationships after completion of orthodontics, fixed restorations in the upper arch, and a lower removable partial denture (**E-I**).

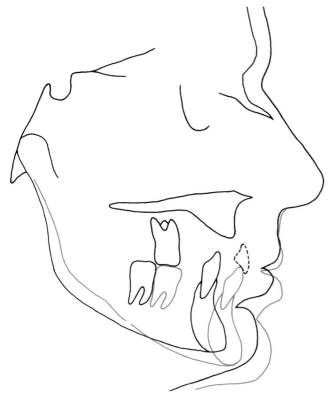

FIGURE 1-10 For the patient shown in Figures 1-8 and 1-9, cephalometric superimposition showing the change in mandibular position created by orthognathic surgery. Note that the mandible was moved forward and rotated downward anteriorly, improving both the anterior-posterior (a-p) and vertical position of the chin, and providing vertical space for appropriate prosthetic rehabilitation.

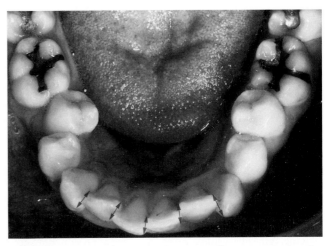

FIGURE 1-11 Incisor irregularity usually is expressed as the irregularity index; the total of the millimeter distances from the contact point on each tooth to the contact point that it should touch.

Major responsibilities of orthodontic practice include the diagnosis, prevention, interception, and treatment of all forms of malocclusion of the teeth and associated alterations in their surrounding structures; the design, application, and control of functional and corrective appliances; and the guidance of the dentition and its supporting structures to attain and maintain optimum relations in physiologic and esthetic harmony among facial and cranial structures.[5]

THE USUAL ORTHODONTIC PROBLEMS: EPIDEMIOLOGY OF MALOCCLUSION

What Angle defined as normal occlusion more properly should be considered the ideal, especially when the criteria are applied strictly. In fact, perfectly interdigitating teeth arranged along a perfectly regular line of occlusion are quite rare. For many years, epidemiologic studies of malocclusion suffered from considerable disagreement among the investigators about how much deviation from the ideal should be accepted within the bounds of normal. As a result, between 1930 and 1965 the prevalence of malocclusion in the United States was variously estimated as 35% to 95%. These tremendous disparities were largely the result of the investigators' differing criteria for normal.

By the 1970s, a series of studies by public health or university groups in most developed countries provided a reasonably clear worldwide picture of the prevalence of various occlusal relationships or malrelationships. In the United States, two large-scale surveys carried out by the Division of Health Statistics of the U.S. Public Health Service (USPHS) covered children ages 6 to 11 between 1963 and 1965 and youths ages 12 to 17 between 1969 and 1970.[6,7] As part of a large-scale national survey of health care problems and needs in the United States in 1989-1994 (National Health and Nutrition Estimates Survey III, abbreviated as NHANES III), estimates of malocclusion again were obtained. This study of some 14,000 individuals was statistically designed to provide weighted estimates for approximately 150 million persons in the sampled racial/ethnic and age groups. The data provide current information for U.S. children and youths and include the first good data set for malocclusion in adults, with separate estimates for the major racial/ethnic groups.[8,9]

The characteristics of malocclusion evaluated in NHANES III included the irregularity index, a measure of incisor alignment (see Figure 1-11), the prevalence of midline diastema >2 mm (see Figure 1-12), and the prevalence of posterior crossbite (see Figure 1-13). In addition, overjet (see Figure 1-14) and overbite/open bite (see Figure 1-15) were measured. Overjet, which reflects Angle's Class II and Class III molar relationships, can be evaluated much more precisely under epidemiologic evaluation conditions, so molar relationship was not evaluated directly.

Current data for these characteristics of malocclusion for children (age 8 to 11), youths (age 12 to 17) and adults (age 18 to 50) in the U.S. population, taken from

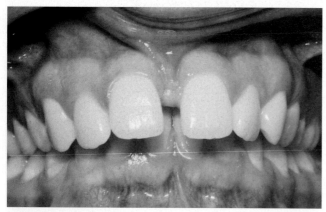

FIGURE 1-12   A space between adjacent teeth is called a **diastema**. A maxillary midline diastema is relatively common, especially during the mixed dentition in childhood. A midline diastema >2 mm rarely closes spontaneously with further development, however.

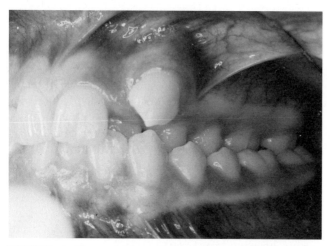

FIGURE 1-13   Posterior crossbite exists when the maxillary posterior teeth are lingually positioned relative to the mandibular teeth, as in this patient. Posterior crossbite most often reflects a narrow maxillary dental arch but can arise from other causes.

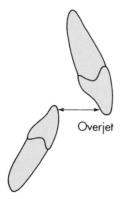

FIGURE 1-14   Overjet is defined as horizontal overlap of the incisors. Normally the incisors are in contact, with the upper incisors ahead of the lower by only the thickness of the upper edges (i.e., 2-3 mm overjet is the normal relationship). If the lower incisors are in front of the upper incisors, the condition is called reverse overjet or anterior crossbite.

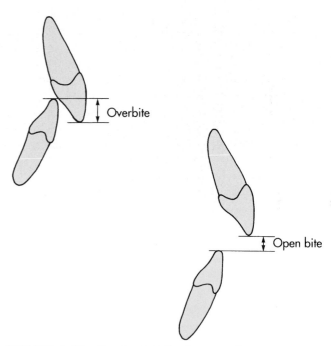

FIGURE 1-15   Overbite is defined as vertical overlap of the incisors. Normally the lower incisal edges contact the lingual surface of the upper incisors at or above the cingulum (i.e., normally there is 1 to 2 mm overbite). In open bite, there is no vertical overlap, and the vertical separation is measured.

NHANES III, are shown in Tables 1-1 and 1-2 and are displayed graphically in Figures 1-16 to 1-19.

Note that just over half of U.S. children age 8 to 11 have well-aligned incisors. The rest have varying degrees of malalignment and crowding. The percent with excellent alignment decreases by age 12 to 17 as the remaining permanent teeth erupt, then remains essentially stable in the upper arch but worsens in the lower arch for adults. Only 34% of adults have well-aligned lower incisors.

Nearly 15% of adolescents and adults have severely or extremely irregular incisors, so that major arch expansion or extraction of some teeth would be necessary to align them. A wide space between the maxillary central incisors (midline diastema) often is present in childhood (26% have >2 mm space). Although this space tends to close, over 6% of youths and adults still have a noticeable diastema. Blacks are more than twice as likely to have a midline diastema than whites or Hispanics (p<.001).

Posterior crossbite reflects deviations from ideal occlusion in the transverse plane of space, overjet or reverse overjet indicate antero-posterior deviations in the Class II/Class III direction, and overbite/open bite indicate vertical deviations from ideal. As Table 1-2 shows, posterior crossbite is relatively rare at all ages. Overjet of 5 mm or more, suggesting Angle's Class II malocclusion, occurs in 23% of children, 15% of youths, and 13% of adults. Reverse overjet, indicative of Class III malocclusion, is much less frequent. This affects about 1% of American children

TABLE 1-1 *Percent of U.S. Population with Incisor Crowding/Malalignment*

Total Population, by Age

Irregularity Index	Age 8-11		Age 12-17		Age 18-50	
	Max	Mand	Max	Mand	Max	Mand
0-1 [ideal]	52.7	54.5	42.3	43.7	43.2	33.7
2-3 [mild crowding]	25.3	25.0	26.8	25.2	26.5	27.3
4-6 [moderate]	13.3	15.9	18.4	18.5	19.7	23.3
7-10 [severe]	6.2	3.5	9.4	8.9	8.0	11.4
>10 [extreme]	2.5	1.2	3.2	3.6	2.7	4.3
Midline diastema >2 mm	26.4		6.6		6.4	

Racial/Ethnic Groups, Ages Combined

Irregularity Index	White		Black		Hispanic		Total	
	Max	Mand	Max	Mand	Max	Mand	Max	Mand
0-1 [ideal]	43.8	35.6	48.1	45.6	35.9	38.8	44.0	37.1
2-3 [mild crowding]	26.3	26.9	27.0	27.2	26.5	23.0	26.4	26.8
4-6 [moderate]	19.1	22.6	15.7	17.1	22.5	23.8	18.8	21.9
7-10 [severe]	8.0	10.8	6.7	7.2	12.1	9.6	8.0	10.3
>10 [extreme]	2.8	4.0	2.5	3.0	3.0	4.8	2.8	3.9
Midline diastema >2 mm	7.0		18.9		6.7		8.5	

Data from NHANES III

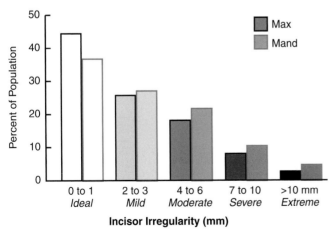

FIGURE 1-16 Incisor irregularity in the U.S. population, 1989-1994. One-third of the population have at least moderately irregular (usually crowded) incisors, and nearly 15% have severe or extreme irregularity.

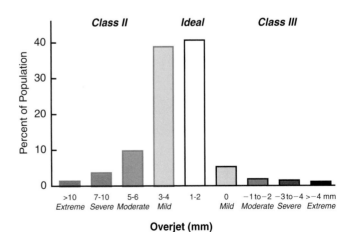

FIGURE 1-17 Overjet (Class II) and reverse overjet (Class III) in the U.S. population, 1989-1994. Only one-third of the population have ideal antero-posterior incisor relationships, but overjet is only moderately increased in another one-third. Increased overjet accompanying Class II malocclusion is much more prevalent than reverse overjet accompanying Class III.

TABLE 1-2   *Percent of U.S. Population with Occlusal Contact Discrepancies*

		8-11*	12-17*	18-50*	White†	Black†	Hispanic†	Total
Posterior Crossbite		7.1	8.8	9.5	9.1	9.6	7.3	9.1
Overjet (mm)								
Class II								
>10	[extreme]	0.2	0.2	0.4	0.3	0.4	0.4	0.3
7-10	[severe]	3.4	3.5	3.9	3.8	4.3	2.2	3.8
5-6	[moderate]	18.9	11.9	9.1	10.1	11.8	6.5	10.6
3-4	[mild]	45.2	39.5	37.7	38.0	39.8	49.0	38.8
Ideal								
1-2		29.6	39.3	43.0	42.4	35.6	33.6	41.1
Class III								
0	[mild]	2.2	4.6	4.8	4.1	6.1	6.7	4.5
–1 to –2	[moderate]	0.7	0.5	0.7	0.5	1.5	0.9	0.6
–3 to –4	[severe]	0.0	0.6	0.2	0.2	0.4	0.4	0.3
> –4	[extreme]	0.0	0.0	0.1	0.1	0.1	0.3	0.2
Overbite (mm)								
Open bite								
> –4	[extreme]	0.3	0.2	0.1	0.1	0.7	0.0	0.1
–3 to –4	[severe]	0.6	0.5	0.5	0.4	1.3	0.0	0.5
0 to –2	[moderate]	2.7	2.8	2.7	2.4	4.6	2.1	2.7
Ideal								
0-2		40.2	45.0	49.0	45.5	56.4	56.5	47.5
Deep bite								
3 - 4	[moderate]	36.2	34.7	32.5	34.0	28.5	32.6	33.1
5 - 7	[severe]	18.8	15.5	13.4	15.7	7.5	8.7	14.2
>7	[extreme]	1.2	1.3	1.8	1.9	0.9	0.0	1.7

Data from NHANES III

*All racial/ethnic groups.

†All ages.

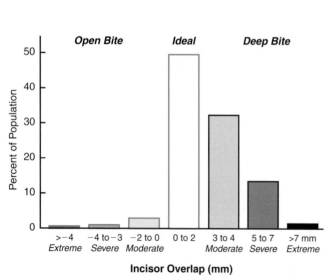

FIGURE 1-18   Open bite/deep bite relationships in the U.S. population, 1989-1994. Half the population have an ideal vertical relationship of the incisors. Deep bite is much more prevalent than open bite. Vertical relationships vary greatly between racial groups (see Table 1-2).

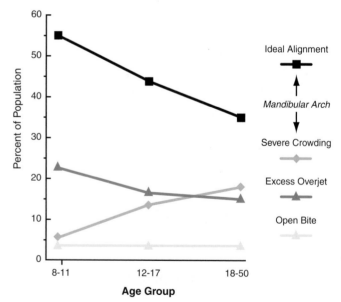

FIGURE 1-19   Changes in the prevalence of types of malocclusion from childhood to adult life, United States, 1989-1994. Note the increase in incisor irregularity and decrease in severe overjet, both of which are related to mandibular growth.

and increases slightly in youths and adults. Severe Class II and Class III problems, at the limit of orthodontic correction, occur in about 4% of the population, with severe Class II much more prevalent. Both severe Class II and Class III are more prevalent in the Hispanic than the white or black groups (p<.03).

Vertical deviations from the ideal overbite of 0-2 mm are less frequent in adults than children but occur in half the adult population, the great majority of whom have excessive overbite. Severe deep bite (overbite ≥ 5 mm) is found in nearly 20% of children and 13% of adults, while open bite (negative overbite >-2 mm) occurs in less than 1%. There are striking differences between the racial/ethnic groups in vertical dental relationships. Severe deep bite is nearly twice as prevalent in whites as blacks or Hispanics (p<.001), while open bite >2 mm is five times more prevalent in blacks than in whites or Hispanics (p<.001). This almost surely reflects the slightly different craniofacial proportions of the black population groups (see Chapter 5 for a more complete discussion). Despite their higher prevalence of antero-posterior problems, vertical problems are less prevalent in Hispanics than either blacks or whites.

From the survey data, it is interesting to calculate the percentage of American children and youths who would fall into Angle's four groups. From this perspective, 30% at most have Angle's normal occlusion. Class I malocclusion (50% to 55%) is by far the largest single group; there are about half as many Class II malocclusions (approximately 15%) as normal occlusion; and Class III (less than 1%) represents a very small proportion of the total.

Differences in malocclusion characteristics between the United States and other countries would be expected because of differences in racial and ethnic composition. Although the available data are not as extensive as for American populations, it seems clear that Class II problems are most prevalent in whites of northern European descent (for instance, 25% of children in Denmark are reported to be Class II), while Class III problems are most prevalent in Asian populations (3% to 5% in Japan, nearly 2% in China with another 2% to 3% pseudo-Class III, [i.e., shifting into anterior crossbite because of incisor interferences]).[10] African populations are by no means homogenous, but from the differences found in the United States between blacks and whites, it seems likely that Class III and open bite are more frequent in African than European populations and deep bite less frequent.

WHY IS MALOCCLUSION SO PREVALENT?

Although malocclusion now occurs in a majority of the population, that does not mean it is normal. Skeletal remains indicate that the present prevalence is several times greater than it was only a few hundred years ago. Crowding and malalignment of teeth was unusual until relatively recently[11] (but not unknown [Figure 1-20]). Because the mandible tends to become separated from the rest of the skull when long-buried skeletal remains are unearthed, it is easier to be sure what has happened to alignment of teeth than to occlusal relationships. The skeletal remains suggest that all members of a group might tend toward a Class III,

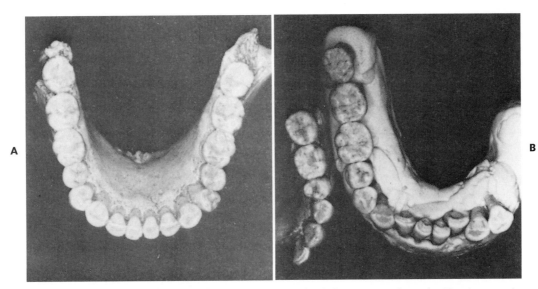

Figure 1-20   Mandibular dental arches from Neanderthal specimens from the Krapina cave in Yugoslavia, estimated to be approximately 100,000 years old. **A,** Note the excellent alignment in the specimen. **B,** Crowding and malalignment are seen in this specimen, which had the largest teeth in this find of skeletal remains from approximately 80 individuals. (From Wolpoff WH: *Paleoanthropology*, New York, 1998, Alfred A Knopf.)

PAST AND PRESENT TOOTH SIZE

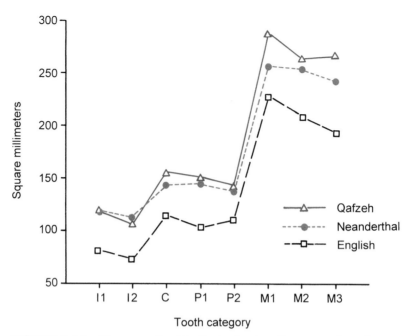

FIGURE 1-21   The generalized decline in the size of human teeth can be seen by comparing tooth sizes from the anthropological site at Qafzeh, dated 100,000 years ago; Neanderthal teeth, 10,000 years ago; and modern human populations. (Redrawn from Kelly MA, Larsen CS (editors): *Advances in dental anthropology*, New York, 1991, Wiley-Liss.)

or less commonly, a Class II jaw relationship. Similar findings are noted in present population groups that have remained largely unaffected by modern development: crowding and malalignment of teeth are uncommon, but the majority of the group may have mild anteroposterior or transverse discrepancies, as in the Class III tendency of South Pacific islanders[12] and buccal crossbite (X-occlusion) in Australian aborigines.[13]

Although 1000 years is a long time relative to a single human life, it is a very short time from an evolutionary perspective. The fossil record documents evolutionary trends over many thousands of years that affect the present dentition, including a decrease in the size of individual teeth, a decrease in the number of the teeth, and a decrease in the size of the jaws. For example, there has been a steady reduction in the size of both anterior and posterior teeth over at least the last 100,000 years (Figure 1-21). The number of teeth in the dentition of higher primates has been reduced compared with the usual mammalian pattern (Figure 1-22). The third incisor and third premolar have disappeared, as has the fourth molar. At present, the human third molar, second premolar, and second incisor often fail to develop, which indicates that these teeth may be on their way out. Compared with primitive peoples, modern human beings have quite underdeveloped jaws.

It is easy to see that the progressive reduction in jaw size, if not well matched to a decrease in tooth size and number, could lead to crowding and malalignment. It is less easy to see why dental crowding should have increased quite recently, but this seems to have paralleled the transition from primitive agricultural to modern urbanized societies. Cardiovascular disease and related health problems appear rapidly when a previously unaffected population group leaves agrarian life for the city and civilization. High blood pressure, heart disease, diabetes, and several other medical problems are so much more prevalent in developed than underdeveloped countries that they have been labeled "diseases of civilization." There is some evidence that malocclusion increases within well-defined populations after a transition from rural villages to the city. Corruccini, for instance, reports a higher prevalence of crowding, posterior crossbite, and buccal segment discrepancy in urbanized youths compared with rural Punjabi youths of northern India.[14] One can argue that malocclusion is another condition made worse by the changing conditions of modern life, perhaps resulting in part from less use of the masticatory apparatus with softer foods now. Under primitive conditions, of course, excellent function of the jaws and teeth was an important predictor of the ability to survive and reproduce. A capable masticatory apparatus was essential to deal with uncooked or partially cooked meat and plant foods.

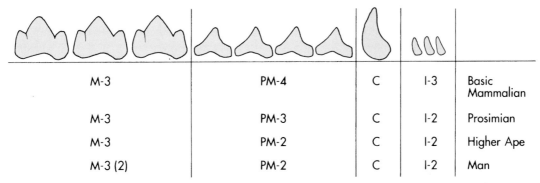

M-3	PM-4	C	I-3	Basic Mammalian
M-3	PM-3	C	I-2	Prosimian
M-3	PM-2	C	I-2	Higher Ape
M-3 (2)	PM-2	C	I-2	Man

FIGURE 1-22 Reduction in the number of teeth has been a feature of primate evolution. In the present human population, third molars are so frequently missing that it appears a further reduction is in progress, and the variability of lateral incisors and second premolars suggests evolutionary pressure of these teeth.

Watching an Australian aboriginal man using every muscle of his upper body to tear off a piece of kangaroo flesh from the barely cooked animal, for instance, makes one appreciate the decrease in demand on the masticatory apparatus that has accompanied civilization (Figure 1-23).

Determining whether changes in jaw function have increased the prevalence of malocclusion is complicated by the fact that both dental caries and periodontal disease, which are rare on the primitive diet, appear rapidly when the diet changes. The resulting dental pathology can make it difficult to establish what the occlusion might have been in the absence of early loss of teeth, gingivitis and periodontal breakdown. The increase in malocclusion in modern times certainly parallels the development of modern civilization, but a reduction in jaw size related to disuse atrophy is hard to document, and the parallel with stress-related diseases can be carried only so far. Although it is difficult to know the precise cause of any specific malocclusion, we do know in general what the etiologic possibilities are, and these are discussed in some detail in Chapter 5.

What difference does it make if you have a malocclusion? Let us consider now the reasons for orthodontic treatment.

NEED AND DEMAND FOR ORTHODONTIC TREATMENT

Need for Orthodontic Treatment

Protruding, irregular, or maloccluded teeth can cause three types of problems for the patient: (1) discrimination because of facial appearance; (2) problems with oral function, including difficulties in jaw movement (muscle incoordination or pain), temporomandibular joint dysfunction (TMD), and problems with mastication, swallowing or speech; and (3) greater susceptibility to trauma, periodontal disease, or tooth decay.

Psychosocial Problems. A number of studies in recent years have confirmed what is intuitively obvious, that severe malocclusion is likely to be a social handicap. The

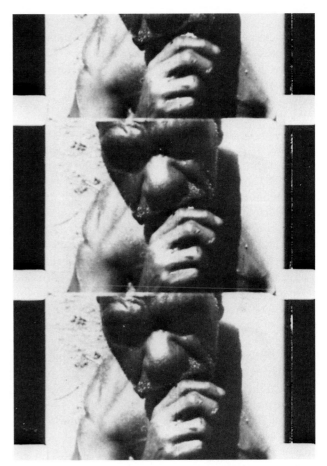

FIGURE 1-23 Sections from a movie of an Australian aboriginal man eating a kangaroo prepared in the traditional fashion. Note the activity of muscles, not only in the facial region, but throughout the neck and shoulder girdle. (Courtesy M.J. Barrett.)

usual caricature of an individual who is none too bright includes extremely protruding teeth. Well-aligned teeth and a pleasing smile carry positive status at all social levels, whereas irregular or protruding teeth carry negative status.[15,16] Appearance can and does make a difference in teachers' expectations and therefore student progress in school, in employability, and in competition for a mate. Tests of the psychologic reactions of individuals to various dental conditions, carried out by showing photographs of various mouths to the individual whose response was being evaluated, show that cultural differences are smaller than might have been anticipated. A dental appearance pleasing to Americans was also judged pleasing in Australia and East Germany, whereas a dental appearance considered in the United States to carry with it some social handicap drew about the same response in these other cultural settings.[17] Protruding incisors are judged unattractive within populations where most individuals have prominent teeth, just as they are within less protrusive groups.[18]

There is no doubt that social responses conditioned by the appearance of the teeth can severely affect an individual's whole adaptation to life. This places the concept of "handicapping malocclusion" in a larger and more important context. If the way you interact with other individuals is affected constantly by your teeth, your dental handicap is far from trivial. It is interesting that psychic distress caused by disfiguring dental or facial conditions is not directly proportional to the anatomic severity of the problem. An individual who is grossly disfigured can anticipate a consistently negative response. An individual with an apparently less severe problem (e.g., a protruding chin or irregular incisors) is sometimes treated differently because of this but sometimes not. It seems to be easier to cope with a defect if other people's responses to it are consistent rather than if they are not. Unpredictable responses produce anxiety and can have strong deleterious effects.[19]

The impact of a physical defect on an individual also will be strongly influenced by that individual's self-esteem (how positively or negatively the person feels about himself). The result is that the same degree of anatomic abnormality can be merely a condition of no great consequence to one individual but a genuinely severe problem to another.[20] It seems clear that the major reason people seek orthodontic treatment is to minimize psychosocial problems related to their dental and facial appearance. These problems are not "just cosmetic."

Oral Function.   A severe malocclusion may compromise all aspects of oral function. Adults with severe malocclusion routinely report difficulty in chewing, and after treatment patients say that masticatory problems are largely corrected.[21] It seems reasonable that poor dental occlusion would be a handicap to function, but there is no good test for chewing ability and no objective way to measure the extent of any functional handicap. Methods to test for jaw function would put this reason for orthodontic treatment on a more scientific basis. Scoring the efficiency of mastication from video tapes of standard tasks now offers the possibility of doing this.[22]

Severe malocclusion may make adaptive alterations in swallowing necessary. In addition, it can be difficult or impossible to produce certain sounds (see Chapter 6), and ef-

fective speech therapy may require some preliminary orthodontic treatment. Even less severe malocclusions tend to affect function, not by making it impossible but by making it difficult, so that extra effort is required to compensate for the anatomic deformity. For instance, everyone uses as many chewing strokes as it takes to reduce a food bolus to a consistency that is satisfactory for swallowing, so if chewing is less efficient in the presence of malocclusion, either the affected individual uses more effort to chew or settles for less well masticated food before swallowing it. Similarly, almost everyone can move the jaw so that proper lip relationships exist for speech, so distorted speech is rarely noted even though an individual may have to make an extraordinary effort to produce normal speech. As methods to quantitate functional adaptations of this type are developed, it is likely that the effect of malocclusion on function will be appreciated more than it has been in the past.

The relationship of malocclusion and adaptive function to temporomandibular dysfunction (TMD), manifested as pain in and around the TM joint, is understood much better now than only a few years ago.[23] The pain may result from pathologic changes within the joint, but more often is caused by muscle fatigue and spasm. Muscle pain almost always correlates with a history of constantly posturing the mandible to an anterior or lateral position, or clenching or grinding the teeth as a response to stressful situations. The excessive muscle activity accompanying clenching or grinding may occur during the day or may be present during sleep.

Some dentists have suggested that even minor imperfections in the occlusion serve to trigger clenching and grinding activities. If this were true, it would indicate a real need for perfecting the occlusion in everyone, to avoid the possibility of developing facial muscle pain. Because the number of people with at least moderate degrees of malocclusion (50% to 75% of the population) far exceeds the number with TMD (5% to 30%, depending on which symptoms are examined), it seems unlikely that occlusal patterns alone are enough to cause hyperactivity of the oral musculature.[24] A reaction to stress usually is involved. Some individuals with poor occlusion have no problem with muscle pain when stressed but develop symptoms in other organ systems. Almost never does an individual have both ulcerative colitis (also a common stress-induced disease) and TMD. Some types of malocclusion (especially posterior crossbite with a shift on closure) correlate positively with TM joint problems while other types do not,[23] but even the strongest correlation coefficients are only 0.3 to 0.4. This means that for the great majority of patients, there is no association between malocclusion and TMD.

On the other hand, if a patient does respond to stress by increased oral muscle activity, improper occlusal relationships may make the problem more severe and harder to control. Therefore malocclusion coupled with pain and spasm in the muscles of mastication may indicate a need for orthodontic treatment as an adjunct to other treatment for

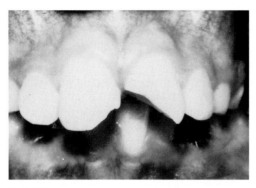

FIGURE 1-24 Fractured maxillary central incisors in a 10-year-old girl. There is almost one chance in three of an injury to a protruding incisor; most of the accidents occur during normal activity, not in sports.

the muscle pain (but orthodontics as the primary treatment almost never is indicated). If the problem is a pathologic process within the joint itself, occlusal therapy may or may not help the patient adapt to the necessarily altered joint function (see Chapter 20).

Relationship to Injury and Dental Disease. Malocclusion, particularly protruding maxillary incisors, can increase the likelihood of an injury to the teeth (Figure 1-24). There is about one chance in three that a child with an untreated Class II malocclusion will experience significant trauma to the upper incisors, resulting in a fracture of the tooth and/or devitalization of the pulp.[25] Reducing the chance of injury when incisors protrude is one argument for early treatment of Class II problems (see Chapter 8). Extreme overbite, so that the lower incisors contact the palate, can cause significant tissue damage, leading to loss of the upper incisors in a few patients. Extreme wear of incisors also occurs in some patients with excessive overbite.

It seems obvious that malocclusion could contribute to both dental decay and periodontal disease, by making it harder to care for the teeth properly or by causing occlusal trauma. Current data indicate, however, that malocclusion has little if any impact on diseases of the teeth or supporting structures. An individual's willingness and motivation determine oral hygiene much more than how well the teeth are aligned, and presence or absence of dental plaque is the major determinant of the health of both the hard and soft tissues of the mouth. If individuals with malocclusion are more prone to tooth decay, the effect is small compared with hygiene status.[26] Occlusal trauma, once thought to be important in the development of periodontal disease, now is recognized to be a secondary, not a primary, etiologic factor.[27]

Two studies carried out in the late 1970s, in which a large number of patients were carefully examined 10 to 20 years after completion of orthodontic treatment, shed some light on long-term relationships between malocclusion and oral health.[28,29] In both studies, comparison of the

patients who underwent orthodontic treatment years earlier with untreated individuals in the same age group showed similar periodontal status, despite the better functional occlusions of the orthodontically treated group. There was only a tenuous link between untreated malocclusion and major periodontal disease later in life. No evidence of a beneficial effect of orthodontic treatment on future periodontal health was demonstrated, as would have been expected if untreated malocclusion had a major role in the cause of periodontal problems.

Patients with a history of orthodontic treatment appear to be more likely to seek later periodontal care than those who were not treated, and thus are over-represented among periodontal patients. Because of this, it has been suggested that previous orthodontic treatment predisposes to later periodontal disease. The long-term studies show no indication that orthodontic treatment increased the chance of later periodontal problems. The association between early orthodontic and later periodontal treatment appears to be only another manifestation of the phenomenon that one segment of the population seeks dental treatment while another avoids it. Those who have had one type of successful dental treatment, like orthodontics in childhood, are more likely to seek another like periodontal therapy in adult life.

In summary, it appears that both psychosocial and functional handicaps can produce significant need for orthodontic treatment. The evidence is less clear that orthodontic treatment reduces the development of later dental disease.

Epidemiologic Estimates of Orthodontic Treatment Need. Psychosocial and facial considerations, not just the way the teeth fit, play a role in defining orthodontic treatment need. For this reason, it is difficult to determine who needs treatment and who does not, just from an examination of dental casts or radiographs. It seems reasonable that the severity of a malocclusion correlates with need for treatment. This assumption is necessary when treatment need is estimated for population groups.

Several indices for scoring how much the teeth deviate from the normal, as indicators of orthodontic treatment need, were proposed in the 1970s. Of these, Grainger's Treatment Priority Index (TPI)[30] is the most prominent because it was used in the 1965-1970 U.S. population surveys. None of the early indices were widely accepted for screening potential patients, however.

More recently, Shaw and co-workers in the United Kingdom developed a scoring system for malocclusion, the Index of Treatment Need (IOTN),[31] that places patients in five grades from "no need for treatment" to "treatment need." The index has a dental health component derived from occlusion and alignment (Box 1-1) and an esthetic component derived from comparison of the dental appearance to standard photographs (Figure 1-25). IOTN usually is calculated from direct examination, but the dental health component also can be determined from dental casts. A

BOX 1-1

IOTN TREATMENT GRADES

Grade 5 (Extreme/Need Treatment)

5.i Impeded eruption of teeth (except third molars) due to crowding, displacement, the presence of supernumerary teeth, retained deciduous teeth, and any pathological cause.

5.h Extensive hypodontia with restorative implications (more than one tooth per quadrant) requiring pre-prosthetic orthodontics.

5.a Increased overjet greater than 9 mm.

5.m Reverse overjet greater than 3.5 mm with reported masticatory and speech difficulties.

5.p Defects of cleft lip and palate and other craniofacial anomalies.

5.s Submerged deciduous teeth.

Grade 4 (Severe/Need Treatment)

4.h Less extensive hypodontia requiring pre-restorative orthodontics or orthodontic space closure (one tooth per quadrant).

4.a Increased overjet greater than 6 mm but less than or equal to 9 mm.

4.b Reverse overjet greater than 3.5 mm with no masticatory or speech difficulties.

4.m Reverse overjet greater than 1 mm but less than 3.5 mm with recorded masticatory or speech difficulties.

4.c Anterior or posterior crossbites with greater than 2 mm discrepancy between retruded contact position and intercuspal position.

4.l Posterior lingual crossbite with no functional occlusal contact in one or both buccal segments.

4.d Severe contact point displacements greater than 4 mm.

4.e Extreme lateral or anterior open bites greater than 4 mm.

4.f Increased and complete overbite with gingival or palatal trauma.

4.t Partially erupted teeth, tipped, and impacted against adjacent teeth.

4.x Presence of supernumerary teeth.

Grade 3 (Moderate/Borderline Need)

3.a Increased overjet greater than 3.5 mm but less than or equal to 6 mm with incompetent lips.

3.b Reverse overjet greater than 1 mm but less than or equal to 3.5 mm.

3.c Anterior or posterior crossbites with greater than 1 mm but less than or equal to 2 mm discrepancy between retruded contact position and intercuspal position.

3.d Contact point displacements greater than 2 mm but less than or equal to 4 mm.

3.e Lateral or anterior open bite greater than 2 mm but less than or equal to 4 mm.

3.f Deep overbite complete on gingival or palatal tissues but no trauma.

Grade 2 (Mild/Little Need)

2.a Increased overjet greater than 3.5 mm but less than or equal to 6 mm with competent lips.

2.b Reverse overjet greater than 0 mm but less than or equal to 1 mm.

2.c Anterior or posterior crossbite with less than or equal to 1 mm discrepancy between retruded contact position and intercuspal position.

2.d Contact point displacements greater than 1 mm but less than or equal to 2 mm.

2.e Anterior or posterior openbite greater than 1 mm but less than or equal to 2 mm.

2.f Increased overbite greater than or equal to 3.5 mm without gingival contact.

2.g Pre-normal or post-normal occlusions with no other anomalies.

Grade 1 (No Need)

1. Extremely minor malocclusions including contact point displacements less than 1 mm.

---

special ruler (Figure 1-26) summarizes the information needed for the dental health component, and after some calibration of examiners, reliable (i.e., reproducible) data are obtained. The significance of various occlusal discrepancies was established by a consensus panel of orthodontists, and the IOTN grades seem to reflect clinical judgments better than previous methods.[32] There is a surprisingly good correlation between treatment need assessed by the dental health and esthetic components of IOTN (i.e., children selected as needing treatment on one of the scales are also quite likely to be selected using the other).

With some allowances for the effect of missing teeth, it is possible to calculate the percentages of U.S. children and youths who would fall into the various IOTN grades from the NHANES III data set.[9] Figure 1-27 shows the number of youths age 12-17 estimated to have mild/moderate/severe treatment need by IOTN. Although the prevalence of malocclusion is similar for the three groups, the percentage of blacks with severe problems is higher. Although the TPI scores of 30 years ago placed more children toward the severe end of the malocclusion spectrum than the current IOTN grades, it seems unlikely that there has been a major change in treatment need. To some extent, the difference may be due to the difference in the indices, but there is another factor. Many more children have orthodontic treatment now. The number of white children who receive treatment is considerably higher than blacks or Hispanics (p<.001). Treatment almost always produces an improvement but may not totally eliminate all the characteristics of malocclusion,[33] so the effect is to move some in-

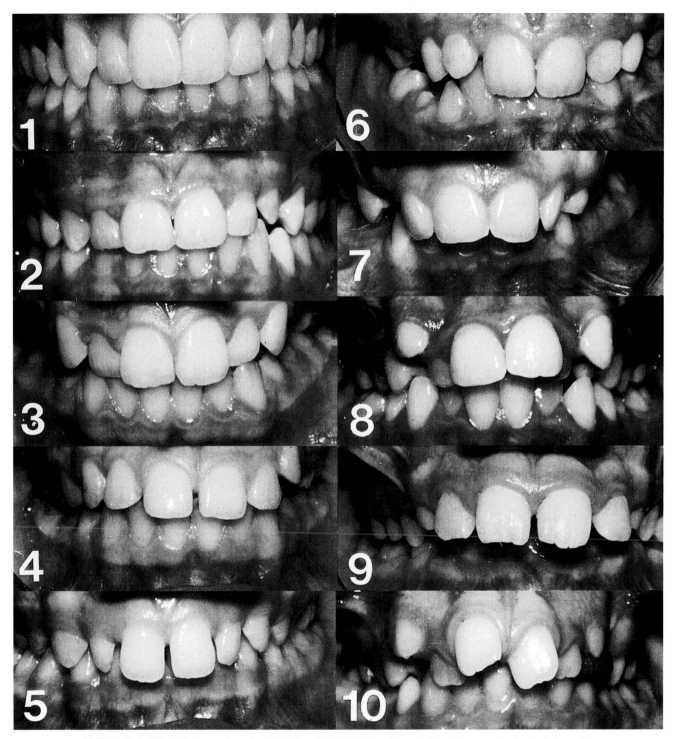

FIGURE 1-25 The stimulus photographs of the IOTN esthetic index. The score is derived from the patient's answer to "Here is a set of photographs showing a range of dental attractiveness. Number 1 is the most attractive and number 10 the least attractive arrangement. Where would you put your teeth on this scale?" Grades 8-10 indicate definite need for orthodontic treatment, 5-7 moderate/borderline need, 1-4 no/slight need.

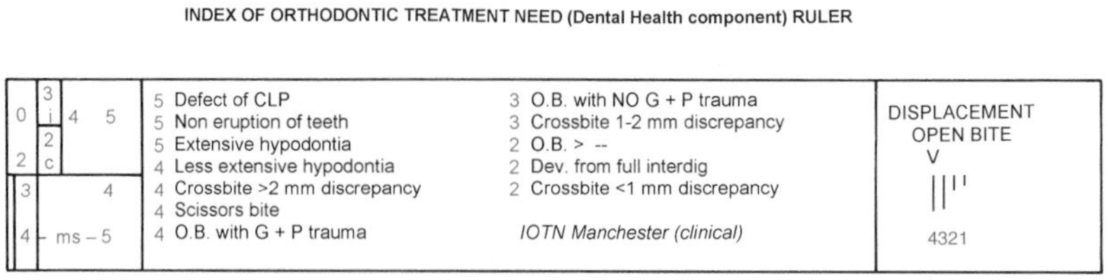

INDEX OF ORTHODONTIC TREATMENT NEED (Dental Health component) RULER

0 i 4 5 2 c 3 4 4 ms – 5	5 Defect of CLP 5 Non eruption of teeth 5 Extensive hypodontia 4 Less extensive hypodontia 4 Crossbite >2 mm discrepancy 4 Scissors bite 4 O.B. with G + P trauma	3 O.B. with NO G + P trauma 3 Crossbite 1-2 mm discrepancy 2 O.B. > -- 2 Dev. from full interdig 2 Crossbite <1 mm discrepancy *IOTN Manchester (clinical)*

DISPLACEMENT OPEN BITE

V

|| |¹

4321

FIGURE 1-26   The IOTN ruler, which makes it easy to measure the key characteristics that determine the score on IOTN's dental health component.

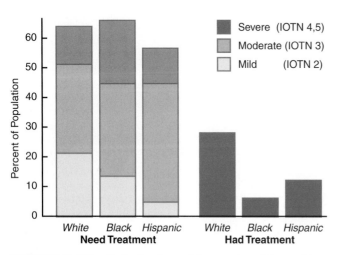

FIGURE 1-27   Orthodontic need by severity of the problem for white, black and Mexican-American youths age 12-17 in the United States 1989-94, and the percent of each group who report receiving orthodontic treatment. The greater number of whites who receive treatment probably accounts for the smaller number of severe problems in the white population.

dividuals from the severe to the mild treatment need categories. The higher proportion of severe malocclusion among blacks, who are much less likely to receive treatment at this point than whites, probably reflects the effect of more treatment in the white group, and may not indicate the presence of more severe malocclusion in the black population.

How do the IOTN scores compare with what parents and dentists think relative to orthodontic treatment need? The (rather weak) existing data suggest that in typical American neighborhoods, about 35% of adolescents are perceived by parents and peers as needing orthodontic treatment (see Figure 1-27). Note that this is larger than the number of children who would be placed in IOTN grades 4 and 5 as severe problems definitely needing treatment but smaller than the total of grades 3, 4, and 5 for moderate and severe problems. Dentists usually judge that only about one-third of their patients have normal occlusion, and they suggest treatment for about 55% (thereby putting about 10% in a category of malocclusion with little need for treatment). It appears that they would include all the children in IOTN grade 3 and some of those in

grade 2 (Table 1-3) in the group who would benefit from orthodontics. Presumably, facial appearance and psychosocial considerations are used in addition to dental characteristics when parents judge treatment need or dentists decide to recommend treatment.

Demand for Orthodontic Treatment

Demand for treatment is indicated by the number of patients who actually make appointments and seek care. Not all patients with malocclusion, even those with extreme deviations from the normal, seek orthodontic treatment. Some do not recognize that they have a problem; others feel that they need treatment but cannot afford it or cannot obtain it.

Both the perceived need and demand vary with social and cultural conditions.[34] More children in urban areas are thought (by parents and peers) to need treatment than children in rural areas. Family income is a major determinant of how many children receive treatment (Figure 1-28). This appears to reflect not only that higher income families can more easily afford orthodontic treatment but also that good facial appearance and avoidance of disfiguring dental conditions are associated with more prestigious social positions and occupations. The higher the aspirations for a child, the more likely the parent is to seek orthodontic treatment for him or her. It is widely recognized that severe malocclusion can affect an individual's entire life adjustment, and every state now provides at least some orthodontic treatment through its Medicaid program, but Medicaid and related programs support only a tiny fraction of the population's orthodontic care. From that perspective it is interesting that even in the lowest income group almost 5% of the youths and over 5% of adults report receiving treatment, with 10-15% treated at intermediate income levels. This probably reflects the importance placed on orthodontic treatment by some families as a factor in social and career progress.

The effect of financial constraints on demand can be seen most clearly by the response to third-party payment plans. When third-party copayment is available, the number of individuals seeking orthodontic treatment rises considerably (but even when all costs are covered, some individuals for whom treatment is recommended do not accept it—see Table 1-3). It seems likely that under optimal economic conditions, demand for orthodontic treat-

TABLE 1-3 *Percent of U.S. Population Estimated to Need Orthodontics, 1965-1970 vs 1989-1994*

	White				Black				Hispanic**	
	Child		Youth		Child		Youth		Child	Youth
Age	6-11	8-11	12-17		6-11	8-11	12-17		8-11	12-17
Year	1965-70	1989-91	1965-70	1989-91	1965-70	1989-91	1965-70	1989-91	1989-91	1989-91
Index	TPI	IOTN	TPI	IOTN	TPI	IOTN	TPI	IOTN	IOTN	IOTN
No treatment need (TPI 0-1, IOTN 1)	28.7	36.5	20.0	43.7	39.7	40.4	24.3	42.2	49.4	41.5
Minimal need (TPI 2-3, IOTN 2)	33.9	16.3	25.1	16.5	28.4	8.8	27.3	9.2	11.7	8.5
Moderate need (TPI 4-6, IOTN 3)	23.7	36.4	25.7	25.3	15.0	37.1	21.0	26.0	29.9	36.8
Definite need (TPI >6, IOTN 4-5)	13.7	10.8	29.2	14.5	16.9	13.7	27.4	22.6	9.0	13.2
Had orthodontic treatment	2.5*	10.5	10.7*	27.4		3.6		6.2	1.4	11.7

Data from NHANES I and III
*White/black combined
**No data for 1965-1970

ment will at least reach the 35% level thought by the public to need treatment. The NHANES III data show that 35%-50% of children and youths in higher socioeconomic areas in the United States already are receiving orthodontic care.[9] A survey of orthodontic specialists showed that over 4 million patients were in orthodontic treatment in the United States in 1996.[35]

As late as the 1960s, 95% or more of all orthodontic patients were children or adolescents. From 1975 to the late 1980s, much of the growth in the orthodontic patient population was adults (age 18 or older). By 1990, 25% of all orthodontic patients were adults (18 or older). Interestingly, the absolute number of adults seeking orthodontic treatment has remained constant since then while the number of younger patients has grown, so in the late 1990s the proportion of adults in the orthodontic patient population had dropped to 20%.[35] Many of these adult patients indicate that they wanted treatment earlier but did not receive it, often because their families could not afford it; now they can. Wearing braces as an adult is more socially acceptable than it was previously, though no one really knows why, and this too has made it easier for adults to seek treatment. Recently, more older adults (40 and over) have sought orthodontics, usually in conjunction with other treatment to save their teeth. As the population ages, this is likely to be the fastest-growing type of orthodontic treatment.

Orthodontics has become a more prominent part of dentistry in recent years and this trend is likely to continue. The vast majority of individuals who had orthodontic treatment feel that they benefited from the treatment and are

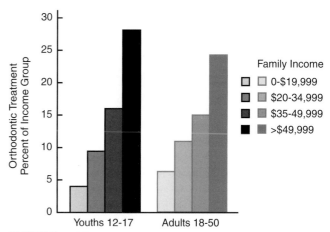

FIGURE 1-28 The percent of the U.S. population 1989-94 who received orthodontic treatment, as a function of family income. Although severe malocclusion is recognized as an important problem and all states offer at least some coverage to low-income children through their Medicaid program, this funds treatment for a very small percentage of the population. Nevertheless, nearly 5% of the lowest income group, and 10%-15% of intermediate income groups, have had some orthodontic treatment. The increasing availability of orthodontics in recent years is reflected in the larger number of youths than adults who report being treated.

pleased with the result. Not all patients have the dramatic changes in dental and facial appearance shown in Figures 1-5 to 1-10, but nearly all recognize an improvement in both dental condition and psychologic well-being.

REFERENCES

1. Corrucini RS, Pacciani E: "Orthodontistry" and dental occlusion in Etruscans, Angle Orthod 59:61-64, 1989.
2. Kingsley NW: Treatise on oral deformities as a branch of mechanical surgery, New York, 1880, Appleton.
3. Angle EH: Treatment of malocclusion of the teeth and fractures of the maxillae, Angle's system, ed 6, Philadelphia, 1900, SS White Dental Mfg Co.
4. Sarver DM: Esthetics orthodontics and orthognathic surgery, St Louis, 1998, Mosby.
5. Glossary of dentofacial orthopedic terms, St Louis, 1996, American Association of Orthodontists.
6. Kelly JE, Sanchez M, Van Kirk LE: An assessment of the occlusion of teeth of children, DHEW Publication No (HRA) 74-1612, Washington, DC, 1973, National Center for Health Statistics.
7. Kelly J, Harvey C: An assessment of the teeth of youths 12-17 years, DHEW Pub No (HRA) 77-1644, Washington, DC, 1977, National Center for Health Statistics.
8. Brunelle JA, Bhat M, Lipton JA: Prevalence and distribution of selected occlusal characteristics in the US population, 1988-91. J Dent Res 75:706-713, 1996.
9. Proffit WR, Fields HW, Moray LJ: Prevalence of malocclusion and orthodontic treatment need in the United States: estimates from the NHANES-III survey, Int J Adult Orthod Orthogn Surg 13:97-106, 1998.
10. El-Mangoury NH, Mostafa YA: Epidemiologic panorama of malocclusion, Angle Orthod 60:207-214, 1990.
11. Larsen CS: Bioarchaeology: interpreting behavior from the human skeleton, 1997, Cambridge, Mass., Cambridge University Press.
12. Baume LJ: Uniform methods for the epidemiologic assessment of malocclusion, Am J Orthod 66:251-272, 1974.
13. Brown T, Abbott AA, Burgess VB: Longitudinal study of dental arch relationships in Australian aboriginals with reference to alternate intercuspation, Am J Phys Anthropol 72:49-57, 1987.
14. Corruccini RS: Anthropological aspects of orofacial and occlusal variations and anomalies. In Kelly MA, Larsen CS (editors), Advances in dental anthropology, New York, 1991, Wiley-Liss.
15. Shaw WC: The influence of children's dentofacial appearance on their social attractiveness as judged by peers and lay adults, Am J Orthod 79:399-415, 1981.
16. Shaw WC, Rees G, Dawe M, Charles CR: The influence of dentofacial appearance on the social attractiveness of young adults, Am J Orthod 87:21-26, 1985.
17. Cons NC, Jenny J, Kohout FJ et al: Perceptions of occlusal conditions in Australia, the German Democratic Republic, and the United States, Int Dent J 33:200-206, 1983.
18. Farrow AL, Zarinnia K, Khosrow A: Bimaxillary protrusion in black Americans—an esthetic evaluation and the treatment considerations, Am J Orthod Dentofac Orthop 104:240-250, 1993.
19. Macgregor FC: Social and psychological implications of dentofacial disfigurement, Angle Orthod 40:231-233, 1979.
20. Kenealy P, Frude N, Shaw W: An evaluation of the psychological and social effects of malocclusion: some implications for dental policy making, Soc Sci Med 28:583-591, 1989.
21. Ostler S, Kiyak HA: Treatment expectations vs outcomes in orthognathic surgery patients, Int J Adult Orthod Orthognath Surg 6:247-256, 1991.
22. Feine JS, Maskawi K, de Grandmont P et al: Within-subject comparisons of implant-supported mandibular prostheses: evaluation of masticatory function, J Dent Res 73:1646-1656, 1994.
23. McNamara JA, Seligman DA, Okeson JP: Occlusion, orthodontic treatment and temporomandibular disorders, J Orofacial Pain 9:73-90, 1995.
24. Greene CS: Etiology of temporomandibular disorders, Seminars Orthod 1:222-228, 1995.
25. Tulloch JFC, Phillips C, Koch G, Proffit WR: The effect of early intervention on skeletal pattern in Class II malocclusion: a randomized clinical trial, Am J Orthod Dentofac Orthop 111:391-400, 1997.
26. Helm S, Petersen PE: Causal relation between malocclusion and caries, Acta Odontol Scand 47:217-221, 1989.
27. Burgett FG: Trauma from occlusion: periodontal concerns, Dent Clin NA 39:301-311, 1995.
28. Sadowsky C, BeGole EA: Long-term effects of orthodontic treatment on periodontal health, Am J Orthod 80:156-172, 1981.
29. Polson AM: Long-term effect of orthodontic treatment on the periodontium. In McNamara JA, Ribbens KA (editors): Malocclusion and the periodontium, Ann Arbor, Mich., 1987, The University of Michigan Press.
30. Grainger RM: Orthodontic treatment priority index, USPHS Publication No 1000-Series 2, No 25, Washington, DC, 1967, National Center for Health Statistics.
31. Brook PH, Shaw WC: The development of an index for orthodontic treatment priority, Eur J Orthod 11:309-332, 1989.
32. Richmond S, Shaw WC, O'Brien KD et al: The relationship between the index of treatment need and consensus opinion of a panel of 74 dentists, Brit Dent J 178:370-374, 1995.
33. Richmond S, Roberts CT, Andrews M: Use of the index of treatment need (IOTN) in assessing the need for orthodontic treatment pre- and post-appliance therapy, Brit J Orthod 21:175-184, 1994.
34. Tulloch JFC, Shaw WC, Underhill C et al: A comparison of attitudes toward orthodontic treatment in British and American communities, Am J Orthod 85:253-259, 1984.
35. Patient census survey results, Bulletin Am Assn Orthod 15:4 July-Aug. 1997.

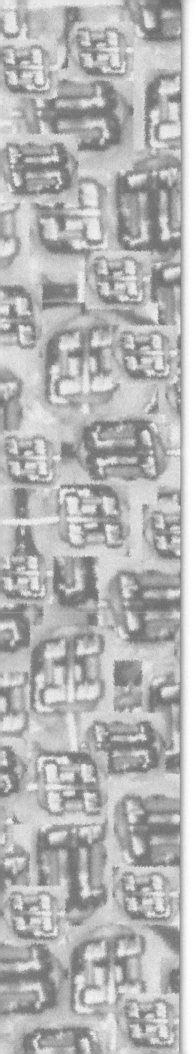

SECTION

II

THE DEVELOPMENT OF ORTHODONTIC PROBLEMS

Malocclusion and dentofacial deformity arise through variations in the normal developmental process, and so must be evaluated against a perspective of normal development. Because orthodontic treatment often involves manipulation of skeletal growth, clinical orthodontics requires an understanding not only of dental development but also of more general concepts of physical growth and of physiologic and psychosocial development.

This section begins in Chapter 2 with a discussion of basic concepts in growth and development. A brief discussion of psychologic development is included, emphasizing emotional and cognitive development, as well as how the dentist can utilize this information to communicate with children and adolescents. Information on physical growth and dental development at the various stages is then presented sequentially in Chapters 3 and 4, beginning with prenatal growth and extending into adult life where developmental changes continue at a slower pace. The etiology of malocclusion and special developmental problems in children with malocclusion and dentofacial deformity are considered in some detail in Chapter 5.

CHAPTER

2

Concepts of Growth and Development

A thorough background in craniofacial growth and development is necessary for every dentist. Even for those who never work with children, it is difficult to comprehend conditions observed in adults without understanding the developmental processes that produced these problems. For those who do interact professionally with children—and almost every dentist does so at least occasionally—it is important to distinguish normal variation from the effects of abnormal or pathologic processes. Since dentists and orthodontists are heavily involved in the development of not just the dentition but the entire dentofacial complex, a conscientious practitioner may be able to manipulate facial growth for the benefit of the patient. Obviously, it is not possible to do so without a thorough understanding of both the pattern of normal growth and the mechanisms that underlie it.

The very terms *growth* and *development* can cause difficulties in understanding. Growth and development, though closely related, are not synonymous. In conversational English, growth usually refers to an increase in size, but tends to be linked more to change than anything else. Only if growth meant change, after all, could someone seriously speak of a period of economic recession as one of "negative economic growth." Since some tissues grow rapidly and then shrink or disappear, a plot of physical growth versus time may include a negative phase. On the other hand, if growth is defined solely as a process of change, the term becomes almost meaningless. As a general term, development connotes an increasing degree of organization, often with unfortunate consequences for the natural environment. In this chapter, the term growth usually refers to an increase in size or number. Occasionally, however, the increase will be in neither size nor number, but in complexity. More often, the term development will be used to refer to an increase in complexity. Development carries an overtone of increasing specialization, so that one price of increased development is a loss of potential. Growth is largely an anatomic phenomenon, whereas development is physiologic and behavioral.

It should be kept in mind that although dentists work with the physical features of the teeth and face, a major reason for orthodontic treatment is its psychosocial effects. Furthermore, patient cooperation is necessary—eliciting it in children of different ages requires a knowledge of social and behavioral development. Both physiologic and psychosocial development are important subjects for this chapter. For convenience, not because they are innately more important, physical growth concepts are presented first and then developmental factors are reviewed.

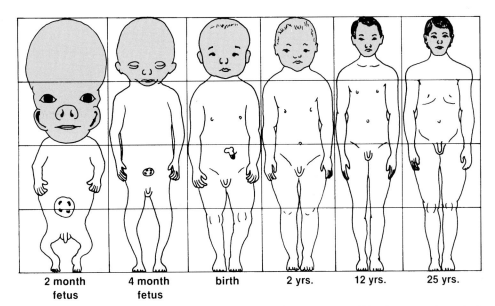

| 2 month fetus | 4 month fetus | birth | 2 yrs. | 12 yrs. | 25 yrs. |

FIGURE 2-1   Schematic representation of the changes in overall body proportions during normal growth and development. After the third month of fetal life, the proportion of total body size contributed by the head and face steadily declines. (Redrawn from Robbins WJ et al: *Growth*, New Haven, 1928, Yale University Press.)

GROWTH: PATTERN, VARIABILITY, AND TIMING

In studies of growth and development, the concept of pattern is an important one. In a general sense, pattern (as in the pattern from which articles of clothing of different sizes are cut) reflects proportionality, usually of a complex set of proportions rather than just a single proportional relationship. Pattern in growth also represents proportionality, but in a still more complex way, because it refers not just to a set of proportional relationships at a point in time, but to the change in these proportional relationships over time. In other words, the physical arrangement of the body at any one time is a pattern of spatially proportioned parts. But there is a higher level pattern, the pattern of growth, which refers to the changes in these spatial proportions over time.

Figure 2-1 illustrates the change in overall body proportions that occurs during normal growth and development. In fetal life, at about the third month of intrauterine development, the head takes up almost 50% of the total body length. At this stage, the cranium is large relative to the face and represents more than half the total head. In contrast, the limbs are still rudimentary and the trunk is underdeveloped. By the time of birth, the trunk and limbs have grown faster than the head and face, so that the proportion of the entire body devoted to the head has decreased to about 30%. The overall pattern of growth thereafter follows this course, with a progressive reduction of the relative size of the head to about 12% of the adult. At birth the legs represent about one third of the total body length, while in the adult they represent about half. As Figure 2-1

illustrates, there is more growth of the lower limbs than the upper limbs during postnatal life. All of these changes, which are a part of the normal growth pattern, reflect the "cephalocaudal gradient of growth." This simply means that there is an axis of increased growth extending from the head toward the feet.

Another aspect of the normal growth pattern is that not all the tissue systems of the body grow at the same rate (Figure 2-2). Obviously, the muscular and skeletal elements grow faster than the brain and central nervous system, as reflected in the relative decrease of head size. The overall pattern of growth is a reflection of the growth of the various tissues making up the whole organism. To put it differently, one reason for gradients of growth is that different tissue systems that grow at different rates are concentrated in various parts of the body.

Even within the head and face, the cephalocaudal growth gradient strongly affects proportions and leads to changes in proportion with growth (Figure 2-3). When the skull of a newborn infant is compared proportionally with that of an adult, it is easy to see that the infant has a relatively much larger cranium and a much smaller face. This change in proportionality, with an emphasis on growth of the face relative to the cranium, is an important aspect of the pattern of facial growth. When the facial growth pattern is viewed against the perspective of the cephalocaudal gradient, it is not surprising that the mandible, being further away from the brain, tends to grow more and later than the maxilla, which is closer.

An important aspect of pattern is its predictability. Patterns repeat, whether in the organization of different

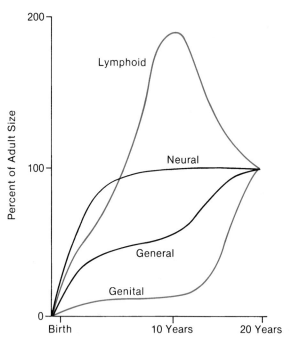

FIGURE 2-2 Scammon's curves for growth of the four major tissue systems of the body. As the graph indicates, growth of the neural tissues is nearly complete by 6 or 7 years of age. General body tissues, including muscle, bone and viscera, show an S-shaped curve, with a definite slowing of the rate of growth during childhood and an acceleration at puberty. Lymphoid tissues proliferate far beyond the adult amount in late childhood, and then undergo involution at the same time that growth of the genital tissues accelerates rapidly. (From Scammon RD: *The measurement of the body in childhood.* In Harris JA (editor): *The measurement of man,* Minneapolis, 1930, University of Minnesota Press.)

colored tiles in the design of a floor or in skeletal proportions changing over time. The proportional relationships within a pattern can be specified mathematically, and the only difference between a growth pattern and a geometric one is the addition of a time dimension. Thinking about pattern in this way allows one to be more precise in defining what constitutes a change in pattern. Change, clearly, would denote an alteration in the predictable pattern of mathematical relationships. A change in growth pattern would indicate some alteration in the expected changes in body proportions.

A second important concept in the study of growth and development is variability. Obviously, everyone is not alike in the way that they grow as in everything else. It can be difficult, but clinically very important, to decide whether an individual is merely at the extreme of the normal variation or falls outside the normal range.

Rather than categorizing people as normal or abnormal, it is more useful to think in terms of deviations from the usual pattern and to express variability quantitatively. One way to do this is to evaluate a given child relative to peers on a standard growth chart (Figure 2-4). Although charts of this type are commonly used for height and weight, the growth of any part of the body can be plotted in this way. The "normal variability," as derived from large-scale studies of groups of children, is shown by the solid lines on the graphs. An individual who stood exactly at the midpoint of the normal distribution would fall along the 50% line of the graph. One who was larger than 90% of the population would plot above the 90% line; one who was smaller than 90% of the population would plot below the 10% line.

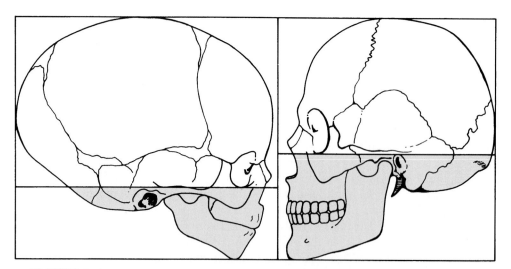

FIGURE 2-3 Changes in proportions of the head and face during growth. At birth, the face and jaws are relatively underdeveloped compared with their extent in the adult. As a result, there is much more growth of facial than cranial structures postnatally. (Redrawn from Lowery GH: *Growth and development of children,* ed 6, Chicago, 1973, Mosby.)

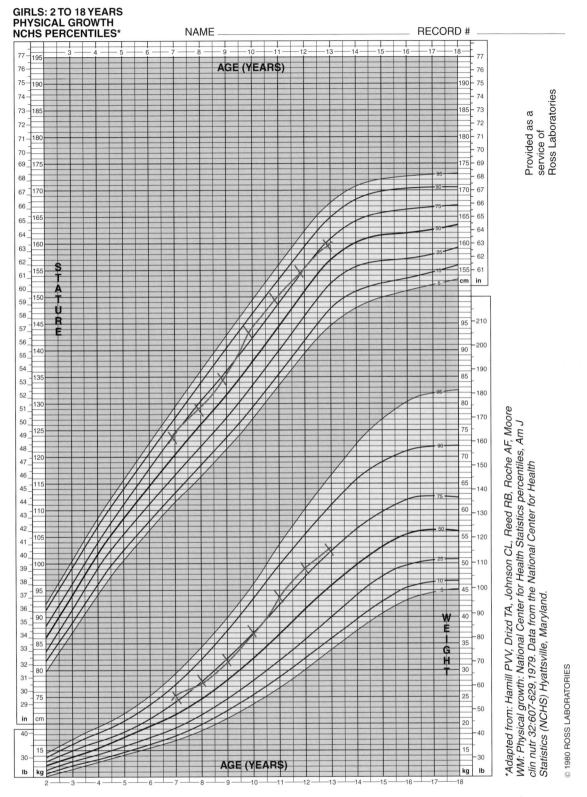

GIRLS: 2 TO 18 YEARS
PHYSICAL GROWTH
NCHS PERCENTILES*

NAME _____   RECORD # _____

*Adapted from: Hamill PVV, Drizd TA, Johnson CL, Reed RB, Roche AF, Moore WM: Physical growth: National Center for Health Statistics percentiles, Am J clin nutr 32:607-629, 1979. Data from the National Center for Health Statistics (NCHS) Hyattsville, Maryland.

Provided as a
service of
Ross Laboratories

FIGURE 2-4   Growth of a normal girl plotted on the female chart. Note that this girl remained at about the seventy-fifth percentile for height and weight over this entire period of observation. (Data from Hamill et al: National Center for Health Statistics, 1979; chart copyright Ross Laboratories, 1980.)

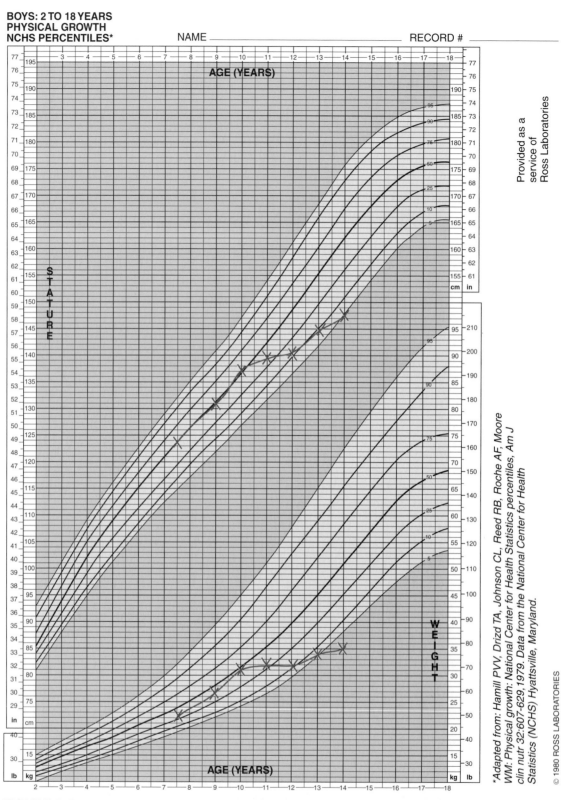

FIGURE 2-5   Growth of a boy plotted on the male chart. Note the change in pattern between age 10 and 11, reflecting the impact of a serious illness on growth beginning at that time, with partial recovery after age 13 but a continuing effect on growth.

These charts can be used in two ways to determine whether growth is normal or abnormal. First, the location of an individual relative to the group can be established. A general guideline is that a child who falls beyond the range of 97% of the population should receive special study before being accepted as just an extreme of the normal population. Second and perhaps more importantly, growth charts can be used to follow a child over time to evaluate whether there is an unexpected change in growth pattern (Figure 2-5). Pattern implies predictability. For the growth charts, this means that a child's growth should plot along the same percentile line at all ages. If the percentile position of an individual relative to his or her peer group changes, especially if there is a marked change, the clinician should suspect some growth abnormality and should investigate further. Inevitably, there is a gray area at the extremes of normal variations, at which it is difficult to determine if growth is normal.

A final major concept in physical growth and development is that of timing. Variability in growth arises in several ways: from normal variation, from influences outside the normal experience (e.g., serious illness), and from timing effects. Variation in timing arises because the same event happens for different individuals at different times—or, viewed differently, the biologic clocks of different individuals are set differently.

Variations in growth and development because of timing are particularly evident in human adolescence. Some children grow rapidly and mature early, completing their growth quickly and thereby appearing on the high side of developmental charts until their growth ceases and their contemporaries begin to catch up. Others grow and develop slowly, and so appear to be behind even though, given time, they will catch up with and even surpass children who once were larger. All children undergo a spurt of growth at adolescence, which can be seen more clearly by plotting change in height or weight (Figure 2-6), but the growth spurt occurs at different times in different individuals.

Growth effects because of timing variation can be seen particularly clearly in girls, in whom the onset of menstruation, often referred to as menarche, gives an excellent indicator of the arrival of sexual maturity. Sexual maturation is accompanied by a spurt in growth. When the growth velocity curves for early, average, and late maturing girls are compared in Figure 2-7, the marked differences in sizes between these girls during growth are apparent. At age 11, the early maturing girl is already past the peak of her adolescent growth spurt, whereas the late maturing girl has not even begun to grow rapidly. This sort of timing variation, which occurs in many ways other than that shown here, can be an important contributor to variability.

Because of time and variability, chronologic age often is not a good indicator of the individual's growth status. Although age is usually measured chronologically as the amount of time since birth or conception, it is also possible to measure age biologically, in terms of progress toward

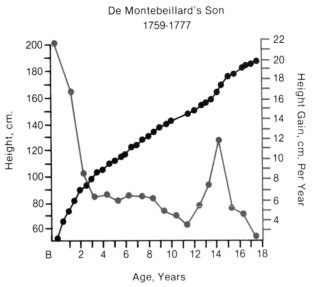

FIGURE 2-6 Growth can be plotted either in height or weight at any age (the black line here) or the amount of change in any given interval (the red line here, showing the same data as the black line). A curve like the black line is called a "distance curve," where the red line is a "velocity curve." Plotting velocity rather than distance makes it easier to see when accelerations and decelerations in the rate of growth occurred. These data are for the growth of one individual, the son of a French aristocrat in the late eighteenth century, whose growth followed the typical pattern. Note the acceleration of growth at adolescence, which occurred for this individual at about age 14. (Redrawn from Tanner JM: *Growth at adolescence*, ed 2, Oxford, 1962, Blackwell Scientific Publications.)

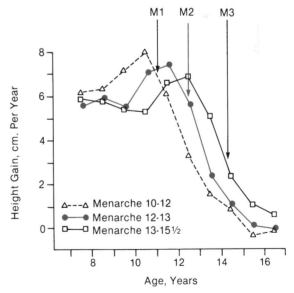

FIGURE 2-7 Growth velocity curves for early, average, and late maturing girls. It is interesting to note that the earlier the adolescent growth spurt occurs, the more intense it appears to be. Obviously, at age 11 or 12, an early maturing girl would be considerably larger than one who matured late. In each case, the onset of menstruation (menarche) (M1, M2, and M3) came after the peak of growth velocity.

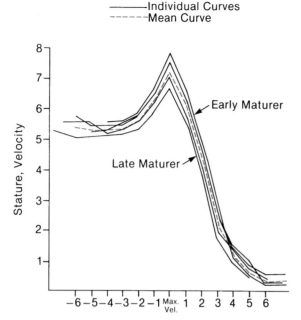

FIGURE 2-8   Velocity curves for four girls with quite different times of menarche, replotted using menarche as a zero time point. It is apparent that the growth pattern in each case is quite similar, with almost all of the variations resulting from timing.

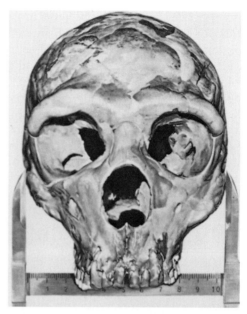

FIGURE 2-9   Craniometric studies are based on measurements between landmarks on dried skulls, typically those found in skeletal remains of early people.

various developmental markers or stages. Timing variability can be reduced by using developmental age rather than chronologic age as an expression of an individual's growth status. For instance, if data for gain in height for girls are replotted, using menarche as a reference time point (Figure 2-8), it is apparent that girls who mature early, average, or late really follow a very similar growth pattern. This graph substitutes stage of sexual development for chronologic time, to produce a biologic time scale, and shows that the pattern is expressed at different times chronologically but not at different times physiologically. The effectiveness of biologic or developmental ages in reducing timing variability makes this approach useful in evaluating a child's growth status.

METHODS FOR STUDYING PHYSICAL GROWTH

Before beginning the examination of growth data, it is important to have a reasonable idea of how the data were obtained. There are two basic approaches to studying physical growth. The first is based on techniques for measuring living animals (including humans), with the implication that the measurement itself does no harm and that the animal will be available for additional measurements at another time. The second approach uses experiments in which growth is manipulated in some way. This implies that the subject of the experiment will be available for

study in some detail, and the detailed study may be destructive. For this reason, such experimental studies are largely restricted to non-human species.

Measurement Approaches

The first of the measurement approaches for studying growth, with which the science of physical anthropology began, is *craniometry*, based on measurements of skulls found among human skeletal remains (Figure 2-9). Craniometry was originally used to study the Neanderthal and Cro-Magnon peoples whose skulls were found in European caves in the eighteenth and nineteenth centuries. From such skeletal material, it has been possible to piece together a great deal of knowledge about extinct populations and to get some idea of their pattern of growth by comparing one skull with another. Craniometry has the advantage that rather precise measurements can be made on dry skulls; it has the important disadvantage for growth studies that, by necessity, all these growth data must be cross-sectional. Cross-sectional means that although different ages are represented in the population, the same individual can be measured at only one point in time.

It is also possible to measure skeletal dimensions on living individuals. In this technique, called *anthropometry*, various landmarks established in studies of dry skulls are measured in living individuals simply by using soft tissue points overlying these bony landmarks. For example, it is possible to measure the length of the cranium from a point at the bridge of the nose to a point at the greatest convexity of the rear of the skull. This measurement can be made on either a dried skull or a living individual, but results would be different because of the soft tissue thickness over-

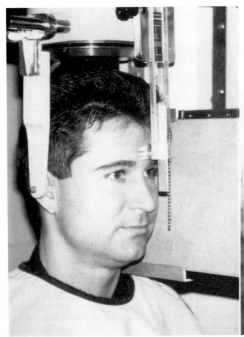
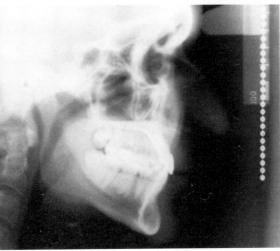

FIGURE 2-10 A cephalometric radiograph merits this name because of the use of a head positioning device to provide precise orientation of the head. This means that valid comparisons can be made between external and internal dimensions in members of the same population group, or that the same individual can be measured at two points in time, because the head orientation is reproducible. This film was taken in natural head position (NHP) (see Chapter 6).

lying both landmarks. Although the soft tissue introduces variation, anthropometry does make it possible to follow the growth of an individual directly, making the same measurements repeatedly at different times. This produces longitudinal data: repeated measures of the same individual. In recent years, Farkas' anthropometric studies have provided valuable new data for human facial proportions and their changes over time.[1]

The third measurement technique, *cephalometric radiology*, is of considerable importance not only in the study of growth but also in clinical evaluation of orthodontic patients. The technique depends on precisely orienting the head before making a radiograph with equally precise control of magnification. This approach can combine the advantages of craniometry and anthropometry. It allows a direct measurement of bony skeletal dimensions, since the bone can be seen through the soft tissue covering in a radiograph (Figure 2-10), but it also allows the same individual to be followed over time. The disadvantage of a cephalometric radiograph is that it produces a two-dimensional representation of a three-dimensional structure, and so even with precise head positioning, not all measurements are possible. To some extent, this can be overcome by making more than one radiograph at different orientations and using triangulation to calculate oblique distances. The general pattern of craniofacial growth was known from craniometric and anthropometric studies before cephalometric radiography was in-

vented, but much of the current picture of craniofacial growth is based on cephalometric studies.

Both anthropometric and cephalometric data can be expressed cross-sectionally rather than longitudinally. Obviously, it would be much easier and quicker to do a cross-sectional study, gathering data once for any individual and including subjects of different ages, rather than spending many years on a study in which the same individuals were measured repeatedly. For this reason, most studies are cross-sectional. When this approach is used, however, variability within the sample can conceal details of the growth pattern, particularly when there is no correction for timing variation (Figure 2-11). Fluctuations in the growth curve that may occur for nearly every individual would be seen in a cross-sectional study only if they occurred at the same time for each person, which is unlikely. Longitudinal studies are efficient in the sense that a great deal of information can be gained from a relatively small number of subjects, fewer than would be needed in a cross-sectional study. In addition, the longitudinal data highlight individual variations, particularly variations caused by timing effects.

Measurement data can be presented graphically in a number of different ways, and frequently it is possible to clarify growth changes by varying the method of display. For example, we have already seen that growth data can be presented by plotting the size attained as a function of age, which is called a "distance" curve, or as a "velocity" curve, showing not the total length but the increment added each year (see

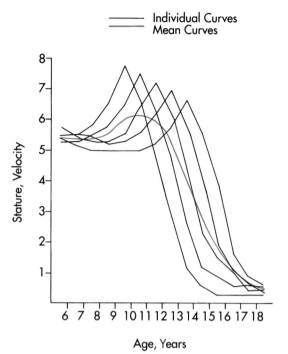

FIGURE 2-11 over image: Individual Curves / Mean Curves (legend); y-axis: Stature, Velocity; x-axis: Age, Years

FIGURE 2-11 If growth velocity data for a group of individuals with a different timing of the adolescent growth spurt are plotted on a chronologic scale, it is apparent that the average curve is not an accurate representation of the pattern of growth for any particular individual. This smoothing of individual variation is a characteristic of cross-sectional data and a major limitation inuse of the cross-sectional method for studies of growth. Only by following individuals through time in a longitudinal study is it possible to see the details of growth patterns.

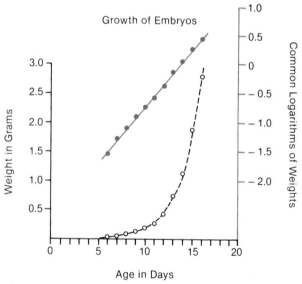

Growth of Embryos (chart title); y-axis left: Weight in Grams; y-axis right: Common Logarithms of Weights; x-axis: Age in Days

FIGURE 2-12 Data for the increase in weight of early embryos, with the raw data plotted in black and the same data plotted after logarithmic transformation in red. At this stage, the weight of the embryo increases dramatically but, as shown by the straight line after transformation, the rate of multiplication of individual cells remains fairly constant. When more cells are present, more divisions can occur, the weight increases faster. (From Lowery GH: *Growth and development of children,* ed 8, Chicago, 1986, Mosby.)

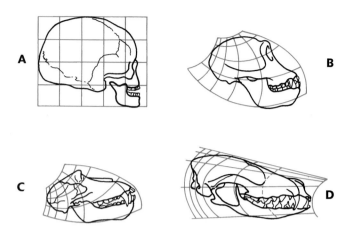

FIGURE 2-13 In the early 1900s, D'Arcy Thompson showed that mathematical transformation of a grid could account for the changes in the shape of the face from man (**A**) to chimpanzee (**B**), monkey (**C**), dog (**D**) or other animals. Application of this method revealed previously unsuspected similarities among various species. (Redrawn from Thompson JT: *On growth and form,* Cambridge, Mass., 1971, Cambridge University Press.)

Figure 2-6). Changes in the rate of growth are much more easily seen in the velocity curve than the distance curve.

Various other mathematical transformations can be used with growth data to make it easier to understand. For instance, the growth in weight of any embryo at an early stage follows a logarithmic or exponential curve, because the growth is based on division of cells; the more cells there are, the more cell divisions can occur. If the same data are plotted using the logarithm of the weight, a straight-line plot is attained (Figure 2-12). This demonstrates that the rate of multiplication for cells in the embryo is remaining more or less constant.

More complex mathematical transformations were used many years ago by D'Arcy Thompson[2] to reveal similarities in proportions and growth changes that had not previously been suspected (Figure 2-13). To correctly interpret data after mathematical transformation, it is important to understand how the data were transformed, but the approach is a powerful one in clarifying growth concepts.

Experimental Approaches

Much has been learned about skeletal growth using the technique called vital staining, in which dyes that stain mineralizing tissues (or occasionally, soft tissues) are injected into an animal. These dyes remain in the bones and teeth and can be detected later after sacrifice of the animal. This method was originated by the great English anatomist John Hunter in the eighteenth century. Hunter observed that the bones of pigs that occasionally were fed textile waste were often stained in an interesting way. He discovered that the active agent was a dye called alizarin, which still is used for vital staining studies (Figure 2-14). Alizarin reacts strongly with calcium at sites where bone calcification is occurring. Since these are the sites of active skeletal growth, the dye marks the locations at which active growth

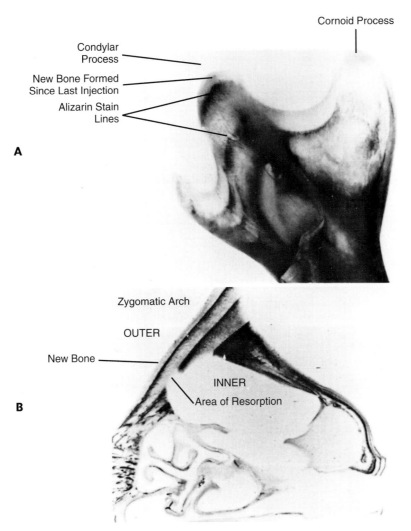

FIGURE 2-14 **A,** The mandible of a rat that received three injections of alizarin at 3-week intervals and was sacrificed 2 weeks after the last injection. Remodeling of the bone as it grows blurs some of the injection lines, but sequential lines in the condylar process can be seen clearly. **B,** Section through the zygomatic arch, from the same animal. The zygomatic arch grows outward by apposition of bone on the outer surface and removal from the inner surface. The interruptions in the staining lines on the inner surface clearly show the areas where bone is being removed. What was the outer surface of the zygomatic arch at one point becomes the inner surface a relatively short time later, and then is removed.

was occurring when it was injected. Bone remodels rapidly, and areas from which bone is being removed also can be identified by the fact that vital stained material has been removed from these locations. Highly-detailed studies of bony changes in craniofacial development in experimental animals now are available.[3]

Although studies using vital stains are not possible in humans, vital staining can occur. Many children born in the late 1950s and early 1960s were treated for recurrent infections with the antibiotic tetracycline. It was discovered too late that tetracycline is an excellent vital stain that binds to calcium at growth sites in the same way as alizarin. The discoloration of incisor teeth that results from tetracycline given when the teeth are mineralizing has been an esthetic disaster for some individuals (Figure 2-15), and therefore tetracycline rarely is used now for infections in children.

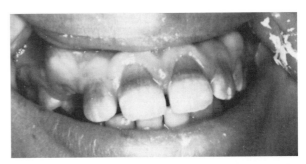

FIGURE 2-15 Tetracycline staining in the teeth of a boy who received large doses of tetracycline because of repeated upper respiratory infections in early childhood. From the location of the staining, it is apparent that tetracycline was not administered in infancy but was given in large doses beginning when the crowns of the central incisors were about half formed, or at approximately 30 months.

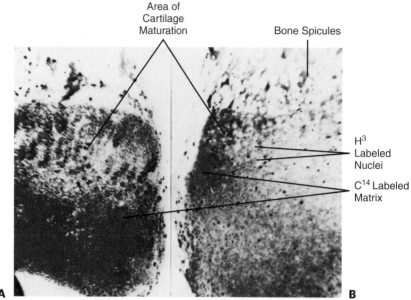

Area of
Cartilage
Maturation

Bone Spicules

H³
Labeled
Nuclei

C¹⁴ Labeled
Matrix

A   **B**

FIGURE 2-16   Autoradiographs of fetal rat bones growing in organ culture, with ^{14}C-proline and ^{3}H-thymidine incorporated in the culture medium. Thymidine is incorporated into DNA, which is replicated when a cell divides, so labeled nuclei are those of cells that underwent mitosis in culture. Because proline is a major constituent of collagen, cytoplasmic labeling indicates areas where proline was incorporated, primarily into extracellularly secreted collagen. **A,** Normal growth in the medium, with many labeled cells and heavy incorporation of proline. **B,** Decreased growth in a bone grown with a small amount of bacterial endotoxin added to the culture.

With the development of radioactive tracers, it has become possible to use almost any radioactively labeled metabolite that becomes incorporated into the tissues as a sort of vital stain. The location is detected by the weak radioactivity given off at the site where the material was incorporated. The gamma-emitting isotope ^{99m}Tc can be used to detect areas of rapid bone growth in humans, but these images are more useful in diagnosis of localized growth problems (see Chapter 21) than for studies of growth patterns. For most studies of growth, radioactively labeled materials in the tissues of experimental animals are detected by the technique of autoradiography, in which a film emulsion is placed over a thin section of tissue containing the isotope and then is exposed in the dark by the radiation. After the film is developed, the location of the radiation that indicates where growth is occurring can be observed by looking at the tissue section through the film (Figure 2-16).

Rapid advances in molecular genetics are providing new information about growth and its control. For example, the whole family of transforming growth-factor beta genes now are known to be important in regulating cell growth and organ development. Bone morphogenetic proteins that directly affect skeletal development and show clinical promise in improving healing after fractures were identified in the mid-1990s,[4] and a gene that controls muscle size was identified recently.[5] Because bone

remodels in response to forces on it, genetic alterations that affect muscle also would affect the skeleton. Experiments that clarify how growth is controlled at the cellular level offer exciting prospects for better control of growth in the future.

Another experimental method, applicable to studies of humans, is implant radiography. In this technique, inert metal pins are placed in bones anywhere in the skeleton, including the face and jaws. These metal pins are well tolerated by the skeleton and become permanently incorporated into the bone without causing any problems (Figure 2-17). If metallic implants are placed in the jaws, a considerable increase in the accuracy of a longitudinal cephalometric analysis of growth pattern can be achieved. This method of study, developed by Professor Arne Bjork and coworkers at the Royal Dental College in Copenhagen, Denmark,[6] and used extensively by workers there (see Chapter 4), has provided important new information about the growth pattern of the jaws. The metal pins stay where they were placed within the bones in the absence of infection or inflammation, which is rarely a problem. Superimposing cephalometric radiographs on the implanted pins allows precise observation of both changes in the position of one bone relative to another and changes in the external contours of individual bones. Before radiographic studies using implants, the extent of remodeling changes in the contours of the jaw bones was underesti-

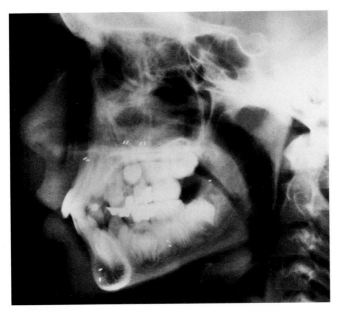

FIGURE 2-17 Lateral cephalometric radiograph from the archives of Bjork's implant studies, showing a subject with six maxillary and five mandibular tantalum implants. (Courtesy Professor Beni Solow, Department of Orthodontics, University of Copenhagen.)

mated, and the rotational pattern of jaw growth described in Chapter 4 was not appreciated. Precise evaluation of dentofacial growth in humans still is done best by implant radiography.[7]

THE NATURE OF SKELETAL GROWTH

At the cellular level, there are only three possibilities for growth. The first is an increase in the size of individual cells, which is referred to as *hypertrophy*. The second possibility is an increase in the number of the cells, which is called *hyperplasia*. The third is for the cells to *secrete extracellular material*, thus contributing to an increase in size independent of the number or size of the cells themselves.

In fact, all three of these processes occur in skeletal growth. Hyperplasia is a prominent feature of all forms of growth. Hypertrophy occurs in a number of special circumstances but is a less important mechanism than hyperplasia in most instances. Although tissues throughout the body secrete extracellular material, this phenomenon is particularly important in the growth of the skeletal system, where extracellular material later mineralizes.

The fact that the extracellular material of the skeleton becomes mineralized leads to an important distinction between growth of the soft or nonmineralized tissues of the body and the hard or calcified tissues. Hard tissues are bones, teeth, and sometimes cartilages. Soft tissues are everything else. In most instances, cartilage, particularly the cartilage significantly involved in growth, behaves like soft tissue and should be thought of in that group, rather than as hard tissue.

Growth of soft tissues occurs by a combination of hyperplasia and hypertrophy. These processes go on everywhere within the tissues, and the result is what is called *interstitial growth*, which simply means that it occurs at all points within the tissue. Secretion of extracellular material can also accompany interstitial growth, but hyperplasia primarily and hypertrophy secondarily are its characteristics. Interstitial growth is characteristic of nearly all soft tissues and of uncalcified cartilage within the skeletal system.

In contrast, when mineralization takes place so that hard tissue is formed, interstitial growth becomes impossible. Hyperplasia, hypertrophy, and secretion of extracellular material all are still possible, but in mineralized tissues, these processes can occur only on the surface, not within the mineralized mass. Direct addition of new bone to the surface of existing bone can and does occur through the activity of cells in the periosteum—the soft tissue membrane that covers bone. Formation of new cells occurs in the periosteum, and extracellular material secreted there is mineralized and becomes new bone. This process is called *direct* or *surface apposition* of bone. Interstitial growth is a prominent aspect of overall skeletal growth because a major portion of the skeletal system is originally modeled in cartilage. This includes the basal part of the skull as well as the trunk and limbs.

Figure 2-18 shows the cartilaginous or chondrocranium at 8 and 12 weeks of intrauterine development. The height of cartilaginous skeletal development occurs during the third month of intrauterine life. A continuous plate of cartilage extends from the nasal capsule posteriorly all the way to the foramen magnum at the base of the skull. It must be kept in mind that cartilage is a nearly avascular tissue whose internal cells are supplied by diffusion through the outer layers. This means, of course, that the cartilage must be thin. At early stages in development, the extremely small size of the embryo makes a chondroskeleton feasible, but with further growth, such an arrangement is no longer possible without an internal blood supply.

During the fourth month in utero, there is an ingrowth of blood vascular elements into various points of the chondrocranium (and the other parts of the early cartilaginous skeleton). These areas become centers of ossification, at which cartilage is transformed into bone, and islands of bone appear in the sea of surrounding cartilage (see Figure 2-18, *B*). The cartilage continues to grow rapidly but is replaced by bone with equal rapidity. The result is that the relative amount of bone increases rapidly and the relative (but not the absolute) amount of cartilage decreases. Eventually, the old chondrocranium is represented only by small areas of cartilage interposed between large sections of bone, which assume the characteristic form of the ethmoid, sphenoid, and basioccipital bones.

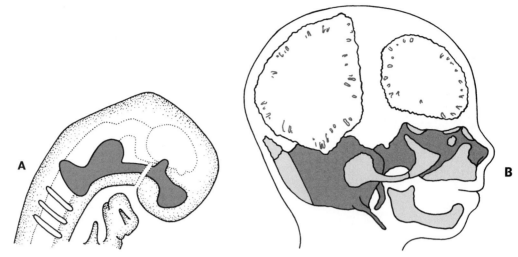

FIGURE 2-18   Development and maturation of the chondrocranium (cartilage: pink; bone: stippled red). **A,** Diagrammatic representation at about 8 weeks. Note that an essentially solid bar of cartilage extends from the nasal capsule anteriorly to the occipital area posteriorly. **B,** Skeletal development at 12 weeks. Ossification centers have appeared in the midline cartilage structures, and in addition, intramembranous bone formation of the jaws and brain case has begun. From this point on, bone replaces cartilage of the original chondrocranium rapidly, so that only the small cartilaginous synchondroses connecting the bones of the cranial base remain.

Growth at these cartilaginous connections between the skeletal bones is similar to growth in the limbs.

In the long bones of the extremities, areas of ossification appear in the center of the bones and at the ends, ultimately producing a central shaft called the *diaphysis* and a bony cap on each end called the *epiphysis.* Between the epiphysis and diaphysis is a remaining area of uncalcified cartilage called the *epiphyseal plate* (Figure 2-19). The epiphyseal plate cartilage of the long bones is a major center for their growth, and in fact this cartilage is responsible for almost all growth in length of these bones. The periosteum on the surface of the bones also plays an important role in adding to thickness and in reshaping the external contours.

Near the outer end of each epiphyseal plate is a zone of actively dividing cartilage cells. Some of these, pushed toward the diaphysis by proliferative activity beneath, undergo hypertrophy, secrete an extracellular matrix, and eventually degenerate as the matrix begins to mineralize and then is rapidly replaced by bone (see Figure 2-19). As long as the rate at which cartilage cells proliferate is equal to or greater than the rate at which they mature, growth will continue. Eventually, however, toward the end of the normal growth period, the rate of maturation exceeds the rate of proliferation, the last of the cartilage is replaced by bone, and the epiphyseal plate disappears. At that point, the growth of the bone is complete, except for surface changes in thickness, which can be produced by the periosteum.

Not all bones of the adult skeleton were represented in the embryonic cartilaginous model, and it is possible for bone to form by secretion of bone matrix directly within

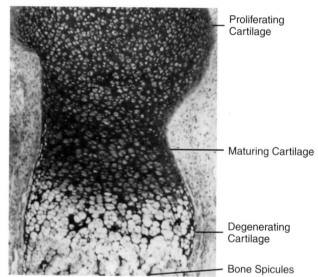

Proliferating Cartilage

Maturing Cartilage

Degenerating Cartilage

Bone Spicules

FIGURE 2-19   Endochondral ossification at an epiphyseal plate. Growth occurs by proliferation of cartilage, occurring here at the top. Maturing cartilage cells are displaced away from the area of proliferation, undergo hypertrophy, degenerate, and are replaced by spicules of bone, as seen in the bottom.

connective tissues, without any intermediate formation of cartilage. Bone formation of this type is called *intramembranous bone formation.* This type of ossification occurs in the cranial vault and both jaws (Figure 2-20).

Early in embryonic life, the mandible of higher animals develops in the same area as the cartilage of the first pharyngeal arch—Meckel's cartilage. It would seem that the mandible should be a bony replacement for this carti-

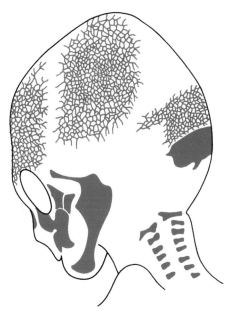

FIGURE 2-20 The bones of the skull of a 12-week-old fetus, drawn from a cleared alizarin-stained specimen. (Redrawn from Langman J: *Medical embryology,* ed 4, Baltimore, 1984, Williams & Wilkins.)

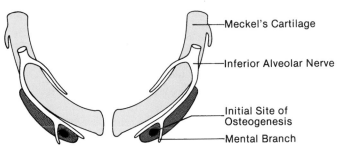

Meckel's Cartilage

Inferior Alveolar Nerve

Initial Site of Osteogenesis

Mental Branch

FIGURE 2-21 Diagrammatic representation of the relation of initial bone formation in the mandible to Meckel's cartilage and the inferior alveolar nerve. Bone formation begins just lateral to Meckel's cartilage and spreads posteriorly along it without any direct replacement of the cartilage by the newly forming bone of the mandible. (Redrawn from Ten Cate AR: *Oral histology,* St. Louis, 1985, Mosby.)

lage in the same way that the sphenoid bone beneath the brain replaces the cartilage in that area. In fact, development of the mandible begins as a condensation of mesenchyme just lateral to Meckel's cartilage and proceeds entirely as an intramembranous bone formation (Figure 2-21). Meckel's cartilage disintegrates and largely disappears as the bony mandible develops. Remnants of this cartilage are transformed into a portion of two of the small bones that form the conductive ossicles of the middle ear but not into a significant part of the mandible. Its perichondrium persists as the sphenomandibular ligament. The condylar cartilage develops initially as an independent secondary cartilage, which is separated by a considerable gap from the body of the mandible (Figure 2-22). Early in fetal life, it fuses with the developing mandibular ramus.

The maxilla forms initially from a center of mesenchymal condensation in the maxillary process. This area is located on the lateral surface of the nasal capsule, the most anterior part of the chondrocranium, but although the growth cartilage contributes to lengthening of the head and anterior displacement of the maxilla, it does not contribute directly to formation of the maxillary bone. An accessory cartilage, the zygomatic or malar cartilage, which forms in the developing malar process, disappears and is totally replaced by bone well before birth, unlike the mandibular condylar cartilage, which persists.

Whatever the location for intramembranous bone formation, interstitial growth within the mineralized mass is impossible, and the bone must be formed entirely by apposition of new bone to free surfaces. Its shape can be changed through removal (resorption) of bone in one area and addition (apposition) of bone in another (see Figure 2-13). This balance of apposition and resorption, with new bone being formed in some areas while old bone is removed in others, is an essential component of the growth process. *Remodeling* of this type is seen at the surfaces of bones that are growing primarily by endochondral replacement as well as in bones that formed directly within a connective tissue membrane.

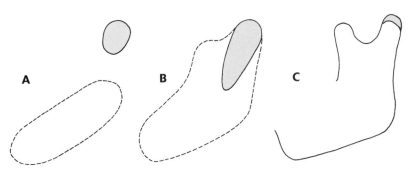

A B C

FIGURE 2-22 The condylar cartilage *(pink)* develops initially as a separate area of condensation from that of the body of the mandible, and only later is incorporated within it. **A,** Separate areas of mesenchymal condensation, at 8 weeks; **B,** fusion of the cartilage with the mandibular body, at 4 months, **C,** situation at birth (reduced to scale).

SITES AND TYPES OF GROWTH IN THE CRANIOFACIAL COMPLEX

To understand growth in any area of the body, it is necessary to understand: (1) the sites or location of growth, (2) the type of growth occurring at that location, and (3) the determinant or controlling factors in that growth.

For the following discussion of sites and types of growth, it is convenient to divide the craniofacial complex into four areas that grow rather differently: (1) the cranial vault, the bones that cover the upper and outer surface of the brain; (2) the cranial base, the bony floor under the brain, which also is the dividing line between the cranium and the face; (3) the nasomaxillary complex, made up of the nose, maxilla, and associated small bones; and (4) the mandible. Determinants or controlling factors, as they are viewed from the perspective of current theories of growth control, are discussed in the following section.

Cranial Vault

The cranial vault is made up of a number of flat bones that are formed directly by intramembranous bone formation, without cartilaginous precursors. From the time that ossification begins at a number of centers that foreshadow the eventual anatomic bony units, the growth process is entirely the result of periosteal activity at the surfaces of the bones. Remodeling and growth occur primarily at the periosteum-lined contact areas between adjacent skull bones, the *cranial sutures*, but periosteal activity also changes both the inner and outer surfaces of these plate-like bones.

At birth, the flat bones of the skull are rather widely separated by relatively loose connective tissues (Figure 2-23). These open spaces, the fontanelles, allow a considerable amount of deformation of the skull at birth. This is important in allowing the relatively large head to pass through the birth canal (see Chapter 3 for more detail). After birth, apposition of bone along the edges of the fontanelles eliminates these open spaces fairly quickly, but the bones remain separated by a thin periosteum-lined suture for many years, eventually fusing in adult life.

Despite their small size, apposition of new bone at these sutures is the major mechanism for growth of the cranial vault. Although the majority of growth in the cranial vault occurs at the sutures, there is a tendency for bone to be removed from the inner surface of the cranial vault, while at the same time new bone is added on the exterior surface. This remodeling of the inner and outer surfaces allows for changes in contour during growth.

Cranial Base

In contrast to the cranial vault, the bones of the base of the skull (the cranial base) are formed initially in cartilage and are later transformed by endochondral ossification to bone. This is particularly true of the midline structures. As one moves laterally, growth at sutures and surface remodeling become more important, but the cranial base is essentially a midline structure. The situation is more complicated, however, than in a long bone with its epiphyseal plates.

As indicated previously, centers of ossification appear early in embryonic life in the chondrocranium, indicating the eventual location of the basioccipital, sphenoid, and ethmoid bones that form the cranial base. As ossification proceeds, bands of cartilage called synchondroses remain between the centers of ossification (Figure 2-24). These important growth sites are the synchondrosis between the sphenoid and occipital bones, or *spheno-occipital synchondrosis*, the *intersphenoid synchondrosis*, between two parts of the

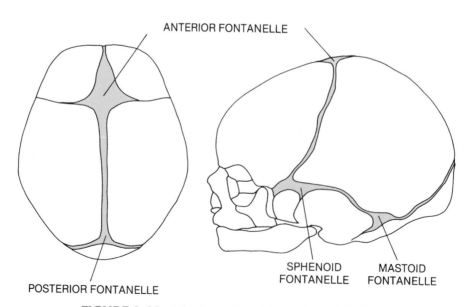

ANTERIOR FONTANELLE

POSTERIOR FONTANELLE

SPHENOID FONTANELLE   MASTOID FONTANELLE

FIGURE 2-23   The fontanelles of the newborn skull *(pink)*.

sphenoid bone, and the *spheno-ethmoidal synchondrosis*, between the sphenoid and ethmoid bones. Histologically, a synchondrosis looks like a two-sided epiphyseal plate (Figure 2-25). The area between the two bones consists of growing cartilage. The synchondrosis has an area of cellular hyperplasia in the center with bands of maturing cartilage cells extending in both directions, which will eventually be replaced by bone.

A significant difference from the bones of the extremities is that immovable joints develop between the bones of the cranial base, in considerable contrast to the highly movable joints of the extremities. The cranial base is thus rather like a single long bone, except that there are multiple epiphyseal plate-like synchondroses. Immovable joints also

occur between most of the other cranial and facial bones, the mandible being the only exception. The periosteum-lined sutures of the cranium and face, containing no cartilage, are quite different from the cartilaginous synchondroses of the cranial base.

Maxilla (Nasomaxillary Complex)

The maxilla develops postnatally entirely by intramembranous ossification. Since there is no cartilage replacement, growth occurs in two ways: (1) by apposition of bone at the sutures that connect the maxilla to the cranium and cranial base and (2) by surface remodeling. In contrast to the cranial vault, however, surface changes in the maxilla are quite dramatic and as important as changes at the sutures.

The growth pattern of the face requires that it grow "out from under the cranium," which means that the maxilla must move through growth a considerable distance downward and forward relative to the cranium and cranial base. As Figure 2-26 illustrates, the sutures attaching the maxilla posteriorly and superiorly are ideally situated to allow its downward and forward repositioning. As the downward and forward movement occurs, the space that would otherwise open up at the sutures is filled in by proliferation of bone at these locations. The sutures remain the same width, and the various processes of the maxilla become longer. Bone apposition occurs on both sides of a suture, so the bones to which the maxilla is attached also become larger. Part of the posterior border of the maxilla is a free surface in the tuberosity region. Bone is added at this surface, creating additional space into which the primary and then the permanent molar teeth successively erupt.

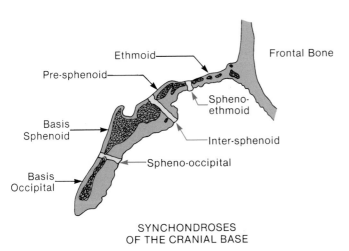

FIGURE 2-24 Diagrammatic representation of the synchondroses of the cranial base, showing the location of these important growth sites.

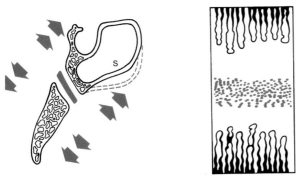

FIGURE 2-25 Diagrammatic representation of growth at the intersphenoid synchondrosis. A band of immature proliferating cartilage cells is located at the center of the synchondrosis, while a band of maturing cartilage cells extends in both directions away from the center, and endochondral ossification occurs at both margins. Growth at the synchondrosis lengthens this area of the cranial base. Even within the cranial base, bone remodeling on surfaces is also important—it is the mechanism by which the sphenoid sinus(es) enlarges, for instance.

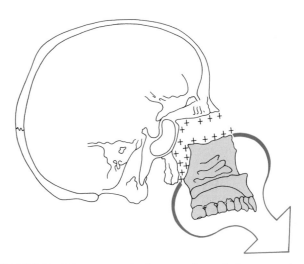

FIGURE 2-26 As growth of surrounding soft tissues translates the maxilla downward and forward, opening up space at its superior and posterior sutural attachments, new bone is added on both sides of the sutures. (Redrawn from Enlow DH, Hans MG: *Essentials of facial growth,* Philadelphia, 1996, W.B. Saunders.)

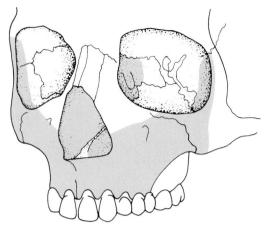

FIGURE 2-27   As the maxilla is carried downward and forward, its anterior surface tends to resorb. Resorption surfaces are shown here in pink. Only a small area around the anterior nasal spine is an exception. (Redrawn from Enlow DH, Hans MG: *Essentials of facial growth*, Philadelphia, 1996, W.B. Saunders.)

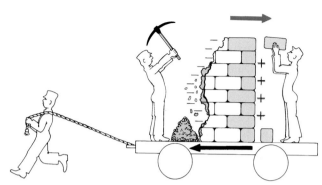

FIGURE 2-28   Surface remodeling of a bone in the opposite direction to that in which it is being translated by growth of adjacent structures creates a situation analogous to this cartoon, in which the wall is being rebuilt to move it backward at the same time the platform on which it is mounted is being moved forward. (Redrawn from Enlow DH, Hans MG: *Essentials of facial growth*, Philadelphia, 1996, W.B. Saunders.)

Interestingly, as the maxilla grows downward and forward, its front surfaces are remodeled, and bone is removed from most of the anterior surface. Note in Figure 2-27 that almost the entire anterior surface of the maxilla is an area of resorption, not apposition. It might seem logical that if the anterior surface of the bone is moving downward and forward, this should be an area to which bone is added, not one from which it is removed. The correct concept, however, is that bone is removed from the anterior surface although the anterior surface is growing forward.

To understand this seeming paradox, it is necessary to comprehend that two quite different processes are going on simultaneously. The overall growth changes are the result of both a downward and forward translation of the maxilla and a simultaneous surface remodeling. The whole bony nasomaxillary complex is moving downward and forward relative to the cranium, being translated in space. Enlow,[8] whose careful anatomic studies of the facial skeleton underlie much of our present understanding, has illustrated this in cartoon form (Figure 2-28). The maxilla is like the platform on wheels, being rolled forward, while at the same time its surface, represented by the wall in the cartoon, is being reduced on its anterior side and built up posteriorly, moving in space opposite to the direction of overall growth.

It is not necessarily true that remodeling changes oppose the direction of translation. Depending on the specific location, translation and remodeling may either oppose each other or produce an additive effect. The effect is additive, for instance, on the roof of the mouth. This area is carried downward and forward along with the rest of the maxilla, but at the same time bone is removed on the nasal side and added on the oral side, thus creating an additional downward and forward movement of the palate (Figure 2-29). Immediately adjacently, however, the anterior part

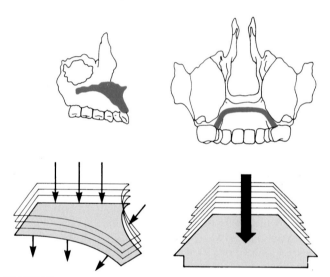

FIGURE 2-29   Remodeling of the palatal vault (which is also the floor of the nose) moves it in the same direction as it is being translated; bone is removed from the floor of the nose and added to the roof of the mouth. On the anterior surface, however, bone is removed, partially canceling the forward translation. As the vault moves downward, the same process of bone remodeling also widens it. (Redrawn from Enlow DH, Hans MB: *Essentials of facial growth*, Philadelphia, 1996, W.B. Saunders.)

of the alveolar process is a resorptive area, so removal of bone from the surface here tends to cancel some of the forward growth that otherwise would occur because of translation of the entire maxilla.

Mandible

In contrast to the maxilla, both endochondral and periosteal activity are important in growth of the mandible. Cartilage covers the surface of the mandibular condyle at the temporomandibular joint. Although this cartilage is not

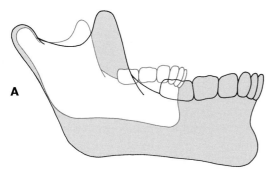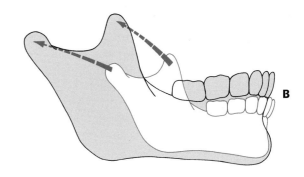

FIGURE 2-30 **A,** Growth of the mandible, as viewed from the perspective of a stable cranial base: the chin moves downward and forward. **B,** Mandibular growth, as viewed from the perspective of vital staining studies, which reveal minimal changes in the body and chin area, while there is exceptional growth and remodeling of the ramus, moving it posteriorly. The correct concept of mandibular growth is that the mandible is translated downward and forward and grows upward and backward in response to this translation, maintaining its contact with the skull.

like the cartilage at an epiphyseal plate or a synchondrosis, hyperplasia, hypertrophy and endochondral replacement do occur there. All other areas of the mandible are formed and grow by direct surface apposition and remodeling.

The overall pattern of growth of the mandible can be represented in two ways, as shown in Figure 2-30. Depending on the frame of reference, both are correct. If the cranium is the reference area, the chin moves downward and forward. On the other hand, if data from vital staining experiments are examined, it becomes apparent that the principal sites of growth of the mandible are the posterior surface of the ramus and the condylar and coronoid processes. There is little change along the anterior part of the mandible. From this frame of reference, Figure 2-30, *B*, is the correct representation.

As a growth site, the chin is almost inactive. It is translated downward and forward, as the actual growth occurs at the mandibular condyle and along the posterior surface of the ramus. The body of the mandible grows longer by periosteal apposition of bone on its posterior surface, while the ramus grows higher by endochondral replacement at the condyle accompanied by surface remodeling. Conceptually, it is correct to view the mandible as being translated downward and forward, while at the same time increasing in size by growing upward and backward. The translation occurs largely as the bone moves downward and forward along with the soft tissues in which it is embedded.

Nowhere is there a better example of remodeling resorption than in the backward movement of the ramus of the mandible. The mandible grows longer by apposition of new bone on the posterior surface of the ramus. At the same time, large quantities of bone are removed from the anterior surface of the ramus (Figure 2-31). In essence, the body of the mandible grows longer as the ramus moves away from the chin, and this occurs by removal of bone from the anterior surface of the ramus and deposition of bone on the posterior surface. On first examination, one might expect a growth center somewhere underneath the

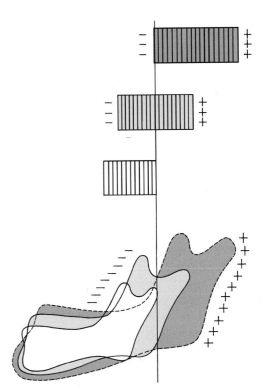

FIGURE 2-31 As the mandible grows in length, the ramus is extensively remodeled, so much so that bone at the tip of the condylar process at an early age can be found at the anterior surface of the ramus some years later. Given the extent of surface remodeling changes, it is an obvious error to emphasize endochondral bone formation at the condyle as the major mechanism for growth of the mandible. (Redrawn from Enlow DH, Hans MG: *Essentials of facial growth*, Philadelphia, 1996, W.B. Saunders.)

teeth, so that the chin could grow forward away from the ramus. But that is not possible, since there is no cartilage and interstitial bone growth cannot occur. Instead, the ramus remodels. What was the posterior surface at one time becomes the center at a later date and eventually may become the anterior surface as remodeling proceeds.

In infancy, the ramus is located at about the spot where the primary first molar will erupt. Progressive posterior remodeling creates space for the second primary molar and then for the sequential eruption of the permanent molar teeth. More often than not, however, this growth ceases before enough space has been created for eruption of the third permanent molar, which becomes impacted in the ramus.

THEORIES OF GROWTH CONTROL

It is a truism that growth is strongly influenced by genetic factors, but it also can be significantly affected by the environment, in the form of nutritional status, degree of physical activity, health or illness, and a number of similar factors. Since a major part of the need for orthodontic treatment is created by disproportionate growth of the jaws, in order to understand the etiologic processes of malocclusion and dentofacial deformity, it is necessary to learn how facial growth is influenced and controlled. Great strides have been made in recent years in improving the understanding of growth control. Exactly what determines the growth of the jaws, however, remains unclear and continues to be the subject of intensive research.

Three major theories in recent years have attempted to explain the determinants of craniofacial growth: (1) bone, like other tissues, is the primary determinant of its own growth; (2) cartilage is the primary determinant of skeletal growth, while bone responds secondarily and passively; and (3) the soft tissue matrix in which the skeletal elements are embedded is the primary determinant of growth, and both bone and cartilage are secondary followers.

The major difference in the theories is the location at which genetic control is expressed. The first theory implies that genetic control is expressed directly at the level of the bone, and therefore its locus should be the periosteum. The second, or cartilage, theory suggests that genetic control is expressed in the cartilage, while bone responds passively to being displaced. This indirect genetic control is called *epigenetic*. The third theory assumes that genetic control is mediated to a large extent outside the skeletal system and that growth of both bone and cartilage is controlled epigenetically, occurring only in response to a signal from other tissues. In contemporary thought, the truth is to be found in some synthesis of the second and third theories, while the first, though it was the dominant view until the 1960s, has largely been discarded.

Level of Growth Control: Sites versus Centers of Growth

Distinguishing between a *site* of growth and a *center* of growth clarifies the differences between the theories of growth control. A site of growth is merely a location at which growth occurs, whereas a center is a location at which independent (genetically controlled) growth occurs. All centers of growth also are sites, but the reverse is not true. A major impetus to the theory that the tissues that form bone carry with them their own stimulus to do so came from the observation that the overall pattern of craniofacial growth is remarkably constant. The constancy of the growth pattern was interpreted to mean that the major sites of growth were also centers. Particularly, the sutures between the membranous bones of the cranium and jaws were considered growth centers, along with the sites of endochondral ossification in the cranial base and at the mandibular condyle. Growth, in this view, was the result of the expression at all these sites of a genetic program. The translation of the maxilla, therefore, was the result of pressure created by growth of the sutures, so that the bones were literally pushed apart.

If this theory were correct, growth at the sutures should occur largely independently of the environment, and it would not be possible to change the expression of growth at the sutures very much. While this was the dominant theory of growth, few attempts were made to modify facial growth because orthodontists "knew" that it could not be done.

It is clear now that sutures, and the periosteal tissues more generally, are not primary determinants of craniofacial growth. Two lines of evidence lead to this conclusion. The first is that when an area of the suture between two facial bones is transplanted to another location (to a pouch in the abdomen, for instance), the tissue does not continue to grow. This indicates a lack of innate growth potential in the sutures. Second, it can be seen that growth at sutures will respond to outside influences under a number of circumstances. If cranial or facial bones are mechanically pulled apart at the sutures, new bone will fill in, and the bones will become larger than they would have been otherwise (see Figure 2-26). If a suture is compressed, growth at that site will be impeded. Thus sutures must be considered areas that react—not primary determinants. The sutures of the maxilla are sites of growth but are not growth centers.

Cartilage as a Determinant of Craniofacial Growth

The second major theory is that the determinant of craniofacial growth is growth of cartilages. The fact that, for many bones, cartilage does the growing while bone merely replaces it makes this theory attractive for the bones of the jaws. If cartilaginous growth were the primary influence, the cartilage at the condyle of the mandible could be considered as a pacemaker for growth of that bone, and the remodeling of the ramus and other surface changes could be viewed as secondary to the primary cartilaginous growth.

One way to visualize the mandible is by imagining that it is like the diaphysis of a long bone, bent into a horseshoe with the epiphyses removed, so that there is cartilage representing "half an epiphyseal plate" at the ends, which represent the mandibular condyles (Figure 2-32). If this were the

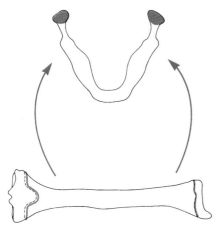

FIGURE 2-32 The mandible was once viewed conceptually as being analogous to a long bone that had been modified by (1) removal of the epiphysis, leaving the epiphyseal plates exposed, and (2) bending of the shaft into a horseshoe shape. If this analogy were correct, of course, the cartilage at the mandibular condyles should behave like true growth cartilage. Modern experiments indicate that, although the analogy is attractive, it is incorrect.

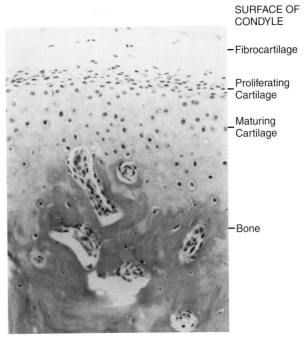

SURFACE OF CONDYLE

—Fibrocartilage

—Proliferating Cartilage

—Maturing Cartilage

—Bone

FIGURE 2-33 Endochondral ossification at the head of the mandibular condyle. A zone of proliferating cartilage is located just beneath the fibrocartilage on the articular surface, and endochondral ossification is occurring beneath this area. Compare the pattern of cellular activity to that of an epiphyseal plate (see Figure 2-18).

true situation, then indeed the cartilage at the mandibular condyle should act as a growth center, behaving basically like an epiphyseal growth cartilage (Figure 2-33).

Growth of the maxilla is more difficult but not impossible to explain on a cartilage theory basis. Although there is no cartilage in the maxilla itself, there is cartilage in the nasal septum, and the nasomaxillary complex grows as a unit. Proponents of the cartilage theory hypothesize that the cartilaginous nasal septum serves as a pacemaker for other aspects of maxillary growth.[9] Note in Figure 2-34 that the cartilage is located so that its growth could easily lead to a downward and forward translation of the maxilla. If the sutures of the maxilla served as reactive areas, as they seem to do, then they would respond to this translation by forming new bone when the sutures were pulled apart by forces from the growing cartilage. Although the amount of nasal septal cartilage reduces as growth continues, cartilage persists in this area throughout life, and the pacemaker role is certainly possible.

Two kinds of experiments have been carried out to test the idea that cartilage can serve as a true growth center. These involve an analysis of the results of transplanting cartilage and an evaluation of the effect on growth of removing cartilage at an early age.

Transplantation experiments demonstrate that not all skeletal cartilage acts the same when transplanted.[10] If a piece of the epiphyseal plate of a long bone is transplanted, it will continue to grow in a new location or in culture, indicating that these cartilages do have innate growth potential. Cartilage from the spheno-occipital synchondrosis of the cranial base also grows when transplanted, but not as well. It is difficult to obtain cartilage from the cranial base to transplant, particularly at an early age when the

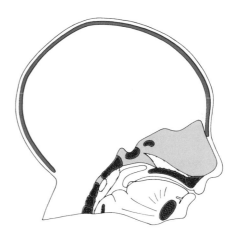

FIGURE 2-34 Diagrammatic representation of the chondrocranium at an early stage of development, showing the large amount of cartilage in the anterior region that eventually becomes the cartilaginous nasal septum.

cartilage is actively growing under normal conditions; perhaps this explains why it does not grow in vitro as much as epiphyseal plate cartilage. In early experiments, transplanting cartilage from the nasal septum gave equivocal results: sometimes it grew, sometimes it did not. In more precise recent experiments, however, nasal septal cartilage was found to grow nearly as well in culture as epiphyseal plate cartilage.[11] Little or no growth was observed when

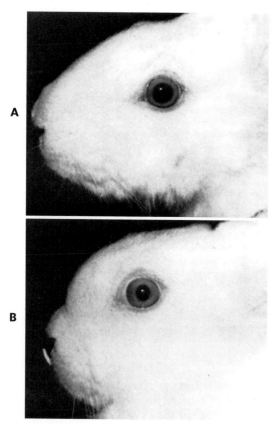

FIGURE 2-35   The effect of removing the cartilaginous nasal septum on forward growth of the snout in the rabbit. **A,** Normal control. **B,** Litter mate in whom the cartilaginous nasal septum was removed soon after birth. The deficient forward growth of the nasomaxillary complex after this surgery is apparent. (From Sarnat BG. In McNamara JA Jr. (editor): *Factors affecting the growth of the midface*, Ann Arbor, Mich., 1976, University of Michigan Center for Human Growth and Development.)

the mandibular condyle was transplanted,[12] and cartilage from the mandibular condyle showed significantly less growth in culture than the other cartilages.[13] From these experiments, the other cartilages appear capable of acting as growth centers, but the mandibular condyle does not.

Experiments to test the effect of removing cartilages are also informative. The basic idea is that if removing a cartilaginous area stops or diminishes growth, perhaps it really was an important center for growth. The impact on a growing rabbit of having a segment of cartilaginous nasal septum removed is shown in Figure 2-35. Obviously, extirpating a young rabbit's septum causes a considerable deficit in growth of the midface. It does not necessarily follow, however, that the entire effect on growth in such experiments results from loss of the cartilage. It can be argued that the surgery itself and the accompanying interference with blood supply to the area, not the loss of the cartilage, cause the growth changes.

There are few reported cases of early loss of the cartilaginous nasal septum in humans. One individual in whom

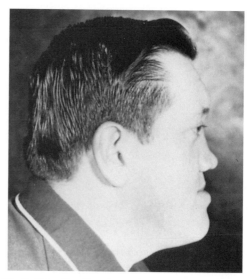

FIGURE 2-36   Profile view of a man whose cartilaginous nasal septum was removed at age 8, after an injury. The obvious midface deficiency developed after the septum was removed.

the entire septum was removed at age 8 after an injury is shown in Figure 2-36. It is apparent that a midface deficiency developed, but one cannot confidently attribute this to the loss of the cartilage. Nevertheless, the loss of growth in experimental animals when this cartilage is removed is great enough to lead most observers to conclude that the septal cartilage does have some innate growth potential, whose loss makes a difference in maxillary growth.

The neck of the mandibular condyle is a relatively fragile area. When the side of the jaw is struck sharply, the mandible often fractures just below the opposite condyle. When this happens, the condyle fragment is usually retracted well away from its previous location by the pull of the lateral pterygoid muscle (Figure 2-37). The condyle literally has been removed when this occurs, and it resorbs over a period of time. Condylar fractures occur relatively frequently in children. If the condyle was an important growth center, one would expect to see severe growth impairment after such an injury at an early age. As recently as the 1960s, it was stated in standard texts that fracture of the mandibular condyle at an early age did invariably lead to severe growth disturbances.

Two excellent studies carried out in Scandinavia disproved this contention. Both Gilhuus-Moe[14] and Lund[15] demonstrated that after fracture of the mandibular condyle in a child, there was an excellent chance that the condylar process would regenerate to approximately its original size and a small chance that it would overgrow after the injury. In experimental animals, after a fracture, all of the original bone and cartilage resorbs, and a new condyle regenerates directly from periosteum at the fracture site. Eventually, a new layer of cartilage forms at the condylar surface. Although there is no direct evidence that the cartilage layer itself regenerates in children after condylar fractures, it is likely that this occurs in humans also.

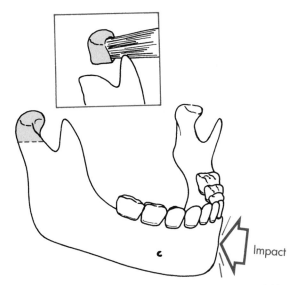

Impact

FIGURE 2-37 A blow to one side of the mandible may fracture the condylar process on the opposite side. When this happens, the pull of the lateral pterygoid muscle distracts the condylar fragment including all the cartilage, and it subsequently resorbs.

However, in 15% to 20% of the Scandinavian children studied who suffered a condylar fracture, there was a reduction in growth after the injury. Similar findings have been reported elsewhere.[16] This growth reduction seems to relate to the amount of trauma to the soft tissues and the resultant scarring in the area. The mechanism by which this occurs is discussed in the following section.

In summary, it appears that epiphyseal cartilages and (probably) the cranial base synchondroses can and do act as independently growing centers, as can the nasal septum (perhaps to a lesser extent). Neither transplantation experiments nor experiments in which the condyle is removed lend any support to the idea that the cartilage of the mandibular condyle is an important center.[17] It appears that the growth at the mandibular condyles is much more analogous to growth at the sutures of the maxilla—entirely reactive—than to growth at an epiphyseal plate.

Functional Matrix Theory of Growth

If neither bone nor cartilage were the determinant for growth of the craniofacial skeleton, it would appear that the control would have to lie in the adjacent soft tissues. This point of view was put formally in the 1960s by Moss, in his "functional matrix theory" of growth, and reviewed and updated recently by him.[18] While granting the innate growth potential of cartilages of the long bones, his theory holds that neither the cartilage of the mandibular condyle nor the nasal septum cartilage is a determinant of jaw growth. Instead, he theorizes that growth of the face occurs as a response to functional needs and neurotrophic influences, and is mediated by the soft tissue in which the jaws are em-

bedded. In this conceptual view, the soft tissues grow, and both bone and cartilage react.

The growth of the cranium illustrates this view of skeletal growth very well. There can be little question that the growth of the cranial vault is a direct response to the growth of the brain. Pressure exerted by the growing brain separates the cranial bones at the sutures, and new bone passively fills in at these sites so that the brain case fits the brain.

This phenomenon can be seen readily in humans in two experiments of nature (Figure 2-38). First, when the brain is very small, the cranium is also very small, and the condition of microcephaly results. In this case, the size of the head is an accurate representation of the size of the brain. A second natural experiment is the condition called hydrocephaly. In this case, reabsorption of cerebrospinal fluid is impeded, the fluid accumulates, and intracranial pressure builds up. The increased intracranial pressure impedes development of the brain, so the hydrocephalic may have a small brain and be mentally retarded; but this condition also leads to an enormous growth of the cranial vault. Uncontrolled hydrocephaly may lead to a cranium two or three times its normal size, with enormously enlarged frontal, parietal, and occipital bones. This is perhaps the clearest example of a "functional matrix" in operation. Another excellent example is the relationship between the size of the eye and the size of the orbit. An enlarged eye or small eye will cause a corresponding change in the size of the orbital cavity. In this instance, the eye is the functional matrix.

Moss theorizes that the major determinant of growth of the maxilla and mandible is the enlargement of the nasal and oral cavities, which grow in response to functional needs. The theory does not make it clear how functional needs are transmitted to the tissues around the mouth and nose, but it does predict that the cartilages of the nasal septum and mandibular condyles are not important determinants of growth and that their loss would have little effect on growth if proper function could be obtained. From the view of this theory, however, absence of normal function would have wide-ranging effects.

We have already noted that in 75% to 80% of human children who suffer a condylar fracture, the resulting loss of the condyle does not impede mandibular growth. The condyle regenerates very nicely. What about the 20% to 25% of children in whom a growth deficit occurs after condylar fracture?[19] Could some interference with function be the reason for the growth deficiency?

The answer seems to be a clear yes. It has been known for many years that mandibular growth is greatly impaired by an ankylosis (Figure 2-39), defined as a fusion across the joint so that motion is prevented or extremely limited. Mandibular ankylosis can develop in a number of ways. For instance, one possible cause is a severe infection in the area of the temporomandibular joint, leading to destruction of tissues and ultimate scarring. Another cause, of course, is trauma, which can result in a growth deficiency if there is

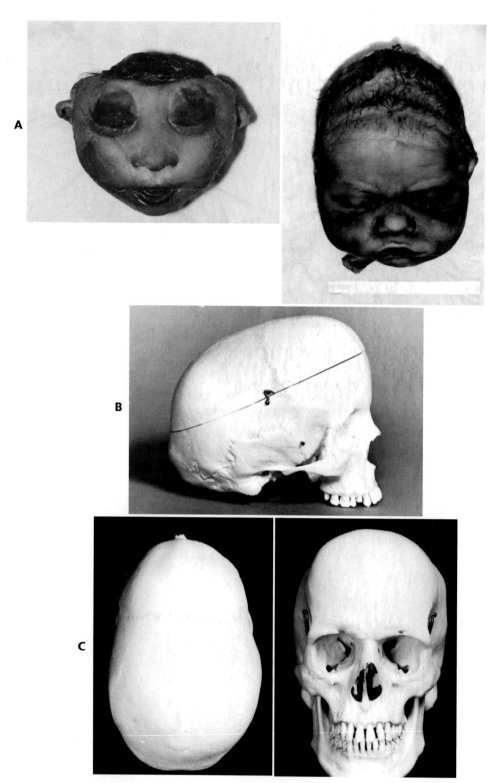

FIGURE 2-38   **A,** The brain case of an anencephalic full-term infant *(left);* in comparison with a facially-normal stillborn infant. Note the failure of the bony covering of the brain to develop in the absence of the brain. If the brain were very small, the brain case would also be small. **B,** The skull of a young child with hydrocephaly. Note the tremendous enlargement of the brain case in response to the increased intracranial pressure. **C,** Superior *(left)* and front *(right)* views of the skull of an individual with scaphocephaly, in which the midsagittal suture fuses prematurely. Note the absence of the midsagittal suture and the extremely narrow width of the cranium. In compensation for its inability to grow laterally, the brain and brain case have become abnormally long posteriorly. **(C** from Proffit WR, White RP: *Surgical-orthodontic treatment,* St. Louis, 1991, Mosby.)

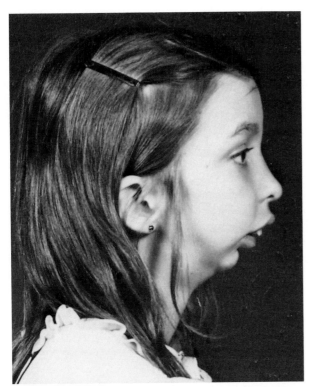

FIGURE 2-39 Profile view of a girl in whom a severe infection of the mastoid air cells involved the temporomandibular joint and led to ankylosis of the mandible. The resulting restriction of mandibular growth is apparent.

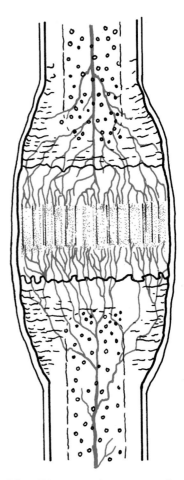

FIGURE 2-40 Diagrammatic representation of distraction osteogenesis in a long bone. The drawing represents the situation after a bone cuts through the cortex, initial healing, and then a few weeks of distraction. In the center, a fibrous radiolucent interzone with longitudinally oriented collagen bundles in the area where lengthening of the bone is occurring. Proliferating fibroblasts and undifferentiated mesenchymal cells are found throughout this area. Osteoblasts appear at the edge of the interzone. On both sides of the interzone, a rich blood supply is present in a zone of mineralization. Beneath that, a zone of remodeling exists. This sequence of formation of a stretched collagen matrix, mineralization, and remodeling is typical of distraction osteogenesis. (Redrawn from Samchukov et al. In McNamara J, Trotman C (editors): *Distraction osteogenesis and tissue engineering*, Ann Arbor, Mich., 1998, University of Michigan Center for Human Growth and Development.)

enough soft tissue injury to lead to severe scarring as the injury heals. It appears that the mechanical restriction caused by scar tissue in the vicinity of the temporomandibular joint impedes translation of the mandible as the adjacent soft tissues grow, and that this is the reason for growth deficiency in some children after condylar fractures.

It is interesting, and potentially quite significant clinically, that under some circumstances bone can be induced to grow at surgically-created sites by the method called *distraction osteogenesis* (Figure 2-40). The Russian surgeon Alizarov discovered in the 1950s that if cuts were made through the cortex of a long bone of the limbs, the arm or leg then could be lengthened by tension to separate the bony segments. Current research shows that the best results are obtained if this type of distraction starts after a few days of initial healing and callus formation and if the segments are separated at a rate of a 0.5-1.5 millimeters per day (see Figure 2-40).[20] Surprisingly large amounts of new bone can form at the surgical site, lengthening the arm or leg by several centimeters in some cases. Distraction osteogenesis now is widely used to correct limb deformities, especially after injury but also in patients with congenital problems.

The bone of the mandible is quite similar in its internal structure to the bone of the limbs,[21] even though its developmental course is rather different. Lengthening the

mandible via distraction osteogenesis clearly is possible (Figure 2-41), but a number of practical problems still must be overcome before this approach can be used to correct mandibular deficiency. The bone of the maxilla and other facial structures is much less like the limb bones, and it is less clear that distraction techniques can be applied to these structures. In a sense, inducing growth by separating cranial and facial bones at their sutures is a distraction method. Manipulating maxillary growth by influencing growth at the sutures has been a major part of orthodontic treatment for many years. At this writing, the differences in reactions to distraction between the facial bones and the bones of the limbs still are being evaluated, but rapid advances in both biologic understanding and distraction mechanisms suggest that distraction osteogenesis will be clinically useful in orthodontics, at least to lengthen the mandible, in the near future.[22] The current status of distraction osteogenesis as a method to correct deficient growth in the face and jaws is reviewed in some detail in Chapter 22.

In summary, it appears that growth of the cranium occurs almost entirely in response to growth of the brain.

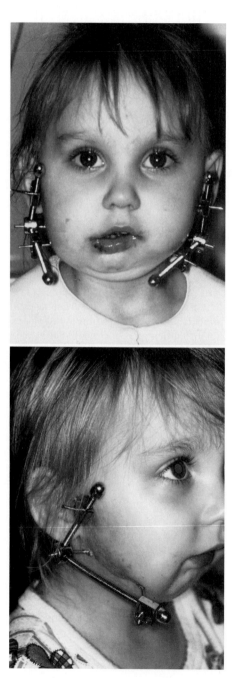

FIGURE 2-41   External fixation for lengthening the mandible by distraction osteogenesis in a child with hemifacial microsomia.

Growth of the cranial base is primarily the result of endochondral growth and bony replacement at the synchondroses, which have independent growth potential but perhaps are influenced by the growth of the brain. Growth of the maxilla and its associated structures occurs from a combination of growth at sutures and direct remodeling of the surfaces of the bone. The maxilla is translated downward and forward as the face grows, and new bone fills in at the sutures. The extent to which growth of cartilage of the nasal septum leads to translation of the maxilla remains unknown, but both the surrounding soft tissues and this cartilage probably contribute to the forward repositioning of the maxilla. Growth of the mandible occurs by both endochondral proliferation at the condyle and apposition and resorption of bone at surfaces. It seems clear that the mandible is translated in space by the growth of muscles and other adjacent soft tissues and that addition of new bone at the condyle is in response to the soft tissue changes.

SOCIAL AND BEHAVIORAL DEVELOPMENT

F.T. McIver and W.R. Proffit

Physical growth can be considered the outcome of an interaction between genetically controlled cell proliferation and environmental influences that modify the genetic program. Similarly, behavior can be viewed as the result of an interaction between innate or instinctual behavioral patterns and behaviors learned after birth. In animals, it appears that the majority of behaviors are instinctive, although even lower animals are capable of a degree of learned behavior. In humans, on the other hand, it is generally conceded that the great majority of behaviors are learned.

For this reason, it is less easy to construct stages of behavioral development in humans than stages of physical development. The higher proportion of learned behavior means that what might be considered environmental effects can greatly modify behavior. On the other hand, there are human instinctual behaviors (e.g., the sex drive), and in a sense, the outcome of behavior hinges on how the instinctual behavioral urges have been modified by learning. Another factor that is emerging as an influence on behavior is temperament. Children early in infancy appear to exhibit temperament that influences their behavior. The impact of temperament on behavior and health is the subject of considerable current investigation. For all these reasons, the older the individual, the more complex the behavioral pattern and the more important the learned overlay of behavior will be.

In this section, a brief overview of social, cognitive, and behavioral development is presented, greatly simplifying a complex subject and emphasizing the evaluation and management of children who will be receiving dental and orthodontic treatment. First, the process by which behavior can be learned is presented. Second, the structural substrate of behavior, which appears to relate both to the organization of the nervous system at various stages and to emotional components underlying the expression of behavior,[23-26] will be reviewed. The relevance of the theoretical areas discussed to the day-to-day treatment of patients is emphasized.

Learning and the Development of Behavior

The basic mechanisms of learning appear to be essentially the same at all ages. As learning proceeds, more complex skills and behaviors appear, but it is difficult to define the process in distinct stages—a continuous flow model appears more appropriate. It is important to remember that this discussion is of the development of behavioral patterns, not the acquisition of knowledge or intellectual skills in the academic sense.

At present, psychologists generally consider that there are three distinct mechanisms by which behavioral responses are learned: (1) classical conditioning, (2) operant conditioning, and (3) observational learning.

Classical Conditioning. Classical conditioning was first described by the Russian physiologist Ivan Pavlov, who discovered in the nineteenth century during his studies of reflexes that apparently unassociated stimuli could produce reflexive behavior. Pavlov's classic experiments involved the presentation of food to a hungry animal, along with some other stimulus, for example, the ringing of a bell. The sight and sound of food normally elicit salivation by a reflex mechanism. If a bell is rung each time food is presented, the auditory stimulus of the ringing bell will become associated with the food presentation stimulus, and in a relatively short time, the ringing of a bell by itself will elicit salivation. Classical conditioning, then, operates by the simple process of association of one stimulus with another. For

that reason, this mode of learning is sometimes referred to as learning by association.[27]

Classical conditioning occurs readily with young children and can have a considerable impact on a young child's behavior on the first visit to a dental office. By the time a child is brought for the first visit to a dentist, even if that visit is at an early age, it is highly likely that he or she will have had many experiences with pediatricians and medical personnel. When a child experiences pain, the reflex reaction is crying and withdrawal. In Pavlovian terms, the infliction of pain is an unconditioned stimulus, but a number of aspects of the setting in which the pain occurs can come to be associated with this unconditioned stimulus.

For instance, it is unusual for a child to encounter people who are dressed entirely in white uniforms or long white coats. If the unconditioned stimulus of painful treatment comes to be associated with the conditioned stimulus of white coats (Figure 2-42), a child may cry and withdraw immediately at the first sight of a white-coated dentist or dental assistant. In this case, the child has learned to associate the conditioned stimulus of pain and the unconditioned stimulus of a white-coated adult, and the mere sight of the white coat is enough to produce the reflex behavior initially associated with pain.

Associations of this type tend to become generalized. Painful and unpleasant experiences associated with medical treatment can become generalized to the atmosphere of a physician's office, so that the whole atmosphere of a waiting room, receptionist, and other waiting children may produce crying and withdrawal after several experiences in the physician's office, even if there is no sign of a white coat.

Because of this association, behavior management in the dentist's office is easier if the dental office looks as little like the typical pediatrician's office or hospital clinic as

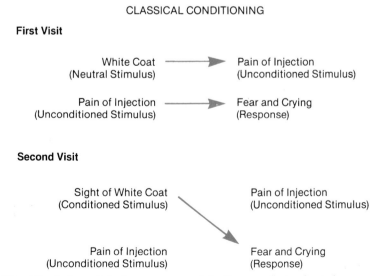

CLASSICAL CONDITIONING

First Visit

White Coat (Neutral Stimulus) ⟶ Pain of Injection (Unconditioned Stimulus)

Pain of Injection (Unconditioned Stimulus) ⟶ Fear and Crying (Response)

Second Visit

Sight of White Coat (Conditioned Stimulus) ⟶ Pain of Injection (Unconditioned Stimulus)

Pain of Injection (Unconditioned Stimulus) ⟶ Fear and Crying (Response)

FIGURE 2-42 Classical conditioning causes an originally neutral stimulus to become associated with one that leads to a specific reaction. If individuals in white coats are the ones who give painful injections that cause crying, the sight of an individual in a white coat soon may provoke an outburst of crying.

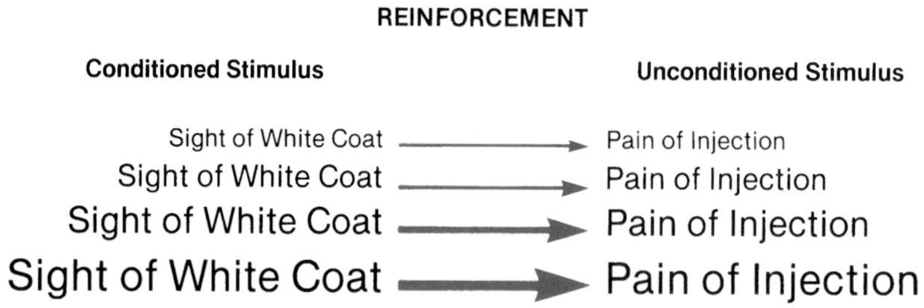

REINFORCEMENT

Conditioned Stimulus   Unconditioned Stimulus

Sight of White Coat ⟶ Pain of Injection
Sight of White Coat ⟶ Pain of Injection
Sight of White Coat ⟶ Pain of Injection
Sight of White Coat ⟶ Pain of Injection

FIGURE 2-43   Every time they occur, the association between a conditioned and unconditioned stimulus is strengthened. This process is called reinforcement.

possible. In practices where the dentist and auxiliaries work with young children, they have found that it is helpful in reducing children's anxiety if their appearance is different from that associated with the physician. It also helps if they can make the child's first visit as different as possible from the previous visits to the physician. Treatment that might produce pain should be avoided if at all possible on the first visit to the dental office.

The association between a conditioned and an unconditioned stimulus is strengthened or reinforced every time they occur together (Figure 2-43). Every time a child is taken to a hospital clinic where something painful is done, the association between pain and the general atmosphere of that clinic becomes stronger, as the child becomes more sure of his conclusion that bad things happen in such a place. Conversely, if the association between a conditioned and an unconditioned stimulus is not reinforced, the association between them will become less strong, and eventually the conditioned response will no longer occur. This phenomenon is referred to as extinction of the conditioned behavior. Once a conditioned response has been established, it is necessary to reinforce it only occasionally to maintain it. If the conditioned association of pain with the doctor's office is strong, it can take many visits without unpleasant experiences and pain to extinguish the associated crying and avoidance.

The opposite of generalization of a conditioned stimulus is discrimination. The conditioned association of white coats with pain can easily be generalized to any office setting. If a child is taken into other office settings that are somewhat different from the one where painful things happen, a dental office, for instance, where painful injections are not necessary, a discrimination between the two types of offices soon will develop and the generalized response to any office as a place where painful things occur will be extinguished.

Operant Conditioning.   Operant conditioning, which can be viewed conceptually as a significant extension of classical conditioning, has been emphasized by the preeminent behavioral theorist of recent years, B.F. Skinner. Skinner contended that the most complex human behaviors can be explained by operant conditioning.[28,29] His theories, which downplay the role of the individual's con-

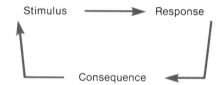

FIGURE 2-44   Operant conditioning differs from classical conditioning in that the consequence of a behavior is considered a stimulus for future behavior. This means that the consequence of any particular response will affect the probability of that response occurring again in a similar situation.

scious determination in favor of unconscious determined behavior, have met with much resistance but have been remarkably successful in explaining many aspects of social behavior far too complicated to be understood from the perspective of classical conditioning.

Since the theory of operant conditioning explains—or attempts to explain—complex behavior, it is not surprising that the theory itself is more complex. Although it is not possible here to explore operant conditioning in any detail, a brief overview is presented as an aid in understanding the acquisition of behavior that older children are likely to demonstrate in the dentist's or orthodontist's office.

The basic principle of operant conditioning is that the consequence of a behavior is in itself a stimulus that can affect future behavior (Figure 2-44). In other words, the consequence that follows a response will alter the probability of that response occurring again in a similar situation. In classical conditioning, a stimulus leads to a response; in operant conditioning, a response becomes a further stimulus. The general rule is that if the consequence of a certain response is pleasant or desirable, that response is more likely to be used again in the future; but if a particular response produces an unpleasant consequence, the probability of that response being used in the future is diminished.

Skinner described four basic types of operant conditioning, distinguished by the nature of the consequence (Figure 2-45). The first of these is *positive reinforcement*. If a pleasant consequence follows a response, the response has been positively reinforced, and the behavior that led to this pleasant consequence becomes more likely in the future. For example, if a child is given a reward such as a toy for be-

	PROBABILITY OF RESPONSE INCREASES	PROBABILITY OF RESPONSE DECREASES
Pleasant Stimulus (S₁)	I S₁ Presented Positive Reinforcement or Reward	III S₁ Withdrawn Omission or Time-Out
Unpleasant Stimulus (S₂)	II S₂ Withdrawn Negative Reinforcement or Escape	IV S₂ Presented Punishment

FIGURE 2-45 The four basic types of operant conditioning.

having well during her first dental visit, she is more likely to behave well during future dental visits; her behavior was positively reinforced.

A second type of operant conditioning, called *negative reinforcement*, involves the withdrawal of an unpleasant stimulus after a response. Like positive reinforcement, negative reinforcement increases the likelihood of a response in the future. In this context, the word negative is somewhat misleading. It merely refers to the fact that the response that is reinforced is a response that leads to the removal of an undesirable stimulus. Note that negative reinforcement is not a synonym for the term *punishment*, discussed at right.

As an example, a child who views a visit to the hospital clinic as an unpleasant experience may throw a temper tantrum at the prospect of having to go there. If this behavior (response) succeeds in allowing the child to escape the visit to the clinic, the behavior has been negatively reinforced and is more likely to occur the next time a visit to the clinic is proposed. The same can be true, of course, in the dentist's office. If behavior considered unacceptable by the dentist and his staff nevertheless succeeds in allowing the child to escape from dental treatment, that behavior has been negatively reinforced and is more likely to occur the next time the child is in the dental office. In dental practice, it is important to reinforce only desired behavior, and it is equally important to avoid reinforcing behavior that is not desired.[30]

The other two types of operant conditioning decrease the likelihood of a response. The third type, *omission* (also called time-out), involves removal of a pleasant stimulus after a particular response. For example, if a child who throws a temper tantrum has his favorite toy taken away for a short time as a consequence of this behavior, the probability of similar misbehavior is decreased. Because children are likely to regard attention by others as a very pleasant stimulus, withholding attention following undesirable behavior is a use of omission that is likely to reduce the unwanted behavior.

The fourth type of operant conditioning, *punishment*, occurs when an unpleasant stimulus is presented after a response. This also decreases the probability that the behavior that prompted punishment will occur in the future. Punishment, like the other forms of operant conditioning, is effective at all ages, not just with children. For example, if the dentist with his new sports car receives a ticket for driving 50 miles per hour down a street marked for 35 miles per hour, he is likely to drive more slowly down that particular street in the future, particularly if he thinks that the same radar speed trap is still operating. Punishment, of course, has traditionally been used as a method of behavior modification in children, more so in some societies than others.

In general, positive and negative reinforcement are the most suitable types of operant conditioning for use in the dental office, particularly for motivating orthodontic patients who must cooperate at home even more than in the dental office. Both types of reinforcement increase the likelihood of a particular behavior recurring, rather than attempting to suppress a behavior as punishment and omission do. Simply praising a child for desirable behavior produces positive reinforcement, and additional positive reinforcement can be achieved by presenting some tangible reward.

Older children are just as susceptible to positive reinforcement as younger ones. Adolescents in the orthodontic treatment age, for instance, can obtain positive reinforcement from a simple pin saying, "World's Greatest Orthodontic Patient" or something similar. A reward system, perhaps providing a T-shirt with some slogan as a prize for three consecutive appointments with good hygiene, is another simple example of positive reinforcement (Figure 2-46).

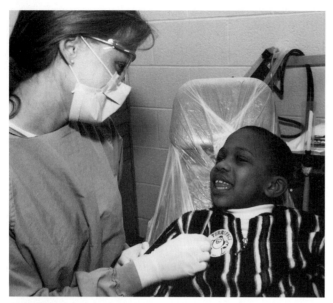

FIGURE 2-46   This 8-year-old boy is being positively reinforced by receiving a "terrific patient" button after his visit to the dentist. The same methods work well for older orthodontic patients, who enjoy receiving a button or T-shirt saying something like, "Braces are beautiful".

Negative reinforcement, which also accentuates the probability of any given behavior, is more difficult to utilize as a behavioral management tool in the dental office, but it can be used effectively if the circumstances permit. If a child is concerned about a treatment procedure but behaves well and understands that the procedure has been shortened because of his good behavior, the desired behavior has been negatively reinforced. In orthodontic treatment, long bonding and banding appointments may go more efficiently and smoothly if the child understands that his helpful behavior has shortened the procedure and reduced the possibility that the procedure will need to be redone.

The other two types of operant conditioning, omission and punishment, should be used sparingly and with caution in the dental office. Since a positive stimulus is removed in omission, the child may react with anger or frustration. When punishment is used, both fear and anger sometimes result. In fact, punishment can lead to a classically conditioned fear response. Obviously, it is a good idea for the dentist and staff to avoid creating fear and anger in a child (or adult) patient, and thus these two types of operant conditioning should be used cautiously.

One mild form of punishment that can be used with children is called "voice control." Voice control involves speaking to the child in a firm voice to gain his (or her) attention, telling him that his present behavior is unacceptable, and directing him as to how he should behave. This technique should be used with care and the child should be immediately rewarded for an improvement in his behavior.

It is most effective when a warm, caring relationship has been established between the dental team and the patient.[31]

There is no doubt that operant conditioning can be used to modify behavior in individuals of any age, and that it forms the basis for many of the behavior patterns of life. Behavioral theorists believe that operant conditioning forms the pattern of essentially all behavior, not just the relatively superficial ones. Whether or not this is true, operant conditioning is a powerful tool for learning of behavior and an important influence throughout life.

Concepts of reinforcement as opposed to extinction, and generalization as opposed to discrimination, apply to operant conditioning as well as to classical conditioning. In operant conditioning, of course, the concepts apply to the situation in which a response leads to a particular consequence, not to the conditioned stimulus that directly controls the conditioned response. Positive or negative reinforcement becomes even more effective if repeated, although it is not necessary to provide a reward at every visit to the dental office to obtain positive reinforcement. Similarly, conditioning obtained through positive reinforcement can be extinguished if the desired behavior is now followed by omission, punishment, or simply a lack of further positive reinforcement.

Operant conditioning that occurs in one situation can also be generalized to similar situations. For example, a child who has been positively reinforced for good behavior in the pediatrician's office is likely to behave well on the first visit to a similarly equipped dentist's office because he or she will anticipate a reward at the dentist's also, based on an assessment of the similarity of the situation. A child who continues to be rewarded for good behavior in the pediatrician's office but does not receive similar rewards in the dentist's office, however, will learn to discriminate between the two situations and may eventually behave better for the pediatrician than for the dentist.

Observational Learning (Modeling).   Another potent way that behavior is acquired is through imitation of behavior observed in a social context. This type of learning appears to be distinct from learning by either classical or operant conditioning. Acquisition of behavior through imitation of the behavior of others, of course, is entirely compatible with both classical and operant conditioning. Some theorists[32] emphasize the importance of learning by imitation in a social context, whereas others, especially Skinner and his followers,[30] argue that conditioning is more important although recognizing that learning by imitation can occur. It certainly seems that much of a child's behavior in a dental office can be learned from observing siblings, other children, or even parents.

There are two distinct stages in observational learning: *acquisition* of the behavior by observing it, and the actual *performance* of that behavior (Figure 2-47). A child can observe many behaviors and thereby acquire the potential to perform them, without immediately demonstrating or performing that behavior. Children are capable of acquiring

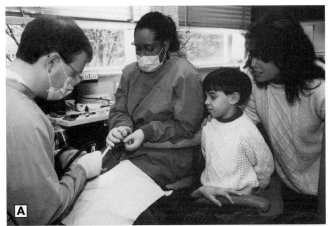

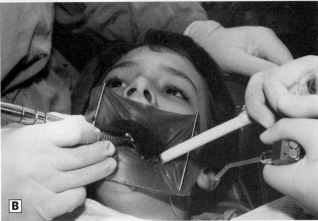

FIGURE 2-47   Observational learning: a child acquires a behavior by first observing it and then actually performing it. For that reason, allowing a younger child to observe an older one calmly receiving dental treatment greatly increases the chance that he will behave in the same way when it is his turn to be treated.

almost any behavior that they observe closely and that is not too complex for them to perform at their level of physical development. A child is exposed to a tremendous range of possible behaviors, most of which he acquires even though the behavior may not be expressed immediately or ever.

Whether a child will actually perform an acquired behavior depends on several factors. Important among these are the characteristics of the role model. If the model is liked or respected, the child is more likely to imitate him or her. For this reason, a parent or older sibling is often the object of imitation by the child. For children in the elementary and junior high school age groups, peers within their own age group, or individuals slightly older, are increasingly important role models, while the influence of parents and older siblings decreases. For adolescents, the peer group is the major source of role models.

Another important influence on whether a behavior is performed is the expected consequences of the behavior. If a child observes an older sibling refuse to obey his father's command and then sees punishment follow this refusal, he

is less likely to defy the father on a future occasion, but he probably still has acquired the behavior, and if he should become defiant, is likely to stage it in a similar way.

Observational learning can be an important tool in management of dental treatment. If a young child observes an older sibling undergoing dental treatment without complaint or uncooperative behavior, he or she is likely to imitate this behavior. If the older sibling is observed being rewarded, the younger child will also expect a reward for behaving well. Because the parent is an important role model for a young child, the mother's attitude toward dental treatment is likely to influence the child's approach.

Research has demonstrated that one of the best predictors of how anxious a child will be during dental treatment is how anxious the mother is. A mother who is calm and relaxed about the prospect of dental treatment teaches the child by observation that this is the appropriate approach to being treated, whereas an anxious and alarmed mother tends to elicit the same set of responses in her child (see Figure 2-47, *A*).[33,34]

Observational learning can be used to advantage in the design of treatment areas. At one time, it was routine for dentists to provide small private cubicles in which all patients, children and adults, were treated. The modern trend, particularly in treatment of children and adolescents but to some extent with adults also, is to carry out dental treatment in open areas with several treatment stations.

Sitting in one dental chair watching the dentist work with someone else in an adjacent chair can provide a great deal of observational learning about what the experience will be like. Direct communication among patients, answering questions about exactly what happened, can add even further learning. Both children and adolescents do better, it appears, if they are treated in open clinics rather than in private cubicles, and observational learning plays an important part in this. The dentist hopes, of course, that the patient waiting for treatment observes appropriate behavior on the part of the patient who is being treated, which will be the case in a well-managed clinical setting.

Several studies have demonstrated that these behavioral guidance principles do work in a dental treatment setting, and that dentists can learn to be more effective in guiding the behavior of children.[35-39]

Stages of Emotional and Cognitive Development

Emotional Development.   In contrast to continuous learning by conditioning and observation, both emotional or personality development and cognitive or intellectual development seem to pass through relatively discrete stages. The contemporary description of emotional development is based on Sigmund Freud's psychoanalytic theory of personality development but has been greatly extended by Erik Erikson.[40] Erikson's work, although connected to Freud's, represents a great departure from psychosexual

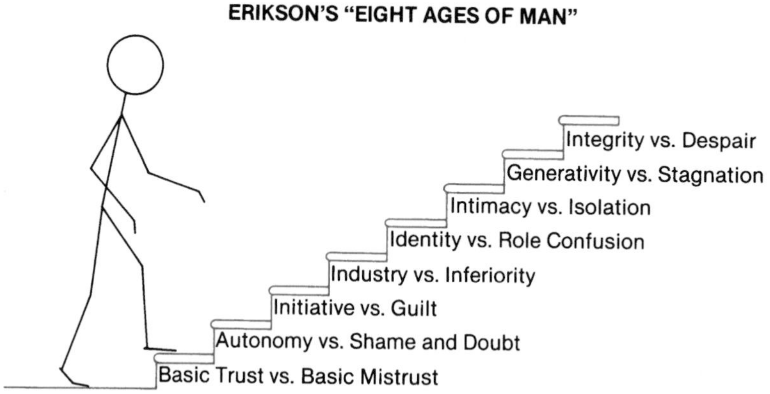

ERIKSON'S "EIGHT AGES OF MAN"

Integrity vs. Despair

Generativity vs. Stagnation

Intimacy vs. Isolation

Identity vs. Role Confusion

Industry vs. Inferiority

Initiative vs. Guilt

Autonomy vs. Shame and Doubt

Basic Trust vs. Basic Mistrust

FIGURE 2-48   Erikson's stages of emotional development: the sequence is more fixed than the time when each stage is reached. Some adults never reach the final steps on the developmental staircase.

stages as proposed by Freud. His "eight ages of man" illustrate a progression through a series of personality development stages. In Erikson's view, "psychosocial development proceeds by critical steps—'critical' being a characteristic of turning points, of moments of decision between progress and regression, integration and retardation." In this view, each developmental stage represents a "psychosocial crisis" in which individuals are influenced by their social environment to develop more or less toward one extreme of the conflicting personality qualities dominant at that stage.

Although chronologic ages are associated with Erikson's developmental stages, as in physical development, the chronologic age varies among individuals but the sequence of the developmental stages is constant. Rather differently from physical development, it is possible and indeed probable that qualities associated with earlier stages may be evident in later stages because of incomplete resolution of the earlier stages.

Erikson's stages of emotional development are as follows (Figure 2-48):

1. Development of Basic Trust (Birth to 18 Months). In this initial stage of emotional development a basic trust—or lack of trust—in the environment is developed. Successful development of trust depends on a caring and consistent mother or mother-substitute, who meets both the physiologic and emotional needs of the infant. There are strongly held theories but no clear answers to exactly what constitutes proper mothering, but it is important that a strong bond develop between parent and child. This bond must be maintained to allow the child to develop basic trust in the world. In fact, physical growth can be significantly retarded unless the child's emotional needs are met by appropriate mothering.

The syndrome of "maternal deprivation," in which a child receives inadequate maternal support, is well recognized though fortunately rare. Such infants fail to gain weight and are retarded in their physical as well as emotional growth (Figure 2-49). The maternal deprivation must be extreme to produce a deficit in physical growth.

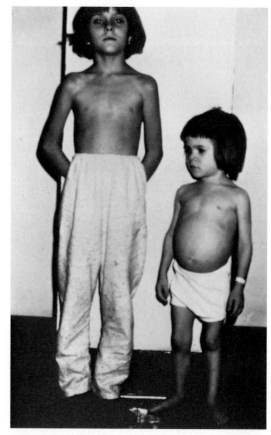

FIGURE 2-49   Both these girls are 7 years old. The one on the left is normal, whereas the one on the right had extreme emotional neglect from a mother who rejected her. The effect on physical growth in this "maternal deprivation syndrome" is obvious; fortunately, this condition is rare. The emotional response probably affects physical growth by altering hormone production, but the mechanism is not fully understood. (Courtesy Dr. F. Debusk.)

Unstable mothering that produces no apparent physical effects can result in a lack of sense of basic trust. This may occur in children from broken families or who have lived in a series of foster homes.

The tight bond between parent and child at this early stage of emotional development is reflected in a strong sense of "separation anxiety" in the child when separated from the parent. If it is necessary to provide dental treatment at an early age, it usually is preferable to do so with the parent present, and if possible, while the child is being held by one of the parents. At later ages, a child who never developed a sense of basic trust will have difficulty entering into situations that require trust and confidence in another person. Such an individual is likely to be an extremely frightened and uncooperative patient who needs special effort to establish rapport and trust with the dentist and staff.

2. Development of Autonomy (18 Months to 3 Years).   Children around the age of 2 often are said to be undergoing the "terrible two's" because of their uncooperative and frequently obnoxious behavior. At this stage of emotional development, the child is moving away from the mother and developing a sense of individual identity or autonomy. Typically, the child struggles to exercise free choice in his life. He or she varies between being a little devil who says no to every wish of the parents and insists on having his own way, and being a little angel who retreats to the parents in moments of dependence. The parents and other adults with whom the child reacts at this stage must protect him against the consequences of dangerous and unacceptable behavior, while providing opportunities to develop independent behavior. Consistently enforced limits on behavior at this time allow the child to further develop trust in a predictable environment (Figure 2-50).

Failure to develop a proper sense of autonomy results in the development of doubts in the child's mind about his ability to stand alone, and this in turn produces doubts about others. Erikson defines the resulting state as one of shame, a feeling of having all one's shortcomings exposed. Autonomy in control of bodily functions is an important part of this stage, as the young child is toilet trained and taken out of diapers. At this stage (and later!), wetting one's pants produces a feeling of shame. This stage is considered decisive in producing the personality characteristics of love as opposed to hate, cooperation as opposed to selfishness, and freedom of expression as opposed to self-consciousness. To quote Erikson, "From a sense of self-control without a loss of self-esteem comes a lasting sense of good will and pride; from a sense of loss of self-control and foreign overcontrol come a lasting propensity for doubt and shame."[40]

A key toward obtaining cooperation with treatment from a child at this stage is to have the child think that whatever the dentist wants was his or her own choice, not something required by another person. For a 2-year-old seeking autonomy, it is all right to open your mouth if you want to, but almost psychologically unacceptable to do it if someone tells you to. One way around this is to offer the child reasonable choices whenever possible, for instance, either a green or a yellow napkin for the neck.

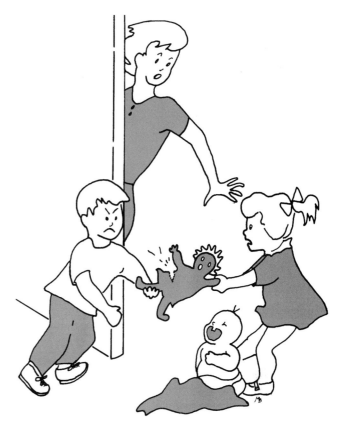

FIGURE 2-50   During the period in which children are developing autonomy, conflicts with siblings, peers, and parents can seem never-ending. Consistently enforced limits on behavior during this stage, often called the "terrible two's", are needed to allow the child to develop trust in a predictable environment.

A child at this stage who finds the situation threatening is likely to retreat to mother and be unwilling to separate from her. Allowing the parent to be present during treatment may be needed for even the simplest procedures. Complex dental treatment of children at this age is quite challenging and may require extraordinary behavior management procedures such as sedation or general anesthesia.

3. Development of Initiative (3 to 6 Years).   In this stage, the child continues to develop greater autonomy, but now adds to it planning and vigorous pursuit of various activities. The initiative is shown by physical activity and motion, extreme curiosity and questioning, and aggressive talking. A major task for parents and teachers at this stage is to channel the activity into manageable tasks, arranging things so that the child is able to succeed, and preventing him or her from undertaking tasks where success is not possible. At this stage, a child is inherently teachable. One part of initiative is the eager modeling of behavior of those whom he respects.

The opposite of initiative is guilt resulting from goals that are contemplated but not attained, from acts initiated but not completed, or from faults or acts rebuked by persons the child respects. In Erikson's view, the child's ultimate ability to initiate new ideas or activities depends on how well he or she is able at this stage to express new thoughts and do new things without being made to feel guilty about expressing a bad idea or failing to achieve what was expected.

For most children, the first visit to the dentist comes during this stage of initiative. Going to the dentist can be constructed as a new and challenging adventure in which the child can experience success. Success in coping with the anxiety of visiting the dentist can help develop greater independence and produce a sense of accomplishment. Poorly managed, of course, a dental visit can also contribute toward the guilt that accompanies failure. A child at this stage will be intensely curious about the dentist's office and eager to learn about the things found there. An exploratory visit with the mother present and with little treatment accomplished usually is important in getting the dental experience off to a good start. After the initial experience, a child at this stage can usually tolerate being separated from the mother for treatment and is likely to behave better in this arrangement, so that independence rather than dependence is reinforced.

4. Mastery of Skills (Age 7 to 11 Years). At this stage, the child is working to acquire the academic and social skills that will allow him or her to compete in an environment where significant recognition is given to those who produce. At the same time, the child is learning the rules by which that world is organized. In Erikson's terms, the child acquires industriousness and begins the preparation for entrance into a competitive and working world. Competition with others within a reward system becomes a reality; at the same time, it becomes clear that some tasks can be accomplished only by cooperating with others. The influence of parents as role models decreases and the influence of the peer group increases.

The negative side of emotional and personality development at this stage can be the acquisition of a sense of inferiority. A child who begins to compete academically, socially, and physically is certain to find that others do some things better and that someone does nearly anything better. Somebody else gets put in the advanced section, is selected as leader of the group, or is chosen first for the team. Failure to measure up to the peer group on a broad scale predisposes toward personality characteristics of inadequacy, inferiority, and uselessness. Again, it is important for responsible adults to attempt to structure an environment that provides challenges, but challenges that have a reasonable chance of being met rather than guarantee failure.

By this stage, a child should already have experienced the first visit to the dentist, although a significant number will not have done so. Orthodontic treatment often begins during this stage of development. Children at this age are trying to learn the skills and rules that define success in any situation, and that includes the dental office. A

key to behavioral guidance is setting attainable intermediate goals, clearly outlining for the child how to achieve those goals, and positively reinforcing success in achieving these goals. Because of the child's drive for a sense of industry and accomplishment, cooperation with treatment can be obtained.

Orthodontic treatment in this age group is likely to involve the faithful wearing of removable appliances (Figure 2-51). Whether a child will do so is determined in large part by whether he or she understands what is needed to please the dentist and parents, whether the peer group is supportive, and whether the desired behavior is reinforced by the dentist.

Children at this stage still are not likely to be motivated by abstract concepts such as "If you wear this appliance your bite will be better." They can be motivated, however, by improved acceptance or status from the peer group. This means that emphasizing how the teeth will look better as the child cooperates is more likely to be a motivating factor than emphasizing a better dental occlusion, which the peer group is not likely to notice.

5. Development of Personal Identity (Age 12 to 17 Years). Adolescence, a period of intense physical development, is also the stage in psychosocial development in which a unique personal identity is acquired. This sense of identity includes both a feeling of belonging to a larger

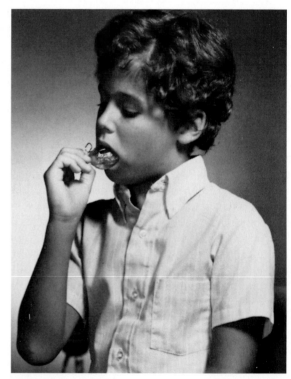

FIGURE 2-51 Instructions for a young child who will be wearing a removable orthodontic appliance must be explicit and concrete. Children at this stage cannot be motivated by abstract concepts but are influenced by improved acceptance or status from the peer group.

group and a realization that one can exist outside the family. It is an extremely complex stage because of the many new opportunities that arise. Emerging sexuality complicates relationships with others. At the same time, physical ability changes, academic responsibilities increase, and career possibilities begin to be defined.[41]

Establishing one's own identity requires a partial withdrawal from the family, and the peer group increases still further in importance because it offers a sense of continuity of existence in spite of drastic changes within the individual (Figure 2-52). Members of the peer group become important role models, and the values and tastes of parents and other authority figures are likely to be rejected. At the same time, some separation from the peer group is necessary to establish one's own uniqueness and value. As adolescence progresses, an inability to separate from the group indicates some failure in identity development. This in turn can lead to a poor sense of direction for the future, confusion regarding one's place in society, and low self-esteem.

Most orthodontic treatment is carried out during the adolescent years, and behavioral management of adolescents can be extremely challenging. Since parental authority is being rejected, a poor psychologic situation is created by orthodontic treatment if it is being carried out primarily because the parents want it, not the child. At this stage, orthodontic treatment should be instituted only if the patient wants it, not just to please the parents.

Motivation for seeking treatment can be defined as internal or external. External motivation is from pressure from others, as in orthodontic treatment "to get mother off my back." Internal motivation is provided by an individual's own desire for treatment to correct a defect that he perceives in himself, not some defect pointed to by authority figures whose values are being rejected anyway. Approval of the peer group is extremely important. At one time, there was a certain stigma attached to being the only one in the group so unfortunate as to have to wear braces. In some areas of the United States now, orthodontic treatment has become so common that there may be a loss of status attached to being one of the few in the group who is not receiving treatment, so that treatment may even be requested in order to remain "one of the crowd."

It is extremely important for an adolescent to actively desire the treatment as something being done *for*, not *to*, him or her. In this stage, abstract concepts can be grasped readily, but appeals to do something because of its impact on personal health are not likely to be heeded. The typical adolescent feels that health problems are concerns of somebody else, and this attitude covers everything from accidental death in reckless driving to development of decalcified areas on carelessly brushed teeth.

6. Development of Intimacy (Young Adult). The adult stages of development begin with the attainment of intimate relationships with others. Successful development of intimacy depends on a willingness to compromise and even to sacrifice to maintain a relationship. Success leads to the establishment of affiliations and partnerships, both with a mate and with others of the same sex in working toward the attainment of career goals. Failure leads to isolation from others and is likely to be accompanied by strong prejudices and a set of attitudes that serve to keep others away rather than bringing them into closer contact.

A growing number of young adults are seeking orthodontic care. Often these individuals are seeking to correct a dental appearance they perceive as flawed. They may feel that a change in their appearance will facilitate attainment of intimate relationships. On the other hand, a "new look" resulting from orthodontic treatment may interfere with previously established relationships.

The factors that affect the development of an intimate relationship include all aspects of each person—appearance, personality, emotional qualities, intellect, and others. A significant change in any of these may be perceived by either partner as altering the relationship. Because of these potential problems, the potential psychologic impact of orthodontic treatment must be fully explained to and explored with the young adult patient before beginning therapy.

7. Guidance of the Next Generation (Adult). A major responsibility of a mature adult is the establishment and guidance of the next generation. Becoming a successful and supportive parent is obviously a major part of this, but another aspect of the same responsibility is service to the group, community, and nation. The next generation is guided, in short, not only by nurturing and influencing one's own children but also by supporting the network of social services needed to ensure the next generation's

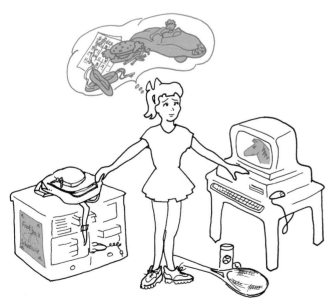

FIGURE 2-52 Adolescence is an extremely complex stage because of the many new opportunities and challenges thrust upon the teenager. Emerging sexuality, academic pressures, earning money, increased mobility, career aspirations and recreational interests combine to produce stress and rewards.

success. The opposite personality characteristic in mature adults is stagnation, characterized by self-indulgence and self-centered behavior.

8. Attainment of Integrity (Late Adult). The final stage in psychosocial development is the attainment of integrity. At this stage, the individual has adapted to the combination of gratification and disappointment that every adult experiences. The feeling of integrity is best summed up as a feeling that one has made the best of this life's situation and has made peace with it. The opposite characteristic is despair. This feeling is often expressed as disgust and unhappiness on a broad scale, frequently accompanied by a fear that death will occur before a life change that might lead to integrity can be accomplished.

Cognitive Development. Cognitive development, the development of intellectual capabilities, also occurs in a series of relatively distinct stages. Like the other psychologic theories, the theory of cognitive development is strongly associated with one dominant individual, in this case the Swiss psychologist Jean Piaget. From the perspective of Piaget and his followers, the development of intelligence is another example of the widespread phenomenon of biologic adaptation. Every individual is born with the capacity to adjust or adapt to both the physical and sociocultural environments in which he or she must live.

In Piaget's view, adaptation occurs through two complementary processes, *assimilation* and *accommodation*.[42] From the beginning, a child incorporates or assimilates events within the environment into mental categories called cognitive structures. A cognitive structure in this sense is a classification for sensations and perceptions.

For example, a child who has just learned the word "bird" will tend to assimilate all flying objects into his idea of bird. When he sees a bee, he will probably say, "Look, bird!" However, for intelligence to develop, the child must also have the complementary process of accommodation. Accommodation occurs when the child changes his or her cognitive structure or mental category to better represent the environment. In the previous example, the child will be corrected by an adult or older child and will soon learn to distinguish between birds and bees. In other words, the child will accommodate to the event of seeing a bee, by creating a separate category of flying objects for bees.

Intelligence develops as an interplay between assimilation and accommodation. Each time the child in our example sees a flying object he or she will try to assimilate it into existing cognitive categories. If these categories do not work, he or she will try to accommodate by creating new ones. However, the child's ability to adapt is limited by the current level of development. The notion that the child's ability to adapt is *age-related* is a crucial concept in Piaget's theory of development.

From the perspective of cognitive development theory, life can be divided into four major stages (Figure 2-53): the *sensorimotor* period, extending from birth to 2 years of age; the *preoperational* period, from 2 to 7 years; the *concrete*

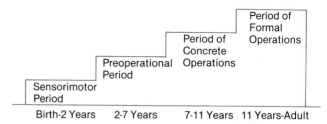

FIGURE 2-53 Cognitive development is divided into four major periods, as diagrammed here.

operational period from about age 7 to puberty; and the period of *formal operations*, which runs from adolescence through adulthood. Like the other developmental stages, it is important to realize that the time frame is variable, especially for the later ones. Some adults never reach the last stage. The sequence of the stages, however, is fixed.

It appears that a child's way of thinking about and viewing the world is quite different at the different stages. A child simply does not think like an adult until the period of formal operations has been reached. Since a child's thought processes are quite different, one cannot expect a child to process and utilize information in the same way that an adult would. To communicate successfully with a child, it is necessary to understand his or her intellectual level and the way in which thought processes work at the various stages.

Considering the cognitive development stages in more detail:

1. Sensorimotor Period. During the first 2 years of life, a child develops from a newborn infant who is almost totally dependent on reflex activities to an individual who can develop new behavior to cope with new situations. During this stage, the child develops rudimentary concepts of objects, including the idea that objects in the environment are permanent; they do not disappear when the child is not looking at them. Simple modes of thought that are the foundation of language develop during this time, but communication between a child at this stage and an adult is extremely limited because of the child's simple concepts and lack of language capabilities. At this stage, a child has little ability to interpret sensory data and a limited ability to project forward or backward in time.

2. Preoperational Period. Because children above the age of 2 begin to use language in ways similar to adults, it appears that their thought processes are more like those of adults than is the case. During the preoperational stage, the capacity develops to form mental symbols representing things and events not present, and children learn to use words to symbolize these absent objects. Because young children use words to symbolize the external appearance or characteristics of an object, however, they often fail to consider important aspects such as function and thus may understand some words quite differently from adults. To an adult, the word "coat" refers to a whole family of external garments that may be long or short, heavy or light, and so on. To a preoperational child, however, the word "coat" is initially associated with only the one he or she wears, and the garment that daddy wears would require another word.

A particularly prominent feature of thought processes of children at this age is the concrete nature of the process and hence, the concrete or literal nature of their language. In this sense, concrete is the opposite of abstract. Children in the preoperational period understand the world in the way they sense it through the five primary senses. Concepts that cannot be seen, heard, smelled, tasted, or felt—for example, time and health—are very difficult for preoperational children to grasp. At this age, children use and understand language in a literal sense and thus understand words only as they have learned them. They are not able to comprehend more than the literal meaning of idioms, and sarcastic or ironic statements are likely to be misinterpreted.

A general feature of thought processes and language during the preoperational period is *egocentrism*, meaning that the child is incapable of assuming another person's point of view. At this stage, his own perspective is all that he can manage—assuming another's view is simply beyond his mental capabilities.

Still another characteristic of thought processes at this stage is *animism*, investing inanimate objects with life. Essentially everything is seen as being alive by a young child, and so stories that invest the most improbable objects with life are quite acceptable to children of this age. Animism can be used to the dental team's advantage by giving dental instruments and equipment life-like names and qualities. For example, the handpiece can be called "Whistling Willie" who is happy while he works at polishing the child's teeth.

At this stage, capabilities for logical reasoning are limited, and the child's thought processes are dominated by the immediate sensory impressions. This characteristic can be illustrated by asking the child to solve a liquid conservation problem. The child is first shown two equal size glasses with water in them. The child agrees that both contain the same amount of water. Then the contents of one glass are poured into a taller, narrower glass while the child watches. Now when asked which container has more water, the child will usually say that the tall one does. Her impressions are dominated by the greater height of the water in the tall glass.

For this reason, the dental staff should use immediate sensations rather than abstract reasoning in discussing concepts like prevention of dental problems with a child at this stage. Excellent oral hygiene is very important when an orthodontic appliance is present (a lingual arch to prevent drift of teeth, for instance). A preoperational child will have trouble understanding a chain of reasoning like the following: "Brushing and flossing remove food particles, which in turn prevents bacteria from forming acids, which cause tooth decay." He or she is much more likely to understand: "Brushing makes your teeth feel clean and smooth," and, "Toothpaste makes your mouth taste good," because these statements rely on things the child can taste or feel immediately.

A knowledge of these thought processes obviously can be used to improve communication with children of this age. A further example would be talking to a 4-year-old about how desirable it would be to stop thumb sucking. The dentist might have little problem in getting the child to accept the idea that "Mr. Thumb" was the problem and that the dentist and the child should form a partnership to control Mr. Thumb who wishes to get into the child's mouth. Animism, in other words, can apply even to parts of the child's own body, which seem to take on a life of their own in this view.

On the other hand, it would not be useful to point out to the child how proud his father would be if he stopped sucking his thumb, since the child would think his father's attitude was the same as the child's (egocentrism). Since the child's view of time is centered around the present, and he or she is dominated by how things look, feel, taste, and sound now, there also is no point in talking to the 4-year-old about how much better his teeth will look in the future if he stops sucking his thumb. Telling him that the teeth will feel better now or talking about how bad his thumb tastes, however, may make an impact, since he can relate to that.

3. Period of Concrete Operations.

As a child moves into this stage, typically after a year or so of preschool and first grade activity, an improved ability to reason emerges. He or she can use a limited number of logical processes, especially those involving objects that can be handled and manipulated (i.e., concrete objects). Thus an 8-year-old could watch the water being poured from one glass to another, imagine the reverse of that process, and conclude that the amount of water remains the same no matter what size the container is. If a child in this stage is given a similar problem, however, stated only in words with no concrete objects to illustrate it, the child may fail to solve it. The child's thinking is still strongly tied to concrete situations, and the ability to reason on an abstract level is limited.

By this stage, the ability to see another point of view develops, while animism declines. Children in this period are much more like adults in the way they view the world but they are still cognitively different from adults. Presenting ideas as abstract concepts rather than illustrating them with concrete objects can be a major barrier to communication. Instructions must be illustrated with concrete objects. "Now wear your retainer every night and be sure to keep it clean," is too abstract. More concrete directions would be: "This is your retainer. Put it in your mouth like this, and take it out like that. Put it in every evening right after dinner before you go to bed, and take it out before breakfast every morning. Brush it like this with an old toothbrush to keep it clean."

4. Period of Formal Operations.   For most children, the ability to deal with abstract concepts and abstract reasoning develops by about age 11. At this stage, the child's thought process has become similar to that of an adult, and the child is capable of understanding concepts like health, disease, and preventive treatment. At this stage, intellectually the child can and should be treated as an adult. It is as great a mistake to talk down to a child who has developed the ability to deal with abstract concepts, using the concrete approach needed with an 8-year-old, as it is to assume that the 8-year-old can handle abstract ideas. Successful communication, in other words, requires a feel for the child's stage of intellectual development.[43]

In addition to the ability to deal with abstractions, teenagers have developed cognitively to the point where they can think about thinking. They are now aware that others think, but usually, in a new expression of egocentrism, presume that they and others are thinking about the same thing. Because young adolescents are experiencing tremendous biologic changes in growth and sexual development, they are preoccupied with these events. When an adolescent considers what others are thinking about, he assumes that others are thinking about the same thing he is thinking about, namely himself. Adolescents assume that others are as concerned with their bodies, actions, and feelings as they themselves are. They feel as though they are constantly "on stage," being observed and criticized by those around them. This phenomenon has been called the "imaginary audience" by Elkind.[44]

The imaginary audience is a powerful influence on young adolescents, making them quite self-conscious and particularly susceptible to peer influence. They are very worried about what peers will think about their appearance and actions, not realizing that others are too busy with themselves to be paying attention to much other than themselves.

The reaction of the imaginary audience to braces on the teeth, of course, is an important consideration to a teenage patient. As orthodontic treatment has become more common, adolescents have less concern about being singled out because they have braces on their teeth, but they are very susceptible to suggestions from their peers about how the braces should look. In some settings, this has led to pleas for tooth-colored plastic or ceramic brackets (to make them less visible); at other times, brightly colored ligatures and elastics have been popular (because everybody is wearing them).

The notion that "others really care about my appearance and feelings as much as I do" leads adolescents to think they are quite unique, special individuals. If this were not so, why would others be so interested in them? As a result of this thought a second phenomenon emerges, which Elkind called the "personal fable." This concept holds that "because I am unique, I am not subject to the consequences others will experience." The personal fable is a powerful motivator that allows us to cope in a dangerous world. It permits us to do things such as travel on airplanes while knowing that "occasionally they crash, but the one I'm on will arrive safely."

While both the imaginary audience and the personal fable have useful functions in helping us develop a social awareness and allowing us to cope in a dangerous environment, they may also lead to dysfunctional behavior and even foolhardy risk-taking. The adolescent may drive too fast thinking "I am unique. I'm especially skilled at driving. Other less skillful drivers may have wrecks, but not I." These phenomena are likely to have significant influence on orthodontic treatment. The imaginary audience, depending on what the adolescent believes, may influence him to accept or reject treatment, and to wear or not wear appliances. The personal fable may make a patient ignore threats to health, such as decalcification of teeth from poor oral hygiene during orthodontic therapy. The thought, of course, is "Others may have to worry about that, but I don't."

The challenge for the dentist is not to try to impose change on reality as perceived by adolescents, but rather to help them more clearly see the actual reality that surrounds them. A teenage patient may protest to his orthodontist that he does not want to wear a particular appliance because others will think it makes him "look goofy." In this situation, telling the patient that he should not be concerned because many of his peers also are wearing this appliance does little to encourage him to wear it. A more useful approach that does not deny the point of view of the patient is to agree with him that he may be right in what others will think, but ask him to give it a try for a specified time. If his peers do respond as the teenager predicts, then a different, but less desirable treatment technique can be discussed. This test of the teenager's perceived reality usually demonstrates that the audience does not respond negatively to the appliance or that the patient can successfully cope with the peer response. Wearing interarch elastics while in public often falls into this category. Encouraging a reluctant teenager to try it and judge his peers' response is much more likely to get him to wear the elastics than telling him everybody else does it so he should too (Figure 2-54).

Sometimes teenage patients have experience with the imaginary audience regarding a particular appliance, but have incorrectly measured the response of the audience. They may require guidance to help them accurately assess the view of the audience. Experience with thirteen-year-old Beth illustrates this point. Following the loss of a maxillary central incisor in an accident, treatment for Beth included a removable partial denture to replace the tooth. She and her parents had been told on several occasions that it would be necessary to wear the removable appliance until enough healing and growth had occurred to permit treatment with a fixed bridge. At a routine recall appointment, Beth asked if the bridge could be placed now. Realizing that this must be a significant concern for Beth, the dentist commented "Beth, wearing this partial must be a problem. Tell me more about it." Beth replied, "It's embarrassing." Inquiring

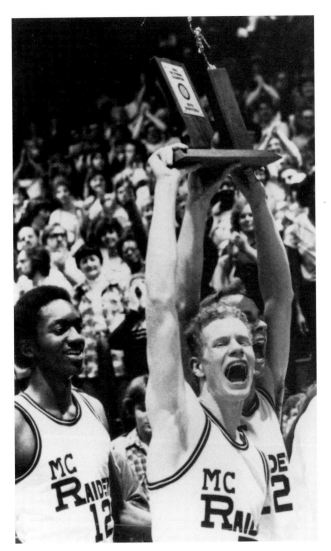

FIGURE 2-54 Wearing your orthodontic elastics during the championship high school basketball game, as this boy obviously was doing, is acceptable to your peers—but the orthodontist is more likely to convince a teenager of that by encouraging him to try it and test their response, than by telling him that he should do it because everybody else does. (Courtesy TP Laboratories.)

further, the dentist asked "When is it embarrassing?" Beth said, "When I spend the night at other girls' homes and have to take it out to brush my teeth." "Well, what is the response of the girls when they see you remove your tooth?" Beth replied, "They think it's neat." Nothing more was said about the tooth and the conversation moved to the vacation that Beth's family was planning.

This illustration indicates how it is possible to provide guidance toward a more accurate evaluation of the attitude of the audience and thus allow teenagers to solve their own problems. This approach on the part of the dentist neither argues with the teenager's reality nor uncritically accepts it. One role of an effective dental professional is to help teenagers test the reality that actually surrounds them.

To be received, the dentist's message must be presented in terms that correspond to the stage of cognitive and psychosocial development that a particular child has reached. It is the job of the dentist to carefully evaluate the development of the child, and adapt his or her language so that concepts are presented in a way that the patient can understand them. The adage "different strokes for different folks" applies strongly to children, whose variations in intellectual and psychosocial development affect the way they receive orthodontic treatment, just as their differing stages of physical development do.

REFERENCES

1. Farkas LG: Anthropometry of the head and face, New York, 1994, Raven Press.
2. Thompson DT: On growth and form, Cambridge, Mass., 1971, Cambridge University Press.
3. Baer MJ, Bosma JF, Ackerman JL: The postnatal development of the rat skull, Ann Arbor, Mich., 1983, The University of Michigan Press.
4. Stone CA: A molecular approach to bone regeneration, Brit J Plast Surg 50:369-73, 1997.
5. McPherron AC, Lawler AM, Lee SJ: Regulation of skeletal muscle mass in mice by a new TGF-beta superfamily member, Nature 387:83-90, 1997.
6. Bjork A: The use of metallic implants in the study of facial growth in children: method and application, Am J Phys Anthropol 29:243-250, 1968.
7. Korn EL, Baumrind S: Transverse development of the human jaws between the ages of 8.5 and 15.5 years, studied longitudinally with use of implants, J Dent Res 69:1298-1306, 1990.
8. Enlow DH, Hans MG: Essentials of Facial Growth, Philadelphia, 1996, Saunders.
9. Latham RA: The septo-premaxillary ligament and maxillary development, J Anat 104:584-586, 1969.
10. Peltomaki T, Kylamarkula S, Vinkka-Puhakka H et al: Tissue separating capacity of growth cartilages, Eur J Orthod 19:473-481, 1997.
11. Copray JC: Growth of the nasal septal cartilage of the rat in vitro, J Anat 144:99-111, 1986.
12. Meikle MC: In vivo transplantation of the mandibular joint of the rat: an autoradiographic investigation into cellular changes at the condyle, Arch Oral Biol 18:1011-1020, 1973.
13. Jansen HW, Duterloo HS: Growth and growth pressure of mandibular condylar and some primary cartilages of the rat in vitro, Am J Orthod Dentofacial Orthop 90:19-28, 1986.
14. Gilhuus-Moe O: Fractures of the Mandibular Condyle in the Growth Period, Stockholm, 1969, Scandinavian University Books, Universitatsforlaget.
15. Lund K: Mandibular growth and remodelling process after mandibular fractures, Acta Odontol Scand 32 (suppl 64), 1974.
16. Sahm G, Witt E: Long-term results after childhood condylar fracture: a CT study, Eur J Orthod 11:154-160, 1990.
17. Copray JC, Dibbets JM, Kantomaa T: The role of condylar cartilage in the development of the temporomandibular joint, Angle Orthod 58:369-380, 1988.

18. Moss ML: The functional matrix hypothesis revisited, Am J Orthod Dentofac Orthop 112: 8-11, 221-226, 338-342, 410-417, 1997.

19. Proffit WR, Vig KWL, Turvey TA: Early fracture of the mandibular condyles: frequently an unsuspected cause of growth disturbances, Am J Orthod 78:1-24, 1980.

20. Yen SLK: Distraction osteogenesis: application to dentofacial orthopedics, Seminars Orthod 3:275-283, 1997.

21. Roberts WE: Bone physiology, metabolism, and biomechanics in orthodontic practice. In Graber TM, Vanarsdall RL, editors: Orthodontics: current principles and techniques, ed 2, St. Louis, Mosby, 1994.

22. Weil TS, Van Sickels JE, Payne CJ: Distraction osteogenesis for correction of transverse mandibular deficiency: a preliminary report, J Oral Maxillofac Surg 55:953-960, 1997.

23. Radis FG, Wilson S, Griffen AL, Coury DL: Temperament as a predictor of behavior during initial dental examination in children, Ped Dent 16:121-127, 1994.

24. Bates JE, Wachs TD, van den Bos GR: Trends in research on temperament, Psychiatric Services 46:661-663, 1995.

25. Santrock JW: Life-span development, Dubuque, Iowa, 1997, Brown and Benchmark.

26. Wallace WA: Theories of personality, Boston, 1993, Allyn and Bacon.

27. Chambers DW: Managing anxieties of young dental patients, J Dent Child 37:363-373, 1970.

28. Skinner BF: Science and human behavior, New York, 1953, Macmillan.

29. Kanfer FH, Goldstein AP: Helping people change, New York, 1986, Pergamon Press.

30. Troutman KC: Behavior of children in the dental office, Update Pediatr Dent 1:1-4, 6-8, 1988.

31. Greenbaum PE, Turner C, Cook EW III, Melamed BG: Dentists' voice control: effects on children's disruptive and affective behavior, Health Psychology 9(5):546-58, 1990.

32. Decker JD, Nathan BR: Behavior modeling training—principles and applications, New York, 1985, Praeger.

33. Folger J: Relationship of children's compliance to mothers' health beliefs and behavior, J Clin Orthod 22:424-426, 1988.

34. Holst A, Schroder U, Ek L et al: Prediction of behavior management problems in children, Scand J Dent Res 96:457-465, 1988.

35. Holst A, Ek L: Effect of systematized "behavior shaping" on acceptance of dental treatment in children, Community Dent Oral Epidemiol 16:349-355, 1988.

36. Weinstein P, Nathan JE: The challenge of fearful and phobic children, Dent Clin North Am 32:667-692, 1988.

37. Greenbaum PE, Melamed BG: Pretreatment modeling: a technique for reducing children's fear in the dental operatory, Dent Clin North Am 32:693-704, 1988.

38. Prins P, Veerkamp J, ter Horst G et al: Behavior of dentists and child patients during treatment, Community Dent Oral Epidemiol 15:253-257, 1987.

39. ter Horst G, Prins P, Veerkamp J, Verhey H: Interactions between dentists and anxious child patients: a behavioral analysis, Community Dent Oral Epidemiol 15:249-252, 1987.

40. Erikson EH: A way of looking at things—selected papers from 1930 to 1980 (S. Schlein, editor), New York, 1987, WW Norton & Co.

41. Oppenheim MN, Spedding RH, Ho CC, York S: Psychosocial pathology and developmental tasks in the adolescent, Pediatr Dent 9:344-346, 1987.

42. Wadsworth BJ: Piaget's theory of cognitive and affective development, New York, 1989, Longman.

43. Waggoner WF, Bougere A: Parenting the adolescent, Pediatr Dent 9:342-343, 1987.

44. Elkind D: The teenager's reality, Pediatr Dent 9:337-341, 1987.

CHAPTER

3

Early Stages of Development

PRENATAL INFLUENCES ON FACIAL DEVELOPMENT

A general understanding of the formation of the face, as presented in the standard embryology texts, is presumed in the discussion that follows. The focus here is on the events in prenatal development that are particularly pertinent to orthodontic problems later in life.

Embryologic Development

In broad overview, nearly all the tissues of the face and neck originate from ectoderm. This includes the muscular and skeletal elements that elsewhere in the body are derived from mesoderm. Most of these tissues develop from neural crest cells that migrate downward beside the neural tube and laterally under the surface ectoderm.[1] After the crest cells have completed their migration, facial growth is dominated by regional growth centers as the organ systems are formed and the final differentiation of tissues occurs.

There are five principal stages in craniofacial development (Table 3-1): (1) germ layer formation and initial organization of craniofacial structures; (2) neural tube formation and initial formation of the oropharynx; (3) origins, migrations, and interactions of cell populations, especially neural crest cells; (4) formation of organ systems, especially the pharyngeal arches and the primary and secondary palates; and (5) final differentiation of tissues

TABLE 3-1 *Stages of Embryonic Craniofacial Development*

Stage	Time (humans) (post-fertilization)	Related syndromes
Germ layer formation and initial organization of structures	Day 17	Fetal alcohol syndrome (FAS)
Neural tube formation	Days 18-23	Anencephaly
Origin, migration, and interaction of cell populations	Days 19-28	Hemifacial microsomia Mandibulofacial dysostosis (Treacher Collins' syndrome) Limb abnormalities
Formation of organ systems		
—Primary palate	Days 28-38	Cleft lip and/or palate, other facial clefts
—Secondary palate	Days 42-55	Cleft palate
Final differentiation of tissues	Day 50-birth	Achondroplasia Synostosis syndromes (Crouzon's, Apert's, etc.)

FACIAL FEATURES OF FETAL ALCOHOL SYNDROME

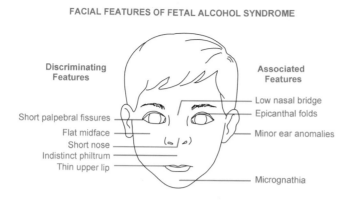

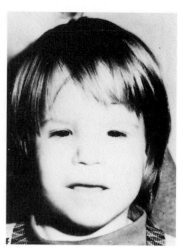

Discriminating Features

Short palpebral fissures
Flat midface
Short nose
Indistinct philtrum
Thin upper lip

Associated Features

Low nasal bridge
Epicanthal folds
Minor ear anomalies

Micrognathia

FIGURE 3-1 The characteristic facial appearance of fetal alcohol syndrome (FAS), caused by exposure to very high blood alcohol levels during the first trimester of pregnancy.

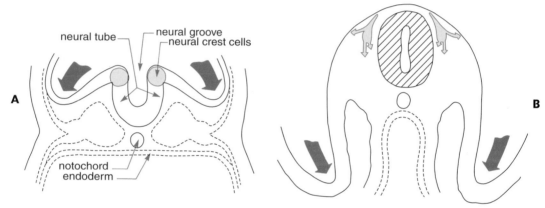

neural tube
neural groove
neural crest cells

notochord
endoderm

A

B

FIGURE 3-2 Diagrammatic lateral sections of embryos at 20 and 24 days, showing formation of the neural folds, neural groove and neural crest. **A,** At 20 days, neural crest cells can be identified at the lips of the deepening neural groove, forerunner of the central nervous system. **B,** At 24 days, the neural crest cells *(pink)* have separated from the neural tube and are beginning their extensive migration beneath the surface ectoderm. The migration is so extensive, and the role of these neural crest cells so important in formation of structures of the head and face, that they can almost be considered a fourth primary germ layer.

(skeletal, muscular, and nervous elements).[2] Some specific abnormalities in facial form and jaw relationships can be traced to the very early first and second stages. For example, the characteristic facies of fetal alcohol syndrome (FAS) (Figure 3-1) is due to deficiencies of midline tissue of the neural plate very early in embryonic development, caused by exposure to very high levels of ethanol. Although such blood levels can be reached only in extreme intoxication in chronic alcoholics, the resulting facial deformity occurs frequently enough to be implicated in many cases of maxillary and midface deficiency.[3]

Many of the problems that result in craniofacial anomalies arise in the third stage of development, neural crest cell origin and migration. Since most structures of the face are ultimately derived from migrating neural crest cells

(Figure 3-2), it is not surprising that interferences with this migration produce facial deformities. At the completion of the migration of the neural crest cells in the fourth week of human embryonic life, they form practically all of the loose mesenchymal tissue in the facial region that lies between the surface ectoderm and the underlying forebrain and eye and most of the mesenchyme in the mandibular arch. Most of the neural crest cells in the facial area later differentiate into skeletal and connective tissues, including the bones of the jaw and the teeth.

The importance of neural crest migration and the possibility of drug-induced impairment has been brought into sharper focus in recent years. In the 1960s and 70s, exposure to thalidomide caused major congenital defects including facial anomalies in thousands of children. In the

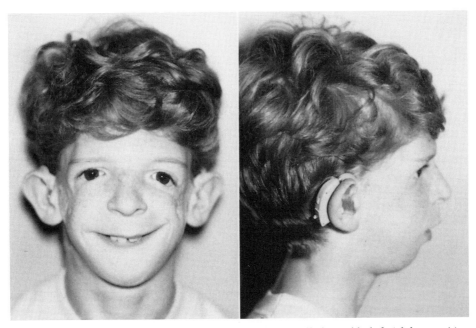

FIGURE 3-3 In the Treacher Collins' syndrome (also called mandibulofacial dysostosis), a generalized lack of mesenchymal tissue in the lateral part of the face is the major cause of the characteristic facial appearance. Note the underdevelopment of the lateral orbital and zygomatic areas. The ears also may be affected.

1980s, severe facial malformations related to the anti-acne drug isotretinoin (Accutane) were reported. The similarities in the defects make it likely that these drugs affect the formation and/or migration of neural crest cells. Fortunately, there was no similar experience in the 1990s.

Altered neural crest development has been implicated in mandibulofacial dysostosis (Treacher Collins' syndrome). In this congenital syndrome, both the maxilla and mandible are underdeveloped as a result of a generalized lack of mesenchymal tissue (Figure 3-3). The best evidence suggests that the problem arises because of excessive cell death (cause unknown) in the trigeminal ganglion, which secondarily affects neural crest-derived cells.[4] Some degree of asymmetry may be present, but both sides are affected.

Hemifacial microsomia, as the name suggests, is primarily a unilateral and always an asymmetrical problem. It is characterized by a lack of tissue on the affected side of the face (Figure 3-4). Typically, the external ear is deformed and both the ramus of the mandible and associated soft tissues (muscle, fascia) are deficient or missing (see Figure 3-4). Until recently it was thought that the defect was due to hemorrhage from the stapedial artery at the time, about 6 weeks after conception, when the maxillary artery takes over the blood supply to the affected area. More recent work suggests that, although hemorrhage at the critical time may be involved, hemifacial microsomia arises primarily from early loss of neural crest cells.[2] Neural crest cells with the longest migration path, those taking a circuitous route to the lateral and lower areas of the face, are most affected, whereas those going to the cen-

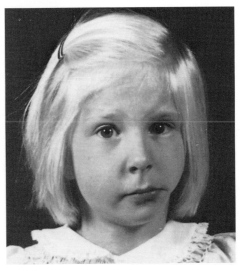

FIGURE 3-4 In hemifacial microsomia, both the external ear and the mandibular ramus are deficient or absent on the affected side.

tral face tend to complete their migratory movement. This explains why midline facial defects including clefts rarely are part of the syndrome. Neural crest cells migrating to lower regions are important in the formation of the great vessels (aorta, pulmonary artery, aortic arch), and they also are likely to be affected. For this reason defects in the great vessels (as in the tetralogy of Fallot) are common in children with hemifacial microsomia. The

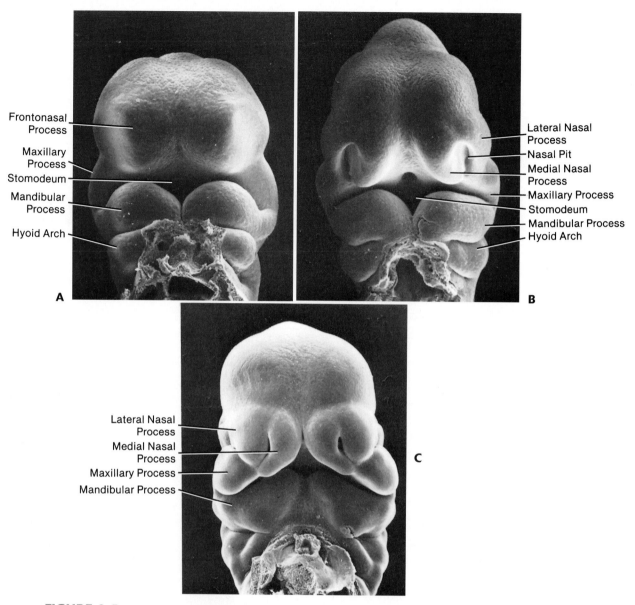

Frontonasal Process
Maxillary Process
Stomodeum
Mandibular Process
Hyoid Arch

A

Lateral Nasal Process
Nasal Pit
Medial Nasal Process
Maxillary Process
Stomodeum
Mandibular Process
Hyoid Arch

B

Lateral Nasal Process
Medial Nasal Process
Maxillary Process
Mandibular Process

C

FIGURE 3-5 Scanning electron micrographs of mouse embryos (which are very similar to human embryos at this stage of development), showing the stages in facial development. **A,** Early formation of the face about 24 days after conception in the human. **B,** At a stage equivalent to about 31 days in the human, the medial and lateral nasal processes can be recognized alongside the nasal pit. **C,** Fusion of the median nasal, lateral nasal, and maxillary processes forms the upper lip, while fusion between the maxillary and mandibular processes establishes the width of the mouth opening. This stage is reached at about 36 days in the human. (Courtesy Dr. K. Sulik.)

spectrum of deformities induced by thalidomide and isotretinoin includes conditions similar to both mandibulofacial dysostosis and hemifacial microsomia.

The most common congenital defect involving the face and jaws, second only to clubfoot in the entire spectrum of congenital deformities, is clefting of the lip, palate, or, less commonly, other facial structures. Clefts arise during the fourth developmental stage. Exactly where they appear is determined by the locations at which fusion of the various facial processes failed to occur (Figures 3-5 and 3-6),

and this in turn is influenced by the time in embryologic life when some interference with development occurred.

Clefting of the lip occurs because of a failure of fusion between the median and lateral nasal processes and the maxillary prominence, which normally occurs in humans during the sixth week of development. At least theoretically a midline cleft of the upper lip could develop because of a split within the median nasal process, but this almost never occurs. Instead, clefts of the lip occur lateral to the midline on either or both sides (Figure 3-7). Since the fusion of

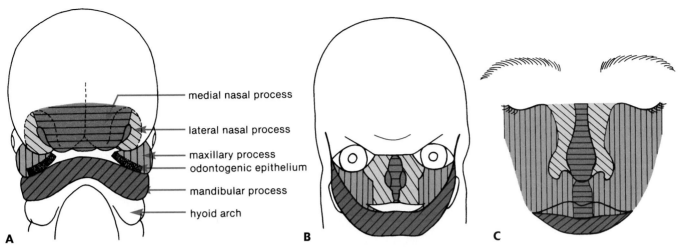

medial nasal process

lateral nasal process

maxillary process
odontogenic epithelium

mandibular process

hyoid arch

A   **B**   **C**

FIGURE 3-6 Schematic representations of fusion of the facial processes. **A,** Diagrammatic representation of structures at 31 days, when fusion is just beginning; **B,** relationships at 35 days, when the fusion process is well-advanced; **C,** schematic representation of the contribution of the embryonic facial processes to the structures of the adult face. The medial nasal process contributes the central part of the nose and the philtrum of the lip. The lateral nasal process forms the outer parts of the nose, and the maxillary process forms the bulk of the upper lip and the cheeks. (**B,** Redrawn from Ten Cate AR: *Oral histology,* ed 3, St Louis, 1989, Mosby; **C,** redrawn from Sulik KK, Johnston MC: *Scan Elect Microsc* 1:309-322, 1982.)

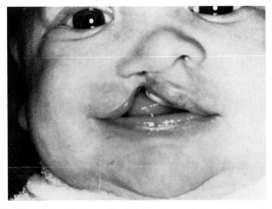

FIGURE 3-7 Unilateral cleft lip in an infant. Note that the cleft is not in the midline, but lateral to the midline.

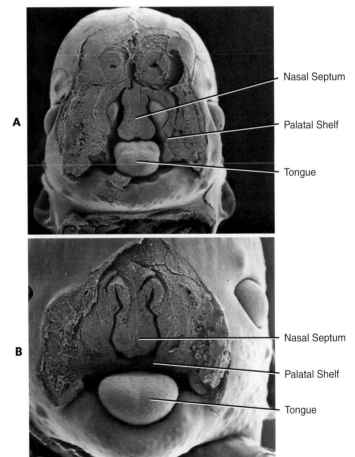

Nasal Septum

Palatal Shelf

Tongue

Nasal Septum

Palatal Shelf

Tongue

FIGURE 3-8 Scanning electron micrographs of mouse embryos sectioned in the frontal plane. **A,** Before elevation of the palatal shelves; **B,** immediately after depression of the tongue and elevation of the shelves. (Courtesy Dr. K. Sulik.)

these processes during primary palate formation creates not only the lip but the area of the alveolar ridge containing the central and lateral incisors, it is likely that a notch in the alveolar process will accompany a cleft lip even if there is no cleft of the secondary palate.

Closure of the secondary palate by elevation of the palatal shelves (Figures 3-8 and 3-9) follows that of the primary palate by nearly 2 weeks, which means that an interference with lip closure that still is present can also affect the palate. About 60% of individuals with a cleft lip also have a palatal cleft (Figure 3-10). An isolated cleft of the secondary palate is the result of a problem that arose after lip closure was completed. Incomplete fusion of the secondary palate, which produces a notch in its posterior

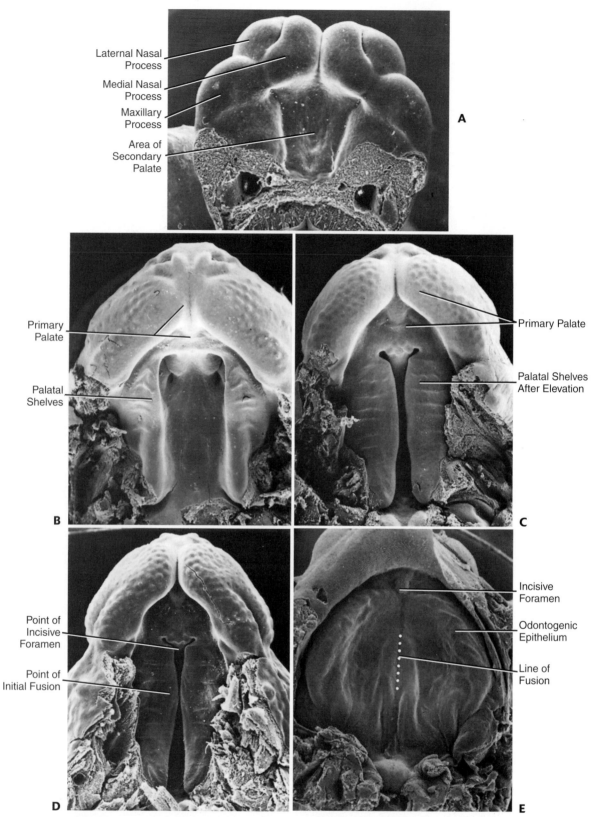

Laternal Nasal Process

Medial Nasal Process

Maxillary Process

Area of Secondary Palate

A

Primary Palate

Palatal Shelves

B

Primary Palate

Palatal Shelves After Elevation

C

Point of Incisive Foramen

Point of Initial Fusion

D

Incisive Foramen

Odontogenic Epithelium

Line of Fusion

E

FIGURE 3-9 Scanning electron micrographs of the stages in palate closure (mouse embryos sectioned so that the lower jaw has been removed), analogous to the same stages in human embryos. **A,** At the completion of primary palate formation; **B,** before elevation of the palatal shelves, equivalent to Figure 3-8, *A*; **C,** shelves during elevation; **D,** initial fusion of the shelves at a point about one third of the way back along their length; **E,** secondary palate immediately after fusion. (Courtesy Dr. K. Sulik.)

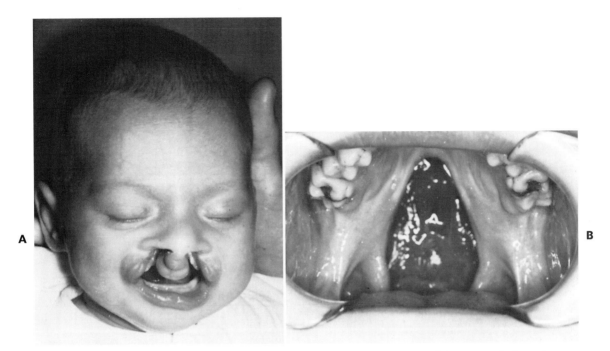

FIGURE 3-10   **A,** Bilateral cleft lip and palate in an infant. The separation of the premaxilla from the remainder of the maxilla is shown clearly; **B,** an unrepaired cleft of the secondary palate in a 12-year-old child. An isolated cleft of the palate can affect all of the secondary palate, as in this individual, or only the posterior portion of it.

extent (sometimes only a bifid uvula), indicates a very late-appearing interference with fusion.

The width of the mouth is determined by fusion of the maxillary and mandibular processes at their lateral extent, and so a failure of fusion in this area could produce an exceptionally wide mouth, or macrostomia. Failure of fusion between the maxillary and lateral processes could produce an obliquely directed cleft of the face. Other patterns of facial clefts are possible, based on the details of fusion.[5] Fortunately, these conditions are rare.

Morphogenetic movements of the tissues are a prominent part of the fourth stage of facial development. As these have become better understood, the way in which clefts of the lip and palate develop has been clarified. For example, it is known now that cigarette smoking by the mother is an etiologic factor in the development of cleft lip and palate.[6] An important initial step in development of the primary palate is a forward movement of the lateral nasal process, which positions it so that contact with the median nasal process is possible. The hypoxia associated with smoking probably interferes with this movement.[7]

Another major group of craniofacial malformations arise considerably later than the ones discussed so far, during the final stage of facial development and in the fetal rather than the embryologic period of prenatal life. These are the synostosis syndromes, which result from early closure of the sutures between the cranial and facial bones.[8] From early in fetal life, normal cranial and facial development is dependent on growth adjustments at the sutures in response to growth of the brain and facial soft tissues. Early closure of a suture, called *synostosis*, leads to characteristic distortions depending on the location of the early fusion.

Crouzon's syndrome is the most frequently occurring member of this group. It is characterized by underdevelopment of the midface and eyes that seem to bulge from their sockets (Figure 3-11). Crouzon's syndrome arises because of prenatal fusion of the superior and posterior sutures of the maxilla, along the wall of the orbit. The premature fusion frequently extends posteriorly into the cranium, producing distortions of the cranial vault as well. If fusion in the orbital area prevents the maxilla from translating downward and forward, the result must be severe underdevelopment of the middle third of the face. The characteristic protrusion of the eyes is largely an illusion—the eyes appear to bulge outward because the area beneath them is underdeveloped. There may be a component of true extrusion of the eyes, however, because when cranial sutures become synostosed, intracranial pressure increases.

Although the characteristic deformity is recognized at birth, the situation worsens as growth disturbances caused by the fused sutures continue postnatally. Surgery to release the sutures is necessary at an early age.

Late Fetal Development and Birth

By the third trimester of intrauterine life, the human fetus weighs approximately 1000 grams and though far from

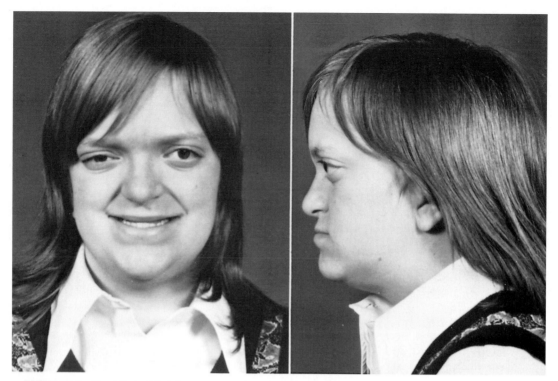

FIGURE 3-11 Typical facial appearance in Crouzon's syndrome of moderate severity. Note the deficiency of the midfacial structures, which usually is coupled with wide separation of the eyes (hypertelorism), as in this individual.

TABLE 3-2 *Chronology of Tooth Development, Primary Dentition*

Tooth	Calcification begins Max.	Calcification begins Mand.	Crown completed Max.	Crown completed Mand.	Eruption Max.	Eruption Mand.	Root completed Max.	Root completed Mand.
Central	14 wk. in utero	14 wk. in utero	1½ mo.	2½ mo.	10 mo.	8 mo.	1½ yr.	1½ yr.
Lateral	16 wk. in utero	16 wk. in utero	2½ mo.	3 mo.	11 mo.	13 mo.	2 yr.	1½ yr.
Canine	17 wk.	17 wk. in utero	9 mo.	9 mo.	19 mo.	20 mo.	3¼ yr.	3¼ yr.
1st Molar	15 wk. in utero	15 wk. in utero	6 mo.	5½ mo.	16 mo.	16 mo.	2½ yr.	2¼ yr.
2nd Molar	19 wk. in utero	18 wk. in utero	11 mo.	10 mo.	29 mo.	27 mo.	3 yr.	3 yr.

ready for life outside the protective intrauterine environment, can often survive premature birth. During the last 3 months of intrauterine life, continued rapid growth results in a tripling of body mass to about 3000 grams. Dental development, which begins in the third month, proceeds rapidly thereafter (Table 3-2). Development of all primary teeth and the permanent first molars starts well before birth.

Although the proportion of the total body mass represented by the head decreases from the fourth month of intrauterine life onward, at birth the head is still nearly half the total body mass and represents the largest impediment to passage of the infant through the birth canal. Making the head longer and narrower obviously would facilitate birth, and this is accomplished by a literal distor-

tion of its shape (Figure 3-12). The change of shape is possible because at birth, relatively large uncalcified fontanelles persist between the flat bones of the brain case. As the head is compressed within the birth canal, the brain case (calvarium) can increase in length and decrease in width, assuming the desired tubular form and easing passage through the birth canal.

The relative lack of growth of the lower jaw prenatally also makes birth easier, since a prominent bony chin at the time of birth would be a considerable problem in passage through the birth canal. Many a young dentist, acutely aware of the orthodontic problems that can arise later because of skeletal mandibular deficiency, has been shocked to discover how incredibly mandibular deficient his or her

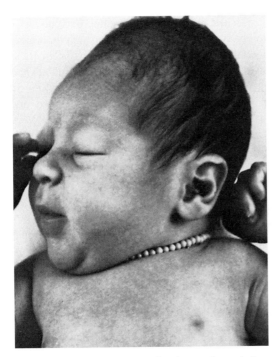

FIGURE 3-12   This photograph of a newborn infant clearly shows the head distortion accompanying passage through the birth canal. Note that the head has been squeezed into a more elliptical or tubular shape, a distortion made possible by the presence of the relatively large fontanelles. (Courtesy Mead Johnson Co.)

own newborn is, and has required reassurance that this is a perfectly normal and indeed desirable phenomenon. Postnatally, the mandible grows more than the other facial structures and gradually catches up, producing the eventual adult proportions.

Despite the physical adaptations that facilitate it, birth is a traumatic process. In the best of circumstances, being thrust into the world requires a dramatic set of physiologic adaptations. For a short period, growth ceases and there may be a small decrease in weight during the first 7 to 10 days of life. Such an interruption in growth produces a physical effect in skeletal tissues that are forming at the time, because the orderly sequence of calcification is disturbed. The result is a noticeable line across both bones and teeth that are forming at the time. However, bones are not visible and are remodeled to such an extent that any lines caused by the growth arrest at birth would soon be covered over at any rate.

Teeth, on the other hand, are quite visible, and the extent of any growth disturbance related to birth can be seen in the enamel, which is not remodeled. Almost every child has a "neonatal line" across the surface of the primary teeth, its location varying from tooth to tooth depending on the stage of development at birth (Figure 3-13). Under normal circumstances, the line is so slight that it can be seen only if the tooth surface is magnified, but if the

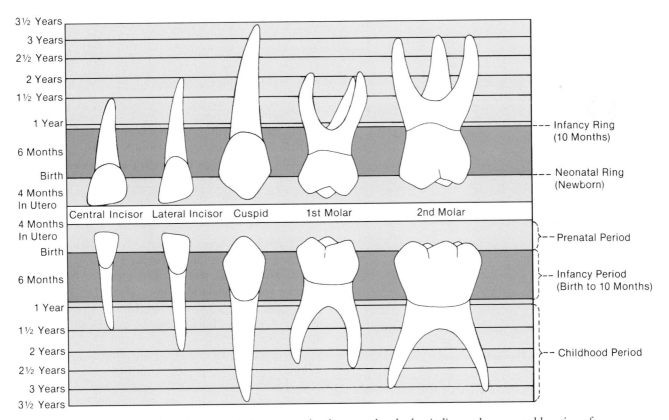

FIGURE 3-13   Primary teeth shown on a developmental scale that indicates the expected location of the neonatal line. From a chart of this type, the timing of illness or traumatic events that led to disturbances of enamel formation can be deduced from the location of enamel lines on various teeth.

neonatal period was stormy, a prominent area of stained, distorted, or poorly calcified enamel can be the result.[9]

Birth is not the only circumstance that can have this effect. As a general rule, it can be anticipated that growth disturbances lasting 1 to 2 weeks or more, such as the one that accompanies birth or a growth cessation caused by a febrile illness later, will leave a visible record in the enamel of teeth forming at the time. Permanent as well as primary teeth can be affected by illnesses during infancy and early childhood.

INFANCY AND EARLY CHILDHOOD: THE PRIMARY DENTITION YEARS

Physical Development in the Preschool Years

The general pattern of physical development after birth is a continuation of the pattern of the late fetal period: rapid growth continues, with a relatively steady increase in height and weight, although the rate of growth declines as a percentage of the previous body size (Figure 3-14).

Three circumstances merit special attention:

1. Premature birth (low birth weight). Infants weighing less than 2500 gm at birth are at greater risk of

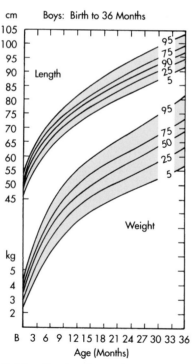

FIGURE 3-14 Graphs of growth in length and weight in infancy for boys (the curves for girls are almost identical at these ages). Note the extremely rapid growth in early infancy, with a progressive slowing after the first 6 months. (Based on data from the National Center for Health Statistics; redrawn from Lowrey GH: *Growth and development of children,* ed 8, Chicago, 1986, Mosby.)

problems in the immediate postnatal period. Since low birth weight is a reflection of premature birth, it is reasonable to establish the prognosis in terms of birth weight rather than estimated gestational age. Until recent years, children with birth weights below 1500 gm often did not survive. Even with the best current specialized neonatal services, the chances of survival for extremely low birth weight infants (less than 1000 gm) are not good, though some now are saved.

If a premature infant survives the neonatal period, however, there is every reason to expect that growth will follow the normal pattern and that the child will gradually overcome the initial handicap (Figure 3-15). Premature infants can be expected to be small throughout the first and into the second years of life. In many instances, by the third year of life premature and normal-term infants are indistinguishable in attainment of developmental milestones.[10]

2. Chronic illness. Skeletal growth is a process that can occur only when the other requirements of the individual have been met. A certain amount of energy is necessary to maintain life. An additional amount is needed for activity, and a further increment is necessary for growth. For a normal child, perhaps 90% of the available energy must be "taken off the top" to meet the requirements for survival and activity, leaving 10% for growth.

Chronic illness alters this balance, leaving relatively less of the total energy available to support growth. Chronically ill children typically fall behind their healthier peers, and if the illness persists, the growth deficit is cumulative. An episode of acute illness leads to a temporary cessation of growth, but if the growth interruption is relatively brief, there will be no long-term effect. The more chronic the illness, the greater the cumulative impact. Obviously, the more severe the illness, the greater the impact at any given time. Children with congenital hormone deficiencies provide an excellent example. If the hormone is replaced, a dramatic improvement in growth and recovery toward normal height and weight often occurs (Figure 3-16). A congenital heart defect can have a similar effect on growth, and similarly dramatic effects on growth can accompany repair of the defect.[11] Psychologic and emotional stress in extreme cases can affect physical growth in somewhat the same way as chronic illness (Figure 3-17).

3. Nutritional status. For growth to occur, there must be a nutritional supply in excess of the amount necessary for mere survival. Chronically inadequate nutrition, therefore, has an effect similar to chronic illness. On the other hand, once a level of nutritional adequacy has been achieved, additional nutritional intake is not a stimulus to more rapid growth. Adequate nutrition, like reasonable overall health, is a necessary condition for normal growth but is not a stimulus to it.

An interesting phenomenon of the last 300 or 400 years, particularly the twentieth century, has been a generalized increase in size of most individuals. There has also

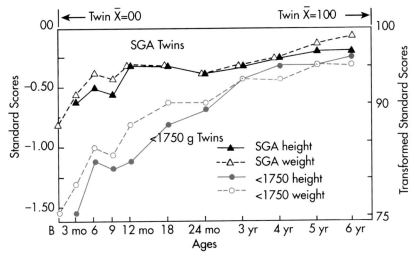

FIGURE 3-15 Growth curves for two groups of at-risk groups of infants: small-for-gestational age (SGA) twins and twins of less than 1750 grams birth weight (premature birth). In this graph, 100 is the expected height and weight for normal, full-term infants. Note the recovery of the low birth weight infants over time. (Redrawn from Lowery GH: *Growth and development of children*, ed 8, Chicago, 1986, Mosby.)

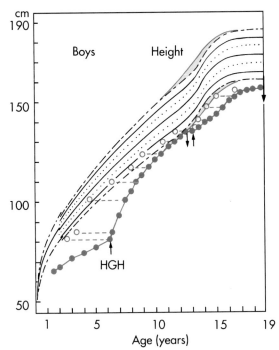

FIGURE 3-16 The curve for growth in height for a boy with isolated growth hormone deficiency. No treatment was possible until he was 6.2 years of age. At that point, human growth hormone (HGH) became available, and it was administered regularly from then until age 19, except for 6 months between 12.5 and 13 years. The beginning and end of HGH administration are indicated by the arrows. The open circles represent height plotted against bone age, thus delay in bone age is represented by the length of each horizontal dashed line. It is 3.5 years at the beginning of treatment, and 0.8 years at 11 to 12 years, when catch-up was essentially complete. Note the very high growth rate immediately after treatment started, equal to the average rate of a 1-year old infant. (Redrawn from Tanner JM, Whitehouse RH: *Atlas of children's growth*, London, 1982, Academic Press.)

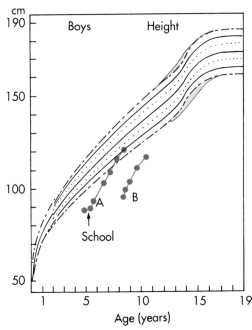

FIGURE 3-17 The effect of a change in social environment on growth of two children who had an obviously disturbed home environment, but no identifiable organic cause for the growth problem. When both children were placed in a special boarding school where presumably their psychosocial stress was lessened, both responded with above-average growth though the more severely affected child was still outside the normal range 4 years later. The mechanism by which psychosocial stress can affect growth so markedly is thought to be induction of a reversible growth hormone deficiency, accompanied by disturbance of the nearby appetite center. (Redrawn from Tanner JM, Whitehouse RH: *Atlas of children's growth*, London, 1982, Academic Press.)

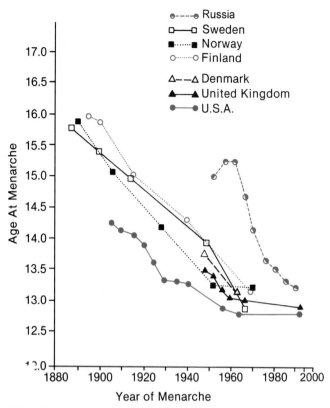

FIGURE 3-18   Age at menarche declined in both the United States and northern European countries in the first half of the 20th century. On the average, children are now larger at any given age than in the early 1900s, and they also mature more quickly. This secular trend seems to have leveled off recently. (Redrawn from Tanner JM: *Foetus into man*, Cambridge, Mass., 1978, Harvard University Press; 1995 U.S. data from Herman-Giddens et al: *Pediatrics* 99:597-598, 1997; 1995 English data from Cooper C et al: *Brit J Obstet Gyn* 103:814-817, 1996; Russian data from Dubrova YE et al: *Human Biology* 67:755-767, 1995.)

been a lowering in the age of sexual maturation, so that children recently have grown faster and matured earlier than they did previously. Since 1900, in the United States the average height has increased 2 to 3 inches, and the average age of girls at first menstruation, the most reliable sign of sexual maturity, has decreased by more than 1 year (Figure 3-18). This "secular trend" toward more rapid growth and earlier maturation has continued until very recently and may still be occurring. The most recent data suggest that signs of sexual maturation now appear in many girls much earlier than the previously-accepted standard dates.[12]

The trend undoubtedly is related to better nutrition, which allows the faster weight gain that by itself can trigger earlier maturation. Because a secular trend also has been observed in populations whose nutritional status does not seem to have improved significantly, nutrition may not be the entire explanation. Exposure to environmental

chemicals that have estrogenic effects (like some pesticides, for instance) may be contributing to earlier sexual maturation. On the other hand, a deficiency in one or two essential nutritional components can serve to limit the rate of growth, even if the diet is generally adequate. Physical growth requires the formation of new protein, and it is likely that the amount of protein may have been a limiting factor for many populations in the past. A generally adequate diet that was low in trace minerals, vitamins, or other minor but important components may have limited the rate of growth in the past, so that even a small change to supply previously deficient items may in some instances have allowed a considerable increase in growth.

Maturation of Oral Function

The principal physiologic functions of the oral cavity are respiration, swallowing, mastication and speech. Although it may seem odd to list respiration as an oral function, since the major portal for respiration is the nose, respiratory needs are a primary determinant of posture of the mandible and tongue.

At birth, if the newborn infant is to survive, an airway must be established within a very few minutes and must be maintained thereafter. To open the airway, the mandible must be positioned downward and the tongue moved downward and forward away from the posterior pharyngeal wall (Figure 3-19). This allows air to be moved through the nose and across the pharynx into the lungs. Newborn infants are obligatory nasal breathers and may not survive if the nasal passage is blocked at birth. Later, breathing through the mouth becomes physiologically possible. At all times during life, respiratory needs can alter the postural basis from which oral activities begin.

Respiratory movements are "practiced" in utero, although of course the lungs do not inflate at that time. Swallowing also occurs during the last months of fetal life, and it appears that swallowed amniotic fluid may be an important stimulus to activation of the infant's immune system.

Once an airway has been established, the newborn infant's next physiologic priority is to obtain milk and transfer it into the gastrointestinal system. This is accomplished by two maneuvers: suckling (not sucking, with which it is frequently confused) and swallowing.

The milk ducts of lactating mammals are surrounded by smooth muscle, which contracts to force out the milk. To obtain milk, the infant does not have to suck it from the mother's breast and probably could not do so. Instead, the infant's role is to stimulate the smooth muscle to contract and squirt milk into his mouth. This is done by suckling, consisting of small nibbling movements of the lips, a reflex action in infants. When the milk is squirted into the mouth, it is only necessary for the infant to groove the tongue and allow the milk to flow posteriorly into the pharynx and esophagus. The tongue, however, must be placed anteri-

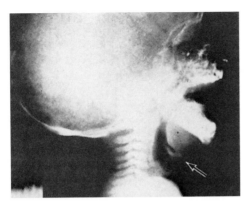

FIGURE 3-19 Radiograph of an infant immediately after birth, during the first breath of life. To breathe, the infant must position the mandible downward and the tongue forward to open up an airway and must maintain this posture thereafter. The arrow indicates the shadow of the tongue, and the open airway behind it is clearly visible. (From Bosma JF: *Am J Orthod* 49:94-104, 1963.)

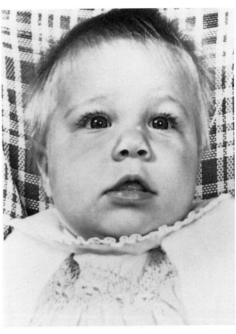

FIGURE 3-20 Characteristic placement of the tongue against the lower lip in an infant of a few months of age. At this stage of development, tongue contact with the lip is maintained most of the time.

orly in contact with the lower lip, so that milk is in fact deposited on the tongue.

This sequence of events defines an infantile swallow, which is characterized by active contractions of the musculature of the lips, a tongue tip brought forward into contact with the lower lip, and little activity of the posterior tongue or pharyngeal musculature. Tongue-to-lower lip apposition is so common in infants that this posture is usually adopted at rest, and it is frequently possible to gently move the infant's lip and note that the tongue tip moves with it, almost as if the two were glued together (Figure 3-20). The suckling reflex and the infantile swallow normally disappear during the first year of life.

As the infant matures, there is increasing activation of the elevator muscles of the mandible as the child swallows. As semisolid and eventually solid foods are added to the diet, it is necessary for the child to use the tongue in a more complex way to gather up a bolus, position it along the middle of the tongue, and transport it posteriorly. The chewing movements of a young child typically involve moving the mandible laterally as it opens, then bringing it back toward the midline and closing to bring the teeth into contact with the food. By the time the primary molars begin to erupt, this sort of juvenile chewing pattern is well established. By this time also, the more complex movements of the posterior part of the tongue have produced a definite transition beyond the infantile swallow.

Maturation of oral function can be characterized in general as following a gradient from anterior to posterior. At birth, the lips are relatively mature and capable of vigorous suckling activity, whereas more posterior structures are quite immature. As time passes, greater activity by the posterior parts of the tongue and more complex motions of the pharyngeal structures are required.

This principle of front-to-back maturation is particularly well illustrated by the acquisition of speech. The first speech sounds are the bilabial sounds , /p/, and /b/—which is why an infant's first word is likely to be "mama" or "papa." Somewhat later, the tongue tip consonants like /t/ and /d/ appear. The sibilant /s/ and /z/ sounds, which require that the tongue tip be placed close to but not against the palate, come later still, and the last speech sound, /r/, which requires precise positioning of the posterior tongue, often is not acquired until age 4 or 5.

Nearly all modern infants engage in some sort of habitual non-nutritive sucking—sucking a thumb, finger, or a similarly shaped object. Some fetuses have been reported to suck their thumbs in utero, and the vast majority of infants do so during the period from 6 months to 2 years or later. This practice is culturally determined to some extent, since children in primitive groups who are allowed ready access to the mother's breast for a long period rarely suck any other object.[13]

After the eruption of the primary molars during the second year, drinking from a cup replaces drinking from a bottle or continued nursing at the mother's breast, and the number of children who engage in non-nutritive sucking diminishes. When sucking activity stops, a continued transition in the pattern of swallow leads to the acquisition of an adult pattern. This type of swallow is characterized by a cessation of lip activity (i.e., lips relaxed, the placement of the tongue tip against the alveolar process behind the upper incisors, and the posterior teeth brought into occlusion during swallowing). As long as sucking habits persist, however, there will not be a total transition to the adult swallow.

Surveys of American children indicate that at age 8, about 60% have achieved an adult swallow, while the remaining 40% are still somewhere in the transition.[14] After sucking habits are extinguished, a complete transition to the adult swallow may require some months. This is complicated, however, by the fact that an anterior open bite, which may well be present if a sucking habit has persisted for a long time, can delay the transition even further because of the physiologic need to seal the anterior space. The relationship of tongue position and the pattern of swallowing to malocclusion is discussed further in Chapter 5.

The chewing pattern of the adult is quite different from that of a typical child: an adult typically opens straight down, then moves the jaw laterally and brings the teeth into contact, whereas a child moves the jaw laterally on opening (Figure 3-21). The transition from the juvenile to adult chewing pattern appears to develop in conjunction with eruption of the permanent canines, at about age 12. Interestingly, adults who do not achieve normal function of the canine teeth because of a severe anterior open bite retain the juvenile chewing pattern.[15]

Eruption of the Primary Teeth

At birth, neither the maxillary nor the mandibular alveolar process is well developed. Occasionally, a "natal tooth" is present, although the first primary teeth normally do not erupt until approximately 6 months of age. The natal tooth may be a supernumerary one, formed by an aberration in the development of the dental lamina, but usually is merely a very early but otherwise normal central incisor. Because of the possibility that it is perfectly normal, such a natal tooth should not be extracted casually.

The timing and sequence of eruption of the primary teeth are shown in Table 3-2. The dates of eruption are relatively variable; up to 6 months of acceleration or delay is within the normal range. The eruption sequence, however, is usually preserved. One can expect that the mandibular central incisors will erupt first, closely followed by the other incisors. After a 3-to-4 month interval, the mandibular and maxillary first molars erupt, followed in another 3 or 4 months by the maxillary and mandibular canines, which nearly fill the space between the lateral incisor and first molar. The primary dentition is usually completed at 24 to 30 months as the mandibular, then the maxillary second molars erupt.

Spacing is normal throughout the anterior part of the primary dentition but is most noticeable in two locations, called the primate spaces. (Most subhuman primates have these spaces throughout life, thus the name.) In the maxillary arch, the primate space is located between the lat-

Chewing Movements At The Central Incisor

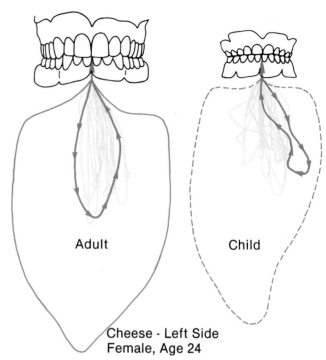

Cheese - Left Side
Female, Age 24

FIGURE 3-21   Chewing movements of an adult contrasted to a child. Children move the jaw laterally on opening, while adults open straight down, then move the jaw laterally. (Redrawn from Lundeen HC, Gibbs CH: *Advances in occlusion*, Boston, 1982, John Wright's PSG, Inc.)

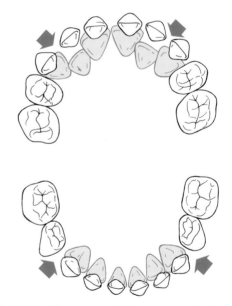

FIGURE 3-22   The crowns of the permanent incisors (*red*) lie lingual to the crowns of the primary incisors (*black*), particularly in the case of the maxillary laterals. Arrows point to the primate spaces.

eral incisors and canines, whereas in the mandibular arch, the space is between the canines and first molars (Figure 3-22). The primate spaces are normally present from the time the teeth erupt. Developmental spaces between the incisors are often present from the beginning, but become somewhat larger as the child grows and the alveolar processes expand. Generalized spacing of the primary teeth is a requirement for proper alignment of the permanent incisors.

LATE CHILDHOOD: THE MIXED DENTITION YEARS

Physical Development in Late Childhood

Late childhood, from age 5 or 6 to the onset of puberty, is characterized by important social and behavioral changes (see Chapter 2) but the physical development pattern of the previous period continues. The normally different rates of growth for different tissue systems, however, must be kept in mind. The maximum disparity in the development of different tissue systems occurs in late childhood (see Figure 2-2).

By age 7, a child has essentially completed his or her neural growth. The brain and the brain case are as large as they will ever be, and it is never necessary to buy a child a larger baseball cap because of growth (unless, of course, the growth is of uncut hair). Lymphoid tissue throughout the body has proliferated beyond the usual adult levels, and large tonsils and adenoids are common. In contrast, growth of the sex organs has hardly begun and general body growth is only modestly advanced. During early childhood the rate of general body growth declines from the rapid pace of infancy, then stabilizes at a moderate lower level during late childhood. Both nutrition and general health can affect the level at which stabilization occurs.

Eruption of the Permanent Teeth

The eruption of any tooth can be divided into several stages. This includes the primary teeth: the physiologic principles underlying eruption that are discussed in this section are not different for the primary teeth, despite the root resorption that eventually causes their loss. The nature of eruption and its control before the emergence of the tooth into the mouth are somewhat different from eruption after emergence, and we will consider these major stages separately.

Preemergent Eruption. During the period when the crown of a tooth is being formed, there is a very slow labial or buccal drift of the tooth follicle within the bone, but this follicular drift is not attributed to the eruption mechanism itself. In fact, the amount of change in the position of the tooth follicle is extremely small, observable only with vital staining experiments and so small that a follicle can be used as a natural marker in radiographic studies of growth. Eruptive movement begins soon after the root begins to form. This supports the idea that metabolic activity within the periodontal ligament is a major part of, if not the only mechanism for, eruption.

Two processes are necessary for preemergent eruption. First, there must be resorption of bone and primary tooth roots overlying the crown of the erupting tooth; second, the eruption mechanism itself then must move the tooth in the direction where the path has been cleared (Figure 3-23). Although the two mechanisms normally operate in concert, in some circumstances they do not. Investigations of the results of a failure of bone resorption, or alternately, of a failure of the eruption mechanism when bone resorption is normal, have yielded considerable insight into the control of preemergent eruption.

Defective bone resorption occurs in a mutant species of mice, appropriately labeled *Ia*, for Incisors absent. In these animals, the deficient bone resorption means that the incisor teeth cannot erupt, and they never appear in the mouth. Failure of teeth to erupt because of a failure of bone

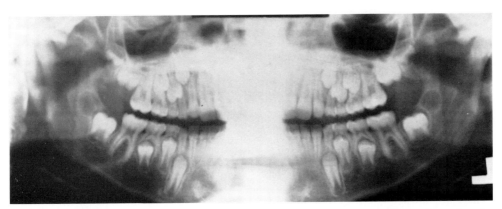

FIGURE 3-23 Panoramic radiograph of normal eruption in a 10-year-old boy. Note that the permanent teeth erupt as resorption of overlying primary teeth and bone occurs. Resorption must occur to make eruption possible.

resorption also occurs in humans, as for instance in the syndrome of cleidocranial dysplasia (Figure 3-24). In children with this condition, not only is resorption of primary teeth and bone deficient, but heavy fibrous gingiva and multiple supernumerary teeth also impede normal eruption. All of these serve to mechanically block the succedaneous teeth (those replacing primary teeth) from erupting. If the interferences are removed, the teeth often erupt and can be brought into occlusion.[16]

It has been demonstrated experimentally in animals that the rate of bone resorption and the rate of tooth eruption are not controlled physiologically by the same mechanism. For instance, if the tooth bud of a dog premolar is wired to the lower border of the mandible, the tooth can no longer erupt because of this mechanical obstruction, but resorption of overlying bone proceeds at the usual rate, resulting in a large cystic cavity overlying the ligated tooth bud.[17]

On at least two occasions, the same experiment has inadvertently been done to a child, in whom an unerupted permanent tooth was inadvertently wired to the lower border of the mandible when a mandibular fracture was repaired (Figure 3-25). The result was the same as in the animal experiments: eruption of the tooth stopped, but bone resorption continued. In a rare but now well documented human syndrome called "primary failure of eruption," affected posterior teeth fail to erupt, presumably because of a defect in the eruption mechanism (see Chapter 5). In these individuals, bone resorption apparently proceeds normally, but the involved teeth simply do not follow the path that has been cleared.

It appears, therefore, that resorption is the rate-limiting factor in preemergent eruption. Normally, the overlying bone and primary teeth resorb, and the eruption mechanism then moves the tooth into the space created by the resorption. Nevertheless, the follicle of the erupting tooth normally signals for the bone resorption that allows eruption, and a misdirected tooth can follow a widely abnormal eruption path because of this. The nature of the signal is unknown: pressure? chemical? something else?

Despite many years of study, the precise mechanism through which the eruption force is generated remains unknown. From animal studies, it seems clear that at least the major eruption mechanism (there may, after all, be more than one) is localized within the periodontal ligament. Substances that interfere with the development of cross-links in maturing collagen interfere with eruption, which makes it tempting to theorize that cross-linking of maturing collagen in the periodontal ligament provides the eruptive force. It is no coincidence that eruptive movements begin when root formation starts and a periodontal ligament begins to develop.

Other possibilities for the eruption mechanism besides collagen maturation are localized variations in blood pressure or flow, forces derived from contraction of fibroblasts, and alterations in the extracellular ground substances of the periodontal ligament similar to those that occur in thixotropic gels (see Marks and Schroeder[18] for a review). A tooth will continue to erupt after its apical area has been removed, so the proliferation of cells associated with lengthening of the root is not an essential part of the mechanism. Normally, the rate of eruption is such that the apical area remains at the same place while the crown moves occlusally, but if eruption is mechanically blocked, the proliferating apical area will move in the opposite direction, inducing resorption where it usually does not occur (Figure 3-26). This often causes a distortion of root form, which is called *dilaceration*.

Postemergent Eruption. Once a tooth emerges into the mouth, it erupts rapidly until it approaches the occlusal level and is subjected to the forces of mastication. At that point, its eruption slows and then as it reaches the occlusal level of other teeth and is in complete function,

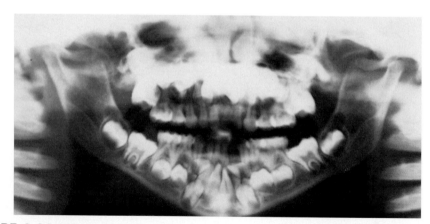

FIGURE 3-24 Panoramic radiograph of an 8-year-old patient with cleidocranial dysplasia, showing the characteristic features of this condition. In cleidocranial dysplasia, the succedaneous teeth do not erupt because of abnormal resorption of both bone and primary teeth, and the eruption of nonsuccedaneous teeth is delayed by fibrotic gingiva. Supernumerary teeth often are also present, as in this patient, creating additional mechanical obstruction.

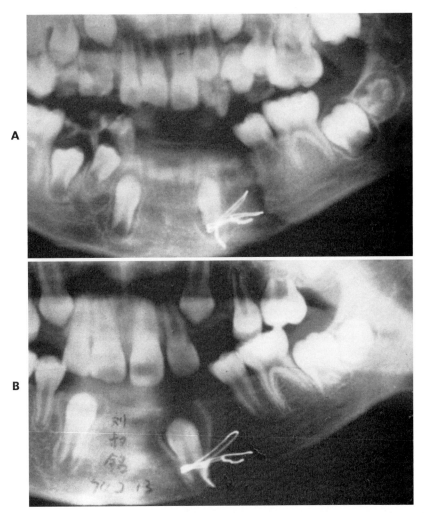

FIGURE 3-25 Radiographs of a boy whose lower jaw was fractured at age 10. **A,** Immediately after the fracture, when osseous wires were placed to stabilize the bony segments. One of the wires inadvertently pinned the mandibular left canine to the bone, simulating Cahill's experiments with animals. **B,** One year later. Note that resorption over the canine has proceeded normally, clearing its eruption path even though it has not moved. (Courtesy Dr. John Lin.)

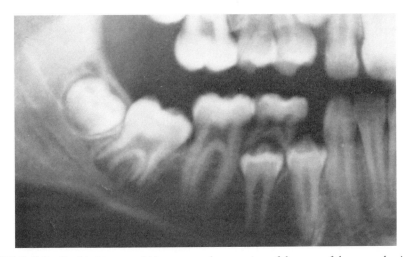

FIGURE 3-26 In this 14-year-old boy, normal resorption of the root of the second primary molar has not occurred, and eruption of the first premolar has been delayed by mechanical obstruction. Note the lengthening of the crypt of this tooth, with resorption at the apical area. Some distortion of root form is probably also occurring.

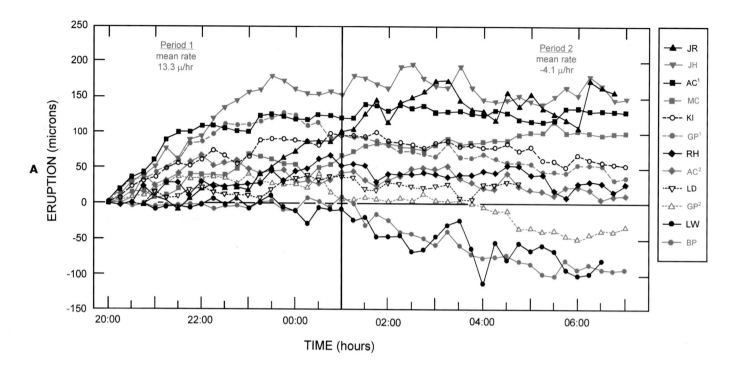

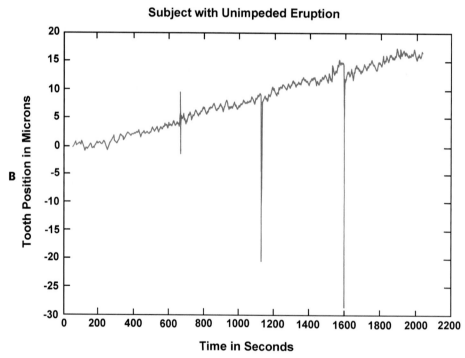

FIGURE 3-27   A, Eruption plots for human second premolars observed via a fiber optic cable to a video microscope, which provides 1-2 micron resolution, from 8 PM (20:00) to 6 AM (06:00). Note the consistent pattern of eruption in the early evening, trailing off to no eruption or intrusion toward midnight, with no further eruption after that. It now is clear that eruption occurs only during a few critical hours in the early evening. (Redrawn from Risinger RK, Proffit WR: *Arch Oral Biol* 41:779-786, 1996.) **B,** Eruption plots for a human second premolar observed via Moire magnification, which provides 0.2 micron resolution, over a 30-minute period in the early evening when force opposing eruption was applied while active eruption was occurring. Note that the tooth erupted nearly 10 microns during this short time. The vertical spikes are movement artefacts produced by the applied force; a short-duration cycle superimposed on the eruption curve (significance unknown) also can be observed. Force applications either have no effect on eruption, as in this subject, or produce a transient depression of eruption that lasts less than 2 minutes. (Redrawn from Gierie WV, Paterson RL, Proffit WR: *Arch Oral Biol* 44:423-428, 1999.)

eruption all but halts. The stage of relatively rapid eruption from the time a tooth first penetrates the gingiva until it reaches the occlusal level is called the *postemergent spurt*, in contrast to the following phase of very slow eruption, termed the *juvenile occlusal equilibrium*.

Recently new instrumentation has made it possible to track the short-term movements of a tooth during the postemergent spurt, and it has been observed that eruption occurs only during a critical period between 8 PM and midnight or 1 AM.[19] During the early morning hours and the day, the tooth stops erupting and often intrudes slightly (Figure 3-27). The day-night differences in eruption seem to reflect an underlying circadian rhythm, probably related to the very similar cycle of growth hormone release. Experiments with the application of pressure against an erupting premolar suggest that eruption is stopped by force for only one to three minutes, so food contacts with the erupting tooth even though it is out of contact with its antagonist, almost surely do not explain the daily rhythm.[20]

The eruption mechanism may be different after emergence—collagen crosslinking in the periodontal ligament is more prominent after a tooth comes into occlusal function, so shortening of collagen fibers as the mechanism seems more likely—and the control mechanism certainly is different (Figure 3-28). It seems obvious that as a tooth is subjected to biting forces that oppose eruption, the overall rate of eruption would be slowed, and in fact exactly this occurs. In humans, after the teeth reach the occlusal level, eruption becomes almost imperceptibly slow although it definitely continues. During the juvenile equilibrium, teeth that are in function erupt at a rate that parallels the rate of vertical

growth of the mandibular ramus (Figure 3-29). As the mandible continues to grow, it moves away from the maxilla, creating a space into which the teeth erupt. Exactly how eruption is controlled so that it matches mandibular growth, however, is not known, and since some of the more

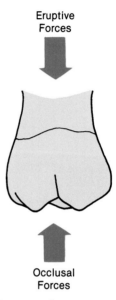

FIGURE 3-28 Diagrammatic representation of the equilibrium between forces promoting eruption and those opposing it, after a tooth has emerged into the oral cavity.

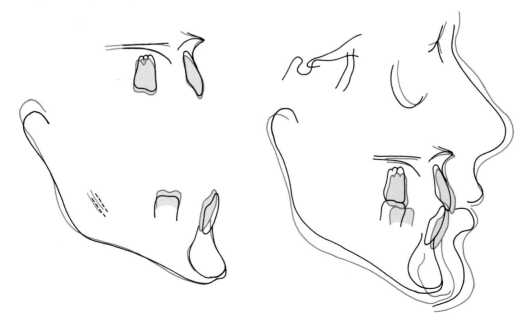

FIGURE 3-29 The amount of tooth eruption after the teeth have come into occlusion equals the vertical growth of the ramus in a patient who is growing normally. Vertical growth increases the space between the jaws, and the maxillary and mandibular teeth normally divide this space equally. Note the equivalent eruption of the upper and lower molars in this patient between age 10 *(black)* and 14 *(red)*. This is a normal growth pattern.

difficult orthodontic problems arise when eruption does not coincide with growth, this is an important area for further study.

The amount of eruption necessary to compensate for jaw growth can best be appreciated by observing what happens when a tooth becomes ankylosed (i.e., fused to the alveolar bone). An ankylosed tooth appears to submerge over a period as the other teeth continue to erupt, while it remains at the same vertical level (Figure 3-30). The total eruption path of a first permanent molar is about 2.5 cm. Of that distance, nearly half is traversed after the tooth reaches the occlusal level and is in function. If a first molar becomes ankylosed at an early age, which fortunately is rare, it can "submerge" to such an extent that the tooth is covered over again by the gingiva as other teeth erupt and the alveolar process increases in height (Figure 3-31).

Since the rate of eruption parallels the rate of jaw growth, it is not surprising that a pubertal spurt in eruption of the teeth accompanies the pubertal spurt in jaw growth. This reinforces the concept that after a tooth is in occlusion, the rate of eruption is controlled by the forces opposing eruption, not those promoting it. After a tooth is in the mouth, the forces opposing eruption are those from chewing, and perhaps in addition, soft tissue pressures from lips, cheeks, or tongue contacting the teeth. If eruption only occurs during quiet periods, the soft tissue pressures (from tongue position during sleep, for instance) probably are more important in controlling eruption than the heavy pressures during chewing. Light pressures of long duration are more important in producing orthodontic tooth movement (see Chapter 10), so it also seems logical that light but prolonged pressures might affect eruption.

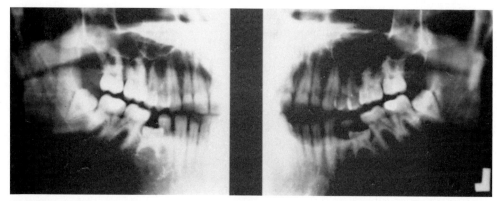

FIGURE 3-30   The mandibular second primary molars in this young adult, whose second premolars were congenitally missing, became ankylosed well before eruption of the other teeth was completed. Their apparant submergence is really because the other teeth have erupted past them. Note that the permanent first molars have tipped mesially over the submerged primary molars.

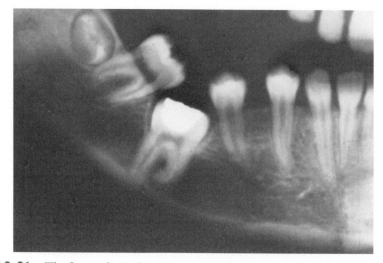

FIGURE 3-31   The first molar in this 15-year-old girl ceased erupting soon after its emergence into the mouth at age 6 or 7. When the dentist placed an occlusal restoration, the tooth was apparently in or near occlusion, well into the oral cavity. This dramatically illustrates the amount of eruption that must occur after the initial occlusal contact of first molars.

When the pubertal growth spurt ends, a final phase in tooth eruption called the *adult occlusal equilibrium* is achieved. During adult life, teeth continue to erupt at an extremely slow rate. If its antagonist is lost at any age, a tooth can again erupt more rapidly, demonstrating that the eruption mechanism remains active and capable of producing significant tooth movement even late in life.

Wear of the teeth may become significant as the years pass. If extremely severe wear occurs, eruption may not compensate for the loss of tooth structure, so that the vertical dimension of the face decreases. In most individuals, however, any wear of the teeth is compensated by additional eruption, and face height remains constant or even increases slightly in the fourth, fifth, and sixth decades of life (see the section on maturation and aging in Chapter 4).

Eruption Sequence and Timing (Table 3-3). The transition from the primary to the permanent dentition begins at about age 6 with the eruption of the first permanent molars, followed soon thereafter by the permanent incisors. The permanent teeth tend to erupt in groups, and it is less important to know the most common eruption sequence than to know the expected timing of these eruption stages. The stages are used in the calculation of dental age, which is particularly important during the mixed dentition years. Dental age is determined from three characteristics. The first is which teeth have erupted. The second and third, which are closely related, are the amount of resorption of the roots of primary teeth and the amount of development of the permanent teeth.

The first stage of eruption of the permanent teeth, at dental age 6, is illustrated in Figure 3-32. The most common eruption sequence is the eruption of the mandibular central incisor, closely followed by the mandibular first permanent molar and the maxillary first permanent molar. These teeth normally erupt at so nearly the same time, however, that it is quite within normal variation for the first molars to slightly precede the mandibular central incisors or vice versa. Usually, the mandibular molar will precede the maxillary molar. The beginning eruption of this group of teeth characterizes dental age 6.

In the second stage of eruption at dental age 7, the maxillary central incisors and the mandibular lateral incisors erupt. The maxillary central incisor is usually a year behind the mandibular central incisor, but erupts simultaneously with the mandibular lateral incisor. At dental age 7, root formation of the maxillary lateral incisor is well

TABLE 3-3 *Chronology of Tooth Development, Permanent Dentition*

Tooth	Calcification begins		Crown completed		Eruption		Root completed	
	Max.	Mand.	Max.	Mand.	Max.	Mand.	Max.	Mand.
Central	3 mo.	3 mo.	4½ yr.	3½ yr.	7¼ yr.	6¼ yr.	10½ yr.	9½ yr.
Lateral	11 mo.	3 mo.	5½ yr.	4 yr.	8¼ yr.	7½ yr.	11 yr.	10 yr.
Canine	4 mo.	4 mo.	6 yr.	5¾ yr.	11½ yr.	10½ yr.	13½ yr.	12¾ yr.
1st Premolar	20 mo.	22 mo.	7 yr.	6¾ yr.	10¼ yr.	10½ yr.	13½ yr.	13½ yr.
2nd Premolar	27 mo.	28 mo.	7¾ yr.	7½ yr.	11 yr.	11¼ yr.	14½ yr.	15 yr.
1st Molar	32 wk. in utero	32 wk. in utero	4¼ yr.	3¾ yr.	6¼ yr.	6 yr.	10½ yr.	10¾ yr.
2nd Molar	27 mo.	27 mo.	7¾ yr.	7½ yr.	12½ yr.	12 yr.	15¾ yr.	16 yr.
3rd Molar	8 yr.	9 yr.	14 yr.	14 yr.	20 yr.	20 yr.	22 yr.	22 yr.

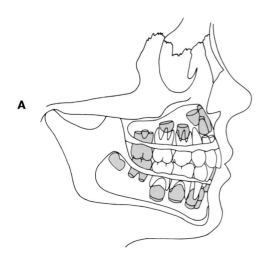

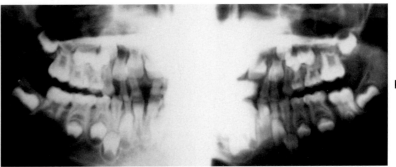

FIGURE 3-32 The first stage of eruption of the permanent teeth, at age 6, is characterized by the near-simultaneous eruption of the mandibular central incisors, the mandibular first molars, and the maxillary first molars. **A,** Drawing of right side; **B,** panoramic radiograph.

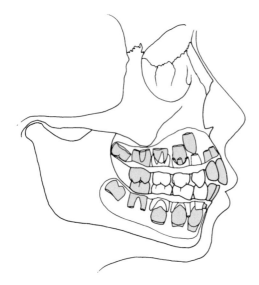

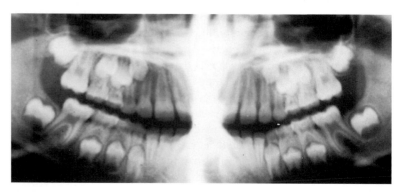

FIGURE 3-33   Dental age 8 is characterized by eruption of the maxillary lateral incisors.

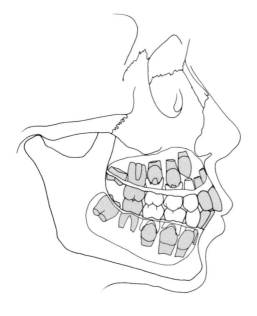

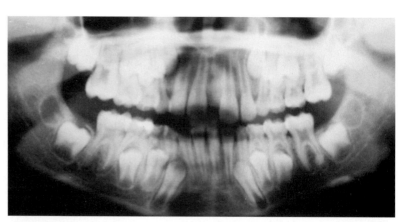

FIGURE 3-34   At dental age 9, the maxillary lateral incisors have been in place for 1 year, and root formation on other incisors and first molars is nearly complete. Root development of the maxillary canines and all second premolars is just beginning, while about one third of the root of the mandibular canines and all of the first premolars have been completed.

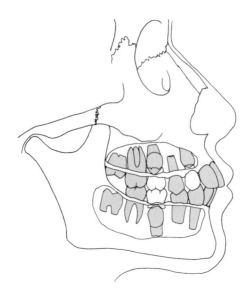

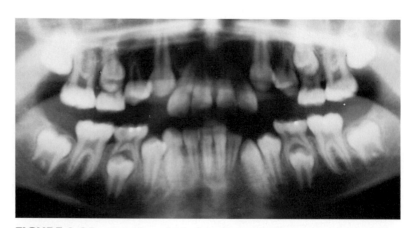

FIGURE 3-35   Dental age 11 is characterized by the more or less simultaneous eruption of the mandibular canines, mandibular first premolars, and maxillary first premolars.

advanced, but it is still about 1 year from eruption, while the canines and premolars are still in the stage of crown completion or just at the beginning of root formation.

Dental age 8 (Figure 3-33) is characterized by the eruption of the maxillary lateral incisors. After these teeth come into the arch, there is a delay of 2 to 3 years before any further permanent teeth appear.

Since no teeth are erupting at that time, dental ages 9 and 10 must be distinguished by the extent of resorption of the primary canines and molars and the extent of root development of their permanent successors. At dental age 9, the primary canines, first molars, and second molars are present. Approximately one third of the root of the mandibular canine and the mandibular first premolar is completed. Root development is just beginning, if it has started at all, on the mandibular second premolar (Figure 3-34). In the maxillary arch, root development has begun on the first premolar but is just beginning, if it is present at all, on both the canine and the second premolar.

Dental age 10 is characterized by a greater amount of both root resorption of the primary canines and molars, and root development of their permanent successors. At dental age 10, approximately one half of the roots of the mandibular canine and mandibular first premolar have been completed; nearly half the root of the upper first premolar is complete; and there is significant root development of the mandibular second premolar, maxillary canine, and maxillary second premolar.

Teeth usually emerge when three fourths of their roots are completed.[21] Thus a signal of the impending eruption of a tooth that has not yet appeared is its root development approaching this level. The roots of the incisors were not complete, of course, when they first erupted. It takes about 2 to 3 years for roots to be completed after a tooth has erupted into occlusion.

Another indicator of dental age 10, therefore, would be completion of the roots of the mandibular incisor teeth and near completion of the roots of the maxillary laterals. By dental age 11, the roots of all incisors and first permanent molars should be well completed.

Dental age 11 (Figure 3-35) is characterized by the eruption of another group of teeth: the mandibular canine, mandibular first premolar, and maxillary first premolar, which all erupt more or less simultaneously. In the mandibular arch, the mandibular canine most often appears just ahead of the first premolar, but the similarity in the time of eruption, not the details of the sequence, is the important point. In the maxillary arch, on the other hand, the first premolar usually erupts well ahead of the canine. At dental age 11, the only remaining primary teeth are the maxillary canine and second molar, and the mandibular second molar.

At dental age 12 (Figure 3-36), the remaining succedaneous permanent teeth erupt. *Succedaneous* refers to permanent teeth that replace primary predecessors; thus a canine is a succedaneous tooth, whereas a first molar is not. In addition, at age 12 the second permanent molars in both arches are nearing eruption. The succedaneous teeth complete their eruption before the emergence of the second molars in most but by no means all normal children. Although mineralization often begins later, it is usually possible to note the early beginnings of the third molars by age 12.

Dental ages 13, 14, and 15 are characterized by the extent of completion of the roots of permanent teeth. By dental age 15 (Figure 3-37), if a third molar is going to form, it should be apparent on the radiographs, and the roots of all other permanent teeth should be complete.

Like all other developmental ages (discussed in more detail in paragraphs following), dental age correlates with chronologic age—but the correlation for dental age is one of the weakest. In other words, the teeth erupt with a considerable degree of variability from the chronologic age standards.[22] It remains true, however, that the teeth erupt in the stages described above. A child who has precocious

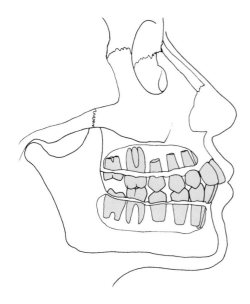

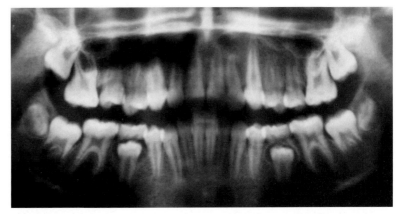

FIGURE 3-36 Dental age 12 is characterized by eruption of the remaining succedaneous teeth (the maxillary canine and the maxillary and mandibular second premolars) and, typically a few months later, the maxillary and mandibular second molars.

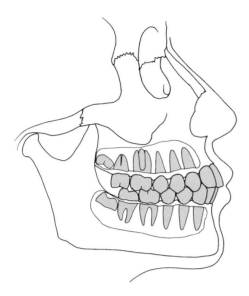

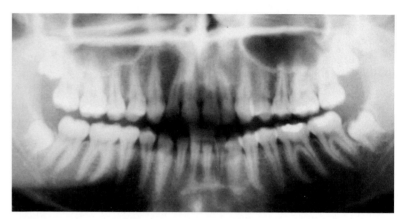

FIGURE 3-37   By dental age 15, the roots of all permanent teeth except the third molars are complete, and crown formation of third molars often has been completed.

dental development might have the mandibular central incisors and first molars erupt at age 5 and could reach dental age 12 by chronologic age 10. A child with slow dental development might not reach dental age 12 until chronologic age 14, which is within the range of normal variation.

A change in the sequence of eruption is a much more reliable sign of a disturbance in normal development than a generalized delay or acceleration. The more a tooth deviates from its expected position in the sequence, the greater the likelihood of some sort of problem. For example, a delay in eruption of maxillary canines to age 14 is within normal variation if the second premolars are also delayed, but if the second premolars have erupted at age 12 and the canines have not, something is probably wrong.

Several reasonably normal variations in eruption sequence have clinical significance and should be recognized. These are: (1) eruption of second molars ahead of premolars in the mandibular arch, (2) eruption of canines ahead of premolars in the maxillary arch, and (3) asymmetries in eruption between the right and left sides.

Early eruption of the mandibular second molars can be unfortunate in a dental arch where room to accommodate the teeth is marginal. The eruption of the second molar before the second premolar tends to decrease the space for the second premolar and may lead to its being partially blocked out of the arch. Some dental intervention may be needed to get the second premolar into the arch when the mandibular second molar erupts early.

If a maxillary canine erupts at about the same time as the maxillary first premolar (remember that this is the normal eruption sequence of the lower arch but is abnormal in the upper), the canine probably will be forced labially. Labial positioning of maxillary canines often occurs when there is an overall lack of space in the arch, because this tooth is the last to erupt normally; but displacement of the canine also can be an unfortunate consequence of an eruption sequence abnormality.

An asymmetry in the rate of eruption on the two sides of the dental arch is a frequent enough variation to approach the bounds of normal. A striking illustration of genetic influences on eruption timing is seen in identical twins, who frequently have mirror-image asymmetries in the dentition at the various stages of eruption. For example, if the premolars erupt a little earlier on the left in one of the twins, they will erupt a little earlier on the right in the other. The normal variation is only a few months, however. As a general rule, if a permanent tooth on one side erupts but its counterpart on the other does not within 6 months, a radiograph should be taken to investigate the cause of the problem. Although small variations from one side to the other are normal, large ones often indicate a problem.

Space Relationships in Replacement of the Incisors

If a dissected skull is examined, it can be seen that in both the maxillary and mandibular arches, the permanent incisor tooth buds lie lingual as well as apical to the primary incisors (Figure 3-38). The result is a tendency for the mandibular permanent incisors to erupt somewhat lingually and in a slightly irregular position, even in children who have normal dental arches and normal spacing within the arches. In the maxillary arch, the lateral incisor is likely to be lingually positioned at the time of its emergence and to remain in that position if there is any crowding in the arch. The permanent canines are positioned to lie more nearly in line with the primary canines. If there are problems in eruption, these teeth can be displaced either lingually or labially, but usually they are displaced labially if there is not enough room to accommodate them within the arch.

The permanent incisor teeth are considerably larger than the primary incisors that they replace. For instance, the mandibular permanent central incisor is about 5.5 mm in width, whereas the primary central it replaces is about 3

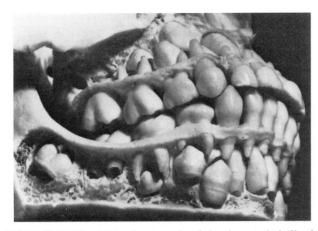

FIGURE 3-38 This photograph of the dissected skull of a child of approximately 6 years of age shows the relationship of the developing permanent tooth buds to the primary teeth. Note that the permanent incisors are positioned lingual to the roots of the primary incisors, while the canines are more labially placed. (From van der Linden FPGM, Duterloo HS: *Development of the human dentition: an atlas,* New York, 1976, Harper & Row.)

mm in width. Because the other permanent incisors and canines are each 2 to 3 mm wider than their primary predecessors, spacing between the primary incisors is not only normal, it is critically important (Figure 3-39). Otherwise, there will not be enough room for the permanent incisors when they erupt.

Spacing in the primary incisor region is normally distributed among all the incisors, not just in the "primate space" locations where permanent spaces exist in most mammalian species (see Figure 3-22). This arrangement of the primary incisor teeth with gaps between them may not be very pretty, but it is normal. All dentists sooner or later meet a mother like Janie's, who is very concerned that her child has crowded permanent incisors. Her frequent comment is, "But Janie had such beautiful baby teeth!" What the mother means is that Janie's primary incisors lacked the normal spacing. An adult appearing smile in a primary dentition child is an abnormal, not a normal finding—the spaces are necessary for alignment of the permanent teeth.

Changes in the amount of space anterior to the canine teeth are shown graphically in Figure 3-40. Note the excess

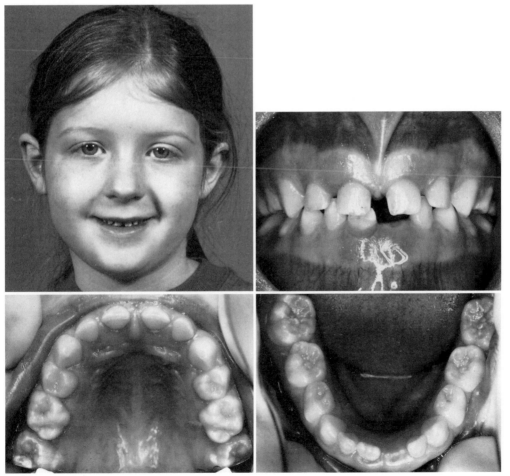

FIGURE 3-39 Spacing of this magnitude between the primary incisors is normal in the late primary dentition and is necessary to provide enough room for alignment of the permanent incisors when they erupt. At age 6 a gap-toothed smile, not a "Hollywood smile" with the teeth in contact, is what you would like to see.

AVAILABLE SPACE · INCISOR SEGMENT

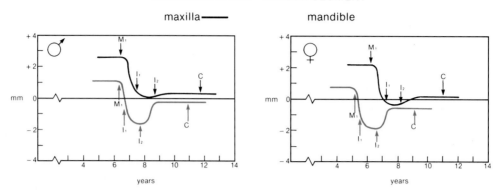

FIGURE 3-40   Graphic representation of the average amount of space available within the arches in boys *(left)* and girls *(right)*. The time of eruption of the first molar (M_1), central and lateral incisors (I_1 and I_2), and canines (C) are shown by arrows. Note that in the mandibular arch in both sexes, the amount of space for the mandibular incisors is negative for about 2 years after their eruption, meaning that a small amount of crowding in the mandibular arch at this time is normal. (From Moorrees CFA, Chadha JM: *Angle Orthod* 35:12-22, 1965.)

space in the maxillary and mandibular arches before the permanent incisors begin to erupt. In the maxillary arch, the primate space is mesial to the canines and is included in the graph. In the mandibular arch, the primate space is distal to the canine, which adds nearly another millimeter to the total available space in the lower arch. The total amount of spacing in the two arches therefore is about the same. The primary molars normally have tight contacts, so there is no additional spacing posteriorly.

When the central incisors erupt, these teeth use up essentially all of the excess space found in the normal primary dentition. With the eruption of the lateral incisors, the space situation becomes tight in both arches. The maxillary arch, on the average, has just enough space to accommodate the permanent lateral incisors when they erupt. In the mandibular arch, however, when the lateral incisors erupt, there is on the average 1.6 mm less space available for the four mandibular incisors than would be required to perfectly align them (see Figure 3-40). This difference between the amount of space needed for the incisors and the amount available for them is called the "incisor liability." Because of the incisor liability, a normal child will go through a transitory stage of mandibular incisor crowding at age 8 to 9 even if there will eventually be enough room to accommodate all the permanent teeth in good alignment (Figure 3-41). In other words, a period when the mandibular incisors are slightly crowded is a normal developmental stage. Continued development of the arches improves the spacing situation, and by the time the canine teeth erupt, space is once again adequate.

Where did the extra space come from to align these mildly crowded lower incisors? Most jaw growth is in the posterior, and there is no mechanism by which the mandible can easily become longer in its anterior region. Rather than from jaw growth per se, the extra space comes from three sources (Figure 3-42)[23]:

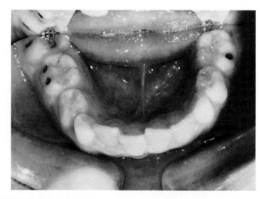

FIGURE 3-41   Mild irregularity of the mandibular incisors, of the magnitude pictured here, is normal at age 7 to 8, when the permanent incisors and first molars have erupted but the primary canines and molars are retained.

1. A slight increase in the width of the dental arch across the canines. As growth continues, the teeth erupt not only upward but also slightly outward. This increase is small, about 2 mm on the average, but it does contribute to the resolution of early crowding of the incisors. More width is gained in the maxillary arch than in the mandibular, and more is gained by boys than by girls. For this reason, girls have a greater liability to incisor crowding, particularly mandibular incisor crowding.
2. Labial positioning of the permanent incisors relative to the primary incisors. The primary incisors tend to stand quite upright. As the permanent incisors replace them, these teeth lean slightly forward, which arranges them along the arc of a larger circle. Although this change is also small, it contributes 1 to 2 mm of additional space in the average child, and thus helps resolve crowding.

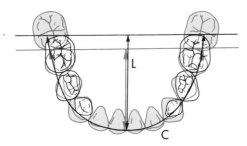

FIGURE 3-42 Tooth sizes and arch dimensions in the transition to the permanent dentition. The additional space to align mandibular incisors, after the period of mild normal crowding, is derived from three sources: (1) a slight increase in arch width across the canines, (2) slight labial positioning of the central and lateral incisors, and (3) a distal shift of the permanent canines when the primary first molars are exfoliated. The primary molars are significantly larger than the premolars that replace them, and the "leeway space" provided by this difference offers an excellent opportunity for natural or orthodontic adjustment of occlusal relationships at the end of the dental transition. Both arch length (*L*), the distance from a line perpendicular to the mesial surface of the permanent first molars to the central incisors, and arch circumference (*C*) tend to decrease during the transition (i.e., some of the leeway space is used by mesial movement of the molars).

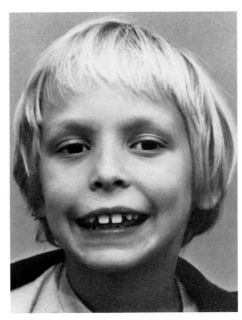

FIGURE 3-43 In some children, the maxillary incisors flare laterally and are widely spaced when they first erupt, a condition often called the "ugly duckling" stage. The spaced incisors tend to improve when the permanent canines erupt, but this condition increases the possibility that the canines will become impacted.

3. Repositioning of the canines in the mandibular arch. As the permanent incisors erupt, the canine teeth not only widen out slightly but move slightly back into the primate space. This contributes to the slight width increase already noted because the arch is wider posteriorly, and it also provides an extra millimeter of space. Since the primate space in the maxillary arch is mesial to the canine, there is little opportunity for a similar change in the anteroposterior position of the maxillary canine.

It is important to note that all three of these changes occur without significant skeletal growth in the front of the jaws. The slight increases in arch dimension during normal development are not sufficient to overcome discrepancies of any magnitude, so crowding is likely to persist into the permanent dentition if it was severe initially. In fact, crowding of the incisors—the most common form of Angle's Class I malocclusion—is by far the most prevalent form of malocclusion.

The mandibular permanent central incisors are almost always in proximal contact from the time that they erupt. In the maxillary arch, however, there may continue to be a space, called a *diastema*, between the maxillary central incisors in the permanent dentition, after the permanent teeth erupt. A central diastema tends to close as the lateral incisors erupt but may persist even after the lateral incisors have erupted, particularly if the primary canines have been lost or if the upper incisors are flared to the labial. This situation is another of the variations in the normal developmental pattern that occur frequently enough to be almost normal. Since the spaced upper incisors are not very esthetic, this is referred to as the "ugly duckling stage" of development (Figure 3-43).

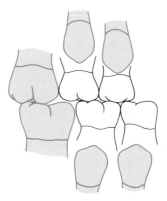

FIGURE 3-44 The size difference between the primary molars and permanent premolars, as would be observed in a panoramic radiograph.

The spaces tend to close as the permanent canines erupt. The greater the amount of spacing, the less the likelihood that a maxillary central diastema will totally close on its own. As a general guideline, a maxillary central diastema of 2 mm or less will probably close spontaneously, while total closure of a diastema initially greater than 2 mm is unlikely.[24]

Space Relationships in Replacement of Canines and Primary Molars

In contrast to the anterior teeth, the permanent premolars are smaller than the primary teeth they replace (Figure 3-44). The mandibular primary second molar is on the average 2 mm larger than the second premolar, while in the maxillary arch, the primary second molar is 1.5 mm larger. The primary first molar is only slightly larger than the first premolar, but does contribute an extra 0.5 mm in the mandible. The result is that each side in the mandibular arch contains about 2.5 mm of what is called *leeway space*, while in the maxillary arch, about 1.5 mm is available on the average.

When the second primary molars are lost, the first permanent molars move forward (mesially) relatively rapidly, using the leeway space. This decreases both arch length and arch circumference, which are related and commonly confused terms. The difference between them is illustrated in Figure 3-42. Even if incisor crowding is present, the leeway space is normally used by mesial movement of the permanent molars. An opportunity for orthodontic treatment is created at this time, since crowding could be relieved by using the leeway space (see Chapters 13 and 14).

Occlusal relationships in the mixed dentition parallel those in the permanent dentition, but the descriptive terms are somewhat different. A normal relationship of the primary molar teeth is the *flush terminal plane* relationship illustrated in Figure 3-45. The primary dentition equivalent of Angle's Class II is the *distal step*. A *mesial step* relationship corresponds to Angle's Class I. An equivalent of Class III is almost never seen in the primary dentition because of the normal pattern of craniofacial growth in which the mandible lags behind the maxilla.

At the time the primary second molars are lost, both the maxillary and mandibular molars tend to shift mesially into the leeway space, but the mandibular molar normally moves mesially more than its maxillary counterpart. This differential movement contributes to the normal transition from a flush terminal plane relationship in the mixed dentition to a Class I relationship in the permanent dentition.

Differential growth of the mandible relative to the maxilla is also an important contributor to the molar transition. As we have discussed, a characteristic of the growth pattern at this age is more growth of the mandible than the maxilla, so that a relatively deficient mandible gradually catches up. Conceptually, one can imagine that the upper and lower teeth are mounted on moving platforms, and that the platform on which the lower teeth are mounted

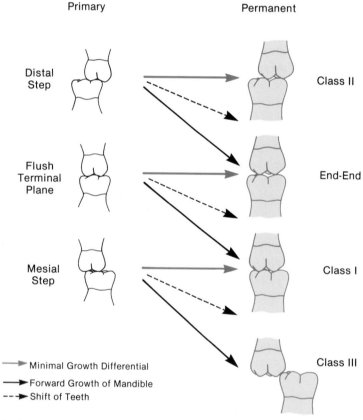

FIGURE 3-45   Occlusal relationships of the primary and permanent molars. The flush terminal plane relationship, shown in the middle left, is the normal relationship in the primary dentition. When the first permanent molars erupt, their relationship is determined by that of the primary molars. The molar relationship tends to shift at the time the second primary molars are lost and the adolescent growth spurt occurs, as shown by the arrows. The amount of differential mandibular growth and molar shift into the leeway space determines the molar relationship, as shown by the arrows as the permanent dentition is completed. With good growth and a shift of the molars, the change shown by the solid black line can be expected. (Adapted from Moyers RE: *Handbook of orthodontics*, ed 3, Chicago, 1973, Mosby.)

moves a bit faster than the upper platform. This differential growth of the jaws carries the mandible slightly forward relative to the maxilla during the mixed dentition.

If a child has a flush terminal plane molar relationship early in the mixed dentition, about 3.5 mm of movement of the lower molar forward relative to the upper molar is required for a smooth transition to a Class I molar relationship in the permanent dentition. About half of this distance must be supplied by differential growth of the lower jaw, carrying the lower molar with it. The other half can be obtained from the leeway space, which allows greater mesial movement of the mandibular than the maxillary molar.

Only a modest change in molar relationship can be produced by this combination of differential growth of the jaws and differential forward movement of the lower molar. It must be kept in mind that the changes described here are those that happen to a child experiencing a normal growth pattern. There is no guarantee in any given individual that differential forward growth of the mandible will occur, nor that the leeway space will close in a way that moves the lower molar relatively forward.

The possibilities for the transition in molar relationship from the mixed to the early permanent dentition are summarized in Figure 3-45. Note that the transition is usually accompanied by a one-half cusp (3 to 4 mm) relative forward movement of the lower molar, accomplished by a combination of differential growth and tooth movement. A child's initial distal step relationship may change during the transition to an end-to-end (one-half cusp Class II) relationship in the permanent dentition but is not likely to be corrected all the way to Class I. It also is possible that the pattern of growth will not lead to greater prominence of the mandible, in which case the molar relationship in the permanent dentition probably will remain a full cusp Class II.

Similarly, a flush terminal plane relationship, which produces an end-to-end relationship of the permanent molars when they first erupt, can change to Class I in the permanent dentition but can remain end-to-end in the permanent dentition if the growth pattern is not favorable.

Finally, a child who has experienced early mandibular growth may have a mesial step relationship in the primary molars, producing a Class I molar relationship at an early age. It is quite possible for this mesial step relationship to progress to a half-cusp Class III during the molar transition and proceed further to a full Class III relationship with continued mandibular growth. On the other hand, if differential mandibular growth no longer occurs, the mesial step relationship at an early age may simply become a Class I relationship later.

For any given child, the odds are that the normal growth pattern will prevail, and that there will be a one-half cusp transition in the molar relationship at the time the second primary molars are lost. It must be understood that although this is the most likely outcome, it is by no means the only one. The possibility that a distal step will become Class II malocclusion or that a flush terminal plane will become end-to-end is very real. Class III malocclusion is much less common than Class II, but a child who has a mesial step relationship at an early age is also at some risk of developing Class III malocclusion as time passes.

Assessment of Skeletal and Other Developmental Ages

As noted previously, dental development correlates reasonably well with chronologic age but occurs relatively independently. Of all the indicators of developmental age, dental age correlates least well with the other developmental indices. Physical growth status also varies from chronologic age in many children but does correlate well with skeletal age, which is determined by the relative level of maturation of the skeletal system. In planning orthodontic treatment it can be important to know how much skeletal growth remains, so an evaluation of skeletal age is frequently needed.

An assessment of skeletal age must be based on the maturational status of markers within the skeletal system. Although a number of indicators could theoretically be used, the ossification of the bones of the hand and the wrist is normally the standard for skeletal development (Figure 3-46).

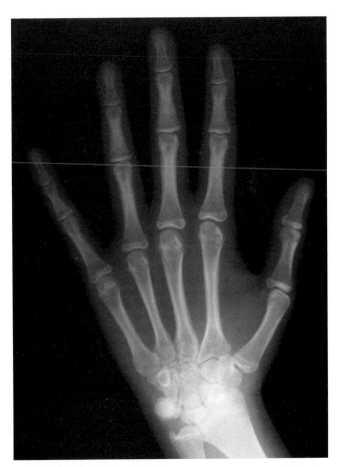

FIGURE 3-46   A radiograph of the hand and wrist can be used to assess skeletal age by comparing the degree of ossification of the wrist, hand, and finger bones to plates in a standard atlas of hand-wrist development.

A radiograph of the hand and wrist provides a view of some 30 small bones, all of which have a predictable sequence of ossification. Although a view of no single bone is diagnostic, an assessment of the level of development of the bones in the wrist, hand, and fingers can give an accurate picture of a child's skeletal development status. To do this, a hand-wrist radiograph of the patient is simply compared with standard radiographic images in an atlas of the development of the hand and wrist.[25] The description is in exactly the same terms as a description of the status of the dentition: skeletal age 10 at chronologic age 12, for instance.

Developmental ages based on any of a large number of criteria can be established, if there is some scale against which a child's progress can be measured. For instance, one could measure a child's position on a scale of behavior, equating behavior of certain types as appropriate for 5-year-olds or 7-year-olds. In fact, behavioral age can be important in the dental treatment of children, since it is difficult to render satisfactory treatment if the child cannot be induced to behave appropriately and cooperate. The assessment of behavioral age is covered more completely in the section on social and behavioral development in Chapter 2.

The correlation between developmental ages of all types and chronologic age is quite good, as biologic correlations go (Figure 3-47).[22] For most developmental indicators, the correlation coefficient between developmental status and chronologic age is about 0.8. The ability to predict one characteristic from another varies as the square of the correlation coefficient, so the probability that one could predict the developmental stage from knowing the chronologic age or vice versa is $(0.8)^2 = 0.64$. The correlation of dental age with chronologic age is not quite as good, about 0.7, which means that there is about a 50% chance of predicting the stage of dental development from the chronologic age.

It is interesting that the developmental ages correlate better among themselves than the developmental ages correlate with chronologic age.[26] Despite the caricature in our society of the intellectually advanced but socially and physically retarded child, the chances are that a child who is advanced in one characteristic—skeletal age, for instance—is advanced in others as well. The mature looking and behaving 8-year-old is likely, in other words, also to have precocious development of the dentition. What will actually occur in any one individual is subject to the almost infinite variety of human variation, and the magnitude of the correlation coefficients must be kept in mind. Unfortunately for those dentists who want to examine only the teeth, the variations in dental development mean that it often is necessary to assess skeletal, behavioral, or other developmental ages in planning dental treatment.

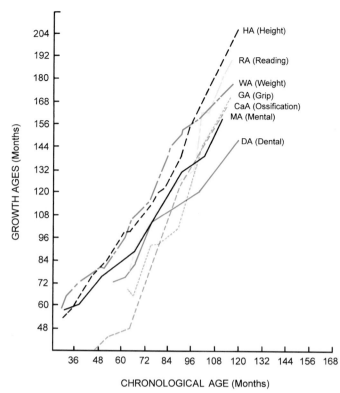

FIGURE 3-47   Changes in various developmental parameters for one normal child. Note that this child was advanced for his chronologic age in essentially all the parameters and that all are reasonably well-correlated. For this individual, as for many children, dental age correlated less well with the group of developmental indicators than any of the others. (Redrawn from Lowery GH: *Growth and development of children*, ed 6, Chicago, 1973, Mosby.)

REFERENCES

1. Johnston MC: Developmental biology of the mouth, palate and pharynx. In Tewfik TL, Derkaloussian VM (editors): Congenital anomalies of the ears, nose and throat, New York, 1997, Oxford University Press.
2. Johnston MC, Bronsky PT: Abnormal craniofacial development: an overview, Crit Rev Oral Biol Med 6:368-422, 1995.
3. Jackson IT, Hussain K: Craniofacial and oral manifestations of fetal alcohol syndrome, Plast Reconstr Surg 85:505-512, 1990.
4. Webster WS, Johnston MC, Lammer EJ, Sulik KK: Isotretinoin embryopathy and the cranial neural crest: an in vivo and in vitro study, J Craniofac Genet Dev Biol 6:211-222, 1986.
5. Tessier P: Anatomical classification of facial, craniofacial and latero-facial clefts, J Maxillofac Surg 4:69-92, 1976.
6. Wyszynski DF, Duffy DL, Beaty TH: Maternal cigarette smoking and oral clefts: a meta-analysis, Cleft Palate Craniofacial J 34:206-210, 1997.

7. Snow MD, Danielson BRG, Walsh DA, Edwards MJ: Facial clefting, teratogenic agents and hypoxia, Teratology, in press.

8. Cohen MM Jr: Craniosynostosis: diagnosis, evaluation and management, New York, 1986, Raven Press.

9. Eli J, Sarnat H, Talmi E: Effect of the birth process on the neonatal line in primary tooth enamel, Pediatr Dent 11:220-223, 1989.

10. Brandt I: Growth dynamics of low-birth-weight infants. In Falkner F, Tanner JM, (editors): Human growth, vol 1, ed 2, New York, 1986, Plenum Publishing.

11. Salzer HR, Haschke F, Wimmer M, et al: Growth and nutritional intake of infants with congenital heart disease, Pediatr Cardiol 10:17-23, 1989.

12. Herman-Giddens ME, Slora EJ, Wasserman RC et al: Secondary sexual characteristics and menses in young girls seen in office practice, Pediatrics 99:505-512, 1997.

13. Larsson EF, Dahlin KG: The prevalence of finger and dummy-sucking habits in European and primitive population groups, Am J Orthod 87:432-435, 1985.

14. Gross AM, Kellum GD, Hale ST et al: Myofunctional and dentofacial relationships in second grade children, Angle Orthod 60:247-253, 1990.

15. Lundeen HC, Gibbs CH: Advances in occlusion, Boston, 1982, John Wright-PSG.

16. Jensen BL, Kreiborg S: Development of the dentition in cleidocranial dysplasia, J Oral Pathol Med 19:89-93, 1990.

17. Marks SC Jr: The basic and applied biology of tooth eruption, Connective Tissue Res 32:149-157, 1995.

18. Marks SC Jr, Schroeder HE: Tooth eruption: theories and facts, Anat Rec 245:374-393, 1996.

19. Risinger RK, Proffit WR: Continuous overnight observation of human premolar eruption, Arch Oral Biol 41:779-789, 1996.

20. Trentini CJ, Proffit WR: High resolution observations of human premolar eruption, Arch Oral Biol 41:63-68, 1996.

21. Gron A: Prediction of tooth emergence, J Dent Res 41:573-585, 1962.

22. Anderson DL, Thompson GW, Popovich F: Interrelationship of dental maturity, skeletal maturity, height and weight from age 4 to 14 years, Growth 39:453-462, 1975.

23. Moorrees CFA, Chadha JM: Available space for the incisors during dental development—a growth study based on physiologic age, Angle Orthod 35:12-22, 1965.

24. Edwards JG: The diastema, the frenum, the frenectomy, Am J Orthod 71:489-508, 1977.

25. Gruelich WW, Pyle SI: Radiographic atlas of skeletal development of the hand and wrist, Palo Alto, Calif., 1959, Stanford University Press.

26. Tanner JM: Use and abuse of growth standards. In Falkner F, Tanner JM, (editors): Human growth, vol 3, ed 2, New York, 1986, Plenum Publishing.

CHAPTER
4
Later Stages of Development

ADOLESCENCE: THE EARLY PERMANENT DENTITION YEARS

Adolescence is a sexual phenomenon. It can be defined as the period of life when sexual maturity is attained. More specifically, it is the transitional period between the juvenile stage and adulthood, during which the secondary sexual characteristics appear, the adolescent growth spurt takes place, fertility is attained, and profound physiologic changes occur. All these developments are associated with the maturation of the sex organs and the accompanying surge in secretion of sex hormones.

This period is particularly important in dental and orthodontic treatment, because the physical changes at adolescence significantly affect the face and dentition. Major events in dentofacial development that occur during adolescence include the exchange from the mixed to the permanent dentition, an acceleration in the overall rate of facial growth, and differential growth of the jaws.

Initiation of Adolescence

The first events of puberty occur in the brain, and although considerable research progress has been made in this area,[1] the precise stimulus for their unfolding remains unknown. For whatever reason, apparently influenced both by an internal clock and external stimuli, brain cells in the hypothalamus begin to secrete substances called releasing factors. Both the cells and their method of action are somewhat unusual. These neuroendocrine cells look like typical neurons, but they secrete materials in the cell body, which are carried by cytoplasmic transport down the axon toward a richly vascular area at the base of the hypothalamus near the pituitary gland (Figure 4-1). The substances secreted by the nerve cells pass into capillaries in this vascular region and are carried the short distance to the pituitary by blood flow. It is unusual in the body for the venous return system to transport substances from one closely adjacent region to another, but here the special arrangement of the vessels seems made to order for this purpose. Accordingly, this special network of vessels, analogous to the venous supply to the liver but on a much smaller scale, is called the *pituitary portal system*.

In the anterior pituitary, the hypothalamic releasing factors stimulate pituitary cells to produce several related but different hormones called *pituitary gonadotropins*. Their function is to stimulate endocrine cells in both the adrenal glands and the developing sex organs to produce sex hormones. In every individual a mixture of male and female sex hormones is produced, and it is a biologic fact as well as an everyday observation that there are feminine males and masculine females. Presumably this represents the balance of the competing male and female hormones. In the male, different cell types in the testes produce both the male sex hormone testosterone and female sex hormones. A different pituitary gonadotropin stimulates each of these cell

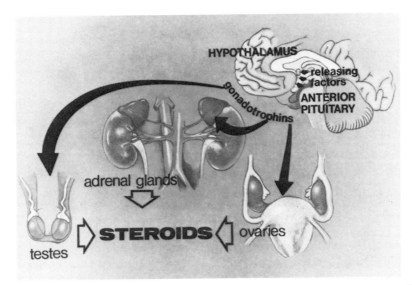

FIGURE 4-1 Diagrammatic representation of the cascade of endocrine signals controlling sexual development. Releasing factors from the hypothalamus are carried via the pituitary portal circulation to the anterior pituitary gland, where they initiate the release of pituitary gonadotropic hormones. These in turn stimulate cells in the testes, ovaries and adrenals, which secrete the steroid sex hormones.

types. In the female, the pituitary gonadotropins stimulate secretion of estrogen by the ovaries, and later progesterone by the same organ. In the female, male sex hormones are produced in the adrenal cortex, stimulated by still another pituitary hormone, and possibly some female hormones are produced in the male adrenal cortex.

Under the stimulation of the pituitary gonadotropins, sex hormones from the testes, ovaries and adrenal cortex are released into the bloodstream in quantities sufficient to cause development of secondary sexual characteristics and accelerated growth of the genitalia. The increasing level of the sex hormones also causes other physiologic changes, including the acceleration in general body growth and shrinkage of lymphoid tissues seen in the classic growth curves described in Chapter 2. Neural growth is unaffected by the events of adolescence, since it is essentially complete by age 6. The changes in the growth curves for the jaws, general body, lymphoid and genital tissues, however, can be considered the result of the hormonal changes that accompany sexual maturation (Figure 4-2).

The system by which a few neurons in the hypothalamus ultimately control the level of circulating sex hormones may seem curiously complex. The principle, however, is one utilized in control systems throughout the body and also in modern technology. Each of the steps in the control process results in an amplification of the control signal, in a way analogous to the amplification of a small musical signal between the tape head and speakers of a stereo system. The amount of pituitary gonadotropin produced is 100 to 1000 times greater than the amount of gonadotropin releasing factors produced in the hypothalamus, and the amount of sex hormones produced is 1000 times greater than the amount of the pituitary hormones

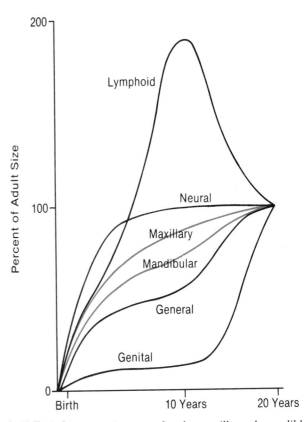

FIGURE 4-2 Growth curves for the maxilla and mandible shown against the background of Scammon's curves. Note that growth of the jaws is intermediate between the neural and general body curves, with the mandible following the general body curve more closely than the maxilla. The acceleration in general body growth at puberty, which affects the jaws, parallels the dramatic increase in development of the sexual organs. Lymphoid involution also occurs at this time.

themselves. The system, then, is a three-stage amplifier. Rather than being a complex biologic curiosity, it is better viewed as a rational engineering design. A similar amplification of controlling signals from the brain is used, of course, in all body systems.

Timing of Puberty

There is a great deal of individual variation, but puberty and the adolescent growth spurt occur on the average nearly 2 years earlier in girls than in boys (Figure 4-3).[2] Why this occurs is not known, but the phenomenon has an important impact on the timing of orthodontic treatment, which must be done earlier in girls than in boys to take advantage of the adolescent growth spurt. Because of the considerable individual variation, however, early maturing boys will reach puberty ahead of slow maturing girls, and it must be remembered that chronologic age has very little to do with where an individual stands developmentally. The stage of development of secondary sexual characteristics provides a physiologic calendar of adolescence that correlates with the individual's physical growth status. Not all the secondary sexual characteristics are readily visible, of course, but most can be evaluated in a normal fully clothed examination, such as would occur in a dental office.

Adolescence in girls can be divided into three stages, based on the extent of sexual development. The first stage, which occurs at about the beginning of the physical growth spurt, is the appearance of breast buds and early stages of the development of pubic hair. The peak velocity for physical growth occurs about 1 year after the initiation of stage I, and coincides with stage II of development of sexual

characteristics (see Figure 4-3). At this time, there is noticeable breast development. Pubic hair is darker and more widespread, and hair appears in the armpits (axillary hair).

The third stage in girls occurs 1 to 1½ years after stage II and is marked by the onset of menstruation. By this time, the growth spurt is all but complete. At this stage, there is noticeable broadening of the hips with more adult fat distribution, and development of the breasts is complete.

The stages of sexual development in boys are more difficult to specifically define than in girls. Puberty begins later and extends over a longer period—about 5 years compared with 3½ years for girls (see Figure 4-3). In boys, four stages in development can be correlated with the curve of general body growth at adolescence.

The initial sign of sexual maturation in boys usually is the "fat spurt." The maturing boy gains weight and becomes almost chubby, with a somewhat feminine fat distribution. This probably occurs because estrogen production by the Leydig cells in the testes is stimulated before the more abundant Sertoli cells begin to produce significant amounts of testosterone. During this stage, boys may appear obese and somewhat awkward physically. At this time also, the scrotum begins to increase in size and may show some increase or change in pigmentation.

At stage II, about 1 year after stage I, the spurt in height is just beginning. At this stage, there is a redistribution and relative decrease in subcutaneous fat, pubic hair begins to appear, and growth of the penis begins.

The third stage occurs 8 to 12 months after stage II and coincides with the peak velocity in gain in height. At this time, axillary hair appears and facial hair appears on the upper lip only. A spurt in muscle growth also occurs, along with a continued decrease in subcutaneous fat and an obviously harder and more angular body form. Pubic hair distribution appears more adult but has not yet spread to the medial of the thighs. The penis and scrotum are near adult size.

Stage IV for boys, which occurs anywhere from 15 to 24 months after stage III, is difficult to pinpoint. At this time, the spurt of growth in height ends. There is facial hair on the chin as well as the upper lip, adult distribution and color of pubic and axillary hair, and a further increase in muscular strength.

The timing of puberty makes an important difference in ultimate body size, in a way that may seem paradoxical at first: the earlier the onset of puberty, the smaller the adult size, and vice versa. Growth in height depends on endochondral bone growth at the epiphyseal plates of the long bones, and the impact of the sex hormones on endochondral bone growth is twofold. First, the sex hormones stimulate the cartilage to grow faster, and this produces the adolescent growth spurt. But the sex hormones also cause an increase in the rate of skeletal maturation, which for the long bones is the rate at which cartilage is transformed into bone. The acceleration in maturation is even greater than the acceleration in growth. Thus during the rapid growth at adolescence, the cartilage is used up faster than it is

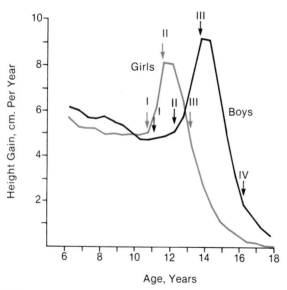

FIGURE 4-3 Velocity curves for growth at adolescence, showing the difference in timing for girls and boys. Also indicated on the growth velocity curves are the corresponding stages in sexual development (see text). (From Marshall WA, Tanner JM: Puberty. In Falkner F, Tanner JM (editors): *Human growth*, vol 2, ed 2, New York, 1986, Plenum Publishing.)

replaced. Toward the end of adolescence, the last of the cartilage is transformed into bone, and the epiphyseal plates close. At that point, of course, growth potential is lost and growth stops.

This early cessation of growth after early sexual maturation is particularly prominent in girls. It is responsible for much of the difference in adult size between men and women. Girls mature earlier on the average, and finish their growth much sooner. Boys are not bigger than girls until they grow for a longer time at adolescence. The difference arises because there is slow but steady growth before the growth spurt, and so when the growth spurt occurs, for those who mature late, it takes off from a higher plateau. The epiphyseal plates close more slowly in males than in females, and therefore the cutoff in growth that accompanies the attainment of sexual maturity is also more complete in girls.

The timing of puberty seems to be affected by both genetic and environmental influences. There are early- and late-maturing families, and individuals in some racial and ethnic groups mature earlier than others. As Figure 4-4 shows, Dutch boys are about 5 cm taller than their American counterparts at age 10, and it is likely that both heredity and environment play a role in producing that considerable difference. In girls, it appears that the onset of menstruation requires the development of a certain amount of body fat. In girls of a slender body type, the onset of

menstruation can be delayed until this level is reached. Athletic girls with low body fat often are slow to begin their menstrual periods, and highly trained female athletes whose body fat levels are quite low may stop menstruating, apparently in response to the low body fat levels.

Seasonal and cultural factors also can affect the overall rate of physical growth. For example, everything else being equal, growth tends to be faster in spring and summer than in fall and winter, and city children tend to mature faster than rural ones, especially in less developed countries. Such effects presumably are mediated via the hypothalamus and indicate that the rate of secretion of gonadotropin-releasing factors can be influenced by external stimuli.

The stages of adolescent development described here were correlated with growth in height. Fortunately, growth of the jaws usually correlates with the physiologic events of puberty in about the same way as growth in height (Figure 4-5). There is an adolescent growth spurt in the length of the mandible, though not nearly as dramatic a spurt as that in body height, and a modest though discernible increase in growth at the sutures of the maxilla. The cephalocaudal gradient of growth, which is part of the normal pattern, is dramatically evident at puberty. More growth occurs in the lower extremity than in the upper, and within the face, more growth takes place in the lower jaw than in the upper. This produces an acceleration in mandibular growth relative to the maxilla and results in the differential jaw growth referred to previously. The maturing face becomes less convex as the mandible and chin become more prominent as a result of the differential jaw growth.

Although jaw growth follows the curve for general body growth, the correlation is not perfect. Longitudinal data from studies of craniofacial growth indicate that a significant number of individuals, especially among the girls, have a "juvenile acceleration" in jaw growth that occurs

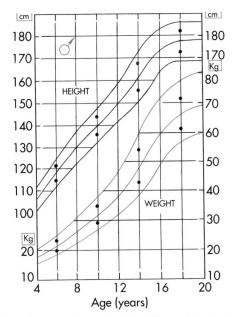

FIGURE 4-4 Growth can be affected by racial, ethnic, national and other variables. As this graph shows, the average 10-year-old boy in the Netherlands (*black lines*) is nearly 5 cm (2 inches) taller than his American counterpart (*red lines*). Cross-sectional data of this type is most useful for one-time comparisons of an individual with the group. Because of the smoothing effect of the averages, these curves do not represent the velocity changes any individual is likely to experience during growth spurts (see Figure 2-7).

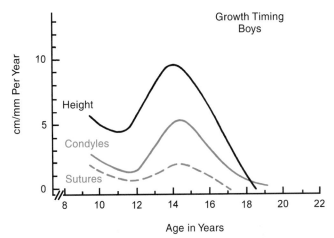

FIGURE 4-5 On the average, the spurt in growth of the jaws occurs at about the same time as the spurt in height, but it must be remembered that there is considerable individual variation. (From Woodside DG: In Salzmann JA: *Orthodontics in daily practice*, Philadelphia, 1974, JB Lippincott.)

1 to 2 years before the adolescent growth spurt (Figure 4-6).[3] This juvenile acceleration can equal or even exceed the jaw growth that accompanies secondary sexual maturation. In boys, if a juvenile spurt occurs, it is nearly always less intense than the growth acceleration at puberty.

Recent research has shown that sexual development really begins much earlier than previously thought.[4] Sex hormones produced by the adrenal glands first appear at age 6 in both sexes, primarily in the form of a weak androgen (dihydroepiandrosterone, [DHEA]). This activation of the adrenal component of the system is referred to as *adrenarche*. DHEA reaches a critical level at about age 10 that correlates with the initiation of sexual attraction. It is likely that a juvenile acceleration in growth is related to the intensity of adrenarche and not surprising that a juvenile acceleration is more prominent in girls because of the greater adrenal component of their early sexual development.

This tendency for a clinically useful acceleration in jaw growth to precede the adolescent spurt, particularly in girls, is a major reason for careful assessment of physiologic age in planning orthodontic treatment. If treatment is delayed too long, the opportunity to utilize the growth spurt is missed. In early-maturing girls, the adolescent growth spurt often precedes the final transition of the dentition, so that by the time the second premolars and second molars erupt, physical growth is all but complete. The presence of a juvenile growth spurt in girls accentuates this tendency for significant acceleration of jaw growth in the mixed dentition. If most girls are to receive orthodontic treatment while they are growing rapidly, the treatment must begin during the mixed dentition rather than after all succedaneous teeth have erupted.

In slow-maturing boys, on the other hand, the dentition can be relatively complete while a considerable amount of physical growth remains. In the timing of orthodontic treatment, clinicians have a tendency to treat girls too late and boys too soon, forgetting the considerable disparity in the rate of physiologic maturation.

GROWTH PATTERNS IN THE DENTOFACIAL COMPLEX

Dimensional Changes

Growth of the Nasomaxillary Complex. Growth of the nasomaxillary area is produced by two basic mechanisms: (1) passive displacement, created by growth in the cranial base that pushes the maxilla forward, and (2) active growth of the maxillary structures and nose (Figure 4-7).[5]

Passive displacement of the maxilla is an important growth mechanism during the primary dentition years but becomes less important as growth at the synchondroses of the cranial base slows markedly with the completion of neural growth at about age 7. Total forward movement of the maxilla and the amount resulting from forward displacement are shown in Table 4-1. Note that during the entire period between ages 7 and 15, about one third of the total forward movement of the maxilla can be accounted for on the basis of passive displacement. The rest is the result of active growth of the maxillary sutures in response to stimuli from the enveloping soft tissues (see Chapter 2).

The effect of surface remodeling must be considered when active growth of the maxilla is considered. Surface

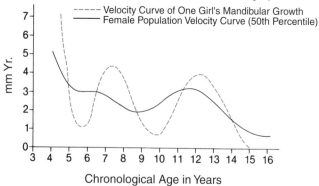

FIGURE 4-6 Longitudinal data for increase in length of the mandible in one girl, taken from the Burlington growth study in Canada, demonstrates an acceleration of growth at about 8 years of age (juvenile acceleration) equal in intensity to the pubertal acceleration between ages 11 and 14. Changes of this type in the pattern of growth for individuals tend to be smoothed out when cross-sectional or group average data are studied. (From Woodside DG: In Salzmann JA: *Orthodontics in daily practice*, Philadelphia, 1974, J.B. Lippincott.)

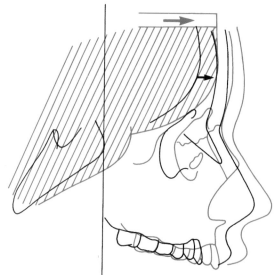

FIGURE 4-7 Diagrammatic representation of a major mechanism for growth of the maxilla: structures of the nasomaxillary complex are displaced forward as the cranial base lengthens and the anterior lobes of the brain grow in size. (Redrawn from Enlow DH, Hans MG: *Essentials of facial growth*, Philadelphia, 1996, W.B. Saunders.)

changes can either add to or subtract from growth in other areas by surface apposition or resorption respectively. In fact, the maxilla grows downward and forward as bone is added in the tuberosity area posteriorly and at the posterior and superior sutures, but the anterior surfaces of the bone are resorbing at the same time (Figure 4-8). For this reason, the distance that the body of the maxilla and the maxillary teeth are carried downward and forward during growth is greater by about 25% than the forward movement of the anterior surface of the maxilla. This tendency for surface

remodeling to conceal the extent of relocation of the jaws is even more prominent when rotation of the maxilla during growth is considered (see the following sections).

The nasal structures undergo the same passive displacement as the rest of the maxilla. However, the nose grows more rapidly than the rest of the face, particularly during the adolescent growth spurt. Nasal growth is produced in part by an increase in size of the cartilaginous nasal septum. In addition, proliferation of the lateral cartilages alters the shape of the nose and contributes to an increase in overall size. The growth of the nose is extremely variable, as a cursory examination of any group of people will confirm. Average increases in nasal dimensions of white Americans are illustrated in Table 4-2. Comparison with Table 4-1 shows that nasal dimensions increase at a rate about 25% greater than growth of the maxilla.

Mandibular Growth. Growth of the mandible continues at a relatively steady rate before puberty. On the average, as Table 4-3 shows, ramus height increases 1 to 2 mm per year and body length increases 2 to 3 mm per year. These cross-sectional data tend to smooth out the juvenile and pubertal growth spurts, which do occur in growth of the mandible (see previous discussion).

TABLE 4-1 *Maxillary Length Changes*

	Total forward movement (mm) (basion-ANS increment)		Forward displacement (mm) (basion-PNS increment)	
Age	Male	Female	Male	Female
7	1.3	2.1	0.0	0.8
8	1.5	1.8	0.9	1.1
9	1.6	0.4	0.4	0.4
10	1.8	2.0	0.8	0.2
11	1.9	1.0	0.2	0.2
12	2.0	1.3	0.4	1.1
13	2.1	1.2	1.0	–0.1
14	1.1	1.5	0.3	0.1
15	1.2	1.1	0.4	0.8

Data from Riolo ML et al: *An atlas of craniofacial growth,* Ann Arbor, Mich., 1974, University of Michigan, Center for Human Growth and Development.

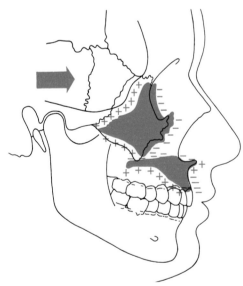

FIGURE 4-8 As the maxilla is translated downward and forward, bone is added at the sutures and in the tuberosity area posteriorly, but at the same time, surface remodeling removes bone from the anterior surfaces (except for a small area at the anterior nasal spine). For this reason, the amount of forward movement of anterior surfaces is less than the amount of displacement. In the roof of the mouth, however, surface remodeling adds bone, while bone is resorbed from the floor of the nose. The total downward movement of the palatal vault, therefore, is greater than the amount of displacement. (Redrawn from Enlow DH, Hans MG: *Essentials of facial growth*, Philadelphia, 1996, WB Saunders.)

TABLE 4-2 *Length and Height of the Nose*

	Nose length (nasion to tip)		Vertical height of nose	
Age	Male	Female	Male	Female
6	43.3	41.1	36.0	34.2
9	47.7	45.2	40.1	37.0
12	51.7	50.2	43.5	41.1
15	54.9	54.4	46.6	44.3
18	60.2	57.8	49.0	46.1

Data from Subtelny JD: Am J Orthod 45:481, 1959.

TABLE 4-3 *Mandibular Length Changes*

	Body length increase (mm) (gonion-pogonion)		Ramus height increase (mm) (condylar-gonion)	
Age	Male	Female	Male	Female
7	2.8	1.7	0.8	1.2
8	1.7	2.5	1.4	1.4
9	1.9	1.1	1.5	0.3
10	2.0	2.5	1.2	0.7
11	2.2	1.7	1.8	0.9
12	1.3	0.8	1.4	2.2
13	2.0	1.8	2.2	0.5
14	2.5	1.1	2.2	1.7
15	1.6	1.1	1.1	2.3
16	2.3	1.0	3.4	1.6

Data from Riolo ML et al: An atlas of craniofacial growth, Ann Arbor, Mich., 1974, University of Michigan, Center for Human Growth and Development.

One feature of mandibular growth is an accentuation of the prominence of the chin. At one time, it was thought that this occurred primarily by addition of bone to the chin, but that is incorrect. Although small amounts of bone are added, the change in the contour of the chin itself occurs largely because the area just above the chin, between it and the base of the alveolar process, is a resorptive area. The increase in chin prominence with maturity results from a combination of forward translation of the chin as a part of the overall growth pattern of the mandible and resorption above the chin that alters the bony contours.

An important source of variability in how much the chin grows forward is the extent of growth changes at the glenoid fossa. If the area of the temporal bone to which the mandible is attached moved forward relative to the cranial base during growth, this would translate the mandible forward in the same way that cranial base growth translates the maxilla. However, this rarely happens. More often, the attachment point moves straight down or posteriorly, thus subtracting from rather than augmenting the forward projection of the chin.[6] In both the patients shown in Figure 4-9, for instance, there was an approximate 7 mm increase in length of the mandible during orthodontic treatment around the time of puberty. In one of the patients, the temporomandibular (TM) joint did not relocate during growth and the chin projected forward 7 mm. In the other patient, the TM joint moved posteriorly, resulting in only a small forward projection of the chin despite the increase in mandibular length.

Timing of Growth in Width, Length, and Height. For the three planes of space in both the maxilla and mandible, there is a definite sequence in which growth is "completed," (i.e., declines to the slow rate that characterizes normal adults). Growth in width is completed first, then growth in length, and finally growth in height. Growth in width of both jaws, including the width of the dental arches, tends to be completed before the adolescent growth spurt and is affected minimally if at all by adolescent growth changes (Figure 4-10). Intercanine width is more likely to decrease than increase after age 12.[7] There is a partial exception to this rule, however. As the jaws grow in length posteriorly, they also grow wider. For the maxilla, this affects primarily the width across the second molars, and if they are able to erupt, the third molars in the region of the tuberosity as well. For the mandible, both molar and bicondylar widths show small increases until the end of growth in length. Anterior width dimensions of the mandible stabilize earlier.

Growth in length and height of both jaws continues through the period of puberty. In girls, the maxilla grows slowly downward and forward to age 14 to 15 on the average (more accurately, by 2 to 3 years after first menstruation), then tends to grow slightly more almost straight forward (Figure 4-11).[8] In both sexes, growth in vertical

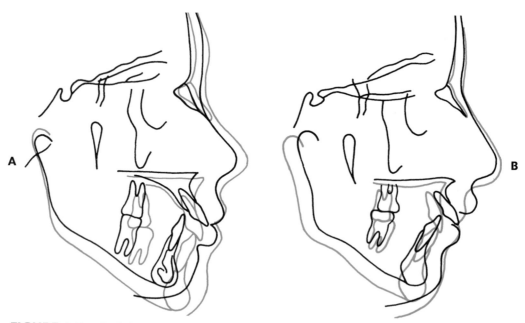

FIGURE 4-9   Cephalometric tracings showing growth in two patients during the orthodontic correction of moderate Class II malocclusion (superimposed on sphenoethmoid triad in cranial base). **A,** Changes from age 11 years 10 months to age 14 years 11 months. In this patient, approximately 7 mm of mandibular growth was expressed entirely as forward movement of the chin, while the area of the temporomandibular (TM) joint remained in the same anteroposterior position relative to the cranial base. **B,** Changes from age 11 years 8 months to age 15 years 0 months. This patient also had approximately 7 mm of mandibular growth, but the TM joint area moved downward and backward relative to the cranial base, so that much of the growth was not expressed as forward movement of the chin. (Courtesy Dr. V. Kokich.)

height of the face continues longer than growth in length, with the late vertical growth primarily in the mandible. Increases in facial height and concomitant eruption of teeth continue throughout life, but the decline to the adult level (which for vertical growth is surprisingly large

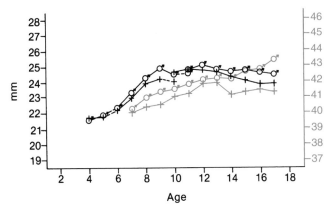

FIGURE 4-10 Average changes in mandibular canine and molar widths in both sexes during growth. Molar widths are shown in red, canine widths in black. (From Moyers RE et al: *Standards of human occlusal development*, Ann Arbor, Mich., 1976, University of Michigan Center for Human Growth and Development.)

[see the following section]) often does not occur until the early twenties in boys, somewhat earlier in girls.

Rotation of Jaws during Growth

Implant Studies of Jaw Rotation. Until longitudinal studies of growth using metallic implants in the jaws were carried out in the 1960s, primarily by Bjork and coworkers in Copenhagen,[9] the extent to which both the maxilla and mandible rotate during growth was not appreciated. The reason is that the rotation that occurs in the core of each jaw, called *internal rotation*, tends to be masked by surface changes and alterations in the rate of tooth eruption. The surface changes produce *external rotation*. Obviously, the overall change in the orientation of each jaw, as judged by the palatal plane and mandibular plane, results from a combination of internal and external rotation.

The terminology for describing these rotational changes is itself confusing. The descriptive terms used here, in an effort to simplify and clarify a complex and difficult subject, are not those Bjork used in the original papers on this subject, or exactly the same as suggested in some previous papers.[9,10] See Table 4-4 for a comparison of terms.

It is easier to visualize the internal and external rotation of the jaws by considering the mandible first. The core

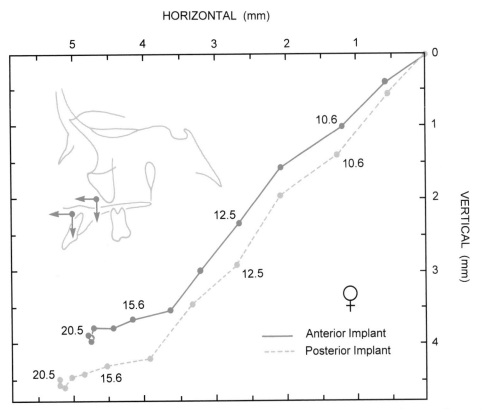

FIGURE 4-11 Mean growth tracks of anterior and posterior maxillary implants relative to the cranial base and its perpendicular, in a group of Danish girls. The two tracks are shown with their origins superimposed to facilitate comparison. Note that the posterior implant moves down and forward more than the anterior one, with growth continuing into the late teens at a slow rate. (Courtesy Dr. B. Solow.)

TABLE 4-4   *Terminolgy, Rotational Changes of the Jaws*

Condition	Bjork	Shudy	
Posterior growth greater than posterior	Backward rotation	Counterclockwise rotation	
Anterior growth greater than anterior	Forward rotation	Clockwise rotation	

	Bjork	Solow, Houston	Proffit
Rotation of mandibular core relative to cranial base	Total rotation	True rotation	Internal rotation
Rotation of mandibular plane relative to cranial base	Matrix rotation	Apparent rotation	Total rotation
Rotation of mandibular plane relative to core of mandible	Intramatrix rotation	Angular remodeling of lower border	External rotation

Proffit: Total rotation = internal rotation – external rotation
Bjork: Matrix rotation = total rotation – intramatrix rotation
Solow: Apparent rotation = true rotation – angular remodeling of lower border

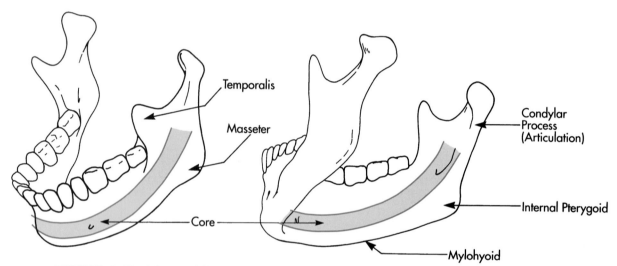

FIGURE 4-12   The mandible can be visualized as consisting of a core of bone surrounding the inferior alveolar neurovascular bundle, and a series of functional processes: the alveolar process, serving the function of mastication; the muscular processes, serving for muscle attachments; and the condylar process, serving to articulate the bone with the rest of the skull.

of the mandible is the bone that surrounds the inferior alveolar nerve. The rest of the mandible consists of its several functional processes (Figure 4-12). These are the alveolar process (bone supporting the teeth and providing for mastication), the muscular processes (the bone to which the muscles of mastication attach), and the condylar process, the function in this case being the articulation of the jaw with the skull. If implants are placed in areas of stable bone away from the functional processes, it can be observed that in most individuals, the core of the mandible rotates during growth in a way that would tend to decrease the mandibular plane angle (i.e., up anteriorly and down posteriorly).

Bjork and Skieller[11] distinguished two contributions to internal rotation (which they called total rotation) of the mandible: (1) matrix rotation, or rotation around the condyle; and (2) intramatrix rotation, or rotation centered within the body of the mandible (Figure 4-13). By convention, the rotation of either jaw is considered "forward" and given a negative sign if there is more growth posteriorly than anteriorly. The rotation is "backward" and given a positive direction if it lengthens anterior dimensions more than posterior ones, bringing the chin downward and backward.

One of the features of internal rotation of the mandible is the variation between individuals, ranging up to 10 to 15 degrees. The pattern of vertical facial development, discussed in more detail later, is strongly related to the rotation of both jaws. For an average individual with normal

CRANIAL BASE

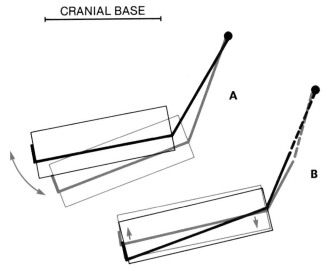

FIGURE 4-13 Internal rotation of the mandible (i.e., rotation of the core relative to the cranial base) has two components: **A,** rotation around the condyle, or matrix rotation; and **B,** rotations centered within the body of the mandible, or intramatrix rotation. (Redrawn from Bjork A, Skieller V: *Eur J Orthod* 5:1-46, 1983.)

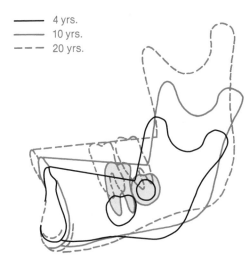

FIGURE 4-14 Superimposition on implants for an individual with a normal pattern of growth, showing surface changes in the mandible from ages 4 to 20 years. For this patient there was -19 degrees internal rotation but only -3 degrees change in the mandibular plane angle. Note how the dramatic remodeling (external rotation) compensates for and conceals the extent of the internal rotation. (From Bjork A, Skieller V: *Eur J Orthod* 5:1-46, 1983.)

vertical facial proportions, however, there is about a -15 degree internal rotation from age 4 to adult life. Of this, about 25% results from matrix rotation and 75% results from intramatrix rotation.

During the time that the core of the mandible rotates forward an average of 15 degrees, the mandibular plane angle, representing the orientation of the jaw to an outside observer, decreases only 2 to 4 degrees on the average. The reason that the internal rotation is not expressed in jaw orientation, of course, is that surface changes (external rotation) tend to compensate. This means that the posterior part of the lower border of the mandible must be an area of resorption, while the anterior aspect of the lower border is unchanged or undergoes slight apposition. Studies of surface changes reveal exactly this as the usual pattern of apposition and resorption (Figure 4-14). On the average, then, there is about 15 degrees of internal, forward rotation and 11 to 12 degrees of external, backward rotation producing the 3 to 4 degree decrease in mandibular plane angle observed in the average individual during childhood and adolescence.

It is less easy to divide the maxilla into a core of bone and a series of functional processes. The alveolar process is certainly a functional process in the classic sense, but there are no areas of muscle attachment analogous to those of the mandible. The parts of the bone surrounding the air passages serve the function of respiration, and the form-function relationships involved are poorly understood. If implants are placed above the maxillary alveolar process, however, one can observe a core of the maxilla that undergoes a small and variable degree of rotation, forward or backward (Figure 4-15).[9,12] This internal rotation is anal-

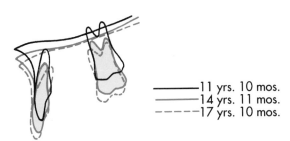

FIGURE 4-15 Superimposition on implants in the maxilla reveals that this patient experienced a small amount of backward internal rotation of the maxilla (i.e., down anteriorly). A small amount of forward rotation is the more usual pattern, but backward rotation occurs frequently. (From Bjork A, Skieller V: *Am J Orthod* 62:357, 1972.)

ogous to the intramatrix rotation of the mandible. Matrix rotation, as defined for the mandible, is not possible for the maxilla.

At the same time that internal rotation of the maxilla is occurring, there also are varying degrees of resorption of bone on the nasal side and apposition of bone on the palatal side in the anterior and posterior parts of the palate. Similar variations in the amount of eruption of the incisors and molars occur. These changes amount, of course, to an external rotation. For most patients, the external rotation is opposite in direction and equal in magnitude to the internal rotation, so that the two rotations cancel and the net change in jaw orientation (as evaluated by the palatal plane) is zero (see Figure 3-29). Until the implant studies were done, rotation of the maxilla during normal growth had not been suspected.

Although both internal and external rotation occur in everybody, variations from the average pattern are common. Greater or lesser degrees of both internal and external rotation often occur, altering the extent to which external changes compensate for the internal rotation. The result is moderate variation in jaw orientation, even in individuals with normal facial proportions. In addition, the rotational patterns of growth are quite different for individuals who have what are called the short face and long face types of vertical facial development.[13]

Individuals of the short face type, who are characterized by short anterior lower face height, have excessive forward rotation of the mandible during growth, resulting from both an increase in the normal internal rotation and a decrease in external compensation. The result is a nearly horizontal palatal plane and mandibular morphology of the "square jaw" type, with a low mandibular plane angle and a square gonial angle (Figure 4-16). A deep bite malocclusion and crowded incisors usually accompany this type of rotation (see following sections).

In long face individuals, who have excessive lower anterior face height, the palatal plane rotates down posteriorly, often creating a negative rather than the normal positive inclination to the true horizontal. The mandible shows an opposite, backward rotation, with an increase in the mandibular plane angle (Figure 4-17). The mandibular changes result primarily from a lack of the normal for-

ward internal rotation or even a backward internal rotation. The internal rotation, in turn, is primarily matrix rotation (centered at the condyle), not intramatrix rotation. This type of rotation is associated with anterior open bite malocclusion and mandibular deficiency (because the chin rotates back as well as down). As one would expect, changes in face height correlate better with changes in the mandibular plane angle (which reflects total rotation) than with changes in the corpus axis (which reflects internal rotation). This is another reflection of the fact that the total change is determined by the interaction between internal and external changes. Backward rotation of the mandible also occurs in patients with abnormalities or pathologic changes affecting the temporomandibular joints. In these individuals, growth at the condyle is restricted. The interesting result in three cases documented by Bjork and Skieller[14] was an intramatrix rotation centered in the body of the mandible, rather than the backward rotation at the condyle that dominated in individuals of the classic long face type. Jaw orientation changes in both the backward-rotating types, however, are similar, and the same types of malocclusions develop.

Interaction between Jaw Rotation and Tooth Eruption.   As we have discussed, growth of the mandible away from the maxilla creates a space into which the teeth erupt.

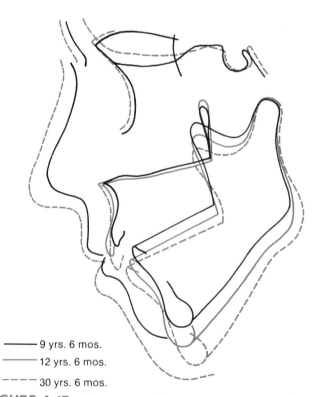

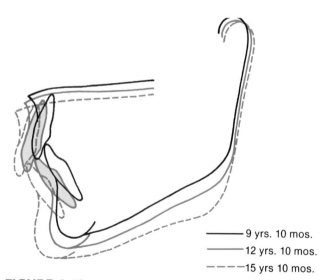

FIGURE 4-16   Cranial base superimposition shows the characteristic pattern of forward mandibular rotation in an individual developing in the "short face" pattern. The forward rotation flattens the mandibular plane and tends to increase overbite. (From Bjork A, Skieller V: *Am J Orthod* 62:344, 1972.)

FIGURE 4-17   The pattern of jaw rotation in an individual with the "long face" pattern of growth (cranial base superimposition). As the mandible rotates backward, anterior face height increases, there is a tendency toward anterior open bite, and the incisors are thrust forward relative to the mandible. (From Bjork A, Skieller V: *Eur J Orthod* 5:29, 1983.)

The rotational pattern of jaw growth obviously influences the magnitude of tooth eruption. To a surprising extent, it can also influence the direction of eruption and the ultimate anteroposterior position of the incisor teeth.

The path of eruption of the maxillary teeth is downward and somewhat forward (see Figure 4-11). In normal growth, the maxilla usually rotates a few degrees forward but frequently rotates slightly backward. Forward rotation would tend to tip the incisors forward, increasing their prominence, while backward rotation directs the anterior teeth more posteriorly than would have been the case without the rotation, relatively uprighting them and decreasing their prominence. Movement of the teeth relative to the cranial base obviously could be produced by a combination of *translocation* as the tooth moved along with the jaw in which it was embedded, and true *eruption*, movement of the tooth within its jaw. As Figure 4-18 shows, translocation contributes about half the total maxillary tooth movement during adolescent growth.

The eruption path of mandibular teeth is upward and somewhat forward. The normal internal rotation of the mandible carries the jaw upward in front. This rotation alters the eruption path of the incisors, tending to direct them more posteriorly than would otherwise have been the case (Figure 4-19). Because the internal jaw rotation tends to upright the incisors, the molars migrate further mesially during growth than do the incisors, and this migration is reflected in the decrease in arch length that normally occurs (Figure 4-20). Since the forward internal rotation of the mandible is greater than that of the maxilla, it is not surprising that the normal decrease in mandibular arch length is somewhat greater than the decrease in maxillary arch length.

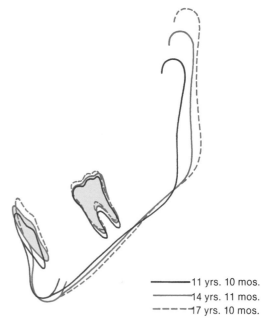

11 yrs. 10 mos.
14 yrs. 11 mos.
17 yrs. 10 mos.

FIGURE 4-19 Superimposition on mandibular implants shows the lingual positioning of the mandibular incisors relative to the mandible that often accompanies forward rotation during growth. (From Bjork A, Skieller V: *Am J Orthod* 62:357, 1972.)

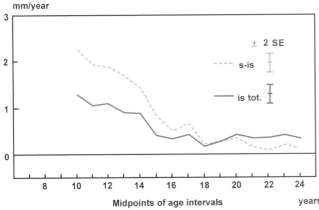

AVERAGE VELOCITY OF CONTINUED ERUPTION
AND TRANSLOCATION OF MAXILLARY INCISORS

mm/year

± 2 SE

s-is

is tot.

Midpoints of age intervals   years

FIGURE 4-18 The average velocity of continued eruption (movement of the incisors relative to implants in the maxilla) and translocation (movement away from the cranial base) of maxillary incisors in Danish girls, from a mixed longitudinal sample. (Redrawn from Solow and Haluk. In Davidovitch S, Norton L (editors): *Biological mechanisms of tooth movement and craniofacial adaptation*, Boston, 1996, Harvard Society for Advancement of Orthodontics.)

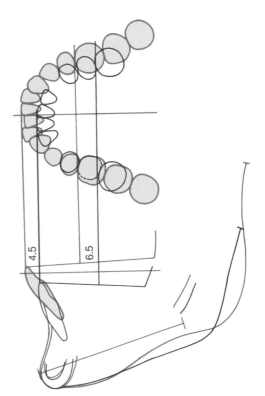

FIGURE 4-20 Superimposition of the mandible at ages 10 years 3 months (*black*) and 21 years 3 months (*red*) for this patient with a relatively small amount of internal rotation (minus 7.5 degrees) shows that the anterior and posterior teeth moved forward on the mandible, but the molars came forward more. (From Bjork A, Skieller V: *Eur J Orthod* 5:15, 1983.)

Note that this explanation for the decrease in arch length that normally occurs in both jaws is different from the traditional interpretation that emphasizes forward migration of the molar teeth. The modern view places relatively greater importance on lingual movement of the incisors and relatively less importance on the forward movement of molars. In fact, the same implant studies that revealed the internal jaw rotation also confirmed that changes in anteroposterior position of the incisor teeth are a major influence on arch length changes.

Given this relationship between jaw rotation and incisor position, it is not surprising that both the vertical and anteroposterior positions of the incisors are affected in short face and long face individuals.[15] When excessive rotation occurs in the short face type of development, the incisors tend to be carried into an overlapping position even if they erupt very little; hence the tendency for deep bite malocclusion in short face individuals (Figure 4-21). The rotation also progressively uprights the incisors, displacing them lingually and causing a tendency toward crowding (Figure 4-22). In the long face growth pattern, on the other hand, an anterior open bite will develop as anterior face height increases unless the incisors erupt for an extreme distance. The rotation of the jaws also carries the incisors forward, creating dental protrusion.

The interaction between tooth eruption and jaw rotation explains a number of previously puzzling aspects of tooth positioning in patients who have vertical facial disproportions. This topic is discussed from an etiologic perspective in Chapter 5 and is reviewed from the point of view of treatment planning in Chapter 8.

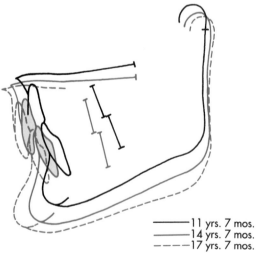

——— 11 yrs. 7 mos.
——— 14 yrs. 7 mos.
- - - - 17 yrs. 7 mos.

FIGURE 4-21 Cranial base superimpositon for a patient with the short face pattern of growth. As the mandible rotates upward and forward, the vertical overlap of the teeth tends to increase, creating a deep bite malocclusion. In addition, even though both the upper and lower teeth do move forward relative to cranial base, lingual displacement of incisors relative to the maxilla and mandible increases the tendency toward crowding. (From Bjork A, Skieller V: *Am J Orthod* 62:355, 1972.)

MATURATIONAL AND AGING CHANGES IN THE DENTAL APPARATUS

Maturational changes in the dentition affect the teeth and their supporting structures and the dental occlusion itself.

Changes in Teeth and Supporting Structures

At the time a permanent tooth erupts, the pulp chamber is relatively large. As time passes, additional dentin slowly deposits on the inside of the tooth, so that the pulp chamber gradually becomes smaller with increasing age (Figure 4-23). This process continues relatively rapidly until the late teens, at which time the pulp chamber of a typical permanent tooth is about half the size that it was at the time of initial eruption. Because of the relatively large pulp chambers of young permanent teeth, complex restorative procedures are more likely to result in mechanical exposures in adolescents than in adults. Additional dentin continues to be produced at a slower rate throughout life, so that in old age, the pulp chambers of some permanent teeth are all but obliterated.

Maturation also brings about greater exposure of the tooth outside its investing soft tissues. At the time a permanent first molar erupts, the gingival attachment is high on the crown. Typically, the gingival attachment is still well above the cementoenamel junction when any permanent tooth comes into full occlusion, and during the next few years more and more of the crown is exposed. This relative apical movement of the attachment (in normal circumstances) results more from vertical growth of the jaws and accompanying eruption of the teeth than from downward migration of the gingival attachment. As we have noted previously in this chapter, vertical growth of the jaws and an increase in face height continue after transverse and anteroposterior growth have been completed. By the time the jaws all but stop growing vertically in the late teens, the gingival attachment is usually near the cementoenamel junction. In the absence of inflammation, mechanical abrasion, or pathologic changes, the gingival attachment should remain at about the same level almost indefinitely. In fact,

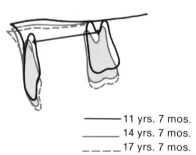

——— 11 yrs. 7 mos.
——— 14 yrs. 7 mos.
- - - - 17 yrs. 7 mos.

FIGURE 4-22 Superimposition on the maxilla reveals uprighting of the maxillary incisors in the short face growth pattern (same patient as Figure 4-21). This decreases arch length and contributes to progressive crowding. (From Bjork A, Skieller V: *Am J Orthod* 62:355, 1972.)

however, most individuals experience some pathology of the gingiva or periodontium as they age, and so further recession of the gingiva is common.

At one time, it was thought that "passive eruption" occurred, defined as an actual gingival migration of the attachment without any eruption of the tooth. It now appears that as long as the gingival tissues are entirely healthy, this sort of downward migration of the soft tissue attachment does not occur. What was once thought to be passive eruption during the teens is really active eruption, compensating for the vertical jaw growth still occurring at that time (Figure 4-24).

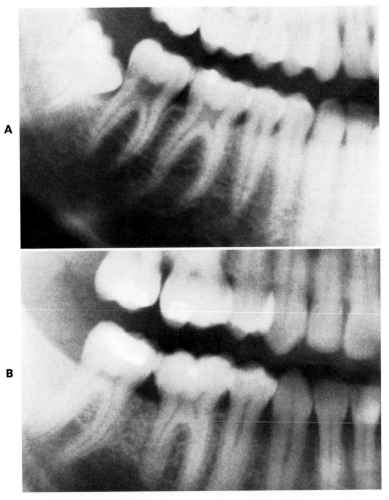

FIGURE 4-23   The size of the pulp chambers of permanent teeth decreases during adolescence then continues to fill in more slowly for the rest of adult life. **A,** Age 16; **B,** Age 26.

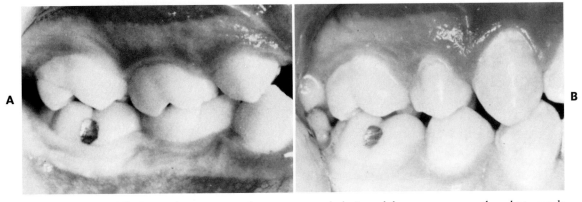

FIGURE 4-24   The increasing exposure of permanent teeth during adolescence was once thought to result from a downward migration of the attachment but now is recognized to occur mostly in response to vertical growth. **A,** Age 10; **B,** Age 16.

Both occlusal and interproximal wear, often to a severe degree, occurred in primitive people eating an extremely coarse diet. The elimination of most coarse particles from modern diets has also largely eliminated wear of this type. With few exceptions (tobacco chewing is one), wear facets on the teeth now indicate bruxism, not what the individual has been eating.

Changes in Alignment and Occlusion

Individuals in primitive societies who experienced wear of the teeth lost tooth substance interproximally as well as from the occlusal surfaces. The alveolar bone bends during heavy mastication, allowing the teeth to move relative to each other (see Chapter 9 for more details). On a coarse diet, this movement causes both interproximal and occlusal wear. The result in many primitive populations was a reduction in arch circumference of 10 mm or more after completion of the permanent dentition at adolescence.

When this type of interproximal wear occurs, spaces do not open up between the posterior teeth, although some spacing may develop anteriorly. Instead, the permanent molars migrate mesially, keeping the contacts reasonably tight even as the contact points are worn off and the mesiodistal width of each tooth decreases.

In modern populations, there is a strong tendency for crowding of the mandibular incisor teeth to develop in the late teens and early twenties, no matter how well aligned the teeth were initially. Mild crowding of the lower incisors tends to develop if the teeth were initially well aligned, or initially mild crowding becomes worse (Figure 4-25). These changes appear as early as age 17 to 18 in some individuals and as late as the mid-twenties in others. Three major theories to account for this crowding have been proposed:

1. Lack of "Normal Attrition" in the Modern Diet. As noted in Chapter 1, primitive populations tend to have a much smaller prevalence of malocclusion than do contemporary populations in developed countries. If a shortening of arch length and a mesial migration of the permanent molars is a natural phenomenon, it would seem reasonable that crowding would develop unless the amount of tooth struc-

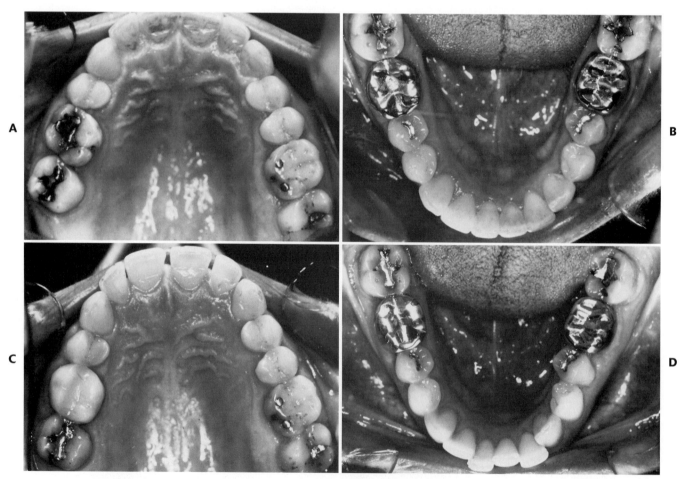

FIGURE 4-25   **A, B,** Age 28; **C, D,** Age 38, in a woman who experienced mandibular growth (because of condylar hyperplasia) during that time. Note the typical pattern of change that accompanies late mandibular growth: spacing of upper incisors and crowding of lower incisors but more crowding in the lower. Late mandibular growth after maxillary growth stops, which often occurs in the late teens, is a major cause of mandibular incisor crowding at that time.

ture was reduced during the final stages of growth. Raymond Begg,[16] a pioneer Australian orthodontist, noted in his studies of the Australian aborigines that malocclusion is uncommon but that large amounts of interproximal and occlusal attrition occurred (Figure 4-26). He concluded that the teeth became crowded when attrition did not occur with soft diets, and advocated widespread extraction of premolar teeth to provide the equivalent of the attrition he saw in aborigines. Unfortunately for this theory, when Australian aborigines change to a modern diet, as happened in most of this group by the late 20th century, occlusal and interproximal wear all but disappears. Late crowding rarely develops,[17] although periodontal disease does become a major problem. It has been observed in other population groups that late crowding may develop even after premolars are extracted and arch length is reduced by modern orthodontic treatment. Thus this theory, though superficially attractive, does not explain late crowding.

2. Pressure From Third Molars. Late crowding develops at about the time the third molars should erupt. In most individuals, these teeth are hopelessly impacted because the jaw length did not increase enough to accommodate them via backward remodeling of the ramus (Figure 4-27). Erupting teeth produce pressure, and it has seemed entirely logical to many dentists that pressure from third molars with no room to erupt is the cause of late incisor crowding. It is difficult to detect such a force, however, even with modern instrumentation that should have found it if it exists.[18] In fact, late crowding of lower incisors can and often does develop in individuals whose lower third molars are congenitally missing. There is some evidence that crowding may be lessened by early removal of second molars, which presumably would relieve pressure from third molars,[19] but pressure from third molars clearly is not the total explanation either.[20]

3. Late Mandibular Growth. As a result of the cephalocaudal gradient of growth discussed in Chapter 2, the mandible can and does undergo more growth in the late teens than the maxilla. Is it possible that late mandibular growth somehow causes late mandibular incisor crowding? If so, how? Bjork's implant studies have provided an understanding of why late crowding occurs and how it indeed relates to the growth pattern of the jaw.

The position of the dentition relative to the maxilla and mandible is influenced by the pattern of growth of the jaws, a concept explored in some detail in previous sections. When the mandible grows forward relative to the maxilla, as it usually does in the late teens as well as earlier, the mandibular incisor teeth tend to be displaced lingually (see Figure 4-19), particularly if any excessive rotation is also present.

In patients with a tight anterior occlusion before late differential mandibular growth occurs, the contact relationship of the lower incisors with the upper incisors must change if the mandible grows forward. In that circumstance,

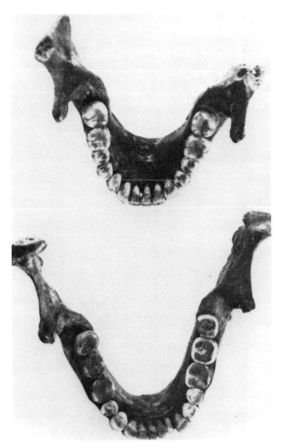

FIGURE 4-26 Mandibles of an adolescent Australian aborigine (*top*) and an adult (*bottom*), taken from prehistoric skeletal remains. Note the attrition of the teeth of the adult, resulting in interproximal as well as occlusal wear. Arch length in this population shortened by 1 cm or more after adolescence because of the extensive interproximal wear. (From Begg PR: *Am J Orthod* 40:298-312, 1954.)

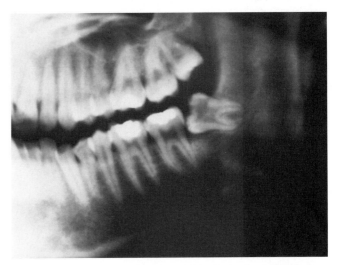

FIGURE 4-27 It seems reasonable that a horizontally impacted third molar would provide pressure against the dental arch, but it is highly unlikely that there is enough pressure from this source to cause the crowding of mandibular incisors that often develops in the late teens.

one of three events must occur: (1) the mandible is displaced distally, accompanied by a distortion of temporomandibular joint function and displacement of the articular disc; (2) the upper incisors flare forward, opening space between these teeth; or (3) the lower incisors displace distally and become crowded.

All three of these phenomena have been reported. The second response, flaring and spacing of the maxillary incisors, is the least common. Posterior displacement of a "trapped mandible" can happen and may occasionally be related to myofascial pain and dysfunction, but despite the claims of some occlusion theorists, this too seems to be quite rare. Distal displacement of the lower incisors, with concomitant crowding and a decrease in the lower intercanine distance, is the most likely response.

It is not even necessary for the incisors to be in occlusal contact for late crowding to develop. This also occurs commonly in individuals who have an anterior open bite and backward, not forward, rotation of the mandible (see Figure 4-20). In this situation, the rotation of the mandible carries the dentition forward, thrusting the incisors against the lip. This creates light but lasting pressure by the lip, which tends to reposition the protruding incisors somewhat lingually, reducing arch length and causing crowding.

The current concept is that late incisor crowding almost always develops as the mandibular incisors, and perhaps the entire mandibular dentition, move distally relative to the body of the mandible late in mandibular growth. This also sheds some light on the possible role of the third molars in determining whether crowding will occur, and how severe it will be. If space were available at the distal end of the mandibular arch, it might be possible for all the mandibular teeth to shift slightly distally, allowing the lower incisors to upright without becoming crowded. On the other hand, impacted third molars at the distal end of the lower arch would prevent the posterior teeth from shifting distally, and if differential mandibular growth occurred, their presence might guarantee that crowding would develop. In this case, the lower third molars could be the "last straw" in a chain of events that led to late incisor crowding. As noted previously, however, late incisor crowding does occur in individuals with no third molars at all, and so the presence of these teeth is not the critical variable. The extent of late mandibular growth is. The more your mandible grows after other growth has essentially stopped, the greater the chance your lower incisors will become crowded.

Facial Growth in Adults

Until recently, although some anthropologists in the 1930s had reported small amounts of growth continuing into middle age, it was generally assumed that growth of the facial skeleton ceased in the late teens or early twenties. In the early 1980s, Behrents[21] succeeded in recalling over 100 individuals who had participated in the Bolton growth study in Cleveland in the 1930s and late 1940s, more than 40 years previously. Most had never had orthodontic treatment; a few did. While they were participants in the study, the growth of these individuals had been carefully evaluated and recorded, by both measurements and serial cephalometric films. The magnification in the radiographs was known precisely, and it was possible to obtain new radiographs more than 4 decades later with known magnification, so that precise measurements of facial dimensions could be made.

The results were surprising but unequivocal: facial growth had continued during adult life (Figure 4-28). There was an increase in essentially all of the facial dimensions, but both size and shape of the craniofacial complex altered with time. Vertical changes in adult life were more prominent than anteroposterior changes, whereas width changes were least evident, and so the alterations observed in the adult facial skeleton seem to be a continuation of the pattern seen during maturation. In a point of particular interest, an apparent deceleration of growth in females in the late teens was followed by a resumption of growth during the twenties. It appears that a woman's first pregnancy often produces some growth of her jaws. Although the magnitude of the adult growth changes, assessed on a millimeters per year basis, was quite small, the cumulative effect over decades was surprisingly large (Figure 4-29).

The data also revealed that rotation of both jaws continued into adult life, in concert with the vertical changes and eruption of teeth. Because implants were not used in these patients, it was not possible to precisely differentiate internal from external rotation, but it seems likely that both internal rotation and surface changes did continue. In general, males showed a net rotation of the jaws in a forward direction, slightly decreasing the mandibular plane angle, whereas females had a tendency toward backward rotation, with an increase in the mandibular plane angle. In both groups, compensatory changes were noted in the dentition, so that occlusal relationships largely were maintained.

Both a history of orthodontic treatment and loss of multiple teeth had an impact on facial morphology in these adults and on the pattern of change. In the smaller group of patients who had orthodontic treatment many years previously, Behrents noted that the pattern of growth associated with the original malocclusion continued to express itself even in adult life. This finding is consistent with previous observations of growth in the late teens but also indicates how a gradual worsening of occlusal relationships could occur in some patients long after the completion of orthodontic treatment.

As expected, changes in the facial soft tissue profile were greater than changes in the facial skeleton. The soft tissue changes involved an elongation of the nose (which often became significantly longer during adult life), flattening of the lips, and an augmentation of the chin. In the light of Behrents' findings, it seems clear that the view of facial growth as a process that ends in the late teens or early twenties must be revised. It is correct, however, to view the

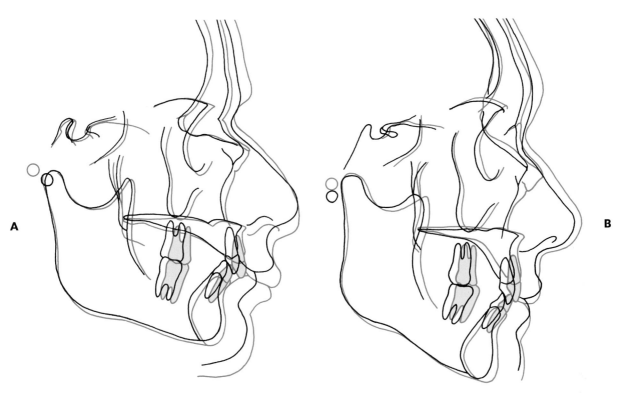

FIGURE 4-28   Growth changes in adults. **A,** Changes in a male from age 37 (*black*) to age 77 (*red*). Note that both the maxilla and mandible grew forward, and the nose grew considerably. **B,** Growth changes in a woman between age 34 (*black*) and 83 (*red*). Note that both jaws grew forward and somewhat downward, and that the nasal structures enlarged. (From Behrents RG: *A treatise on the continuum of growth in the aging craniofacial skeleton*, Ann Arbor, Mich., 1984, University of Michigan Center for Human Growth and Development.)

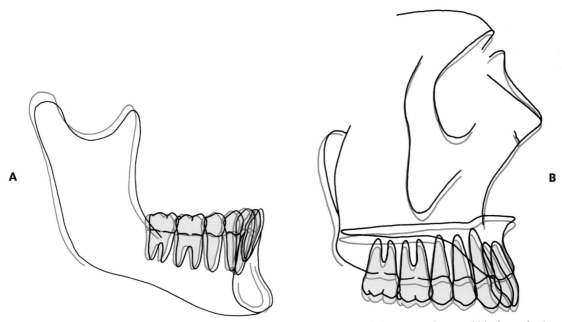

FIGURE 4-29   Growth changes in adults. **A,** Mean dimensional changes in the mandible for males in adult life. It is apparent that the pattern of juvenile and adolescent growth continues at a slower but ultimately significant rate. **B,** The mean positional changes in the maxilla during adult life, for both sexes combined. Note that the maxilla moves forward and slightly downward, continuing the previous pattern of growth. (From Behrents RG: *A treatise on the continuum of growth in the aging craniofacial skeleton*, Ann Arbor, Mich., 1984, University of Michigan Center for Human Growth and Development.)

growth process as one that declines to a basal level after the attainment of sexual maturity, that continues to show a cephalocaudal gradient (i.e., more mandibular than maxillary changes in adult life), and that affects the three planes of space differently. Growth in width is not only the first to drop to adult levels, usually reaching essential completion by the onset of puberty, but the basal or adult level observed thereafter is quite low.[22] Anteroposterior growth continues at a noticeable rate for a longer period, declining to basal levels only after puberty, with small but noticeable changes continuing throughout adult life. Vertical growth, which had previously been observed to continue well after puberty in both males and females, continues at a moderate level throughout adult life. The existing data are not adequate to answer the question of whether growth rates are greater in early than late adult life, but even if they are, skeletal growth comes much closer to being a process that continues throughout life than most observers had previously suspected.

REFERENCES

1. Veldhuis JD: Neuroendocrine mechanisms mediating awakening of the human gonadotrophic axis in puberty, Pediatric Nephrology 10:304-317, 1997.
2. Marshall WA, Tanner JM: Puberty. In Falkner F, Tanner JM (editors): Human growth, vol 2, ed 2, New York, 1986, Plenum Publishing.
3. Anderson DL, Thompson GW, Popovich F: Interrelationship of dental maturity, skeletal maturity, height and weight from age 4 to 14 years, Growth 39:453-462, 1975.
4. McClintock MK, Herdt G: Rethinking puberty: the development of sexual attraction, Current Directions Psychological Science 5:178-183, 1996.
5. Enlow DH, Hans MG: Essentials of facial growth, Philadelphia, 1996, Saunders.
6. Agronin KJ, Kokich VG: Displacement of the glenoid fossa: a cephalometric evaluation of growth during treatment, Am J Orthod Dentofacial Orthop 91:42-48, 1987.
7. Bishara SE, Jakobsen JR, Treder J, Nowak A: Arch width changes from 6 weeks to 45 years of age, Am J Orthod Dentofac Orthop 111:401-409, 1997.
8. Solow B, Iseri H: Maxillary growth revisited: an update based on recent implant studies. In Davidovitch Z, Norton LA (editors): Biological mechanisms of tooth movement and craniofacial adaptation, Boston, 1996, Harvard Society for Advancement of Orthodontics.
9. Bjork A: The use of metallic implants in the study of facial growth in children: method and application, Am J Phys Anthropol 29:243-254, 1968.
10. Solow B, Houston WJ: Mandibular rotations: concept and terminology, Eur J Orthod 10:177-179, 1988.
11. Bjork A, Skieller V: Normal and abnormal growth of the mandible: a synthesis of longitudinal cephalometric implant studies over a period of 25 years, Eur J Orthod 5:1-46, 1983.
12. Bjork A, Skieller V: Postnatal growth and development of the maxillary complex. In McNamara JA (editor): Factors affecting growth of the midface, Ann Arbor, Mich., 1976, University of Michigan Center for Human Growth and Development.
13. Houston WJ: Mandibular growth rotations—their mechanisms and importance, Eur J Orthod 10:369-373, 1988.
14. Bjork A, Skieller V: Contrasting mandibular growth and facial development in long face syndrome, juvenile rheumatoid arthritis and mandibulofacial dysostosis, J Craniofac Genet Dev Biol (suppl) 1:127-138, 1985.
15. Nanda SK: Growth patterns in subjects with long and short faces, Am J Orthod Dentofacial Orthop 98:247-258, 1990.
16. Begg PR: Stone age man's dentition, Am J Orthod 40:298-312, 373-383, 462-475, 517-531, 1954.
17. Corruccini RS: Australian aboriginal tooth succession, interproximal attrition and Begg's theory, Am J Orthod Dentofacial Orthop 97:349-357, 1990.
18. Southard TE, Southard KA, Weeda LW: Mesial force from unerupted third molars, Am J Orthod Dentofacial Orthop 99:220-225, 1991.
19. Richardson M, Mills K: Late lower arch crowding: the effect of second molar extraction, Am J Orthod Dentofacial Orthop 98:242-246, 1990.
20. Richardson ME: The etiology of late lower arch crowding alternative to mesially directed forces: a review, Am J Orthod Dentofac Orthop 105:592-597, 1994.
21. Behrents RG: A treatise on the continuum of growth in the aging craniofacial skeleton, Ann Arbor, Mich., 1985, University of Michigan Center for Human Growth and Development.
22. Harris EF: A longitudinal study of arch size and form in untreated adults, Am J Orthod Dentofacial Orthop 111:419-427, 1997.

CHAPTER
5

The Etiology of Orthodontic Problems

Malocclusion is a developmental condition. In most instances, malocclusion and dentofacial deformity are caused, not by some pathologic process, but by moderate distortions of normal development. Occasionally a single specific cause is apparent, as for example, mandibular deficiency secondary to a childhood fracture of the jaw or the characteristic malocclusion that accompanies some genetic syndromes. More often these problems result from a complex interaction among multiple factors that influence growth and development, and it is impossible to describe a specific etiologic factor (Figure 5-1).

Although it is difficult to know the precise cause of most malocclusions, we do know in general what the possibilities are, and these must be considered when treatment is considered. In this chapter, we examine etiologic factors for malocclusion under three major headings: specific causes, hereditary influences, and environmental influences. The chapter concludes with a perspective on the interaction of hereditary and environmental influences in the development of the major types of malocclusion.

SPECIFIC CAUSES OF MALOCCLUSION

Disturbances in Embryologic Development

Defects in embryologic development usually result in death of the embryo. As many as 20% of early pregnancies terminate because of lethal embryologic defects, often so early that the mother is not even aware of conception. Only a relatively small number of recognizable conditions that produce orthodontic problems are compatible with long-term survival. The more common of these conditions and their embryologic origins are discussed briefly and illustrated in Chapter 3. Further details are provided in current texts on facial syndromes[1] and dentofacial deformity.[2,3]

A variety of causes exist for embryologic defects, ranging from genetic disturbances to specific environmental insults. Chemical and other agents capable of producing embryologic defects if given at the critical time are called *teratogens.* Most drugs do not interfere with normal development or, at high doses, kill the embryo without producing defects, and therefore are not teratogenic. Teratogens typically cause specific defects if present at low levels but if given in higher doses, do have lethal effects. Teratogens known to produce orthodontic problems are listed in Table 5-1.

Problems that can be traced to embryologic defects, though devastating to the affected individual, fortunately are relatively rare. The best estimate is that fewer than 1% of children who need orthodontics had a disturbance in embryologic development as a major contributing cause.

113

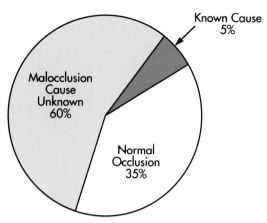

FIGURE 5-1   From a broad perspective, only about one third of the U.S. population has normal occlusion, while two thirds have some degree of malocclusion. In the malocclusion group, a small minority have problems attributable in a specific known cause; the remainder are the result of a complex and poorly-understood combination of hereditary and environmental influences.

TABLE 5-1   *Teratogens Affecting Dentofacial Development*

Teratogens	Effect
Aminopterin	Anencephaly
Aspirin	Cleft lip and palate
Cigarette smoke (hypoxia)	Cleft lip and palate
Cytomegalovirus	Microcephaly, hydrocephaly, microphthalmia
Dilantin	Cleft lip and palate
Ethyl alcohol	Central mid-face deficiency
6-Mercaptopurine	Cleft palate
13-cis Retinoic acid (Accutane)	Retinoic acid syndrome: malformations virtually same as hemifacial microsomia, Treacher Collins' syndrome
Rubella virus	Microphthalmia, cataracts, deafness
Thalidomide	Malformations similar to hemifacial microsomia, Treacher Collins syndrome
Toxoplasma	Microcephaly, hydrocephaly, microphthalmia
X-radiation	Microcephaly
Valium	Cleft lip and palate
Vitamin D excess	Premature suture closure

Skeletal Growth Disturbances

Fetal Molding and Birth Injuries.   Injuries apparent at birth fall into two major categories: (1) intrauterine molding and (2) trauma to the mandible during the birth process, particularly from the use of forceps in delivery.

Intrauterine Molding.   Pressure against the developing face prenatally can lead to distortion of rapidly growing areas. Strictly speaking, this is not a birth injury, but because the effects are noted at birth, it is considered in that category. On rare occasions an arm is pressed across the face in utero, resulting in severe maxillary deficiency at birth (Figure 5-2). Occasionally a fetus' head is flexed tightly against the chest in utero, preventing the mandible from growing forward normally. This is related to a decreased volume of amniotic fluid, which can occur for any of several reasons. The result is an extremely small mandible at birth, usually accompanied by a cleft palate because the restriction on displacement of the mandible forces the tongue upward and prevents normal closure of the palatal shelves.

This extreme mandibular deficiency at birth is the Pierre Robin syndrome. The reduced volume of the oral cavity can lead to respiratory difficulty at birth, and it may be necessary to suture the tongue forward temporarily or even perform a tracheostomy so the infant can breathe.[4]

Because the pressure against the face that caused the growth problem would not be present after birth, one would predict normal growth thereafter and perhaps eventually a complete recovery. Some children with Pierre Robin syndrome at birth do have favorable mandibular growth thereafter. For that reason, early aggressive treatment to lengthen the mandible should be avoided. Others never make up the deficit (Figure 5-3) and surgical intervention is needed. It has been estimated that about one-third of the Pierre Robin patients have a defect in cartilage formation and can be said to have Stickler syndrome. Not surprisingly, this group have limited growth potential. Catch-up growth is most likely when the original problem was mechanical growth restriction that no longer existed after birth.[5]

Birth Trauma to the Mandible.   Many deformity patterns now known to result from other causes once were blamed on injuries during birth. Many parents, despite explanations from their doctors, will refer to their child's facial deformity as being caused by a birth injury even if a congenital syndrome pattern is evident. No matter what the parents say later, Treacher Collins syndrome or Crouzon's syndrome (see Chapter 3) obviously did not arise because of birth trauma.

In some difficult births, however, the use of forceps to the head to assist in delivery might damage either or both the temporomandibular joints. At least in theory, heavy pressure in the area of the temporomandibular joints could cause internal hemorrhage, loss of tissue, and a subsequent underdevelopment of the mandible. At one time this was a common explanation for mandibular deficiency. If the cartilage of the mandibular condyle were an important growth center, of course, the risk from damage to a presumably critical area would seem much greater. In light of the contemporary understanding that the condylar cartilage is not critical for proper growth of the mandible, it is not as easy to blame underdevelopment of the mandible on birth injuries.

It is interesting to note that although the use of forceps in deliveries has decreased considerably over the last 50 years, the prevalence of Class II malocclusion as a result of mandibular deficiency has not decreased. In short, injury to

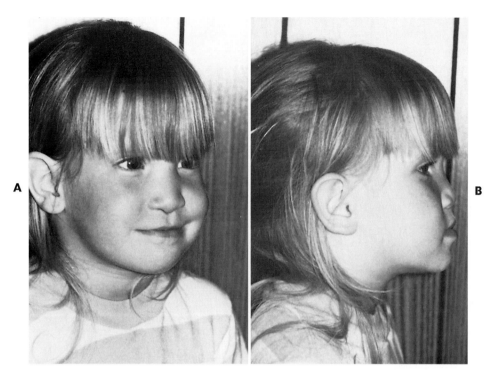

FIGURE 5-2   A and **B,** Midface deficiency in a 3-year-old, still apparent though much improved from the severe deficiency that was present at birth because of intrauterine molding.

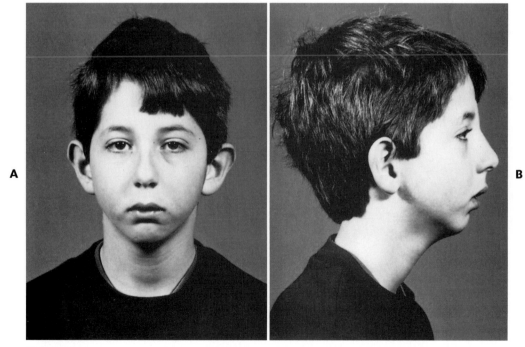

FIGURE 5-3   A and **B,** Severe mandibular deficiency in a 9-year-old boy, who was noted at birth to have a very small mandible and cleft palate and was diagnosed as having Pierre Robin syndrome. Despite considerable postnatal growth of the mandible, mandibular deficiency has persisted. (From Proffit WR, White RP Jr: *Surgical-orthodontic treatment*, St Louis, 1991, Mosby.)

the mandible during a traumatic delivery appears to be a rare and unusual cause of facial deformity. Children with deformities involving the mandible are much more likely to have a congenital syndrome.

Childhood Fractures of the Jaw.   The falls and impacts of childhood can fracture jaws just like other parts of the body. The condylar neck of the mandible is particularly vulnerable, and fractures of this area in childhood are relatively common. Fortunately, the condylar process tends to regenerate well after early fractures. The best human data suggest that about 75% of children with early fractures of the mandibular condylar process have normal mandibular growth, and therefore do not develop malocclusions that they would not have had in the absence of such trauma (see

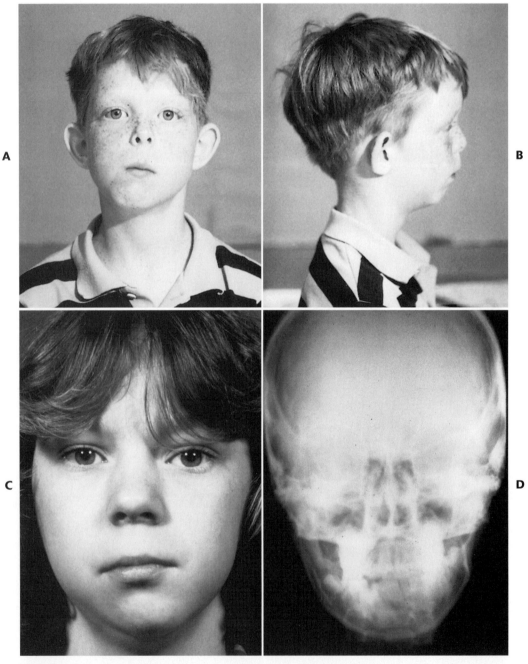

FIGURE 5-4   **A** and **B,** Mandibular asymmetry in an 8-year-old boy, due to deficient growth on the affected side after fracture of the left condylar process, probably at age 2. For this patient, growth was normal until mandibular growth began to be restricted at age 6; then facial asymmetry developed rapidly. **C** and **D,** Mandibular asymmetry in a 10-year-old girl due to rheumatoid arthritis that has affected the temporomandibular (TM) joint on the left side. Note the shortening of the left ramus because of resorption at the condyle. An old fracture is the most likely cause of asymmetric mandibular deficiency in a child, but other destructive processes also can produce this problem.

Chapter 2). Interestingly, the prognosis is better the earlier the condylar fracture occurs, perhaps because the growth potential is greater early in life. From the number of children with later growth problems whose original fracture was not diagnosed, it appears that many early fractures of the condylar process go completely unnoticed. It seems to be relatively common for a child to crash the bicycle, chip a tooth and fracture a condyle, cry a bit, and then continue to develop normally, complete with total regeneration of the condyle.

When a problem does arise following condylar fracture, it usually is asymmetric growth, with the previously injured side lagging behind (Figure 5-4). A survey of patients seen in the Dentofacial Clinic at the University of North Carolina indicates that only about 5% of patients referred for evaluation of severe mandibular deficiency have clinical and/or historical evidence of an early fracture of the jaw.[6] This suggests that childhood jaw fractures, though potentially a cause of severe orthodontic problems, do not make a large contribution to the total pool of patients with malocclusion.

It is important to understand the mechanism by which trauma can produce a distortion in subsequent growth. The maxilla normally grows downward and forward because of a combination of push from behind by the lengthening cranial base (which is largely complete at an early age) and pull from in front by anteriorly positioned tissue elements (probably including but not limited to the cartilaginous nasal septum). The mandible seems to be almost entirely pulled forward by the soft tissue matrix in which it is embedded. After an injury, growth problems arise when there is enough scarring in the area to restrict the normal growth movements, so that the maxilla or, more frequently, the mandible cannot be pulled forward along with the rest of the growing face. If there is more scarring and restriction on one side, subsequent growth will be asymmetric.

This concept is highly relevant to the management of condylar fractures in children. It suggests, and clinical experience confirms, that there would be little if any advantage from surgical open reduction of a condylar fracture in a child. The additional scarring produced by surgery could make things worse. The best therapy therefore is conservative management at the time of injury and early mobilization of the jaw to minimize any restriction on movement.

An old condylar fracture is the most likely cause of asymmetric mandibular deficiency in a child, but other destructive processes that involve the temporomandibular joint such as rheumatoid arthritis (See Figure 5-4), or a congenital absence of tissue as in hemifacial microsomia (see Chapter 3), also can produce this problem.

Muscle Dysfunction

The facial muscles can affect jaw growth in two ways. First, the formation of bone at the point of muscle attachments depends on the activity of the muscle; second, the musculature is an important part of the total soft tissue matrix whose growth normally carries the jaws downward and forward. Loss of part of the musculature can occur from unknown causes in utero or as a result of a birth injury, but is most likely to result from damage to the motor nerve (the muscle atrophies when its motor nerve supply is lost). The result would be underdevelopment of that part of the face (Figure 5-5).

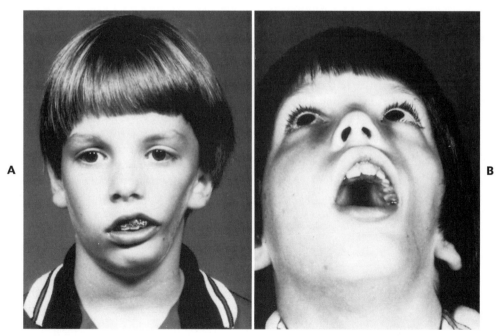

FIGURE 5-5 **A** and **B,** Facial asymmetry in an 11-year-old boy whose masseter muscle was largely missing on the left side. The muscle is an important part of the total soft tissue matrix; in its absence growth of the mandible in the affected area also is deficient.

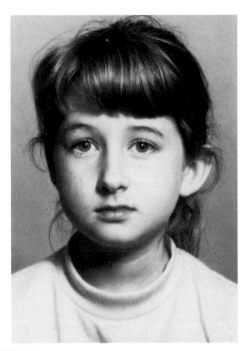

FIGURE 5-6 Facial asymmetry in a 6-year-old girl with torticollis. Excessive muscle contraction can restrict growth in a way analogous to scarring after an injury. Despite surgical release of the contracted neck muscles at age 1, moderate facial asymmetry developed in this case, and a second surgical release of the muscles was performed at age 7. Note that the asymmetry affects the entire side of the face, not just the mandible.

Excessive muscle contraction can restrict growth in much the same way as scarring after an injury. This effect is seen most clearly in torticollis, a twisting of the head caused by excessive tonic contraction of the neck muscles on one side (primarily the sternocleidomastoid) (Figure 5-6). The result is a facial asymmetry because of growth restriction on the affected side, which can be quite severe unless the contracted neck muscles are surgically detached at an early age.[7] Conversely, the decrease in tonic muscle activity that occurs in muscular dystrophy, some forms of cerebral palsy, and various muscle weakness syndromes allow the mandible to drop downward away from the rest of the facial skeleton. The result is increased anterior face height, distortion of facial proportions and mandibular form, excessive eruption of the posterior teeth, narrowing of the maxillary arch and anterior open bite (Figure 5-7).[8]

Acromegaly and Hemimandibular Hypertrophy

In acromegaly, which is caused by an anterior pituitary tumor that secretes excessive amounts of growth hormone, excessive growth of the mandible may occur, creating a skeletal Class III malocclusion in adult life (Figure 5-8). Often (but not always—sometimes the mandible is unaffected) mandibular growth accelerates again to the levels seen in the adolescent growth spurt, years after adolescent

growth was completed.[9] The condylar cartilage proliferates, but it is difficult to be sure whether this is the cause of the mandibular growth or merely accompanies it. Although the excessive growth stops when the tumor is removed or irradiated, the skeletal deformity persists and orthognathic surgery to reposition the mandible is likely to be necessary (see Chapter 22).

Occasionally, unilateral excessive growth of the mandible occurs in individuals who seem metabolically normal. Why this occurs is entirely unknown. It is most likely in girls between the ages of 15 and 20, but may occur as early as age 10 or as late as the early 30s in either sex. The condition formerly was called *condylar hyperplasia*, and proliferation of the condylar cartilage is a prominent aspect; however, because the body of the mandible also is affected (Figure 5-9), *hemimandibular hypertrophy* now is considered a more accurate descriptive term.[10] The excessive growth may stop spontaneously, but in severe cases removal of the affected condyle and reconstruction of the area is necessary.

Disturbances of Dental Development

Disturbances of dental development may accompany major congenital defects but are most significant as contributors to isolated Class I malocclusion. Significant disturbances include:

Congenitally Missing Teeth. Congenital absence of teeth results from disturbances during the initial stages of formation of a tooth—initiation and proliferation. *Anodontia*, the total absence of teeth, is the extreme form. The term *oligodontia* refers to congenital absence of many but not all teeth, whereas the rarely used term *hypodontia* implies the absence of only a few teeth. Since the primary teeth give rise to the permanent tooth buds, there will be no permanent tooth if its primary predecessor was missing. It is possible, however, for the primary teeth to be present and for some or all the permanent teeth to be absent.

Anodontia or oligodontia, the absence of all or most of the permanent teeth, is usually associated with an unusual but mild systemic abnormality, *ectodermal dysplasia*. Individuals with ectodermal dysplasia have thin, sparse hair and an absence of sweat glands in addition to their characteristically missing teeth (Figure 5-10). Occasionally, oligodontia occurs in a patient with no apparent systemic problem or congenital syndrome. In these children, it appears as if there is a random pattern to the missing teeth.

Anodontia and oligodontia are rare, but hypodontia is a relatively common finding. As a general rule, if only one or a few teeth are missing, the absent tooth will be the most distal tooth of any given type. If a molar tooth is congenitally missing, it is almost always the third molar; if an incisor is missing, it is nearly always the lateral; if a premolar is missing, it almost always is the second rather than the first. Rarely is a canine the only missing tooth.

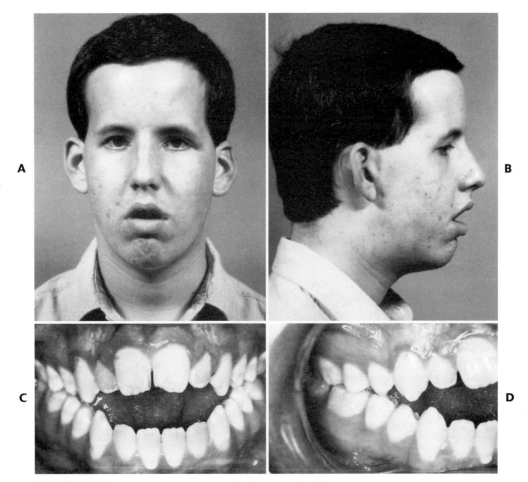

FIGURE 5-7 **A** and **B,** Lengthening of the lower face typically occurs in patients with muscle weakness syndromes, as in this 15-year-old boy with muscular dystrophy. **C** and **D,** Anterior open bite, as in this patient, usually (but not always) accompanies excessive face height.

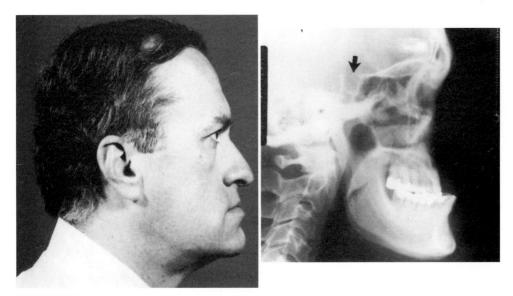

FIGURE 5-8 Profile view and cephalometric radiograph of a 45-year-old man with acromegaly, which was diagnosed 3 years previously after he went to his dentist because his lower jaw was coming forward. After irradiation of the anterior pituitary area, elevated growth hormone levels dropped and mandibular growth ceased. Note the enlargement of sella turcica and loss of definition of its bony outline in the cephalometric radiograph *(arrow)*, reflecting the secretory tumor in that location. (From Proffit WR, White RP Jr: *Surgical-orthodontic treatment*, St Louis, 1991, Mosby.)

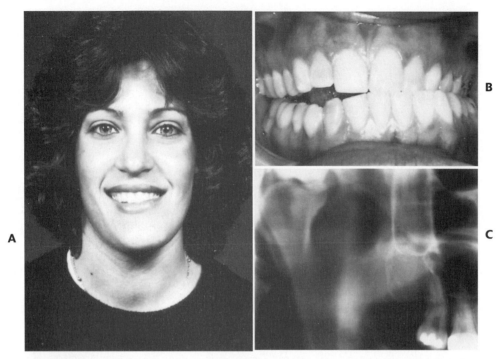

FIGURE 5-9   A, Facial asymmetry in this 21-year-old woman developed gradually in her late teens, after orthodontic treatment of Class II malocclusion between ages 12 and 14, due to excessive growth of the mandible on the right side. **B,** The dental occlusion shows open bite on the affected right side, reflecting the vertical component of the excessive growth. **C,** Note the grossly enlarged mandibular condyle on the right side. Why this type of excessive but histologically normal growth occurs, and why it is seen predominantly in females, is unknown.

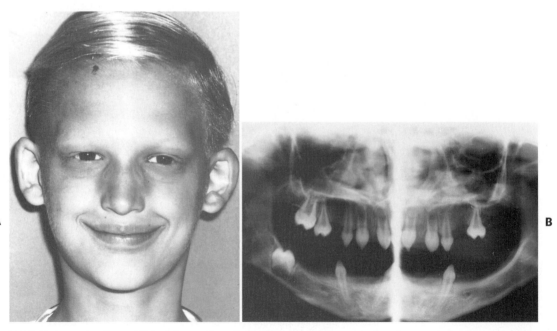

FIGURE 5-10   A, a child with ectodermal dysplasia, in addition to the characteristic thin and light-colored hair, is likely to have an overclosed appearance because of lack of development of the alveolar processes; **B,** panoramic radiograph of the same boy, showing the multiple missing teeth. Oligodontia of this extent is almost pathognomonic of ectodermal dysplasia.

Malformed and Supernumerary Teeth. Abnormalities in tooth size and shape result from disturbances during the morphodifferentiation stage of development, perhaps with some carryover from the histodifferentiation stage. The most common abnormality is a variation in size, particularly of maxillary lateral incisors (Figure 5-11) and second premolars. About 5% of the total population have a significant "tooth size discrepancy" because of disproportionate sizes of the upper and lower teeth. Unless the teeth are matched for size, normal occlusion is impossible. As might be expected, the most variable teeth, the maxillary lateral incisors, are the major culprits. The diagnosis of tooth size discrepancy, discussed in Chapter 6, is based on comparison of the widths of teeth to published tables of expected tooth sizes.

Occasionally, tooth buds may fuse or geminate (partially split) during their development. Fusion results in teeth with separate pulp chambers joined at the dentin, whereas gemination results in teeth with a common pulp chamber (Figure 5-12). The differentiation between gemination and fusion can be difficult and is usually confirmed by counting the number of teeth in an area. If the other central and both lateral incisors are present, a bifurcated central incisor is the result of either gemination or, less probably, fusion with a supernumerary incisor. On the other hand, if the lateral incisor on the affected side is missing, the problem probably is fusion of the central and lateral incisor buds. Normal occlusion, of course, is all but impossible in the presence of geminated, fused, or otherwise malformed teeth.

Supernumerary or extra teeth also result from disturbances during the initiation and proliferation stages of dental development. The most common supernumerary tooth appears in the maxillary midline and is called a *mesiodens*. Supernumerary lateral incisors also occur; extra premolars occasionally appear; a few patients have fourth as well as third molars. The presence of an extra tooth obviously has great potential to disrupt normal occlusal development (Figure 5-13), and early intervention to remove it is usually required to obtain reasonable alignment and occlusal relationships. Multiple supernumerary teeth are most often seen in the congenital syndrome of cleidocranial dysplasia

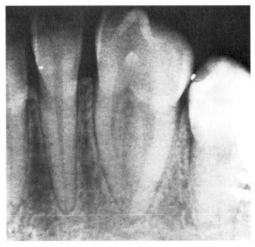

FIGURE 5-12 Fusion of a mandibular lateral incisor and canine.

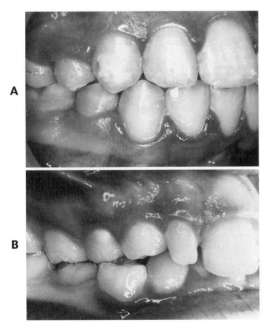

FIGURE 5-11 Disproportionately large (**A**) or small (**B**) maxillary lateral incisors are relatively common. This creates a tooth-size discrepancy that makes normal alignment and occlusion almost impossible. It is easier to build up small laterals than reduce the size of large ones—the lateral incisors for the patient in (**A**) already have been reduced as much as possible without going through the enamel.

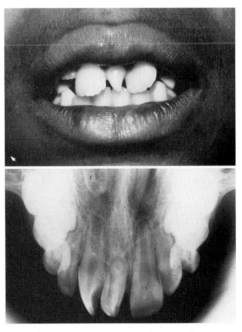

FIGURE 5-13 The maxillary midline is the most common location for a supernumerary tooth, which can be of almost any shape. The supernumerary may block the eruption of one or both the central incisors, or may separate them widely and also displace the lateral incisors, as in this girl.

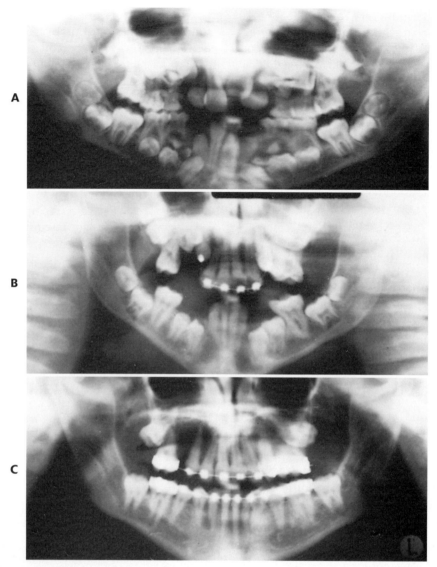

FIGURE 5-14   Sequence of panoramic radiographs of a patient with cleidocranial dysplasia (same patient as Figure 3-24, which shows the pretreatment condition). **A,** Age 10, after surgical removal of primary and supernumerary incisors and uncovering of the permanent incisors. There has been some spontaneous eruption of the permanent teeth. **B,** Age 14, after orthodontic treatment to bring the incisors into the mouth and surgical removal of primary canines and molars, as well as supernumerary teeth in that area. **C,** Age 16, toward the completion of orthodontic treatment to bring the unerupted teeth into occlusion. The maxillary right second premolar became ankylosed, but other teeth responded satisfactorily to treatment.

(see Figure 3-24), which is characterized by missing clavicles (collar bones), many supernumerary and unerupted teeth, and failure of the succedaneous teeth to erupt (see further discussion following).

Interference with Eruption.   For a permanent tooth to erupt, the overlying bone as well as the primary tooth roots must resorb, and the tooth must make its way through the gingiva. Supernumerary teeth, sclerotic bone, and heavy fibrous gingiva can obstruct eruption.

All of these interferences are present in cleidocranial dysplasia. The multiple supernumerary teeth contribute an element of mechanical interference. More seriously, children with this condition have a defect in bone resorption, and the gingiva is quite heavy and fibrous.[11] If the eruption path can be cleared, the permanent teeth will

erupt (Figure 5-14). To accomplish this, it is necessary not only to extract any supernumerary teeth that may be in the way but also to remove the bone overlying the permanent teeth and reflect the gingiva so that the teeth can break through into the mouth.

In patients with less severe interferences with eruption, delayed eruption of some permanent teeth contributes to malocclusion only when other teeth drift to improper positions in the arch. In 5% to 10% of U.S. children, at least one primary molar becomes ankylosed (fused to the bone) before it finally resorbs and exfoliates. Although this delays eruption of its permanent successor, there is usually no lasting effect.[12]

Ectopic Eruption.   Occasionally, malposition of a permanent tooth bud can lead to eruption in the wrong place. This condition is called *ectopic eruption* and is most likely to occur in the eruption of maxillary first molars.[13] If the eruption path of the maxillary first molar carries it too far mesially at an early stage, the permanent molar is unable to erupt, and the root of the second primary molar may be damaged (Figure 5-15). The mesial position of the permanent molar means that the arch will be crowded unless the child receives treatment.

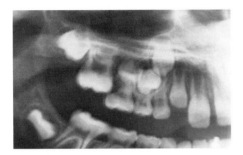

FIGURE 5-15 Ectopic eruption of the permanent maxillary first molar apparently results from mesial position or inclination of the tooth bud. This causes the eruptive path of the first molar to contact the root of the primary second molar. Delay in eruption of the first molar and root resorption of the second primary molar usually result, as shown here in an 8-year-old boy. Loss of space can cause crowding in the arch. Crowding of the permanent teeth is inevitable without treatment.

Ectopic eruption of other teeth is rare but can result in transposition of teeth or bizarre eruption positions. Mandibular second premolars sometimes erupt distally and can end up in the ramus (Figure 5-16).[13] A poor eruption direction of other teeth, especially maxillary canines, usually is due to the eruption path being altered by a lack of space.

Early Loss of Primary Teeth. When a unit within the dental arch is lost, the arch tends to contract and the space to close. At one time, this space closure was attributed entirely to mesial drift of posterior teeth, which in turn was confidently ascribed to forces from occlusion. Although a mesially-directed force can accompany occlusion,[14] it probably is not a major factor in closure of spaces within the dental arches.

The contemporary view is that mesial drift is a phenomenon of the permanent molars only. The major reason these teeth move mesially when a space opens up is their mesial inclination, so that they erupt mesially as well as occlusally. Experimental data suggest that, rather than causing mesial drift, forces from occlusion actually retard it.[15] In other words, a permanent molar is likely to drift mesially more rapidly in the absence of occlusal contacts than if they are present.

Mesial drift of the permanent first molar after a primary second molar is lost prematurely (Figure 5-17) can

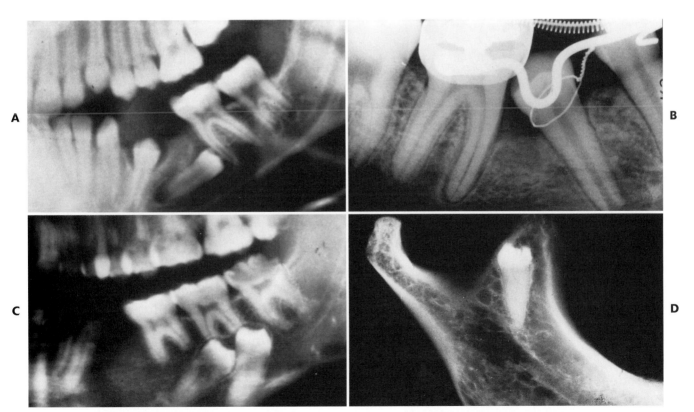

FIGURE 5-16 Mandibular second premolars tend to erupt tipped distally, and are prone to horizontal impaction, especially if the first molar is lost prematurely (**A**), but orthodontic correction is possible (**B**). Rarely, the premolars migrate distally beneath the permanent molars (**C**), and extreme migration into the mandibular ramus, even to the point that a premolar is found at the top of the coronoid process, is possible (**D**), as in this specimen from a sixteenth century burial site. (**D**, Courtesy Dr. K. Mitchell.)

significantly contribute to the development of crowding in the posterior part of the dental arch. This has been a significant cause of crowding and malalignment of premolars in the past. For this reason, maintenance of the space after a primary second molar has been lost is indicated (see Chapter 13).

When a primary first molar or canine is lost prematurely, there is also a tendency for the space to close. This occurs primarily by distal drift of incisors, not by mesial drift of posterior teeth (Figure 5-18). The impetus for distal drift appears to have two sources: force from active contraction of transseptal fibers in the gingiva, and pressures from the lips and cheeks.[16] The pull from transseptal fibers probably is the more consistent contributor to this space closure tendency, whereas lip pressure adds a variable component (see the following section on equilibrium). If a primary canine or first molar is lost prematurely on only one side, the permanent teeth drift distally only on that side, leading to an asymmetry in the occlusion as well as a tendency toward crowding.

From this description, it is apparent that early loss of primary teeth can cause crowding and malalignment within the dental arches. Is this a major cause of Class I crowding problems? The impact of fluoridation and other caries-preventive treatment on the prevalence of malocclusion indicates that it is not. Although fluoridation greatly reduced caries and early loss of primary teeth in typical U.S. communities, there was little or no impact on the prevalence of malocclusion. Even without fluoridation, in other words, most crowding problems are not caused by early loss of primary teeth.

Traumatic Displacement of Teeth.   Almost all children fall and hit their teeth during their formative years. Occasionally, the impact is intense enough to knock out or severely displace a primary or permanent tooth. Dental trauma can lead to the development of malocclusion in three ways: (1) damage to permanent tooth buds from an injury to primary teeth, (2) drift of permanent teeth after premature loss of primary teeth, and (3) direct injury to permanent teeth.

Trauma to a primary tooth can displace the permanent tooth bud underlying it. There are two possible results. First, if the trauma occurs while the crown of the permanent tooth is forming, enamel formation will be disturbed and there will be a defect in the crown of the permanent tooth.

Second, if the trauma occurs after the crown is complete, the crown may be displaced relative to the root. Root formation may stop, leaving a permanently shortened root. More frequently, root formation continues, but the remaining portion of the root then forms at an angle to the traumatically displaced crown (Figure 5-19). This distortion of root form is called *dilaceration*, defined as a distorted root form. Dilaceration may result from mechanical interference with eruption (as from an ankylosed primary tooth that does not resorb), but its usual cause, particularly in permanent incisor teeth, is trauma to primary teeth that also displaced the permanent buds.

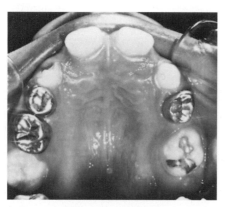

FIGURE 5-17   In this 8-year-old child, the space once occupied by the primary maxillary left second molar (on the right side in this mirror-image photograph) has almost totally closed as the permanent first molar drifted mesially.

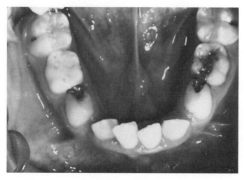

FIGURE 5-18   Premature loss of primary canines leads to closure of space, not by mesial drift of the primary posterior teeth but by distal drift of the permanent incisors.

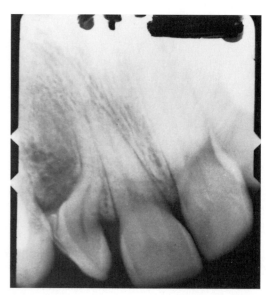

FIGURE 5-19   Distortion of the root (termed dilaceration) of this lateral incisor resulted from trauma at an earlier age that displaced the crown relative to the forming root.

If distortion of root position is severe enough, it is almost impossible for the crown to assume its proper position—that might require the root to extend out through the alveolar bone. For this reason, it may be necessary to extract a severely dilacerated tooth. Traumatically displaced tooth buds in children should be repositioned as early as possible, so that when root formation does resume, distortion of the root position will be minimized. This topic is discussed in more detail in Chapter 13.

Permanent teeth are often displaced by trauma. If the tooth is knocked labially or lingually, the root of the tooth is sometimes damaged, but there always is a fracture of the alveolar process. Immediately after the accident, an intact tooth usually can be moved back to its original position rapidly and easily, so early treatment is indicated (see Chapter 14). After healing (which takes 2 to 3 weeks), it is difficult to reposition the tooth, and ankylosis may develop that makes it impossible.

GENETIC INFLUENCES

A strong influence of inheritance on facial features is obvious at a glance—it is easy to recognize familial tendencies in the tilt of the nose, the shape of the jaw, and the look of the smile. It is apparent that certain types of malocclusion run in families. The Hapsburg jaw, the prognathic mandible of the German royal family, is the best known example, but dentists see repeated instances of similar malocclusions in parents and their offspring. The pertinent question for the etiologic process of malocclusion is not whether there are inherited influences on the jaws and teeth, because obviously there are, but whether malocclusion is often caused by inherited characteristics.

Malocclusion could be produced by inherited characteristics in two major ways. The first would be an inherited disproportion between the size of the teeth and the size of the jaws, which would produce crowding or spacing. The second would be an inherited disproportion between size or shape of the upper and lower jaws, which would cause improper occlusal relationships. The more independently these characteristics are determined, the more likely that disproportions could be inherited. Could a child inherit large teeth but a small jaw, for instance, or a large upper jaw and a small lower one? That would be quite possible if jaw and tooth sizes were inherited independently, but if dentofacial characteristics tended to be linked, an inherited mismatch of this type would be unlikely.

Primitive human populations in which malocclusion is less frequent than in modern groups are characterized by genetic isolation and uniformity. If everyone in a group carried the same genetic information for tooth size and jaw size, there would be no possibility of a child inheriting discordant characteristics. In the absence of processed food, one would expect strong selection pressure for traits that produced good masticatory function. Genes that introduced disturbances into the masticatory system would tend to be eliminated from the population (unless they conferred some other advantage). The result should be exactly what is seen in primitive populations: individuals in whom tooth size-jaw size discrepancies are infrequent, and groups in which everyone tends to have the same jaw relationship. Different human groups have developed impressive variations in facial proportions and jaw relationships. What happens, then, when there is outbreeding between originally distinct human population groups?

One of the characteristics of civilization is the collection of large groups of people into urban centers, where the opportunities for mating outside one's own small population group are greatly magnified. If inherited disproportions of the functional components of the face and jaws were frequent, one would predict that modern urban populations would have a high prevalence of malocclusion and a great variety of orthodontic problems. The United States, reflecting its role as a "genetic melting pot," should have one of the world's highest rates of malocclusion—which it does. In the 1930s and 1940s, as knowledge of the new science of genetics developed, it was tempting to conclude that the great increase in outbreeding that occurred as human populations grew and became more mobile was the major explanation for the increase in malocclusion in recent centuries.

This view of malocclusion as primarily a genetic problem was greatly strengthened by breeding experiments with animals carried out in the 1930s. By far the most influential individual in this regard was Professor Stockard, who methodically crossbred dogs and recorded the interesting effects on body structure.[17] Present-day dogs, of course, come in a tremendous variety of breeds and sizes. What would happen if one crossed a Boston terrier with a collie? Might the offspring have the collie's long, pointed lower jaw and the terrier's diminutive upper jaw? Could unusual crowding or spacing result because the teeth of one breed were combined in the offspring with the jaw of the other? Stockard's experiments indicated that dramatic malocclusions did occur in his crossbred dogs, more from jaw discrepancies than from tooth size-jaw size imbalances (Figure 5-20). These experiments seemed to confirm that independent inheritance of facial characteristics could be a major cause of malocclusion and that the rapid increase in malocclusion accompanying urbanization was probably the result of increased outbreeding.

These dog experiments turned out to be misleading, however, because many breeds of small dogs carry the gene for achondroplasia. Animals or humans affected by this condition have deficient growth of cartilage. The result is extremely short extremities and an underdeveloped midface. The dachshund is the classic achondroplastic dog, but most terriers and bulldogs also carry this gene. Achondroplasia is an autosomal dominant trait. Like many dominant genes, the gene for achondroplasia sometimes has only partial penetrance, meaning simply that the trait will

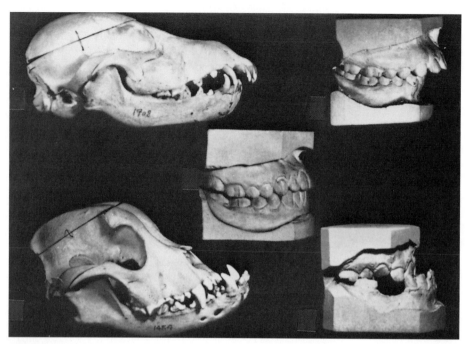

FIGURE 5-20   In breeding experiments with dogs in the 1930s, Professor Stockard demonstrated that severe malocclusions could be developed by crossing morphologically different breeds. His analogy to human malocclusion was a powerful influence in the rejection of the prevailing belief of the 1920s that improper jaw function caused malocclusion. (From Stockard CR, Johnson AL: *Genetic and endocrinic basis for differences in form and behavior,* Philadelphia, 1941, The Wistar Institute of Anatomy and Biology.)

be expressed more dramatically in some individuals than in others. Most of the unusual malocclusions produced in Stockard's breeding experiments can be explained not on the basis of inherited jaw size but by the extent to which achondroplasia was expressed in that animal.

Achondroplasia is rare in humans, but it does occur, and it produces the expected changes (Figure 5-21). In addition to short limbs, the cranial base does not lengthen normally because of the deficient growth at the synchondroses, the maxilla is not translated forward to the normal extent, and a relative midface deficiency occurs. In a number of relatively rare genetic syndromes like achondroplasia, influences on the form of the face, jaws, and teeth can be discerned,[1] but those cause only a small percentage of orthodontic problems.

A careful examination of the results of outbreeding in human populations also casts doubt on the hypothesis that independently inherited tooth and jaw characteristics are a major cause of malocclusion. The best data are from investigations carried out in Hawaii by Chung et al.[18] Before its discovery by the European explorers of the eighteenth century, Hawaii had a homogeneous Polynesian population. Large scale migration to the islands by European, Chinese and Japanese groups, as well as the arrival of smaller numbers of other racial and ethnic groups, resulted in an exceptionally heterogeneous modern population. Tooth size, jaw size, and jaw proportions were all rather different for the Polynesian, Oriental, and European contributors to the

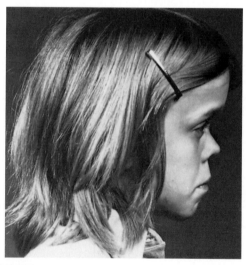

FIGURE 5-21   Characteristic facial appearance in an individual with achondroplasia. Note the deficient midface, particularly at the bridge of the nose. This results from decreased growth of cartilage in the cranial base, with a resulting lack of forward translation of the maxilla.

Hawaiian melting pot. Therefore if tooth and jaw characteristics were inherited independently, a high prevalence of severe malocclusion would be expected in this population. The prevalence and types of malocclusion in the current Hawaiian population, though greater than the prevalence of malocclusion in the original population, do not support this concept. The effects of interracial crosses appear to be more additive than multiplicative. For example, about 10% of the Chinese who migrated to Hawaii had Class III malocclusion, whereas about 10% of the Polynesians had crowded teeth. The offspring of this cross seem to have about a 10% prevalence of each characteristic, but there is no evidence of dramatic facial deformities like those seen in the crossbred dogs. In other words, if malocclusion or a tendency to malocclusion is inherited, the mechanism is not the independent inheritance of discrete morphologic characteristics like tooth and jaw sizes.

The classic way to determine to what extent a characteristic is determined by inheritance is to compare monozygotic (identical) with dizygotic (fraternal) twins. Monozygotic twins occur because of the early division of a fertilized egg, so each individual has the same chromosomal deoxyribonucleic acid (DNA) and the two are genetically identical. Any differences between them should be solely the result of environmental influences. Twins also occur when two eggs are released at the same time and fertilized by different spermatozoa. These dizygotic twins are not more similar than ordinary siblings except that they have shared the same intrauterine and family environment.

By comparing identical twins, fraternal twins, and ordinary siblings, an estimate of the heritability of any characteristic can be determined. That is, the proportion of the variability in that characteristic due to heredity can be estimated. Studies of this type are limited in several ways not only because it is difficult to obtain the twin pairs for study but also because it can be difficult to establish zygosity and confirm that the environments were in fact the same for both members of a twin pair. Lauweryns et al,[19] summarizing a number of research investigations of this type, concluded that about 40% of the dental and facial variations that lead to malocclusion can be attributed to hereditary factors. Corruccini and coworkers[20,21] argue that with appropriate corrections for unsuspected environmental differences within twin pairs, the heritability for some dental characteristics such as overjet is almost zero.

The other classic method of estimating the influence of heredity is to study family members, observing similarities and differences between mother-child, father-child, and sibling pairs. For most measurements of facial skeletal dimensions (i.e., length of the mandible), correlation coefficients for parent-child pairs are about 0.5, which is the theoretical upper limit of the genetic contribution for a first-degree relative. For dental characteristics, the parent-child correlations are lower, ranging from a maximum of nearly 0.5 for overjet to a minimum of 0.15 for overbite.[22,23] When parent-child correlations are used to assist in predicting facial growth, errors are reduced, which in itself strongly indicates the hereditary influence on these dimensions.[24]

From an examination of longitudinal cephalometric radiographs and dental casts of siblings who participated in the Bolton-Brush growth study (carried out between the late 1930s and the early 1970s), Harris and Johnson[25] concluded that the heritability of craniofacial (skeletal) characteristics was relatively high, but that of dental (occlusal) characteristics was low. For skeletal characteristics, the heritability estimates increased with increasing age; for dental characteristics, the heritability estimates decreased, indicating an increasing environmental contribution to the dental variation. To the extent that the facial skeleton determines the characteristics of a malocclusion, therefore, a hereditary component is likely to be present, but purely dental variation seems to be much more environmentally determined.

The influence of inherited tendencies is particularly strong for mandibular prognathism. In one study, one third of a group of children who presented with severe Class III malocclusion had a parent with the same problem, and one sixth had an affected sibling.[26] The long face pattern of facial deformity seems to be the second most likely type of deformity to run in families. In general, siblings are likely to have severe malocclusions, perhaps because their genetically influenced facial types and growth patterns lead to similar responses to environmental factors.[27]

The extent to which other types of malocclusion are related to genetic influences is less clear. Let us now examine the role of the environment in the etiology of malocclusion.

ENVIRONMENTAL INFLUENCES

Environmental influences during the growth and development of the face, jaws, and teeth consist largely of pressures and forces related to physiologic activity. Function must adapt to the environment. For example, how you chew and swallow will be determined in part by what you have to eat; pressures against the jaws and teeth will occur during both activities and could affect how jaws grow and teeth erupt.

A relationship between anatomic form and physiologic function is apparent in all animals. Over evolutionary time, adaptations in the jaws and dental apparatus are prominent in the fossil record. Form-function relationships at this level are controlled genetically and, though important for a general understanding of the human condition, have little to do with any individual's deviation from the current norm.

On the other hand, there is every reason to suspect that form-function relationships during the lifetime of an individual may be significant in the development of malocclusion. Although the changes in body form are minimal, an individual who does heavy physical work as an adolescent has both heavier and stronger muscles and a sturdier skeletal system than one who is sedentary. If function could affect the growth of the jaws, altered function would be a major cause of malocclusion, and it would be logical for chewing exercises and other forms of physical therapy to be an important part of orthodontic treatment. But if function makes little or no difference in the individual's pattern of development, altering his or her jaw function would have little if any impact, etiologically or therapeutically. Because of its importance in contemporary orthodontics, particular emphasis is placed here on evaluating potential functional contributions to the etiology of malocclusion and to possible relapse after treatment.

Equilibrium Theory and Development of the Dental Occlusion

Equilibrium theory, as applied in engineering, states that an object subjected to unequal forces will be accelerated and thereby will move to a different position in space (Figure 5-22). It follows that if any object is subjected to a set of forces but remains in the same position, those forces must be in balance or equilibrium. From this perspective, the dentition is obviously in equilibrium, since the teeth are subjected to a variety of forces but do not move to a new location under usual circumstances. Even when teeth are moving, the movements are so slow that a static equilibrium can be presumed to exist at any instant in time.

The effectiveness of orthodontic treatment is itself a demonstration that forces on the dentition are normally in equilibrium. Teeth normally experience forces from masticatory effort, swallowing, and speaking but do not move. If a tooth is subjected to a continuous force from an orthodontic appliance, it does move. From an engineering point of view, the force applied by the orthodontist has altered the previous equilibrium, resulting in tooth movement. The nature of the forces necessary for tooth movement is discussed in detail in Chapter 9.

Equilibrium considerations also apply to the skeleton, including the facial skeleton. Skeletal alterations occur all the time in response to functional demands and are magnified under unusual experimental situations. As discussed in Chapter 2, the bony processes to which muscles attach are especially influenced by the muscles and the location of the attachments. The form of the mandible, because it is largely dictated by the shape of its functional processes, is particularly prone to alteration. The density of the facial bones, like the skeleton as a whole, increases when heavy work is done and decreases in its absence.

Equilibrium Effects on the Dentition.   Equilibrium effects on the dentition can be understood best by observing the effect of various types of pressures. Although one might think that force multiplied by duration would explain the effects, this is not the case. The duration of a force, because of the biologic response, is more important than its magnitude.

This important point is made clearer by examining the response to the forces applied during chewing. When heavy masticatory forces are applied to the teeth, the fluid-filled periodontal ligament acts as a shock absorber, stabilizing the tooth for an instant while alveolar bone bends and the tooth is displaced for a short distance along with the bone. If the heavy pressure is maintained for more than a few seconds, increasingly severe pain is felt, and so the biting force is released quickly. This type of heavy intermittent pressure has no impact on the long-term position of a tooth (see Chapter 9 for more detail). A number of pathologic responses to heavy intermittent occlusal contacts on a tooth may occur, including increased mobility and pain, but as long as the periodontal apparatus is intact, forces from occlusion are rarely prolonged enough to move the tooth to a new position in which the occlusal trauma is lessened.

A second possible contributor to the equilibrium that governs tooth position is pressure from the lips, cheeks, and tongue. These pressures are much lighter than those from masticatory function, but are also much greater in duration. Experiments suggest that even very light forces are successful in moving teeth, if the force is of long enough duration.

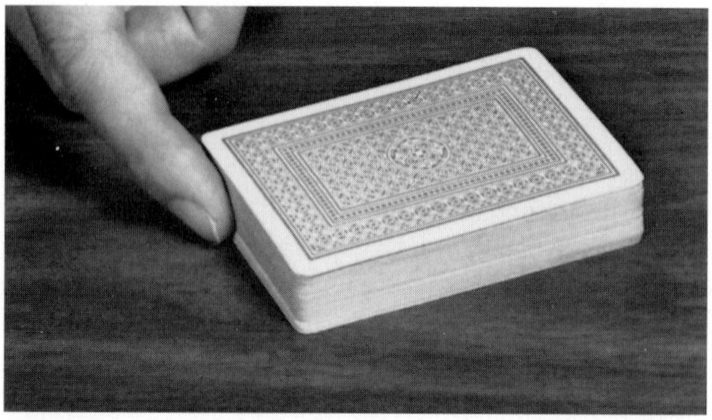

FIGURE 5-22   If you push lightly against a deck of cards on a table top, the cards do not move initially because there is an equilibrium between the force applied by your finger and frictional resistance. When the force of the finger exceeds the friction, however, the cards must move. Tooth movement occurs only when the equilibrium against the dentition is unbalanced.

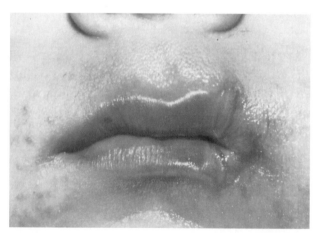

FIGURE 5-23   Scarring of the corner of the mouth in this child is related to a burn at an early age from biting an electrical cord. From equilibrium theory, one would expect a distortion in the form of the dental arch in the region of the contracting scar, and exactly this occurs.

The duration threshold seems to be approximately 6 hours in humans. Since the light pressures from lips, cheeks, and tongue at rest are maintained most of the time, one would expect these pressures to affect tooth position.

It is easy to demonstrate that this is indeed the case. For example, if an injury to the soft tissue of the lip results in scarring and contracture, the incisors in this vicinity will be moved lingually as the lip tightens against them (Figure 5-23). On the other hand, if restraining pressure by the lip or cheek is removed, the teeth move outward in response to unopposed pressure from the tongue (Figure 5-24). Pressure from the tongue, whether from an enlargement of the tongue from a tumor or other source or because its posture has changed, will result in labial displacement of the teeth even though the lips and cheeks are intact, because the equilibrium is altered (Figure 5-25).

These observations make it plain that, in contrast to forces from mastication, light sustained pressures from lips, cheeks, and tongue at rest are important determinants of tooth position. It seems unlikely, however, that the intermittent short-duration pressures created when the tongue and lips contact the teeth during swallowing or speaking would have any significant impact on tooth position.[28] As with masticatory forces, the pressure magnitudes would be great enough to move a tooth, but the duration is inadequate (Table 5-2).

Another possible contributor to the equilibrium could be pressures from external sources, of which various habits

TABLE 5-2 *Possible Equilibrium Influences: Magnitude and Duration of Force Against the Teeth During Function*

Possible equilibrium influence	Force magnitude	Force duration
Tooth contacts		
Mastication	Very heavy	Very short
Swallowing	Light	Very short
Soft tissue pressures of lip, cheek, and tongue		
Swallowing	Moderate	Short
Speaking	Light	Very short
Resting	Very light	Long
External pressures		
Habits	Moderate	Variable
Orthodontics	Moderate	Variable
Intrinsic pressures		
PDL fibers	Light	Long
Gingival fibers	Variable	Long

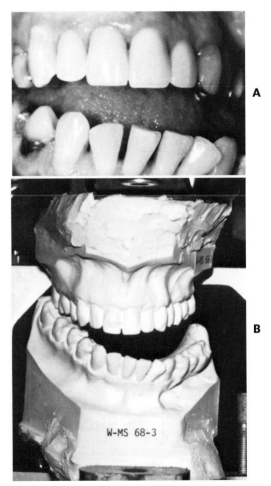

A

B

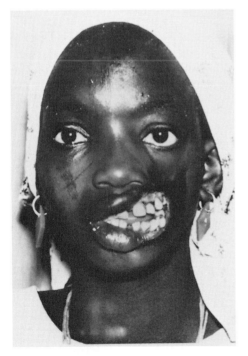

FIGURE 5-24 In this unfortunate patient, a large portion of the cheek has been lost because of a tropical infection. The outward splaying of the teeth when the restraining force of the cheek is lost illustrates the effect of a change in equilibrium. (From Moss JP, Picton DCA: *Arch Oral Biol* 12:1313-1320, 1967.)

FIGURE 5-25 After a paralytic stroke in this patient, the side of the tongue rested against the mandibular left posterior teeth. **A,** Intraoral view; **B,** casts mounted on an articulator. The extreme displacement of teeth in this adult resulted from the increased tongue pressure, altering the equilibrium. (Courtesy Dr. T. Wallen.)

and orthodontic appliances would be most prominent. As an example, an orthodontic appliance that created light pressure on the inside of the dental arch might be used to expand the teeth laterally and anteriorly, creating enough space to bring all teeth into alignment. After a certain amount of arch expansion, cheek and lip pressure begins to increase. One could expect that as long as the appliance remained in place, even though it no longer exerted any active force, it would serve as a retainer to counter these increased forces. When the appliance was removed, however, the equilibrium would again be unbalanced, and the teeth would collapse lingually until a new position of balance was reached.

Whether a habit can serve in the same way as an orthodontic appliance to change the position of the teeth has been the subject of controversy since at least the first century AD, when Celsus recommended that a child with a crooked tooth be instructed to apply finger pressure against it so that it would be moved to its proper position. From our present understanding of equilibrium, we would expect that this would work, *if* the child kept the finger pressure against the tooth for 6 hours or more per day.

The same reasoning can be applied to other habits: if a habit like thumbsucking created pressure against the teeth for more than the threshold duration (6 hours or more per day), it certainly could move teeth (Figure 5-26). On the other hand, if the habit had a shorter duration little or no effect would be expected, no matter how heavy the pressure. Whether a behavior pattern is essential or nonessential, innate or learned, its effect on the position of the teeth is determined not by the force that it applies to the teeth but by how long that force is sustained.

This concept also makes it easier to understand how playing a musical instrument might relate to the development of a malocclusion. In the past, many clinicians have suspected that playing a wind instrument might affect the position of the anterior teeth, and some have prescribed instruments as part of orthodontic therapy. Playing a clarinet, for instance, might lead to increased overjet because of the way the reeds are placed between the incisors, and this instrument could be considered both a potential cause of a Class II malocclusion and a therapeutic device for treatment of Class III. String instruments like the violin and viola require a specific head and jaw posture that affects tongue vs lip/cheek pressures and could produce asymmetries in arch form. Although the expected types of displacement of teeth are seen in professional musicians,[29] even in this group the effects are not dramatic, and little or no effect is observed in most children.[30] It seems quite likely that the duration of tongue and lip pressures associated with playing the instrument is too short to make any difference, except in the most devoted musician.

Another possible contributor to the dental equilibrium is the periodontal fiber system, both in the gingival tissues and within the periodontal ligament. We have already noted that if a tooth is lost, the space tends to close, in part because of force created by the transseptal fibers in the gingiva. The importance of this force has been demonstrated experimentally in monkeys by extracting a tooth and then making repeated incisions in the gingiva so that the transseptal fiber network is disrupted and cannot reestablish continuity. Space closure is almost completely abolished under these circumstances.[31]

The same gingival fiber network stretches elastically during orthodontic treatment and tends to pull the teeth back toward their original position. Clinical experience has shown that after orthodontic treatment, it is often wise to eliminate this force by making gingival incisions that sever the stretched transseptal fibers, thereby allowing them to heal with the teeth properly aligned (see Chapter 18). In the absence of a space created by extraction or orthodontic

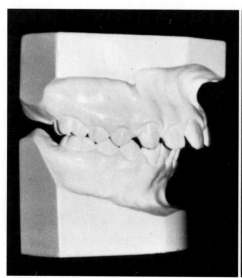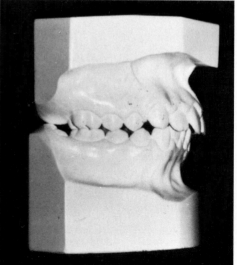

FIGURE 5-26 Dental casts from 11-year-old identical twins, one of whom (**A**) continued to suck her thumb several hours per day while the other (**B**) stopped at age 6. Displacement of the anterior teeth in the thumbsucker is obvious. (Courtesy Dr. T. Wallen.)

tooth movement, however, the gingival fiber network apparently has minimal effects on the dental equilibrium.

The periodontal ligament itself can contribute to the forces that make up the dental equilibrium. Exactly how the eruption mechanism works is still not completely understood, but it seems clear now that the eruptive force is generated within the periodontal ligament. This force is large enough and sustained enough to move a tooth. It seems likely that the same metabolic activity can and does produce forces that serve as a part of "active stabilization" for teeth, directly contributing to the equilibrium. The extent to which this occurs in teeth that are not erupting is not known. It is known, however, that the eruption mechanism remains at least potentially active throughout life, since a tooth can begin to erupt again many years after eruptive movements have apparently ceased, if its antagonist is extracted. Thus there is at least the potential for metabolic activity in the periodontal ligament to affect equilibrium.

Consideration of eruptive forces leads to a final aspect of the dental equilibrium: the effect of forces against the teeth must be considered, not only in the anteroposterior and transverse planes of space that relate to the position of a tooth within the arch, but also vertically in relation to how much or how little a tooth erupts. The vertical position of any tooth, of course, is determined by the equilibrium between the forces that produce eruption and those that oppose it. Forces from mastication are the primary ones opposing eruption, but lighter, more sustained forces from soft tissues such as the tongue interposed between the teeth probably are more important, just as they are for the horizontal equilibrium.

Equilibrium Effects on Jaw Size and Shape. The jaws, particularly the mandible, can be thought of as consisting of a core of bone to which functional processes are attached (see Figure 4-12). The functional processes of bones will be altered if the function is lost or changed. For example, the bone of the alveolar process exists only to support the teeth. If a tooth fails to erupt, alveolar bone never forms in the area it would have occupied, and if a tooth is extracted, the alveolus in that region resorbs until finally it completely atrophies. When one of a pair of opposing teeth is extracted, the other usually begins to erupt again, and even as bone is resorbing in one jaw where the tooth was lost, new alveolar bone forms in the other as the erupting tooth brings bone with it. The position of the tooth, not the functional load on it, determines the shape of the alveolar ridge.

The same is true for the muscular processes: the location of the muscle attachments is more important in determining bone shape than mechanical loading or degree of activity. Growth of the muscle, however, determines the position of the attachment, and so muscle growth can produce a change in shape of the jaw, particularly at the coronoid process and angle of the mandible.

If the condylar processes of the mandible can be considered functional processes serving to articulate the mandible with the rest of the facial skeleton, as apparently

they can, the intriguing possibility is raised that altering the position of the mandible might alter mandibular growth. The idea that holding the mandible forward or pressing it backward would change its growth has been accepted, rejected, and partially accepted again during the past century. Obviously, this theory has important implications for the etiology of malocclusion. For example, if a child positions his mandible forward on closure because of incisor interferences or because his tongue is large, will this stimulate the mandible to grow larger and ultimately produce a Class III malocclusion? Would allowing a young child to sleep on his stomach, so that the weight of the head rested on the chin, cause underdevelopment of the mandible and a Class II malocclusion?

The effect of force duration is not as clear for equilibrium effects on the jaws as for the teeth. It appears, however, that the same principle applies: the magnitude of force is less important than its duration. Positioning the jaw forward only when the teeth are brought into occlusion means that most of the time, when the mandible is in its rest position, there is no protrusion. We would expect no effects on a functional process from repeated intermittent force because of the short total duration, and the condylar process seems to respond in accordance with this principle. Neither experimental nor clinical evidence suggests that mandibular growth is any different because of occlusal interferences (though it should be kept in mind that tooth eruption, and thereby the final position of the teeth, can be altered).

If the mandible were protruded at all times, as might well be the case if the tongue were unusually large, the duration threshold could be surpassed, and growth effects might be observed. On clinical examination, individuals who appear to have a large tongue almost always have a well-developed mandible, but it is very difficult to establish tongue size. Only in extreme cases, as with a patient with early-onset thyroid deficiency, is it possible to be reasonably sure that an enlarged tongue contributed to excessive growth of the mandible (Figure 5-27). This is unlikely to be a major cause of mandibular prognathism.[32]

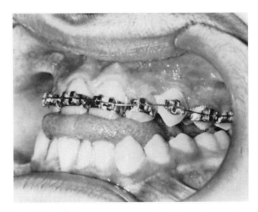

FIGURE 5-27 A large tongue, as in this patient with a history of thyroid deficiency from infancy onward, may contribute to the development of mandibular prognathism by causing the mandible to be positioned forward at all times.

Although it was widely believed in Edward Angle's era that pressures against the mandible from various habits, particularly sleeping on the stomach, interfered with growth and caused Class II malocclusion, little or no evidence supports this contention. Growth of the soft tissue matrix that moves the mandible forward and creates a space between the condyle and the temporal fossa is the normal mechanism by which growth occurs. Inhibition of mandibular growth by pressure is not a feature of normal development and is much harder to achieve, if indeed it is possible at all.

From the perspective of equilibrium theory, then, we can conclude that intermittent pressures or forces have little if any effect on either the position of the teeth or the size and shape of the jaws. Density of bone in the alveolar process and throughout the basal areas of the jaws should differ as a function of masticatory forces, but shape should not. Neither masticatory forces nor soft tissue pressures during swallowing and speaking should have any major influence on tooth position.

Major equilibrium influences for the teeth should be the light but long-lasting pressures from tongue, lips, and cheeks at rest. In addition, significant equilibrium effects should be expected from the elasticity of gingival fibers and from metabolic activity within the periodontal ligament (see Table 5-2). These equilibrium influences would affect the vertical as well as horizontal position of the teeth and could have a profound effect on how much tooth eruption occurred as well as where a tooth was positioned within the dental arch. The major equilibrium influences on the jaws should be positional changes affecting the functional processes, including the condylar process.

In the remainder of this section, functional patterns and habits that might produce malocclusion are examined as potential etiologic agents from the perspective of equilibrium theory.

Functional Influences on Dentofacial Development

Masticatory Function.   The pressures generated by chewing activity potentially could affect dentofacial development in two ways: (1) greater use of the jaws, with higher and/or more prolonged biting force, could increase the dimensions of the jaws and dental arches. Less use of the jaws might then lead to underdeveloped dental arches, and to crowded and irregular teeth; (2) decreased biting force could affect how much the teeth erupt, thereby affecting lower face height and overbite/open bite relationships. Let us now examine both possibilities in more detail.

Function and Dental Arch Size.   Equilibrium theory, as reviewed earlier, suggests that the size and shape of the muscular processes of the jaws should reflect muscle size and activity. Enlargement of the mandibular gonial angles can be seen in humans with hypertrophy of the mandibular elevator muscles (Figure 5-28), and changes in the form of the coronoid processes occur in children when temporalis muscle function is altered after injuries, so there is no doubt that the muscular processes of the jaws are affected by muscle function in humans. Equilibrium theory also suggests that heavy intermittent forces produced during mastication should have little direct effect on tooth positions, and therefore that size of the dental arches would be affected by function only if their bony base were widened. Does the extent of masticatory activity affect the width of the base of the dental arches?

It seems likely that differences between human racial groups, to some extent, reflect dietary differences and the accompanying masticatory effort. The characteristic cran-

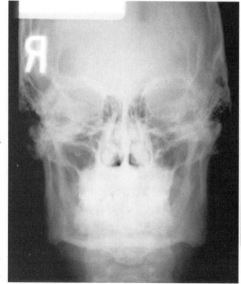
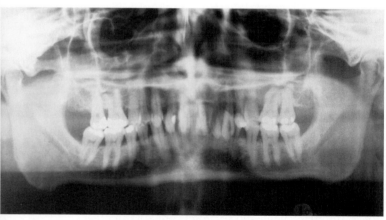

FIGURE 5-28   Hypertrophy of the masseter muscles leads to excessive bone formation at the angles of the mandible, as would be expected in a bony area that responds to muscle attachment.

iofacial morphology of Eskimos, which includes broad dental arches, is best explained as an adaptation to the extreme stress they place on jaws and teeth,[33] and changes in craniofacial dimensions from early to modern human civilizations have been related to the accompanying dietary changes.[34] A number of studies by physical anthropologists indicate that changes in dental occlusion, and an increase in malocclusion, occur along with transitions from a primitive to modern diet and lifestyle, to the point that Corrucini labels malocclusion a "disease of civilization".[35] In the context of adaptations to changes in diet over even a few generations, it appears that dietary changes probably have played a role in the modern increase in malocclusion.

Whether masticatory effort influences the size of the dental arches and the amount of space for the teeth during the development of a single individual is not so clear. Vertical jaw relationships clearly are affected by muscular activity (the effect on tooth eruption is discussed below); the effect on arch width is not so clear.[36]

Animal experiments with soft versus hard diets show that morphologic changes can occur within a single generation when diet consistency is altered. When a pig, for instance, is raised on a soft rather than a normal diet, there are changes in jaw morphology, the orientation of the jaws to the rest of the facial skeleton, and in dental arch dimensions.[37] Whether similar effects exist in humans remains unclear. If dietary consistency affects dental arch size and the amount of space for the teeth as an individual develops, it must do so early in life, because dental arch dimensions are established early. The intercanine distance, the key dimension for the alignment or crowding of incisors that is the major component of non-skeletal malocclusion, increases only modestly after the primary canines erupt at age 2 and tends to decrease after the permanent canines erupt (see Chapter 4). Is it possible that a child's masticatory effort plays a major role in determining dental arch dimensions? That seems unlikely. Genetic drift toward smaller jaw sizes, accelerated by the dietary changes that have occurred, is a more plausible explanation, but the precise relationship remains unknown.

Biting Force and Eruption. Patients who have excessive overbite or anterior open bite usually have posterior teeth that are infra- or supra-erupted, respectively. It seems reasonable that how much the teeth erupt should be a function of how much force is placed against them during function. Is it possible that differences in muscle strength, and therefore in biting force, are involved in the etiology of short- and long-face problems?

It was noted some years ago that short-face individuals have higher, and long-face persons lower, maximum biting forces than those with normal vertical dimensions. The difference between long-face and normal-face patients is highly significant statistically for occlusal tooth contacts during swallow, simulated chewing, and maximum biting (Figure 5-29).[38] Such an association between facial morphology and occlusal force does not prove a

cause-and-effect relationship. In the rare muscle weakness syndromes discussed earlier, there is a downward and backward rotation of the mandible associated with excessive eruption of the posterior teeth, but this is almost a caricature of the more usual long-face condition, not just an extension of it. If there were evidence of decreased occlusal forces in children who were showing the long-face pattern of growth, a possible causative relationship would be strengthened.

It is possible to identify a long-face pattern of growth in pre-pubescent children. Measurement of occlusal forces in this group produces a surprising result: there are no differences between children with long faces and normal faces, nor between either group of children and long-face adults.[39] All three groups have forces far below those of normal adults (Figure 5-30). Therefore it appears that the differences in occlusal force arise at puberty, when the normal group gains masticatory muscle strength and the long-face group does not. Because the long-face growth pattern can be identified before the differences in occlusal force appear, it seems more likely that the different biting force is an effect rather than a cause of the malocclusion.

These findings suggest that the force exerted by the masticatory muscles is not a major environmental factor in controlling tooth eruption and not an etiologic factor for most patients with deep bite or open bite. The effect of muscular dystrophy and related syndromes shows that there can be definite effects on growth if the musculature is abnormal, but in the absence of syndromes of this type, there is no reason to believe that how a patient bites is a major determinant of either dental arch size or vertical dimensions.

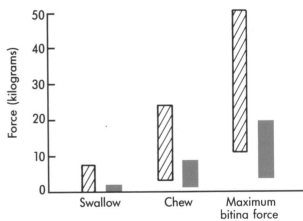

FIGURE 5-29 Comparison of occlusal force for swallowing, simulated chewing, and maximum effort at 2.5 mm molar separation in normal-face (*black*) and long-face (*red*) adults. Note that the normal subjects have much greater occlusal force during swallowing and chewing as well as at maximum effort. The differences are highly significant statistically. (From Proffit WR, Fields HW, Nixon WL: Occlusal forces in normal and long face adults, *J Dent Res* 62:566-571, 1983.)

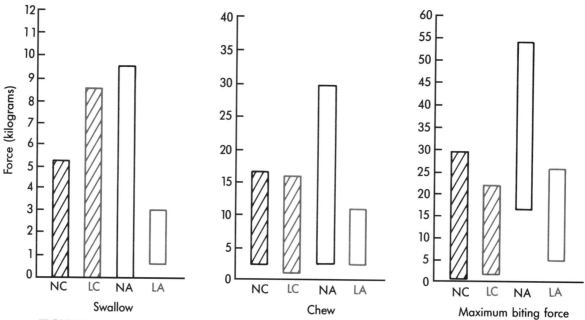

FIGURE 5-30 Comparison of occlusal forces in normal-face children (*NC*, black crosshatch), long-face children (*LC*, red crosshatch), normal-face adults (*NA*, black), and long-face adults (*LA*, red). Values for both groups of children and the long-face adults are similar; values for normal adults are significantly higher than any of the other three groups. The implication is that the differences in occlusal force in adults result from failure of the long-face group to gain strength during adolescence, not to the long condition itself. (From Proffit WR, Fields HW: Occlusal forces in normal and long face children, *J Dent Res* 62:571-574, 1983.)

Sucking and Other Habits. Although almost all normal children engage in non-nutritive sucking, prolonged sucking habits can lead to malocclusion. As a general rule, sucking habits during the primary dentition years have little if any long-term effect. If these habits persist beyond the time that the permanent teeth begin to erupt, however, malocclusion characterized by flared and spaced maxillary incisors, lingually positioned lower incisors, anterior open bite, and a narrow upper arch is the likely result (see Figure 5-26). The characteristic malocclusion associated with sucking arises from a combination of direct pressure on the teeth and an alteration in the pattern of resting cheek and lip pressures.

When a child places a thumb or finger between the teeth, it is usually positioned at an angle so that it presses lingually against the lower incisors and labially against the upper incisors (Figure 5-31). This direct pressure is presumably responsible for the displacement of the incisors. There can be considerable variation in which teeth are affected and how much, depending on which teeth are contacted. How much the teeth are displaced should correlate better with the number of hours per day of sucking than with the magnitude of the pressure. Children who suck vigorously but intermittently may not displace the incisors much if at all, whereas others who produce 6 hours or more of pressure, particularly those who sleep with a thumb or finger between the teeth all night, can cause a significant malocclusion.

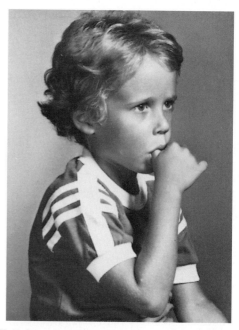

FIGURE 5-31 A child sucking his thumb usually places it as shown here, causing pressure that pushes the lower incisors lingually and the upper incisors labially. In addition, the jaw is positioned downward, providing additional opportunity for posterior teeth to erupt, and cheek pressure is increased while the tongue is lowered vertically away from the maxillary posterior teeth, altering the equilibrium that controls width dimensions. If the thumb is placed asymmetrically, the symmetry of the arch may be affected.

The anterior open bite associated with thumbsucking arises by a combination of interference with normal eruption of incisors and excessive eruption of posterior teeth. When a thumb or finger is placed between the anterior teeth, the mandible must be positioned downward to accommodate it. The interposed thumb directly impedes incisor eruption. At the same time, the separation of the jaws alters the vertical equilibrium on the posterior teeth, and as a result, there is more eruption of posterior teeth than might otherwise have occurred. Because of the geometry of the jaws, 1 mm of elongation posteriorly opens the bite about 2 mm anteriorly, so this can be a powerful contributor to the development of anterior open bite (Figure 5-32).

Although negative pressure is created within the mouth during sucking, there is no reason to believe that this is responsible for the constriction of the maxillary arch that usually accompanies sucking habits. Instead, arch form is affected by an alteration in the balance between cheek and tongue pressures. If the thumb is placed between the teeth, the tongue must be lowered, which decreases pressure by the tongue against the lingual of upper posterior teeth. At the same time, cheek pressure against these teeth is increased as the buccinator muscle contracts during sucking (Figure 5-33). Cheek pressures are greatest at the corners of the mouth, and this probably explains why the maxillary arch tends to become V-shaped, with more constriction across the canines than the molars. A child who sucks vigorously is more likely to have a narrow upper arch than one who just places the thumb between the teeth.

Although sucking habits can be a powerful contributor to malocclusion, sucking by itself does not create a severe malocclusion unless the habit persists well into the mixed dentition years. Mild displacement of the primary incisor teeth is often noted in a 3- or 4-year-old thumbsucker, but if sucking stops at this stage, normal lip and cheek pressures soon restore the teeth to their usual positions. If the habit persists after the permanent incisors begin to erupt, orthodontic treatment may be necessary to overcome the resulting tooth displacements. The constricted maxillary arch is the aspect of the malocclusion least likely to correct spontaneously. In many children, if the maxillary arch is expanded transversely, both the incisor protrusion and anterior open bite will improve spontaneously (see Chapter 13). There is no point in beginning orthodontic therapy, of course, until the habit has stopped.

Many other habits have been indicted as causes of malocclusion. As noted previously, a "sleeping habit" in which the weight of the head rested on the chin once was thought to be a major cause of Class II malocclusion. Facial asymmetries have been attributed to always sleeping on one side of the face or even to "leaning habits," as when an inattentive child leans the side of his face against one hand to doze without falling out of the classroom chair.

It is not nearly as easy to distort the facial skeleton as these views implied. Sucking habits often exceed the time threshold necessary to produce an effect on the teeth, but even prolonged sucking has little impact on the underlying form of the jaws. On close analysis most other habits have such a short duration that dental effects, much less skeletal effects, are unlikely.

Tongue Thrusting. Much attention has been paid at various times to the tongue and tongue habits as possible etiologic factors in malocclusion. The possible deleterious effects of "tongue thrust swallowing" (Figure 5-34), defined as placement of the tongue tip forward between the incisors during swallowing, received particular emphasis in the 1950s and 1960s.

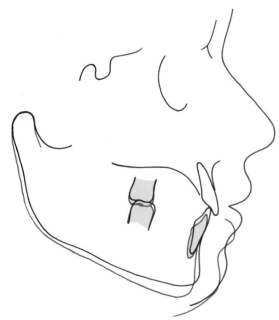

FIGURE 5-32 Cephalometric tracing showing the effects of posterior eruption on the extent of anterior opening. The only difference between the red and black tracings is that the first molars have been elongated 2 mm in the red tracing. Note that the result is 4 mm of separation of the incisors, because of the geometry of the jaw.

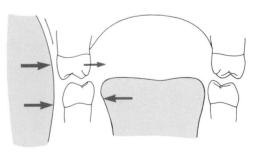

FIGURE 5-33 Diagrammatic representation of soft tissue pressures in the molar region in a child with a sucking habit. As the tongue is lowered and the cheeks contract during sucking, the pressure balance against the upper teeth is altered, and the upper but not the lower molars are displaced lingually.

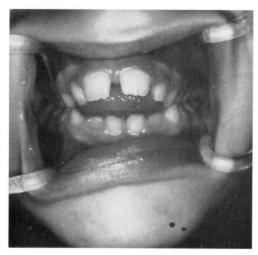

FIGURE 5-34 The typical appearance of a "tongue thrust swallow," with the tongue tip between the incisors protruding forward to put in contact with the elevated lower lip.

Laboratory studies indicate that individuals who place the tongue tip forward when they swallow usually do not have more tongue force against the teeth than those who keep the tongue tip back; in fact, tongue pressure may be lower.[40] The term *tongue thrust* is therefore something of a misnomer, since it implies that the tongue is forcefully thrust forward. Swallowing is not a learned behavior, but is integrated and controlled physiologically at subconscious levels, so whatever the pattern of swallow, it cannot be considered a habit in the usual sense. It is true, however, that individuals with an anterior open bite malocclusion place the tongue between the anterior teeth when they swallow while those who have a normal incisor relationship usually do not, and it is tempting to blame the open bite on this pattern of tongue activity.

Maturation of oral activities, including swallowing, has been discussed in some detail in Chapter 2. The mature or adult swallow pattern appears in some normal children as early as age 3, but is not present in the majority until about age 6 and is never achieved in 10% to 15% of a typical population. Tongue thrust swallowing in older patients superficially resembles the infantile swallow (described in Chapter 3), and sometimes children or adults who place the tongue between the anterior teeth are spoken of as having a retained infantile swallow. This is clearly incorrect. Only brain damaged children retain a truly infantile swallow in which the posterior part of the tongue has little or no role.

Since coordinated movements of the posterior tongue and elevation of the mandible tend to develop before protrusion of the tongue tip between the incisor teeth disappears, what is called "tongue thrusting" in young children is often a normal transitional stage in swallowing. During the transition from an infantile to a mature swallow, a child can be expected to pass through a stage in which the swallow is characterized by muscular activity to bring the lips

together, separation of the posterior teeth, and forward protrusion of the tongue between the teeth. This is also a description of the classic tongue thrust swallow. A delay in the normal swallow transition can be expected when a child has a sucking habit.

When there is an anterior open bite and/or upper incisor protrusion, as often occurs from sucking habits, it is more difficult to seal off the front of the mouth during swallowing to prevent food or liquids from escaping. Bringing the lips together and placing the tongue between the separated anterior teeth is a successful maneuver to close off the front of the mouth and form an anterior seal. In other words, a tongue thrust swallow is a useful physiologic adaptation if you have an open bite, which is why an individual with an open bite also has a tongue thrust swallow. The reverse is not true—a tongue thrust swallow is often present in children with good anterior occlusion. After a sucking habit stops, the anterior open bite tends to close spontaneously, but the position of the tongue between the anterior teeth persists for a while as the open bite closes. Until the open bite disappears, an anterior seal by the tongue tip remains necessary.

The modern viewpoint is, in short, that tongue thrust swallowing is seen primarily in two circumstances: in younger children with reasonably normal occlusion, in whom it represents only a transitional stage in normal physiologic maturation; and in individuals of any age with displaced incisors, in whom it is an adaptation to the space between the teeth. The presence of overjet (often) and anterior open bite (nearly always) conditions a child or adult to place the tongue between the anterior teeth. A tongue thrust swallow therefore should be considered the result of displaced incisors, not the cause. It follows, of course, that correcting the tooth position should cause a change in swallow pattern, and this usually happens. It is neither necessary nor desirable to try to teach the patient to swallow differently before beginning orthodontic treatment.

This is not to say that the tongue has no etiologic role in the development of open bite malocclusion. From equilibrium theory, light but sustained pressure by the tongue against the teeth would be expected to have significant effects. Tongue thrust swallowing simply has too short a duration to have an impact on tooth position. Pressure by the tongue against the teeth during a typical swallow lasts for approximately 1 second. A typical individual swallows about 800 times per day while awake but has only a few swallows per hour while asleep. The total per day therefore is usually under 1000. One thousand seconds of pressure, of course, totals only a few minutes, not nearly enough to affect the equilibrium.

On the other hand, if a patient has a forward resting posture of the tongue, the duration of this pressure, even if very light, could affect tooth position, vertically or horizontally. Tongue tip protrusion during swallowing is sometimes associated with a forward tongue posture. If the position from which tongue movements start is different from

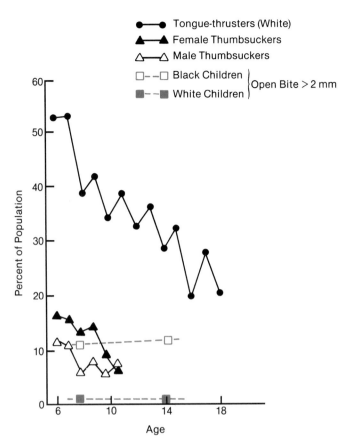

FIGURE 5-35 Prevalence of anterior open bite, thumbsucking, and tongue thrust swallowing as a function of age. Open bite occurs much more frequently in blacks than in whites. Note that the prevalence of anterior open bite at any age is only a small fraction of the prevalence of tongue thrust swallowing and is also less than the prevalence of thumbsucking. (Data from Fletcher SG et al, *J Speech Hear Disord* 26:201-208, 1961; Kelly JE et al: DHEW Pub No [HRA] 77-144, 1977.)

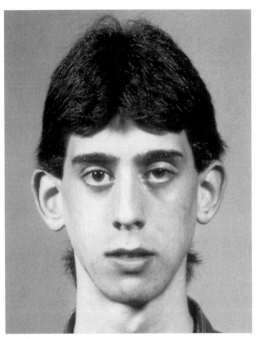

FIGURE 5-36 The classic "adenoid facies," consisting of narrow width dimensions, protruding teeth, and lips separated at rest, has often been attributed to mouth breathing. Since it is perfectly possible to breathe through the nose with the lips separated, simply by creating an oral seal posteriorly with the soft palate, the facial appearance is not diagnostic of the respiratory mode. On careful study, many of these patients are found not to be obligatory mouth breathers.

normal, so that the pattern of resting pressures is different, there is likely to be an effect on the teeth, whereas if the postural position is normal, the tongue thrust swallow has no clinical significance.

Perhaps this point can best be put in perspective by comparing the number of children who have an anterior open bite malocclusion with the number of children of the same age reported to have a tongue thrust swallow. As Figure 5-35 shows, at every age above 6, the number of children reported to have a tongue thrust swallow is about 10 times greater than the number reported to have an anterior open bite. Thus there is no reason to believe that a tongue thrust swallow always implies an altered rest position and will lead to malocclusion. The odds are approximately 10 to 1 that this is not the case for any given child. In a child who has an open bite, tongue posture may be a factor, but the swallow itself is not.

Respiratory Pattern. Respiratory needs are the primary determinant of the posture of the jaws and tongue (and of the head itself, to a lesser extent). Therefore it

seems entirely reasonable that an altered respiratory pattern, such as breathing through the mouth rather than the nose, could change the posture of the head, jaw, and tongue. This in turn could alter the equilibrium of pressures on the jaws and teeth and affect both jaw growth and tooth position. In order to breathe through the mouth, it is necessary to lower the mandible and tongue, and extend (tip back) the head. If these postural changes were maintained, face height would increase, and posterior teeth would super-erupt; unless there was unusual vertical growth of the ramus, the mandible would rotate down and back, opening the bite anteriorly and increasing overjet; and increased pressure from the stretched cheeks might cause a narrower maxillary dental arch.

Exactly this type of malocclusion often is associated with mouth breathing (note its similarity to the pattern also blamed on sucking habits and tongue thrust swallow). The association has been noted for many years: the descriptive term *adenoid facies* has appeared in the English literature for at least a century, probably longer (Figure 5-36). Unfortunately, the relationship between mouth breathing, altered posture, and the development of malocclusion is not so clear-cut as the theoretical outcome of shifting to oral respiration might appear at first glance.[41] Recent experimental studies have only partially clarified the situation.

In analyzing this, it is important to understand first that although humans are primarily nasal breathers, everyone breathes partially through the mouth under certain physiologic conditions, the most prominent being an increased need for air during exercise. For the average individual, there is a transition to partial oral breathing when ventilatory exchange rates above 40 to 45 L/min are reached.[42] At maximum effort, 80 or more L/min of air are needed, about half of which is obtained through the mouth. At rest, minimum airflow is 20 to 25 L/min, but heavy mental concentration or even normal conversation lead to increased airflow and a transition to partial mouth breathing.

During resting conditions, greater effort is required to breathe through the nose than through the mouth—the tortuous nasal passages introduce an element of resistance to airflow as they perform their function of warming and humidifying the inspired air. The increased work for nasal respiration is physiologically acceptable up to a point, and indeed respiration is most efficient with modest resistance present in the system. If the nose is partially obstructed, the work associated with nasal breathing increases, and at a certain level of resistance to nasal airflow, the individual switches to partial mouth breathing. This crossover point varies among individuals, but is usually reached at resistance levels of about 3.5 to 4 cm H-2-O/L/min.[43] The swelling of the nasal mucosa accompanying a common cold occasionally converts all of us to mouth breathing at rest by this mechanism.

Chronic respiratory obstruction can be produced by prolonged inflammation of the nasal mucosa associated with allergies or chronic infection. It can also be produced by mechanical obstruction anywhere within the nasorespiratory system, from the nares to the posterior nasal choanae. Under normal conditions, the size of the nostril is the limiting factor in nasal airflow. The pharyngeal tonsils or adenoids normally are large in children, and partial obstruction from this source may contribute to mouth breathing in children. Individuals who have had chronic nasal obstruction may continue to breathe partially through the mouth even after the obstruction has been relieved. In this sense, mouth breathing can sometimes be considered a habit.

If respiration had an effect on the jaws and teeth, it should do so by causing a change in posture that secondarily altered long-duration pressures from the soft tissues. Experiments with human subjects have shown that a change in posture does accompany nasal obstruction.[44] For instance, when the nose is completely blocked, usually there is an immediate change of about 5 degrees in the craniovertebral angle (Figure 5-37). The jaws move apart, as much by elevation of the maxilla because the head tips back, as by depression of the mandible. When the nasal obstruction is removed, the original posture immediately returns. This physiologic response occurs to the same extent, however, in individuals who already have some nasal obstruction, which indicates that it may not totally result from respiratory demands.

Experiments with growing monkeys show that totally obstructing the nostrils for a prolonged period in this species leads to the development of malocclusion but not of the type commonly associated with mouth breathing in humans.[45] Instead, the monkeys tend to develop some degree of mandibular prognathism, although their response shows considerable variety (Figure 5-38). Placing a block in the roof of a monkey's mouth, which forces a downward position of the tongue and mandible, also produces a variety of malocclusions. It seems clear that altered posture is the mechanism by which growth changes were produced. The variety of responses in the monkeys suggests that the type of malocclusion is determined by the individual animal's pattern of adaptation.

In evaluating these experiments, it must be kept in mind that mouth breathing of any extent is completely

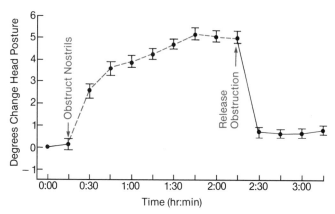

FIGURE 5-37 Data from an experiment with dental students, showing the immediate change in head posture when the nostrils are totally blocked: the head tips back about 5 degrees, increasing the separation of the jaws. When the obstruction is relieved, head posture returns to its original position. (From Vig PS et al: *Am J Orthod* 77:258-268, 1980.)

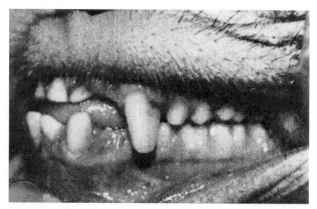

FIGURE 5-38 Malocclusion in a monkey who underwent several months of total nasal obstruction during growth. Note the mandibular prognathism, the most common response in this series of experiments. (From Harvold EP et al: *Am J Orthod* 79:359-372, 1981.)

unnatural for monkeys, who will die if the nasal passages are obstructed abruptly. To carry out the experiments, it was necessary to gradually obstruct their noses, giving the animals a chance to learn how to survive as mouth breathers. Total nasal obstruction is also extremely rare in humans.

There are only a few well-documented cases of facial growth in children with long-term total nasal obstruction, but it appears that under these circumstances the growth pattern is altered in the way one would predict (Figure 5-39). Because total nasal obstruction in humans is so rare, the important clinical question is whether partial nasal obstruction, of the type that occurs occasionally for a short time in everyone and chronically in some children, can lead to malocclusion; or more precisely, how close to total obstruction does partial obstruction have to come before it is clinically significant?

The question is difficult to answer, primarily because it is difficult to know what the pattern of respiration really is at any given time in humans. Observers tend to equate lip separation at rest with mouth breathing (see Figure 5-36), but this is simply not correct. It is perfectly possible for an individual to breathe through the nose while the lips are apart. To do this, it is only necessary to seal off the mouth by placing the tongue against the palate. Since some lip separation at rest (lip incompetence) is normal in children, many children who appear to be mouth breathers may not be.

Simple clinical tests for mouth breathing can also be misleading. The highly vascular nasal mucosa undergoes cycles of engorgement with blood and shrinkage. The cycles alternate between the two nostrils: when one is clear, the other is usually somewhat obstructed. For this reason, clinical tests to determine whether the patient can breathe freely through both nostrils nearly always show that one is at least partially blocked. One partially obstructed nostril should not be interpreted as a problem with normal nasal breathing.

The only reliable way to quantify the extent of mouth breathing is to establish how much of the total airflow goes through the nose and how much through the mouth, which requires special instrumentation to simultaneously measure nasal and oral airflow. This allows the percentage of nasal or oral respiration (nasal/oral ratio) to be calculated, for the length of time the subject can tolerate being continuously monitored. It seems obvious that a certain percentage of oral respiration, maintained for a certain percentage of the time, should be the definition of significant mouth breathing, but despite years of effort such a definition has not been produced.

The best current experimental data for the relationship between malocclusion and mouth breathing are derived from studies of the nasal/oral ratio in normal versus long-face children.[46] The relationship is not nearly as clear-cut as theory might predict. It is useful to represent the data as in Figure 5-40, which shows that both normal and long-face children are likely to be predominantly nasal breathers under laboratory conditions. A minority of the long-face children had less than 40% nasal breathing, while none of the normal children had such low nasal percentages. When adult long-face patients are examined, the findings are similar: the number with evidence of nasal obstruction is increased in comparison to a normal population, but the majority are not mouth breathers in the sense of predominantly oral respiration.

It seems reasonable to presume that children who require adenoidectomy and/or tonsillectomy for medical purposes, or those diagnosed as having chronic nasal allergies, would have some degree of nasal obstruction (although it must be kept in mind that this has not been documented). Allergic children tend to have increased anterior face height and the increased overjet/decreased overbite that accompanies it.[47] Studies of Swedish children who underwent adenoidectomy showed that on the average, children in the adenoidectomy group had a significantly longer anterior face height than control children (Figure 5-41). They also had a tendency toward maxillary constriction and more upright incisors.[48] Furthermore, when children in the adenoidectomy group were followed after their treatment, they tended to return toward the mean of the control group, though the

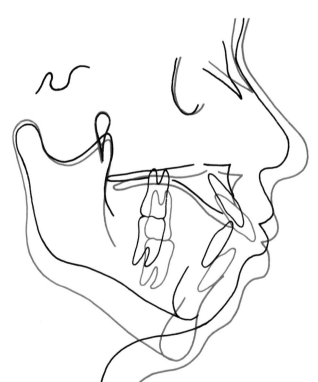

FIGURE 5-39 Cephalometric superimposition showing the effect of total nasal obstruction produced by a pharyngeal flap operation (for cleft palate speech) that sealed off the nose posteriorly. From age 12 (*black*) to 16 (*red*), the mandible rotated downward and backward as the patient experienced considerable growth. (Redrawn from McNamara JA: Influences of respiratory pattern on craniofacial growth, *Angle Orthod* 51:269-300, 1981.)

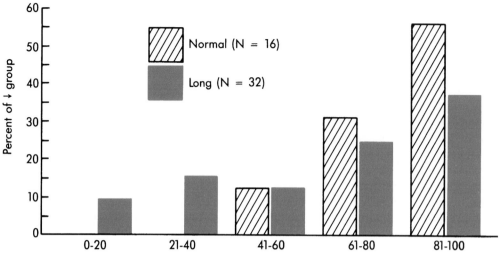

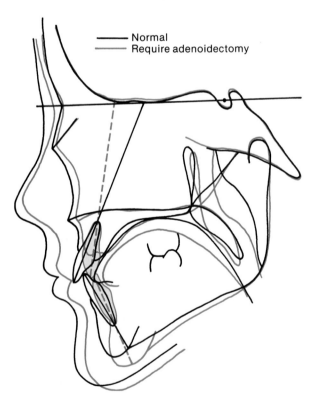

FIGURE 5-40   Comparison of the percentage of nasal respiration in long-face versus normal-face adolescents. About a third of the long-face group have less than 50% nasal respiration, whereas none of the normal-face group have such a low nasal percentage. But most of the long-face group are predominantly nasal breathers. The data suggest that impaired nasal respiration may contribute to the development of the long-face condition but is not the sole or even the major cause. (Data redrawn from Fields HW, Warren DW, Black BK, Phillips C: Relationship between vertical dentofacial morphology and respiration in adolescents, *Am J Orthod Dentofac Orthop* 99:147-154, 1991.)

FIGURE 5-41   Average cephalometric tracings for a group of Swedish children requiring adenoidectomy for medical purposes, compared with a group of normal controls. The adenoidectomy group had statistically significantly greater anterior face height and steeper mandibular plane angles than the controls, but the differences were quantitatively not large. (From Linder-Aronson S: *Acta Otolaryngol Scand* [suppl 265], 1970.)

differences persisted (Figure 5-42). Similar differences from normal control groups were seen in other groups requiring adenoidectomy and/or tonsillectomy.[49]

Although the differences between normal children and those in the allergy or adenoidectomy groups were statistically significant and undoubtedly real, they were not large. Face height on the average was about 3 mm greater in the adenoidectomy group. Earlier English workers indicated that the percentage of children with various malocclusions was about the same in a group being seen in an ear, nose, and throat clinic as in controls without respiratory problems.[50]

It appears therefore that research to this point on respiration has established two opposing principles, leaving a large gray area between them: (1) total nasal obstruction is highly likely to alter the pattern of growth and lead to malocclusion in experimental animals and humans, and individuals with a high percentage of oral respiration are over-represented in the long-face population; but (2) the majority of individuals with the long-face pattern of deformity have no evidence of nasal obstruction and must therefore have some other etiologic factor as the principal cause. Perhaps the alterations in posture associated with partial nasal obstruction and moderate increases in the percentage of oral respiration are not great enough by themselves to create a severe malocclusion. Mouth breathing, in short, may contribute to the development of orthodontic problems but is difficult to indict as a frequent etiologic agent.

It is interesting to consider the other side of this relationship: can malocclusion sometimes cause respiratory

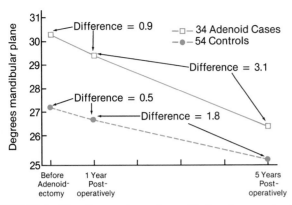

FIGURE 5-42 Comparison of mandibular plane angles in a group of postadenoidectomy children compared with normal controls. Note that the differences existing at the time of adenoidectomy decreased in size but did not totally disappear. (From Linder-Aronson S: In Cook JT (editor): *Transactions of the Third International Orthodontic Congress*, St Louis, 1975, Mosby.)

obstruction? Sleep apnea has been recognized recently as a more frequent problem than had been appreciated, and it is apparent that mandibular deficiency can contribute to its development.[51] Its etiology, however, is by no means determined just by orofacial morphology—obesity, age/gender, and cephalometric characteristics seem to be important, in that order.[52]

ETIOLOGY IN CONTEMPORARY PERSPECTIVE

Changing Views of Etiologic Possibilities

Part of the philosophy of the early orthodontists was their belief in the perfectibility of man. Edward Angle and his contemporaries, influenced by the romanticized view of primitive peoples commonly held 100 years ago, took it for granted that malocclusion was a disease of civilization and blamed it on improper function of the jaws under the "degenerate" modern conditions. Changing jaw function in order to produce proper growth and change facial proportions was an important goal of treatment—which unfortunately proved difficult to achieve.

Classical (Mendelian) genetics developed rapidly in the first part of the twentieth century, and a different view of malocclusion gradually replaced the earlier one. This new view was that malocclusion is primarily the result of inherited dentofacial proportions, which may be altered somewhat by developmental variations, trauma, or altered function, but which are basically established at conception. If that were true, the possibilities for orthodontic treatment also would be rather limited. The orthodontist's role would be to adapt the dentition to the existing facial structures, with little hope of producing underlying changes.

In the1980s, there was a strong swing back toward the earlier view, as the failure of heredity to explain most vari-

ation in occlusion and jaw proportions was appreciated and as the new theories of growth control indicated how environmental influences could operate by altering posture. The earlier concept that jaw function is related to the development of malocclusion was revived and strengthened, both by the evidence against simple inheritance and by a more optimistic view of the extent to which the human skeleton can be altered. Clinical applications, some already recognized as unfortunate, reflected extreme optimism about arch expansion and growth modification.

As the 21st century begins, a more balanced view seems to be emerging. Contemporary research has refuted the simplistic picture of malocclusion as resulting from independent inheritance of dental and facial characteristics, but the research findings consistently have shown also that there are no simple explanations for malocclusion in terms of oral function. Mouth breathing, tongue thrusting, soft diet, sleeping posture—none can be regarded as the sole or even the major reason for most malocclusions. Along the same lines, it is fair to say that the research has not yet clarified the precise role of heredity as an etiologic agent for malocclusion. The relatively high heritability of craniofacial dimensions and the relatively low heritability of dental arch variations now has been established, but exactly how this relates to the etiologic process of malocclusions that have both skeletal and dental components remains unknown. Conclusions about the etiology of most orthodontic problems are difficult, because several interacting factors probably played a role.

The following summary discussion is an attempt to synthesize present knowledge into a contemporary overview and is offered in full awareness that the facts do not yet allow definite conclusions.

Etiology of Crowding and Malalignment

Crowding of the teeth, the most common type of malocclusion at present, undoubtedly is related in part to the continuing reduction in jaw and tooth size in human evolutionary development, but that cannot be a major factor in the increased crowding of quite recent years. Increased outbreeding can explain at least part of the increase in crowding in recent centuries. The additive effects on malocclusion seen in the Hawaiian studies indicate how outbreeding could lead to an increased prevalence of malocclusion even if independent inheritance of dentofacial characteristics did not occur. Jaw dimensions do seem to have a strong genetic control, and the transverse dimensions directly affect the amount of space for the teeth.

Environmental factors must have played some role in the recent increase in crowding of the dental arches, however, and it is not clear what these are. There is no theoretical explanation of how a coarser diet and more powerful jaw function could significantly alter the dimensions of the dental arches. Perhaps the relatively recent alterations in diet, which without question have reduced the functional demands on the jaws, have accelerated the trend toward reduction in jaw size that was already occurring. Mouth breathing might conceivably contribute to crowding by altering the tongue-lip/cheek equilibrium as the mandible rotated down and back but obviously is not a major cause.

The judgment that inherited characteristics contribute to crowding is an important one in planning orthodontic therapy, for it implies that a significant number of patients will continue to require extractions to provide space for aligning the remaining teeth. Physical therapy to make the dental apparatus grow larger seems an unlikely alternative. In the era when all malocclusions were attributed to a degenerate environment, extraction of teeth was never recommended, and orthodontic expansion was the routine treatment. At the height of enthusiasm for inherited characteristics as determinants of malocclusion, the majority of patients were treated with extractions. In contemporary perspective, the truth—and the extraction percentage—is somewhere in between.

Other types of Class I (nonskeletal) problems—crossbites, individual tooth malalignments—appear to arise from an interaction between the initial position of tooth buds and the pressure environment that guides eruption of the teeth. Forces from the lips, cheek, tongue, fingers, or other objects can influence tooth position, both vertically and horizontally, if the pressures are maintained for a long enough time. A small increment of continuous pressure can be quite effective in displacing teeth. Any individual tooth or all teeth in a section of the arch can be displaced buccally or lingually, or caused to erupt more or less than might otherwise have been the case. The conclusion is, therefore, that minor Class I problems, especially nonskeletal crossbites, often are caused primarily by alterations in function. Major problems usually have an additional genetic or developmental component.

Etiology of Skeletal Problems

Skeletal orthodontic problems, those resulting from malpositions or malformations of the jaws rather than just from irregularity of the teeth, can arise from a number of causes. Inherited patterns, defects in embryologic development, trauma, and functional influences can and apparently do contribute. Specific genetic syndromes or congenital defects involving the jaws are rare, as are malocclusions caused primarily by trauma. The fact that ideal occlusion does not necessarily occur in primitive populations suggests that variations from an idealized occlusal scheme are quite compatible with normal function. Perhaps greater variations in the jaws are tolerated now, with the change in diet, than were once compatible with long-term survival and reproductive success.

It seems reasonable to view the majority of moderate skeletal malocclusions as being the result of an inherited pattern which, although not constant with our concept of ideal occlusion, is compatible with acceptable function.

Fifteen percent to 20% of the contemporary U.S. and northern European population have a Class II malocclusion, and it is likely that for most of these individuals, there is an inherited tendency toward retrognathic facial proportions. Only a few Class II malocclusions are caused by some specific interference with growth, and there is little reason to believe that any significant number are the result of functional causes alone—which is not to say that functional alterations in equilibrium cannot accentuate Class II tendencies when they are present. The more severe cases probably fall into this category of inherited tendencies made worse by environmental effects.

There is a definite familial and racial tendency to mandibular prognathism. Excessive mandibular growth could arise because of mandibular posture, since constant distraction of the mandibular condyle from the fossa may be a stimulus to growth. Functional mandibular shifts affect only tooth position, but constant posturing because of respiratory needs, tongue size or pharyngeal dimensions may affect the size of the jaw. In the final analysis it may not matter whether the inherited tendency is for a large mandible primarily, or for a large tongue or other characteristics that lead secondarily to a large mandible. Why maxillary deficiency occurs is almost entirely unknown, but a simple environmental cause appears unlikely, and like Class II problems, the majority of Class III problems are related to inherited jaw proportions.

Altered function has traditionally been associated with vertical growth problems, especially anterior open bite. A child with an anterior open bite of moderate severity should be presumed to have a sucking habit until proved otherwise. Open bite also may be related to tongue posture, although not to tongue activity during swallowing. The postural changes dictated by partial nasal obstruction may also play a role. Excessive eruption of posterior teeth predisposes any individual to anterior open bite, and downward posturing of the mandible and tongue can allow excessive posterior eruption. However, vertical jaw proportions are inherited just as are anteroposterior proportions, with very similar heritability. Anterior open bite is much more common in blacks than whites, whereas deep bite is much more common in whites (see Chapter 1). It seems reasonably clear that this reflects a different inherent facial morphology rather than environmental influences. Perhaps posture and the associated equilibrium effects interact with inherited jaw proportions to produce open bite or deep bite in some individuals.

A final word on etiology: whatever the malocclusion, it is nearly always stable after growth has been completed. If an orthodontic problem is corrected in adult life, which can be difficult because so much of treatment depends on growth, a surprising amount of change is also stable. The etiologic agents, in other words, are usually no longer present when growth is completed. Malocclusion, after all, is a developmental problem.

REFERENCES

1. Gorlin RJ, Pindborg JJ, Cohen MM: Syndromes of the head and neck, ed 2, New York, 1990, McGraw Hill.
2. Proffit WR, White RP Jr: Surgical-orthodontic treatment, St Louis, 1991, Mosby.
3. Epker BN, Stella JP, Fish LC: Dentofacial deformities: integrated orthodontic and surgical correction, ed 2, St Louis, 1998, Mosby.
4. Perkins JA, Sie KC, Milczuk H, Richardson MA: Airway management in children with craniofacial anomalies, Cleft Palate-Craniofacial J 34:134-150, 1997.
5. Randall P: The Robin anomalad: micrognathia and glossoptosis with airway obstruction. In Converse JM (editor): Reconstructive plastic surgery, Philadelphia, 1987, W.B. Saunders.
6. Proffit WR, Vig KWL, Dann C IV: Who seeks surgical-orthodontic treatment? The characteristics of patients evaluated in the UNC Dentofacial Clinic, Int J Adult Orthod Orthogn Surg 5: 153-160, 1990.
7. Ferguson JW: Surgical correction of the facial deformities secondary to untreated congenital muscular torticollis, J Cranio-Maxillo-Facial Surg 21:137-142, 1993.
8. Kiliaridis S, Mejersjo C, Thilander B: Muscle function and craniofacial morphology: a clinical study in patients with myotonic dystrophy, Eur J Orthod 11:131-138, 1989.
9. Lamberts SWJ, Melmed S: New developments in the management of acromegaly, J Endocrinol 155 (Suppl 1), 1997.
10. Obwegeser HL, Makek MS: Hemimandibular hypertrophy, hemimandibular elongation, J Maxillofac Surg 14:183-208, 1986.
11. Becker A, Lustmann J, Shteyer A: Cleidocranial dysplasia: Part 1—General principles of the orthodontic and surgical treatment modality,. Am J Orthod Dentofac Orthop 111: 28-33, 1997; Part 2—Treatment protocol for the orthodontic and surgical modality, Am J Orthod Dentofac Orthop 111:173-183, 1997.
12. Messer LB, Cline JT: Ankylosed primary molars: results and treatment recommendations from an eight-year longitudinal study, Pediatr Dent 2:37-47, 1980.
13. Matteson SR, Kantor ML, Proffit WR: Extreme distal migration of the mandibular second bicuspid, Angle Orthod 52:11-18, 1982.
14. Southard TE, Behrents RG, Tolley EA: The anterior component of occlusal force. I. Measurement and distribution, Am J Orthod Dentofacial Orthop 96:493-500, 1989.
15. Moss JP, Picton DCA: Experimental mesial drift in adult monkeys (Macaca irus), Arch Oral Biol 12:1313-1320, 1967.
16. Moss JP: The soft tissue environment of teeth and jaws: an experimental and clinical study, Br J Orthod 7:107-137, 1980.
17. Stockard CR, Johnson AL: Genetic and endocrinic basis for differences in form and behavior, Philadelphia, 1941, The Wistar Institute of Anatomy and Biology.
18. Chung CS, Niswander JD, Runck DW et al: Genetic and epidemiologic studies of oral characteristics in Hawaii's schoolchildren. II. Malocclusion, Am J Human Genet 23:471-495, 1971.
19. Lauweryns I, Carels C, Vlietinck R: The use of twins in dentofacial genetic research, Am J Orthod Dentofac Orthop 103:33-38, 1993.
20. Corruccini RS, Sharma K, Potter RHY: Comparative genetic variance and heritability of dental occlusal variables in U.S. and northwest Indian twins, Am J Phys Anthropol 70:293-299, 1986.
21. Corruccini RS, Townsend GC, Richards LC, Brown T: Genetic and environmental determinants of dental occlusal variation in twins of different nationalities, Human Biol 62:353-367, 1990.
22. Lobb WK: Craniofacial morphology and occlusal variation in monozygous and dizygous twins, Angle Orthod 57:219-233, 1987.
23. Harris EF, Smith RJ: A study of occlusion and arch widths in families, Am J Orthod 78:155-163, 1980.
24. Suzuki A, Takahama Y: Parental data used to predict growth of craniofacial form, Am J Orthod Dentofacial Orthop 99:107-121, 1991.
25. Harris EF, Johnson MG: Heritability of craniometric and occlusal variables: a longitudinal sib analysis, Am J Orthod Dentofacial Orthop 99:258-268, 1991.
26. Litton SF, Ackerman LV, Isaacson RJ, Shapiro B: A genetic study of Class III malocclusion, Am J Orthod 58:565-577, 1970.
27. King L, Harris EF, Tolley EA: Heritability of cephalometric and occlusal variables as assessed from siblings with overt malocclusions, Am J Orthod Dentofac Orthop 104: 121-131, 1993.
28. Proffit WR: Equilibrium theory revisited, Angle Orthod 48:175-186, 1978.
29. Kovero O, Kononen M, Pirinen S: The effect of professional violin and viola playing on the bony facial structures, Eur J Orthod 19:39-45, 1997.
30. Kindisbacher I, Hirschi U, Ingervall B, Geering A: Little influence on tooth position from playing a wind instrument, Angle Orthod 60:223-228, 1990.
31. Picton DCA, Moss JP: The part played by the trans-septal fibre system in experimental approximal drift of the cheek teeth of monkeys (Macaca irus), Arch Oral Biol 18:669-680, 1973.
32. Yoo E, Murakami S, Takada K et al: Tongue volume in human female adults with mandibular prognathism, J Dent Res 75:1957-1962, 1996.
33. Hylander WL: The adaptive significance of Eskimo craniofacial morphology. In Dahlberg AA, Graber TM (editors): Orofacial growth and development, Paris, 1977, Mouton.
34. Larsen CS: Bioarchaeology: interpreting behavior from the human skeleton, Cambridge, Mass., 1997, Cambridge University Press.
35. Corruccini RS: Anthropological aspects of orofacial and occlusal variations and anomalies. In Kelly MA, Larsen CS (editors): Advances in dental anthropology, New York, 1991, Wiley-Liss.
36. Kiliaridis S: Masticatory muscle influence on craniofacial growth, Acta Odontol Scand 53:196-202, 1995.
37. Ciochon RL, Nisbett RA, Corrucini RS: Dietary consistency and craniofacial development related to masticatory function in minipigs, J Craniofac Genetics Dev Biol 17:96-102, 1997.
38. Proffit WR, Fields HW, Nixon WL: Occlusal forces in normal and long face adults, J Dent Res 62:566-571, 1983.
39. Proffit WR, Fields HW: Occlusal forces in normal and long face children, J Dent Res 62:571-574, 1983.

40. Proffit WR: Lingual pressure patterns in the transition from tongue thrust to adult swallowing, Arch Oral Biol 17:555-563, 1972.

41. Vig KWL: Nasal obstruction and facial growth: the strength of evidence for clinical assumptions, Am J Orthod Dentofac Orthop 113:603-611, 1998.

42. Niinimaa V, Cole P, Mintz S, Shephard RJ: Oronasal distribution of respiratory airflow, Respir Physiol 43:69-75, 1981.

43. Warren DW, Mayo R, Zajac DJ, Rochet AH: Dyspnea following experimentally induced increased nasal airway resistance, Cleft Palate-Craniofac J 33:231-235, 1996.

44. Tourne LLCPM, Schweiger J: Immediate postural responses to total nasal obstruction, Am J Orthod Dentofac Orthop 111:606-611, 1997.

45. Harvold EP, Tomer BS, Vargervik K, Chierici G: Primate experiments on oral respiration, Am J Orthod 79:359-372, 1981.

46. Fields HW, Warren DW, Black K, Phillips C: Relationship between vertical dentofacial morphology and respiration in adolescents, Am J Orthod Dentofac Orthop 99:147-154, 1991.

47. Trask GM, Shapiro GG, Shapiro PS: The effects of perennial allergic rhinitis and dental and skeletal development: a comparison of sibling pairs, Am J Orthod Dentofacial Orthop 92:286-293, 1987.

48. Linder-Aronson S: Adenoids: their effect on mode of breathing and nasal airflow and their relationship to characteristics of the facial skeleton and dentition, Acta Otolaryngol Scand (supp 265), 1970.

49. Woodside DG, Linder-Aronson S, Lundstrom A, McWilliam J: Mandibular and maxillary growth after changed mode of breathing, Am J Orthod Dentofac Orthop 100:1-18, 1991.

50. Leech HL: A clinical analysis of orofacial morphology and behavior of 500 patients attending an upper respiratory research clinic, Dent Practitioner 9:57-68, 1958.

51. Battagel J: Obstructive sleep apnea—fact not fiction, Brit J Orthod 23:315-324, 1996.

52. Lowe AA, Ozbek MM, Miyamoto K et al: Cephalometric and demographic characteristics of obstructive sleep apnea, Angle Orthod 67:143-154, 1997.

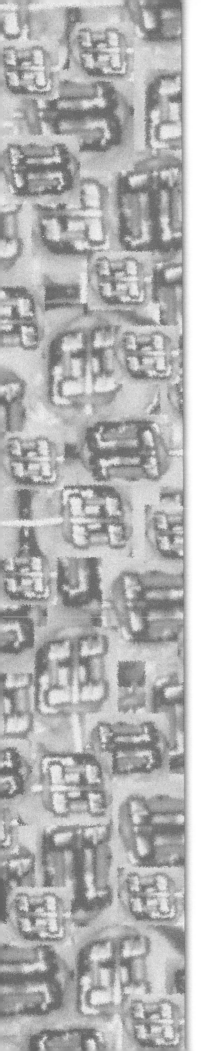

SECTION III

DIAGNOSIS AND TREATMENT PLANNING

The process of orthodontic diagnosis and treatment planning lends itself well to *the problem-oriented approach*. Diagnosis in orthodontics, as in other disciplines of dentistry and medicine, requires the collection of an adequate database of information about the patient and the distillation from that database of a comprehensive but clearly stated list of the patient's problems. It is important to recognize that both the patient's perceptions and the doctor's observations are needed in formulating the problem list. Then the task of treatment planning is to synthesize the possible solutions to these specific problems (often there are many possibilities) into a specific treatment strategy that would provide maximum benefit for this particular patient.

Keep in mind that diagnosis and treatment planning, though part of the same process, are different procedures with fundamentally different goals. In the development of a database and formulation of a problem list, the goal is *truth*—the goal of scientific inquiry. At this stage there is no room for opinion or judgment. Instead, a totally factual appraisal of the situation is required. On the other hand, the goal of treatment planning is not scientific truth, but *wisdom*—the plan that a wise and prudent clinician would follow to maximize benefit for the patient. For this reason, treatment planning inevitably is something of an art form. Diagnosis must be done scientifically; for all practical purposes, treatment planning cannot be science alone. Judgment by the clinician is required as problems are prioritized and as alternative treatment possibilities are evaluated. Wise treatment choices, of course, are facilitated if no significant points have been overlooked previously and if it is realized that treatment planning is an interactive process, requiring that the patient be given a role in the decision-making process.

We recommend carrying out diagnosis and treatment planning in a series of logical steps. The first two steps constitute diagnosis:

1. Development of an adequate diagnostic database
2. Formulation of a problem list—the diagnosis—from the database. Both pathologic and developmental problems may be present. If so, pathologic problems should be separated from the developmental ones so that they can receive priority for treatment—not because they are more important but because pathologic processes must be under control before treatment of developmental problems begins. The diagnostic process is outlined in detail in Chapter 6.

Once a patient's orthodontic problems have been identified and prioritized, four issues must be faced in determining the optimal treatment plan: (1) the timing of treatment, (2) the complexity of the treatment that would be required, (3) the predictability of success with a given treatment approach, and (4) the patient's (and parents') goals and desires. Considering these briefly in turn:

Orthodontic treatment can be carried out at any time during a patient's life and can be aimed at a specific problem or be comprehensive. Usually it is comprehensive (i.e., with a goal of the best possible occlusion, facial esthetics, and stability) and is done in adolescence, as the last permanent teeth are erupting. There are good reasons for this choice. At this point, for most patients there is sufficient growth remaining to potentially improve jaw relationships, and all permanent teeth including the second molars can be controlled and placed in a more or less final position. From a psychosocial point of view, patients in this age group often are reaching the point of self-motivation for treatment, which is evident in their improved ability to cooperate during appointments and in appliance and oral hygiene care. A reasonably short course of treatment in early adolescence, as opposed to two stages of early and later treatment, fits well within the cooperative potential of patients and families. Even though not all patients respond well to treatment during adolescence, treatment at this time remains the "gold standard" against which other approaches must be measured. For a child with obvious malocclusion, does it really make sense to start treatment early in the preadolescent years? Obviously, that will depend on the specific problems. Issues in the timing of treatment are reviewed in detail in Chapter 8.

The complexity of the treatment that would be required affects treatment planning especially in the context of who should do the treatment. In orthodontics as in all areas of dentistry, it makes sense that the less complex cases would be selected for treatment in general or family practice, while the more complex cases would be referred to a specialist. The only difference in orthodontics is that traditionally the family practitioner has referred a larger number of orthodontic cases. In family practice, an important issue is how you rationally select patients for treatment or referral. Chapter 7 includes a formal scheme for separating patients most appropriate for treatment in family practice from those more likely to require complex treatment.

The third special issue is the predictability of treatment with any particular method. If alternative methods of treatment are available—as usually is the case—which one should be chosen? Data gradually are accumulating to allow choices to be based on evidence of outcomes rather than anecdotal reports and the claims of advocates of particular approaches. Existing data for treatment outcomes, as a basis for deciding what the best treatment approach might be, are emphasized in Chapter 8.

Finally, treatment planning must be an interactive process. No longer can the doctor decide, in a paternalistic way, what is best for a patient. Both ethically and practically, patients must be involved in the decision-making process. Ethically, patients have the right to control what happens to them in treatment—treatment is something done for them, not to them. Practically, the patient's compliance is likely to be a critical issue in success or failure, and there is little reason to select a mode of treatment that the patient would not support. Informed consent, in its modern form, requires the involvement of the patient in the treatment planning process. This is emphasized in the procedure for presenting treatment recommendations to patients in Chapter 7.

The logical sequence for treatment planning, with these issues in mind, is:

1. Prioritization of the items on the orthodontic problem list, so that the most important problem receives highest priority for treatment
2. Consideration of possible solutions to each problem, with each problem evaluated for the moment as if it were the only problem the patient had
3. Evaluation of the interactions among possible solutions to the individual problems
4. Development of alternative treatment approaches, with consideration of benefits to the patient vs. risks, costs, and complexity
5. Determination of a final treatment concept, with input from the patient and parent, and selection of the specific therapeutic approach (appliance design, mechanotherapy) to be used.

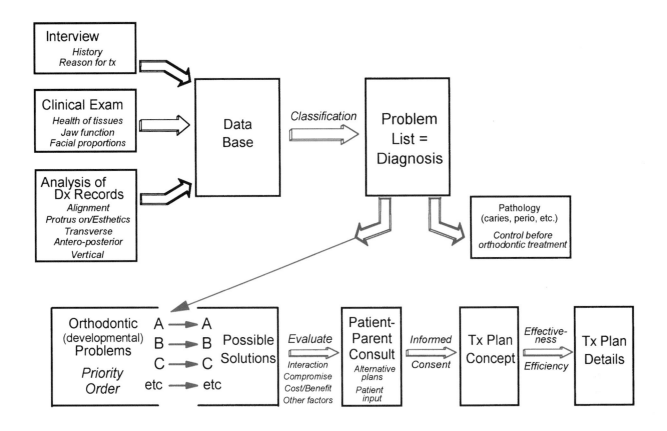

This process culminates with a level of patient-parent understanding of the treatment plan that provides informed consent to treatment. In most instances, after all, orthodontic treatment is elective rather than required. Rarely is there a significant health risk from no treatment, so functional and esthetic benefits must be compared to risks and costs. Interaction with the patient is required to develop the plan in this way.

This diagnosis and treatment planning sequence is illustrated diagrammatically in the figure above.

The chapters of this section address both the important issues and the procedures of orthodontic diagnosis and treatment planning. Chapter 6 focuses on the diagnostic database and the steps in developing a problem list. Chapter 7 addresses the issues of timing and complexity, reviews the principles of treatment planning and evaluates treatment possibilities for preadolescent, adolescent and adult patients. Chapters 6 and 7 provide an overview of orthodontic diagnosis and treatment planning that every dentist needs. Chapter 8 goes into greater depth relative to decisions that often are made in specialty practice. In it, we examine the quality of evidence on which clinical decisions are based, discuss controversial areas in current treatment planning with the goal of providing a consensus judgment to the extent this is possible, and outline treatment for patients with special problems related to injury or congenital problems like cleft lip and palate.

CHAPTER

6

Orthodontic Diagnosis: The Development of a Problem List

THE PROBLEM-ORIENTED APPROACH

In diagnosis, whether in orthodontics or other areas of dentistry or medicine, it is important not to concentrate so closely on one aspect of the patient's overall condition that other significant problems are overlooked. In a medical context, if a patient has an acute infection, it nevertheless is important to detect that he or she is also suffering from diabetes. In an orthodontic context, it is important not to characterize the dental occlusion while overlooking a jaw discrepancy, developmental syndrome, periodontal prob-lem, or systemic disease. The natural bias of any specialist (and one does not have to be a dental specialist to already take a very specialized point of view) is to characterize problems in terms of his or her own special interest. This bias must be recognized and consciously resisted. Diagnosis, in short, must be comprehensive, not focused only on a single aspect of what in many instances can be a complex situation. Orthodontic diagnosis requires a broad overview of the patient's situation.

The problem-oriented approach to diagnosis and treatment planning has been widely advocated in medicine and dentistry as a way to overcome the tendency to concentrate on only one part of a patient's problem. The essence of the problem-oriented approach is the development of a comprehensive database of pertinent information so that no problems will be overlooked. From this database, the list of problems that is the diagnosis is abstracted.

For orthodontic purposes, the database may be thought of as derived from three major sources: (1) patient questioning, (2) clinical examination of the patient, and (3) evaluation of diagnostic records, including dental casts, radiographs, and photographs. Since all possible diagnostic records will not be obtained for all patients, one of the goals of clinical examination is to determine what additional information is required. The steps in assembling an adequate database are presented below in sequence. A discussion of which diagnostic records are needed is included.

At all stages of the diagnostic evaluation, a specialist may seek more detailed information than would a generalist, and in fact this is a major reason for referring a patient to a specialist. The specialist is particularly likely to obtain more extensive diagnostic records, which may not be readily available to a generalist. In orthodontics, cephalometric radiographs are an example. Nevertheless, the basic approach is the same. A competent generalist will follow the same sequence of steps in evaluating a patient, as well as in planning treatment, if he or she will provide that aspect of the patient's care.

In the material that follows, the minimum examination that any generalist should employ for any patient with an orthodontic problem is indicated, and then supplemental information likely to be needed by specialists is discussed. Because direct input into computers is rapidly replacing traditional written chart entries, the information is organized as it might be for computer entry, and illustrations of computer screens (which also could be printed pages) are shown in several instances.

QUESTIONNAIRE/INTERVIEW

The first step in the interview process should be to establish the patient's chief complaint, usually by a direct question to the patient or parent. In orthodontic specialty practice, it can be quite helpful to use a form to begin the process of finding out exactly why this particular patient has sought consultation, especially if facial esthetics may be a concern (Figure 6-1). Further information should be sought in three major areas: (1) medical and dental history, (2) physical growth status, and (3) motivation, expectations, and other sociobehavioral factors.

Patient Name: Date:

Are you interested in: (Please indicate all that apply)
[ ] Information
[ ] Treatment at this time
[ ] Clarification of previously received or conflicting information

If your child's teeth were to be changed, how would you like them changed?
[ ] Upper teeth   Forward/Backward
[ ] Lower teeth   Forward/Backward
[ ] Upper teeth up because gums show too much
[ ] Close spaces   Upper/Lower
[ ] Straighten crowded teeth   Upper/Lower
[ ] Improve the appearance of chipped/cracked/stained/dark/pointed teeth

Do you realize that growth has a strong influence on the success of orthodontic treatment?
Yes _____ No _____

Is it likely that your son or daughter will be an early maturer or late maturer?
Early _____ Late _____

How tall do you think this child will be when growth is completed? ___ ft ___ inches

Are you aware that orthodontic treatment can to some extent alter facial appearance?
Yes _____ No _____

If any features of the face could be changed, what would you like to see:
[ ] Upper lip   Forward/Backward
[ ] Lower lip   Forward/Backward
[ ] Upper jaw   Forward/Backward
[ ] Lower jaw   Forward/Backward
[ ] Chin   Larger/Smaller
[ ] Nose   Larger/Smaller/Different Shape

Would you prefer that facial appearance NOT be discussed in front of your child?
Yes _____ No _____

Is there any significant family history of jaw or teeth problems?

Are you interested in improving the appearance of the teeth at this time even if more treatment will be needed later? Yes _____ No _____

_____   _____
          Signature   Relationship to Patient

FIGURE 6-1 "Why are you here" and "Why now" are important questions at the initial orthodontic interview. A form of this type that patients or parents fill out in advance can be very helpful in determining what they really want. (Adapted from Dr. Alan Bloore.)

Chief Complaint

There are two logical reasons for patient concern about the alignment and occlusion of the teeth: impaired dentofacial esthetics that can lead to psychosocial problems and impaired function. It is important to establish their relative importance to the patient. The dentist should not assume that esthetics is the patient's major concern just because the teeth appear unesthetic. Nor should the dentist focus on the functional implications of, for instance, a crossbite with a lateral shift without appreciating the patient's concern about what seems to be a trivial space between the maxillary central incisors. A series of leading questions, beginning with, "Tell me what bothers you about your face or your teeth," may be necessary to clarify what is important to the patient. The dentist may or may not agree with the patient's assessment—that judgment comes later. At this stage the objective is to find out what is important to the patient.

Medical and Dental History

Orthodontic problems are almost always the culmination of a developmental process, not the result of a pathologic process. As the discussion in Chapter 5 illustrates, often it is difficult to be certain of the etiologic process, but it is important to establish the cause of malocclusion if this can be done, and at least to rule out some of the possible causes. A careful medical and dental history is needed for orthodontic patients both to provide a proper background for understanding the patient's overall situation and to evaluate specific orthodontically related concerns.

The outline of an appropriate medical and dental history is presented in Figure 6-2. A number of the items are annotated to explain their implications for an orthodontic patient.

Two areas deserve a special comment. First, although most children with condylar fractures recover uneventfully, remember that a growth deficit related to an old condylar injury is the most probable cause of facial asymmetry (Figure 6-3). It has become apparent in recent years that early fractures of the condylar neck of the mandible occur more frequently than was previously thought (see Chapter 5). A mandibular fracture in a child often is overlooked in the aftermath of an accident that caused other trauma, so a jaw injury may not have been diagnosed at the time. Although old jaw fractures have particular significance, trauma to the teeth may also affect the development of the occlusion and should not be overlooked.

Second, it is important to note whether the patient is on long-term medication of any type, and if so, for what purpose. This may reveal systemic disease or metabolic problems that the patient did not report in any other way. Chronic medical problems in adults or children do not contraindicate orthodontic treatment if the medical problem is under control, but special precautions may be necessary if orthodontic treatment is to be carried out. For example, or-

thodontic treatment would be possible in a patient with controlled diabetes but would require especially careful monitoring, since the periodontal breakdown to which these individuals are susceptible might be accentuated by orthodontic forces (see Chapter 8). In adults being treated for arthritis or osteoporosis, high doses of prostaglandin inhibitors or resorption-inhibiting agents may impede orthodontic tooth movement (see Chapter 10).

Physical Growth Evaluation

A second major area that should be explored by questions to the patient or parents is the individual's physical growth status. This is important for a number of reasons, not the least of which is the gradient of facial growth discussed in Chapters 2 to 4. Rapid growth during the adolescent growth spurt facilitates tooth movement, but significant growth modification may not be possible in a child who is beyond the peak of the growth spurt.

Growth Charts.   For normal youths who are approaching puberty, questions about how rapidly the child has grown recently, whether clothes sizes have changed, whether there are signs of sexual maturation, and when sexual maturation occurred in older siblings usually provide the necessary information about where the child is on the growth curve. Valuable information can also be obtained from clinical examination, particularly from observing the stage of secondary sexual characteristics (see below). In many instances, height-weight records and the child's progress on standard growth charts (see Figures 2-4 and 2-5) can be obtained from the pediatrician. If a child is being followed for referral to an orthodontist at the optimum time, or by an orthodontist for observation of growth before beginning treatment, recording height and weight changes in the dental office provides important insight into growth status. Occasionally, a more precise assessment of whether a child has reached the adolescent growth spurt is needed, and a radiograph of the hand and wrist to assess the patient's stage of bone ossification can be helpful.

Hand-Wrist Radiographs.   Hand-wrist radiographs have been used for the calculation of skeletal age for many years (see Figure 3-46). The ossification and development of the carpal bones of the wrist, the metacarpals of the hands, and the phalanges of the fingers form a chronology of skeletal development. A satisfactory hand-wrist radiograph can be made utilizing a standard cephalometric cassette and a dental x-ray or the cephalometric x-ray source. In use, the overall pattern observed in the hand-wrist film is compared with age standards in a reference atlas[1] to obtain a skeletal age for the patient. In addition, the status of certain specific landmarks such as the ulnar sesamoid or hamate bones can be used to obtain an estimate of the timing of the adolescent growth spurt.[2]

The primary indication for a hand-wrist film is a child with a skeletal Class II problem whose chronologic age suggests that adolescence should be well advanced, but who

MEDICAL HISTORY
(Child/Adolescent)

PATIENT NAME: _____   DATE: _____

BIRTH DATE: _____

Name of your child's physician: _____   Office Phone: _____

Address of your child's physician: _____   Date of last exam: _____

1.   Is your child in good health? .... Yes   No   Don't know

2.   Does your child have a health problem? .... Yes   No   Don't know

      If yes, explain: _____

3.   Has your child ever been hospitalized, had general anesthesia, or emergency room

      visits? .... Yes   No   Don't know

      If yes, explain: _____

4.   Are your child's immunizations up to date? .... Yes   No   Don't know

5.   Does your child have allergies to medications (drugs), medical products (latex), or the environment

      (dust, mites, pollen, mold)? .... Yes   No   Don't know

      If yes, please list: _____

6.   List past medications taken by child: _____

7.   List daily medications child is now taking: _____

8.   Has your child ever had or been treated by a physician for:

Check one for each condition

Yes	No	?		Yes	No	?	
			a. Problems at birth				p. Cancer
			b. Heart murmur				q. Cerebral palsy
			c. Heart disease				r. Seizures
			d. Rheumatic fever				s. Asthma
			e. Anemia				t. Cleft lip/palate
			f. Sickle cell anemia				u. Speech or hearing problems
			g. Bleeding/hemophilia				v. Eye problems/contact lenses
			h. Blood transfusion				w. Skin problems
			i. Hepatitis				x. Tonsil/adenoid/sinus problems
			j. AIDS or HIV+				y. Sleep problems
			k. Tuberculosis				z. Emotional/behavior problems
			l. Liver disease				aa. Radiation therapy
			m. Kidney disease				bb. Growth problems
			n. Diabetes				cc. Attention deficit disorders
			o. Arthritis				

9.   Has your child had any recent rapid growth? _____ If so, how much? _____

10.   Parents: (Father) Ht: _____ Wt: _____   (Mother) Ht: _____ Wt: _____

11.   Older brothers and sisters: (1) Ht: _____ Wt: _____ (2) Ht: _____ Wt: _____ (3) Ht: _____ Wt: _____

12.   Females: Has menstruation begun? _____ If yes, when? _____ Pregnant? _____

      Using birth control pills? _____

13.   If yes to any above, please explain this or any other problem:_____

      _____

14.   Child's grade in school: _____ Child's school: _____

15.   Do you consider your child to be (check one): Advanced in learning ___   Progressing normally ___

      Slow learner ___

FIGURE 6-2   Form for obtaining medical/dental history for young orthodontic patients. A separate but similar form is needed for adult patients. Annotated comments, explaining why some of the questions are asked, are placed immediately below the form and are keyed by number to the question to which they refer.

Continued

DENTAL HISTORY

16.   What is your main concern about your child's dental condition? _____

17.   Has your child been to a dentist before? No Yes If yes, date of last visit: _____

18.   Regular dentist's name: _____

19.   Check one for each condition:

Yes	No	?	
			a. Has your child ever had dental x-rays? Date of last x-rays? _____
			b. Will your child be uncooperative? If yes, explain: _____
			c. Has your child experienced any complications following dental treatment? If yes, explain: _____
			d. Has your child had cavities and / or toothaches?
			e. Are your child's teeth sensitive to temperature or food?
			f. Did you or your child ever get instructions in brushing?
			g. Do your child's gums bleed when brushed?
			h. Does your child use fluoride products: rinses, drops, tabs?
			i. Does or has your child had any clicking or pain in the jaw joint?
			j. Does or has your child had any problems opening or closing their mouth?
			k. Has your child inherited any family facial or dental characteristics? If yes, explain: _____
			l. Has your child ever injured his/her teeth?
			m. Has your child ever injured his/her jaws or face?
			n. Does or did your child use a pacifier?
			o. Does or did your child suck his/her fingers or thumb?

20.   Does your child have any other dental problems we should know about? _____ Please explain: ___
_____

21.   Whom may we thank for referring you to our office? _____

22.   PERSON COMPLETING THIS FORM: Signature _____
          Relationship to patient: _____

ANNOTATIONS ON SELECTED QUESTIONS

2. This helps establish the patient's social-emotional status.

3. This helps establish a history of trauma.

4. In the instance of oral-facial trauma the DPT status is critical. Soft tissue injury is increased with appliances in place.

5. This helps identify allergies to all types of allergens. One must also consider latex used in dental treatment gloves and elastics. This sensitivity is increasing rapidly in the population.

8b,c,d,f: These patients need antibiotic coverage during banding and debanding procedures.

8g,h,i,j,k. With modern infection control procedures, these patients can be treated, but the treatment may need to be modified.

8o. This may relate to mandibular growth and development.

8p. This will help determine treatments using radiation or chemotherapy that can alter dental development, jaw growth, or somatic growth, depending on the site of the lesion and the treatment.

8x. This can help with evaluation of respiratory problems and tooth sensitivity.

8aa. Radiation therapy to the jaws can greatly alter local dental and skeletal development. The risks of osteoradioecrosis is also a risk in these patients depending on the radiation dosage and the type of treatment under consideration.

8bb. Some children with growth problems may be treated with growth hormones, which can have implications for growth modification treatment timing. In some cancer patients, growth hormones can be part of the post-radiation treatment regime. This, too, can affect treatment timing.

8cc. Attention Deficit Disorders can be treated with numerous drugs. The affect on growth of some of these medications is unclear.

9-12. These questions help establish growth status and timing. Birth control pills can be rendered ineffective by antibiotics used for SBE prevention and oral infections. Patients should be alerted to this problem.

16. The chief complaint is critical to determine why the patient is seeking care. This must be considered carefully in the planning of the treatment.

19a. Reduction in unnecessary radiation is critical to the highest quality care. Many practitioners will request films as part of the examination procedures. Patients seeking second opinions often have already had some records obtained.

19g. Orthodontic treatment in the face of periodontal disease, either acute or chronic, is contraindicated until the disease stage is either controlled or reversed.

19i. A previous history of TMJ problems or treatment merits pretreatment investigation.

19j. Limitations or problems with opening or closing can indicate TMJ problems.

19k. Familial tendency is indicated in some skeletal patterns, and missing teeth have a documented genetic component.

19l. Dental trauma may have implications during tooth movement due to the increased possibility of root resorption.

19n,o. Habits may explain some aspects of the malocclusion.

22. This helps establish the authenticity of the historian.

FIGURE 6-2, cont'd

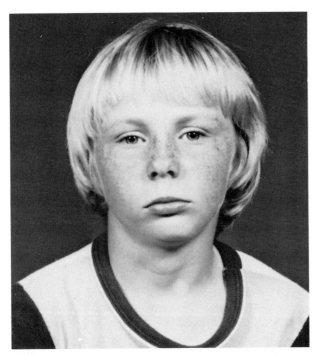

FIGURE 6-3 Facial asymmetry developed in this boy after fracture of the left mandibular condylar process at age 5, because scarring in the fracture area prevented normal translation of the mandible on that side during growth (see Chapter 2). Trauma is a frequent cause of asymmetry of this type.

is somewhat immature sexually and who would benefit from orthodontic treatment to modify growth if that were possible (i.e, if the child had not yet reached the peak of the adolescent growth spurt). If the hand-wrist film shows delayed skeletal development, the growth spurt probably still is in the future; if the skeletal age indicates considerable maturity, adolescent growth of the jaws probably has already occurred. Hand-wrist radiographs are less useful in establishing other factors that sometimes are important clinically, such as a patient's position on the growth curve before or after puberty, or whether jaw growth has subsided to adult levels in a teenager with mandibular prognathism. Serial cephalometric radiographs offer the most accurate way to determine whether growth has stopped or is continuing.

Social and Behavioral Evaluation

Social and behavioral evaluation should explore several related areas: the patient's motivation for treatment, what he or she expects as a result of treatment, and how cooperative or uncooperative the patient is likely to be.

Motivation for seeking treatment can be classified as external or internal. External motivation is that supplied by pressure from another individual, as with a reluctant child who is being brought for orthodontic treatment by a determined mother or an older patient who is seeking alignment of incisor teeth because her boyfriend (or his

girlfriend) wants the teeth to look better. Internal motivation, on the other hand, comes from within the individual and is based on his or her own assessment of the situation and desire for treatment. Even quite young children can encounter difficulties in their interaction with others because of their dental and facial appearance,[3] which sometimes produces a strong internal desire for treatment. Other children with apparently similar malocclusions seem to perceive no problem, and therefore are less motivated internally.[4] Older patients usually are aware of functional or psychosocial difficulties related to their malocclusion, and so are likely to have some component of internal motivation.[5,6]

It is rare to find purely internal motivation, especially in children who do many things because a dominant adult requires it. Self-motivation for treatment often develops at adolescence. Nevertheless, even in a child it is important for a patient to have a component of internal motivation. Cooperation is likely to be much better if the child genuinely wants treatment for himself or herself, rather than just putting up with it to please a parent. The child or adult who feels that the treatment is being done *for* him will be a much more receptive patient than one who views the treatment as something being done *to* him. Often it is necessary to follow up the questions, "Do you think you need braces?" and "Why?" to establish what the motivation really is. In doing this, of course, it is important to keep in mind the psychosocial developmental stages described in Chapter 2. Establishing motivation in a preadolescent child, mid-adolescent teenager, and adult requires different styles of communication.

What the patient expects from treatment is very much related to the type of motivation and should be explored carefully with adults, especially those with primarily cosmetic problems. If the incisor teeth are irregular, and it turns out that the young adult expects social adjustment problems to be solved after the teeth are straight, he or she may be a poor risk for orthodontic treatment. It is one thing to undertake to correct a diastema between the maxillary incisors to improve the patient's appearance and dental function, and something else to do this so the patient will now experience greater social or job success. If the social problems continue after treatment, as is quite likely, the orthodontic treatment may become a focus for resentment.

Cooperation is more likely to be a problem with a child than an adult. Two factors are important in determining this: (1) the extent to which the child sees the treatment as a benefit, as opposed to something else he or she is required to undergo; and (2) the degree of parental control. A resentful and rebellious adolescent, particularly one with ineffective parents, is especially likely to become a problem in treatment. It is important to take the time to understand what the patient perceives his or her problems to be, and if necessary, to help the patient appreciate the reality of the situation (see the final section of Chapter 2).

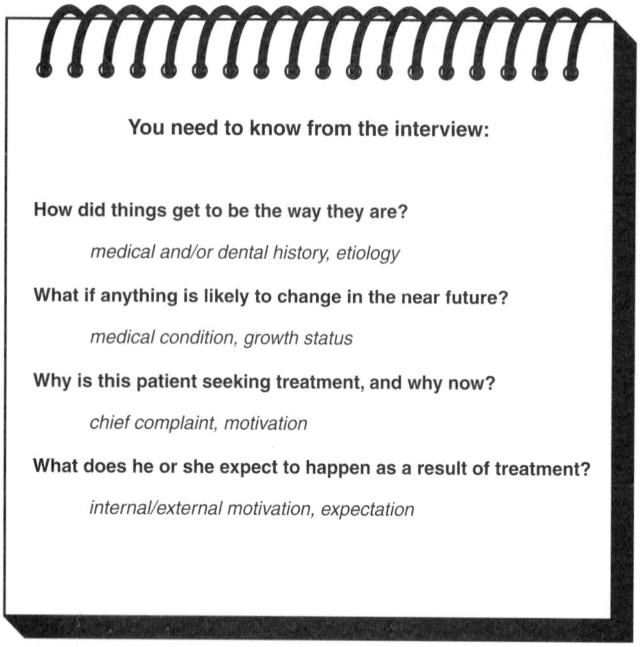

FIGURE 6-4 The key points for investigation during the initial orthodontic interview.

The important points to be evaluated at the interview of a prospective orthodontic patient are summarized in Figure 6-4.

CLINICAL EVALUATION

There are two goals of the orthodontic clinical examination: (1) to evaluate and document oral health, jaw function, and facial esthetics; and (2) to decide which diagnostic records are required.

Evaluation of Oral Health

The health of oral hard and soft tissues must be assessed for potential orthodontic patients as for any other. The general guideline is that any problems of disease or pathology must be under control before orthodontic treatment of developmental problems begins. This includes medical problems, dental caries or pulpal pathology, and periodontal disease.

It sounds trivial to say that the dentist should not overlook missing teeth—and yet almost every dentist, concentrating on details rather than the big picture, has done just that on some occasion. It is particularly easy to fail to notice a missing or supernumerary lower incisor. At some point in the evaluation, count the teeth to be sure they are all there.

In the periodontal evaluation, there are two major points of interest: indications of active periodontal disease and potential or actual mucogingival problems. Any orthodontic examination should include gentle probing through the gingival sulci, not to establish pocket depths but to detect any areas of bleeding. Bleeding on probing indicates

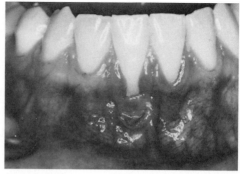

FIGURE 6-5 Dehiscence of soft tissue around a lower incisor after orthodontic alignment of the previously irregular teeth. This is likely to occur when there is inadequate attached gingiva and is much easier to prevent with a free gingival graft or other periodontal therapy than to correct later.

active disease, which must be brought under control before other treatment is undertaken. Inadequate attached gingiva around crowded incisors indicates the possibility of tissue dehiscence developing when the teeth are aligned, especially with nonextraction (arch expansion) treatment (Figure 6-5). The interaction between periodontic and orthodontic treatment for both children and adults is discussed in Chapter 8.

Evaluation of Jaw and Occlusal Function

Three aspects of function require evaluation: mastication (including but not limited to swallowing), speech and the presence or absence of temporomandibular (TM) joint problems. It is important to note in the beginning whether the patient has normal coordination and movements. If not, as in an individual with cerebral palsy or other types of gross incoordination, normal adaptation to the changes in tooth position produced by orthodontics may not occur, and the equilibrium effects discussed in Chapter 5 may lead to post-treatment relapse.

Patients with malocclusion often have difficulty in normal mastication. In severe cases patients often have learned to avoid certain foods that are hard to incise and chew, and cheek and lip biting may occur during mastication. More often, a greater degree of effort is required to allow the individual to chew effectively. If asked, patients report such problems and indicate that after orthodontic treatment they can chew better. Unfortunately, there are almost no reasonable diagnostic tests to evaluate function in this sense, so it is difficult to be quantitative about the degree of masticatory handicap and difficult to document functional improvement. Swallowing is almost never affected by malocclusion. It has been suggested that lip and tongue weakness may indicate problems in normal swallowing, but there is no evidence to support this contention (see Chapter 5). Measuring lip strength or how hard the patient can push with the tongue therefore adds little or nothing to the diagnostic evaluation.

Speech problems can be related to malocclusion, but normal speech is possible in the presence of severe anatomic

TABLE 6-1 *Speech Difficulties Related to Malocclusion*

Speech sound	Problem	Related malocclusion
/s/, /z/ (sibilants)	Lisp	Anterior open bite, large gap between incisors
/t/, /d/ (linguoalveolar stops)	Difficulty in production	Irregular incisors, especially lingual position of maxillary incisors
/f/, /v/ (labiodental fricatives)	Distortion	Skeletal Class III
th, sh, ch (linguodental fricatives) (voiced or voiceless)	Distortion	Anterior open bite

---

BOX 6-1

SCREENING EXAM FOR JAW FUNCTION (TMJ)

Jaw function/TM joint
  complaint now: [] No   [] Yes
  If yes, specify: _____
History of pain: [] No   [] Yes _____duration
History of sounds: [] No   [] Yes _____duration
TM joint tenderness
  to palpation: [] No   [] Yes   [] Right
                                               [] Left
Muscle tenderness to palpation: [] No   [] Yes
  If yes, where? _____
Range of Motion: Maximum opening_____mm
                       Right excursion _____mm
                       Left excursion   _____mm
                       Protrusion   _____mm

---

distortions. Speech difficulties in a child, therefore, are unlikely to be solved by orthodontic treatment. Specific relationships are outlined in Table 6-1. If a child has a speech problem and the type of malocclusion related to it, a combination of speech therapy and orthodontics may help. If the speech problem is not listed as related to malocclusion, orthodontic treatment may be valuable in its own right but is unlikely to have any impact on speech.[7]

Sleep disorders may be related to severe mandibular deficiency, and occasionally this functional problem is the reason for seeking orthodontic consultation. The relationship is discussed briefly in Chapter 5. Both the diagnosis and management of sleep disorders requires an interdisciplinary team and should not be attempted independently in a dental office setting.[8]

Jaw function is more than TM joint function, but evaluation of the TM joints is an important aspect of the diagnostic workup. A form for recording routine clinical examination of TM joint function is shown in Box 6-1. As a general guideline, if the mandible moves normally, its function is not severely impaired, and by the same token, restricted movement usually indicates a functional problem.[9] For that reason, the most important single indicator of joint function is the amount of maximum opening. Palpating the muscles of mastication and TM joints should be a routine part of any dental examination, and it is important to note any signs of TM joint problems such as joint pain, noise, or limitation of opening.

For orthodontic purposes, any lateral or anterior shifts of the mandible on closure are of special interest. Because the articular eminence is not well developed in children, it can be quite difficult to find the sort of positive "centric relation" position that can be determined in adults. Nevertheless, it is important to note whether the mandible shifts laterally or anteriorly when a child closes. A child with an apparent unilateral crossbite usually has a bilateral narrowing of the maxillary arch, with a shift to the unilateral crossbite position. It is vitally important to verify this during the clinical examination, or to rule out a shift and confirm a true unilateral crossbite. Similarly, many children and adults with a skeletal Class II relationship and an underlying skeletal Class II jaw relationship will position the mandible forward in a "Sunday bite," making the occlusion look better than it really is. Sometimes an apparent Class III relationship results from a forward shift to escape incisor interferences in what is really an end-to-end relationship (Figure 6-6). These patients are said to have pseudo-Class III malocclusion.

Occlusal interferences with functional mandibular movements, though of interest, are less important than they would be if treatment to alter the occlusion were not being contemplated. Balancing interferences, presence or absence of canine protection in lateral excursions, and other such factors take on greater significance if they are still present when the occlusal changes produced by orthodontic treatment are nearing completion.

Evaluation of Facial Proportions

The first step in evaluating facial proportions is to take a good look at the patient, examining him or her for developmental characteristics and a general impression. With faces as with everything else, looking too quickly at the details carries the risk of missing the big picture.

Assessment of Developmental Age. During the examination of the face, in a step particularly important for children around the age of puberty when most orthodontic treatment is carried out, the patient's developmental age should be assessed. Everyone becomes a more or less accurate judge of other people's ages—we expect to come

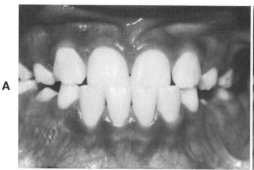 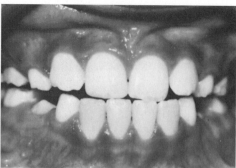

FIGURE 6-6   The anterior crossbite in this 10-year-old child (**A**) results largely from an anterior shift of the mandible because of incisor interferences (**B**). This shift into anterior crossbite is often referred to as a pseudo-Class III relationship because it frequently is not a reflection of a true Class III jaw relationship.

within a year or two simply by observing the other person's facial appearance. Occasionally, we are fooled, as when we say that a 12-year-old girl looks 15, or a 15-year-old boy looks 12. With adolescents, the judgment is of physical maturity. This is valuable information when orthodontic treatment is contemplated because the stage of physical maturity correlates well with how much jaw growth remains. Before sexual maturity, continuing growth can be expected; after sexual maturity, much less growth is anticipated.

The attainment of recognizable secondary sexual characteristics for girls and boys and the correlation between stages of sexual maturation and facial growth are discussed in Chapter 4, and are summarized in Table 6-2. The degree of physical development is much more important than chronologic age in determining how much growth remains.

In some children, it is apparent that a discrepancy between chronologic and maturational age exists, but it is not clear where on the developmental scale the child should be placed. Remember that dental age often differs from the other developmental ages, and so it can happen that the stage of dental development is quite different from chronologic age or the other developmental ages. In this circumstance, as discussed above in the interview section of this chapter, a hand-wrist radiograph can be used to establish the child's skeletal age more clearly.

Facial Esthetics vs. Facial Proportions.   Because a major reason for orthodontic treatment is to overcome psychosocial difficulties relating to facial and dental appearance, evaluating esthetics is an important part of the clinical examination. Esthetics, unfortunately, is very much in the eye of the beholder. It helps to recast the purpose of this part of the clinical evaluation as an evaluation of facial proportions, not esthetics per se. Distorted and asymmetric facial features are a major contributor to facial esthetic problems, whereas proportionate features are acceptable if not always beautiful. An appropriate goal for the facial examination therefore is to detect disproportions.

TABLE 6-2   *Adolescent Growth Stages vs. Secondary Sexual Characteristics*

Girls Total duration of adolescent growth: 3½ years	

Stage 1
Beginning of
    adolescent growth
	Appearance of breast buds,
	    initial pubic hair

Stage 2 *(about 12 months later)* Peak velocity in height	Noticeable breast development, axillary hair, darker/more abundant pubic hair
Stage 3 *(12-18 months later)* Growth spurt ending	Menses, broadening of hips with adult fat distribution, breasts completed

Boys Total duration of adolescent growth: 5 years	

Stage 1
Beginning of
    adolescent growth
	"Fat spurt" weight gain,
	    feminine fat distribution

Stage 2 *(about 12 months later)* Height spurt beginning	Redistribution/reduction in fat, pubic hair, growth of penis
Stage 3 *(8-12 months later)* Peak velocity in height	Facial hair appears on upper lip only, axillary hair, muscular growth with harder/more angular body form
Stage 4 *(15-24 months later)* Growth spurt ending	Facial hair on chin and lip, adult distribution/color of pubic and axillary hair, adult body form

Frontal Examination.   The first step in analyzing facial proportions is to examine the face in frontal view for proportional widths of the eyes/nose/mouth (Figure 6-7) and for bilateral symmetry (Figure 6-8). A small degree of bilateral facial asymmetry exists in essentially all normal individuals. This can be revealed most readily by comparing the real full face photograph with composites consisting of two right or two left sides (Figure 6-9). This "normal asymmetry," which usually results from a small size difference between the two sides, should be distinguished from a chin or nose that deviates to one side, which can produce severe disproportion and esthetic problems (see Figure 6-3). Similarly, mild deviations in vertical proportions often occur but should be distinguished from disproportionate shortness or length of the middle or lower thirds of the face.

Prior to the advent of cephalometric radiography, dentists and orthodontists often used anthropometric measurements (i.e., measurements made directly during the clinical examination) to help establish facial proportions. Although this method was largely replaced by cephalometric analysis, it still can be quite useful. Clinical anthropometry (Figure 6-10) has undergone a revival recently because of Farkas' studies of Canadians of northern European origin,[10] which provided the data for Tables 6-3 and 6-4.

Note that some of the measurements in Table 6-3 could be made on a cephalometric film, but many could not. When there are questions about facial proportions, it is better to make the measurements clinically rather than waiting for the cephalometric analysis, because soft-tissue as well as hard-tissue distances can be important.

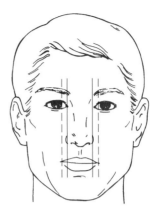

FIGURE 6-7   For ideal proportions from the frontal view, the width of the base of the nose should be approximately the same as the interinnercanthal distance (*solid line*), while the width of the mouth should approximate the distance between the irises (*dotted line*).

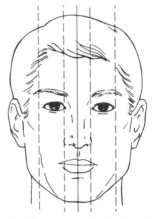

FIGURE 6-8   Facial symmetry in the frontal plane.

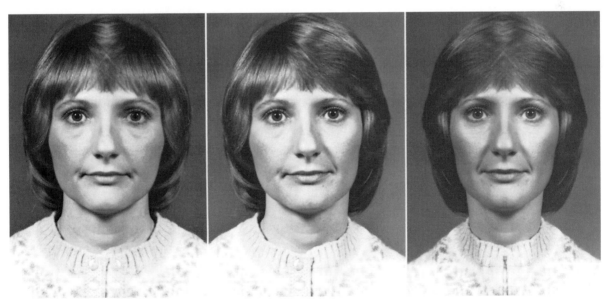

FIGURE 6-9   Composite photographs to indicate normal facial asymmetry. The true photograph is in the center. On the right is a composite of the two right sides, while on the left is a composite of the two left sides. This technique dramatically illustrates the difference in the two sides, which occurs normally.

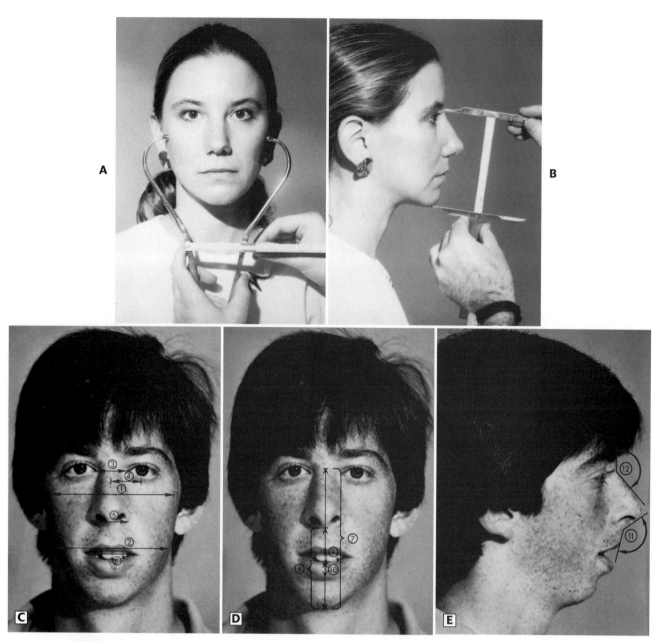

FIGURE 6-10   Facial measurements for anthropometric analysis are made with either bow calipers (**A**) or straight calipers (**B**). **C** to **E**, Frequently-used facial anthropometric measurements (numbers are keyed to Table 6-3).

The proportional relationship of height and width (the facial index), more than the absolute value of either height or width, establishes the overall facial type. A patient with an anterior open bite and a large lower face height may or may not have too long a lower face, depending on facial width. The normal values for the facial index and other proportions that may be clinically useful are shown in Table 6-4. Differences in facial types and body types obviously must be taken into account when facial proportions are assessed, and variations from the average ratios can be compatible with good facial esthetics. An important point, however, is to avoid treatment that would change the ratios in

the wrong direction—for example, treatment with interarch elastics that could rotate the mandible downward in a patient whose face already is too long for its width.

Another important point for the full face examination is the relationship of the dental midline of each arch to the skeletal midline of that jaw (i.e., the lower incisor midline related to the midline of the mandible, and the upper incisor midline related to the midline of the maxilla). Dental casts will show the relationship of the midlines to each other if the casts are trimmed to represent the occlusion but provide no information about the dental-skeletal midlines. This must be recorded during the clinical examination.

TABLE 6-3 *Facial Anthropometric Measurements (Young Adults)*

Parameter	Male	Female
1. Zygomatic width (zy-zy) (mm)	137 (4.3)	130 (5.3)
2. Gonial width (go-go)	97 (5.8)	91 (5.9)
3. Intercanthal distance	33 (2.7)	32 (2.4)
4. Pupil-midfacial distance	33 (2.0)	31 (1.8)
5. Nasal base width	35 (2.6)	31 (1.9)
6. Mouth width	53 (3.3)	50 (3.2)
7. Face height (N-gn)	121 (6.8)	112 (5.2)
8. Lower face height (subnasale-gn)	72 (6.0)	66 (4.5)
9. Upper lip vermilion	8.9 (1.5)	8.4 (1.3)
10. Lower lip vermilion	10.4 (1.9)	9.7 (1.6)
11. Nasolabial angle (degrees)	99 (8.0)	99 (8.7)
12. Nasofrontal angle (degrees)	131 (8.1)	134 (1.8)

Data from Farkas LG: *Anthropometry of the head and face in medicine,* New York, 1981, Elsevier Science Publishing Co.
Measurements are illustrated in Figure 6-10.
Standard deviation is in parenthesis.

TABLE 6-4 *Facial Indices (Young Adults)*

Index	Measurements	Male	Female
Facial	n-gn/zy-zy	88.5 (5.1)	86.2 (4.6)
Mandible-face width	go-go/zy-zy	70.8 (3.8)	70.1 (4.2)
Upper face	n-sto-/zy-zy	54.0 (3.1)	52.4 (3.1)
Mandibular width— face height	go-go/n-gn	80.3 (6.8)	81.7 (6.0)
Mandibular	sto-gn/go-go	51.8 (6.2)	49.8 (4.8)
Mouth-face width	ch-ch × 100/zy-zy	38.9 (2.5)	38.4 (2.5)
Lower face— face height	sn-gn/n-gn	59.2 (2.7)	58.6 (2.9)
Mandible-face height	sto-gn/n-gn	41.2 (2.3)	40.4 (2.1)
Mandible-upper face height	sto-ng/n-sto	67.7 (5.3)	66.5 (4.5)
Mandible-lower face height	sto-ng/sn-gn	69.6 (2.7)	69.1 (2.8)
Chin-face height	sl-gn × 100/sn-gn	25.0 (2.4)	25.4 (1.9)

From Farkas LG, Munro JR: *Anthropometric facial proportions in medicine,* Springfield, Ill, 1987, Charles C Thomas.
Standard deviation is in parenthesis.

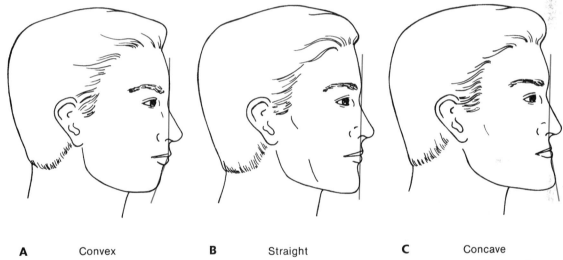

A Convex   **B** Straight   **C** Concave

FIGURE 6-11 Profile convexity or concavity results from a disproportion in the size of the jaws, but does not by itself indicate which jaw is at fault. A convex facial profile (**A**) indicates a Class II jaw relationship, which can result from either a maxilla that projects too far forward or a mandible too far back. A concave profile (**C**) indicates a Class III relationship, which can result from either a maxilla that is too far back or a mandible that protrudes forward.

Profile Analysis. A careful examination of the profile yields the same information, though in less detail, as that obtained from analysis of lateral cephalometric radiographs. For diagnostic purposes, particularly to separate out patients with severe disproportions, careful clinical evaluation is adequate. For this reason, the technique of facial profile analysis has sometimes been called the "poor man's cephalometric analysis." This is a vital diagnostic technique for all dentists. It must be mastered by all those who will see patients for primary care in dentistry, not just by orthodontists.

There are three goals of facial profile analysis, approached in three clear and distinct steps. These are:
1. Establishing whether the jaws are proportionately positioned in the anteroposterior plane of space. This step requires placing the patient in natural head position—either sitting upright or standing, but not reclining in a dental chair, and looking at a distant object. With the head in this position, note the relationship between two lines, one dropped from the bridge of the nose to the base of the upper lip, and a second one extending from that point downward to the chin (Figure 6-11). These line

segments should form a nearly straight line. An angle between them indicates either profile convexity (upper jaw prominent relative to chin) or profile concavity (upper jaw behind chin). A convex profile therefore indicates a skeletal Class II jaw relationship, whereas a concave profile indicates a skeletal Class III jaw relationship.

If the profile is approximately straight, it does not matter whether it slopes either anteriorly (anterior divergence) or posteriorly (posterior divergence) (Figure 6-12). Divergence of the face (the term was coined by the eminent orthodontist-anthropologist Milo Hellman[11]) is influenced by the patient's racial and ethnic background. American Indians and Orientals, for example, tend to have an anteriorly divergent face, whereas whites of northern European ancestry are likely to be posteriorly divergent. A straight profile line, regardless of whether the face is divergent, does not indicate a problem. Convexity or concavity does.

2. Evaluation of lip posture and incisor prominence. Detecting excessive incisor protrusion (which is relatively

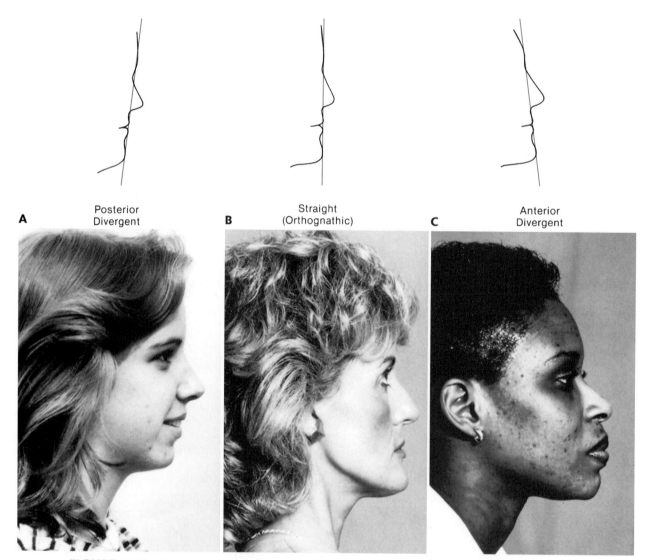

A Posterior Divergent   **B** Straight (Orthognathic)   **C** Anterior Divergent

FIGURE 6-12   Divergence of the face is defined as an anterior or posterior inclination of the lower face relative to the forehead. Divergence of a straight profile line does not indicate facial or dental disproportions. To some extent, this is a racial and ethnic characteristic. It must be distinguished from the profile convexity or concavity that does indicate disproportions. **A,** A girl of northern European descent with a posteriorly divergent profile. She has only minimal overjet and no complaints about facial esthetics. **B,** A woman of eastern European descent with a very straight profile, producing a strong chin but with normal dental occlusion and acceptable facial esthetics. **C,** A woman of African descent with an anteriorly divergent profile (which is not uncommon among both blacks and Orientals), again with normal occlusion and acceptable esthetics. (**B** and **C,** From Proffit WR, White RP: *Surgical-orthodontic treatment,* St Louis, 1991, Mosby.)

common) or retrusion (which is rare) is important because of the effect on space within the dental arches. If the incisors protrude, they align themselves on the arc of a larger circle as they lean forward, whereas if the incisors are upright or retrusive, less space is available (Figure 6-13). In the extreme case, incisor protrusion can produce ideal alignment of the teeth instead of severely crowded incisors, at the expense of lips that protrude and are difficult to bring into function over the protruding teeth. This is *bimaxillary dentoalveolar protrusion*, meaning simply that in both jaws the teeth protrude (Figure 6-14). Dentists often refer to the condition as just *bimaxillary protrusion*, a simpler term but a misnomer since it is not the jaws but the teeth that protrude. (Physical anthropologists use bimaxillary protrusion to describe faces in which both jaws are prominent relative to the cranium. Such a face would have an anteriorly divergent profile if jaw sizes were proportional.)

Determining how much incisor prominence is too much can be difficult but is simplified by understanding the relationship between lip posture and the position of the incisors. The teeth protrude excessively if (and only if) two conditions are met: (1) the lips are prominent and everted, and (2) the lips are separated at rest by more than 3 to 4 mm (which is sometimes termed *lip incompetence*). In other words, excessive protrusion of the incisors is revealed by prominent lips that are separated when they are relaxed, so that the patient must strain to bring the lips together over the protruding teeth (Figure 6-15). For such a patient, retracting the teeth tends to improve both lip function and facial esthetics. On the other hand, if the lips are prominent but close over the teeth without strain,

the lip posture is largely independent of tooth position. For that individual, retracting the incisor teeth would have little effect on lip function and would produce little or no change in lip prominence.

Like facial divergence, lip prominence is strongly influenced by racial and ethnic characteristics. Whites of northern European backgrounds often have relatively thin lips, with minimal lip and incisor prominence. Whites of southern European and middle eastern origin normally have more lip and incisor prominence than their northern cousins. Greater degrees of lip and incisor prominence normally occur in Orientals and in blacks. This difference simply means that a degree of lip and incisor prominence normal for many whites would be considered retrusive for many Orientals or blacks, while a lip and tooth position normal for blacks would be excessively protrusive for most whites.

Lip posture and incisor prominence should be evaluated by viewing the profile with the patient's lips relaxed. This is done by relating the upper lip to a true vertical line passing through the concavity at the base of the upper lip (soft tissue point A) and by relating the lower lip to a similar true vertical line through the concavity between the lower lip and chin (soft tissue point B) (see Figure 6-14). If the lip is significantly forward from this line, it can be

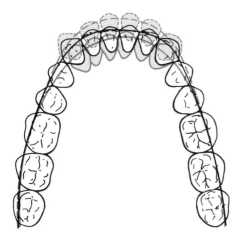

FIGURE 6-13 If the incisors flare forward, they can align themselves along the arc of a larger circle, which provides more space to accommodate the teeth and alleviates crowding. Conversely, if the incisors move lingually, there is less space, and crowding becomes worse. For this reason, crowding and protrusion of incisors must be considered two aspects of the same thing: how crowded and irregular the incisors are reflects both how much room is available and where the incisors are positioned relative to supporting bone.

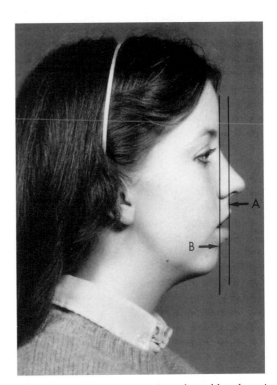

FIGURE 6-14 Lip prominence is evaluated by observing the distance that each lip projects forward from a true vertical line through the depth of the concavity at its base (soft tissue points A and B) (i.e., a different reference line is used for each lip, as shown here). Lip prominence of more than 2 to 3 mm in the presence of lip incompetence (excessive separation of the lips at rest), as in this girl, indicates dentoalveolar protrusion.

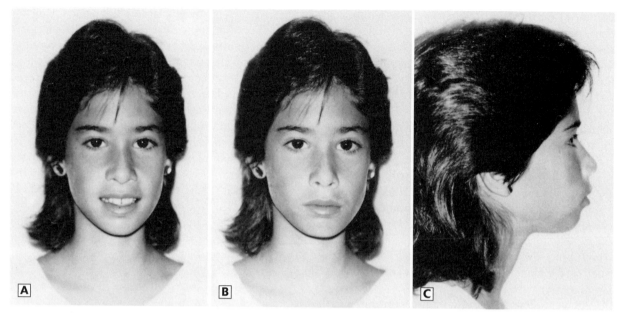

FIGURE 6-15 Bimaxillary dentoalveolar protrusion is seen in the facial appearance in three ways: **A,** excessive separation of the lips at rest (lip incompetence). The general guideline is that lip separation at rest should be not more than 4 mm; **B,** excessive effort to bring the lips into closure (lip strain): and **C,** prominence of lips in the profile view. Remember that all three characteristics must be present to make the diagnosis of dental protrusion, not just the lip protrusion—different people have different degrees of lip prominence, independent of tooth position.

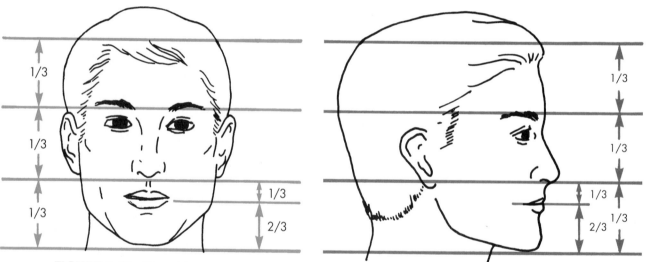

FIGURE 6-16 Vertical facial proportions in the frontal and lateral views. The vertical height of the mid-face, from the supraorbital ridges to the base of the nose, should equal the height of the lower face. Within the lower face, the mouth should be about one third of the way between the base of the nose and the chin.

judged to be prominent; if the lip falls behind the line, it is retrusive. If the lips are both prominent and incompetent (separated by more than 3 to 4 mm), the anterior teeth are excessively protrusive.

Note that this important information cannot be obtained from measurements on cephalometric radiographs, because it is not determined by the relationship of the teeth to their supporting bone, but instead by soft tissue relationships that must be evaluated clinically.

3. Evaluation of vertical facial proportions and mandibular plane angle. Vertical proportions can be observed during the full face examination but sometimes can be seen more clearly in profile. A well-proportioned face can be divided into vertical thirds as shown in Figure 6-16. In the clinical examination, the inclination of the mandibular plane to the true horizontal should be noted. This is important because a steep mandibular plane angle correlates with long anterior facial vertical dimensions and

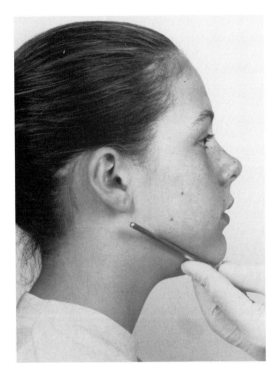

FIGURE 6-17 The mandibular plane angle can be visualized clinically by placing a mirror handle or other instrument along the border of the mandible. For this patient the mandibular plane angle is normal, neither too steep nor too flat.

anterior open bite malocclusion, while a flat mandibular plane angle correlates with short anterior facial height and deep bite malocclusion. The mandibular plane is visualized readily by placing a finger or mirror handle along the lower border (Figure 6-17).

Facial form analysis carried out this way takes only a couple of minutes but provides information that simply is not present from dental radiographs and casts. Such an evaluation by the primary care practitioner is an essential part of the evaluation of every prospective orthodontic patient.

Which Diagnostic Records Are Needed?

Orthodontic diagnostic records are taken for two purposes: to document the starting point for treatment (after all, if you don't know where you started, it's hard to tell where you're going), and to add to the information gathered on clinical examination. The records fall into three major categories: those for (1) evaluation of the teeth and oral structures, (2) evaluation of the occlusion, and (3) evaluation of facial and jaw proportions. The (relatively rare) indications for a hand-wrist radiograph to evaluate skeletal age are discussed previously.

Records for Evaluation of the Teeth and Oral Structures. A major purpose of intraoral photographs, which should be obtained routinely for patients receiving complex orthodontic treatment, is to document the initial condition of the hard and soft tissues. Five standard intraoral photographs are suggested: right, center, and left views with the

TABLE 6-5 *U.S. Public Health Service Guidelines: Dental Radiographic Examination for Pathology*

Condition	Recommended radiographs
Regular dental care No previous caries No obvious pathology History of fluoridation	Panoramic film only
Previous caries Obvious caries	Add bitewings
Deep caries Periodontal disease	Add periapicals, affected area only

From *The selection of patients for x-ray examination: dental radiographic examination,* HHS Pub FDA 88-8273, Rockville, Md, 1987, U.S. Food and Drug Administration, Center for Devices and Radiologic Health.

teeth in occlusion, and maxillary and mandibular occlusal views (see Figure 6-58). Maximum retraction of the cheeks and lips is needed. If there is a special soft-tissue problem (e.g., no attached gingiva in the lower anterior), an additional photograph of that area may be needed.

A panoramic intraoral radiograph is valuable for orthodontic evaluation at any age. The panoramic film has two significant advantages over a series of intraoral radiographs: it yields a broader view and thus is more likely to show any pathologic lesions and supernumerary or impacted teeth, and the radiation exposure is much lower. It also gives a view of the mandibular condyles, which can be helpful, both in its own right and as a screening film to determine if other TM joint radiographs are needed.

The panoramic film should be supplemented with periapical and bitewing radiographs only when their greater detail is required. Current recommendations for dental radiographic screening for pathology are shown in Table 6-5. In addition, for children and adolescents, periapical views of incisors are indicated if there is evidence or suspicion of root resorption. The principle is that periapical films to supplement the panoramic radiograph are ordered only if there is a specific indication for doing so.

Radiographs of the temporomandibular joint should be reserved for patients who have symptoms of dysfunction of that joint that may be related to internal joint pathology. In that case, CT or MRI scans are likely to be more useful than transcranial or laminagraphic TM joint films. Routine TM joint radiographs simply are not indicated for orthodontic patients. Imaging of the TM joint, and recommendations for current practice, are covered in detail by a recent review.[12]

Records for Occlusal Evaluation. Evaluation of the occlusion requires impressions for dental casts or for digitization into computer memory and a record of the occlusion so that the casts or images can be related to each other. For orthodontic diagnosis, maximum displacement of soft tissues, created by maximum extension of the impression, is desired. The inclination of the teeth, not just the location of the crown, is important. If the impression is not well extended, important diagnostic information may be missing.

At the minimum, a wax bite or polysiloxane record of the patient's usual interdigitation (centric occlusion) should be made, and a check should be made to be sure that this does not differ significantly from the retruded position. An anterior shift of 1 to 2 mm from the retruded position is of little consequence, but lateral shifts or anterior shifts of greater magnitude should be noted carefully and a wax bite in an approximate centric relation position should be made for these patients. After the casts are poured, the wax bite is used to trim them so that when the casts are placed on their back, the teeth are in proper occlusion.

Dental casts for orthodontic purposes are usually trimmed so that the bases are symmetric (Figure 6-18) and then are polished. There are two reasons for doing this: (1) If the casts are trimmed so that a symmetric base is oriented to the midline of the palate, it is much easier to analyze arch form and detect asymmetry within the dental arches; (2) Neatly trimmed and polished models are more acceptable for presentation to the patient, as will be necessary during any consultation about orthodontic treatment.

Whether it is necessary or even desirable to mount casts on an articulator as part of an orthodontic diagnostic evaluation is a matter of continuing debate. There are two reasons for mounting casts on articulators. The first is to record and document any discrepancy between the occlusal relations at the initial contact of the teeth (centric relation [CR]) and the relations at the patient's full or habitual occlusion (centric occlusion, [CO]). The second is to record the lateral and excursive paths of the mandible, documenting these and making the tooth relationships during excursions more accessible for study.

Knowing the occlusal relationship in CR, when the condyles are positioned "correctly," obviously is important for orthodontic diagnostic purposes if there is a significant CR-CO difference. Unfortunately, there is no current agreement as to what the "correct" CR position is, though the "muscle-guided" position (the most superior position to which a patient can bring the mandible using his or her own musculature), seems most appropriate for orthodontic purposes. It is now generally accepted that in normal individuals this neuromuscular position is anterior to the most retruded condylar position.[13] Lateral shifts or large anterior shifts are not normal and should be recorded. Articulator-mounted casts are one way, but not the only way, to do that.

The second reason for mounting casts—to record the excursive paths—is very important when restorative dentistry is being planned because the contours of the replacement or restored teeth must accommodate the path of movement. This is less important when tooth positions and jaw relationships will change during treatment.

The current consensus is that for preadolescent and early adolescent patients (i.e., those who have not completed their adolescent growth spurt), there is little point in an articulator mounting. In these young patients, the contours of the TM joint are not fully developed, so that condylar guidance is much less prominent than in adults. The shape of the temporal fossa in an adult reflects function during growth. Thus until mature canine function is reached and the chewing pattern changes from that of the child to the normal adult, completion of the articular eminence and the medial contours of the joint should not be expected (see Chapter 3). In addition, the relationships between the dentition and the joint that are recorded in articulator mountings change rapidly while skeletal growth is continuing and tend to be only of historic interest after orthodontic treatment.

The situation is different when growth is complete or largely complete. In adults with symptoms of temporomandibular dysfunction (clicking, limitation of motion, pain), articulator-mounted casts may be useful to document significant discrepancies between habitual and relaxed mandibular positions. These patients often need therapy to reduce muscle spasm and splinting before the articulator mounting is done. An articulator mounting may also be needed for surgical treatment planning (see Chapter 22).

Records for Evaluation of Facial Proportions.   For any orthodontic patient, facial and jaw proportions, not just dental occlusal relationships, must be evaluated. This can

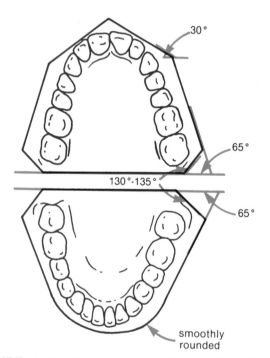

30°
65°
130°-135°
65°
smoothly rounded

FIGURE 6-18   Orthodontic casts have traditionally been trimmed with symmetric bases. The backs are trimmed perpendicular to the midsagittal line, most easily visualized as the midpalatal raphe for most patients. The angles shown for the casts are suggested values; symmetry is more important than the precise angulation.

be done by a careful clinical evaluation of the patient's face, with a recording of positive findings, or by cephalometric radiographs if indicated.

The clinical examination described above provides a record of facial proportions in the form of judgments about frontal and profile relationships. Facial photographs document these findings.

Like all radiographic records, cephalometric films should be taken only when they are indicated. Comprehensive orthodontic treatment almost always requires a lateral cephalometric film, because it is rare that jaw relationships and incisor positions would not be altered during the treatment, and the changes cannot be understood without cephalometric superimpositions. It is irresponsible to undertake growth modification treatment in a child without a pretreatment lateral cephalometric film. For treatment of minor problems in children, or for adjunctive treatment procedures in adults, cephalometric radiographs usually are not required, simply because jaw relationships and incisor positions would not be changed significantly. The major indication for a frontal (posteroanterior, not anteroposterior) cephalometric film is facial asymmetry—routine posteroanterior cephalometric films are not recommended.

Minimal diagnostic records for any orthodontic patient consist of dental casts trimmed to represent the oc-clusal relationship, a panoramic radiograph supplemented with appropriate periapical radiographs, and data from facial form analysis. A lateral cephalometric film is needed for all patients except those with minor or adjunctive treatment needs.

ANALYSIS OF DIAGNOSTIC RECORDS

Comments on the analysis of intraoral radiographs appear in the previous section on clinical evaluation, as does information about intraoral and facial clinical findings that were recorded photographically. In this section, the focus is on evaluation of space and symmetry within the dental arches by dental cast analysis and on cephalometric analysis of dentofacial relationships.

Cast Analysis: Symmetry and Space

Symmetry.   An asymmetric position of an entire arch should have been detected already in the facial/esthetic examination. An asymmetry of arch form also may be present even if the face looks symmetric. A transparent ruled grid placed over the upper dental arch and oriented to the mid-palatal raphe can make it easier to see a distortion of arch form (Figure 6-19).

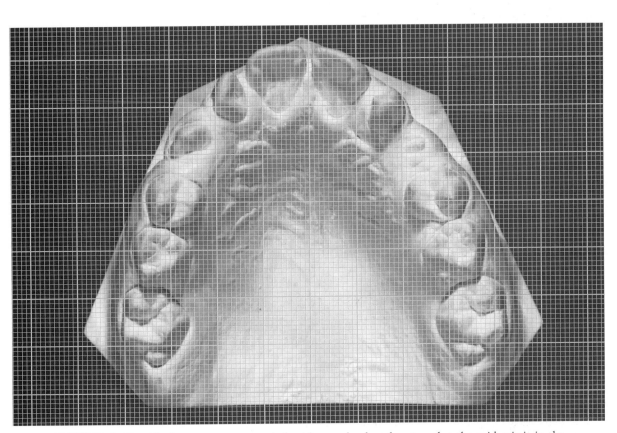

FIGURE 6-19   Placing a transparent ruled grid over the dental cast so that the grid axis is in the midline makes it easier to spot asymmetries in arch form (wider on the patient's left than right, in this example) and in tooth position (molars drifted forward on the right).

Asymmetry within the dental arch, but with symmetric arch form, also can occur. It usually results either from lateral drift of incisors or from drift of posterior teeth unilaterally. The ruled grid also helps in seeing where drift of teeth has occurred. Lateral drift of incisors occurs frequently in patients with severe crowding, particularly if a primary canine was lost prematurely on one side. This often results in one permanent canine being blocked out of the arch while the other canine is nearly in its normal position, with all the incisors shifted laterally. Drift of posterior teeth is usually caused by early loss of a primary molar, but sometimes develops even when primary teeth were exfoliated on a normal schedule.

Alignment (Crowding): Space Analysis. It is important to quantify the amount of crowding within the arches, because treatment varies depending on the severity of the crowding. Space analysis, using the dental casts, is required for this purpose.

Principles of Space Analysis. Since malaligned and crowded teeth usually result from lack of space, this analysis is primarily of space within the arches. Space analysis requires a comparison between the amount of *space available* for the alignment of the teeth and the amount of *space required* to align them properly (Figure 6-20).

The analysis can be done either directly on the dental casts or by computer after appropriate digitization of the arch and tooth dimensions. The dental cast analysis is two-dimensional, and if a computer method is preferred, it is easier and more practical to use an office copying machine to obtain a two-dimensional image of the occlusal view of the dental casts, then digitize from that. A readable and surprisingly accurate image can be obtained by simply placing the casts on the center of the copying machine, avoiding the edges of its image area, where distortions often appear.

Whether the analysis is done manually or in the computer, the first step in space analysis is calculation of space available. This is accomplished by measuring arch perimeter from one first molar to the other, over the contact points of posterior teeth and incisal edge of anteriors. There are two basic ways to accomplish this: (1) by dividing the dental arch into segments that can be measured as straight line approximations of the arch (Figure 6-21), or (2) by contouring a piece of wire (or a curved line on the computer screen) to the line of occlusion and then straightening it out for measurement. The first method is preferred for manual calculation because of its greater reliability. Either method can be used with an appropriate computer program.

The second step is to calculate the amount of space required for alignment of the teeth. This is done by measuring the mesiodistal width of each tooth from contact point to contact point, and then summing the widths of the individual teeth (Figure 6-22). If the sum of the widths of the permanent teeth is greater than the amount of space available, there is an arch perimeter space deficiency and

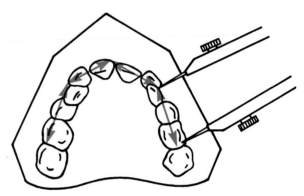

FIGURE 6-21 Space available can be measured most easily by dividing the dental arch into 4 straight line segments as shown. Each segment is measured individually with a sharp-pointed measuring instrument (dividers, as used in architectural drafting, are best; a sharpened Boley gauge is acceptable).

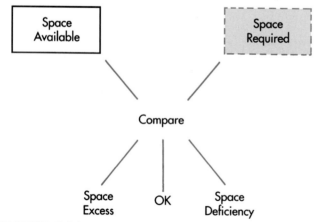

FIGURE 6-20 A comparison of space available versus space required establishes whether a deficiency of space within the arch will ultimately lead to crowding, whether the correct amount of room is available to accommodate the teeth, or whether excess space will result in gaps between the teeth.

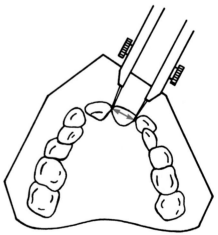

FIGURE 6-22 Space required is the sum of the mesiodistal widths of all individual teeth, measured from contact point to contact point.

crowding would occur. If available space is larger than the space required (excess space), gaps between some teeth would be expected.

Space analysis carried out in this way is based on two important assumptions: (1) the anteroposterior position of the incisors is correct (i.e., the incisors are neither excessively protrusive nor retrusive), and (2) the space available will not change because of growth. Neither assumption can be taken for granted.

With regard to the first assumption, it must be remembered that incisor protrusion is relatively common and that retrusion, though uncommon, does occur. There is an interaction between crowding of the teeth and protrusion or retrusion: if the incisors are positioned lingually (retruded), this accentuates any crowding; but if the incisors protrude, the potential crowding will be at least partially alleviated (see Figure 6-13). Crowding and protrusion are really different aspects of the same phenomenon. In other words, if there is not enough room to properly align the teeth, the result can be crowding, protrusion, or (most likely) some combination of the two. For this reason, information about how much the incisors protrude must be available from clinical examination to evaluate the results of space analysis. This information comes from facial form analysis (or from cephalometric analysis if available).

The second assumption, that space available will not change during growth, is valid for adults but may not be for children. In a child with a well-proportioned face, there is little or no tendency for the dentition to be displaced relative to the jaw during growth, but the teeth often shift anteriorly or posteriorly in a child with a jaw discrepancy. For this reason, space analysis is less accurate and less useful for children with skeletal problems (Class II, Class III, long face, short face) than in those with good facial proportions. This important topic is reviewed in detail in Chapter 4 (see Figures 4-16 to 4-22 for illustrations of the interaction between jaw growth pattern and the relationship of the teeth to the jaw).

Even in children with well-proportioned faces, the position of the permanent molars changes when primary molars are replaced by the premolars (see Chapter 3 for a detailed review). If space analysis is done in the mixed dentition, it is necessary to adjust the space available measurement to reflect the shift in molar position that can be anticipated.

Mixed Dentition Space Analysis: Estimating the Size of Unerupted Permanent Teeth.
For space analysis in the mixed dentition, it also is necessary to estimate the size of the unerupted permanent teeth to calculate the space required. There are three basic approaches for doing this:

1. Measurement of the teeth on radiographs. This requires an undistorted radiographic image, which is more easily achieved with individual periapical films than with panoramic films. Even with individual films, it is often difficult to obtain an undistorted view of the canines, and this inevitably reduces the accuracy. With any type

of radiograph, it is necessary to compensate for enlargement of the radiographic image. This can be done by measuring an object that can be seen both in the radiograph and on the casts, usually a primary molar tooth (Figure 6-23). A simple proportional relationship can then be set up:

$$\frac{\text{True width of primary molar}}{\text{Apparent width of primary molar}} = \frac{\text{True width of unerupted premolar}}{\text{Apparent width of unerupted premolar}}$$

Accuracy is fair to good depending on the quality of the radiographs and their position in the arch. The technique can be used in maxillary and mandibular arches for all ethnic groups.

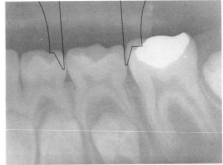
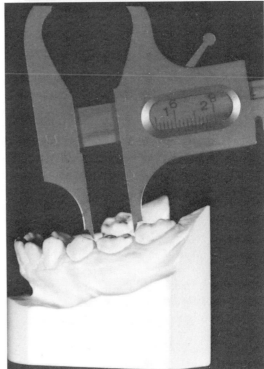

FIGURE 6-23 To correct for magnification in films, the same object is measured on the cast and on the film, which will yield the percentage of magnification. This ratio is used to correct for magnification on unerupted teeth.

TABLE 6-6   *Moyers Prediction Values (75% level)*

Total Mandibular-Incisor Width		19.5	20.0	20.5	21.0	21.5	22.0	22.5	23.0
Predicted width of canine and premolars	Maxilla	20.6	20.9	21.2	21.3	21.8	22.0	22.3	22.6
	Mandible	20.1	20.4	20.7	21.0	21.3	21.6	21.9	22.2

From Moyers RE: *Handbook of orthodontics,* ed 3, Chicago, 1973, Mosby.

BOX 6-2

TANAKA AND JOHNSTON PREDICTION VALUES

One half of the mesiodistal width of the four lower incisors	+ 10.5 m =	estimated width of mandibular canine and premolars in one quadrant
	+ 11.0 mm =	estimated width of maxillary canine and premolars in one quadrant

From Tanaka MM, Johnston LE: *J Am Dent Assoc* 88:798, 1974.

2. Estimation from proportionality tables. There is a reasonably good correlation between the size of the erupted permanent incisors and the unerupted canines and premolars. These data have been tabulated for white American children by Moyers (Table 6-6). To utilize the Moyers prediction tables, the mesiodistal width of the *lower* incisors is measured and this number is used to predict the size of *both* the lower and upper unerupted canines and premolars. The size of the lower incisors correlates better with the size of the upper canines and premolars than does the size of the upper incisors, because upper lateral incisors are extremely variable teeth. Despite a tendency to overestimate the size of unerupted teeth, accuracy with this method is fairly good for the northern European white children on whose data it is based. No radiographs are required, and it can be used for the upper or lower arch.

   Tanaka and Johnston developed another way to use the width of the lower incisors to predict the size of unerupted canines and premolars (Box 6-2). The method has good accuracy despite a small bias toward overestimating the unerupted tooth sizes. It requires neither radiographs nor reference tables (once the method is memorized), which makes it very convenient.

3. Combination of radiographic and prediction table methods. Since the major problem with using radiographic images comes in evaluating the canine teeth, it would seem reasonable to use the size of permanent incisors measured from the dental casts and the size of unerupted premolars measured from the films to predict the size of unerupted canines. A graph developed by Staley and Kerber from Iowa growth data (Figure 6-24) allows canine width to be read directly from the sum of incisor and premolar widths. This method can be used only for the mandibular arch and, of course, requires periapical radiographs. For white children, it is quite accurate.

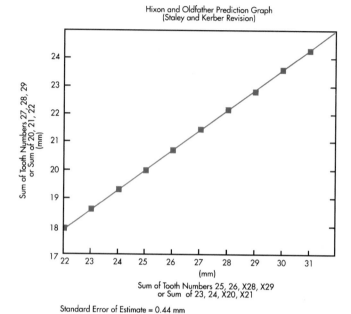

FIGURE 6-24   Graph showing relationship between size of lower incisors measured from cast plus lower first and second premolars measured from radiographs (*x-axis*) and size of canine plus premolars (*y-axis*). (Redrawn from Staley RN, Kerber RE: *Am J Orthod* 78:296-302, 1980.)

Which of these methods is best for an individual patient depends on the circumstances. The prediction tables work surprisingly well when applied to the population group from which they were developed. The Moyers, Tanaka-Johnston, and Staley-Kerber predictions are all based on data from white school children of northern European descent. If the patient fits this population group, the Staley-Kerber method will give the best prediction, followed by the Tanaka-Johnston and Moyers approaches. These methods are superior to measurement from radiographs. On balance, the Tanaka-Johnston method probably is most practical because no radiographs are required and the simple calculation can be printed right on the space analysis form, so that no reference tables must be consulted.

On the other hand, if the patient does not fit the population group, as a black or Oriental would not, direct measurement from the radiographs is the best approach. In addition, if obvious anomalies in tooth size or form are seen in the radiographs, the correlation methods (which assume normal tooth size relationships) should not be used.

A contemporary form for mixed dentition space analysis is shown in Figure 6-25. Note that: (1) a correction for

23.5	24.0	24.5	25.0	25.5	26.0	26.5	27.0	27.5	28.0	28.5	29.0
22.9	23.1	23.4	23.7	24.0	24.2	24.5	24.8	25.0	25.3	25.6	25.9
22.5	22.8	23.1	23.4	23.7	24.0	24.3	24.6	24.8	25.1	25.4	25.7

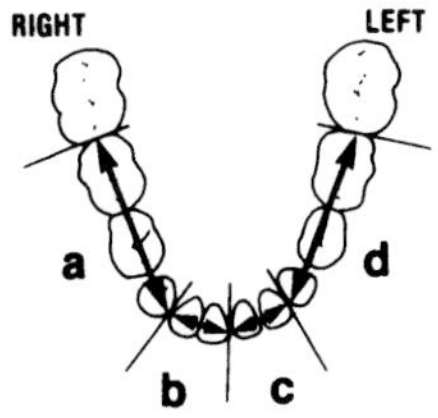

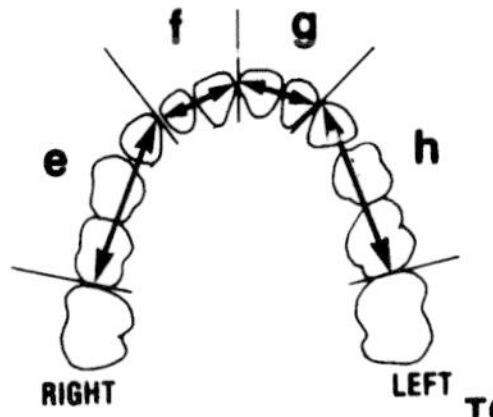

FIGURE 6-25 Space analysis form.

mesial movement of the lower molars following the exchange of the dentition is included, (2) the Tanaka-Johnston method for predicting the size of unerupted canines and premolars is used, and (3) the result from facial form analysis is requested to check for appropriateness of the entire method and for interpretation of the results. This or a similar form can be completed easily and almost automatically on a computer, after appropriate digitization of the arch and tooth measurements.

Tooth Size Analysis.   For good occlusion, the teeth must be proportional in size. If large upper teeth are combined with small lower teeth, as in a denture setup with mismatched sizes, there is no way to achieve ideal occlusion. Although the natural teeth match very well in most individuals, approximately 5% of the population have some degree of disproportion among the sizes of individual teeth. This is defined as *tooth size discrepancy.* An anomaly in the size of the upper lateral incisors is the most common cause, but variation in premolars or other teeth may be present. Occasionally, all the upper teeth will be too large or too small to fit properly with the lower teeth.

Tooth size analysis, sometimes called Bolton analysis after its developer,[14] is carried out by measuring the mesiodistal width of each permanent tooth. A standard table (Table 6-7) is then used to compare the summed widths of the maxillary to the mandibular anterior teeth and the total width of all upper to lower teeth (excluding second and third molars). One advantage of digitizing tooth dimensions for space analysis is that the computer then can quickly provide a tooth size analysis.

A quick check for anterior tooth size discrepancy can be done by comparing the size of upper and lower lateral incisors. Unless the upper laterals are larger, a discrepancy almost surely exists. A quick check for posterior tooth size

discrepancy is to compare the size of upper and lower second premolars, which should be about equal size. A tooth size discrepancy of less than 1.5 mm is rarely significant, but larger discrepancies create treatment problems and must be included in the orthodontic problem list.

Cephalometric Analysis

The introduction of radiographic cephalometrics in 1934 by Hofrath in Germany and Broadbent in the United States provided both a research and a clinical tool for the study of malocclusion and underlying skeletal disproportions (Figure 6-26). The original purpose of cephalomet-

TABLE 6-7   *Tooth Size Relationships*

Maxillary anterior sum of 3-3	Mandibular anterior sum of 3-3	Maxillary total sum of 6-6	Mandibular total sum of 6-6
40	30.9	86	78.5
41	31.7	88	80.3
42	32.4	90	82.1
43	33.2	92	84.0
44	34.0	94	85.8
45	34.7	96	87.6
46	35.5	98	89.5
47	36.3	100	91.3
48	37.1	102	93.1
49	37.8	104	95.0
50	38.6	106	96.8
51	39.4	108	98.6
52	40.1	110	100.4
53	40.9		
54	41.7		
55	42.5		

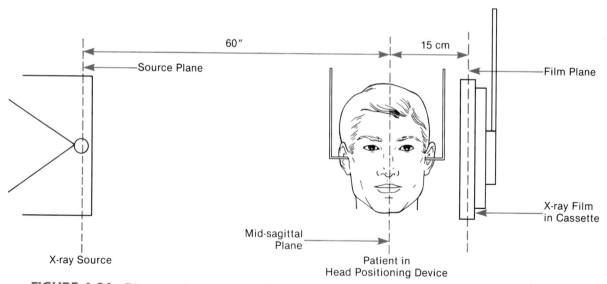

FIGURE 6-26   Diagrammatic representation of the American standard cephalometric arrangement. By convention, the distance from the x-ray source to the subject's midsagittal plane is 5 feet. The distance from the midsagittal plane to the cassette can vary in many machines but must be the same for each patient every time.

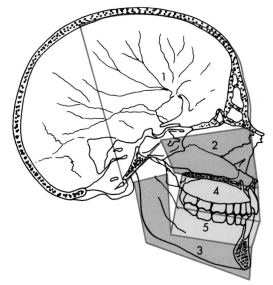

FIGURE 6-27 The functional components of the face, shown superimposed on the anatomic drawing. The cranium and cranial base (*1*), the skeletal maxilla and nasomaxillary complex (*2*), and the skeletal mandible (*3*) are parts of the face that exist whether or not there is a dentition. The maxillary teeth and alveolar process (*4*) and the mandibular teeth and alveolar process (*5*) are independent functional units, which can be displaced relative to the supporting bone of the maxilla and mandible, respectively. The goal of cephalometric analysis is to establish the relationship of these functional components in both the anteroposterior and vertical planes of space.

rics was research on growth patterns in the craniofacial complex. The concepts of normal development presented in Chapters 2 and 3 were largely derived from such cephalometric studies.

It soon became clear, however, that cephalometric films could be used to evaluate dentofacial proportions and clarify the anatomic basis for a malocclusion. The orthodontist needs to know how the major functional components of the face (cranial base, jaws, teeth) are related to each other (Figure 6-27). Any malocclusion is the result of an interaction between jaw position and the position the teeth assume as they erupt, which is affected by the jaw relationships (see Chapter 4 for a discussion of dental compensation or adaptation). For this reason, two apparently similar malocclusions as evaluated from the dental casts may turn out to be quite different when evaluated more completely, using cephalometric analysis to reveal differences in dentofacial proportions.

Another way that radiographic cephalometrics is useful clinically is in recognizing and evaluating changes brought about by orthodontic treatment. Serial cephalometric radiographs taken at intervals before, during, and after treatment can be superimposed to study changes in jaw and tooth positions retrospectively (Figure 6-28). The observed changes result from a combination of growth and

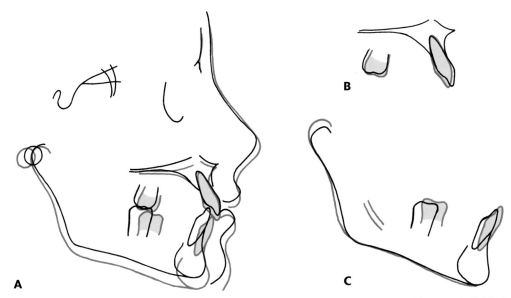

FIGURE 6-28 The three major cephalometric superimpositions showing tracings of the same individual at an earlier (*black*) and later (*red*) time. **A,** Superimposition on the anterior cranial base along the SN line. This superimposition shows the overall pattern of changes in the face, which result from a combination of growth and orthodontic treatment in children receiving orthodontic therapy. Note in this patient that the lower jaw grew downward and forward, while the upper jaw moved straight down. This allowed the correction of the patient's Class II malocclusion. **B,** Superimposition on the maxilla. This view shows changes of the maxillary teeth relative to the maxilla. In this patient's case, minimal changes occurred, the most notable being a forward movement of the upper first molar when the second primary molar was lost. **C,** Superimposition on the mandible, specifically on the inner surface of the mandibular symphysis and the outline of the mandibular canal and unerupted third molar crypts. This superimposition shows both changes of the mandible and changes of the mandibular teeth relative to the mandible. Note that the mandibular ramus increased in length posteriorly, while the condyle grew upward and backward. As would be expected, the mandibular molar teeth moved forward as the transition from the mixed to the early permanent dentition occurred.

treatment (except in nongrowing adults). It is all but impossible to know what is really occurring during treatment of a growing patient without reviewing cephalometric superimpositions, which is the reason that cephalometric radiographs are required for comprehensive orthodontic treatment of children and adolescents.

Cephalometric radiographs are not taken as a screen for pathology, but the possibility of observing pathologic changes on these films should not be overlooked. Occasionally, previously-unsuspected degenerative changes or anomalies in the cervical spine are revealed in a cephalometric radiograph (Figure 6-29; also see Chapter 22), and sometimes other pathologic changes in the skull, jaws, or cranial base can be observed.[15]

For diagnostic purposes, the major use of radiographic cephalometrics is in characterizing the patient's dental and skeletal relationships. In this section, we focus on the use of cephalometric analysis to compare a patient to his or her peers, using population standards. The use of cephalometric predictions to estimate orthodontic and surgical treatment effects is covered in Chapter 8.

Development of Cephalometric Analysis.   Cephalometric analysis is commonly carried out, not on the radiograph itself, but on a tracing or digital model that emphasizes the relationship of selected points. In essence, the tracing or model is used to reduce the amount of information on the film to a manageable level. The common cephalometric landmarks and a typical tracing are shown in Figures 6-30 and 6-31.

Cephalometric landmarks can be represented as a series of points whose coordinates are specified, making it possible to enter cephalometric data in a computer-compatible format. There is an increasing trend to use computers to assist in cephalometric analysis. The increasing power and decreasing cost of small computer systems suggest that computer analysis may be routine in the near future. An adequate digital model is required, which means that 50 to 100 landmark locations should be specified (Figure 6-32).

The principle of cephalometric analysis, however, is not different when computers are used. The goal is to compare the patient with a normal reference group, so that differences between the patient's actual dentofacial relationships and those expected for his or her racial or ethnic group are revealed. This type of cephalometric analysis was first popularized after World War II in the form of the Downs analysis, developed at the University of Illinois and based on skeletal and facial proportions of a reference group of 25 untreated adolescent whites selected because of their ideal dental occlusions.[16]

From the very beginning, the issue of how to establish the normal reference standards was difficult. It seems obvious that patients with severe cranial disproportions

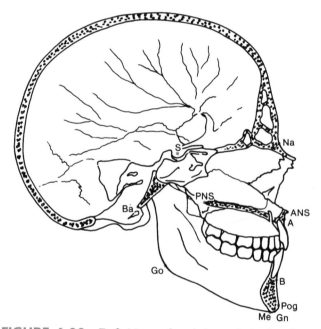

FIGURE 6-30   Definitions of cephalometric landmarks (as they would be seen in a dissected skull): *Point A*, the innermost point on the contour of the premaxilla between anterior nasal spine and the incisor tooth. *ANS* (anterior nasal spine), the tip of the anterior nasal spine (sometimes modified as the point on the upper or lower contour of the spine where it is 3 mm thick: see Harvold analysis). *Point B*, the innermost point on the contour of the mandible between the incisor tooth and the bony chin; *Ba* (basion), the lowest point on the anterior margin of foramen magnum, at the base of the clivus; *Gn* (gnathion), the center of the inferior point on the mandibular symphysis (i.e., the bottom of the chin); *Na* (nasion), the anterior point of the intersection between the nasal and frontal bones; *PNS* (posterior nasal spine), the tip of the posterior spine of the palatine bone, at the junction of the hard and soft palates; *Pog* (Pogonion), the most anterior point on the contour of the chin.

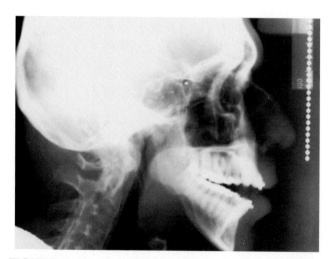

FIGURE 6-29   Cephalometric radiographs of a woman with rheumatoid arthritis who has degenerative changes in both the condylar process of the mandible and the cervical spine. Note the collapse of the upper cervical vertebrae. Cephalometric films should be reviewed routinely for pathologic changes in the head and neck.

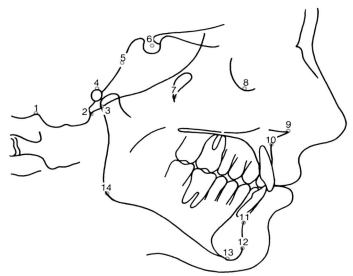

FIGURE 6-31 Definitions of cephalometric landmarks (as seen in a lateral cephalometric tracing): *1. Bo* (Bolton point), the highest point in the upward curvature of the retrocondylar fossa of the occipital bone; *2. Ba* (basion), the lowest point on the anterior margin of the foramen magnum, at the base of the clivus; *3. Ar* (articular), the point of intersection between the shadow of the zygomatic arch and the posterior border of the mandibular ramus; *4. Po* (porion), the midpoint of the upper contour of the external auditory canal (anatomic porion); or, the midpoint of the upper contour of the metal ear rod of the cephalometer (machine porion); *5. SO* (sphenoccipital synchondrosis), the junction between the occipital and basisphenoid bones (if wide, the upper margin); *6. S* (sella), the midpoint of the cavity of sella turcica; *7. Ptm* (pterygomaxillary fissure), the point at the base of the fissure where the anterior and posterior walls meet; *8. Or* (orbitale), the lowest point on the inferior margin of the orbit; *9. ANS* (anterior nasal spine), the tip of the anterior nasal spine (sometimes modified as the point on the upper or lower contour of the spine where it is 3 mm thick; see Harvold analysis); *10. Point A*, the innermost point on the contour of the premaxilla between anterior nasal spine and the incisor tooth; *11. Point B*, the innermost point on the contour of the mandible between the incisor tooth and the bony chin; *12. Pog* (pogonion), the most anterior point on the contour of the chin; *13. Me* (menton), the most inferior point on the mandibular symphysis (i.e., the bottom of the chin); *14. Go* (gonion), the midpoint of the contour connecting the ramus and body of the mandible.

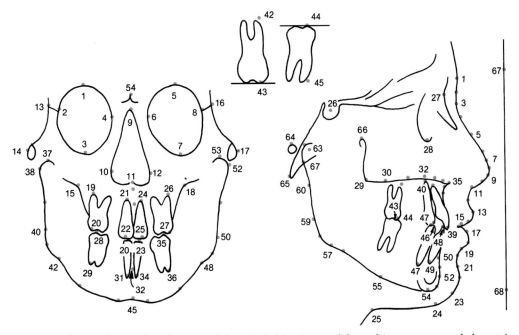

FIGURE 6-32 The standard lateral and frontal digitization models used in a current cephalometric analysis and prediction program (Dentofacial Planner [DFP]). Like other modern programs, DFP allows customization of the digitization model. It provides up to 180 points, more than enough for acceptable analytic accuracy and superimposition.

should be excluded from a normal sample. Since normal occlusion is not the usual finding in a randomly selected population group, one must make a further choice in establishing the reference group, either excluding only obviously deformed individuals while including most malocclusions, or excluding essentially all those with malocclusion to obtain an ideal sample. In the beginning, the latter approach was chosen. Comparisons were made only with patients with excellent occlusion and facial proportions, as in the 25 individuals chosen for the Downs standards. Perhaps the extreme of selectivity in establishing a reference standard was exemplified by Steiner, whose original ideal measurements were reputedly based on one Hollywood starlet. Although the story is apocryphal, if it is true, Dr. Steiner had a very good eye, because recalculation of his original values based on much larger samples produced only minor changes.

The standards developed for the Downs analysis are still useful but have largely been replaced by newer standards based on less rigidly selected groups. A major database for contemporary analysis is the Michigan growth study, carried out in Ann Arbor and involving a typical group of children including those with mild and moderate malocclusions.[17] Other major sources are the Burlington (Ontario) growth study,[18] the Bolton study in Cleveland,[19] and several smaller growth studies, along with numerous specific samples collected in university projects to develop standards for specific racial and ethnic groups.[20]

It can be helpful to conceptualize the goal of cephalometric analysis as evaluating the relationships, both horizontally and vertically, of the five major functional components of the face (see Figure 6-27): the cranium and cranial base, the skeletal maxilla (described as the portions of the maxilla that would remain if there were no teeth and alveolar processes), the skeletal mandible (similarly defined), the maxillary dentition and alveolar process, and the mandibular dentition and alveolar process. In this sense, any cephalometric analysis is a procedure designed to yield a description of the relationships among these functional units.

There are two basic ways to approach this goal. One is the approach chosen originally in the Downs analysis and followed by most workers in the field since that time. This is the use of selected linear and angular measurements to establish the appropriate comparisons. The other is to express the normative data graphically rather than as a series of measurements and to compare the patient's dentofacial form directly with the graphic reference (usually called a template). Then any differences can be observed without making measurements.

Both approaches are employed in contemporary cephalometric analysis. In the sections following, contemporary measurement approaches are discussed first, and then cephalometric analysis via direct comparison with a reference template is presented.

Measurement Analysis

Choice of a Horizontal Reference Line.   In any technique for cephalometric analysis, it is necessary to establish a reference area or reference line. The same problem was faced in the early anthropometric and craniometric studies of the nineteenth century. By the late 1800s, skeletal remains of human beings had been found at many locations and were under extensive study. An international congress of anatomists and physical anthropologists was held in Frankfort, Germany in 1882, with the choice of a horizontal reference line for orientation of skulls an important item for the agenda. At the conference, the Frankfort plane, extending from the upper rim of the external auditory meatus (porion) to the inferior border of the orbital rim (orbitale), was adopted as the best representation of the natural orientation of the skull (Figure 6-33). This Frankfort plane was employed for orientation of the patient from the beginning of cephalometrics and remains commonly used for analysis.

In cephalometric use, however, the Frankfort plane suffers from two difficulties. The first is that both its anterior and posterior landmarks, particularly porion, can be difficult to locate reliably on a cephalometric film. A radiopaque marker is placed on the rod that extends into the external auditory meatus as part of the cephalometric head positioning device, and the location of this marker, referred to as "machine porion" is often used to locate porion. The shadow of the auditory canal can be seen on cephalometric films, usually located slightly above and posterior to machine porion. The upper edge of this canal can also be used to establish "anatomic porion," which gives a slightly different (occasionally, quite different) Frankfort plane (Figure 6-34).

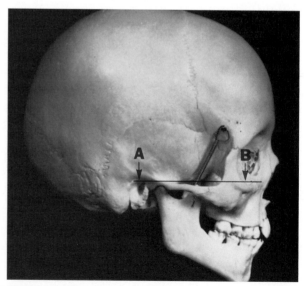

FIGURE 6-33   The Frankfort plane as originally described for orientation of dried skulls. This plane extends from the upper border of the external auditory canal (*A*) (*porion*) anteriorly to the upper border of the lower orbital rim (*orbitale*) (*B*).

An alternative horizontal reference line, easily and reliably detected on cephalometric films, is the line from sella turcica (S) to the junction between the nasal and frontal bones (N). In the average individual, the SN plane is oriented at 6 to 7 degrees to the Frankfort plane. Another way to obtain a Frankfort line is simply to draw it at a specific inclination to SN, usually 6 degrees. However, although this increases reliability and reproducibility, it decreases accuracy.

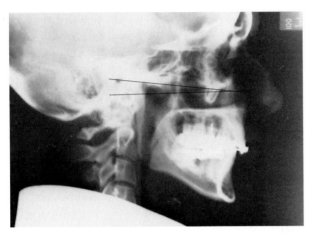

FIGURE 6-34   Using "machine porion," the upper surface of the ear rod of the cephalometric headholder, can give a different Frankfort plane than using "anatomic porion," the upper surface of the shadow of the auditory canal. Both porion and orbitale, the landmarks for the Frankfort plane, are difficult to locate accurately on cephalometric films, making Frankfort a relatively unreliable reference for cephalometric analysis.

The second problem with the Frankfort plane is more fundamental. It was chosen as the best anatomic indicator of the true or physiologic horizontal line. Everyone orients his or her head in a characteristic position, which is established physiologically, not anatomically. As the anatomists of a century ago deduced, for most patients the true horizontal line closely approximates the Frankfort plane. Some individuals, however, show significant differences, up to 10 degrees.

For their long-dead skulls, the anatomists had no choice but to use an anatomic indicator of the true horizontal. For living patients, however, it is possible to use a "true horizontal" line, established physiologically rather than anatomically, as the horizontal reference plane. This approach requires that cephalometric radiographs be taken with the patient in natural head position (i.e., with the patient holding his head level as determined by the internal physiologic mechanism.) This position is obtained when relaxed individuals look at a distant object or into their own eyes in a mirror. The natural head position can be reproduced within 1 or 2 degrees.[21]

In contemporary usage, cephalometric films should be taken in the natural head position (NHP), so that the physiologic true horizontal plane is established (Figure 6-35). Although NHP is not as precisely reproducible as orienting the head to the Frankfort plane, the potential errors from lower reproducibility are smaller than those from inaccurate head orientation.[22] The inclination of SN to the true horizontal plane (or to the Frankfort plane if true horizontal plane is not known) should always be noted, and if the inclination of SN differs significantly from 6 degrees,

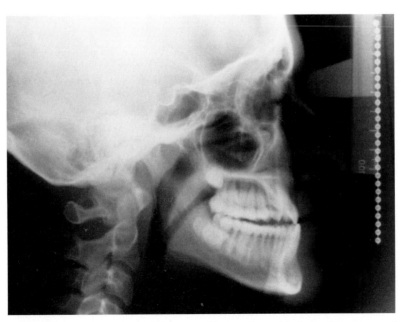

FIGURE 6-35   If the cephalometric film is taken with the patient in natural head position (NHP), a line perpendicular to the true vertical (shown by the image of the freely-suspended chain that is seen on the edge of the film) is the true (physiologic) horizontal line. NHP is preferred in modern cephalometrics to anatomic head positioning.

any measurements based on SN should be corrected by this difference.

Steiner Analysis. The Steiner analysis, developed and promoted by Cecil Steiner in the 1950s,[23] can be considered the first of the modern cephalometric analyses for two reasons: it displayed measurements in a way that emphasized not just the individual measurements but their interrelationship into a pattern, and it offered specific guides for use of cephalometric measurements in treatment planning. Elements of it remain useful today.

In the Steiner analysis, the first measurement is the angle SNA, which is designed to evaluate the anteroposterior position of the maxilla relative to the anterior cranial base (Figure 6-36). The "norm" for SNA is 82 ± 2 degrees. Thus if a patient's SNA were greater than 84 degrees, this would be interpreted as maxillary protrusion, while SNA values of less than 80 degrees would be interpreted as maxillary retrusion. Similarly, the angle SNB is used to evaluate the anteroposterior position of the mandible, for which the norm is 78 ± 2 degrees. This interpretation is valid only if the SN plane is normally inclined to the true horizontal (or if the value is corrected as described above) and the position of N is normal.

The difference between SNA and SNB—the ANB angle—indicates the magnitude of the skeletal jaw discrepancy, and this to Steiner was the measurement of real interest. One can argue, as he did, that which jaw is at fault is of mostly theoretical interest: what really matters is the magnitude of the discrepancy between the jaws that must be overcome in treatment, and this is what the ANB angle measures.

The magnitude of the ANB angle, however, is influenced by two factors other than the anteroposterior difference in jaw position. One is the vertical height of the face. As the vertical distance between nasion and points A and B increases, the ANB angle will decrease. The second is that if the anteroposterior position of nasion is abnormal, the size of the angle will be affected (Figure 6-37). The validity of these criticisms has led to use of different indicators of jaw discrepancy in the later analyses presented in the following sections.

The next step in the Steiner analysis is to evaluate the relationship of the upper incisor to the NA line and both the lower incisor and the chin to the NB line, thus establishing the relative protrusion of the dentition (Figure 6-38). Tweed had earlier suggested that the lower incisor should be positioned at 65 degrees to the Frankfort plane, thus compensating in the incisor position for the steepness of the mandibular plane.[24] In the Steiner analysis, both the angular inclination of each incisor and the millimeter distance of the incisal edge from the vertical line are measured. The millimeter distance establishes how prominent the incisor is relative to its supporting bone, while the inclination indicates whether the tooth has been tipped to its position or has moved there bodily. The prominence of the chin (pogonion) compared with the prominence of the lower incisor establishes the balance between them: the more prominent the chin, the more prominent the incisor can be, and vice versa. This impor-

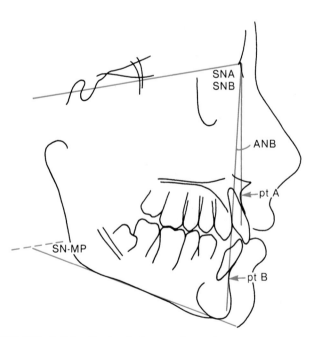

FIGURE 6-36 In the Steiner analysis, the angles *SNA* and *SNB* are used to establish the relationship of the maxilla and mandible to the cranial base, while the *SN-MP* (mandibular plane) angle is used to establish the vertical position of the mandible.

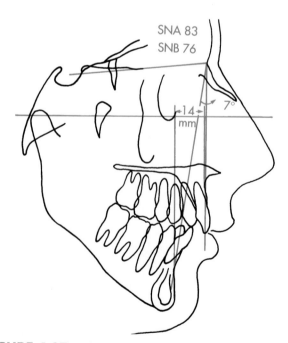

FIGURE 6-37 The *ANB* angle can be misleading when nasion is displaced anteriorly, as in this individual. Note that the *ANB* angle is only 7 degrees, but the *A-B* difference projected to the true horizontal is 14 mm. *ANB*, at best, is an indirect measurement of the *A-B* difference, and must be used with full awareness of its limitations.

tant relationship is often referred to as the *Holdaway ratio*. The final measurement included in the Steiner analysis is the inclination of the mandibular plane to SN, its only indicator of the vertical proportions of the face (see Figure 6-36). Tabulated standard values for five racial groups are given in Table 6-8.

The various measurements incorporated in the Steiner analysis from the beginning were represented graphically as "Steiner sticks," a convenient shorthand for presenting the measurements. Steiner calculated what compromises in

incisor positions would be necessary to achieve normal occlusion when the ANB angle was not ideal. This was a major step in applying cephalometrics to routine treatment planning. The Steiner compromises, and the method for establishing them for any given patient, are illustrated in Figure 6-39. These figures can be helpful in establishing how much tooth movement is needed to correct any malocclusion.

However, it should not be overlooked that relying on tooth movement alone to correct skeletal malocclusion, particularly as the skeletal discrepancies become large, is not necessarily the best approach to orthodontic treatment. It is usually better to correct skeletal discrepancies at their source than to attempt only to achieve a dental compromise or camouflage (see Chapter 8 for further discussion of this important point). It is fair to say that the Steiner compromises reflect the prevailing attitude of Steiner's era, that the effects of orthodontic treatment are almost entirely limited to the alveolar process.

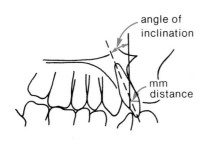

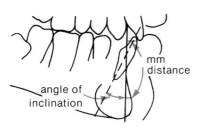

FIGURE 6-38 In the Steiner analysis, the relationship of the upper incisor to the NA line is used to establish the position of the maxillary dentition relative to the maxilla. Both the millimeter distance that the labial surface of the incisor is in front of the line and the inclination of the long axis of the incisor to the line are measured. The position of the lower incisor relative to the mandible is established by similar measurements to the line NB. In addition, the prominence of the chin is established by measuring the millimeter distance from the NB line to pogonion, the most prominent point on the bony chin.

TABLE 6-8 *Cephalometric Values for Selected Groups (All Values in Degrees Except As Indicated)*

	American white	American black	Israeli	Chinese (Taiwan)	Japanese
SNA	82	85	82	82	81
SNB	80	81	78	79	77
ANB	2	4	4	3	4
1-NA	4 mm	7 mm	5 mm	5 mm	6 mm
	22	23	24	24	24
1̄-NB	4 mm	10 mm	6 mm	6 mm	8 mm
	25	34	29	27	31
1 to 1̄	131	119	124	126	120
GoGn-SN	32	32	35	32	34
1̄-MnPl	93	100	93	93	96
1̄-FH	62	51	57	57	57
Y axis	61	63	61	61	62

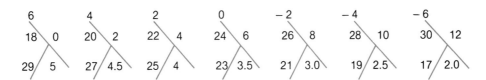

FIGURE 6-39 In the Steiner analysis, the ideal relationship of the incisors is expected when the ANB angle is 2 degrees, as indicated in the third diagram from the left. The inclination of the upper incisor to the NA line in degrees and its prominence in millimeters are shown on the second vertical line (22 degrees and 4 mm for an ANB of 2 degrees). The inclination of the lower incisor to the NB line and its prominence in millimeters are shown on the third line (25 degrees and 4 mm for an ANB of 2 degrees). If the ANB angle is different from 2 degrees, the different positioning of the incisors given by the inclination and protrusion figures will produce a dental compromise that leads to correct occlusion despite the jaw discrepancy. The fact that this degree of compensation in tooth position for jaw discrepancy can be produced by orthodontic treatment does not, of course, indicate that these compromises are necessarily the best possible treatment results.

Sassouni Analysis.   The Sassouni analysis was the first cephalometric method to emphasize vertical as well as horizontal relationships and the interaction between vertical and horizontal proportions.[25] Sassouni pointed out that the horizontal anatomic planes—the inclination of the anterior cranial base, Frankfort plane, palatal plane, occlusal plane, and mandibular plane—tend to converge toward a single point in well-proportioned faces. The inclination of these planes to each other reflects the vertical proportionality of the face (Figure 6-40).

If the planes intersect relatively close to the face and diverge quickly as they pass anteriorly, the facial proportions are long anteriorly and short posteriorly, which predisposes the individual to an open bite malocclusion. Sassouni coined the term *skeletal open bite* for this anatomic relationship. If the planes are nearly parallel, so that they converge far behind the face and diverge only slowly as they pass anteriorly, there is a skeletal predisposition toward anterior deep bite, and the condition is termed *skeletal deep bite*.

In addition, an unusual inclination of one of the planes stands out because it misses the general area of intersection. Rotation of the maxilla down in back and up in front may contribute to skeletal open bite, for instance. The tipped palatal plane reveals this clearly (Figure 6-41).

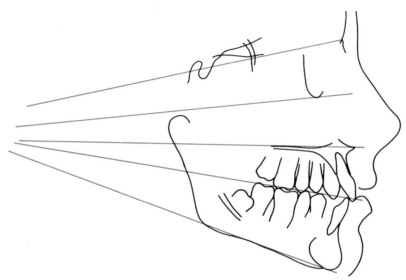

FIGURE 6-40   Sassouni[23] contributed the idea that if a series of horizontal planes are drawn from the SN line at the top to the mandibular plane below they will project toward a common meeting point in a well-proportioned face.

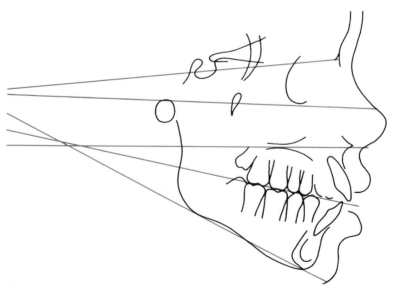

FIGURE 6-41   Inspection of the horizontal planes for this patient makes it clear that the maxilla is rotated downward posteriorly and the mandible rotated downward anteriorly. These rotations of the jaws contribute to an open bite tendency, so the skeletal pattern revealed here is often referred to as "skeletal open bite."

Sassouni evaluated the anteroposterior position of the face and dentition by noting the relationship of various points to arcs drawn from the area of intersection of the planes. In a well-proportioned face, the anterior nasal spine (representing the anterior extent of the maxilla), the maxillary incisor, and the bony chin should be located along the same arc. As with vertical proportions, it could be seen visually if a single point deviated from the expected position, and in what direction. Unfortunately, as a face becomes more disproportionate, it is more and more difficult to establish the center for the arc, and the anteroposterior evaluation becomes more and more arbitrary.

Although the total arcial analysis described by Sassouni is no longer widely used, Sassouni's analysis of vertical facial proportions has become an integral part of the overall analysis of a patient. In addition to any other measurements that might be made, it is valuable in any patient to analyze the divergence of the horizontal planes and to examine whether one of the planes is clearly disproportionate to the others.

Harvold Analysis, Wits Analysis. Both the Harvold and Wits analyses are aimed solely at describing the severity or degree of jaw disharmony. Harvold, using data derived from the Burlington growth study, developed standards for the "unit length" of the maxilla and mandible.[26] The maxillary unit length is measured from the posterior border of the mandibular condyle to the anterior nasal spine, while the mandibular unit length is measured from the same point to the anterior point of the chin (Figure 6-42). The difference between these numbers provides an indication of the size discrepancy between the jaws. In analyzing the difference between maxillary and mandibular

unit lengths, it must be kept in mind that the shorter the vertical distance between the maxilla and mandible, the more anteriorly the chin will be placed for any given unit difference, and vice versa. The position of the teeth has no influence on the Harvold figures (Table 6-9).

The Wits analysis[27] was conceived primarily as a way to overcome the limitations of ANB as an indicator of jaw discrepancy. It is based on a projection of points A and B to the occlusal plane, along which the linear difference between these points is measured. If the anteroposterior position of the jaws is normal, the projections from points A and B will intersect the occlusal plane at very nearly the same point. The magnitude of a discrepancy in the Class II direction can be estimated by how many millimeters the point A projection is in front of the point B projection, and vice versa for Class III.

The Wits analysis, in contrast to the Harvold analysis, is influenced by the teeth both horizontally and vertically—horizontally because points A and B are somewhat influenced by the dentition and vertically because the occlusal plane is determined by the vertical position of the teeth. It is important for Wits analysis that the functional occlusal plane, drawn along the maximum intercuspation of the posterior teeth, be used rather than an occlusal plane influenced by the vertical position of the incisors. Even so, this approach fails to distinguish skeletal discrepancies from problems caused by displacement of the dentition, and if it is used, this limitation must be kept in mind.

The cephalometric approach developed by Ricketts in the 1960s was used in the original computer cephalometric system, and was widely employed at one time. Its greatest weakness was that the normative data for many of the measurements were based on unspecified samples collected by Ricketts. In the half-century that cephalometrics has been used clinically, dozens if not hundreds of other patterns of measurements have been published as named analyses.[20,28] In some of these methods, it is apparent what relationship the measurements are supposed to estimate, and it is clear where the normative data came from. In others both the measurements and the norms take on almost mystical properties. Unless one is careful, it is easy to lose sight of the goal of cephalometric analysis: to estimate the relationships, vertically and horizontally, of the jaws to the cranial base and to each other, and the relationships of the teeth to their supporting bone.

McNamara Analysis. The McNamara analysis, originally published in 1983,[29] still represents the state of the art in cephalometric measurement analysis reasonably well. It combines elements of previous approaches (Ricketts and Harvold) with original measurements to attempt a more precise definition of jaw and tooth positions. In this method, both the anatomic Frankfort plane and the basion-nasion line are used as reference planes. The anteroposterior position of the maxilla is evaluated with regard to its position relative to the "nasion perpendicular," a vertical line extending downward from nasion perpendicular to the

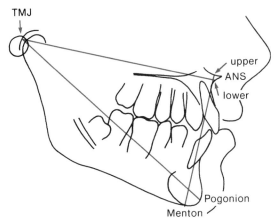

FIGURE 6-42 Measurements used in the Harvold analysis. Maxillary length is measured from *TMJ*, the posterior wall of the glenoid fossa, to lower *ANS*, defined as the point on the lower shadow of the anterior nasal spine where the projecting spine is 3 mm thick. Mandibular length is measured from *TMJ* to prognathion, the point on the bony chin contour giving the maximum length from the temporomandibular joint (close to *pogonion*), while lower face height is measured from *upper ANS*, the similar point on the upper contour of the spine where it is 3 mm thick, to *menton*.

TABLE 6-9 *Harvold Standard Values (mm)*

	Age	Male Mean value	Male Standard deviation	Female Mean value	Female Standard deviation
Maxillary length (temporomandibular point to ANS) (see Figure 6-40)	6	82	3.2	80	3.0
	9	87	3.4	85	3.4
	12	92	3.7	90	4.1
	14	96	4.5	92	3.7
	16	100	4.2	93	3.5
Mandibular length (temporomandibular point to prognathion)	6	99	3.9	97	3.6
	9	107	4.4	105	3.9
	12	114	4.9	113	5.2
	14	121	6.1	117	3.6
	16	127	5.3	119	4.4
Lower face height (ANS-Me)	6	59	3.6	57	3.2
	9	62	4.3	60	3.6
	12	64	4.6	62	4.4
	14	68	5.2	64	4.4
	16	71	5.7	65	4.7

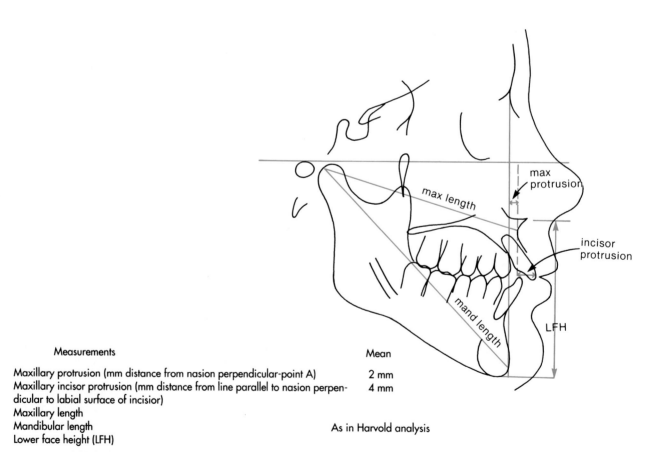

Measurements	Mean
Maxillary protrusion (mm distance from nasion perpendicular-point A)	2 mm
Maxillary incisor protrusion (mm distance from line parallel to nasion perpendicular to labial surface of incisior)	4 mm
Maxillary length	
Mandibular length	As in Harvold analysis
Lower face height (LFH)	

FIGURE 6-43   Measurements used in the McNamara analysis: Maxillary protrusion (mm distance from nasion perpendicular-point A), mean is 2 mm; maxillary incisor protrusion (mm distance from line parallel to nasion perpendicular to labial surface of incisor), mean is 4 mm; maxillary length, mandibular length, and lower face height (LFH) as in Harvold analysis.

Frankfort plane (Figure 6-43). The maxilla should be on or slightly ahead of this line. The second step in the procedure is a comparison of maxillary and mandibular length, using Harvold's approach. The mandible is positioned in space utilizing the lower anterior face height (ANS-menton). The upper incisor is related to the maxilla using a line through point A perpendicular to the Frankfort plane, similar to but slightly different from Steiner's relationship of the incisor to the NA line. The lower incisor is related as in the Ricketts analysis, primarily using the A-pogonion line (Figure 6-44).

The McNamara analysis has two major strengths: (1) It relates the jaws via the nasion perpendicular, in essence projecting the difference in anteroposterior position of the jaws to an approximation of the true vertical line. (Using a true vertical line, perpendicular to the true horizontal rather than anatomic Frankfort, would be better yet; the major reason for not doing so in constructing the analysis is that the cephalometric films from which the normative data were derived were not taken in NHP.) (2) The normative data are based on the well-defined Bolton sample, which is also available in template form, meaning that the McNamara measurements are highly compatible with preliminary analysis by comparison with the Bolton templates.

A major problem with any analysis based on individual measurements is that any one measurement is affected by others within the same face. Not only are the measurements not independent, it is quite possible for a deviation in one relationship to be compensated wholly or partially by changes in other relationships. This applies to both skeletal and dental relationships. Compensatory changes in the dentition to make the teeth fit in spite of the fact that the jaws do not are well known, and often are the goal of orthodontic treatment. Compensatory changes in skeletal components of the face are less well known, but occur frequently, and can lead to incorrect conclusions from measurements if not recognized.

The basic idea of interrelated dimensions leading to an ultimately balanced or unbalanced facial pattern was expressed well by Enlow in the 1960s, in his "counterpart analysis".[30] As Enlow et al pointed out, both the dimensions and alignment of craniofacial components are important in determining the overall facial balance. Consider dimensions first (Figure 6-45). If anterior face height is long, facial balance and proper proportion are preserved if posterior face height and mandibular ramus height also are relatively large. On the other hand, short posterior face height can lead to a skeletal open bite tendency even if anterior face height is normal, because the proportionality is disturbed. The same is true for anteroposterior dimensions. If both maxillary and mandibular lengths are normal but the cranial base is long, the maxilla will be carried forward relative to the mandible and maxillary protrusion will result. By the same token, a short maxilla could compensate perfectly for a long cranial base. Alignment would affect both the vertical and a-p position of the various skeletal units and could compensate for or worsen a tendency toward imbalance. For example, if the maxilla were rotated down

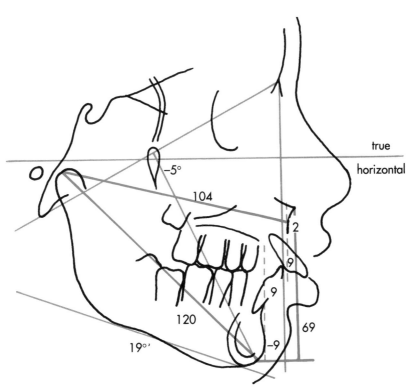

FIGURE 6-44 Analysis of a 12-year-old male, using the McNamara approach.

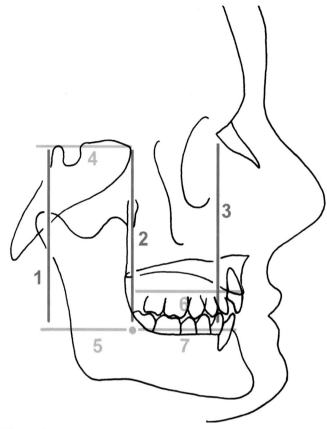

FIGURE 6-45 Enlow's counterpart analysis emphasizes the way changes in proportions in one part of the head and face can either add to increase a jaw discrepancy or compensate so that the jaws fit correctly even though there are skeletal discrepancies. For example, if the maxilla is long (measurement 6), there is no problem if the mandible (7) also is long, but malocclusion will result if the mandibular body length is merely normal. The same would be true for anterior vs posterior vertical dimensions (1-3). If these dimensions match each other, there is no problem, but if they do not, whether short or long, malocclusion will result.

posteriorly, a long ramus and acute gonial angle would compensate and allow normal facial proportions and normal occlusion, but even a slightly short ramus would produce downward-backward mandibular rotation and a long face-open bite tendency.

One way to bring the insights of counterpart analysis into clinical practice is from examination of the patient's proportions versus those of a "normal" template (see at right). Another, developed in Norway[31] and increasingly popular in the 1990s,[32] is the use of "floating point" norms for measurements. The idea is to use standards derived from the individual's facial type rather than relating individual cephalometric values to population means, taking advantage of the correlations between the individual values. Rather than judging normality or abnormality based on individual values, the judgment then would be based on how the values were related to each other—some combinations would be acceptable as normal even if the individual measurements were outside the normal range. Other combinations could be judged as reflecting an abnormal pattern even though the individual measurements were within the

normal range. Assessing skeletal relationships in this way is particularly valuable for patients who are candidates for growth modification therapy or orthognathic surgery.

Template Analysis. In the early years of cephalometric analysis, it was recognized that representing the norm in graphic form might make it easier to recognize a pattern of relationships. The "Moorrees mesh," which was developed in the 1960s but not widely accepted initially because the normative relationships were not clearly established, presents the patient's disproportions as the distortion of a grid. It remains in use at present.[33,34] In recent years, direct comparison of patients with templates derived from the various growth studies has become a reliable method of analysis,[20,28] with the considerable advantage that compensatory skeletal and dental deviations within an individual can be observed directly.

One of the objectives of any analytic approach is to reduce the practically infinite set of possible cephalometric measurements to a manageably small group that can be compared with specific norms and thereby provide useful diagnostic information. From the beginning it was recognized that the measurements for comparison with the norms should have several characteristics. The following were specifically desired: (1) the measurements should be useful clinically in differentiating patients with skeletal and dental characteristics of malocclusion; (2) the measurements should not be affected by the size of the patient (i.e., proportions should be preserved between small and large individuals.) This meant an emphasis on angular rather than linear measurements; and (3) the measurements should be unaffected, or at least minimally affected, by the age of the patient. Otherwise, a different table of standards for each age would be necessary to overcome the effects of growth.

As time passed, it became apparent that a number of measurements that fulfilled the first criterion of diagnostic usefulness did not meet either the second or third criteria. Linear measurements could be used as proportions to make them size-invariant, but more and more linear measurements not used proportionally crept into diagnostic use. Note, for instance, the increasing proportion of linear measurements in the transition from Steiner to Harvold/Wits to McNamara analysis. As excellent samples of children who had participated in growth studies became available and were used for the construction of cephalometric reference standards, it was observed that some relationships previously thought to be invariant with age changed during growth. Like it or not, it was inappropriate with compare cephalometric standards for a 9-year-old child with those of adults, or vice versa. There was obviously an advantage in using standards that changed at various ages, because this allowed a number of clinically useful linear as well as angular measurements to be included.

Any individual cephalometric tracing easily can be represented as a series of coordinate points on an (*x,y*) grid (which is what is done when a film is digitized for computer analysis). But of course cephalometric data from any group also could be represented graphically by calculating the average coordinates of each landmark point, then connecting the points. The resulting average or composite tracing often is referred to as a template.

Templates of this type have been prepared using the data from the major growth studies,[17-20] showing changes in the face and jaws with age. At present, templates exist in two forms: *schematic* (Michigan, Burlington) and *anatomically complete* (Broadbent-Bolton, Alabama). The schematic templates show the changing position of selected landmarks with age on a single template. The anatomically complete templates, a different one for each age, are particularly convenient for direct visual comparison of a patient with the reference group while accounting for age. The Bolton templates, which are readily available (Dept. of Orthodontics, Case-Western Reserve School of Dentistry, Cleveland, Ohio 44106) are most often used for template analysis.

The first step in template analysis, obviously, is to pick the correct template from the set of age-different ones that represent the reference data. Two things must be kept in mind: (1) the patient's physical size and (2) developmental

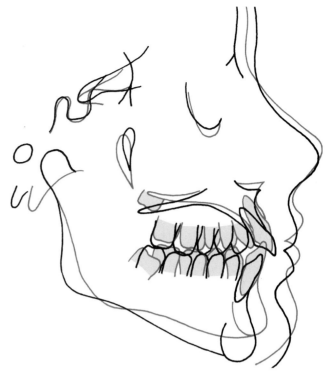

FIGURE 6-46 Cranial base superimposition of the standard Bolton template for age 14 (*red*) on the tracing of a 13-year-old boy. The age 14 template was chosen because it matches cranial base length. Note that from a comparison of the template with this patient, the considerable increase in the lower face height and downward rotation of the mandible can be seen clearly. It also is apparent that the patient's maxilla is rotated down posteriorly. This comparison of a patient's tracing to a template is a direct approach toward describing the relationship of functional facial units.

age. The best plan usually is to select the reference template initially so that the length of the anterior cranial base (of which the SN distance is a good approximation) is approximately the same for the patient and the template and then to consider developmental age, moving forward or backward in the template age if the patient is developmentally quite advanced or retarded. In almost all instances, correcting for differences between developmental and chronologic age also leads to the selection of a template that more nearly approximates the anterior cranial base length.

Analysis using a template is based on a series of superimpositions of the template over a tracing of the patient being analyzed. The sequence of superimpositions follows:

1. Cranial base superimposition, which allows the relationship of the maxilla and mandible to the cranium to be evaluated (Figure 6-46). In general, the most useful approach is to superimpose on the SN line, registering the template over the patient's tracing at nasion rather than sella if there is a difference in cranial base length. (For growth prediction with templates, it is important to use the posterior superimposition points described with the prediction method. For analysis, registering SN at N is usually preferable.)

With the cranial base registered, the anteroposterior and vertical position of maxilla and mandible can be observed and described. It is important at this stage to look, not at the position of the teeth, but at the position of the landmarks that indicate the skeletal units (i.e., anterior nasal spine and point A for the anterior maxilla, posterior nasal spine for the posterior maxilla; point B, pogonion and gnathion for the anterior mandible, and gonion for the posterior mandible). The object is to evaluate the position of the skeletal units. The template is being used to see directly how the patient's jaw positions differ from the norm. Compensations within the individual's skeletal pattern are observed directly.

2. The second superimposition is on the maximum contour of the maxilla to evaluate the relationship of the maxillary dentition to the maxilla (Figure 6-47). Again, it is important to evaluate the position of the teeth both vertically and anteroposteriorly. The template makes it easy to see whether the teeth are displaced vertically, information often not obtained in measurement analysis techniques.

3. The third superimposition is on the symphysis of the mandible along the lower border, to evaluate the relationship of the mandibular dentition to the mandible (Figure 6-48). If the shadow of the mandibular canal is shown on the templates, a more accurate orientation can be obtained by registering along this rather than the lower border posteriorly. Both the vertical and the anteroposterior positions of the anterior and posterior teeth should be noted.

Template analysis in this fashion has two advantages: first, it allows the easy use of age-related standards and second, it quickly provides an overall impression of the way in which the patient's dentofacial structures are related. Sometimes, the reason for making measurements, which is to gain an overall understanding of the pattern of the patient's facial relationships, is overlooked in a focus on acquiring the numbers themselves. Comparing the patient to a template is an excellent way to overcome this hazard and be sure that one does not miss the forest while observing the trees.

Template analysis often is thought of as somehow less scientific than making a series of measurements, but really that is not so. Remember that the template contains exactly the same information as a table of measurements from the same data base (for the anatomic templates, very extensive tables). The information is just expressed in a different way. The difference is that with the template method, there is greater emphasis on the clinician's individual assessment of whatever about the patient may be abnormal, and a corresponding deemphasis of specific criteria.

Templates easily can be used with computer analysis as well. The technique would be to store the templates in computer memory and then pull up the appropriate template for comparison and use the computer to make the series of superimpositions. The clinician, looking at the superimpositions, should be stimulated to make his own assessment of interactions among the various components of the face, incorporating the insights of counterpart analysis and floating norms at that point.

Summary of Contemporary Cephalometric Methodology. In its early years, cephalometric analysis was correctly criticized as being just a "numbers game," leading to orthodontic treatment aimed at producing certain numbers on a cephalometric film that might or might not represent the best treatment result for that patient. Totally accepting the Steiner compromises and setting treatment goals solely in terms of producing these numbers could certainly be criticized on that basis. At present, competent clinicians use cephalometric analysis to better understand the underlying basis for a malocclusion. To do this, they look not just at individual measurements compared with a norm but at the pattern of relationships, including soft tissue relationships. Any measurements are a means to this end, not the end in itself.

Whatever the later steps (measurement or template superimposition), the place to begin cephalometric analysis is by drawing the Sassouni horizontal planes and examining

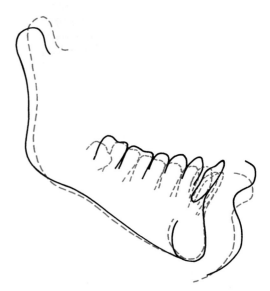

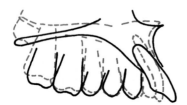

FIGURE 6-47 Superimposition of the Bolton template on the maxilla (primarily, the anterior palatal contour) of the patient shown in Figure 6-46. This superimposition clearly reveals the forward protrusion of the maxillary incisors but shows that the vertical relationship of the maxillary teeth to the maxilla for this patient is nearly ideal.

FIGURE 6-48 Superimposition of the Bolton template on the mandible of the patient in Figure 6-46. This superimposition indicates that the patient's mandible is longer than the ideal, but the ramus is shorter and inclined posteriorly. All the mandibular teeth have erupted more than normal, especially the incisors.

their interrelationships. This simple step highlights rotations of the jaws (remember that both the maxilla and mandible can be rotated) and makes vertical proportions more apparent.

At that point, the analysis should turn to analysis of the anteroposterior relationships of the jaws and the dentition of each jaw. Superimposition of Bolton (or other) templates is one way to do that. The same information can be obtained by using a true vertical line across the front of the face as a reference, as in McNamara analysis, which is a straightforward way to establish skeletal relationships without having the measurements affected by tooth position. Moving the true vertical line so that it passes through point A, and then through point B, reveals the amount of dental protrusion or retrusion of the maxillary and mandibular teeth respectively.

Finally, any other measurements needed to clarify relationships that are not clear should be made. Often this includes measurements of face height, maxillary and mandibular unit lengths or other components of the various analyses that have been discussed. The goal of modern cephalometrics is to evaluate the relationship of the functional units shown in Figure 6-27 and to do whatever is necessary to establish the position, horizontally and vertically, of each of those units. Because what is required amounts to pattern analysis, almost never can any single measurement be viewed in isolation. Instead, the interrelationship among various measurements and observed relationships must be taken into account. In a measurement analysis system, the appropriate floating norms always should be employed.

ORTHODONTIC CLASSIFICATION

Classification has traditionally been an important tool in the diagnosis-treatment planning procedure. An ideal classification would summarize the diagnostic data and imply the treatment plan. In our concept of diagnosis, classification can be viewed as the (orderly) reduction of the database to a list of the patient's problems (Figure 6-49).

Development of Classification Systems

The first useful orthodontic classification, still important now, was Angle's classification of malocclusion into Classes I, II, and III (see Chapter 1). The basis of the Angle classification was the relationship of the first molar teeth and the alignment (or lack of it) of the teeth relative to the line of occlusion. Angle's classification thus created four groups:

Normal occlusion	Normal (Class I) molar relationship, teeth on line of occlusion
Class I malocclusion	Normal (Class I) molar relationship, teeth crowded, rotated, etc.
Class II malocclusion	Lower molar distal to upper molar, relationship of other teeth to line of occlusion not specified
Class III malocclusion	Lower molar mesial to upper molar, relationship of other teeth to line of occlusion not specified

The Angle system was a tremendous step forward, not only because it provided an orderly way to classify malocclusion but also because for the first time it provided a simple definition of normal occlusion, and thereby a way to distinguish normal occlusion from malocclusion.

From an early stage, it was recognized that the Angle classification was not complete, because it did not include important characteristics of the patient's problem. In 1912 a committee of the British Orthodontic Society chaired by Norman Bennett suggested that although the Angle system was an adequate classification of anteroposterior relationships, it did not include information about the transverse and vertical planes and should be extended to do so.

The deficiencies in the original Angle system led to a series of informal additions at an early stage. A series of subdivisions of Class I were proposed by Martin Dewey, initially Angle's protégé but later his rival. Gradually Angle's classification numbers were extended to refer to four distinct but related characteristics: the classification of

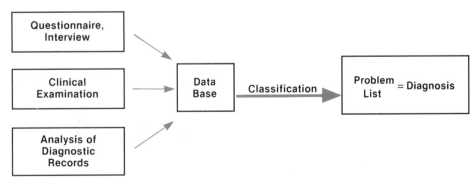

FIGURE 6-49 Conceptually, classification can be viewed as an orderly way to derive a list of the patient's problems from the database.

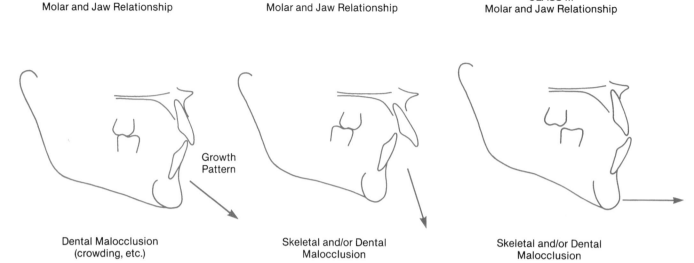

CLASS I
Molar and Jaw Relationship

CLASS II
Molar and Jaw Relationship

CLASS III
Molar and Jaw Relationship

Growth Pattern

Dental Malocclusion
(crowding, etc.)

Skeletal and/or Dental
Malocclusion

Skeletal and/or Dental
Malocclusion

FIGURE 6-50   The Angle classification has come to describe four different characteristics: the type of malocclusion, the molar relationship, the jaw relationship, and the pattern of growth, as shown here diagrammatically. Although the jaw relationship and growth pattern correlate with the molar relationship, the correlations are far from perfect. It is not unusual to observe a Class I molar relationship in a patient with a Class II jaw relationship or to find that an individual with a Class I molar and jaw relationship grows in a Class III pattern, which ultimately will produce a Class III malocclusion.

malocclusion, as in the original plan; the molar relationship; the skeletal jaw relationship; and the pattern of growth (Figure 6-50). Thus a Class II jaw relationship meant the mandible was positioned distally relative to the maxilla. This was usually found in connection with a Class II molar relationship but occasionally could be present despite a Class I molar relationship. Similarly, a Class II growth pattern was defined as a downward and backward growth direction of the mandible, which would tend to create and maintain Class II jaw and molar relationships. Class I and Class III growth patterns show balanced and disproportionate forward mandibular growth, respectively.

In the 1930s the German orthodontist Simon proposed a new system of classification based on a specific recording of the vertical orientation of the jaws to the cranium by what Simon called "gnathostatic" casts. In addition, Simon included an evaluation of the anteroposterior position of the incisors by specifying canine position relative to the orbits. The development of cephalometric radiology made it easier to evaluate both skeletal proportions and incisor protrusion. With the introduction of cephalometric radiology into orthodontic practice in the 1950s, Simon's concepts were incorporated into routine orthodontic diagnosis although his method of gnathostatic casts was abandoned.

In the 1960s, Ackerman and Proffit formalized the system of informal additions to the Angle method by identifying five major characteristics of malocclusion that should be considered and systematically described in classification (Figure 6-51).[35] Experience has confirmed that a minimum of five characteristics must be considered in a complete diagnostic evaluation. Although the elements of

the Ackerman-Proffit scheme are often not combined exactly as originally proposed, this classification by five major characteristics is now widely used. The approach overcomes the major weaknesses of the Angle scheme. Specifically, it (1) incorporates an evaluation of crowding and asymmetry within the dental arches and includes an evaluation of incisor protrusion, (2) recognizes the relationship between protrusion and crowding, (3) includes the transverse and vertical as well as the anteroposterior planes of space, and (4) incorporates information about skeletal jaw proportions at the appropriate point, that is, in the description of relationships in each of the planes of space.

To utilize this classification method, diagnostic information is required about the dentition itself, occlusal relationships, and skeletal jaw relationships. This is derived from clinical examination; panoramic and (if needed) intraoral radiographs; and clinical, photographic, or cephalometric evaluation of dental and facial proportions. Examining five major characteristics in sequence provides a convenient way of organizing the diagnostic information to be sure that no important points are overlooked.

Classification by the Characteristics of Malocclusion

Step 1: Evaluation of Facial Proportions and Esthetics.
This step is carried out during the clinical examination, while facial asymmetry, anteroposterior and vertical facial proportions, and lip prominence as related to incisor protrusion are evaluated. The clinical findings can be checked against the facial photographs and lateral cephalometric film, which should confirm the clinical judgment.

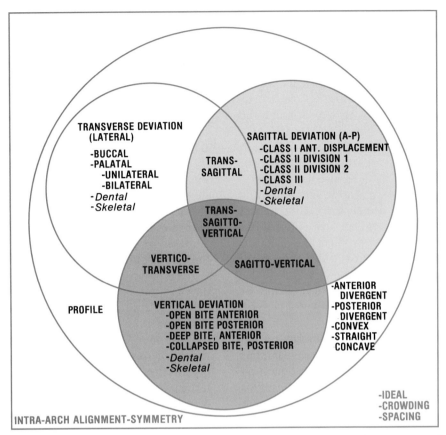

FIGURE 6-51 Ackerman and Proffit represented the five major characteristics of malocclusion via a Venn diagram. The sequential description of the major characteristics, not their graphic representation, is the key to this classification system; but the interaction of the tooth and jaw relationships with facial appearance must be kept in mind.

Step 2: Evaluation of Alignment and Symmetry Within the Dental Arches. This step is carried out by examining the dental arches from the occlusal view, evaluating first the symmetry within each dental arch and second, the amount of crowding or spacing present. Space analysis quantitates crowding or spacing, but these figures must be interpreted in the light of other findings in the total evaluation of the patient. A major point is the presence or absence of excessive incisor protrusion, which cannot be evaluated without knowledge of lip separation at rest.

Step 3: Evaluation of Skeletal and Dental Relationships in the Transverse Plane of Space. At this stage, the casts are brought into occlusion and the occlusal relationships are examined, beginning with the transverse (posterior crossbite) plane of space. The objectives are to accurately describe the occlusion and to distinguish between skeletal and dental contributions to malocclusion.

Posterior crossbite is described in terms of the position of the upper molars (Figure 6-52). Thus a bilateral maxillary lingual (or palatal) crossbite means that the upper molars are lingual to their normal position on both sides, whereas a unilateral mandibular buccal crossbite would mean that the mandibular molars were buccally positioned on one side. This terminology specifies which teeth (maxillary or mandibular) are displaced from their normal position.

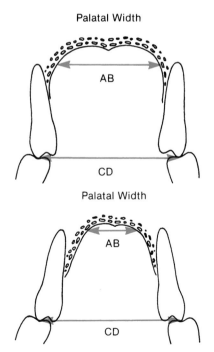

FIGURE 6-52 Posterior crossbite can be either *dental,* as in a patient with adequate palatal width (i.e., distance *AB* approximately equals distance *CD*), or *skeletal* because of inadequate palatal width (i.e., distance *CD* is considerably larger than distance *AB*).

It is also important to evaluate the underlying skeletal relationships, to answer the question, "Why does this crossbite exist?" in the sense of the location of the anatomic abnormality. If a bilateral maxillary palatal crossbite exists, for instance, is the basic problem that the maxilla itself is narrow, thus providing a skeletal basis for the crossbite, or is it that the dental arch has been narrowed although the skeletal width is correct?

The width of the maxillary skeletal base can be seen by the width of the palatal vault on the casts. If the base of the palatal vault is wide, but the dentoalveolar processes lean inward, the crossbite is dental in the sense that it is caused by a distortion of the dental arch. If the palatal vault is narrow and the maxillary teeth lean outward but nevertheless are in crossbite, the problem is skeletal in that it basically results from the narrow width of the maxilla. Just as there are dental compensations for skeletal deformity in the anteroposterior and vertical planes of space, the teeth can compensate for transverse skeletal problems.

Transverse displacement of the lower molars on the mandible is rare, so the question of whether the mandibular arch is too wide can be used both to answer the question of whether the mandible or maxilla is at fault in a posterior crossbite and to implicate skeletal mandibular development if the answer is positive. Tabulated data for normal molar and canine widths are shown in Table 6-10. If there is a crossbite and measurements across the arch show that the mandible is wide while the maxillary arch is normal, a skeletal mandibular discrepancy is probably present.

Step 4: Evaluation of Skeletal and Dental Relationships in the Anteroposterior Plane of Space.   Examining the dental casts in occlusion will reveal any anteroposterior problems in the buccal occlusion or in the anterior relationships. The Angle classification, in its extended form, describes this well. Occasionally the molar occlusion is Class II on one side, and Class I on the other. Angle called this a Class II subdivision right or left, depending on which was the Class II side. In modern classification the subdivision label is only moderately useful—the asymmetric molar relationship reflects either an asymmetry within one or both the dental arches, or a transverse skeletal problem. These must be distinguished and should be addressed in the first or third steps discussed here.

It is important to ask whether an end-to-end, Class II, or Class III buccal segment relationship, or excessive overjet or reverse overjet of the incisors, is caused by a jaw (skeletal) discrepancy, displaced teeth on well-proportioned jaws (dental Class II or III), or a combination of the two, as is often the case. A jaw discrepancy almost always produces an occlusal discrepancy as well, but if the jaw discrepancy is the cause, the problem should be described as a *skeletal* Class II or Class III. The terminology simply means that the skeletal or jaw relationship is the cause of the Class II dental occlusion. The distinction between dental and skeletal is important, because the

---

TABLE 6-10   *Arch Width Measurements**

Age	Male			Female		
	Canine	First premolar	First molar	Canine	First premolar	First molar
Maxillary arch						
6	27.5[†]	32.3[†]	41.9	26.9[†]	31.7[†]	41.3
8	29.7[†]	33.7[†]	43.1	29.1[†]	33.0[†]	42.4
10	30.5[†]	34.4[†]	44.5	29.8[†]	33.6[†]	43.5
12	32.5	35.7	45.3	31.5	35.1	44.6
14	32.5	36.0	45.9	31.3	34.9	44.3
16	32.3	36.6	46.6	31.4	35.2	45.0
18	32.3	36.7	46.7	31.2	34.6	43.9
Mandibular arch						
6	23.3[†]	28.7[†]	40.2	22.2[†]	28.4[†]	40.0
8	24.3[†]	29.7[†]	40.9	24.0[†]	29.5[†]	40.3
10	24.6[†]	30.2[†]	41.5	24.1[†]	29.7[†]	41.0
12	25.1	32.5	42.1	24.8	31.6	41.8
14	24.8	32.3	42.1	24.4	31.0	41.1
16	24.7	32.3	42.8	23.9	31.0	41.5
18	24.8	32.8	43.0	23.1	30.8	41.7

Data from Moyers RE et al: *Standards of human occlusal development,* Monograph 5, Craniofacial Growth Series. Ann Arbor, Mich., 1976, University of Michigan, Center for Human Growth and Development.

*mm distance between centers of teeth.

[†]Primary predecessor.

treatment for a skeletal Class II relationship in a child or adult will be different from treatment for a dental Class II problem. Cephalometric analysis is needed to be precise about the nature of the problem. The object is to accurately evaluate the underlying anatomic basis of the malocclusion (Figure 6-53).

Step 5: Evaluation of Skeletal and Dental Relationships in the Vertical Plane of Space. With the casts in occlusion, vertical problems can be described as anterior open bite (failure of the incisor teeth to overlap), anterior deep bite (excessive overlap of the anterior teeth), or posterior open bite (failure of the posterior teeth to occlude, unilaterally or bilaterally). As with all aspects of malocclusion, it is important to ask, "Why does the open bite (or other problem) exist?" Since vertical problems, particularly anterior open bite, can result from environmental causes or habits, the "why" in this instance has two important components: at what anatomic location is the discrepancy, and can a cause be identified?

It is obvious that if the posterior teeth erupt a normal amount but the anterior teeth do not, an anterior open bite will result. This is possible but rarely is the major reason for an anterior open bite. Instead, anterior open bite patients usually have at least some excessive eruption of posterior teeth. If the anterior teeth erupt a normal amount but the posterior teeth erupt too much, anterior open bite is inevitable. Excessive eruption of posterior

teeth requires a compensatory downward and backward rotation of the mandible. Perhaps more accurately, if the mandible rotates downward and backward, space is created into which the posterior teeth can erupt, allowing excessive posterior eruption.

This leads to an important but sometimes difficult concept: a patient with a *skeletal* open bite will usually have an anterior bite malocclusion that is characterized by excessive eruption of posterior teeth, downward rotation of the mandible and maxilla, and normal (or even excessive) eruption of anterior teeth (Figure 6-54). This facial and dental pattern is sometimes called the "long face syndrome." The reverse is true in a short face, skeletal deep bite relationship (Figure 6-55). In that circumstance, one would expect to see a normal amount of eruption of incisor teeth but rotation of both jaws in the opposite direction and insufficient eruption of the posterior teeth. The skeletal component is revealed by the rotation of the jaws, reflected in the palatal and mandibular plane angles. If the angle between the mandibular and palatal planes is low, there is a skeletal deep bite tendency (i.e., a jaw relationship that predisposes to an anterior deep bite, regardless of whether one is present). Similarly, if the mandibular-palatal angle is high, there is a skeletal open bite tendency.

It is important to remember that if the mandibular plane angle is unusually flat or steep, correcting an

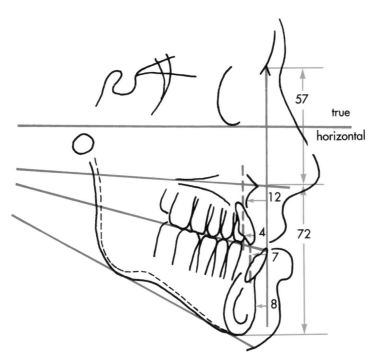

FIGURE 6-53 Cephalometric analysis combining elements of the measurement approaches presented earlier. A description in words of this patient's problems would be that the maxilla is quite deficient relative to the mandible and the cranial base, but the maxillary teeth are reasonably well related to the maxilla. The mandible is fairly well related in the anteroposterior plane of space to the cranial base, but the mandibular teeth protrude relative to the mandible. Vertical proportions are good.

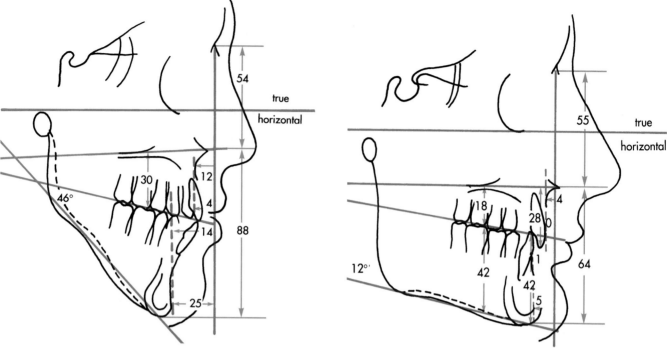

FIGURE 6-54   Cephalometric analysis for a patient with severe vertical problems. Note that the Sassouni lines clearly indicate the skeletal open bite pattern and that the measurements confirm both long anterior facial dimensions and severe mandibular deficiency related to downward and backward rotation of the mandible. Measurements of the distance from the upper first molar mesial cusp to the palatal plane confirms that excessive eruption of the upper molar has occurred.

FIGURE 6-55   Cephalometric analysis of a patient with short anterior vertical dimensions. The measurements show excessive eruption of the lower molar compared with the upper molar and document the distal displacement of the lower incisor relative to the mandible. Note that the Sassouni planes are almost parallel, confirming the skeletal deep bite tendency.

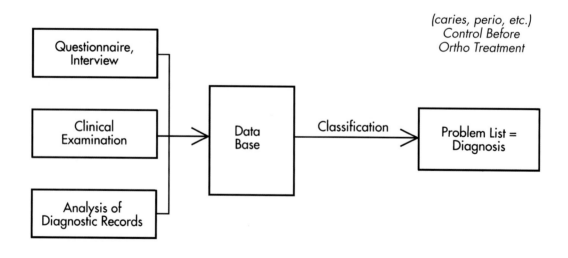

FIGURE 6-56   As a final step in diagnosis, the patient's problems related to pathology should be separated from the developmental problems, so that the pathology can be treated first.

accompanying deep bite or open bite may require an alteration in the vertical position of posterior teeth so that the mandible can rotate to a more normal inclination. Cephalometric analysis is required for evaluation of patients with skeletal vertical problems, again with the goal of accurately describing skeletal and dental relationships. As the tracings in this chapter illustrate, most published analyses do a much better job of identifying antero-posterior than vertical problems. Adequate analysis of long- or short-face patients requires additional measurements to meet the needs of the specific case, or careful superimposition of templates and inspection of the relationships.

DEVELOPMENT OF A PROBLEM LIST

If positive findings from a systematic description of the patient are recorded (i.e., if the procedure described above is used), the automatic and important result is a list of the patient's problems. The step-by-step procedure is designed to ensure that the important distinctions have been made and that nothing has been overlooked.

The problem list often includes two types of problems: (1) those relating to disease or pathologic processes and (2) those relating to disturbances of development that have created the patient's malocclusion (Figure 6-56). The set of developmental abnormalities related to malocclusion is the orthodontic problem list. A developmental problem is just that (e.g., mandibular deficiency), not the findings that indicate its presence (e.g., posterior divergence, increased facial convexity, and increased ANB angle all are findings, not problems).

For efficient clinical application of the method, it is important to group different aspects of the same thing into a single major problem area related to the Ackerman-Proffit classification. This means that it would be impossible for a patient to have more than five major developmental problems, though several sub-problems within a major category would be quite possible. For instance, lingual position of the lateral incisors, labial position of the canines, and rotation of the central incisors all are problems, but they can and should be lumped under the general problem of incisor crowding/malalignment. Similarly, anterior open bite, rotation of the maxilla down posteriorly and rotation of the mandible down anteriorly, and extreme lip incompetence are all aspects of skeletal open bite. Where possible, the problems should be indicated quantitatively, or at least classified as mild, moderate, or severe (i.e., 5 mm mandibular incisor crowding or severe mandibular deficiency).

The development of a problem list for a patient with moderately severe orthodontic problems (Figures 6-57 to 6-60) is shown in Boxes 6-3 to 6-6. Similar diagnostic work-ups for patients with more severe problems are briefly reviewed in Chapters 21 and 22.

With the completion of a problem list, the diagnostic phase of diagnosis and treatment planning is completed, and the more subjective process of treatment planning begins. Thorough diagnostic evaluation means that all problems have been identified and characterized at this stage, omitting nothing of significance. The steps in treatment planning and the outcome of treatment for the patient shown in Figures 6-57 to 6-60 are presented in Chapter 7.

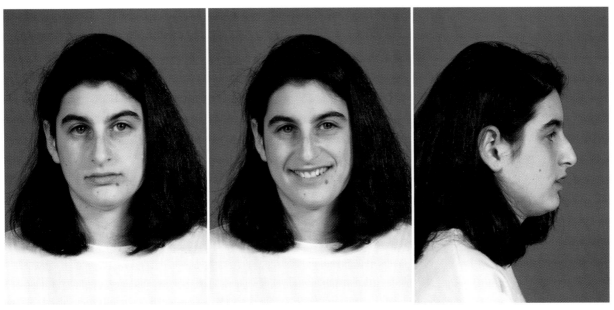

FIGURE 6-57   Patient age 14-11 (Patient F.P.), facial views prior to treatment.

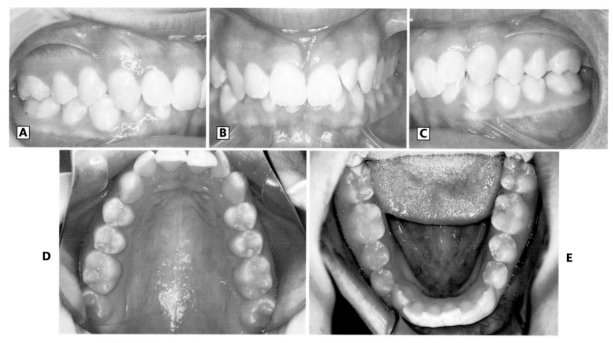

FIGURE 6-58   Patient age 14-11 (Patient F.P.), intraoral views prior to treatment.

PATIENT F.P.: INTERVIEW DATA

Chief complaint
"My front teeth are crooked and my smile is ugly."

History
- Good health, regular medical and/or dental care, wears contact lenses
- Post-menarche > 24 months
- Orthodontic treatment planned earlier, delayed because family moved

Motivation
- Largely internal, wants treatment very much
- Good attitude, understands treatment procedures because friends have been treated

Expectation
- Better appearance, less social stress (no concerns about function), seems realistic

Other pertinent information
- Lives with both parents, good school performance, no apparent social problems

PATIENT F.P.: CLINICAL EXAMINATION DATA

Health of hard and soft tissues
- No caries, no restorations
- Tissue irritation around erupting mandibular right second molar, occasional pain there
- Minimal attached gingiva, mandibular anterior, mandibular incisor region

Jaw function
- Maximum voluntary opening is 40 mm
- Normal lateral and/or protrusive movements
- No joint sounds, no pain on palpation

Facial proportions
- Generally symmetric but chin slightly to left
- Lower third vertically short
- Profile: mildly mandibular deficient, relatively large nose and chin, deep labiomental fold

Diagnostic records needed
- Panoramic radiograph, no other intraoral films
- Lateral cephalometric radiograph (no P-A ceph)
- Dental casts
- Intraoral and extraoral photographs

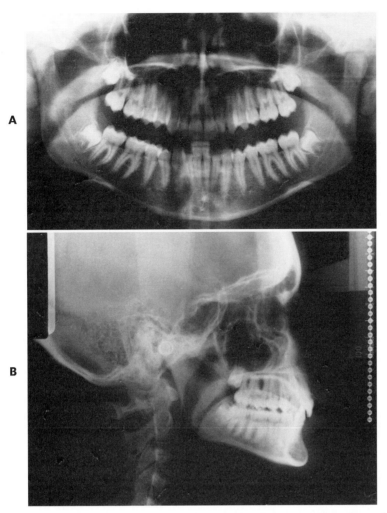

FIGURE 6-59   Patient F.P. age 14-11, panoramic (**A**) and cephalometric (**B**) radiographs prior to treatment.

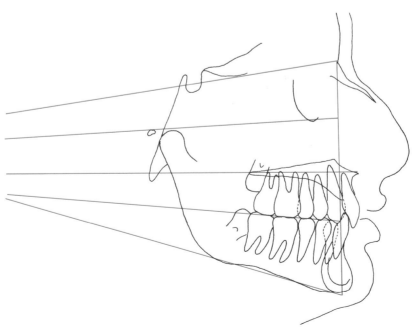

FIGURE 6-60   Patient F.P. age 14-11, cephalometric tracing prior to treatment. This set of horizontal and vertical reference lines is recommended.

BOX 6-5

PATIENT F.P.:
ANALYSIS OF DIAGNOSTIC RECORDS*

1. Facial proportions and esthetics
Short face
Relatively large nose/chin for lips

2. Dental alignment/symmetry
Mild mandibular, moderate maxillary crowding

3. Transverse relationships
No problems

4. Anteroposterior relationships
Class II (½ cusp)
 • Mild mandibular deficiency
 • Angle Class II, division 2

5. Vertical relationships
Extreme overbite, skeletal/dental
 • Short facial height
 • Elongation of maxillary mandibular incisors

using the Ackerman-Proffit classification

BOX 6-6

PATIENT F.P.:
PROBLEM LIST (DIAGNOSIS)

 • Tissue irritation, minimal attached gingiva
 • Moderate maxillary, mild mandibular crowding
 • Mild mandibular deficiency, Class II, division 2 pattern
 • Deep bite, short face, elongated maxillary and/or mandibular incisors

REFERENCES

1. Greulich WW, Pyle SL: Radiographic atlas of skeletal development of the hand and wrist, ed 2, Palo Alto, Calif., 1959, Stanford University Press.
2. Grave KC, Brown T: Skeletal ossification and the adolescent growth spurt, Am J Orthod 69:611-619, 1976.
3. Shaw WC: The influence of children's dentofacial appearance on their social attractiveness as judged by peers and lay adults, Am J Orthod 79:399-415, 1981.
4. Birkeland K, Boe OE, Wisth PJ: Orthodontic concern among 11-year-old children and their parents compared with orthodontic treatment need assessed by index of orthodontic treatment need, Am J Orthod Dentofac Orthop 110:197-205, 1997.
5. Kenealy P, Frude N, Shaw W: An evaluation of the psychological and social effects of malocclusion: some implications for dental policy making, Social Sci Med 28:583-591, 1989.
6. Kerouso H, Hausen H, Laine T, Shaw WC: The influence of incisal malocclusion on the social attractiveness of young adults in Finland, Eur J Orthod 17:505-512, 1995.
7. Bateman HE, Mason RM: Applied anatomy and physiology of the speech and hearing mechanism, Springfield Ill., 1984, Thomas.
8. Battagel JM: Obstructive sleep apnea: fact not fiction, Brit J Orthod 23:315-324, 1996.
9. Okeson JP: Management of temporomandibular disorders and occlusion, ed 4, St Louis, 1997, Mosby.
10. Farkas LG: Anthropometry of the head and face in medicine, ed 2, New York, 1994, Raven Press.
11. Hellman M: Variations in occlusion, Dental Cosmos 63:608-619, 1921.
12. Brooks SA, Brand JW, Gibbs SJ et al: Imaging of the temporomandibular joint—a position paper of the American Academy of Oral and Maxillofacial Radiology, Oral Surg, Oral Med, Oral Path 83:609-618, 1997.
13. Tripodakis AP, Smulow JB, Mehta NR, Clark RE: Clinical study of location and reproducibility of three mandibular positions in relation to body posture and muscle function, J Pros Dent 73:190-198, 1995.
14. Bolton WA: The clinical application of a tooth-size analysis, Am J Orthod 48:504-529, 1962.
15. Kantor ML, Norton LA: Normal radiographic anatomy and common anomalies seen in cephalometric films, Am J Orthod Dentofacial Orthop 91:414-426, 1987.
16. Downs WB: Variations in facial relationships: their significance in treatment and prognosis, Am J Orthod 34:812, 1948.
17. Riolo ML et al: An atlas of craniofacial growth, monograph 2, craniofacial growth series, Ann Arbor, Mich., 1974, University of Michigan, Center for Human Growth and Development.
18. Popovich F, Thompson GW: Craniofacial templates for orthodontic case analysis, Am J Orthod 71:406-420, 1977.
19. Broadbent BH, Sr, Broadbent BH, Jr, Golden WH: Bolton standards of dentofacial developmental growth, St Louis, 1975, Mosby.
20. Jacobson A: Radiographic cephalometry: from basics to videoimaging, Chicago, 1995, Quintessence.
21. Cooke MS: Five-year reproducibility of natural head posture: a longitudinal study, Am J Orthod Dentofacial Orthop 97:487-494, 1990.
22. Lundstrom A, Lundstrom F, Lebret LM, Moorrees CF: Natural head position and natural head orientation: basic considerations in cephalometric analysis, Eur J Orthod 17:111-120, 1995.
23. Steiner CC: The use of cephalometrics as an aid to planning and assessing orthodontic treatment, Am J Orthod 46:721-735, 1960.
24. Tweed CH: The Frankfort-mandibular incisor angle (FMIA) in orthodontic diagnosis, treatment planning and prognosis, Angle Orthod 24:121-169, 1954.
25. Sassouni VA: A classification of skeletal facial types, Am J Orthod 55:109-123, 1969.
26. Harvold EP: The activator in orthodontics, St Louis, 1974, Mosby.
27. Jacobson A: The "Wits" appraisal of jaw disharmony, Am J Orthod 67:125-138, 1975.

28. Athanasiou AE: Orthodontic cephalometry, Chicago, 1995, Mosby.

29. McNamara JA Jr: A method of cephalometric analysis. In Clinical alteration of the growing face, monograph 12, craniofacial growth series, Ann Arbor, Mich., 1983, University of Michigan, Center for Human Growth and Development.

30. Enlow DH, Moyers RE, Hunter WS, McNamara JA: A procedure for the analysis of intrinsic facial form and growth, Am J Orthod 56:6-14, 1969.

31. Segner D: Floating norms as a means to describe individual skeletal patterns, Eur J Orthod 11:214-220, 1989.

32. Franchi L, Baccetti T, McNamara JA: Cephalometric floating norms for North American adults, Angle Orthod 68:497-502, 1998.

33. Faustini MM, Hale C, Cisneros GJ: Mesh diagram analysis: developing a norm for African Americans, Angle Orthod 67:121-128, 1997.

34. Evanko AM, Freeman K, Cisneros GJ: Mesh diagram analysis: developing a norm for Puerto Rican Americans, Angle Orthod 67:381-388, 1997.

35. Ackerman JL, Proffit WR: The characteristics of malocclusion: a modern approach to classification and diagnosis, Am J Orthod 56:443, 1969.

CHAPTER

7

Orthodontic Treatment Planning: From Problem List to Specific Plan

Orthodontic diagnosis is complete when a comprehensive list of the patient's problems has been developed and pathologic and developmental problems have been separated. At that point, the objective in treatment planning is to design the strategy that a wise and prudent clinician, using his or her best judgment, would employ to address the problems while maximizing benefit to the patient and minimizing cost and risk.

It is important to view the goal of treatment in that way. Otherwise, an inappropriate emphasis on some aspect of the case is likely, whether the proposed treatment is medical, dental, or just orthodontics. For example, consider a patient who seeks dental care in a family practice setting because she is concerned about the status of old restorations. For that individual, controlling periodontal breakdown might be more important than replacing old amalgams, and should receive the emphasis in planning treatment, even though the patient initially sought restorative treatment. The same principle applies when orthodontic treatment is planned. The orthodontic treatment plan should be developed to do what, on balance, would be best for that individual patient.

When a group of dentists and dental specialists meet to plan treatment for a patient with complex problems, important orthodontic questions often asked are, "Could you retract the incisors enough to correct the overjet?" or "Could you develop incisal guidance for this patient?" To a question phrased as, "Could you...?" the answer often is yes, given an unlimited commitment to treatment. The more appropriate question is not "Could you...?" but "Should you...?" or "Would it be best for the patient to...?" Cost-benefit and risk-benefit analyses are introduced appropriately when the question is rephrased.

A treatment plan in orthodontics, as in any other field, may be less than optimal if it does not take full advantage of the possibilities or if it is too ambitious. There is always a temptation to jump to conclusions and proceed with a superficially obvious plan without considering all the pertinent factors. The treatment planning approach advocated here is specifically designed to avoid both missed opportunities (the false negative or under-treatment side of treatment planning) and excessive treatment (the false positive or overtreatment side), while appropriately involving the patient in the planning process. The patient whose diagnostic evaluation was outlined at the end of Chapter 6 (Patient F.P.) continues as the illustrative patient (progress and treatment completion are shown in the color section (Figures 7-1 to 7-4).

THE SEQUENCE OF STEPS IN PLANNING ORTHODONTIC TREATMENT

Diagnosis results in a comprehensive list of the patient's problems. Although any number of pathologic problems might be noted, if the five characteristics of malocclusion are used to structure the problem list, there can be a maximum of five major developmental problems. Most patients will not have that many. As the problem list is developed, the findings related to malocclusion can and should be grouped as the classification scheme suggests, to make the treatment planning process work efficiently. Having too many overlapping problems on the problem list only creates confusion.

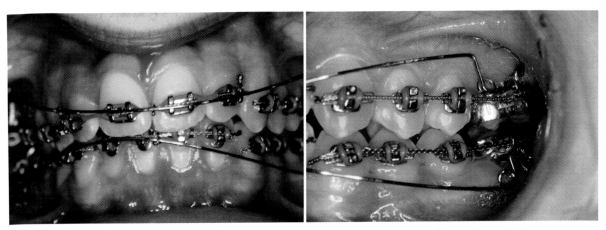

FIGURE 7-1   Example patient (Patient F.P.; see Figures 6-57 to 6-59) maxillary and mandibular intrusion arches in place.

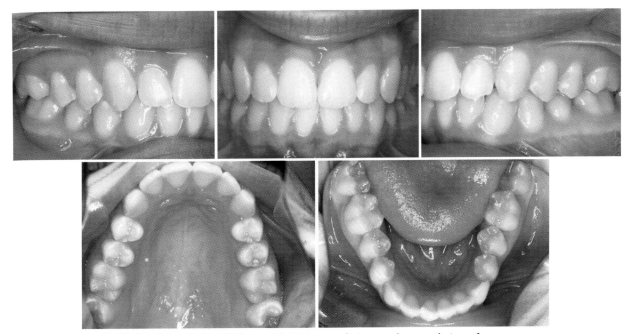

FIGURE 7-2   Patient F. P., age 16-11, intraoral views at the completion of treatment.

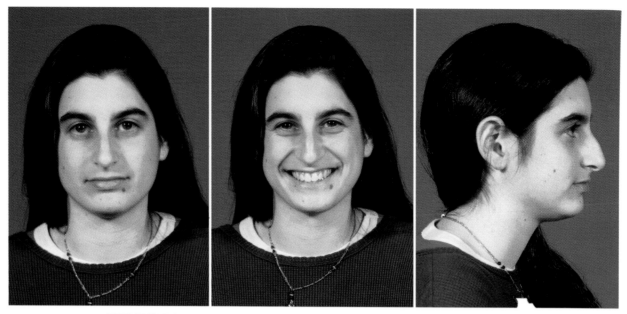

FIGURE 7-3   Patient F.P., age 16-11, facial views at the completion of treatment.

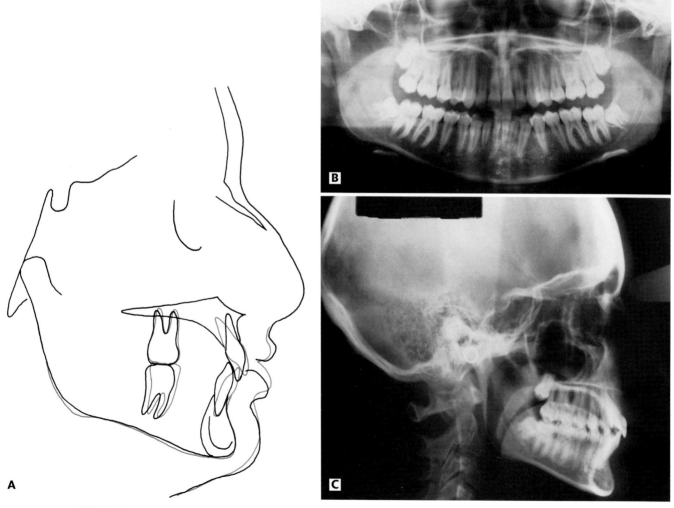

FIGURE 7-4   Patient F.P,. age 16-11, **A,** cephalometric superimposition showing changes relative to cranial base, maxilla and mandible; **B,** panoramic and; **C,** cephalometric radiographs at the completion of treatment.

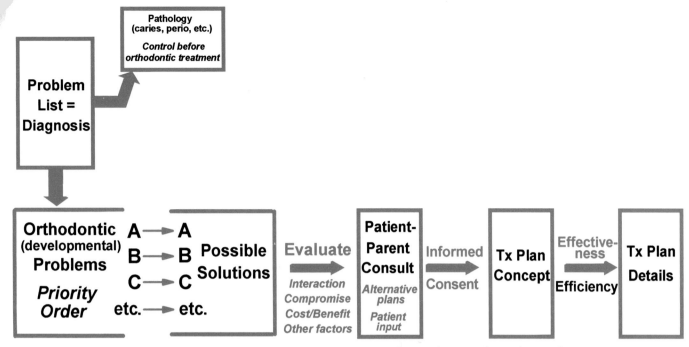

FIGURE 7-5   The treatment planning sequence. In treatment planning, the goal is wisdom, not scientific truth—judgment is required. Interaction with the patient and parent, so that they are involved in the decisions that lead to the final plan, is the key to informed consent.

The first step in planning orthodontic treatment is to separate any pathologic problems from the orthodontic (developmental) problems (Figure 7-5). Then the treatment planning process should proceed through the following steps:

- put the orthodontic problems in priority order
- note the treament possibilities, being sure to be complete
- evaluate the possible solutions, considering factors that can affect the probable result
- establish the treatment plan concept in an interactive session with the patient and parents
- develop the detailed plan of clinical steps and procedures.

Let us now consider this sequence, and the logic behind it, in some detail.

Pathologic vs. Developmental Problems

An important principle is that a patient does not have to be in perfect health to have orthodontic treatment, but any problems related to disease and pathology must be under control (i.e., the progression of any acute or chronic conditions must be stopped). For this reason, pathologic problems must be addressed before treatment of orthodontic (developmental) problems can begin. Thus in a treatment sequence, orthodontic treatment must appear after control of systemic disease, periodontal treatment (at least to the extent of bringing periodontal disease under control), and restoration of dental lesions.

BOX 7-1

PATIENT F.P.: PATHOLOGIC PROBLEMS/PLAN

Inflamed flap over lower second molar
Plan: irrigation, observe

Minimal attached gingiva, lower anterior
Plan: no treatment now, observe

The sequencing of orthodontics with other types of treatment and the implications of certain types of systemic and oral pathology are discussed in Chapter 8. Multi-disciplinary treatment of adults with complex problems is illustrated in Chapters 20 to 22.

Even when pathologic problems are as mild as the gingivitis and minimal attached gingiva in the girl whose diagnostic evaluation is presented at the end of Chapter 6 (see Figures 6-57 to 6-60), they must not be overlooked in the treatment plan. For this patient (Box 7-1), the plan for the pathologic problems would be oral hygiene instruction and monitoring of the gingival attachment during subsequent orthodontic treatment. For patients with more complex disease-related problems, the plan often is appropriate referral to another practitioner, which must be done in a timely manner.

Setting Priorities for the Orthodontic Problem List

Putting the patient's orthodontic (developmental) problems in priority order is the most important single step in the entire treatment planning process. In order to maximize benefit to the patient, the most important problems must be identified, and the treatment plan must focus on what is most important for that particular patient. The patient's perception of his or her condition is important in setting these priorities. For example, if a patient's major reason for seeking dental treatment is protruding and irregular incisors, this condition probably should receive higher priority than missing molar teeth needing prosthetic replacement. On the other hand, if the protruding and irregular incisors are no problem to the patient but occlusal function is, replacing the missing teeth should receive higher priority.

It is always difficult for the clinician to avoid imposing his or her own feelings at this stage, and it is not totally inappropriate to do so; but ignoring the patient's chief complaint can lead to serious errors in planning treatment. For instance, consider the patient who complains of a protruding chin and who has a Class III malocclusion. If the clinician formulates the problem as Class III malocclusion and concentrates on bringing the teeth into correct occlusion while ignoring the chin, it is not likely that the patient will be happy with the treatment result. The plan did not deal with the patient's problem.

The prioritized problem list for the patient whose case we have been following is shown in Box 7-2. Note that on the prioritized list, the most important problem is not the one the patient and her parents identified as their chief complaint. For this patient, correcting the elongation of the incisors is the key to treatment, and that must be recognized at the planning stage. The doctor does not have to agree with the patient's initial thoughts as to what is most important. Indeed, often it is necessary to educate the patient about the nature of the problems. But the importance of various problems must be discussed, and informed consent to treatment has not been obtained unless the patient agrees that the focus of the plan is what he or she wants (see below).

Treatment Possibilities

The next step in the planning process is to list the possibilities for treatment of each of the problems, beginning with the highest priority problem. At this stage each problem is considered individually, and for the moment the possible solutions are examined as if this problem were the only one the patient had. Broad possibilities, not details of treatment procedures, are what is sought at this stage. The more complex the total situation, the more important it is to be sure no possibilities are overlooked.

As we continue our example and review the possibilities for correcting her problems (Box 7-3), references to aspects of treatment that have not yet been presented in the text are inevitable. The first-time reader is urged to follow the logic rather than concentrate on details that will be discussed more fully in the following chapters.

Consider the possible solutions to this patient's most important problem, her extreme overbite and the relatively short face and super-eruption of the maxillary and mandibular incisors that create it. This will require leveling the extreme curve of Spee in the lower arch and correcting the reverse curve in the upper arch. There are three ways this can be done (Figure 7-6): (1) absolute intrusion of the upper and lower incisors, moving their root apices closer to the nose and lower border of the mandible respectively; (2) relative intrusion of the incisors, keeping them where they are while the mandible grows and the posterior teeth erupt; and (3) extrusion of the posterior teeth, which would rotate the mandible downward and backward. Relative intrusion of incisors and extrusion of posterior teeth are identical in terms of the tooth movement. The difference is

---

BOX 7-2

**PATIENT F.P.*:
PRIORITIZED PROBLEM LIST**

1. Severe deep bite, skeletal/dental
2. Moderate maxillary, mild mandibular crowding
3. ½ cusp Class II, II/2 pattern

*See Figures 6-57 to 6-59.

BOX 7-3

PATIENT F.P.: POSSIBLE SOLUTIONS TO PROBLEMS

Severe deep bite, skeletal/dental
Elongate posterior teeth, hold incisors:
- continuous arch wires,
- relative intrusion (requires vertical growth), *or*
- extrusion (would rotate mandible down-back)

Intrude incisors with minimal elongation of molars:
- segmented arch wires
- absolute intrusion (little or no growth expected)

Incisor crowding: moderate max, mild mand
Expand both arches
- would bring incisors forward

Extract upper first premolar
- would require bringing upper molars forward

Extract upper first, lower second premolars
- might retract incisors in both arches: undesirable

Class II tendency
Favorable mandibular growth (?)

Orthognathic surgery: mandibular advancement (??)

Bring lower arch forward: Class II elastics

whether vertical growth of the ramus compensates for the increase in molar height (i.e., whether the mandibular plane angle is maintained [relative intrusion] or increases as the mandible rotates downward and backward [extrusion]).

At age 17, little or no vertical growth can be expected, so absolute intrusion or extrusion are the possibilities. It is significant that in the absence of growth, leveling the arches by extrusion of posterior teeth would cause the mandible to rotate downward and backward, accentuating a Class II tendency (Figure 7-7), which would be undesirable for the patient. So intrusion of the incisors appears to be the best solution to her deep bite, even though that

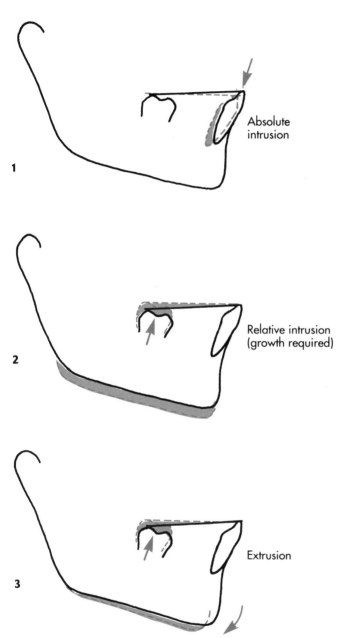

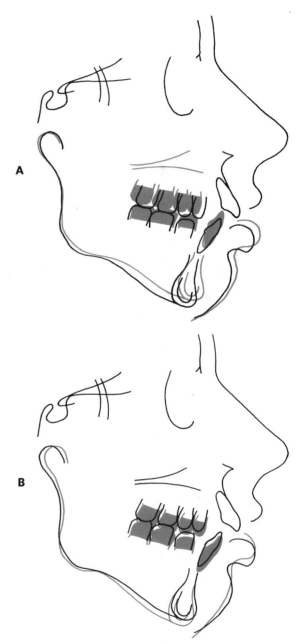

FIGURE 7-6   There are three possible ways to level out a lower arch with an excessive curve of Spee: (1) absolute intrusion; (2) relative intrusion, achieved by preventing eruption of the incisors while growth provides vertical space into which the posterior teeth erupt; and (3) elongation of posterior teeth, which causes the mandible to rotate downward in the absence of growth. Note that the difference between (2) and (3) is whether the mandible rotates downward and backward, which is determined by whether the mandibular ramus grows longer while the tooth movement is occurring.

FIGURE 7-7   There is a strong interaction between the vertical position of the maxilla and both the anteroposterior and vertical positions of the mandible, because the mandible rotates backward as it moves downward (**A**) and forward as it moves upward (**B**). The superimposition in **A** is the actual growth of this particular patient in whom excessive vertical growth of the maxilla and downward-backward rotation of the mandible occurred. The superimposition in **B** shows what would happen if the maxilla were moved upward (this would require surgery). Note that this would improve the apparent mandibular deficiency.

would require the more complex treatment approach of segmented arch mechanics.

The second problem is the crowding of the incisors, severe in the upper arch, mild in the lower. In determining whether expansion of the arches or premolar extraction would be the best choice, the final position of the incisors must be considered. She has a relatively prominent nose and chin, and could benefit esthetically from having more incisor prominence. It would be esthetically undesirable to retract the incisors because that would make the nose look larger, so if extraction spaces were created, space closure by bringing posterior teeth forward would be necessary. The anchorage for intruding the upper incisors would be incompatible with this pattern of space closure. Therefore, if intrusion of the incisors would be best, arch expansion also appears the best choice.

The third problem, the Class II tendency, would be improved by mandibular growth, but for this mature girl, that is extremely unlikely. Jaw surgery could increase mandibular prominence, but is not warranted by this relatively minor problem. (Note that if the Class II tendency were judged to be the most important problem, surgical correction might well be indicated—an indication of the importance of prioritizing the problem list correctly. Often, the same problem list prioritized differently results in a different treatment plan). For this patient, some use of Class II elastics to bring the mandibular arch forward slightly could be considered and might be necessary. But these elastics tend to extrude lower molars and could rotate the mandible down and back, so their use would have to be limited.

The objective at this stage of treatment planning is to be sure that no reasonable possibilities are overlooked. It is easy to develop the mindset that "For this problem, we always . . ." Sometimes an alternate approach would be better, but is overlooked unless a conscious effort is made to keep an open mind. In this patient's case, if continuous arch wires that extrude premolars always are selected to level the arches, an optimal treatment result is unlikely.

Factors in Evaluating Treatment Possibilities

Four additional factors that are pertinent in evaluating treatment possibilities now must be considered:

Interaction Among Possible Solutions. The interaction among possible solutions to the patient's various problems is much easier to see when the possibilities are listed as described above. As in the case of the girl above, it will be clear for nearly every patient that some possible solutions to a high-priority problem would also solve other problems, while others would not and might even make other things worse.

One important interaction to keep in mind, the one that was critical in our case example, is the relationship between vertical and horizontal changes in the position of the mandible (see Figure 7-7). Consider the opposite situation to girl above, the patient with an anterior open bite. Often

this problem is due, not to decreased eruption of incisors, but to excessive eruption of posterior teeth and downward-backward rotation of the mandible. If so, using vertical elastics to elongate the anterior teeth is not a solution. Treatment should be aimed at depressing the elongated posterior teeth, or preventing them from erupting further while everything else grows (relative intrusion). This would allow the mandible to rotate upward, bringing the incisor teeth together. But if the mandible rotates upward, it also will come forward—which would be good if the patient had a skeletal Class II malocclusion to begin with but bad if the malocclusion was Class I or Class III.

Another important interaction, which also came into play in the case example, is the relationship between incisor protrusion and the extraction-expansion decision. Expansion of the arches to bring crowded teeth into alignment, even if most of the expansion is transverse rather than antero-posterior, tends to make the incisors more prominent. There may be esthetic advantages, as in the preceding case, but the tooth alignment is likely to be less stable than if the incisors had been retracted.

Compromise. In patients with many problems, it may not be possible to solve them all. This type of compromise has nothing to do with the clinician's skill. In some cases, no plan of treatment will solve all of the patient's problems. Then careful setting of priorities from the problem list is particularly important.

In a broad sense, the major goals of orthodontic treatment are ideal occlusion, ideal facial esthetics, and ideal stability of result. Often it is impossible to maximize all three. In fact, attempts to achieve an absolutely ideal dental occlusion (if this is taken to prohibit extractions) can diminish both facial esthetics and stability after treatment. In the same way, efforts to achieve the most stable result after orthodontic treatment may result in less than optimal occlusion and facial esthetics, and positioning the teeth to produce ideal facial esthetics may detract from occlusion and stability.

One way to avoid having to face compromises of this type, of course, is to emphasize one of the goals at the expense of the others. In the early twentieth century, Edward Angle, the father of modern orthodontics, solved this problem by focusing solely on the occlusion and declaring that facial esthetics and stability would take care of themselves. Unfortunately, they did not. Echoes of Angle's position are encountered occasionally even now, particularly among dentists strongly committed to avoiding extraction at all costs.

As important as dental occlusion is, it is not the most important consideration for all patients. Sometimes ideal occlusion must be altered, by extraction or otherwise, to gain acceptable esthetics and stability. Adjustments in the other goals also may be needed. It often is the case that placing the teeth for optimal facial esthetics may require permanent retention because they are not stable in that position, or alternatively, that placing the teeth in a position of maximum stability will diminish facial esthetics.

If various elements of a treatment plan are incompatible, benefit to the patient is greatest if any necessary compromises are made so that the patient's most important problems are solved, while less important problems are deferred or left untreated. If all of the three major goals of orthodontic treatment cannot be reached, those of greatest importance to that patient should be favored. Doing this successfully requires judgment and thought on the part of the clinician and input from the patient and parent. For our example patient, would better facial esthetics with more prominent incisors be worth possibly decreased stability of the result?

Cost-Risk/Benefit Analysis. Practical considerations related to the difficulty of various treatment procedures compared with the benefit to be gained from them also must be considered in evaluating treatment possibilities. The difficulty should be considered in both risk and cost to the patient (not just in money, but also in cooperation, discomfort, aggravation, time, and other factors that can be collectively labeled as the "burden of treatment"). These must be contrasted to the probable benefit from that procedure.

For instance, for a patient with anterior open bite, jaw surgery to decrease face height must rank higher in cost and risk than elastics to elongate the incisors or occlusal reduction of the posterior teeth, two other possibilities for correcting the bite relationship. But if the simpler and less risky procedures would provide little real benefit to the patient, while jaw surgery would provide considerable benefit, the cost-risk/benefit analysis might still favor the more difficult procedure. "Is it worth it?" is a question that must be answered not only from the point of view of what is involved, but in terms of the benefit to the patient.

Other Considerations. At this stage, it is important to take into account any pertinent special considerations about the individual patient. Should the treatment time be minimized because of possible exacerbation of periodontal disease? Should treatment options be left open as long as possible because of uncertainty of the pattern of growth? Should visible orthodontic appliances be avoided because of the patient's vanity, even if it makes treatment more difficult? Such questions must be addressed from the perspective of the individual patient. Rational answers can be obtained only when the treatment possibilities and other important factors influencing the treatment plan have been considered.

For our example patient, interactions, thoughts about necessary compromises, and other considerations (which in her case are quite minor) are shown in Box 7-4. The information now has been assembled and treatment possibilities are ready to be discussed with the patient and parents in order to finalize the treatment plan (Box 7-5).

Patient-Parent Consultation: Obtaining Informed Consent

Not so long ago, it was taken for granted that the doctor should analyze the patient's situation and should prescribe what he or she had determined to be the best treatment—with little or no regard for whether that treatment was what

---

BOX 7-4

PATIENT F.P.: INTERACTIONS OF TREATMENT POSSIBILITIES

In the absence of vertical growth, increasing facial height will cause the mandible to rotate downward and backward, making the mandibular deficiency worse.

Expanding the arches will bring incisors forward, improving lip support but creating overjet.

Extraction in either arch would decrease lip support and make the nose and chin look more prominent.

Class II elastics would tend to elongate the lower molars and could rotate the mandible downward and backward.

Other considerations in planning treatment:

- The nose is relatively large and the chin reasonably prominent.
- Little or no growth can be expected at this level of maturity.
- The patient is motivated and likely to cooperate well.

---

the patient desired. This is best described as a paternalistic approach to patient care: the doctor, as a father figure, knows best and makes the decisions.

At present, that approach is not defensible, ethically and legally or practically.[1-3] From an ethical perspective, patients have the right to determine what is done to them in treatment, and increasingly they demand that right. It is unethical not to inform patients of the alternatives, including the likely outcome of no treatment, that are possible in their case. The modern doctrine of informed consent has made the ethical imperative a legal one as well. Legally, the doctor now is liable for problems arising from failure to fully inform the patient about the treatment that is to be performed. Informed consent is not obtained just from a discussion of the risks of treatment. Patients must be told what their problems are, what the treatment alternatives are, and what the possible outcomes of treatment or no treatment are likely to be.

The problem-oriented method of diagnosis and treatment planning lends itself very well to the patient involvement that the modern approach requires.[4] A discussion with the patient and parents should begin with an outline of the patient's problems, and patient involvement begins with the prioritization of the problem list. Perhaps the doctor's single most important question in obtaining informed consent is, "Your most important problem, as I see it, is .... Do you agree?" When problems related to informed consent for orthodontic treatment arise, almost always they result from treatment that failed to address what was most important to the patient, or from treatment that focused on what was not an important problem to the patient.

The problem-oriented method requires examining the possible solutions to the patient's problems, starting with the most important one, and this also is exactly the way in which a discussion with the patient and parents is structured most effectively (see Box 7-5). Interactions, unavoidable compromises and practical considerations must not only be considered by the doctor, they must be shared with the patient as the treatment plan is developed. Under most circumstances, there are advantages and disadvantages to the possible treatment approaches. The doctor's role is to clarify this to the best of his or her ability, involving the patient in the final decision as to the treatment approach that will be employed.

From a practical perspective, involving the patient and parents in decisions about treatment has important advantages. It places the responsibility where it belongs, on a patient who has been led to understand the uncertainties involved. The problems, after all, belong to the patient, not the doctor. A patient who "owns" the problems and recognizes that this is the case, is more likely to be cooperative and oriented toward helping with his or her treatment, than someone who takes the attitude that it's all up to the doctor.

Several specific situations in orthodontics particularly require interaction between the doctor and the patient and parent in choosing the final treatment plan. Perhaps the most frequent revolves around the issue of arch expansion versus extraction in solving crowding problems. From the beginning of the specialty, orthodontists have debated whether the advantages of extraction outweigh the disadvantages. A disadvantage is the loss of a tooth or teeth; an

advantage is likely to be greater stability of the result; and there may be positive or negative effects on facial esthetics. But in fact for any individual patient the decision is a value judgment. It is not only appropriate but necessary to discuss the pros and cons with the patient and parent before making the extraction-nonextraction decision. One option is to attempt the more conservative nonextraction treatment, and evaluate the treatment response before making what is an irreversible decision to remove teeth.[5] Obviously, this would be an important item for discussion with our example patient and her parents.

A second frequent problem requiring input from the patient is the treatment of Class II malocclusion in a pre-adolescent child. In this situation, two aspects must be discussed: the efficacy of beginning treatment early versus waiting for adolescence, and if early treatment is chosen, the mode of treatment. There is no doubt that successful Class II treatment for most patients is possible either by beginning early or waiting. Current data, reviewed below in this chapter and in detail in Chapter 8, suggest that the benefits of early treatment are not compelling in many cases, but there are some definite advantages (primarily, avoidance of trauma to protruding maxillary incisors) and other possible ones (better psychosocial development, greater skeletal change). The disadvantage is a longer treatment time, with greater demands on cooperation and often greater cost. The child's desire for treatment and potential cooperation also

---

BOX 7-5

PATIENT F.P.—OUTLINE OF CASE PRESENTATION

(Goal: to appropriately involve patient/parent in decisions, obtain informed consent)

General and oral health
Two minor problems:
- some tissue irritation around the erupting lower molar
- mild gingivitis

(Both to be controlled with better hygiene)

Orthodontic problems
- mild crowding lower teeth, more severe crowding of upper teeth
- extreme overbite with potential damage to tissue
- tendency for lower jaw and teeth to be behind upper

(To be corrected with full braces)

Benefits from treatment
Functional:
- facilitate lateral jaw movement

Esthetic:
- dental appearance, facial proportions

Most important problem
- deep overbite
- do you agree?

Plan to correct the overbite:
- growth not enough, must intrude incisors

Two ways to correct the crowded upper teeth and Class II tendency
- expand, moving the front teeth forward as well as up
- remove one tooth on each side, pull the teeth back, and align the rest

Advantages/disadvantages of alternative approaches
- esthetics
- stability, retention
- certainty or uncertainty of outcome

(Could show computer predictions at this point)

Then it is agreed that the treatment plan should be . . .
- nonextraction or extraction
- review details of plan, cooperation needs, treatment time

Risks of treatment
- decalcification
- root resorption, especially of maxillary incisors
- any other pertinent items

(A signed form acknowledging this discussion is preferred but not required if this is documented in the chart.)

Treatment schedule, costs, etc.

must be taken into account. This affects both the decision as to treat now or wait and the selection of the appliance to be used if early treatment is chosen. There is little reason to proceed with headgear or functional appliance treatment for a child who has no intention of wearing the device. Treatment results with the two methods are not precisely the same but can be considered more similar than different, and if the child would wear one but not the other, it would be wise to select the one the child would prefer.

A third frequent issue for discussion with the patient and parents is whether orthodontic treatment alone would produce an acceptable result for a skeletal malocclusion, or whether orthognathic surgery should be selected. Sometimes this difficult decision revolves around whether jaw function would be satisfactory with displacement of the in-cisor teeth to compensate for a jaw malrelationship, versus function with the jaws in the correct position. In most instances, however, it is primarily an esthetic decision. Facial esthetics are likely to be better if the jaw relationship is corrected. Is that improvement worth the additional risk, cost and morbidity of surgery? In the final analysis, only the patient and parents can—or should—make that decision.

Recent advances in computer prediction of alternative outcomes, so that the likely effects on facial appearance from various treatment procedures can be simulated, have made it easier to communicate with patients. Especially in decisions like surgery versus orthodontic camouflage but also in deciding whether to expand the dental arches or extract, a picture is worth a thousand words (Figure 7-8). Good evidence now shows that communication is improved

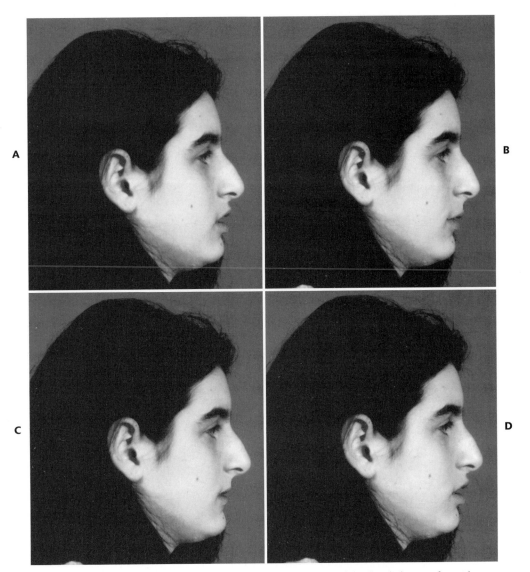

FIGURE 7-8   Patient F.P., age 16-11, computer predictions of the facial changes from alternative treatment plans: **A,** the initial facial profile; **B,** nonextraction orthodontics with incisor intrusion; **C,** premolar extraction; **D,** surgical mandibular advancement. Predictions of this type are most accurate in patients who will have little or no growth; they can be very helpful in getting patients to really understand the esthetic impact of alternative approaches. Compare the prediction (in this case, **B**) to the actual treatment result (see Figure 7-3). (Prediction software: Dentofacial Planner.)

when video images of the likely outcome of alternative treatment procedures are shown to the patient.[4,6,7] Video image predictions are much more accurate when growth is not involved, but this method can help parents understand the options for children and adolescents as well. These prediction techniques also are discussed below.

Sometimes involving patients in treatment planning decisions is interpreted as allowing the patient and parent to make all the decisions. Clearly this is not the case. It is the doctor's responsibility to explain the options to the patient and parents, and to negotiate with them the final treatment plan. It is not the doctor's responsibility to do anything the patient wants. Just as any patient has the right to refuse to accept treatment, the doctor has the right to refuse to supply treatment that he or she considers not in the patient's best interest. At one time, the doctor decided what was to be done, and that was that. Now, establishing the final treatment plan is, and must be, an interactive process between the doctor and the patient.

The patient described earlier and her parents understood the importance of the deep bite, accepted the suggestion that arch expansion would be better than premolar extraction even though long-term stability might be somewhat compromised, and acknowledged that a change in the treatment plan to include extraction or even orthognathic surgery might be needed if the patient did not respond well to the more conservative initial treatment plan. They also reviewed the anticipated risks of treatment in her case (Box 7-6), the primary concerns being root resorption (especially of the maxillary incisors) and the possibility of damage to the teeth from inadequate hygiene. The result was both informed consent in the broad (and correct) sense and the treatment plan concept (Box 7-7).

The Detailed Plan: Specifying Orthodontic Mechanotherapy

What is established in the patient-parent consultation is the treatment plan in conceptual form—Class II treatment by growth modification with a functional appliance, for instance, or the intrusion/arch expansion plan for our example patient. The final step in planning treatment is specification of the treatment method—in orthodontics, the mechanotherapy—that is to be used. For the Class II functional appliance patient, the mechanotherapy might be a bionator with an initial mandibular advancement of 4 mm, the mandibular incisors capped, mandibular posterior teeth free to erupt, and the maxillary teeth blocked vertically.

The detailed plan for our example patient is shown in Box 7-7. Note that for this patient, the conceptual plan leads directly to the mechanotherapy—which usually is the case. For any patient, the selected treatment procedures must meet two criteria: *effectiveness* in producing the desired result and *efficiency* in doing so without wasting either doctor or patient time. Progress and completion of this case are shown in Figures 7-1 to 7-4.

For a relatively simple treatment plan, the associated mechanotherapy is also reasonably simple or at least straightforward. Nevertheless, choices must be made and clearly specified in the treatment plan. For example, if the plan is to expand a narrow maxillary arch, it would be possible to do this with springs on a removable appliance, an expansion lingual arch, or an expansion labial arch. The treatment plan must specify which, and the effectiveness and efficiency of the various possibilities must be considered. There is a time and a place for everything, and this last step is the place for these practical considerations of which appliance to use.

The most serious errors in orthodontic treatment planning are those that result from first thinking of which appliance to use, not what the appliance is supposed to accom-

---

BOX 7-6

PATIENT F.P.: RISKS OF ORTHODONTIC TREATMENT

(Include in disclosure form)
- Discomfort after appliance adjustment
- Decalcification related to poor hygiene
- Root resorption
- Pulp degeneration in previously traumatized teeth
- Return of teeth toward initial position
- Problems related to disproportionate jaw growth
- TMJ problems
- Variations in estimated treatment time

BOX 7-7

PATIENT F.P.: FINAL TREATMENT PLAN (NONEXTRACTION PREFERRED)

Treatment Concept:
- correct overbite by incisor intrusion
- correct crowding by arch expansion
- minimize tendency for mandible to rotate down-back

Mechanotherapy:
1. Band molars, bond other teeth; maxillary transpalatal lingual arch
2. Align anterior segments, stabilize posterior segments
3. Intrude incisors, segmented arch mechanics
4. Minimal Class II elastics to correct anteroposterior relationships

Retention: maintain alignment, bite opening; maxillary removable with lower incisor contact, mandible fixed or removable

plish. The treatment mechanics should not be allowed to determine the treatment result. It is an error to establish the treatment mechanics before establishing the broader goal of treatment. The treatment procedures should be manipulated to produce the desired result, not the other way around.

CRITICAL ISSUES IN TREATMENT PLANNING

In order to plan treatment appropriately, decisions must be made about three critical issues: (1) what treatment is needed, (2) who should do it, and (3) when is the best time to do it. These issues establish the environment for the orthodontic treatment planning process. They must be reviewed before specific points about treatment planning in various circumstances are considered.

Need for Treatment

There are two aspects to the question of what treatment is needed: whether treatment is indicated at all, and if so, what treatment procedures should be used.

Indications for Orthodontic Treatment.   Since no one dies of untreated malocclusion, from that perspective orthodontic treatment always is elective. There are clear benefits, however, from treatment to correct some types of problems, while the benefit from other types of treatment is not so clear. In broad terms, there are four reasons for orthodontic treatment, in the order of their importance: (1) to remove, or at least alleviate, the social handicap created by an unacceptable dental and/or facial appearance; (2) to maintain as normal a developmental process as possible; (3) to improve jaw function and correct problems related to functional impairment; and (4) to reduce the impact on the dentition of trauma or disease. These are discussed in some detail in Chapter 1, and references to the appropriate literature are provided there. The goal here is to summarize what is known about need for orthodontic treatment.

Psychosocial Indications.   Because the research literature makes a reasonably secure case for the impact of the teeth on facial esthetics, self-image and the reactions of others, treatment is justifiable on this basis when the appearance of the face and/or teeth creates a problem for the patient (see Chapter 1). Although the severity of the malocclusion correlates with its psychosocial effect, measuring how much the teeth protrude or how irregular they are is not sufficient to determine individual treatment need. This is case-, patient-, and parent-specific. A malocclusion that is not a problem for one individual can be a significant problem for another. Malocclusion has little or no psychosocial impact on preadolescent children unless it is extremely severe, so for most children there is little or no need to begin treatment early from concern about their social development.

Developmental Indications.   Problems related to the development of the dentition occur relatively frequently,

and often orthodontic treatment is needed to maintain dental health and continue normal development. For example, it is much better to create space to prevent a displaced tooth from erupting through mucosa than to let this periodontal problem develop and plan gingival grafts later. Treatment to control the attrition of tooth structure than can occur when a tooth is out of position, or to control loss of space if a tooth is missing or lost, also is easily justified. Problems of dental development almost always should be corrected when noticed.

Distortions of facial growth that produce jaw discrepancies also are indications for treatment, but the timing of treatment for skeletal problems is not so obvious. Because a major reason for correcting jaw discrepancies is their psychosocial effect, delaying treatment until adolescence may be appropriate even though (for example) protruding upper incisors and excessive overjet were obvious much earlier.

Functional Indications.   It is obvious that severe malocclusion must affect function, at least to the extent of making it more difficult for the affected individual to breathe, incise, chew, swallow, and speak. The reverse also is true: alterations or adaptations in function can be etiologic factors for malocclusion, by influencing the pattern of growth and development (see Chapter 5). The extent to which improved function justifies orthodontic treatment remains poorly defined. Current thinking can be summarized as follows:

- Respiration—There seem to be numerous weak relationships between respiratory mode and malocclusion, but the more refined and rigorous the investigations, the more questionable specific links become. The evidence does not support orthodontic referrals of children for surgery to open the nasal airway (by removing adenoids, turbinates, or other presumed obstacles to nasal airflow), because the effect on the future facial growth pattern is unpredictable. For the same reason, expanding the maxillary dental arch by opening the midpalatal suture, which also widens the nasal passages, cannot be supported as an effective way of changing the respiratory pattern toward nasal breathing and away from mouth breathing.
- Chewing, jaw function, and temporomandibular joint dysfunction(TMD)—It seems obvious that chewing should be easier and more efficient if the dental occlusion is good, but individuals expend the effort necessary to accomplish important tasks like chewing, and there is little evidence to support any impact of malocclusion on nutritional status. Except for the most extreme malocclusions, the effects of malocclusion on chewing appear to be increased work to prepare a satisfactory bolus for swallowing. Masticatory effort is difficult to measure accurately, so there are no good data for how much difference it makes to have mild, moderate, or severe malocclusion.

It is possible that functional problems related to malocclusion would appear as temporomandibular dysfunction. Little or no data support the idea that orthodontic treatment is needed at any age to prevent the development of TMD. Weak correlations exist between some types of malocclusion and the prevalence of TMD, but they are not strong enough to explain even a small fraction of TMD problems.

- Swallowing/speech—Both the pattern of activity in swallowing and tongue-lip function during speech are affected by the presence of the teeth. The most effective way to reduce the prominence of the tongue during swallowing is to retract protruding incisors and close an open bite, so orthodontics can have an effect on swallowing, but rarely is this a reason for orthodontic treatment. Normal speech is possible in the presence of extreme anatomic deviations. Certain types of malocclusion are related to difficulty with specific sounds (see Table 6-1), and occasionally a reason for orthodontic treatment is that it would facilitate speech therapy. Usually, however, speech problems are not a reason for orthodontics.

Trauma/Disease Control Indications.　At one time it was thought that malocclusion contributed to the development of periodontal disease, but this link is so tenuous that almost never is it a reason for orthodontic treatment. In older patients, orthodontics as an adjunct to periodontal therapy may be indicated. In children and adolescents, orthodontics cannot be justified for disease control.

Trauma is another story. There is ample evidence that protruding incisors are more likely to be injured, which can be a valid reason for trying to correct this problem soon after the permanent teeth erupt. There also is good evidence that contact of the lower incisors with the palatal mucosa, which often occurs in deep overbite, leads to periodontal defects long-term. Correcting tissue impingement by the teeth is a good reason for treatment at any age.

The bottom line: orthodontic treatment almost always is elective, but it can produce significant benefits in psychosocial well-being, normal development, jaw function and dental/oral health. Treatment is needed if it would produce these benefits—and not needed if it would not.

Type of Treatment: Evidence-Based Selection.　If treatment is needed, how do you decide what sort of treatment should be provided? The present trend in health care is strongly toward evidence-based treatment, that is, treatment procedures should be chosen on the basis of clear evidence that the selected method is the most successful approach to that particular patient's problem(s).[8] The better the evidence, of course, the better the decision.

The problem-oriented approach to diagnosis and treatment planning is built around identifying the patient's problems, then considering and evaluating the possible solutions to those specific problems. The best way to evaluate alternative treatment methods is with a randomized clinical trial, in which great care is taken to control variables that might affect the outcomes, so that differences

attributable to the treatment procedures become apparent. A second acceptable way to replace opinion with evidence is from careful study of treatment outcomes under well-defined conditions. Clinical trial data are just becoming available in orthodontics, and not all decisions about alternative treatment possibilities can be based on good evidence of any type. In Chapter 8, the quality of clinical evidence relative for current orthodontic procedures is examined in detail. In this and the subsequent chapters, recommendations for treatment are based insofar as possible on solid clinical evidence. Where this is not available, the authors' current opinions are provided and labeled as such.

Orthodontic Triage: Distinguishing Moderate from Complex Treatment Problems

The second basic decision in planning orthodontic treatment, typically faced by the family dentist seeing a child who needs orthodontic intervention now, is who should do the treatment. Does this patient warrant referral to a specialist?

In military and emergency medicine, triage is the process used to separate casualties by the severity of their injuries. Its purpose is twofold: to separate patients who can be treated at the scene of the injury from those who need transportation to specialized facilities, and to develop a sequence for handling patients so that those most likely to benefit from immediate treatment will be treated first. Since orthodontic problems almost never are an emergency, the process of sorting orthodontic problems by their severity is analogous to triage in only one sense of the word. On the other hand, it is very important for the primary care dentist to be able to distinguish moderate from complex problems, because this process determines which patients are appropriately treated within family practice and which are most appropriately referred to a specialist.

As with all components of dental practice, a generalist's decision of whether to include orthodontic treatment as a component of his or her services is an individual one. The principle that the less severe problems are handled within the context of general practice and the more severe problems are referred should remain the same, however, regardless of the practitioner's interest in orthodontics. Only the cutoff points for retention of a patient in the general practice or referral should change.

This section presents a logical scheme for orthodontic triage for children, to select children for referral on the basis of the severity of their malocclusion and the likely complexity of their evaluation and treatment. It is based on the diagnostic approach developed in Chapter 6 and incorporates the principles of determining treatment need that are discussed above. An adequate database and a thorough problem list, of course, are necessary to carry out the triage process. A cephalometric radiograph is not required, but appropriate dental radiographs are needed (usually, a panoramic film; occasionally, bitewings supplemented with anterior occlusal radiographs). A flow chart illustrating the steps in the triage sequence accompanies this section.

Syndromes and Developmental Abnormalities. The first step in the triage process is to separate out patients with facial syndromes and similarly complex problems (Figure 7-9). From physical appearance, the medical and dental histories, and an evaluation of developmental status, nearly all such patients are easily recognized. Examples of these disorders are cleft lip or palate, Treacher-Collins' syndrome, hemifacial microsomia, and Crouzon's syndrome (see Chapter 3). The multidisciplinary treatment approach now considered as the standard of care for these patients should lead to their referral to a craniofacial team of specialists at a regional medical center for evaluation and treatment. The American Cleft Palate Association publishes a directory of these teams,[9] who now cover the whole spectrum of craniofacial problems, not just cleft palate.

A similar route of referral and medical evaluation is recommended for patients who appear to be developing either above the 97th or below the third percentiles on standard growth charts. Growth disorders may demand that any orthodontic treatment be carried out in conjunction with endocrine, nutritional, or psychological therapy. For these patients and those with diseases that affect growth, such as juvenile rheumatoid arthritis, the proper orthodontic therapy must be combined with identification and control of the disease process.

Facial Disproportions and Asymmetries

Facial Asymmetry. Patients with significant skeletal asymmetry (not necessarily those whose asymmetry results from only a functional shift of the mandible) always fall into the severe problem category (see Figure 7-9). These patients could have a developmental problem or the growth anomaly could be the result of injury. They require evaluation including posteroanterior and lateral cephalometric radiographs. Treatment is likely to involve surgery in addition to comprehensive orthodontics. Timing of intervention is affected by whether the cause of the asymmetry is deficient or excessive growth (Chapter 8), but early comprehensive evaluation is indicated even if treatment ultimately is deferred, and early treatment usually is needed.

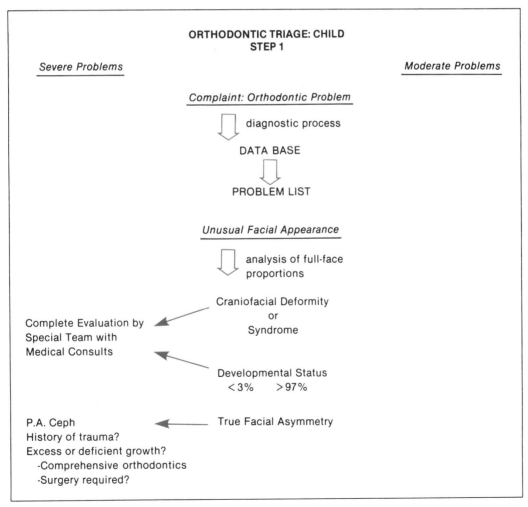

FIGURE 7-9 Orthodontic triage, step 1.

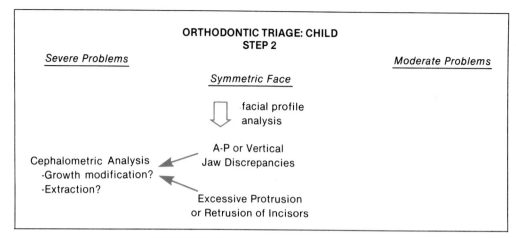

FIGURE 7-10 Orthodontic triage, step 2.

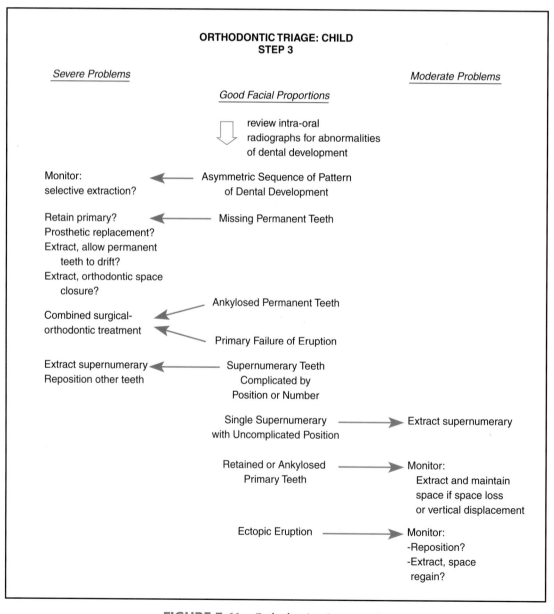

FIGURE 7-11 Orthodontic triage, step 3.

Anteroposterior and Vertical Problems. Skeletal Class II and Class III problems and vertical deformities of the long face and short face types, regardless of their cause, require thorough cephalometric evaluation to plan appropriate treatment and must be considered complex problems (Figure 7-10). As with asymmetry, early evaluation is indicated even if treatment would be deferred, so early referral is appropriate. Issues in treatment planning for growth modification are discussed in Chapter 8, and the appropriate treatment techniques are described in Chapter 15.

Excessive Dental Protrusion or Retrusion. Severe dental protrusion or retrusion, which also is a complex treatment problem, should be recognized during the facial profile analysis (see Figure 7-10). Excessive protrusion or retrusion of incisor teeth often accompanies skeletal jaw discrepancies, and if protrusion is present in a patient who also has a skeletal problem, this should be subordinated to the skeletal problem in planning treatment. It is also possible, however, for an individual with good skeletal proportions to have protrusion of incisor teeth rather than crowding. When this occurs, the space analysis will show a small or nonexistent discrepancy, because the incisor protrusion has compensated for the potential crowding.

Excessive protrusion of incisors (bimaxillary protrusion, not excessive overjet) is usually an indication for premolar extraction and retraction of the protruding incisors. This is complex and prolonged treatment. Because of the profile changes produced by adolescent growth, it is better for most children to defer extraction to correct protrusion until late in the mixed dentition or early in the permanent dentition. It is definitely an error to begin extraction early and then allow the permanent molars to drift forward, because this will make effective incisor retraction impossible. Techniques for controlling the amount of incisor retraction are described in Chapter 17.

Problems Involving Dental Development. Unlike the more complex skeletal problems and problems related to protruding incisors, problems involving dental development usually need treatment as soon as they are discovered, typically during the early mixed dentition, and often can be handled in family practice (Figure 7-11).

Asymmetric Dental Development. An abnormal sequence of dental development should be planned for treatment only after a careful determination of the underlying cause. Asymmetric eruption (one side ahead of the other) is significant if the difference is 6 months or more. Appropriate treatment involves careful monitoring of the situation, and in the absence of outright pathology, often requires selective extraction of primary or permanent teeth. Early intervention to promote more symmetric development of the dental arches, as for example the early extraction of the right mandibular primary canine after the left canine has been lost prematurely, can circumvent the need for treating a severe asymmetry problem at a later time, but such a step must be taken only after careful consideration of the total problem list for an individual patient.

A few patients with asymmetric dental development have a history of childhood radiation therapy to the head and neck. These patients often have extremes of delayed or asymmetric dental development (Figure 7-12). Surgical and orthodontic treatment for these patients must be planned and timed carefully with their medical treatment providers and definitely falls into the complex category.

Missing Permanent Teeth. A congenitally missing permanent tooth is an actual (if the primary predecessor is missing or lost) or potential (if the primary tooth is still

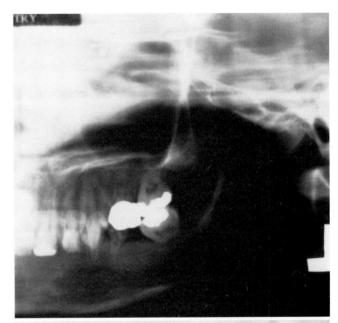

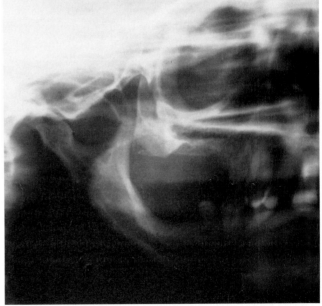

FIGURE 7-12 Radiation to the jaws, as in treatment of a tumor, can significantly reduce the size of developing teeth. This child had significant radiation to the jaw in the treatment of a pharyngeal malignancy; note the effect on the teeth.

present) problem of arch asymmetry. The permanent teeth most likely to be missing are the mandibular second premolars and the maxillary lateral incisors, but the treatment possibilities are the same whatever the missing tooth: (1) maintenance of the primary tooth or teeth; (2) replacement of the missing teeth prosthetically or perhaps by transplantation or implant; (3) extraction of the overlying primary teeth, and then allowing the permanent teeth to drift; or (4) extraction of the primary teeth followed by immediate orthodontic treatment. As with other growth problems, early evaluation and planning is essential, even if the decision is against aggressive treatment at that time, so early referral is indicated. Making the correct decision requires a careful assessment of facial profile, incisor position, space requirements, and the status of the primary teeth. Treatment of missing tooth problems in mixed dentition children is discussed in more detail in Chapter 14.

For all practical purposes, ankylosed permanent teeth at an early age or teeth that fail to erupt for other reasons (like primary failure of eruption) fall into the same category as missing teeth. Usually there is little choice but to extract the affected teeth, and then the choices are orthodontic space closure (if enough alveolar bone exists to allow it) or prosthetic replacement (more likely).

Supernumerary Teeth.   Ninety percent of all supernumerary teeth are found in the anterior part of the maxilla. Multiple or inverted supernumeraries and those that are malformed often displace adjacent teeth or cause problems in eruption.[10] The presence of multiple supernumerary teeth indicates a complex problem and perhaps a syndrome or congenital abnormality like cleidocranial dysplasia. Early removal is indicated, but this must be done carefully to minimize damage to adjacent teeth. If the permanent teeth have been displaced, surgical exposure, adjunctive periodontal surgery, and possibly mechanical traction are likely to be required to bring them into the arch after the supernumerary has been removed.

Single supernumeraries that are not malformed often erupt spontaneously, causing crowding problems. If these teeth can be removed before they cause distortions of arch form, or if the supernumerary tooth erupts outside the line of the arch, extraction may be all that is needed.

Other Eruption Problems.   Ectopic eruption and ankylosed primary teeth should be monitored carefully. Space maintenance or space regaining may be required in their aftermath. Both are moderate problems in the absence of a broader space deficiency. Ankylosed permanent teeth or permanent teeth that fail to erupt, however, are severe problems that often require a combination of surgery and orthodontics if indeed the condition can be treated satisfactorily at all.

Space Problems.   Orthodontic problems in a child with good facial proportions must involve crowding, irregularity, or malposition of the teeth (Figure 7-13). At this stage, regardless of whether crowding is apparent, the results of space analysis are essential for planning treatment. The presence or absence of adequate space for the teeth must be taken into account when other treatment is planned.

In interpreting the results of space analysis for patients of any age, remember that if space to align the teeth is inadequate, either of two conditions may develop. One possibility is for the incisor teeth to remain upright and well positioned over the basal bone of the maxilla or mandible, and then rotate or tip labially or lingually. In this instance, the potential crowding is expressed as actual crowding and is difficult to miss. The other possibility, however, is for the crowded teeth to align themselves completely or partially at the expense of the lips, displacing the lips forward and separating them at rest. Even if the space discrepancy and therefore the potential crowding are extreme, the teeth can always align themselves at the expense of the lip, interfering with lip closure. This must be detected on profile examination. If the incisors are upright and crowding is moderate, a few millimeters of arch expansion can often be carried out to solve the crowding problem. On the other hand, if there is already a degree of protrusion in addition to the crowding, it is safe to presume that the natural limits of anterior displacement of incisors have been reached.

Space discrepancies greater than 4 mm, with or without incisor protrusion, or discrepancies smaller than 4 mm in the presence of incisor protrusion, constitute complex treatment problems. Depending on the circumstances, the appropriate response to space deficiencies of 4 mm or less can be treatment to regain lost space after early loss of a primary molar or ectopic eruption, management of transitional crowding and repositioning of the permanent incisors during the mixed dentition, or deferral of treatment until adolescence. Treatment planning for these moderate problems is outlined below in the preadolescent section of this chapter.

Other Occlusal Discrepancies

Whether other problems of dental alignment and occlusion should be classified as moderate or severe is determined for most children by the facial form and space analysis results (Figure 7-14). A skeletal posterior crossbite, revealed by a narrow palatal vault, is a severe problem, but a dental posterior crossbite falls into the moderate category if no other complicating factors (like severe crowding) are present. In a skeletal posterior crossbite, it is possible to widen the maxilla itself by opening the midpalatal suture, provided the patient is young enough to allow suture opening. This topic is discussed further in Chapter 8. If the crossbite is caused by maxillary posterior teeth that are tipped lingually, it is possible to tip the teeth outward into proper position with a variety of simple appliances (see Chapters 13 and 14).

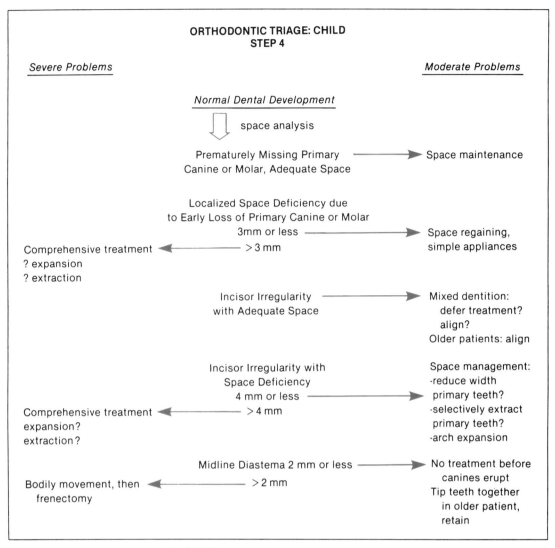

FIGURE 7-13 Orthodontic triage, step 4.

Anterior crossbite usually reflects a jaw discrepancy but can arise by lingual tipping of the incisors as they erupt. Treatment planning for the use of removable versus fixed appliances to correct these simple crossbites is discussed later under mixed dentition treatment. Excessive overjet, with the upper incisors flared and spaced, often reflects a skeletal problem but also can develop in patients with good jaw proportions. If adequate vertical clearance is present, the teeth can be tipped lingually and brought together with a simple removable appliance when the child is at almost any age. If a deep overbite is present, however, the protruding maxillary incisors can be retracted only if adequate vertical clearance is provided. Remember that deep overbite may reflect a skeletal vertical problem even if antero-posterior facial proportions are normal. Even if skeletal vertical also is normal, mixed dentition treatment usually involves placing a fixed orthodontic appliance on both maxillary and mandibular incisors and can rapidly become complex.

Anterior open bite in a young child with good facial proportions usually needs no treatment, because there is a good chance of spontaneous correction. A complex open bite (one with skeletal involvement or posterior manifestations), or any open bite in an older patient, is a severe problem, as is deep bite at all ages.

Traumatically displaced incisors pose a special problem because of the risk of ankylosis after healing occurs. Immediate treatment is needed, and the long-term prognosis must be guarded. Treatment planning after trauma is discussed later in the preadolescent section of this chapter.

This triage scheme is oriented toward helping the family practitioner decide which children with orthodontic problems to treat and which to refer. A triage scheme to help distinguish moderate from severe orthodontic problems in adults is presented in Chapter 20. Now let us review the final question that forms a background for orthodontic treatment planning—the best time for treatment.

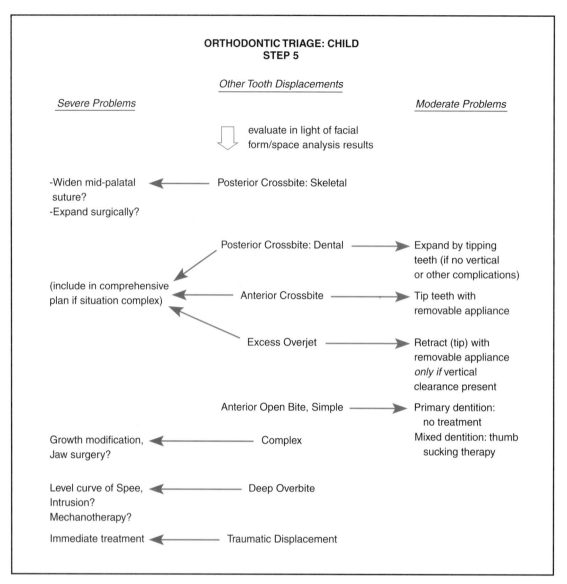

FIGURE 7-14 Orthodontic triage, step 5.

Timing of Treatment

Questions about the timing of orthodontic treatment relate almost totally to the question of whether to begin treatment for a child with obvious malocclusion early, during the primary or mixed dentition, or whether to wait for the adolescent growth spurt and the eruption of the permanent teeth.

From the beginning of comprehensive orthodontic treatment, most patients have been treated during a single stage of treatment during early adolescence, beginning in the late mixed dentition or early permanent dentition and lasting about 24 months. There are good reasons for focusing most treatment then. The child has reached a stage at which self-motivation for treatment is more likely, which is evident in improved ability to cooperate during appointments and in appliance care and hygiene but still remains dependent and compliant in some regards. Usually enough growth remains so that it is possible to change antero-posterior jaw relationships, and adolescent growth provides vertical space that makes it easier to reposition the teeth. All teeth including the second molars can be controlled to bring treatment to a semblance of finality, even though some growth remains after treatment is completed. The relatively limited duration of treatment is within the tolerance of most patients and their families. Acceptable results can be obtained for most patients.

The stability of the results from this traditional timing of treatment have been highly variable. Despite this notable shortcoming, one-stage treatment in early adolescence remains the "gold standard" for contemporary care. To be justified, early or two-stage treatment that takes longer and costs more should offer a clear advantage in esthetic, developmental, functional, or trauma-prevention terms. A different timing of treatment should be based on scientific data for effectiveness and on a logical rationale for the timing choice, not on the availability of the patient and a general feeling that earlier is better. The following overview of the advantages and disadvantages of early versus later treatment is provided to put the timing issue in broad perspective, before we review treatment planning at various ages in more detail.

Treatment during the primary dentition offers the advantage of rapid change in skeletal and dental structures because of relatively rapid growth and because at that age, even moderate biomechanical forces are quite effective. Significant improvement in jaw relationships often can be obtained quite quickly during the preschool years, especially with skeletal Class II problems. Unfortunately, continued rapid growth can easily erase the treatment effects unless active retention, which quickly can become unreasonably extended treatment, is employed. Child behavior can be challenging both during and between appointments, which may test practitioners and parents. For treatment to be justified during this period, the effects should be both dramatic and long lasting. Only treatment that offers significant current and future esthetic and functional advantages, or limited treatment to deal with immediate developmental problems, should be considered.

Parents rarely seek treatment for their children during the primary dentition, but eruption of the permanent incisors makes malocclusion obvious, and orthodontic advice often is sought in the early mixed dentition. The real controversy is whether beginning treatment then, which carries with it the implication of a second phase of permanent dentition treatment later, offers enough advantages to justify it. It is safe to say that two stages of treatment will take longer than one and that two-stage treatment is very likely to be more costly.

There is no doubt that many children do need orthodontics during the mixed dentition. Some developmental problems with the succedaneous teeth are much easier to control by early intervention than to correct later, and there can be functional advantages in correcting interferences with normal jaw movements. There is good evidence that the increased overjet associated with Class II malocclusion increases the chance of preadolescent incisor trauma and that this risk is reduced by overjet reduction. Girls mature earlier than boys, and this can become an important factor in the timing of treatment—by the time the premolars erupt, there may be too little growth remaining for optimal treatment of some girls.

On the other hand, if growth modification is done early, adolescent growth in the original pattern can cause the skeletal problem to recur, so that much of the initial change is lost, and there is little or no psychosocial benefit from correcting the problem early. Early treatment for patients with very severe skeletal problems or problems that are becoming progressively worse (e.g., post-traumatic ankylosis) clearly is indicated. It is difficult to justify early treatment of routine Class II problems because the data (see Chapter 8 for a review of the pertinent literature) indicate that there is little or no difference in the outcomes of two-stage and one-stage treatment.

Whether arch expansion procedures are more effective if done during the mixed dentition is debatable. Good data to resolve this are not yet available. The key question, of course, is not whether the expansion can be accomplished early—clearly it can—but whether there is any long-term advantage in doing it that way. Unfortunately, it takes a long time to get a clear answer. As better data for outcomes become available, it is likely that the indications for early treatment will be focused more clearly and that two-stage treatment will be reserved for patients with special characteristics.

The timing of treatment for adults, interestingly enough, also requires careful thought—not because of growth considerations, as in children, but because orthodontic treatment often must be coordinated with other treatment to control dental disease and replace missing teeth.

In the remainder of this chapter, we review orthodontic treatment planning for preschool children, preadolescents, adolescents and adults in some detail. For children and preadolescents, the objective is to highlight indications for early treatment that are known to provide significant benefit. For adolescents and adults, the goal is to outline treatment possibilities that are discussed in detail in subsequent chapters.

TREATMENT PLANNING FOR PRESCHOOL CHILDREN (PRIMARY DENTITION)

The same diagnostic process used for all other patients is applicable to preschool children: an adequate database should be assembled and utilized to develop a problem list. The triage approach described previously can be applied without difficulty and those with complex problems referred to specialists or treatment teams for evaluation.

Systematic description of a malocclusion in the primary dentition also follows the same five steps as for any other malocclusion, and the comments in this and the following sections of this chapter follow the sequence in the Ackerman-Proffit approach: alignment and symmetry within the arch are examined first and the impact of the dentition on facial esthetics is considered, then problems related to the occlusal and jaw relationships in the three planes of space are noted.

Alignment Problems

In the normal primary dentition, especially by age 5 and 6, spacing between the incisors is normal and in fact is necessary if the permanent incisors are to be properly aligned when they erupt, because growth does not provide much in the way of additional space for the larger permanent teeth (see Chapter 4). If the primary incisors contact each other proximally, one can confidently predict that the permanent incisors will be crowded and irregular (Figure 7-15). Significant crowding in the primary dentition is rare. When this is observed, extremely severe crowding will be present later in the permanent dentition. The child with an adult-appearing

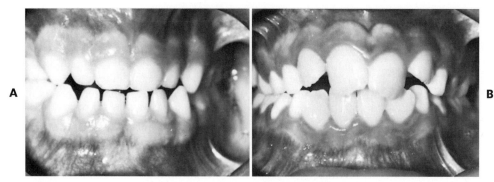

FIGURE 7-15   A "Hollywood smile" in the primary dentition, with no spaces between the primary incisors, guarantees insufficient room for the permanent incisors when they erupt and therefore, severe crowding. **A,** Age 5: **B,** Age 8. (See Figure 3-39 for normal spacing of primary incisors.)

smile at age 5 has space problems in his or her future, and the family dentist should inform the parents of this.

Some dentists have theorized that when future crowding is obvious, very early expansion of the arches, in the primary dentition, would produce more stable long-term results than later expansion. The idea is that expanding the primary teeth would cause the permanent teeth to erupt in already-expanded positions, and that the teeth are stable in their eruption position. Unfortunately, no data exist to support this theory, and in the presence of severe crowding, further orthodontic treatment is certain to be required even if very early expansion is carried out. This type of treatment cannot be recommended.

When a preschool child loses primary teeth prematurely because of caries or trauma, there can be an impact on the position of the permanent teeth when they erupt, and crowding or malalignment may occur. At one time it was thought that the primary teeth were stable in their arch position until forces produced by erupting permanent teeth, such as those generated by permanent first molars, were encountered. This is not the case.[11] Treatment planning guidelines for very early loss of a primary tooth are as follows.

1. Loss of a primary incisor. In most children, spaces are present between the primary incisors, and the early loss of an incisor will cause little if any change in the dentition. Therefore space maintenance is not necessary. On the other hand, prosthetic replacement of the teeth for esthetic reasons may need to be considered, especially since the eruption of the permanent incisors will probably be delayed if a primary incisor is lost at a very early age.

2. Loss of a primary canine. When a primary canine is lost, the incisor teeth tend to shift laterally into this space, creating a midline deviation and dental asymmetry. This tendency is accelerated at the time the permanent incisors begin to erupt but can develop within the primary dentition. Fortunately, these teeth are infrequently lost because of caries or trauma.

3. Loss of a primary first molar. Although space closure after early loss of a first primary molar does not always occur, development of asymmetry within the arch and

space loss are possible. When this happens, mesial movement of posterior teeth in the maxillary arch and a lateral and posterior shift of incisors in the mandibular arch usually are responsible. For this reason, space maintenance should be considered for a child who has lost a primary first molar in the preschool years.

4. Loss of a primary second molar. The primary second molar not only reserves space for the permanent second premolars but its distal root also guides the erupting permanent first molar into position. If the primary second molar is lost prematurely, the permanent first molar will usually migrate mesially within the bone even before it emerges into the oral cavity. A space-maintaining device is needed that will both guide eruption of the permanent first molar before its emergence and then hold the first molar in proper position after occlusion is established (see Chapter 13).

Incisor Protrusion-Retrusion

Sucking habits often persist throughout the primary dentition period and may cause displacement of the incisors, typically forward in the upper arch and backward in the lower. The incisor displacement produced by sucking habits is usually self-correcting if the habit stops before permanent teeth erupt. Rarely if ever is it necessary to plan any orthodontic treatment to reposition the primary incisors.

Anterior crossbite occasionally occurs in the primary dentition because of incisor interferences that cause an anterior shift of the mandible. If this occurs, it should be corrected in an effort to avoid hypertrophy of facial muscles that can contribute to facial soft tissue asymmetry. Usually this correction can be made merely by removing the interference, by either occlusal grinding or extracting the primary incisor if it is already near exfoliation (Figure 7-16).

Posterior Crossbite

Transverse problems, usually manifest as posterior crossbite from a narrow upper arch, are relatively common in the primary dentition. Sucking habits tend to produce constriction of the upper arch, more in the primary canine than

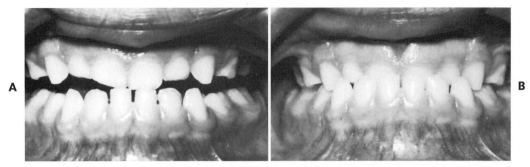

FIGURE 7-16   Anterior crossbite in the primary dentition often is caused by incisor interference and a forward shift: **A,** initial contact position, **B,** habitual occlusion, after forward shift.

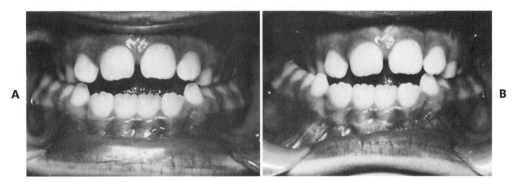

FIGURE 7-17   If the maxillary arch is relatively narrow, it is likely that a child will shift the jaw laterally upon closure, producing an apparent unilateral crossbite. The basic problem is usually a symmetric narrowing of the maxillary arch: **A,** initial contact position, **B,** habitual occlusion.

in the molar region, and occlusal interferences may then lead to a functional shift of the mandible anteriorly and laterally (Figure 7-17).

A unilateral crossbite in a preschool child almost always results, not from a true skeletal or dental asymmetry, but from a symmetrically narrow maxilla combined with a functional shift. Since preschool children do not have well enough developed temporomandibular joints to have the equivalent of the adult's centric relation position, it can be time consuming and frustrating to try to determine where the child would occlude if the mandible were not shifted laterally. Usually a reproducible position can be identified, but if this proves impossible, it is best to simply place the mandible so that the midlines are correct and plan treatment from this point. If intermolar width is satisfactory, grinding the primary canines to eliminate deflective contacts may be the only treatment required. If both molar and canine widths are narrow, expansion of the upper arch is indicated (see Chapter 13). This will provide additional space in the maxillary arch and simplify future evaluation of the occlusion because the functional shift has been eliminated.

Anteroposterior Discrepancies

Primary molar relationships are classified according to the relationship of the distal surfaces of the upper and lower second primary molars: *flush terminal plane*, the normal re-

lationship; *distal step*, with the lower molar distally positioned relative to the upper molar; and *mesial step*, with the lower molar mesially positioned (see Chapter 3). Although the mesial step relationship corresponds to a Class I molar relationship in the permanent dentition, its presence at an early age indicates the possibility of excessive mandibular or deficient maxillary development. A distal step relationship correlates with a skeletal Class II jaw relationship, which in most children with mandibular deficiency can be recognized by age 3.

By using growth modification treatment, it is possible to correct distal step or mesial step dental relationships in most primary dentition children relatively easily. Unfortunately, as growth continues, the discrepancy tends to recur as quickly as it was corrected. For this reason, except in the most severe cases, it is unwise to begin treatment for a skeletal Class II or Class III problem in the primary dentition. There is an adequate amount of growth remaining to obtain the necessary correction if treatment is deferred until the mixed dentition years.

Vertical Problems

Both deep bite and open bite malocclusions occur in the primary dentition. Deep bite is usually associated with the skeletal proportions that predispose to this condition: a relatively short face with a square gonial angle and flat mandibular plane. Open bite, on the other hand, is often seen in children who have good skeletal proportions but sucking habits. If skeletal proportions are good, there is a strong tendency for the anterior open bite to correct spontaneously when the sucking habit ends. Vigorous efforts to prevent a preschool child from sucking (using dental appliances or other coercive approaches) are not warranted in most cases. Up to age 5 or so, sucking habits are unlikely to cause any long-term problems in children with good skeletal jaw relationships. The use of orthodontic appliances to actively close an open bite is not indicated in the primary dentition. There is no reason to place an appliance, either to alter a habit or to move teeth, if the situation is likely to correct itself without any treatment. It is also possible that an open bite is due to a skeletal discrepancy of the long face type, characterized by increased lower anterior facial height. Spontaneous correction of an open bite is not likely to occur in these children. Growth modification treatment, however, is not indicated for the same reasons as for skeletal Classes II and III: if the problem is corrected in the primary dentition, it is likely to recur relatively quickly when the active treatment is discontinued. The same is true, of course, for skeletal deep bite relationships.

In summary: in the primary dentition:

- malposed, crowded and irregular incisors are uncommon, but the absence of spaces between primary incisors often indicates that there will be crowding when permanent incisors erupt. No treatment is indicated until the mixed dentition
- space should be maintained for missing primary molars, but no anterior teeth
- posterior crossbites, particularly those with a lateral shift of the mandible upon closure, should be treated in the primary dentition, either by occlusal adjustment or by maxillary expansion
- anterior crossbites caused by a forward mandibular shift should also be treated early
- although skeletal anteroposterior and vertical problems can be detected in the primary dentition, treatment is indicated only for the most severe problems

TREATMENT PLANNING FOR PREADOLESCENTS (EARLY MIXED DENTITION)

In contrast to the restricted number of indications for orthodontic treatment of preschool children, there are many indications for orthodontic treatment in the mixed dentition. For moderate problems, mixed dentition treatment may be all that is necessary, and this type of treatment often can be provided in the family practice. Children with complex problems whose treatment begins early usually require two phases of treatment, one in the mixed dentition and a second in the early permanent dentition. This treatment usually requires the expertise of a specialist.

Moderate Problems

Moderate problems in mixed dentition children, by our definition, are those selected by the triage scheme described previously. These consist entirely of dental problems resulting from misplaced permanent teeth, with skeletal problems and severe crowding problems excluded. Treatment planning for these non-skeletal problems is discussed in this section, and treatment procedures are described in Chapter 13.

Space Problems

Missing Primary Teeth with Adequate Space: Space Maintenance.   If a primary first or second molar is missing, if there will be more than a 6-month delay before the permanent premolar erupts, and if there is adequate space (because there has been no space loss or because space regaining has been completed) (see later in this section); then space maintenance is needed. Otherwise the space is likely to close spontaneously before the premolar can come into position.

Although space maintenance can be done with either fixed or removable appliances, fixed appliances are preferred in most situations because they eliminate the factor of patient cooperation. If the space is unilateral, it can be managed by a unilateral fixed appliance (Figure 7-18). If molars on both sides have been lost and the lateral incisors have erupted, it is usually better to place a lingual arch rather than two unilateral appliances.

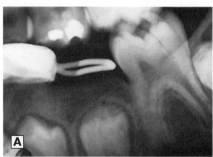 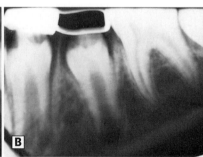 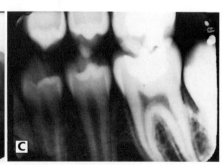

FIGURE 7-18   Space maintenance after early loss of a second primary molar. **A,** Band and loop space maintainer at age 8; **B,** same patient, age 11; **C,** same patient, age 12.

Early loss of a single primary canine in the mixed dentition requires space maintenance or extraction of the contralateral tooth to eliminate midline changes and the loss of arch symmetry (Figure 7-19). In this circumstance, arch length shortens as the incisor teeth drift distally and lingually. If the contralateral canine is extracted, a lingual arch space maintainer may still be needed to prevent lingual movement of the incisors.

Localized Space Loss (3 mm or less): Space Regaining. Potential space problems can be created by drift of permanent incisors or molars after premature extraction of primary canines or molars. In children who meet the criteria for moderate problems (i.e., no skeletal or dentofacial involvement), lost space can be regained by repositioning the teeth that have drifted. Then, after the space discrepancy has been reduced to zero, a space maintainer is necessary to prevent further drift and space loss until the succedaneous teeth have erupted. A space maintainer alone is not adequate treatment for a space deficiency.

Space regaining is most likely to be needed when primary maxillary or mandibular second molars have been lost prematurely because of decay (Figure 7-20) or, rarely, because of ectopic eruption of the permanent first molar. The permanent first molar usually migrates mesially quite rapidly when the primary second molar has been lost, and in the extreme case may totally close the primary second molar extraction site. If the primary second molar has been lost prematurely in a single quadrant, up to 3 mm of space may be regained by tipping the molar back distally. If space

loss is bilateral, the limit of space regaining is about 4 mm for the total arch, or 2 mm per quadrant.

Space regaining also may be indicated after early loss of one mandibular primary canine, because space tends to close as the incisors drift lingually and toward the affected side (see Figure 7-19). Asymmetric activation of a lower lingual arch usually is the best approach. Loss of a primary canine usually occurs because of root resorption caused by erupting lateral incisors without enough space, so it is important to be aware of the overall space deficiency, which should not exceed 4 mm.

Techniques for using space regaining appliances are presented in Chapter 13.

Generalized Moderate Crowding. A child with a generalized arch length discrepancy of 2-4 mm and no prematurely missing primary teeth can be expected to have moderately crowded incisors. Unless the incisors are severely protrusive, the long-term plan would be generalized expansion of the arch to align the teeth. The major advantage of doing this in the mixed dentition is esthetic, and the benefit is largely for the parents, not the child.

If the parents strongly desire early treatment, in the mandibular arch, an adjustable lingual arch is the appliance of choice for simple expansion. In the maxilla, either a removable appliance or a lingual arch can be employed. Keep in mind, however, that rotated incisors usually will not correct spontaneously even if space is provided, so early correction would require bonded attachments for these teeth.

Irregular/Malpositioned Incisors

Spaced and Flared Maxillary Incisors. In children with spaced and flared maxillary incisors who have Class I molar relationships and good facial proportions, space analysis should show that the space available is excessive rather than deficient. Retracting the incisors reduces the chance of trauma to these teeth, and these children may benefit esthetically.

If the upper incisors are flared forward and there is no contact with the lower incisors (Figure 7-21), the protruding upper incisors can be retracted quite satisfactorily with a simple removable appliance. This condition often is found in the mixed dentition after prolonged thumbsucking

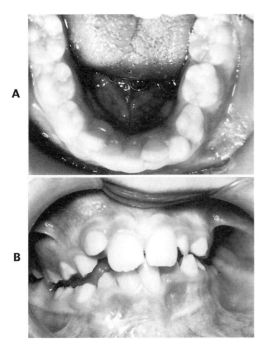

FIGURE 7-19 Premature loss of one primary canine (for this child the mandibular right primary canine) leads to drift of the permanent incisors toward the affected side, creating an asymmetry within the arch (**A**) and a midline discrepancy (**B**).

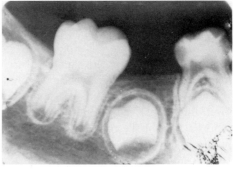

FIGURE 7-20 After early loss of a primary second molar, mesial drift of the permanent first molar nearly always occurs rapidly, as in this child.

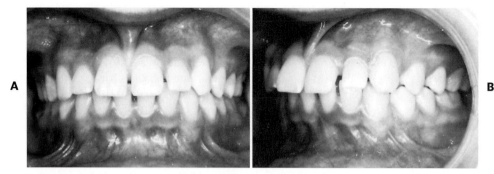

FIGURE 7-21   Flared and spaced maxillary incisors in a child with vertical clearance (i.e., open bite or incomplete overbite [no occlusal contact of the incisors even if they overlap]) can be corrected by tipping the incisors lingually with a removable appliance. If there is occlusal contact, however, even if there is not a deep overbite, a fixed appliance that gives vertical control of the incisors is needed to close the spaces.

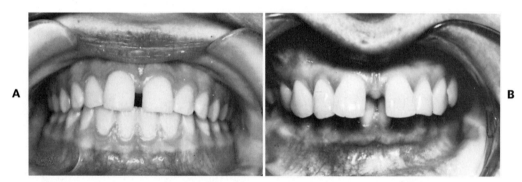

FIGURE 7-22   **A,** A maxillary central diastema of more than 2 mm is unlikely to completely close spontaneously, but the space often decreases when the permanent canines erupt. Surgical revision of the frenal attachment may or may not be required. The preferred treatment is to move the teeth together at about the time the permanent canines are erupting and decide about frenum surgery at that point. **B,** Closing a diastema of this severity requires correction of the deep overbite before the separated teeth can be brought together. A surgical frenectomy would be required as part of the treatment plan for this patient but is most effective if done after the teeth have been brought together.

and frequently occurs in connection with some narrowing of the maxillary arch. A thumb or finger habit should be eliminated before attempting to retract the incisors. Physiologic adaptation to the space between the anterior teeth requires that the tongue be placed in this area to seal off the gap for successful swallowing and speech. This "tongue thrust" is not the cause of the protrusion or open bite and should not be the focus of therapy. If the teeth are retracted, the tongue thrust will disappear.

On the other hand, if there is a deep overbite anteriorly, protruding upper incisor teeth cannot be retracted until it is corrected. The lower incisors biting against the lingual of the upper incisors prevents the upper teeth from being moved lingually. Even if antero-posterior jaw relationships are Class I, a skeletal vertical problem may be present, and complex treatment is likely to be required.

Maxillary Midline Diastema.   A maxillary midline diastema (Figure 7-22) can pose a special management problem. Small spaces between the maxillary incisors are normal before eruption of the maxillary canines (see Chapter 4 and the discussion of the "ugly duckling" stage of development). In the absence of deep overbite, these spaces normally close spontaneously. If the space between the maxillary central incisors is greater than 2 mm, however, spontaneous closure is unlikely.[12] Persistent spacing between the incisors correlates with a cleft in the alveolar process between the central incisors into which fibers from the maxillary labial frenum insert. For larger diastemas, it may be necessary to surgically remove the frenal attachment to obtain a stable closure of the midline diastema.

The best approach, however, is to do nothing until the permanent canines erupt unless crowding is an issue. If the space does not close spontaneously at that time, an appliance can be used to move the teeth together, and a frenectomy should be considered then if there is excessive tissue bunched up in the midline. Early frenectomy should be avoided.

Anterior Crossbite.   Anterior crossbite, particularly crossbite of all the incisors, is rarely found in children who do not have a skeletal Class III jaw relationship. A crossbite relationship of one or two anterior teeth, however, may develop in a child who has good facial proportions. The maxillary lateral incisors tend to erupt to the lingual and may be trapped in that location, especially if there is not enough space (Figure 7-23). In this situation, extracting the adjacent primary canine prior to complete eruption of the lateral incisor usually leads to spontaneous correction of the crossbite. Lingually positioned incisors limit lateral jaw movements and they or their mandibular counterparts sometimes suffer significant incisal abrasion, so early correction of the crossbite is indicated.

It is important to evaluate the space situation before attempting to correct any anterior crossbite. The prognosis for successfully pushing a 7 mm maxillary lateral incisor into a 4 mm space is not good. Frequently, even if there is enough space overall within the arch, it is necessary to remove the maxillary primary canines prematurely to bring lateral incisors out of crossbite. If enough space is available, a maxillary removable appliance to tip the upper incisor(s) facially is usually the best mechanism to correct a simple anterior crossbite. A space maintainer will be required until the remaining permanent teeth erupt. Rotational changes and bodily movement are not effectively produced by removable appliances and require fixed appliance therapy.

Posterior Crossbite. Posterior crossbites in mixed dentition children usually result from a narrowing of the maxillary arch and are often observed in children who have had prolonged sucking habits. If the child shifts on closure, early correction is indicated. If not, there is no compelling reason for early correction. Especially if other problems suggest that comprehensive orthodontics will be needed later, treatment can be deferred until adolescence.

Both removable and fixed appliances can be effective in correcting posterior crossbites (Figure 7-24). Whether a fixed or removable appliance is used, the maxillary arch should be slightly overexpanded and then held passively in this overexpanded position for approximately 3 months before the appliance is removed. Techniques for both removable and fixed appliances to expand the maxillary arch are illustrated in Chapter 13.

Anterior Open Bite. A simple anterior open bite is one that is limited to the anterior region in a child with good facial proportions. The major cause of such an open bite is prolonged thumbsucking, and the most important step in obtaining correction is to stop sucking habits if they are present. For this purpose, behavior modification techniques are appropriate. Several approaches are possible (see Chapter 13). If an intra-oral appliance is needed, the preferred method is a maxillary lingual arch with an anterior crib device, making it extremely difficult for the child to

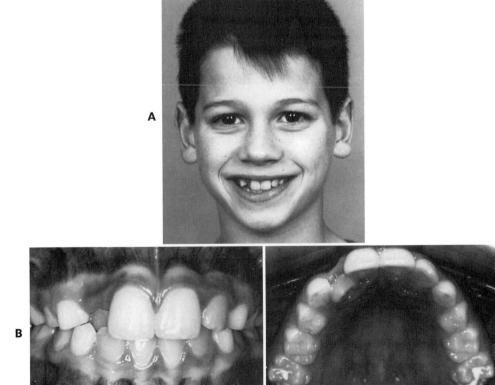

FIGURE 7-23 Anterior crossbite, in the absence of a jaw discrepancy, usually arises as maxillary lateral incisors erupt somewhat lingually, then are deflected further to the lingual because of lack of enough space to move facially into their normal space in the arch. The effect on facial (**A**) and dental (**B, C**) esthetics, as in this child at age 8, often is enough to lead the parents to seek orthodontic advice.

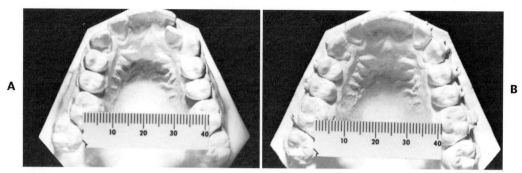

FIGURE 7-24   For this patient, 5 mm lateral expansion of the maxillary molars allowed correction of the posterior crossbite and also produced an increase in arch circumference that assisted in alignment of the crowded incisors (**A,** Pretreatment; **B,** posttreatment). For most patients, lateral expansion of the molars is stable, but whether this can be done for an individual patient depends on the characteristics of the malocclusion.

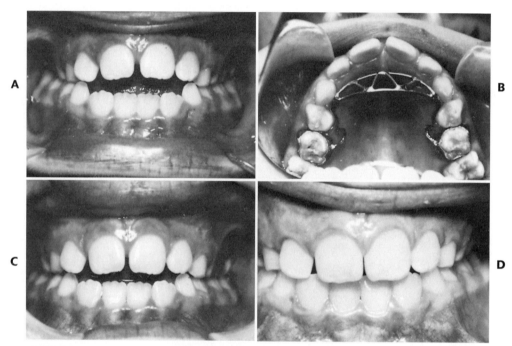

FIGURE 7-25   Correction of anterior open bite after cessation of thumbsucking. **A,** Open bite in an 8-year old thumbsucking girl before treatment; **B,** crib appliance in place, **C,** improvement in open bite after 3 months; **D,** correction of open bite and crib removed after 6 months.

place the thumb or other object in the mouth (Figure 7-25). It is important to present such a device to the child as an aid, not as a punishment, and to provide psychological support to help him or her adjust to it.

In about half of the children for whom such a crib is made, thumbsucking stops immediately and the anterior open bite usually begins to close relatively rapidly thereafter. In the remaining children, thumbsucking persists for a few weeks, but the crib device is eventually effective in extinguishing thumbsucking in 85% to 90% of patients.[13] It is a good idea to leave the crib in place for 3 to 6 months after the habit has apparently been eliminated. Further details on fabrication and use of this appliance are provided in Chapter 13.

Over-Retained Primary Teeth and Ectopic Eruption.   The eruption of a permanent tooth can be delayed if its primary predecessor is retained too long. When this happens, the obvious treatment is to remove the primary tooth. As a general guideline, a permanent tooth should erupt when approximately three-fourths of its root is completed. If root formation of the permanent successor has reached this point while a primary tooth still has considerable root remaining, the primary tooth should be extracted. This problem is most likely to arise when the permanent tooth bud is slightly displaced away from its primary predecessor (as in the canine ectopic eruption problems discussed next). In some children, the pace of resorption of the primary

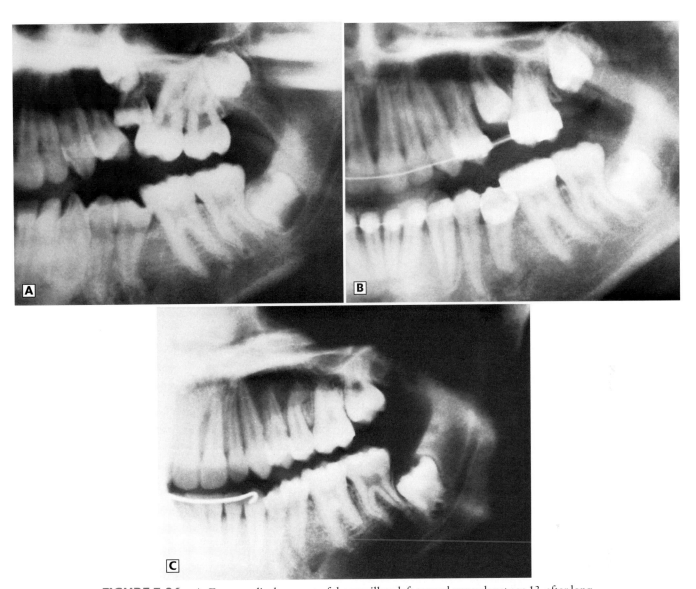

FIGURE 7-26   A, Extreme displacement of the maxillary left second premolar at age 13, after long-term ankylosis of the secondary primary molar. Note the space loss as the first molar has tipped mesially over the extraction of the ankylosed primary molar. **B,** The upper left second molar has been extracted to allow the first molar to be moved distally, opening space for the premolar now erupting; **C,** second premolar in place at age 15, despite the root dilaceration.

teeth is slow, for whatever reason, and occasionally almost all the primary teeth have to be removed to allow timely eruption of their permanent successors.

If a primary tooth is removed quite prematurely, a layer of relatively dense bone and soft tissue may form over the unerupted permanent tooth (see Figures 7-18 and 7-19). This usually delays but does not prevent the eruption of the permanent tooth, and intervention is rarely indicated. If eruption of a permanent tooth has been delayed until its root formation is complete, it may still erupt on its own and should be given a chance to do so. It may be necessary, however, to place an attachment on it and gently pull it into the arch (Figure 7-26) (see Chapter 14).

The eruption of permanent molars and canines can be delayed by malposition of the permanent tooth (ectopic eruption). The most common site is the maxillary molar region, where the second primary molar blocks the first permanent molar and suffers root resorption in the process (Figure 7-27).[14] If the permanent molar does not self-correct (and it usually does), it should be repositioned as described in Chapter 13 or, if all else fails, the primary molar extracted. If the primary molar is extracted, rapid space loss will result in a need for space regaining or premolar extraction.

Ectopic eruption of maxillary canines, which occurs relatively frequently, can permanently damage the roots of

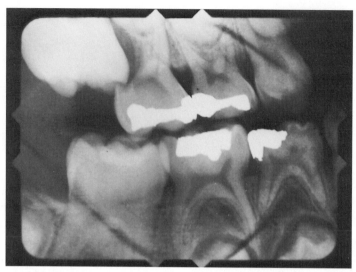

FIGURE 7-27   Ectopic eruption of the permanent first molar produces resorption of the distal root of the primary second molar.

lateral incisors (Figure 7-28). The abnormal eruption path may also leave the unerupted canine in a lingual position nearer the midline than normal. It is much easier to prevent these problems than to correct them later. Research has shown that extracting the maxillary primary canines when radiographs disclose that the permanent canines are overlapping the permanent lateral incisor roots is likely to have a positive influence on the permanent tooth's eruption path (although the more the overlap, the less the chance of eventual normal eruption).[15]

Severe Problems

Severe problems in mixed dentition children fall into three major categories: (1) skeletal discrepancies, (2) dentofacial problems related to incisor protrusion, and (3) space discrepancies of 5 mm or more. These patients usually require a second stage of treatment after permanent teeth erupt, so mixed dentition treatment is aimed at improving rather than comprehensively treating the severe problems.

Skeletal Problems.   Children with jaw discrepancies often can be helped considerably by application of growth modification techniques. The key to growth modification is treatment while adequate growth remains, which does not necessarily mean that mixed dentition treatment is needed. Girls mature faster than boys and must be treated earlier. Treatment planning for growth modification is discussed in Chapter 8, and the appropriate treatment techniques are described in Chapter 15.

Dentofacial Problems Related to Incisor Protrusion.
Excessive protrusion of incisors (bimaxillary protrusion, not excessive overjet) is usually an indication for premolar extraction and retraction of the protruding incisors. Because of the profile changes produced by adolescent growth, it is better for most children to defer extraction to correct protrusion until late in the mixed dentition or early in the permanent dentition. It is definitely an error to begin extraction

early and then allow the permanent molars to drift forward, because this will make effective incisor retraction impossible. A further discussion of this topic is presented in Chapter 8, as part of the discussion of "the great extraction controversy." Techniques for controlling the amount of incisor retraction are described in Chapter 17.

Space Discrepancies of 5 mm or More.   Common sense indicates that the larger the space discrepancy, the greater the chance that extraction of some teeth will be necessary to align the remaining ones. It is not possible to say with certainty that any given amount of arch length discrepancy is the borderline between extraction and nonextraction treatment. As a general guideline, however, one can say that:

- Space discrepancies up to 4 mm usually can be resolved without extraction (except for third molars)
- Discrepancies in the 5 to 9 mm range sometimes are best treated without extraction but often require extraction of some teeth other than third molars
- Children with space discrepancies of 10 mm or greater almost always require premolar extraction, regardless of what happens to third molars at a later date

The decision as to whether more than 4 mm of arch expansion is likely to be acceptably stable must be made on the basis of the patient's potential for lateral as well as anterior arch expansion. One possibility for arch expansion is to round out the arch form, expanding in the premolar region of the arch. Obviously, therefore, a patient with a narrow, V-shaped arch would have more potential for lateral expansion than an individual who already had oval arches. Growth potential also should be considered, since individuals who develop a rather large nose and chin can tolerate greater anterior expansion, in terms of the effect on esthetics, than those who do not.

It can be argued that arch expansion is more successful if it is done relatively early in the mixed dentition,[16] and

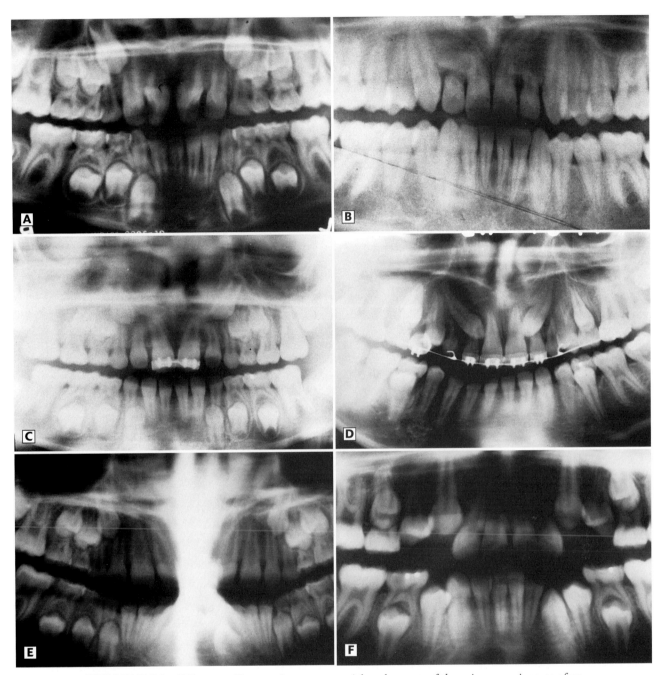

FIGURE 7-28 When maxillary canines erupt mesial to the roots of the primary canines, as often occurs, there is a risk of damage to the lateral incisors. Early extraction of the primary canines is recommended when the permanent canines are mesial to the midline of the primary canine crowns. **A,** Age 8, **B,** age 12 in a child who had no intervention until the erupting canines had severely damaged the lateral incisors; **C,** age 8; **D,** age 10 in a child in whom mesial movement of the permanent canines continued and led to severe damage; **E,** age 9, mesial position of canines that indicates early extraction of the primary canines; **F,** age 11 in same patient, showing reasonably normal eruption of the canines without damage to the lateral incisors, after the early extraction of the primary canines. (*A-D,* courtesy Dr. K. Lieberman.)

this treatment approach became popular in the 1990s. No good documentation of long-term results exists, however. It is possible to maintain the leeway space (the difference in size between primary second molars and second premolars) when the primary molars are exfoliated,[17] and if arch expansion is the plan for moderate crowding, it seems wise to begin in the late mixed dentition to be sure leeway space is not lost.

In some instances, it may be difficult to make the decision between arch expansion and premolar extraction for crowded cases. Treatment planning for such patients should consist of an initial though relatively conservative attempt to expand the arches, while evaluating the result. If the patient tolerates arch expansion well and does not develop excessive incisor protrusion, expansion treatment ultimately may be successful in spite of a relatively large discrepancy. On the other hand, if the expansion proceeds with difficulty and the signs of excessive arch expansion (primarily incisor protrusion and labial tipping of the teeth) begin to appear, uncertainty about the correctness of a decision to extract teeth has been removed (Figure 7-29). Extraction versus nonextraction treatment and how treat-

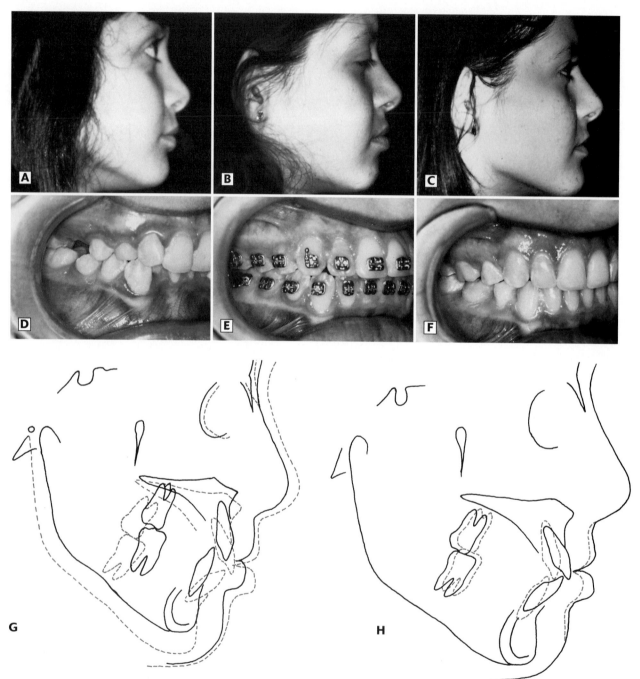

FIGURE 7-29   A patient with moderate crowding and protrusion in whom nonextraction treatment was attempted initially, and then premolars were extracted to reduce excessive protrusion. **A, D,** Prior to treatment; **B, E,** after nearly 2 years of treatment, with the arches aligned. The excessive dental protrusion is apparent in the facial appearance. This is both unesthetic and unstable, and it was clear that premolar extraction was required for better esthetics and stability; **C, F,** At the completion of treatment; **G, H,** cephalometric superimpositions from the beginning of treatment to the extraction decision, and from that point to the completion of treatment. (Courtesy Dr. J.L. Ackerman.)

ment response can be used to improve the chance of a correct decision in borderline situations are discussed in some detail in Chapter 8.

Serial Extraction.   Since the extraction of primary canines eliminates crowding of permanent incisors in the mixed dentition, it is tempting to extract these teeth when early incisor crowding develops. After the primary canines are removed, if permanent first premolars can be extracted before the permanent canines and second premolars erupt, the permanent canines will erupt distally and the extraction spaces may all but close spontaneously. This approach, called "serial extraction," was developed in Europe in the 1930s and at times has been widely advocated as a simple way of dealing with severe space problems.

In its classic form, serial extraction applies to patients who meet the following criteria: (1) no skeletal disproportions, (2) Class I molar relationship, (3) normal overbite, and (4) large arch perimeter deficiency (10 mm or more). The procedure consists of four steps:

- Extraction of primary lateral incisors as the permanent central incisors erupt (if necessary, since this often happens spontaneously in severely crowded cases)
- Extraction of primary canines as the permanent laterals erupt
- Extraction of primary first molars, usually 6 to 12 months before their normal exfoliation, at the point when the underlying premolars have one half to two thirds of their roots formed
- Extraction of the permanent first premolars before eruption of the permanent canines (Figure 7-30)[18]

Because an average first premolar is 7 to 8 mm wide, premolar extraction creates 14 to 16 mm of space in the arch. Only with extremely severe crowding of 10 mm or more is there a chance of a reasonably satisfactory result from serial extraction alone. After serial extraction, the incisors tend to drift lingually, and posterior teeth tend to drift mesially to some extent, typically leading to 2 to 3 mm of space closure in each quadrant or 4 to 6 mm total. The

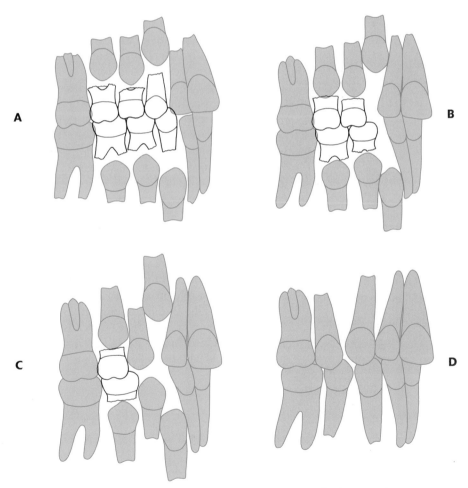

FIGURE 7-30   Stages in serial extraction. **A,** Extraction of primary canines as permanent laterals erupt. **B,** Extraction of primary first molars 6 to 12 months before normal exfoliation. **C,** Extraction of first premolars as they are just emerging before the canines erupt. **D,** Spontaneous space closure as the canines erupt distally and molars/premolars drift mesially. The goal is to transfer the incisor crowding posteriorly to the premolar extraction site, and the key to success is extraction of the first premolars before the canines erupt.

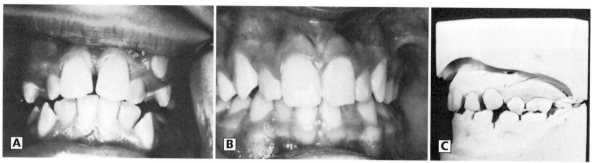

FIGURE 7-31 Results of early premolar extraction: **A**, severe crowding with maxillary and mandibular canines nearly blocked out of the arch; **B**, improvement in alignment after extraction of first premolars; **C**, lateral view of casts, showing failure of the extraction spaces to close completely despite the severity of the crowding. Note also the deepening of the bite anteriorly. Excellent occlusion is unlikely to develop in a patient who has only extractions, despite the significant improvement in alignment that may occur.

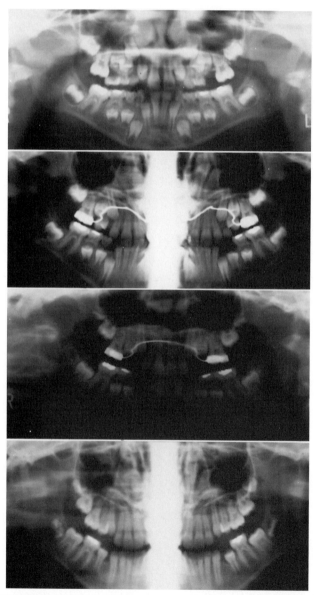

FIGURE 7-32 Sequential panoramic films in a child with severe crowding treated by serial extraction. Note the distal movement of the canines into the first premolar extraction spaces.

remainder of the space, approximately 10 mm, is available for resolution of the crowding. Residual spaces will remain at the extraction sites if the original discrepancy was much smaller than that.

If it is clear that extraction is required, serial extraction in a patient with a relatively small discrepancy may simplify later treatment, even though closing residual spaces with fixed appliances certainly will be required (Figure 7-31). If the space discrepancy is large enough and if everything can be timed perfectly, serial extraction can produce total space closure and reasonably good alignment of the teeth without any orthodontic appliance therapy at all (Figure 7-32). However, such a favorable outcome is rare, and cannot be relied on. Even with large discrepancies the vast majority of patients undergoing serial extraction require a period of fixed appliance treatment to achieve good alignment, interdigitation, and root paralleling.

In rare instances, a child with good skeletal proportions will have a Class II molar relationship and severe maxillary but not mandibular incisor crowding. This condition arises, of course, when upper posterior teeth have slipped mesially. In this circumstance, a modification of the serial extraction procedure to encompass only the maxillary arch can be helpful.[19] Serial extraction should be avoided in any child who has a skeletal Class II jaw discrepancy.

TREATMENT PLANNING FOR ADOLESCENTS (LATE MIXED AND EARLY PERMANENT DENTITION)

Orthodontic treatment traditionally has been carried out in early adolescence, soon after the succedaneous teeth have erupted. This is the ideal time for comprehensive treatment of dental crowding and malalignment, but highly developed clinical judgment and skill in the use of fixed appliances are required. Most of this treatment, therefore, is done by orthodontic specialists.

Alignment Problems

Crowding and Protrusion.   When there is crowding in the early permanent dentition, an accurate space analysis can be carried out directly, without the necessity for predicting the size of unerupted teeth. In this age group, however, it remains true that it is necessary to evaluate the amount of protrusion as well as the amount of crowding to totally evaluate the space situation. Crowding and protrusion in the permanent dentition are interrelated, just as they are in the mixed dentition.

A significant difference between mixed dentition and early permanent dentition patients is that the simple appliances that can be used to solve space problems in the mixed dentition are no longer effective after the permanent teeth have erupted. Whether a patient in the early permanent dentition is to be treated by arch expansion or by extraction, a bonded or banded fixed appliance is needed to position the teeth correctly. Removable appliances of all types, along with lingual arches and other round wire or partially fixed appliances, are effective only for tipping teeth to new positions. If the permanent teeth have been allowed to erupt completely while still malaligned, it is rare that a satisfactory result can be obtained without using an orthodontic appliance that can change root positions. Just tipping the crowns to a new location is not enough. If extraction is required to provide enough space, root movement is required to satisfactorily close the space.

With the possible exception of the maxillary central incisors, any tooth can be chosen for extraction to provide space for others. The amount of space available to correct crowding is greatest when a first premolar, canine, or incisor is extracted, because crowding usually occurs in the anterior part of the dental arch. If a more posterior tooth is selected for extraction, greater amounts of space will inevitably be lost as molars slip forward rather than canines and premolars moving distally. The amount of space available for relief of crowding after the extraction of various teeth is summarized in Table 7-1. Note that extraction space can be used either to relieve crowding or to retract protruding incisors. Examination of the table shows that extraction of first premolars provides the greatest flexibility in terms of closing space from the front posteriorly or from the rear anteriorly, which of course is a major reason for this being the most frequent extraction. In contrast, little useful space for either purpose is provided by second molar extraction. The general topic of extraction treatment is discussed in more detail in Chapter 8.

Tooth Size Discrepancies.   Data from tooth size analysis become available for the first time when the succedaneous teeth erupt. A tooth size discrepancy of less than 1.5 mm is usually insignificant, but larger discrepancies create a problem that must be solved in the development of a treatment plan. There are five possible approaches:[20] (1) compensate for a small size differential by changing the inclination of the incisors; (2) reduce the width of some teeth by interproximal stripping of enamel; (3) build up the width of an anomalously small tooth or teeth by adding composite resin or a crown; (4) alter the normal extraction plan to compensate for size discrepancies (for instance, by extracting anomalously large lower second premolars rather than first premolars in what would otherwise be a first premolar extraction case); or (5) accept a small space in one of the arches, usually distal to the lateral incisors.

Before one of the possible plans is accepted, it is important to determine whether the discrepancy is caused by a variation in one of the teeth or a generalized size difference between upper and lower teeth. This determination can be accomplished by Bolton analysis (see Chapter 6). The usual culprits in tooth size problems are the upper lateral incisors, but second premolars in both arches also vary in size. Reducing or building up lateral incisors, if these are the source of the discrepancy, is the best approach. It is less easy to alter the width of premolars, and one of the other solutions may be required. A diagnostic setup (Figure 7-33) (i.e., resetting the teeth after cutting them off the cast and modifying them) is usually needed to verify that a proposed treatment plan for tooth size discrepancy can succeed.

Transverse Problems

Transverse problems in the adolescent age group, as in younger patients, are most likely the result of a narrow maxillary arch. The necessary maxillary expansion may be approached either skeletally or dentally, depending on the anatomic basis of the problem. The basis of skeletal maxillary expansion is opening the midpalatal suture by applying heavy force across the suture, stimulating the formation of additional bone at that location. This can produce skeletal changes either rapidly (days) or more slowly (weeks). This form of growth modification treatment is discussed in more detail in Chapter 8.

The maxillary arch also can be widened by dental expansion with fixed or removable appliances. Whenever a removable appliance is used for arch expansion, it is extremely important to retain it tightly with excellent clasps.

TABLE 7-1   *Space from Various Extractions**

Extraction	Relief of incisor crowding	Incisor retraction[†] Max.	Incisor retraction[†] Min.	Posterior forward[†] Max.	Posterior forward[†] Min.
Central incisor	5	3	2	1	0
Lateral	5	3	2	1	0
Canine	6	5	3	2	0
First premolar	5	5	2	5	2
Second premolar	3	3	0	6	4
First molar	3	2	0	8	6
Second molar	2	1	0	—	—

*Values given in millimeters.
[†]Anteroposterior plane of space in absence of crowding.

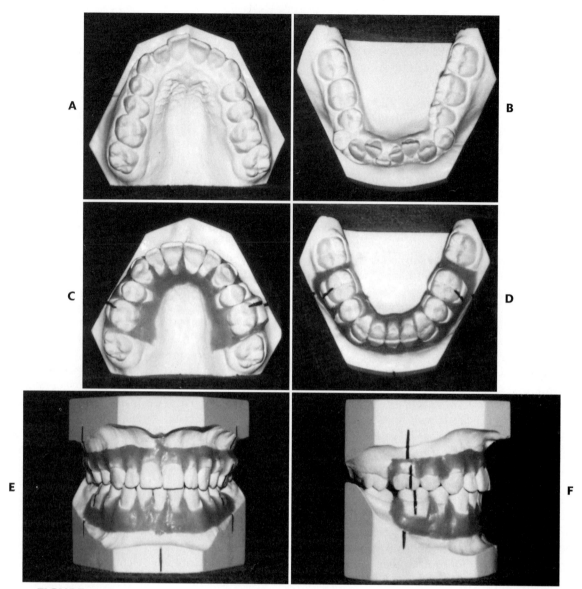

FIGURE 7-33   Resetting the teeth to directly evaluate how they would fit together usually is needed to verify that a plan for correcting tooth size discrepancy could succeed. For this patient with dental protrusion, mandibular but not maxillary incisor crowding, and a tooth size discrepancy due to small maxillary incisors (**A** and **B**), a setup showed that good occlusion could be obtained with extraction of one lower incisor and four first premolars (**C** to **F**). Note that the terminal molars have been left in place on the setup casts, so that the planned amount of forward movement of the posterior teeth can be seen.

Although a screw device in a removable appliance can widen the arch, this will occur largely by tipping the teeth facially and should not be considered a substitute for the fixed expansion devices used for palatal expansion. Better control of dental expansion is usually achieved with a relatively flexible lingual arch.

Single tooth crossbites or true unilateral asymmetries of the dental arch are usually best corrected by cross elastics (i.e., elastics from the lingual of one arch to the buccal of the other) in the affected area (Figure 7-34), provided that there is not a skeletal vertical problem that the elastics could aggravate. Reciprocal tooth movement will result if one tooth is pitted against another. Differential unilateral

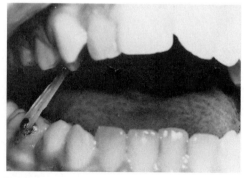

FIGURE 7-34   Cross-elastics from the maxillary lingual to the mandibular labial can be used to correct a single-tooth crossbite.

maxillary expansion can be achieved by placing a lower fixed appliance and using cross elastics from the stabilized lower arch to the maxillary teeth on the affected side. This concept of anchorage reinforcement for differential tooth movement is discussed in more detail in Chapter 10.

True skeletal asymmetries in the adolescent age group pose an extremely difficult problem. A possible plan for moderately severe asymmetry is a hybrid functional appliance (see Chapter 15), but surgery is often required.

Anteroposterior Problems

The preferred treatment for skeletal problems, whatever the plane of space, is always growth modification. For greatest success, growth modification treatment should begin before the adolescent growth spurt, and the amount of remaining growth must be evaluated carefully before treatment is planned for an adolescent. Girls mature earlier than boys, and it is possible that by the time a girl's permanent teeth have erupted, it is too late for effective growth modification. A second plan for correcting anteroposterior discrepancies is to camouflage them by differential movement of upper and lower incisors. If the problem is severe, a third option is surgical repositioning of the jaws. These possibilities are discussed in Chapter 8.

Occasionally a patient who has neither a skeletal jaw discrepancy nor space problems may have excessive overjet because of maxillary incisor protrusion combined with mandibular incisor retrusion. Such cases are rare, unfortunately, since they can be described as "the orthodontist's dream." Essentially any appliance ever invented, coupled with Class II elastics or their equivalent, is capable of correcting such problems. The cases used to illustrate the wonder of many simplistic appliances will be found on close examination to fall into this category.

Vertical Problems

The major vertical problems of adolescents are anterior open bite and anterior deep bite, both of which are likely to be seen in combination with some anteroposterior problem. As a child becomes older, it is more and more likely that malocclusion in the vertical plane of space, as in the anteroposterior plane of space, is related to skeletal jaw proportions and not just to displacement of the teeth. Eruption problems are also likely to be more serious in this age group.

Anterior Open Bite.   The skeletal indications of anterior open bite are increased anterior face height and a steep mandibular plane, both of which reflect excessive vertical growth of the maxilla and rotation of the mandible; and excessive eruption of posterior teeth.[21] Because of the downward and backward rotation of the mandible, the patient is likely to have a Class II jaw relationship in addition to the vertical problem. Growth modification treatment, discussed in more detail in Chapter 8, focuses on controlling both the vertical maxillary growth and eruption in both arches.

In younger children, the major cause of anterior open bite is sucking habits or other environmental influences. Spontaneous correction of open bites caused by these habits often occurs during the mixed dentition and can be facilitated by relatively simple treatment. By the time adolescence is reached, however, environmental causes of anterior open bite are less important than skeletal factors (Figure 7-35). It is rare for anterior open bite in an adolescent to be due solely to some habit, or for the open bite to correct spontaneously at this age after a habit has been corrected.

In the past, tongue thrust swallowing was blamed for many anterior open bites in this age group, and efforts at training the patient to swallow correctly were used in an attempt to control anterior open bite problems. Contemporary research, however, makes it clear that tongue thrust swallow is more an adaptation to the open bite than the cause of it (see Chapter 3). Myofunctional therapy for tongue thrusting, for that reason, is ineffectual and not recommended. The appropriate growth modification therapy is discussed in Chapter 8.

Deep Overbite.   Anterior deep bite problems may result from an upward and forward rotation of the mandible, or from excessive eruption of mandibular incisor teeth. Super-eruption of lower incisors often accompanies a Class II malocclusion, because when there is excessive overjet, the lower incisors tend to erupt until they contact the palatal mucosa. In comprehensive orthodontic treatment, usually it is necessary to correct this elongation of the lower incisors, by leveling out an excessive curve of Spee in the lower arch. In an adolescent whose face height is still increasing, it is only necessary to prevent further

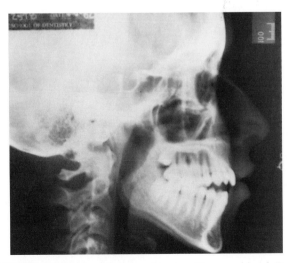

FIGURE 7-35   Anterior open bite in a 13-year-old girl. Every individual with this degree of anterior open bite uses the tongue to seal the anterior opening, and therefore can be labeled as having a tongue thrust swallow. It is unlikely in this age group that an open bite problem results primarily from a habit. Note the signs of skeletal vertical dysplasia, including the steep mandibular plane angle, rotation of the maxilla, and increased lower face height.

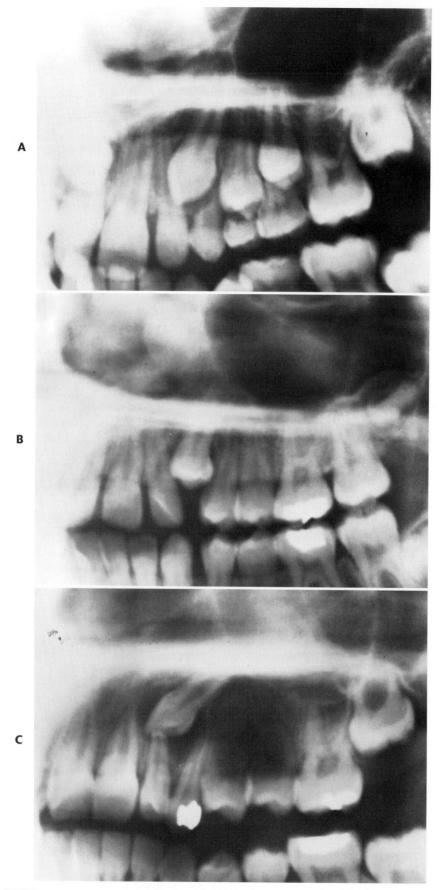

FIGURE 7-36 Impacted maxillary canines: **A,** mild displacement with good prognosis, especially if the primary canine is extracted now; **B,** impaction with minimal displacement from space shortage, with good prognosis; **C,** severe displacement with guarded prognosis for orthodontic correction. Immediate extraction of the primary canine is indicated in this patient.

eruption of the lower incisors as vertical growth continues to achieve a relative intrusion (see Figure 7-6). Continuous arch mechanics are appropriate. In the absence of growth, however, absolute intrusion is required, and segmented arch mechanics must be used to achieve this (see Figures 7-1 to 7-4, and the discussion of treatment procedures in Chapters 10, 16, and 21).

Correction of skeletal deep bite problems requires rotating the mandible downward, thereby increasing the mandibular plane angle and anterior face height. One must keep in mind that in a patient with short anterior facial dimensions and a skeletal deep bite, rotating the mandible downward to correct the deep bite will reveal a skeletal mandibular deficiency. Thus the growth modification techniques necessary to deal with this problem are typically those for correction of mandibular deficiency.

Eruption Problems.   Failure of a permanent tooth to erupt creates a severe orthodontic problem. A localized problem is typically created either by displacement of a permanent tooth from its normal eruption path so that the tooth becomes impacted (usually a maxillary canine) (Figure 7-36) or by trauma that leads to ankylosis (usually a maxillary incisor) (Figure 7-37). A generalized problem implies an abnormality in the eruption mechanism.

Impacted Teeth.   An impacted canine or other tooth in a teenage patient can usually be brought into the arch by orthodontic traction after being surgically exposed.[22] In older patients, there is an increasing risk that the impacted tooth has become ankylosed. Even adolescents have a risk that surgical exposure of a tooth will lead to ankylosis.

In planning treatment for an impacted permanent tooth, three principles should be followed: (1) The prognosis should be based on the extent of displacement and the surgical trauma required for exposure. As a rule, the greater the displacement and the greater the trauma, the poorer the prognosis. Extraction of a severely impacted tooth and orthodontic space closure or prosthetic replacement may be better judgment than heroic efforts to bring the tooth into the arch. (2) During surgical exposure, flaps should be reflected so that the tooth is ultimately pulled into the arch

through keratinized tissue, not through alveolar mucosa. (3) Adequate space should be provided in the arch before attempting to pull the impacted tooth into position.

If a tooth is severely impacted, surgical transplantation is a possible treatment approach. This involves removing the tooth, creating a socket at the appropriate site in the arch, and replanting the tooth in its correct position. External root resorption often ensues after transplantation and is the major cause of failure. Approximately two thirds of transplanted teeth are functional for 5 years, but only about one third are retained for 10 years.[23] Orthodontic movement is preferable if it is possible.

Generalized Eruption Failure.   An eruption delay that affects several teeth in an adolescent patient is an ominous sign. If the problem is a mechanical interference with eruption (see Chapter 4), the obvious treatment plan is to remove the interference and proceed with orthodontic therapy.

The condition called "primary failure of eruption"[24] (Figure 7-38) results from a failure of the eruption mechanism itself (see Chapter 3). Unfortunately, not only do the involved teeth not erupt spontaneously, they do not respond to orthodontic force and cannot be pulled into the arch. Since prosthetic replacement is the only practical solution, it is fortunate that the condition is rare.

Traumatic Dental Displacement and Ankylosis

Trauma to the face can create orthodontic problems that require immediate treatment. Displacement of a traumatized tooth occurs because the alveolar bone moves and takes the teeth with it, usually as fractures occur within the alveolar process. In addition to possible root fractures and loss of pulp vitality, trauma to incisor teeth carries with it a significant risk of ankylosis. If even a small part of the periodontal ligament is obliterated during subsequent healing so that cementum of the root fuses to bone, neither further eruption nor orthodontic tooth movement will be possible.

The best treatment after traumatic displacement is to use orthodontic force to gently reposition the tooth or teeth, bringing them back into position over a period of a few days, so that the bone heals with the teeth in proper

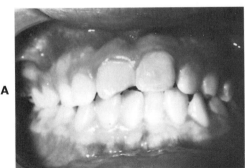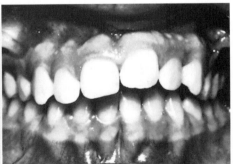

FIGURE 7-37   Ankylosis of maxillary incisors after trauma. **A,** At age 11; **B,** at age 13. Note the failure of the upper left central and lateral incisors to erupt. The fractured right central has been restored.

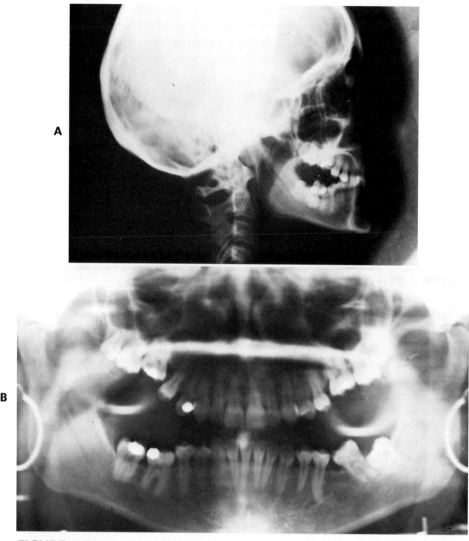

FIGURE 7-38 Primary failure of eruption in all four quadrants. **A,** Cephalometric film showing marked posterior open bite; **B,** panoramic film showing failure of teeth to erupt despite the lack of any obvious mechanical obstruction. Because their periodontal ligament is abnormal, the involved teeth cannot be moved orthodontically.

position.[25] Because of the risk of ankylosis, the repositioning should be completed within two weeks. This treatment is discussed further in Chapter 14.

If the traumatized teeth do become ankylosed, extraction followed by prosthetic replacement usually is the only choice. The one possible alternative, which often is not feasible, is a small segment osteotomy to reposition both the ankylosed tooth and the adjacent alveolar bone (see Chapter 20). This procedure should not be done until growth is completed.

TREATMENT PLANNING FOR ORTHODONTIC PROBLEMS IN ADULTS

Orthodontic treatment for adults can be either comprehensive in scope or limited in its objectives (adjunctive to other treatment). Adjunctive treatment is often within the scope of general dental practice and can be of considerable importance in the management of adults with periodontal disease and restorative needs.

Adjunctive vs. Comprehensive Treatment

The same triage approach used for children applies to adults for whom comprehensive orthodontic treatment is contemplated: those with skeletal discrepancies should be separated from those with dental problems, and the dental problems should be evaluated by their severity.

In adults, however, some orthodontic treatment may be needed as a part of restorative and periodontal treatment, regardless of whether major changes in the occlusion are desired. Adjunctive procedures for adults can be defined as those aimed at improving a specific occlusal characteristic, as part of an overall treatment plan usually involving major components of periodontal and restorative

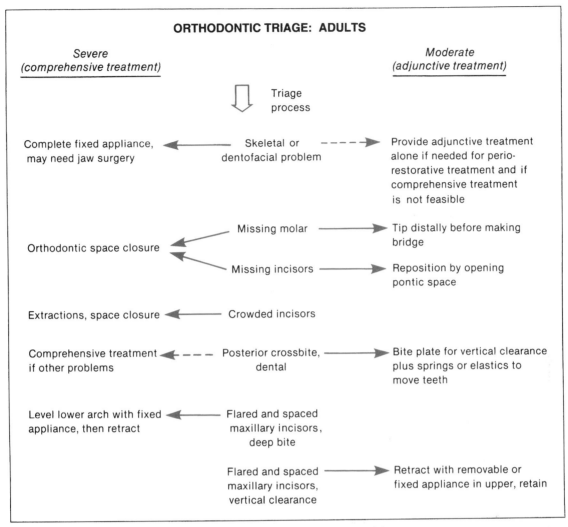

FIGURE 7-39 Steps in orthodontic triage, adults.

treatment. Relatively simple orthodontic appliances are typically involved and applied only to a specific part of the arch. Comprehensive orthodontic treatment, in contrast, nearly always involves a complete fixed appliance.

It is an error in treatment planning to overlook adjunctive treatment because the patient does not wish more comprehensive correction of malocclusion. On the other hand, the patient should receive a thorough evaluation and should be informed of treatment possibilities, including comprehensive correction if a severe malocclusion is present. As a general guideline (Figure 7-39), most adjunctive procedures for adults are appropriately included in general practice, while comprehensive treatment of adults is usually better handled by a specialist. Adjunctive treatment, including a detailed review of treatment techniques, is discussed in Chapter 20. Special considerations in comprehensive adult treatment are covered in Chapter 21.

The major indication for adjunctive orthodontic treatment in adults is drift of potential abutment teeth for bridges. If a permanent first molar is extracted during childhood, there is likely to be considerable mesial drift of the second molar and distal drift of premolars in the succeeding years. Periodontal defects are likely to occur on the mesial of the tipped second molar and may also be found between separated premolar teeth on the distal of the tipped molar (Figure 7-40). If an implant is desired, there is no choice but to orthodontically reposition the teeth. Even if a fixed bridge is planned, in most cases it is desirable to use a partial fixed appliance to upright the mesially tipped second molar and reposition the premolars. This improves the periodontal situation for most patients (Figure 7-41) and also makes it possible to fabricate a more ideal bridge. Early loss of teeth other than the first permanent molar is less common, but drift of other permanent teeth will follow extraction of a tooth at any point in the arch. Because of this, most patients who wait to have a prosthetic replacement made until long after a tooth has been extracted will need orthodontic repositioning of abutment teeth.

If the second molar has drifted mesially, as a general rule it is preferable to upright it by tipping its crown distally and opening up space for a pontic replacing the missing first molar, rather than attempting to move the second molar mesially and close the extraction space. This is true even if the first molar space is nearly closed.

There are two reasons for this rule. The first is that it is relatively easy to tip the second molar distally but much harder to upright the second molar by moving its roots mesially. The second reason is that if a long time has elapsed since the first molar was lost, there is almost always considerable atrophy of the alveolar ridge in the area of the original extraction site, producing a very narrow alveolar ridge. It is always difficult, and frequently impossible, to close the space and bring the second molar into good contact with the second premolar when this atrophy has occurred. Tipping the second molar distally, however, does

require extraction of the third molar in most patients. When the second molar is put into its original position in the arch, there is no room for the third molar, which would have been impacted if it had not drifted mesially.

The second most common indication for repositioning abutment teeth before fabricating a fixed bridge is probably in patients with missing or malformed maxillary lateral incisors. This condition often leads to spacing between the maxillary central incisors, and the position of the maxillary canines may also be abnormal (Figure 7-42). Adults with this problem are best treated with a fixed appliance, using an arch wire with coil springs to open space for the missing lateral incisors while simultaneously closing the central diastema. Realignment of the teeth in other areas of the dental arch, should this be indicated, would be carried out in the same way, using a fixed appliance to open space for the pontic. Closing space is considerably more difficult and falls into the category of comprehensive treatment.

Correction of crossbites in adults may also be needed as an adjunctive procedure. Since the occlusion in adults often locks teeth into a crossbite relationship, it is necessary to disengage the teeth to make tooth movement possible. This can be done either by having the patient wear a bite plate of some type to prevent occlusal contact until the orthodontic tooth movement has been completed, or by occlusal grinding to reduce interferences that would prevent the desired tooth movement.

In some adults, it is desirable to rearrange spaced or flared incisors before bonding composite resins to improve dental esthetics. If there is adequate vertical clearance, redistributing space among the incisors is a straightforward procedure with a bonded fixed appliance (Figure 7-43). If there is a deep overbite, however, it is simply not possible to retract flared and spaced upper incisors without also moving the lower incisors so that there will be proper incisor function at the end of treatment. In the presence of

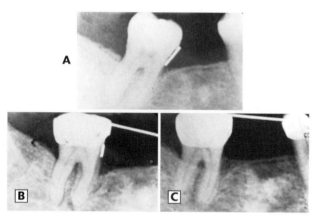

FIGURE 7-40   **A,** Radiograph with silver point in place to the depth of the gingival sulcus before molar uprighting; **B,** silver point to the depth of the gingival sulcus immediately upon completion of molar uprighting; **C,** 3 months after uprighting, showing area of new bone fill-in on the mesial of the uprighted molar.

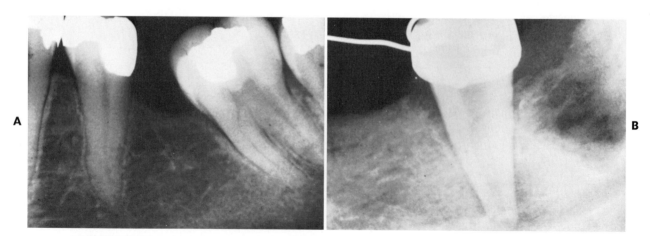

FIGURE 7-41   Changes in the alveolar bony architecture associated with molar uprighting. **A,** Before uprighting; **B,** after extraction of the third molar and uprighting of the second. Note the extent to which new bone has filled in on the mesial of the uprighted second molar and the upward extension of the bony attachment.

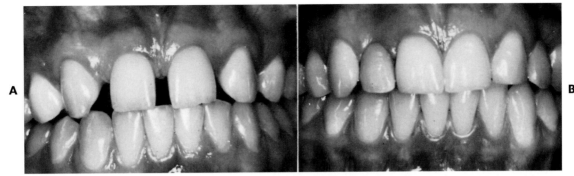

FIGURE 7-42 **A,** Missing maxillary lateral incisors, with drift of the central incisors and canines making esthetic restorations impossible; **B,** same patient 1 year later, with restorations in place after adjunctive orthodontics to reposition the incisors. When lateral incisors are missing and the canines have drifted mesially to partially close the space, there are two possibilities: (1) open the lateral incisor space, placing a pontic there; or (2) bring the canine mesially into the lateral incisor space, and use a pontic in the canine space. Note that for this patient, both solutions have been used. The decision as to which would be the better treatment is based on the position of the teeth initially. For this girl, the right canine was in its proper position, but the left canine was almost totally forward into the lateral incisor position at the beginning of treatment.

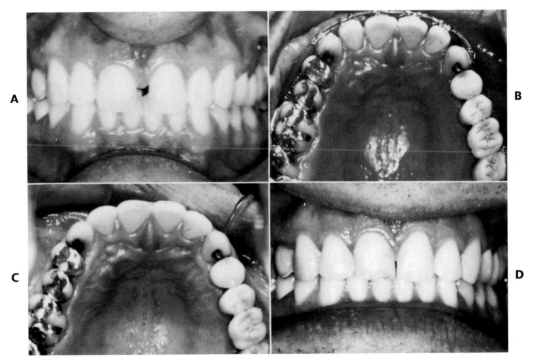

FIGURE 7-43 If a maxillary central diastema is related to small teeth that create a tooth-size discrepancy (usually the lateral incisors are the culprits), composite build-ups are an excellent solution, but satisfactory esthetics may require redistribution of the space before the restorations are placed, as in this patient. **A** and **B,** Prior to treatment. The midline diastema reflects the extra space in the upper arch caused by the small maxillary lateral incisors; **C,** redistribution of the space using a fixed appliance with coil springs on an archwire. Note the space has been created mesial and distal to the lateral incisors so that these teeth can be built up. The restoration should be done immediately upon removal of the orthodontic appliance (the same day); **D,** completed restorations. Note the reduction of the initial overbite, which was necessary to close some of the space and gain ideal relationships. This was accomplished with the fixed appliance.

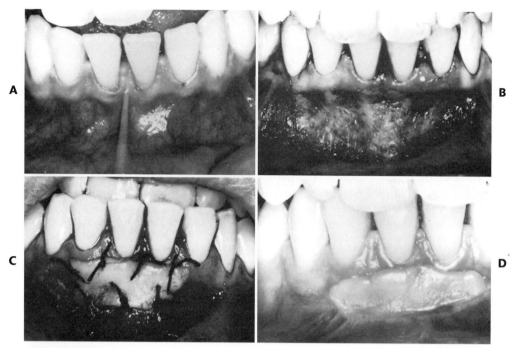

FIGURE 7-44   Free gingival grafts to create adequate attached gingiva may be needed before orthodontic treatment, particularly in the lower incisor area in adults. **A,** Inadequate attached gingiva and high frenum attachment create the possibility that loss of attachment will occur; **B,** preparation of a bed for free gingival graft from the palate; **C,** graft sutured into place; **D,** graft healing 6 weeks later.

overbite, successful treatment almost always requires an upper and lower fixed appliance and a relatively prolonged treatment time. These patients, whose orthodontic problems may look simple at first glance, can be extremely difficult to treat and should be placed in the category of comprehensive treatment.

Periodontal Considerations

When either comprehensive or adjunctive orthodontics for an adult is planned, the periodontal management of the patient must be kept in mind. The incidence of periodontal disease rises sharply in older population groups. A number of studies have indicated that by age 30, a majority of patients have some periodontal problems, and by age 40 this is true for more than 75% of all patients.[26] Beginning or even advanced periodontal breakdown does not contraindicate orthodontic treatment, but the periodontal situation must be kept in mind whenever orthodontic treatment for adults is planned.[27]

Periodontal findings in potential orthodontic patients are of two major types: (1) mucogingival problems, usually inadequate attached gingiva, and (2) inflammatory lesions of the gingiva or periodontium. Before any orthodontic treatment, it is important that adequate attached gingiva to withstand the stress of orthodontic tooth movement be created, if there are areas of deficiency (Figure 7-44). Inflammatory lesions must be brought under control. Adult

patients undergoing orthodontic treatment should have careful scaling on an accelerated schedule, typically at twice the frequency they would require without orthodontic treatment. In other words, an adult who might be seen for scaling and polishing at 6-month intervals without orthodontic treatment probably should be seen at 3-month intervals while being treated orthodontically, while one who required care at 3-month intervals should be seen every 6 weeks while undergoing orthodontics.

Further details of periodontal management for adult orthodontic patients are provided in Chapters 20 and 21.

REFERENCES

1. Kukafka AL: Informed consent in law and medicine: autonomy vs paternalism, J Law and Ethics in Dent 2:132-142, 1989.
2. Baergen R, Baergen C: Paternalism, risk and patient choice, J Am Dent Assn 128:481-484, 1997.
3. Ozar ST, Schiedermayer DL, Siegler M: Value categories in clinical dental ethics, J Am Dent Assoc 116:365-368, 1988.
4. Ackerman JL, Proffit WR: Communication in orthodontic treatment planning: bioethical and informed consent issues, Angle Orthod 65:253-262, 1995.
5. Ackerman JL, Proffit WR: Treatment response as an aid in orthodontic diagnosis and treatment planning, Am J Orthod 57:490-496, 1970.

6. Grubb JE, Smith T, Sinclair PM: Clinical and scientific applications/advances in video imaging, Angle Orthod 66: 407-416, 1996.

7. Le TN, Sameshima GT, Grubb JE, Sinclair PM: The role of computerized video imaging in predicting adult extraction treatment outcomes, Angle Orthod 68:391-400, 1998.

8. Sackett DL: On identifying the best therapy. In Trotman CA, McNamara JA (editors): Orthodontic treatment: outcome and effectiveness, Ann Arbor, Mich., 1995, University of Michigan Center for Human Growth and Development.

9. American Cleft Palate Association: Membership-Team Directory, Chapel Hill, NC, 1998, ACPA/ACPEF National Office, 104 S. Estes Drive, Suite 204.

10. Primosch R: Anterior supernumerary teeth—assessment and surgical intervention in children, Pediatr Dent 3:204-215, 1981.

11. Christensen JC, Fields HW: Space maintenance in the primary dentition. In Pinkham JR (editor): Pediatric dentistry: infancy through adolescence, ed 2, Philadelphia, 1994, W.B. Saunders.

12. Edwards JC: The diastema, the frenum, the frenectomy: a clinical study, Am J Orthod 71:489-508, 1977.

13. Villa NL, Cisneros GJ: Changes in the dentition secondary to palatal crib therapy in digit-suckers, Pediatric Dent 19:323-326, 1997.

14. Teel TT, Henderson HZ: Ectopic eruption of first permanent molars, J Dent Child 56:467-470, 1989.

15. Ericson S, Kurol J: Resorption of maxillary lateral incisors caused by ectopic eruption of the canines, Am J Orthod Dentofacial Orthop 94:504-513, 1988.

16. Spillane LM, McNamara JA: Maxillary adaptation to expansion in the mixed dentition, Sem Orthod 1:176-187, 1995.

17. Gianelly AA: Leeway space and the resolution of crowding in the mixed dentition, Sem Orthod 1:188-194, 1995.

18. Dale JG: Guidance of occlusion: serial extraction. In Graber TM, Vanarsdall RL (editors): Orthodontics: current principles and techniques, ed 2, St Louis, 1994, Mosby.

19. Hotz R: Orthodontics in daily practice, Baltimore, 1974, Williams & Wilkins.

20. Fields HW: Orthodontic-restorative treatment for relative mandibular anterior excess tooth-size problems, Am J Orthod 79:176-183, 1981.

21. Fields HW, Proffit WR, Nixon WL et al: Facial pattern and differences in long face children and adults, Am J Orthod 85:217-223, 1984.

22. Becker A: The orthodontic treatment of impacted teeth, St Louis, 1998, Mosby.

23. Moss JP: The unerupted canine, Dent Pract 22:241-248, 1972.

24. Proffit WR, Vig KWL: Primary failure of eruption: a possible cause of posterior open bite, Am J Orthod 80:173-190, 1981.

25. Andreasen, JO: Textbook of traumatic injuries of the teeth, ed 3, St. Louis, 1993, Mosby.

26. Brown LJ, Brunelle JA, Kingman A: Periodontal status in the United States, 1988-91, J Dent Res 75:672-683, 1996.

27. Boyd RL, Leggott PJ, Quinn RS et al: Periodontal implications of orthodontic treatment in adults with reduced or normal periodontal tissues versus those of adolescents, Am J Orthod Dentofacial Orthop 96:191-198, 1988.

CHAPTER

8

Orthodontic Treatment Planning: Limitations, Controversies, and Special Problems

THE EVIDENCE FOR CLINICAL DECISIONS

Orthodontics traditionally has been a specialty in which the opinions of leaders were important, to the point that professional groups coalesced around a strong leader. Angle, Begg and Tweed societies still exist, and new ones whose primary purpose is to promulgate its leader's opinions were formed as late as the 1980s. As any professional group comes of age, however, there must be a trend toward evidence-based rather than opinion-based decisions. The current trend in orthodontics in that direction is an encouraging indication of professional maturity. It still is the case in orthodontics that some important clinical decisions must be made without solid data on which to base them. In that circumstance the clinician must use his or her best judgment, which requires some understanding of the quality of existing data. This important subject is reviewed in some detail immediately below.

Study Designs

Retrospective vs. Prospective Data. Decisions about treatment are based on some combination of a theoretical understanding of the patient's circumstances (whether or not the theory is correct) and knowledge of the outcome of previous treatment in similar cases. Poorly-conceived views of how the patient's condition developed lead to poor treatment decisions, which is why it is so important to obtain and use the best information about the nature of the clinical problems we treat. The other part of the equation is equally important: we need to know as thoroughly as possible what really happens when various treatment procedures are used. Theories are tested and refined through clinical experience but only if the experience is analyzed logically, carefully, and thoughtfully.

As Box 8-1 illustrates, a hierarchy of quality exists in the evidence on which clinical decisions are based. Clinical data become available as reports of treatment outcomes. In the simplest form this is a case report, showing (usually in considerable detail) what happened in the treatment of a particular patient. A case series requires distilling the information, to separate the general trend among the patients from individual idiosyncrasies. The more patients for whom information is available, the more accurately the general trend can be discerned—if the sample of patients being reported is a reasonable representation of the larger population who might receive treatment of that type and if the data are analyzed appropriately. The hierarchy of quality in clinical data reflects, more than anything else, the probability that an accurate conclusion can be drawn from the group of patients who have been studied.

The unsupported opinion of an expert is the weakest form of clinical evidence. Often the expert opinion is supported by a series of cases that were selected retrospectively from practice records. The problem with that, of course, is that the cases are likely to have been selected because they show the expected outcome. A clinician who becomes an advocate of a treatment method is naturally tempted to select illustrative cases that show the desired outcome, and if even he or she tries to be objective, it is difficult to avoid introducing bias. When outcomes are variable, picking the cases that came out the way they were supposed to and discarding the ones that didn't is a great way to make your point. Information based on highly selected cases, therefore, must be viewed with considerable reserve.

It's much better, if retrospective cases are used in a clinical study, to select them on the basis of their characteristics when treatment began rather than how they responded to treatment. It's better yet to select the cases prospectively before treatment begins. Even then, it is quite possible to bias the sample so that the "right" patients are chosen. In

fact, it is difficult not to bias the sample in a prospective study. After experience with a treatment method, doctors tend to learn subtle indications that a particular patient is or is not likely to respond well, although they may have difficulty verbalizing exactly what criteria they used. But identifying the criteria associated with success is extremely important if the treatment method is to work well in the hands of others, and a biased sample makes that impossible.

For this reason, the gold standard for evaluating clinical procedures is the randomized clinical trial, in which patients are randomly assigned in advance to alternative treatment procedures. The great advantage of this method is that random assignment, if the sample is large enough, should result in a similar distribution of all variables between (or among) the groups. Even variables that were not recognized in advance should be controlled by this type of patient assignment—and in clinical work, often important variables are identified only after the treatment has been started or even completed.

An important aspect of any prospective study is keeping track of *all* the patients once they have been assigned to a treatment regimen. The other major source of bias in prospective studies comes from drop-outs, who are likely to be the very patients who were not responding well to the treatment. Unless these less successful patients are accounted for, the same bias produced by initially selecting only the "good" patients arises. Random assignment of patients, as in a randomized clinical trial, avoids the first source of selection bias but does nothing to control the second one. Data from randomized trials, therefore, must be reviewed on an "intent to treat" basis that includes all the subjects, using statistical techniques to estimate data for the ones who dropped out.

Data from randomized clinical trials now determines many clinical approaches in medicine and is beginning to do so in dentistry. The first clinical trials in orthodontics are being reported now and will be referred to in some detail later in this book. Many important clinical questions, however, do not lend themselves to clinical trial methodology, and inevitably many issues must be evaluated without randomized controls and/or from retrospective data. Let's now consider some important issues in evaluating such data.

Historical Control Groups. The best way to know—often the only way to know—whether a treatment method really works is to compare treated patients with an untreated control group. For such a comparison to be valid, the two groups must be equivalent before treatment starts. If the groups were different to start with, you cannot with any confidence say that differences afterward were due to the treatment.

There are a number of difficulties in setting up control groups for orthodontic treatment. The principal ones are that the controls must be followed over a long period of time, equivalent to the treatment time, and that sequential radiographs usually are required for the controls and the

---

BOX 8-1

EVIDENCE OF CLINICAL EFFECTIVENESS: A HIERARCHY OF QUALITY

Randomized clinical trial
|
Prospective study, non-random assignment
|
Retrospective study, inclusion based only on pre-treatment characteristics
|
Retrospective study, inclusion based on treatment response
|
Case report(s)
|
Unsupported opinion of expert

patients. Radiation exposure for untreated children is problematic. At present it is very difficult to get permission to expose children to x-rays that will be of no benefit to them personally. The growth studies carried out in the 1935-65 era in Burlington (Ontario) in association with the University of Toronto, Ann Arbor by the University of Michigan, and Cleveland by the Bolton Foundation provide reasonably large archives of sequential radiographs of untreated children (some of whom had malocclusion). Several smaller data bases from the same time period also exist.

This historical material is still being used as control data for evaluations of orthodontic treatment procedures, especially those involving growth modification. How valid is this? Are children seeking orthodontic treatment 50 years later, especially in other areas of the United States or even in other countries, really comparable with these historical samples? Probably not as much as one would like. The composition of current population groups often differs from the relatively homogenous growth study groups, especially when a current project focuses on children with a particular type of malocclusion but the comparison is with the mostly-normal growth study groups. In addition, the secular trend in growth over 50 years almost surely has affected expected growth increments. When historical controls are the best that is available, it is better to have them than nothing, but the limitations must be kept in mind.

Sample Sizes and Composition. How many subjects does it take to demonstrate a treatment effect? That depends, of course, on the size of the effect to be detected. The bigger the difference between two groups, the fewer the subjects that are needed to show it (if variability remains the same). Statistical analysis calculates the probability that differences are due to chance alone when the null hypothesis is true. When that probability becomes small enough, we accept the hypothesis that the groups are different.

In orthodontics, the data for clinical decisions often are from cephalometric analysis. The differences created by orthodontic treatment usually are not very large and are about the same magnitude as the variability within the sample. For this reason, although small cephalometric samples can be analyzed, conclusions based on sample sizes under 15 must be regarded with considerable suspicion, regardless of the statistics. With sample sizes of 25-30 patients, often it is possible to discern differences that would be important clinically, and almost always such differences can be demonstrated in sample sizes of 50 or so.

Sample size becomes particularly important when the composition of the groups being studied is not homogenous. Heterogeneity of the group can relate to age, gender, maturity, racial/ethnic origin, and other demographic characteristics. It also can relate to characteristics of the malocclusion being treated. Heterogeneity tends to increase the observed variability, making it more difficult to detect differences of clinical interest within a small sample. Angle classification is inadequate not only for orthodontic

diagnosis but also for sorting research subjects. If you're studying Class II malocclusion, for example, it's not enough to just select Class II subjects. It will be important to note face height as an important variable, because subjects with short and long faces grow differently and are likely to respond differently to treatment aimed at the overjet and Class II occlusion they share (Figure 8-1). Since face height differences increase the variability of changes in overjet or related criteria as a response, the greater the variability in face heights included in a Class II sample, the larger the sample would need to be to discern a treatment effect on these characteristics, and vice versa. Other characteristics of the malocclusion also may need to be controlled if sample sizes are to be kept reasonably small.

Issues in Data Analysis

Clinical vs. statistical significance. Statistical analysis can never flatly confirm or reject the truth of an experimental hypothesis. It merely calculates the odds that the null hypothesis should be accepted or rejected. If the analysis shows less than a 5% chance that a difference between groups could have arisen due to random variation ($p < .05$), the research hypothesis often is accepted (or, in terms of the test procedure, the null form of that hypothesis is not accepted).

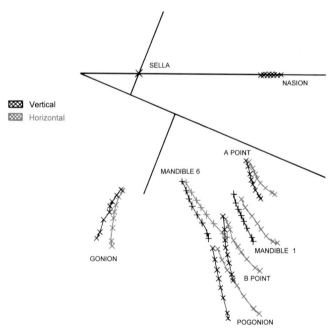

FIGURE 8-1 The varying growth direction of selected maxillary and mandibular landmarks is shown in this drawing derived from the templates of the Burlington (Ontario) growth study. The mean tracks for patients with a vertical vs. a horizontal growth pattern show clearly that both the direction and magnitude of growth at various locations are quite different, and the track for individuals with the usual horizontal-vertical pattern is intermediate between these two. For accuracy in growth prediction it would be important to place the patient in the correct group—which, unfortunately, can be quite difficult.

There are many possible sources of error in statistical analysis. For clinical studies, the most likely error arises from applying statistics based on the normal distribution to a data set that is not distributed like this bell-shaped curve. Wrongly-applied statistics tend to generate incorrect probability values that can lead to incorrect interpretations—in other words, bad statistics lead to bad conclusions. Transforming the data before analyzing it (by performing the same mathematical operation on each datum, for instance, taking the logarithm of each number) often can make normal-distribution (parametric) statistics more applicable. Many clinical studies, however, require statistics not based on the normal distribution (often called non-parametric statistics because the data are non-continuous).

Orthodontics is an excellent example of a clinical area in which both the theoretical framework for treatment and most of the treatment procedures have changed dramatically during the last 25 years. Similar progress has been made in statistics, especially in the analysis of clinical data. At this point, the use only of t-tests in a clinical study would be analogous to orthodontic treatment using gold bands and archwires—not wrong but not the best you could do. The modern clinician should be suspicious of conclusions based on superficial testing. Fortunately, clinical journals increasingly demand adequate statistical analysis, but that cannot be taken for granted, and the statistics that appear in some non-reviewed presentations (prominent on the Internet but not limited to it) must be examined carefully indeed.

It is important to remember that statistical significance and clinical significance are not the same. Tests of statistical significance ask questions like, "Is it probable that the difference between these groups is due only to chance?". Clinical significance asks, "Does that make any difference in treatment outcome?". Sometimes studies demonstrate statistically significant differences that are small enough to have no clinical significance. For example, studies of the size of the mandible with or without treatment aimed at stimulating its growth almost always show small differences in the ultimate size of the jaws (Table 8-1). In some publications the differences are reported as statistically significant, in others as not significant. At that level, the argument is over whether average differences of 1-2 mm in the size of a 12 cm mandible are treatment-related. The more important consideration is whether it would make any difference if they were. The clinician's question is, "Can you stimulate mandibular growth?". The answer has to be based on the magnitude of the changes as well as the statistical analysis. It seems to be, "If you can, not much."

Can clinically significant differences escape detection by statistical analysis? Certainly that is possible, especially when samples are small and/or not well selected. The likelihood is in the other direction, however. If statistical analysis fails to confirm what the clinician is convinced is true, the clinician probably is wrong. It's a human characteristic to remember the unusual, not the usual. Reports of treatment outcomes tend to focus on very good or very poor results, making most doctors think both extremes are more frequent than they really are. Reports of statistically significant differences that may not be clinically significant are more frequently encountered in the literature than clinically significant differences missed statistically.

Variability in Outcomes and the Presentation of Data. How do you report what happened to a group of patients? Almost always, by reporting the central tendency of the data set (the average, or perhaps the median) and by presenting some measure of the dispersion of the group (standard deviation or percentile spread, range). The focus tends to be on the central tendency, so a typical report says, "On average, group A showed significantly [whatever] compared with group B."

The problem with that type of data reporting can be illustrated by comparing Table 8-1 and Figure 8-2, which show exactly the same data but produce (for most clinicians, at least) a different sense of what is happening with this treatment. The data are taken from a randomized clinical trial of early Class II treatment, from which children with abnormally long or short faces were excluded. (This important study is reviewed further and in Chapter 15). Many doctors, looking at the table, would conclude that as they expected, nothing happened to the untreated children. The table shows that headgear produced some reduction in overjet but no change in overbite, while the functional appliance produced nearly twice as much change in overjet and also reduced overbite.

TABLE 8-1 *UNC Class II Clinical Trial: Changes During Phase I (15 months)*

	Control	Funct.	Headg.
Overjet (mm)	−0.1	−2.6	−1.5
s.d.	1.0	1.9	1.4
range	−2.6 1.9	−7.9 0.2	−5.1 1.1
Overbite (mm)	0.4	−1.4	0.0
s.d.	1.1	2.1	1.1
range	−2.4 3.8	−7.0 2.3	−2.3 3.6

TABLE 8-2 *Class II RCT: Skeletal Effects: ANB Angle (S.D.)*

Visit	Control	Bionator	Headgear
Initial	6.29 (1.98)	6.26 (2.06)	6.04 (1.82)
End Ph 1	6.11 (1.90)	5.14 (1.99)	4.72 (1.82)
Ph 1 Change	−0.17	−1.12	−1.31
End Ph 2	4.28 (2.04)	3.93 (1.94)	4.10 (1.97)
Ph 2 Change	−1.83	−1.21	−0.62
Total Change	−2.00	−2.33	−1.93

Figure 8-2 confirms that is true, on the average, but shows the variability within the groups as clearly as the central tendency. The variability was shown in the table too, but the standard deviation and range numbers just do not have the same impact, at least to the untrained eye. What you see in the figure is that many of the untreated children had a reduction in overjet, and about the same number had an increase, so that the average was zero although most children had changes. Some of the headgear patients had great improvement, while others had no response and a few got worse. There also was great variability among the functional appliance patients. It's important to comprehend the variations in response to treatment procedures, not just the average change, and particularly important not to be seduced into thinking that the average response is what you ought to expect to happen for every patient. The graphic form for presenting data (this type is called a 5-box plot) helps clinicians perceive the variability as well as the average changes.

Syndrome Recognition: Sensitivity vs. Specificity in Diagnostic Records.
By definition, a syndrome is a set of concurrent things that form an identifiable pattern. Many syndromes of developmental abnormalities have been recognized, and new ones are being noted all the time. Syndrome recognition is important in clinical studies, because patients who can be grouped by identifiable patterns are more predictable than those who have not been classified at that level. For example, you're much more likely to obtain a useful answer to the question, "How do patients with Crouzon syndrome respond to reverse-pull headgear?" than to the question, "How do patients with maxillary deficiency respond to reverse-pull headgear?", simply because there are several types of maxillary deficiency, Crouzon syndrome being one, that are likely to differ in their response.

Clinical progress requires the recognition of patterns of abnormalities, whether or not they are formally grouped as named syndromes. We already have commented on the importance of going beyond the Angle classification in orthodontic diagnosis. One way to view the Ackerman-Proffit classification is that in grouping patients by their five major characteristics, it places them in more homogenous and therefore more predictable groups.

From that perspective, it is important to consider two additional scientific terms, *sensitivity* and *specificity*, as they apply to diagnostic criteria and criteria for evaluating treatment response. Sensitivity refers to the ability of a given criterion (ANB angle, for example) to differentiate degrees of severity or extent of change (for ANB: diagnostically, the severity of a Class II jaw relationship; as an indicator of treatment response, the amount of improvement or worsening of the Class II condition). Specificity refers to the extent to which the criterion reflects only what it is supposed to, vs. being influenced by other things—in the case of the ANB angle, how well it shows the anteroposterior jaw relationships without being influenced by the vertical position of the jaws, protrusion or retrusion of the incisor teeth, or other factors. An extremely sensitive measure is always positive in the presence of the condition. Specificity sometimes particularly refers to how well a criterion can separate normal (acceptable) from abnormal (unacceptable)—for ANB, its ability to separate skeletal Class II from normal jaw relationships. An extremely specific measure is always negative in the absence of the condition.

Why are these distinctions important? From what you know about ANB, you could deduce that it is sensitive to changes in the anteroposterior jaw relationship (i.e., only small changes in the anteroposterior position of either jaw will produce a measurable change in ANB). Its specificity is not so good, because the ANB angle changes as face height shortens or lengthens even though the anteroposterior position of the jaws stays the same. It also can change if the incisor teeth are moved forward or back because of bone remodeling in the area of points A and B. Could you uncritically accept changes in the ANB angle as showing skeletal change in Class II patients undergoing alternative types of treatment? Only if you could be sure that there were no major vertical changes and no changes in the position of the roots of the anterior teeth. Obviously, the same type of thinking applies to whatever the major indicators are, in any clinical study. The more sensitive and more specific the indicators, the easier it is to interpret the results—and vice versa. No single criterion is likely to be both sensitive and specific enough to indicate all you'd want to know about patient groupings or treatment response.

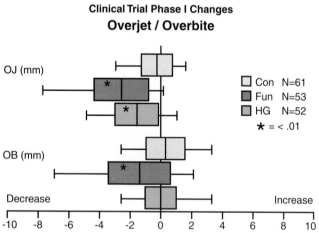

Clinical Trial Phase I Changes
Overjet / Overbite

OJ (mm)

OB (mm)

Decrease   Increase

-10 -8 -6 -4 -2 0 2 4 6 8 10

Con N=61
Fun N=53
HG   N=52
★ = < .01

FIGURE 8-2   In this graphic display (called a 5-box plot) of data from the UNC Class II clinical trial, the median value for each group is shown as the line toward the center of each box; the box dimensions reflect the 25th and 75th percentiles for the group; and the line shows the range. The variability within the groups can be appreciated more readily from a display of this type than from a table (see Table 8-2). Note that although the median change in overjet without treatment was almost zero, some children in the untreated control group had a reduction in overjet while others had an increase. Although the decrease in overjet in both treated groups was statistically significant compared with the controls, not all treated children responded favorably.

Computer Records and the Possibility of Meta-analysis. Clinical data exist in the form of careful records of treatment outcomes in many if not most private practices, not just in university or other clinical settings. Getting enough data about enough patients always is difficult in clinical studies. The widespread use of computers for storage of practice information, and the growing trend in orthodontics toward placing diagnostic as well as practice management information into electronic memory, offers an opportunity to widen the horizons of clinical research in a way that was hardly imaginable only a few years ago.

Most practitioners have had two problems in putting together data from their practices to obtain an honest answer to clinical questions: it was difficult and time-consuming to pull information from handwritten charts, manually analyze radiographs, and take measurements from dental casts or other records; and for most people, there was no clear protocol showing how to do this properly.

Computerization has the potential to solve both problems. If electronic entries replace chart notes and these are stored using a standard protocol (as most will be, because the format is established by the supplier of the practice software), and if x-rays, photographs, and casts are scanned for entry into the computer system (as they are, more and more, so they are accessible for communication with referring dentists as well as for analysis), then the information becomes readily available instead of having to be dug out of charts. One of the greatest problems with most existing data sets is the selective nature of the patients who are included. Often a major reason for selecting only some patients is that it is too much work to include everyone who was treated. But with routine electronic entry for all patients, there would be no reason to include only specially selected patients. In addition, it would be quite possible for a standard protocol for data collection to be established by a research group at a central facility, to which data could be transferred electronically from private practice. It would even be possible to add data to the research file via the Internet at the same time the clinical files were updated, and in fact this already is being done in a few studies in medicine as "Internet trials." Only with this type of cooperative input of data from multiple practice locations will it be possible to pull together enough data to answer many important clinical questions. By the same token, the very availability of the data will make it almost unconscionable not to seek solid answers to questions that have drawn only opinion for so long.

An additional way to gain better data for treatment responses is to group the data from several studies of the same phenomenon. This draws on the recently-developed method of meta-analysis, which allows statistical techniques to be applied across multiple studies.[1] Orthodontic research is an excellent example of an area in which numerous small studies have been carried out toward similar ends, often with protocols that were at least somewhat similar but different enough to make comparisons difficult.

Meta-analysis is no substitute for new data collected with precise protocols, but applying it to the clinical questions has considerable potential to reduce uncertainty about the best treatment methods.

The era of orthodontics as an opinion-driven specialty clearly is at an end. In the future, it will be evidence-driven—which is all for the best. In the meantime, clinical decisions still must be made using the best information currently available. When the latest new method appears with someone's strong recommendation and a series of case reports in which it worked very well, it is wise to remember the aphorism "Enthusiastic reports tend to lack controls; well-controlled reports tend to lack enthusiasm."

REDUCING UNCERTAINTY IN PLANNING TREATMENT

Even when excellent data from clinical trials are available, it is difficult to predict how any one individual will respond to a particular plan of treatment. Variability must be expected. In orthodontics, two interrelated factors contribute most of the variability: the patient's growth pattern and the effect of treatment on the expression of growth. At present, in the absence of growth, treatment responses are reasonably predictable. Growth is not.

Growth Prediction

Because predicting facial growth would be of great benefit in planning orthodontic treatment, repeated efforts have been made to develop methods to do this from cephalometric radiographs. Successful prediction requires specifying both the *amount* and the *direction* of growth, in the context of a baseline or reference point. The serial cephalometric radiographs obtained during the Burlington, Michigan, and Bolton growth studies have been treated statistically to allow their use in growth prediction, by grouping the data to provide a picture of average, normal growth changes. A convenient way to show average growth changes is with templates that show the expected direction and increment of growth at specified points or ages, or as a series of complete templates from which change at given points can be deduced (the same templates that also can be used diagnostically—see Chapter 6).

The more the individual whose growth one is attempting to predict is representative of the sample from which the average changes were derived, the more accurate one would expect the prediction to be, and vice versa. Ideally, separate growth standards would be established for the two sexes, the major racial groups, and important subgroups within each of the major categories (such as patients with skeletal Class II or Class III malocclusions). The existing data sets simply are too small to allow this sort of subdivision, and because it is no longer ethically acceptable to take repeated x-rays of children who will not be treated, it is unlikely that the necessary quantity of data ever will be available.

Data from the Bolton study[2] are not subdivided in any way. The Michigan data[3] are subdivided by sex, providing different male and female predictive values; the Burlington data[4] have been subdivided on the basis of facial pattern, with different growth predictions for individuals with short, normal, and long vertical facial dimensions (see Figure 8-1). All three data sets are derived from whites of northern European descent.

The major difficulty with growth prediction based on average changes is that a patient may have neither the average amount nor direction of growth, and thus there is the possibility of significant error. The growth samples were composed mostly of normal children. In clinical application, growth prediction is really needed for a child who has a skeletal malocclusion. His or her problem developed because of growth that deviated from the norm, and for such a child, deviant growth is likely to continue in the future—which means that average increments and directions are unlikely to be correct. Our ability to predict facial growth, therefore, is poorest for the very patients in whom it would be most useful.

The new clinical trial data offer hope of some improvement in this regard, in that the control groups do provide serial cephalometric radiographs of untreated children with specific types of malocclusion. It may be possible to detect characteristics that predict certain favorable or unfavorable patterns of growth. At present, however, accurate growth predictions simply are not possible for the children who need it most.

Predicting Treatment Outcomes

Visualized Treatment Objectives. A visualized treatment objective (VTO) is a cephalometric tracing representing the changes that are expected (desired) during treatment. In the 1980s, manually-prepared VTOs (Figure 8-3) were advocated as a treatment planning tool. For a child, the VTO would have to incorporate the expected growth, any growth changes induced by treatment, and any repositioning of the teeth from orthodontic tooth movement. In a child with normal facial proportions, average growth increments are reasonably likely and growth modification is not likely to be part of treatment, so growth changes can be predicted fairly well. The effects of tooth movement of various types are much more predictable than growth, although assumptions about the orthodontic therapy are required. For a skeletally normal child, preparing a VTO using average growth increments can be quite helpful in understanding the amount of tooth movement needed to correct the malocclusion. For a child with a skeletal problem, given the uncertainty of both the growth pattern and the response to treatment, a VTO often is more a presentation of what is hoped than what is likely to happen.

When the variables associated with growth are not present, as in treatment for adults and late adolescents with little or no remaining growth, predicting treatment effects becomes easier and more reliable. Cephalometric prediction of possible outcomes of orthodontic camouflage and orthognathic surgery have been used routinely since the early 1980s. Although these are not usually called VTOs, there is no real difference except that growth is not considered.

With modern computer technology, it is possible to link cephalometric tracings and digital facial images, so that when the teeth or jaws are repositioned on the tracing, a corresponding change in the facial appearance is produced. At this point, manual cephalometric predictions or VTOs have been superseded by computer prediction programs.

Computer Cephalometrics and Video Image Predictions. Placing cephalometric information into computer memory is conveniently accomplished by digitizing points on the cephalometric tracing (see Chapter 6). Automatic recognition of cephalometric landmarks already can be accomplished by experimental computer programs and is likely to replace manual identification of landmarks in the future.

The first computer cephalometric programs were used primarily for planning surgical treatment for adults. Their principal advantage was that this made it easy to produce multiple cephalometric predictions from the digitized tracings. Now all the commercially available programs allow superimposition of profile images (either direct digital images or conventional images digitized by scanning) onto the tracing, so that the doctor and patient can more readily visualize treatment effects (Figure 8-4) (see also Figure 7-3, compare with Figure 7-4). Computer images of this type have an important patient education benefit in addition to facilitating treatment planning.[5] Although presenting computer simulations to patients heightens their esthetic goals for treatment, it does not seem to create unrealistic expectations.[6]

It is possible to match changes in hard tissue positions to changes in the soft tissue image because studies of previously-treated patients have shown reasonably consistent relationships between hard and soft tissue changes. For example, when the upper incisors are retracted (orthodontically or surgically) the upper lip typically drops back about two-thirds the distance that the incisors were moved back. Information of that type is incorporated into the computer program and is used to produce the changes in the soft tissue image when retraction of the incisors is simulated. Not surprisingly, the accuracy of the soft tissue simulations is better in some areas than others. Computer predictions of changes in the position of the upper lip and chin are more accurate than changes in the lower lip, especially when face height is lengthened or shortened. The computing algorithms for predictions of surgical or orthodontic changes in the absence of growth have improved remarkably in the last few years, and probably will continue to do so.

Does this mean that computerization will solve the problems of growth prediction? No, because the data on which the growth-prediction algorithms would have to be based simply do not exist. There is no reason to believe that the same kind of prediction that can be done with adults will be possible for children any time soon.

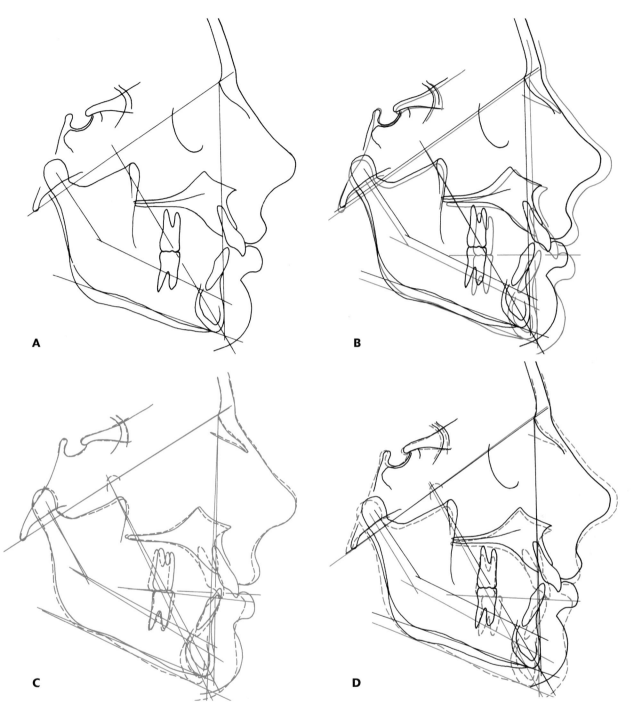

FIGURE 8-3   Preparation of a visual treatment objective (VTO) using the method of Ricketts. **A,** Cephalometric tracing of a 13-year-old boy with maxillary dental crowding and Class II malocclusion with mandibular deficiency. **B,** Growth prediction (*red*) for the next 2 years superimposed on the original tracing. The growth prediction is based on lengthening the basion-nasion line 2 mm per year (1 mm increment at basion and nasion), and on lengthening the mandibular condylar axis and corpus axis 2 mm per year. The maxilla is predicted to move down and forward two thirds as much as the mandible (for details of the prediction method, see Ricketts RM: *Bioprogressive Therapy*, Denver, 1977, Rocky Mountain). **C,** VTO (*dashed red*) superimposed on growth prediction. The guideline for rotation of the mandible (changes in the facial axis): a 1 degree opening of the facial axis (*arrow*) can be expected for each 3 mm of molar correction, 4 mm of overbite reduction, and/or 5 mm convexity reduction. A reduction in point A can be achieved with headgear (maximum 8 mm) or Class II elastics for Class II correction was projected, without extractions, producing the changes shown here. **D,** VTO superimposed on the original tracing, showing the estimated combined effect of growth and treatment. Unfortunately, the accuracy of this approach leaves a great deal to be desired because of variations in both growth and treatment response.

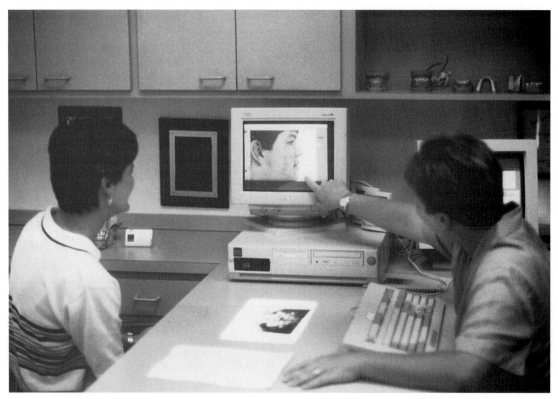

FIGURE 8-4   Presenting a computer-generated simulation of the post-treatment profile can greatly help patients understand the differences between alternative treatment approaches. Although showing patients these simulations heightens their esthetic awareness, it does not seem to create unrealistic expectations.[6] (Courtesy Dr. David Sarver.)

Treatment Response as an Aid in Treatment Planning

A practical problem in treatment planning for children, then, is how to reduce the uncertainty related to growth. What do you do, for instance, with a rather mature 12-year-old boy with a moderately severe skeletal Class II problem? Should you use the estimates underlying a VTO or computer prediction to make the decision, ignoring the possibility of serious error? Proceed with growth modification, regardless of a questionable prognosis? Go ahead with extractions for camouflage, on the theory that this would assure success whatever the patient's growth? Each of these approaches has been advocated seriously by respected orthodontic clinicians, but each has limitations. Growth prediction works satisfactorily for average patients but not so well for the ones whose growth has already produced an orthodontic problem—the chance of error can be distressingly large. Attempted growth modification in a poorly growing patient produces an unstable and generally unsatisfactory result. Camouflage can provide an acceptable result in a poorly growing patient, but extractions for this purpose in a patient with good growth are undesirable esthetically and functionally.

One way to reduce the amount of uncertainty in planning treatment for children whose growth is somewhat unpredictable is to use the initial treatment response as an aid in treatment planning, deferring the adoption of a definitive treatment plan until some experience has been achieved with the patient. This approach, sometimes called "therapeutic diagnosis," allows a better evaluation of both growth response and cooperation with treatment than can be obtained by prediction alone.

In practice, the therapeutic diagnosis approach involves implementing a conservative (i.e., nonextraction) treatment plan initially and scheduling a reevaluation of the patient after 6 to 9 months to observe the response to this treatment. Typically, a child with a skeletal Class II malocclusion might be placed on a functional appliance or extraoral force to the maxilla, with minimal use of fixed appliances for tooth movement. If a good response is observed after 6 to 9 months, this treatment approach is continued, with the odds of long-term success greatly improved. On the other hand, if a poor response is observed, whether because of poor cooperation or poor growth, the growth modification therapy might be dropped in favor of extractions and a fixed appliance, camouflage-oriented approach. The disadvantage of the evaluation period in the latter instance is that treatment may take longer than it would have if the extraction decision had been made initially. The advantage is a decrease in the number of incorrect decisions.

No method of pretreatment prediction is as accurate for establishing the appropriate treatment plan as an observation of the actual response to treatment. Whatever the treatment plan, it is important at all stages of all types of treatment to carefully monitor the patient's response and make appropriate adjustments in the original plan to deal with variations in response. Acknowledging uncertainties and testing the patient's response to treatment before making irrevocable decisions is a logical way to improve the percentage of patients in whom the correct decision is made.

In the sections of this chapter immediately below, the goal is to review what is known about controversial areas, put it into perspective based on the quality of available data, and draw the best conclusions about treatment possibilities that are possible today. Better data in the not-too-distant future should allow a more confident emphasis on specific treatment approaches.

EXTRACTION IN THE TREATMENT OF MALOCCLUSION

"To extract or not to extract" may not have quite the significance of "To be or not to be," but for 100 years it has been a key question in planning orthodontic treatment. In orthodontics, there are two major reasons to extract teeth: (1) to provide space to align the remaining teeth in the presence of severe crowding, and (2) to allow teeth to be moved (usually, incisors to be retracted) so protrusion can be reduced or so skeletal Class II or Class III problems can be camouflaged. The alternative to extraction in treating dental crowding is to expand the arches; the alternative for skeletal problems is to correct the jaw relationship, by modifying growth or surgery. All other things being equal, it is better not to extract—but in some cases extraction provides the best treatment. Opinions as to the indications for extraction have changed remarkably over the years, from one extreme to the other and back (Figure 8-5), and it seems likely that this particular pendulum still is swinging.

The Great Extraction Controversy of the 1920s

As the occlusal concepts that culminated in his definition of normal occlusion were developed, Edward Angle struggled with both facial esthetics and stability of result as potential complications in his efforts to achieve an idealized normal occlusion.[7] It is difficult to recreate the thought processes of a brilliant man many years ago, but it seems clear that Angle was influenced by both the philosophy of Rousseau and the biologic concepts of his time. Rousseau emphasized the perfectibility of man. His strong belief that many of the ills of modern man could be traced to the pernicious influences of civilization struck a responsive chord in Angle, who joined other progressive young dentists of the 1890s in their reaction to the casual attitude of that time toward extraction of teeth. In an era when teeth could be saved by dental treatment, extraction of teeth for orthodontic purposes seemed particularly inappropriate,

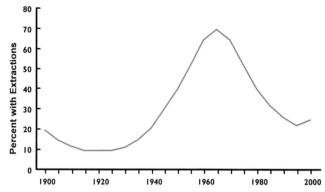

FIGURE 8-5   In general, extraction of teeth for orthodontic purposes was rare in the early 20th century, peaked in the 1960s with extraction occurring in a majority of orthodontic patients, and declined to about the levels of the early 1900s by the 1990s. An increase probably will occur in the early 2000s.

especially if man was inherently capable of having a perfect dentition. Perfection, it appeared, required only diligent efforts to achieve it. It became an article of faith for Angle and the early orthodontists that every person had the potential for an ideal relationship of all 32 natural teeth, and therefore that extraction for orthodontic purposes was never needed.

Secondly, Angle was impressed by the discovery that the architecture of bone responds to the stresses placed on that part of the skeleton. In the early 1900s, the German physiologist Wolff demonstrated that bone trabeculae were arranged in response to the stress lines on the bone (the internal architecture of the head of the femur is the classic example, but the condylar process of the mandible shows the same effect of "Wolff's law of bone") (Figure 8-6). This led Angle to two key concepts. The first was that skeletal growth could be influenced readily by external pressures. If bone remodeled when stressed, the etiology of Class II or Class III problems must be abnormal stresses on the jaws, but different patterns of pressure associated with treatment could change growth so as to overcome the problem. Angle came to believe that skeletal structures were so adaptable that just rubber bands connecting the upper to the lower teeth could overcome improper jaw relationships, stimulating growth where it was needed.

The second concept was that proper function of the dentition would be the key to maintaining teeth in their correct position. Angle reasoned that if the teeth were placed in proper occlusion, forces transmitted to the teeth would cause bone to grow around them, thus stabilizing them in their new position even if a great deal of arch expansion had occurred. He soon saw that merely tipping the teeth to a new position might be inadequate and sought ways to move the teeth bodily. He described his edgewise appliance, the first appliance capable of fully controlling root position (see Chapter 12), as the "bone growing appliance."

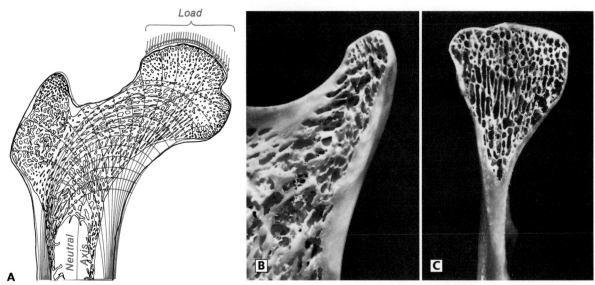

FIGURE 8-6 **A,** Bone trabeculae in the head of the femur follow the calculated stress lines. This observation by the German physiologist Wolff at the end of the 19th century led to "Wolff's law of bone" that the internal architecture of bones represents the stress pattern on them. **B,** Frontal section through the head of the mandibular condyle. **C,** Sagittal section through the head of the condyle. Note the arrangement of bony trabeculae, indicating a similar arrangement for resistance to stress as seen in the head of the femur. (**B** and **C,** From DuBrul EL: *Sicher's oral anatomy*, ed 7, St Louis, 1980, Mosby.)

To Angle and his followers, relapse after expansion of the arches or rubber bands to correct overjet and overbite meant only that an adequate occlusion had not been achieved. This too became an article of faith: if a correct occlusion had been produced, the result would be stable; therefore if the orthodontic result was not stable, the fault was that of the orthodontist, not the theory.

Finally, the problem of dentofacial esthetics was solved, at least for Angle, through his interaction with a famous artist of the day, Professor Wuerpel. Early in his career, Angle devoted much effort to a search for the ideal facial form, in parallel with his search for the ideal dental occlusion (Figure 8-7). When he consulted the art professor for advice about the perfect face, he was ridiculed—the artist's response was that the tremendous variety in human faces makes it impossible to specify any one facial form as the ideal. Reflecting on this, Angle had a moment of insight: the relationship of the dentition to the face, and with it the esthetics of the lower face, would vary, but for each individual, ideal facial esthetics would result when the teeth were placed in ideal occlusion. Whether the patient liked the outcome or not, by definition the best facial appearance for him or her would be achieved when the dental arches had been expanded so that all the teeth were in ideal occlusion.

Therefore, for Angle, proper orthodontic treatment for every patient involved expansion of the dental arches and rubber bands as needed to bring the teeth into occlusion, and extraction was not necessary for stability of result or esthetics. These concepts did not go unchallenged. An-

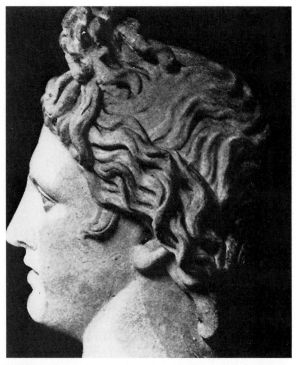

FIGURE 8-7 Angle sought an ideal profile, in parallel to his search for an ideal occlusion, and initially favored this classic Greek profile, which is often incompatible with non-extraction treatment. (From Angle EH: *Treatment of malocclusion of the teeth*, ed 7, Philadelphia, 1907, SS White Manufacturing Co.)

gle's great professional rival, Calvin Case, argued that although the arches could always be expanded so that the teeth could be placed in alignment, neither esthetics nor stability would be satisfactory in the long term for many patients. The controversy culminated in a widely publicized debate between Angle's student Dewey and Case, carried out in the dental literature of the 1920s.[8]

Reading these papers from a current perspective leaves the impression that Case had the better argument by far. Yet Angle's followers won the day, and extraction of teeth for orthodontic purposes essentially disappeared from the American orthodontic scene in the period between World Wars I and II. Even those who did not agree with Angle's appliance systems, particularly in the American South where removable (Crozat) or partially banded appliances (labiolingual, twin wire) were commonly used, accepted the non-extraction approach and its philosophic underpinnings.

The Re-introduction of Extraction in Mid-Century

By the 1930s, relapse after non-extraction treatment was frequently observed. At this time soon after Angle's death, one of his last students, Charles Tweed, decided to re-treat with extraction a number of his patients who had experienced relapse. Four first premolar teeth were removed and the teeth were aligned and retracted. After the re-treatment, Tweed observed that the occlusion was much more stable. Tweed's dramatic public presentation of consecutively treated cases with premolar extraction caused a revolution in American orthodontic thinking and led to the widespread reintroduction of extraction into orthodontic therapy by the late 1940s. Independently of Tweed but simultaneously, another of Angle's students, Raymond Begg in Australia, also concluded that non-extraction treatment was unstable. Like Tweed, he modified the Angle-designed appliance he was using, adapting it for extraction treatment and producing what is now called the Begg appliance (see Chapter 12).

The acceptance of extraction and the repudiation of Angle's ideas were made easier by an intellectual climate in which the limitations of human adaptation both socially and physically, were emphasized. Breeding experiments with animals, of which Stockard's widely publicized results from crossbreeding dogs were most influential, seemed to show conclusively that malocclusion could be inherited (see Chapter 5). Rather than developing the (non-existent) potential within each patient, it appeared that it was necessary for the orthodontist to recognize genetically determined disparities between tooth size and jaw size, or to acknowledge that the lack of proximal wear on teeth produced tooth size-jaw size discrepancies during development. In either case, extraction was frequently necessary.

By the early 1960s, more than half the American patients undergoing orthodontic treatment had extraction of some teeth, usually but not always first premolars. Since the accepted concept was that orthodontic treatment could not affect facial growth, extraction was considered necessary to accommodate the teeth to discrepancies in jaw position as well as to overcome crowding caused by tooth-jaw discrepancies, and was done for either or both purposes.

Recent Trends Toward Non-extraction

Extraction rates always have varied among doctors and regions, so no specific example of changes in extraction patterns can be taken totally as typical. Experience in the orthodontic clinic at the University of North Carolina (Figure 8-8), however, shows well the type of change over time that has occurred widely. At its inception in the 1950s, treatment in the clinic was strongly influenced by attitudes like Angle's. By the 1960s the Tweed/Begg view had been accepted, and extraction rates increased dramatically. From then until the early 1990s there was a continuing decline in extraction rates, which has stabilized or increased slightly recently.

The UNC patients can be grouped into three extraction categories: four first premolars, the usual extraction pattern for treatment of Class I crowding/protrusion (sometimes used also for Class II camouflage); upper first premolars only or upper first-lower second premolars, a pattern that indicates Class II camouflage; and all other extraction patterns (asymmetric extractions, impossibly impacted teeth, one lower incisor, etc.). As Figure 8-8 illustrates, the change over the years occurred mostly in the four first premolar group, with smaller changes in the camouflage extraction rate. For the "other" group, the rate was remarkably constant over the period of 45 years. Decisions in this clinic always have been made by individual attending faculty. It is clear, therefore, that this group of orthodontists (a mix of full- and part-time faculty) showed remarkable changes in their decisions about extraction in the treatment of dental crowding, with much less change in extraction for other reasons. Why?

The reasons for the increase in extraction have been discussed above, but it is important to put this in perspective: premolar extraction was, more than anything else, a search for stability. In the earlier nonextraction era, collapse of expanded arches and relapse into crowding were frequently observed (but, it must be said, not well documented scientifically), and it became clear that perfection of the occlusion did not necessarily lead to stability. Extraction as a strategy was adopted, however, without evidence beyond selected cases that it produced stable results. Why the decline in extraction rates more recently? There are several reasons. Experience has shown that premolar extraction does not necessarily guarantee stability of tooth alignment,[9-11] and one could argue that if the results are not very stable either way, there is no reason to sacrifice teeth. (It also can be argued that even if extraction cases often are unstable, non-extraction would be worse. Nothing remotely like a randomized clinical trial of extraction vs

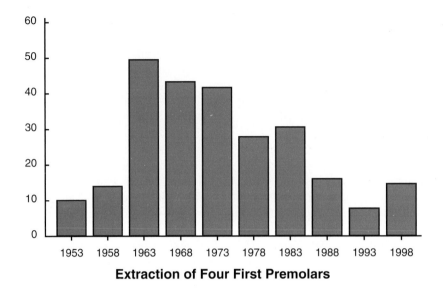

Extraction of Four First Premolars

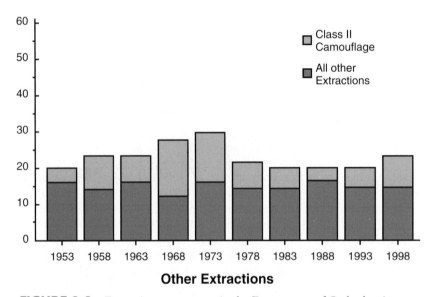

Other Extractions

FIGURE 8-8 Extraction percentages in the Department of Orthodontics at the University of North Carolina, 1953-1998. Extraction of first premolars usually is done for treatment of crowding/protrusion; extraction of upper first or upper first/lower second premolars indicates Class II camouflage; other extractions are done for a variety of purposes related to impaction, asymmetry and tooth-size discrepancy. Note that the number of patients with extraction of four first premolars increased sharply in the 1960s, declined to the 1953 level in 1993, and showed a slight increase recently. The number of patients with extraction for Class II camouflage also increased in the 1960s, decreased in the 1980s, and increased again more recently, but did not change nearly as much. The number of patients with other all other extractions has been remarkably constant for 45 years.

nonextraction treatment of Class I crowding has ever been done, and there are simply no good data that really allow comparison of the stability extraction and non-extraction treatment in similar groups of patients.)

In addition, dentists have realized that the general public often prefer fuller and more prominent lips than the orthodontic standards of the 1950s and 1960s. The facial appearance in "borderline cases" generally is considered better without extraction by both dentists and others. The change from fully banded to largely bonded appliances made it easier to expand the arches by eliminating the need for band space. In the 1980s, claims were made that temporomandibular dysfunction (TMD) problems could be attributed to extraction of upper first premolars, and although this association has been refuted, for a time it also affected extraction rates, at least by some doctors.

The result, however, is two-fold: it is possible, perhaps even likely, that non-extraction treatment once again is being carried to an extreme, so that stability problems once more are likely to become prominent; and controversy over the role of extraction continues because there are no good data to settle the issue. At present every shade of opinion and practice relative to extraction can be found. These range from an absolute rejection of the possibility of a need for extraction, supported by arguments that seem taken word-for-word from Angle's era, to a rejection of the possibilities of arch expansion and growth guidance along with a continued high percentage of extraction. The amount of change in treatment of dental crowding, the most frequent orthodontic problem—in the almost total absence of data—illustrates how far orthodontics still has to go in becoming an evidence-driven specialty. In this, as with so much else, it is necessary to understand the pertinent history to avoid repeating it.

A Contemporary Perspective: Recommendations for Expansion vs. Extraction

In a rational contemporary view, the majority of patients can be treated without removal of teeth but by no means all. In addition to those who fall into the rather constant "other" category described above, some will require extraction to compensate for crowding, incisor protrusion that affects facial esthetics, or jaw discrepancy. Their number varies, depending on the population being treated. Extraction for camouflage is considered separately later in the chapter. The section immediately below is a discussion of the limits of expansion, and therefore the indications for extraction, for patients with normal jaw relationships.

Esthetic Considerations. If the major factors in extraction decisions are stability and esthetics, it is worthwhile to review existing data that relate these factors to expansion and extraction. Consider esthetics first. The conceptual relationship between expansion/extraction and esthetics is illustrated in Figure 8-9. All other things being equal, expansion of the arches moves the patient in the direction of more prominent teeth, while extraction tends to reduce the prominence of the teeth. Facial esthetics can become unacceptable on either the too-protrusive or too-retrusive side.

At what point have the incisors been moved too far forward, so that esthetics is compromised? The answer is found in soft tissue, not hard tissue relationships: when the prominence of the incisors creates excessive lip separation at rest, so that the patient must strain to bring the lips together, the teeth are too protrusive, and retracting the incisors improves facial esthetics (Figure 8-10). As a general guideline, more than 4 mm lip separation at rest is unesthetic. Note that this has nothing to do with the prominence of the teeth relative to the supporting bone. An individual with thick, full lips looks good with incisor prominence that would not be acceptable in someone with thin, tight lips. Cephalometric measurements of incisor position that attempt to establish the esthetic limits of protrusion go all the way back to Tweed, but there is no way to determine the esthetic limit of expansion from tooth-bone relationships alone.

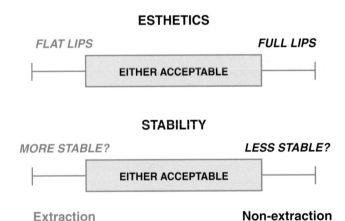

FIGURE 8-9 Expansion of the dental arches tends to make the teeth more prominent and extraction makes them less prominent. The choice between extraction and non-extraction (expansion) treatment is a critical esthetic decision for some patients who are toward the extremes of incisor protrusion or retrusion initially, but because there is an acceptable range of protrusion, many if not most can be treated with satisfactory esthetics either way. This is especially true if expansion is managed so as not to produce too much protrusion, or space closure after extraction is controlled so as not to produce too much incisor retraction. Similarly, expansion tends to make arches less stable and extraction favors stability, but the extraction–non-extraction decision probably is a critical factor in stability largely for patients who are toward the extremes of the protrusion-retrusion distribution. There are no data to show the number of patients who could be treated satisfactorily with either approach, versus the number for whom the extraction–non-extraction decision is critical in determining a satisfactory outcome.

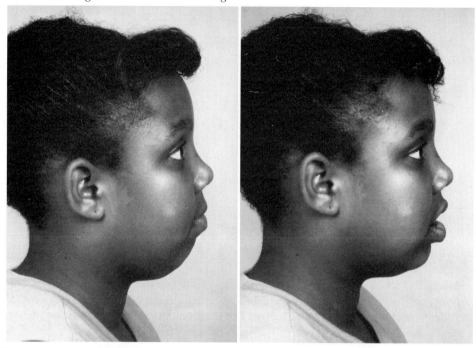

FIGURE 8-10   Excessive protrusion of incisors requires lip strain to close the lips over the teeth, as in this patient, and therefore also is characterized by excessive lip separation at rest (lip incompetence). As a general guideline, more than 4 mm lip separation at rest is considered excessive. The amount of incisor protrusion that is acceptable is determined by soft tissue relationships, whatever the racial or ethnic groups.

The size of the nose and chin has a profound effect on relative lip prominence. For a patient with a large nose and/or a large chin, if the choices are to treat without extraction and move the incisors forward, or extract and retract the incisors at least somewhat, moving the incisors forward is better, provided it does not diminish the labiomental sulcus too much. Lack of a well-defined labiomental sulcus, which usually is related to lip strain in gaining lip seal, can be due either to increased lower face height or protrusion of the teeth, and this also can be taken as evidence that the incisors are too prominent.

At what point are the incisors retracted to the point of adversely affecting facial esthetics? That too depends largely on the soft tissues. A concave profile with thinning of the lips, so that there is little vermilion border, is an unesthetic trait. In a patient with thin lips, proclining the incisors tends to create fuller lips with more vermilion show, and this is likely to be perceived as more attractive. Since the face tends to flatten with age and the lips become less full with aging, retracting teeth in a patient with thin lips can prematurely age the face. The upper incisors are too far lingually if the upper lip inclines backward—it should be slightly forward from its base at soft tissue point A (Figure 8-11, *A*). For best esthetics, the lower lip should be at least as prominent as the chin. Another cause of a poorly-defined labiomental sulcus is retroclined mandibular incisors (Figure 8-11, *B*). Variations in chin morphology may put the proper incisor-chin relationship beyond the control of orthodontics alone, in which case chin surgery

perhaps should be considered (see the section on Class II camouflage below, and Chapter 22).

The extraction–non-extraction decision is one determinant of incisor position, but it is not the only one. Where the incisors end up is also very much influenced by the way the orthodontic treatment is managed. If extraction spaces can be closed without retracting the incisors too much, there is no esthetic liability from the extractions; and if non-extraction treatment can be carried out without protruding the incisors too much, there also would be no esthetic difficulty.

Stability Considerations.   For stable results, how much can arches be expanded? The lower arch is more constrained than the upper, and so its limitations for stable expansion may be somewhat tighter than the upper arch. Current guidelines for the limits of expansion of the lower arch, admittedly based on limited data, are presented in Figure 8-12. The 2 mm limitation for forward movement of the incisors obviously is subject to considerable individual variation, but makes sense in light of the observation that lip pressure increases sharply 2 mm out into space usually occupied by the lip (see Chapter 5). If lip pressure is the limiting factor in forward movement, as it probably is, the initial position of the incisors relative to the lip would be a consideration in how much movement could be tolerated. This suggests, and clinical observation seems to confirm (again, limited data!) that incisors that are tipped lingually away from the lip can be moved further forward than upright incisors. Incisors that are tipped labially and crowded

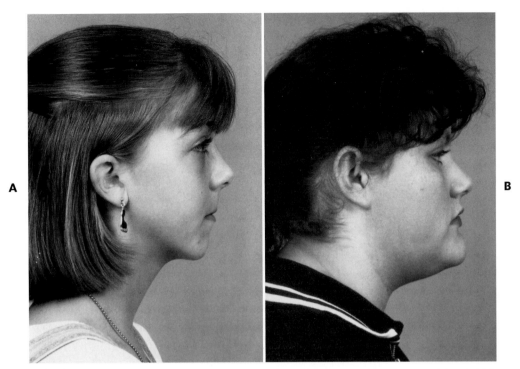

FIGURE 8-11 **A,** An upper lip that inclines backward relative to the true vertical line, which can result from retraction of upper incisors to correct excessive overjet, tends to compromise facial esthetics, as does a poorly-defined labiomental sulcus when lip strain is required to bring the lips together. **B,** Retroclined mandibular incisors, as in this patient with a prominent chin, are another cause of a poorly-defined labiomental sulcus.

probably represent the equivalent of a titrated end point in a chemical reaction, in that they have already become as protrusive as the musculature will allow. Moving them any further forward carries great risk of instability.

Figure 8-12 suggests that there is more opportunity to expand transversely than anteroposteriorly—but only behind the canines. Numerous reports show that transverse expansion across the canines is almost never maintained. In fact, intercanine dimensions typically decrease as patients mature, whether or not they had orthodontic treatment, probably because of lip pressures at the corners of the mouth. Expansion across the premolars and molars is much more likely to be maintained, presumably because of the relatively low cheek pressures.

One approach to arch expansion is to expand the upper arch by opening the midpalatal suture. If the maxillary base is narrow, that is appropriate treatment (see the discussion of transverse maxillary deficiency, on p. 256). Some clinicians theorize (with no supporting evidence) that generously expanding the upper arch by opening the suture, temporarily creating a buccal crossbite, allows the lower arch then to be expanded more than otherwise would have been possible. If the limiting factor is cheek pressure, it seems unlikely that the method of expansion would make any difference. Because sutural expansion typically is achieved with about 50% skeletal change and 50% tooth movement (see further discussion below in this chapter),

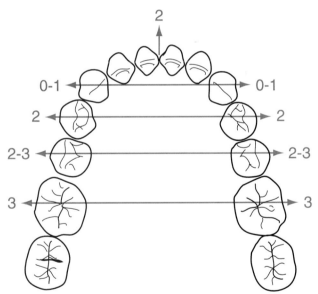

FIGURE 8-12 Because the lower arch is more constrained, the limits of expansion for stability seem to be tighter for it than the maxillary arch. The available data suggest that moving lower incisors forward more than 2 mm is problematic for stability, probably because lip pressure seems to increase sharply at about that point. A considerable body of data shows that expansion across the canines is not stable, even if the canines are retracted when they are expanded. Expansion across the premolars and molars, in contrast, can be stable.

excessive expansion carries the risk of fenestration of pre-molar and molar roots through the alveolar bone. For example, 12 mm total expansion across the maxillary dentition would be achieved with 6 mm widening of the suture and 3 mm per side of dental expansion. There is an increasing risk of fenestration beyond 3 mm of transverse tooth movement (Figure 8-13).[12]

Summary of Contemporary Extraction Guidelines. Contemporary guidelines for orthodontic extraction in Class I crowding and/or protrusion can be summarized as follows:

- Less than 4 mm arch length discrepancy: extraction rarely indicated (only if there is severe incisor protrusion or in a few instances, a severe vertical discrepancy).
- Arch length discrepancy 5 to 9 mm: non-extraction or extraction treatment possible. The extraction/non-extraction decision depends on both the hard- and soft-tissue characteristics of the patient and on how the final position of the incisors will be controlled; any of several different teeth could be chosen for extraction. Non-extraction treatment usually requires transverse expansion across the molars and premolars.
- Arch length discrepancy 10 mm or more: extraction almost always required to obtain enough space. The extraction choice is four first premolars or perhaps upper first premolars and mandibular lateral incisors; second premolar or molar extraction rarely is satisfactory.

This aspect of the extraction–non-extraction decision is discussed further in Chapter 14, as it applies to preadolescent (mixed dentition) children with severe crowding problems.

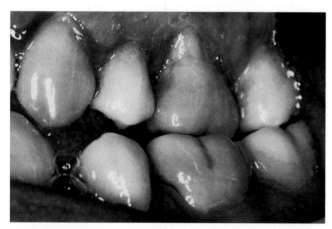

FIGURE 8-13   Excessive transverse expansion can lead to fenestration of roots through the lateral wall of the alveolar process. As a teenager this patient with Class III malocclusion and maxillary deficiency had major expansion of the maxilla via a jackscrew to open the mid-palatal suture, which produces about 50% skeletal expansion and 50% tooth movement. In young adult life, he has experienced gingival recession after developing gingivitis and early periodontal disease. Note the root exposure of the maxillary first molar, which probably is related to the sutural expansion treatment.

Guidelines for extraction to camouflage jaw discrepancies are presented below, in the discussion of that approach to skeletal problems.

GROWTH MODIFICATION IN THE TREATMENT OF SKELETAL PROBLEMS

The best way to correct a jaw discrepancy would be to get the patient to grow out of it. Because the pattern of facial growth is established early in life and rarely changes significantly (see Chapter 2), this is unlikely without treatment. The important questions in planning treatment are the extent to which growth can be modified, and how advantageous it is to start treatment early. The answers are almost as controversial as extraction–non-extraction. In the section of this chapter immediately below, growth modification possibilities and the timing of treatment for the most frequent types of skeletal problems are reviewed. Additional information on methods for early treatment of these problems is presented in Chapter 15.

Transverse Maxillary Deficiency

Narrow skeletal width of the maxilla is indicated by narrow width of the palatal vault (see Figure 6-52). This is one of the few jaw dimensions that can be assessed accurately from dental casts. Remember that a narrow maxillary dental arch may or may not reflect narrow skeletal dimensions.

Maxillary deficiency in the transverse plane of space may occur in children with otherwise normal jaw proportions, but often it accompanies excessive vertical development in a patient with skeletal Class II malocclusion, or is part of a three-dimensional maxillary deficiency in a Class III patient. Isolated transverse maxillary deficiency is discussed in this section. Transverse deficiency accompanying anteroposterior or vertical problems is discussed under those headings.

It is appropriate to discuss maxillary deficiency at the beginning of this discussion of skeletal problems because of its relationship to the extraction–non-extraction decision that was just reviewed. In a child with dental crowding, a diagnosis of deficient maxillary width can become a convenient rationale for enough transverse expansion to align the teeth. Some efforts have been made in the past to calculate what the width of the maxilla ought to be, based on the size of the teeth. For instance, Pont's index from the early 1900s purports to relate the width of the maxillary first premolars to the proper width of the maxilla. This has been resurrected on several occasions to justify rather extreme maxillary expansion.[13] Why the size of the teeth should determine the proper size of the jaw remains unexplained and is unexplainable without applying Angle's logic that function would somehow make the bone grow around the teeth.

Widening the maxillary dental arch may or may not be a justifiable response to crowding, depending on other circumstances of the case; skeletal maxillary expansion certainly should not become a routine response to an intermolar distance that is less than the population average.

If the maxilla is narrow relative to the rest of the face, so that the patient is in posterior crossbite and the teeth are not obviously tipped to produce the crossbite, a diagnosis of transverse maxillary deficiency is justified and skeletal expansion probably is appropriate. If formation of bone really can be stimulated by separating sutures, as current theory suggests (see Chapter 2), opening up the mid-palatal suture should provide a way to widen a narrow maxilla. This is in fact the case: new bone can be induced to form in the palate by separation of the mid-palatal suture, which can be done conveniently by placing heavy force across the maxillary dental arch (Figure 8-14). Like extraoral force to the maxilla, this method was known in the late 1800s, but was abandoned as unnecessary and po-tentially damaging. After demonstration of its potential in experimental animals, the method was reintroduced in the United States in the early 1960s[14] and has been widely used since.

The age of the patient definitely is a factor in obtaining separation of the suture. Growth in width of the jaws and face is completed before anteroposterior and vertical growth, and usually is complete at about the time of the adolescent growth spurt. Like all craniofacial sutures, the mid-palatal suture becomes more tortuous and interdigitated with increasing age (see Figure 9-17). Almost any expansion device (a lingual arch, for example) will tend to separate the mid-palatal suture in addition to moving the molar teeth in a child up to age nine or ten. By adolescence, relatively heavy force from a rigid jackscrew device is needed to separate the partially interlocked suture. After adolescence, there is an increasing chance with advancing age that bone spicules will have interlocked the suture to such an extent that skeletal expansion becomes impossible. Opening the suture for patients in their twenties is unlikely but not impossible.[15]

Expansion across the suture can be done in two ways: (1) rapid expansion, the original (1960s) method; and (2) slow expansion at the rate of approximately 1 mm per week, the method advocated more recently. With both methods, the teeth are used as points of attachment. When force is applied across the maxillary dental arch, some tooth movement occurs but the two halves of the maxilla separate, widening the mid-palatal suture and leading to bone apposition. Compensatory adjustments also occur at the lateral maxillary and frontonasal sutures. It is important to realize that heavy force and rapid expansion should not be used in preschool children because of the risk of producing undesirable changes in the nose at that age (Figure 8-15).

One goal of growth modification always is to maximize the skeletal changes and minimize the dental changes produced by treatment. The object of maxillary expansion is to widen the maxilla, not just expand the dental arch by moving the teeth relative to the bone. Originally, rapid expansion at the mid-palatal suture was recommended to help meet this goal. The theory was that with rapid force application to the posterior teeth, there would not be enough time for tooth movement, the force would be transferred to the suture, and the suture would open up while the teeth moved only minimally relative to their supporting bone. Typically, rapid palatal expansion (RPE) is done with a jackscrew that is activated at 0.5 to 1 mm per day. Although force levels can build up to 10 to 20 pounds as the jackscrew is turned at that rate,[16] the patient rarely experiences pain. Occlusal radiographs make it clear that the mid-palatal suture does open, and the expansion is obvious clinically because a diastema appears between the maxillary central incisors (Figure 8-16). A centimeter or more of expansion is obtained in 2 to 3 weeks, with most of the movement being separation of the two halves of the maxilla.

The space created at the mid-palatal suture is filled initially by tissue fluids and hemorrhage. After completion of

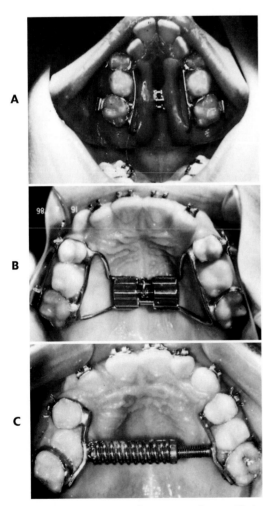

FIGURE 8-14   Transverse force across the maxilla in children and adolescents can open the mid-palatal suture. The expansion force is usually delivered with a jackscrew mechanism fixed to maxillary teeth. **A,** Haas-type expander, with plastic flanges contacting the palatal mucosa; **B,** Hyrax expander, with metal framework and jackscrew; **C,** Minn-expander, which incorporates a spring to smooth the force application.

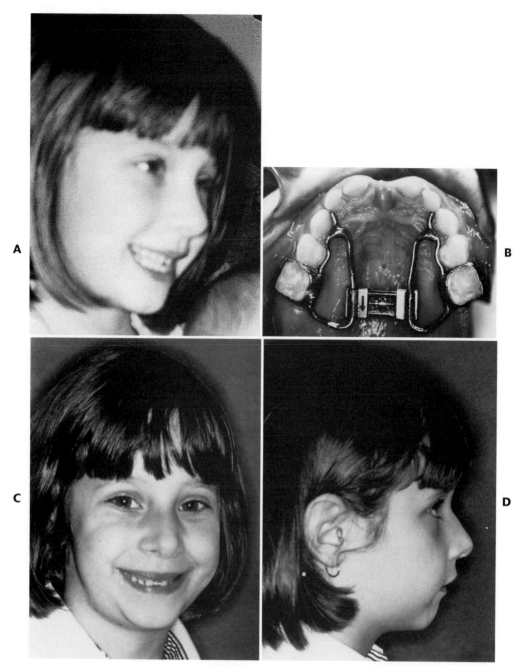

FIGURE 8-15   Rapid palatal expansion in young children can lead to undesirable changes in the nose, as in this 5-year-old who had expansion at the rate of ½ mm/day (2 turns/day of the jackscrew). **A,** Nasal contours before treatment; **B,** jackscrew appliance after activation over a 10-day period; **C,D,** nasal hump and paranasal swelling, which developed after the child complained of discomfort related to the expansion. (Courtesy Dr. D. Patti.)

the expansion, a fixed retainer, usually the expansion device itself stabilized so that it cannot screw itself back shut, is used for 3 to 4 months. By then, new bone has filled in the space at the suture, and the expansion is complete. The midline diastema decreases and may disappear during this time.

The aspect of rapid expansion that was not appreciated initially was that orthodontic tooth movement continues after the expansion is completed, until bone stability is achieved. In most orthodontic treatment, the teeth move relative to a stable bony base. It is possible, of course, for tooth movement to allow bony segments to reposition themselves while the teeth are held in the same relationship to each other, and this is what occurs during the approximately 3 months required for bony fill-in at the suture after rapid expansion. During this time, the dental expansion is maintained, but the two halves of the maxilla move back toward each other, which is possible because at the same time the teeth move laterally on their supporting bone.

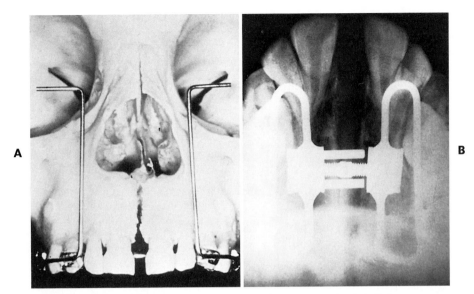

FIGURE 8-16 **A,** Opening of the mid-palatal suture on a dried skull demonstrates the increase in width of the roof of the mouth and the floor of the nose. The maxilla opens as if on a hinge, with its apex at the bridge of the nose. **B,** The suture also opens on a hinge anteroposteriorly, separating more anteriorly than posteriorly, as shown in this radiograph of a patient.

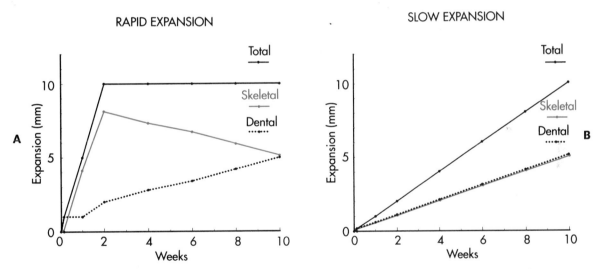

FIGURE 8-17 Diagrammatic representation of the typical skeletal and dental response to rapid (**A**) vs. slow (**B**) palatal expansion. Rapid expansion was recommended when the technique was reintroduced in the 1960s because it was thought that this produced more skeletal than dental change. As the graph indicates, this is true initially—the teeth cannot respond, and the suture is opened. With 10 mm of expansion in 2 weeks, there might be 8 mm of skeletal change and only 2 mm of tooth movement at the time the expansion is completed. It was not appreciated at first that during the next 8 weeks, while bone is filling in, orthodontic tooth movement continues and allows skeletal relapse, so that although the total expansion is maintained, the percentage due to tooth movement increases and the skeletal expansion decreases. With slow expansion at the rate of 1 mm per week, the total expansion is about half skeletal/half dental from the beginning. The outcome of rapid vs. slow expansion looks very different at 2 weeks but quite similar at 10 weeks.

If the changes were represented graphically, the plot would look like Figure 8-17, *A.* Note that when the expansion was completed, 10 mm of total expansion would have been produced by 8 mm of skeletal expansion and only 2 mm of tooth movement. At 4 months, the same 10 mm of dental expansion would still be present, but at that point there would be only 5 mm of skeletal expansion, and tooth movement would account for 5 mm of the total expansion.

If force across the mid-palatal suture is applied more slowly, total force buildup is less. It appears that approximately

1 mm per week is the maximum rate at which the tissues of the midpalatal suture can adapt, so that tissue damage and hemorrhage are minimized. To produce expansion at this rate, 2 to 4 pounds of force appear optimal, depending on the age of the patient.[17] The higher level is needed for older patients. From the beginning, the ratio of dental to skeletal expansion is about 1 to 1, so that 10 mm of expansion over a 10-week period, at the rate of 1 mm per week, would consist of 5 mm of dental and 5 mm of skeletal expansion (Figure 8-17, *B*). A large midline diastema never appears. With expansion at this rate, the situation at the completion of active expansion is approximately analogous to RPE 2 to 3 months after expansion is completed, when bone fill-in has occurred. Thus the overall result of rapid vs. slow expansion is similar, but with slower expansion a more physiologic response is obtained.

Slow expansion can be accomplished either by activating a special spring to give the desired 2 to 4 pounds of force or, more practically, by turning the typical palate separation jackscrew less frequently. Expansion lingual arches that deliver force in the 1 to 2 pound range also open the suture in young children, but in adolescents these appliances produce more dental than skeletal expansion.

Since tooth movement in addition to skeletal expansion is inevitable when the mid-palatal suture is widened, the ideal patient for this treatment should have:

- Full-cusp crossbite with a skeletal component
- Some degree of dental as well as skeletal constriction initially
- No pre-existing dental expansion

If expansion is necessary in a long face-open bite patient, it is advantageous to use a bonded expansion appliance that incorporates bite blocks. This controls the increase in face height that otherwise can be expected.[18]

Following expansion, a retainer is needed even after bone fill-in seems complete. The active expansion appliance will need to be in place for 3 to 4 months, whether the expansion was done rapidly or slowly, and then can be replaced with a removable retainer or other retention device.

Class II Problems

Changing Views of Class II Treatment. In the early years of the 20th century, it was all but taken for granted that pressure against the growing face could change the way it grew. Extraoral force to the maxilla (headgear) was utilized by the pioneer American orthodontists of the late 1800s (Figure 8-18), who found it reasonably effective. This method of treatment was later abandoned, not because it did not work, but because Angle and his contemporaries thought that Class II elastics (from the lower molars to the upper incisors) would cause the mandible to be positioned forward and therefore to grow, and that this would produce an easier and better correction. At a later stage in the United States, guide planes consisting of a wire framework extending down from an upper lingual arch were used to force patients to advance the mandible upon closure, also with the idea of stimulating mandibular growth.[14]

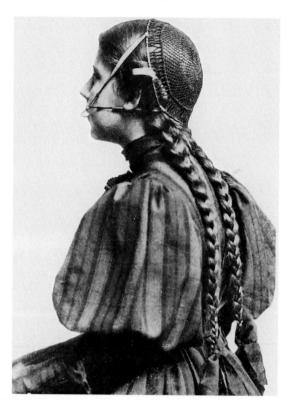

FIGURE 8-18   Extraoral force to the maxilla was used in the late 1800s, then abandoned, not because of ineffectiveness, but because it was thought that intraoral elastics produced the same effect. (From Angle EH: *Treatment of malocclusion of the teeth*, ed 7, Philadelphia, 1907, SS White Manufacturing Co.)

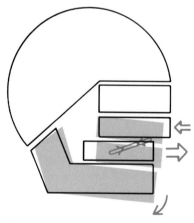

FIGURE 8-19   In a patient who is growing minimally, Class II elastics move the maxillary teeth back somewhat, slip the mandibular teeth forward on the mandibular base, and rotate the occlusal and mandibular planes downward. Stimulation of mandibular growth is not a consistent response.

With the advent of cephalometric analysis, it became clear that both elastics and guide planes corrected Class II malocclusion much more by displacing the mandibular teeth mesially than by stimulating mandibular growth (Figure 8-19). Even if the lack of desired change in jaw relationships is overlooked, correcting a skeletal Class II

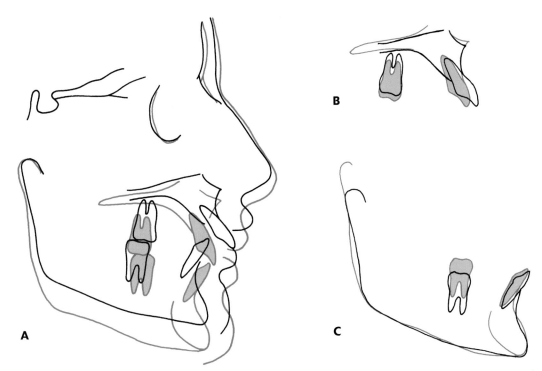

FIGURE 8-20 Cephalometric superimposition showing growth modification produced by extraoral force to the maxilla (straight-pull initially, then high-pull). In the cranial base superimposition (**A**), note that the maxilla has moved downward and backward, not in the downward and forward direction that would have been expected (and that was shown by the mandible). From the maxillary superimposition (**B**) it can be seen that the protruding and spaced upper incisors were retracted, but there was very little posterior movement of the upper molars. In the mandibular superimposition (**C**), note that the lower molars erupted more than the upper molars (i.e., good vertical control of the upper molars was maintained).

problem in this way is undesirable because the resulting mandibular dental protrusion often is unstable. As the protruding lower incisors tend to upright after treatment, lower incisor crowding and overjet return. Because of this, these methods and with them the idea of mandibular growth stimulation fell into disrepute in the United States.

Although headgear was reintroduced in the 1940s and came to be widely used in Class II treatment, it was seen primarily as a tooth-moving device until cephalometric studies in the late 1950s clearly demonstrated not only retraction of upper teeth but also effects on maxillary growth (Figure 8-20).[19] Even then, American orthodontists were slow to accept the idea that mandibular as well as maxillary growth could be manipulated clinically. They recognized that the success of headgear treatment depends on mandibular growth—restraining maxillary growth succeeds in producing a differential in favor of mandibular growth only if the mandible grows spontaneously—but continued to doubt that mandibular growth could be stimulated. As headgear for growth modification became increasingly important, concerns that treated patients might show more downward and less forward mandibular growth (Figure 8-21) led to less use of cervical (neck-strap) force and more use of straight-pull and high-pull devices.

In Europe, efforts to stimulate mandibular growth led to the development of a family of "functional appliances."

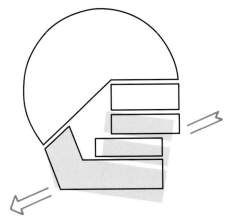

FIGURE 8-21 If extraoral force to the maxilla moves it downward, mandibular growth will be expressed more vertically and less horizontally, impeding the successful correction of a Class II problem. In the extreme case, with minimal mandibular growth, the downward and backward rotation of the mandible can actually cause a worsening of the problem, as in the possible response to low-pull headgear shown diagrammatically here. For this reason, an upward and backward direction of pull is usually needed.

These appliances hold a deficient mandible forward in a position that approximates normal occlusion. Their prototype was Robin's monobloc, first described in 1907, but

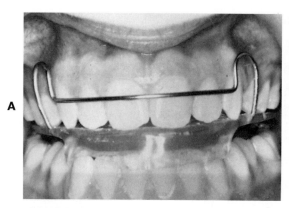
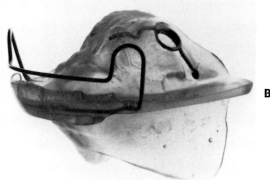

FIGURE 8-22   The activator appliance consists of a single block of plastic, constructed so that the lingual flanges on the lower cause the mandible to be positioned forward. Typically, the mandibular incisor teeth are capped so that forward movement is resisted, while the mandibular posterior teeth are free to erupt. **A,** Appliance in position intraorally; **B,** appliance out of the mouth.

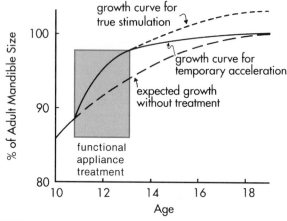

FIGURE 8-23   The difference between growth acceleration in response to a functional appliance and true growth stimulation can be represented using a growth chart. If growth occurs at a faster-than-expected rate while a functional appliance is being worn, and then continues at the expected rate thereafter so that the ultimate size of the jaw is larger, true stimulation has occurred. If faster growth occurs while the appliance is being worn, but slower growth thereafter ultimately brings the patient back to the line of expected growth, there has been an acceleration, not a true stimulation. Although there is a great deal of individual variation, the response to a functional appliance most often is similar to the solid line in this graph.

Andresen's activator of the early 1930s and similar appliances used thereafter in Switzerland and Germany popularized this approach and provided the name (Figure 8-22).[20] The idea was that forcing the patient to function with the lower jaw forward would stimulate mandibular growth and thereby correct the Class II malocclusion. The basic concept was thus quite similar to that of the guide plane. The activator and its successors differed from the fixed guide plane in being removable, but more importantly, they provided a greater area of contact with mandibular teeth and lingual mucosa and thus were more

effective in stimulating the patient to hold the mandible forward constantly. In addition, the plastic framework provided contact with all teeth, giving better resistance to forward displacement of lower incisors and allowing control of eruption. These appliances, which were felt to successfully modify mandibular growth, were the mainstay of European orthodontics in the mid-20th century, at a time when the possibility of changing jaw growth was largely rejected in the United States.

By the 1980s clinical success with functional appliances, including impressive amounts of mandibular growth in some cases, had been clearly demonstrated on both sides of the Atlantic, but questions about whether they could really stimulate mandibular growth continued. Growth stimulation can be defined in two ways: (1) as the attainment of a final size larger than would have occurred without treatment, or (2) as the occurrence of more growth during a given period than would have been expected without treatment. Figure 8-23 is a hypothetical plot of the response to functional appliance treatment, illustrating the difference between (1) absolute stimulation (larger as an adult) and (2) temporal stimulation (acceleration of growth). As the figure suggests, an acceleration of growth often occurs when a functional appliance is used to treat mandibular deficiency,[21] but the final size of the mandible is little if any larger than it would have been without the treatment.[22] Cephalometric superimposition analysis often shows more mandibular growth in the first months that a child wears a well-designed functional appliance than would have been expected (Figure 8-24). This is likely to be followed by a decrease in growth later, so that although the mandible grew faster than normal for a while, later growth was slower than would have been expected and the ultimate size of the mandible in treated and untreated patients is similar.

If that view of their effect on mandibular growth is correct, functional appliances must do something else besides stimulate mandibular growth. Otherwise, the Class II

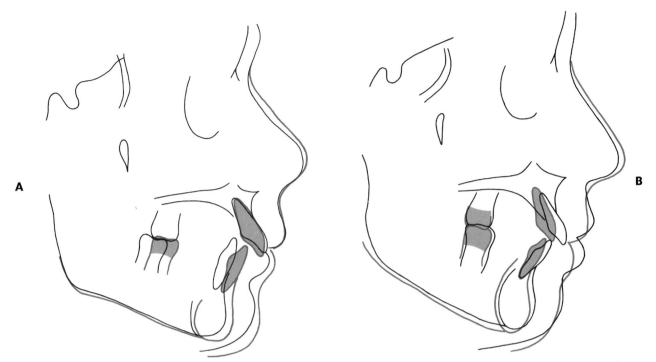

FIGURE 8-24 **A,** Cephalometric superimposition during activator treatment, showing excellent downward and forward mandibular growth between ages 11 and 13; **B,** cephalometric superimpositions for same patient between ages 13 and 15, during fixed appliance therapy for final positioning of teeth. For this patient, the growth response to the activator was much more an acceleration than a true stimulation, as revealed by more growth than expected at first, and less growth later; yet the activator phase of treatment was quite successful in improving the jaw relationship.

malocclusion would never be corrected or would not stay corrected. In fact, these appliances also can affect the maxilla and the teeth in both arches. When the mandible is held forward, the elastic stretch of soft tissues produces a reactive effect on the structures that hold it forward. If the appliance contacts the teeth, this reactive force produces an effect like Class II elastics, moving the lower teeth forward and the upper teeth back, and rotating the occlusal plane (see Figure 8-19). In addition, even if contact with the teeth is minimized, soft tissue elasticity can create a restraining force on forward growth of the maxilla, so that a "headgear effect" is observed (see Figure 8-24). Any combination of these effects can be observed after functional appliance treatment.

By the late1980s, although growth modification possibilities were understood much better than any time previously, it was clear that data were needed to document the chances of success with growth modification and to answer the often-heated question as to which was more effective, headgear or functional appliance. With support from the National Institute of Dental Research, a series of randomized clinical trials of alternative approaches to Class II treatment were carried out in the 1990s. Although all the data from these studies are not yet analyzed and published, the new information has both confirmed some previous concepts and led to revision of others.

The Randomized Clinical Trials of the 1990s. Three major projects using randomized clinical trial methodology were carried out at the University of North Carolina, University of Florida and University of Pennsylvania.[23-28] Although there were differences in the precise goals of these studies and in the procedures, the major objective in each case was to compare the outcome of treatment using either a functional appliance to posture the mandible forward or headgear to restrain maxillary growth, to no treatment. The results provide by far the best data that ever have been available for the response to early Class II treatment.

These data show that, on average, children treated with either headgear or a functional appliance had a small but statistically significant improvement in their jaw relationship, while the untreated children did not. One of the striking findings, however, was the great variation within both the treated and the control groups. Data for cephalometric changes in the UNC trial are shown in Figure 8-2 and in Figure 8-25; the data from the other two studies are similar. Although on average there was no change in the jaw discrepancy of the untreated children, the graphs make it clear that without treatment, some children improved, one or two quite impressively, while an equal number got worse. On average, both the treated groups showed an improvement in jaw relationship. Although the decrease in ANB and related measures was quite similar for headgear

Clinical Trial Phase I Changes
SNA / SNB Relationships

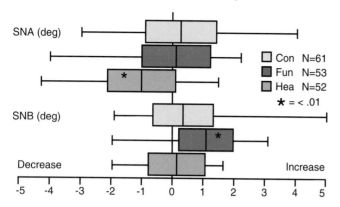

Clinical Trial Phase I Changes
A to N Perp / B to N Perp

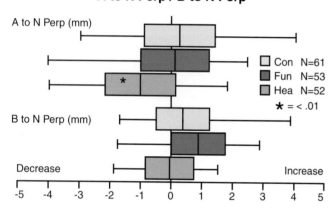

Clinical Trial Phase I Changes
Mx / Md Incisor to N Perp

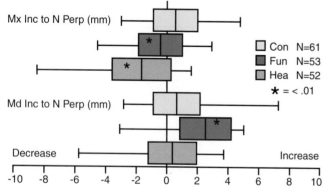

FIGURE 8-25   Changes in the anteroposterior positions of points A and B, and of the maxillary and mandibular incisors, during phase 1 of the UNC clinical trial. Headgear reduced the prominence of point A (maxilla), while functional appliance treatment had a greater effect on point B (mandible), but there was considerable variation in the skeletal growth response among the children in all three groups. Note that both types of treatment tended to reduce the prominence of the upper incisors. Functional treatment tended to bring the lower incisors forward. The wide range of changes in the untreated control group, not surprisingly, was mirrored in the treated children.

and functional appliance, the mechanism by which this occurred usually was different.

In theory, functional appliance therapy should increase mandibular growth, while headgear should primarily restrain maxillary growth. The clinical trial data show that, as a rule, this is what happened. During their preadolescent treatment, on average the children with a functional appliance had a greater increase in mandibular length and a greater increase in the SNB angle than either the controls or the headgear patients. The headgear patients showed greater effects on the maxilla (though the Florida trial did not show statistically significant restraint of maxillary growth with their somewhat unusual protocol for headgear wear).

By no means all the children in the clinical trials responded as might have been expected. The number of children with highly favorable, favorable, zero, and negative growth changes in the UNC study is shown in Figure 8-26. Note that with both headgear and functional appliance treatment, about 75% of the children showed a favorable response, with 25%-30% showing a highly favorable response. In the context of Figure 8-23, there was a 75% chance of mandibular growth acceleration with a functional appliance. The other one-fourth of the children did not respond to treatment.

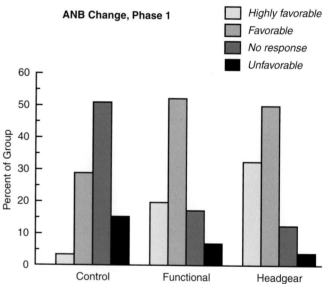

FIGURE 8-26   The percentage of children with highly favorable to unfavorable annualized changes in the ANB angle during phase 1 of the UNC clinical trial. A reduction of 1.5° or more in the ANB angle and a decrease in overjet was considered highly favorable; a decrease in ANB >0.5° was considered favorable; a change in ANB less than ±0.5° was considered no response; and an increase in ANB >0.5° or an increase in overjet was considered unfavorable. Note that two children (3.8%) in the control group had a highly favorable response, while 15% got worse. In the functional group 20% had a highly favorable response, and in the headgear group 30%. In both treated groups 75%-80% responded favorably to treatment. Cooperation undoubtedly was a factor in the failure of the others to respond but is not a total explanation.

Why did some children respond well while others did not? And why did some children improve even without treatment while others got worse? The second question is easier to answer than the first—some of the untreated children simply had a favorable growth pattern, while others did not—but the answer sheds some light on the variation in response of the treated children as well. The better a child cooperates with treatment by wearing the appliance as prescribed, the better the result should be and vice versa. There is no doubt that cooperation is an important factor in establishing the results of treatment. But the clinical trials strongly suggest that cooperation alone does not explain the variability in outcomes. It seems likely that the most favorable responses to treatment are achieved in children who tend to be growing favorably anyway, and that some unfortunate children who grow unfavorably do not respond well even though they were reasonably cooperative.

It is interesting that psychologic testing showed no differences between the children who were treated in the mixed dentition and those who were not. The psychosocial impact of malocclusion seems to become important as sexual development and awareness occur during puberty. There also are no differences in periodontal status between children who received early treatment and those who did not. The chance of trauma to incisors decreases in the treated children, perhaps because of the reduction in overjet.

If the first question about growth modification treatment is, "Does it really modify growth?", the answer now can be, "Yes, though not always or to a large extent." The second question then must be, "Does early treatment really make any difference in the long run, compared with treatment during adolescence?" After two years of treatment, the Florida trial followed their subjects for six months of "retention," with the headgear or functional appliance worn only at night, and for another six months without any treatment. They reported that the skeletal changes produced in the treatment period usually were maintained, while the dental changes relapsed—but the short follow-up time on which this conclusion was based must be noted. The UNC trial was extended into a second phase of treatment for all the children, to compare early two-stage with later one-stage treatment more completely. Both the former controls and the two groups who had preadolescent growth modification treatment received comprehensive fixed appliance orthodontics when their permanent teeth erupted, during adolescence.

These data show that changes in skeletal relationships created during early treatment were likely to be at least partially reversed by later compensatory growth, in both the headgear and functional appliance groups. As Table 8-2 shows, at the end of phase 2, on average, much of the skeletal difference between the former controls and the early treatment groups had been lost. PAR scores, which reflect the alignment and occlusion of the teeth, also were not different at the end of phase 2 between the children who had early treatment and those who did not (Table 8-3).

One advantage of early treatment might be a reduction in the number of patients requiring premolar extraction or orthognathic surgery. In theory, if growth modification were successful, fewer extractions for camouflage of the underlying skeletal Class II relationship would be needed and fewer patients would need surgery to improve the jaw relationship. In the UNC clinical trial, the number of control and headgear patients requiring extractions or surgery during phase 2 were quite similar (Table 8-4). Functional appliance treatment appeared to increase rather than decrease the need for extractions. Although surgery was discussed more often with the control than the early treatment patients, it was not performed more often (Table 8-5).

TABLE 8-3 *Class II RCT: PAR Scores*

	Control n=36	Functional Appliance n=35	Headgear n=35
Change during treatment: median (range)			
Visit 1	31	27	31
Initial	(22-49)	(14-51)	(18-47)
Visit 2	34	24	28
End Ph 1	(19-49)	(1-44)	(5-49)
Visit 4	5.5	6	4
End Ph 2	(0-31)	(1-27)	(0-22)
Distribution end phase 2: number of patients			
5 or less	18	16	20
Ideal			
6-10	7	11	7
Good			
10 or more	11	8	8
Fair			

TABLE 8-4 *Class II RCT: Extractions by Doctor and Group*

	Total treated	Number of extractions			Total extracted
		Control	Bionator	Headgear	
Dr. P	40	3	3	2	8 (20%)
Dr. T	40	3	6	4	13 (32%)
Dr. B	35	3	3	1	7 (20%)
Dr. S	32	0	2	0	2 (5%)
Total	147	9 (17%)	14 (31%)	7 (14%)	30 (20%)

TABLE 8-5 *Class II RCT: Phase 2 Surgery*

	Total	Control	Bionator	Headgear
Started Phase 2	147	52	45	50
Surgery Completed	6 4.1%	3 5.8%	0	3 6.0%
Undecided re: surg	7 4.8%	4 7.7%	1 2.2%	2 4.0%
Total Percent	8.8%	13.5%	2.2%	10.0%

From these studies, what can be concluded about the success of attempts to modify growth in Class II children and the benefits of early treatment for Class II problems? It appears that:

- Skeletal changes are likely to be produced but tend to be diminished or eliminated by subsequent growth
- Alignment and occlusion are very similar in children who did not have early treatment and those who did,

and the percentage of children with excellent, good, and less favorable outcomes also is very similar

- The chances of trauma to protruding upper incisors are decreased by early treatment (a statistically significant difference in the UNC study)
- Signs of TMD are reduced by early treatment (a significant difference in the Florida study but based on relatively short follow-up)

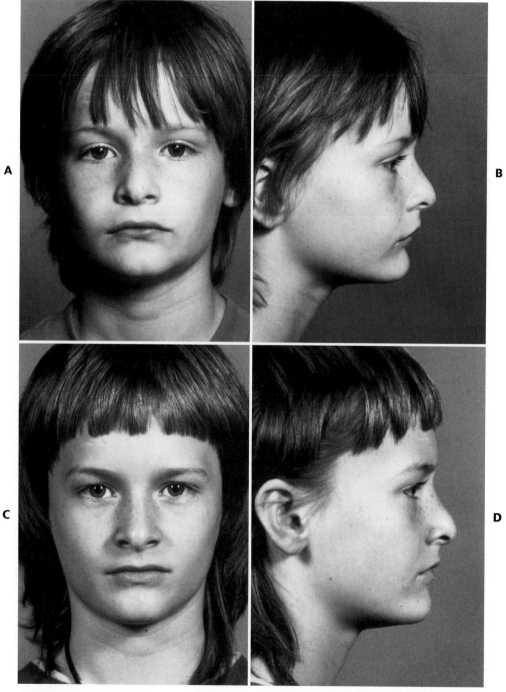

FIGURE 8-27   Facial changes produced by functional appliance treatment in a boy with a short face, skeletal deep bite malocclusion. **A,B,** Age 10 prior to treatment; **C,D,** age 12 after 26 months of treatment. Note the increase in anterior face height and decrease in the labiomental fold.

Based on these results, it seems likely that enthusiasm will diminish for two-phase treatment of Class II problems. The likely outcome will be a better definition of the circumstances in which a first phase of growth modification treatment is most useful, and clearer indications for specific procedures. Perhaps two-phase treatment will be seen to be indicated only for children with esthetic complaints or a propensity for traumatic injury (which would tend to be those with the more severe skeletal problems), and perhaps when it is used in the future, the optimum timing can be better defined. Chapter 15 focuses on the various methods for growth modification and attempts to put them in the perspective of the current studies.

There is a major interaction between the vertical and horizontal anteroposterior characteristics of malocclusion. Although the existing data do not provide clear-cut comparisons of the sort derived from clinical trials, it seems likely that the approach to growth modification should be different in children with short, normal, and long faces. Because children with vertical skeletal deviations of any severity were screened out of the recent clinical trial groups, the quality of the existing data for control of vertical growth problems is less than one would wish. The recommendations that follow for treatment of Class II children with varying face heights are based on our review of what is known at present.

Short Face (Skeletal Deep Bite) Class II. For any child with a skeletal Class II problem, the objective of treatment is to obtain differential growth of the jaws, so that the mandible catches up with the maxilla and the skeletal problem improves or disappears. The additional goals for a short face, deep bite child are, as the child grows, to:

- block eruption of the incisor teeth
- control eruption of the upper posterior teeth
- facilitate eruption of the lower posterior teeth

The goal is to increase face height and correct the deep bite, while allowing more eruption of the lower than the upper teeth so that the occlusal plane rotates up posteriorly, in the direction that facilitates Class II correction (see Chapter 15 for a more complete explanation of how occlusal plane rotation can facilitate or impede the desired occlusal changes).

This pattern of change is produced most effectively with a functional appliance. Although cervical headgear tends to open the bite anteriorly and therefore would help to correct a deep bite problem, it differentially erupts the upper rather than the lower molars and does not produce the desired change in orientation of the occlusal plane. Functional appliances of the activator-bionator type are particularly useful in patients of this type (Figures 8-27 and 8-28), but other types of functionals also can be employed. Because fixed functionals of the Herbst type tend to depress upper molars, usually they are not recommended for short face patients.

Class II Children with Normal Face Height. The clinical trial data make it clear that Class II children with normal face height (many of whom have anterior deep bite because of excessive eruption of lower incisors) can be treated with approximately equal success with two-stage treatment using either headgear or a functional appliance in stage 1, or with one-stage treatment during early adolescence. Retrospective data indicate that for children with normal face height, functional appliances and cervical

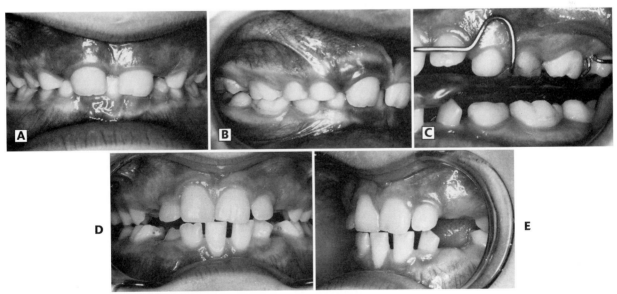

FIGURE 8-28 Dental changes, (same patient as Figure 8-27). **A,B,** Prior to treatment. Note the gingival inflammation around the maxillary right central incisor resulting from palatal trauma from the deep bite. **C,** Deep bite bionator, constructed to allow eruption of lower posterior teeth and block eruption of incisors and upper posterior teeth. **D,E,** Dental relationships at the conclusion of phase 1 treatment, age 12. A second stage of treatment will be needed when the remaining succedaneous teeth erupt.

headgear produce nearly identical vertical changes and growth increments,[29] so the type of headgear also may not be a critical variable in the skeletal response, but if molars are moved distally and extruded, the mandibular plane angle tends to increase.[30]

Within the normal face height group, if the decision is to proceed with mixed dentition treatment rather than wait, current data do not provide solid indications for one treatment approach over another. The current guidelines can be summarized as:

- Either headgear or almost any type of functional appliance is acceptable
- Straight-pull or high-pull headgear is preferred over cervical headgear, to reduce elongation of maxillary molars and better control the inclination of the mandibular plane
- Functional appliance types that minimize tooth movement are preferred, to obtain maximal skeletal effects and minimize compensatory tooth movement

Further comments and recommendations about the advantages and disadvantages of various types of fixed and removable functional appliances, and suggestions for effective use of headgear, are provided in Chapter 15.

Long Face (Skeletal Open Bite) Class II.   Skeletal open bite is characterized by excessive anterior face height. The major diagnostic criteria, either or both of which may be present (see Chapter 6), are a short mandibular ramus and a rotation of the palatal plane down posteriorly. The typical growth pattern shows vertical growth of the maxilla, often more posteriorly than anteriorly, coupled with downward-backward rotation of the mandible and excessive eruption of maxillary and mandibular teeth (Fig-

ure 8-29). Only two-thirds of this patient group actually have an open bite—in the others excessive eruption of incisors keeps the bite closed—but rotation of the mandible produces Class II malocclusion even if the mandible is normal size and severe Class II if the mandible is small.

It follows logically from the description that the keys to successful growth modification would be restraining vertical development and encouraging anteroposterior mandibular growth, while controlling the eruption of teeth in both jaws. Of the several strategies available (Box 8-2), high pull headgear to the maxillary first molars is the least effective because it does not control the eruption of other teeth. High-pull headgear to a maxillary splint is better[31] but still does not control the eruption of the lower teeth, and if they can continue to erupt, face height can continue to increase. Eruption of lower teeth is controlled most readily with interocclusal bite blocks, which are easily incorporated into a functional appliance that also postures the mandible forward (Figure 8-30). If the bite block separates the teeth more than the freeway space, force is created against both upper and lower teeth that opposes eruption. Vertically-directed extraoral force to the functional appliance gives better control of maxillary growth (Figure 8-31), so the most effective treatment is a combination of a functional appliance with bite blocks and high-pull headgear.[32]

BOX 8-2

HIERARCHY OF EFFECTIVENESS IN LONG-FACE CLASS II TREATMENT

HP headgear to functional with bite blocks
|
Bite blocks on functional appliance
|
High-pull headgear to maxillary splint
|
High-pull headgear to molars

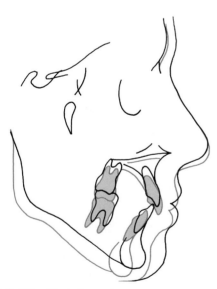

FIGURE 8-29   Cephalometric superimposition for a patient who experienced significant vertical maxillary growth after the completion of orthodontic treatment, without equivalent mandibular growth so that the mandible rotated downward and backward. *Black* = age 14; *red* = age 19. The effect was to produce Class II malocclusion by rotating the mandible down and back.

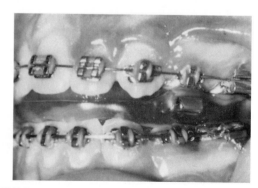

FIGURE 8-30   Functional appliance with bite blocks between the teeth, being used in this case with high-pull headgear in a long-face patient who also required premolar extractions and fixed-appliance treatment.

As with all treatment of this type, cooperation is important. It is asking more of a child to wear both a functional appliance and a headgear than to wear either alone. For treatment planning purposes, it is wise to keep in mind the prognosis is not as good as with less complex problems, even in a cooperative child. This type of treatment is discussed in some detail in Chapter 15.

In an older patient whose face height exceeds acceptable adult dimensions, it is not enough to prevent further eruption of posterior teeth; intrusion is needed. Bite blocks produce a light-force intrusive force by stretching the soft tissues, and some intrusion can result but not enough for successful treatment in most instances. It is tempting to think that more force would be better, and some clinicians have advocated the use of magnets in upper and lower splints oriented so that the magnets repel each other as the splints come together (Figure 8-32). There are both theoretical and practical problems with

this approach.[33] Successful intrusion requires very light prolonged force (see Chapter 10), so it is questionable whether more force should be better. The size of the magnets makes the splints hard to wear and tends to induce poor cooperation. The available evidence suggests that, although intrusion is observed in some patients, the effect of magnets is not greater than could be achieved with bite blocks alone. Most older long-face patients will need orthognathic surgery.

The long face patient described as "Class III rotated to Class I" is a particularly difficult problem, and the one who is still Class III although the mandible is rotated even worse. Any treatment that decreases the excess face height tends to make the Class III condition worse by rotating the mandible upward and forward. Conversely, almost all therapy to control Class III growth tends to increase face height. It is not surprising that most of these patients eventually require orthognathic surgery.

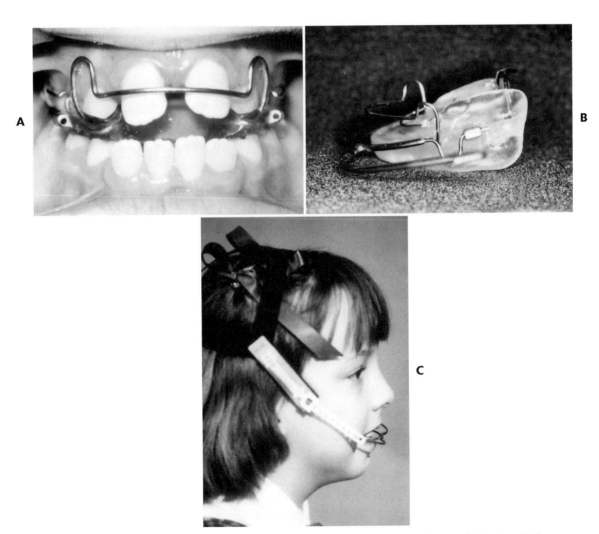

FIGURE 8-31   **A,** Functional appliance with bite blocks and tubes for attachment of a facebow; **B,** facebow inserted into tubes, with the appliance outside the mouth; **C,** patient with high-pull headgear attached to the functional appliance. Note the short outer bow on the facebow, so that the line of force is directed through the point of attachment.

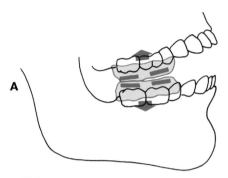
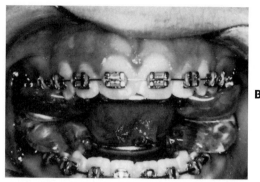

FIGURE 8-32   Magnetic splints for intrusion of posterior teeth. **A,** Diagrammatic representation of maxillary and mandibular splints containing two magnets in each splint on each side; **B,** clinical photograph of splints of this design.

Class III Problems

Growth modification for Class III problems is just the reverse of Class II: what is needed is differential growth of the maxilla relative to the mandible. Edward Angle's concept was that Class III malocclusion was due exclusively to excessive mandibular growth. In fact, almost any combination of deficient maxillary growth and excessive mandibular growth can be found in Class III patients, and maxillary deficiency and mandibular excess are about equally likely. The realization that maxillary deficiency is so frequently a component of skeletal Class III, and new possibilities for correcting it, have led recently to a great increase in treatment aimed at promoting maxillary growth. Unfortunately, data from randomized clinical trials are not available, and treatment recommendations must be based on reports from small and often poorly controlled studies.

Horizontal-vertical Maxillary Deficiency.   If headgear force compressing the maxillary sutures can inhibit forward growth of the maxilla, reverse (forward-pull) headgear separating the sutures should stimulate growth (Figure 8-33). The response of the midpalatal suture to expansion confirms that bone formation at the sutures can be induced. Until recently, however, efforts to stimulate maxillary growth in the anteroposterior and vertical planes of space were impressive mainly for their lack of success. The usual effect of reverse headgear was forward movement of maxillary teeth, with little or no skeletal effect on the maxilla, along with downward and backward rotation of the mandible. In the late 1970s, Delaire and coworkers in France showed that forward positioning of the skeletal maxilla could be achieved with reverse headgear, *if* treatment was begun at an early age.[34] The French results suggested that successful forward repositioning of the maxilla can be accomplished before age 8, but after that orthodontic tooth movement usually overwhelms skeletal change. Subsequent clinical experience suggests that skeletal change can be produced in older children, perhaps up to adolescence.[35] The best data, however, indicate that an increase in maxillary growth only occurs in young patients (below age 10).[36] For this reason, a child with maxillary de-

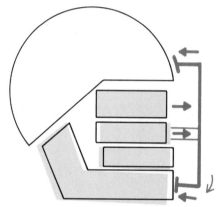

FIGURE 8-33   Forward traction against the maxilla typically has three effects: (1) some forward movement of the maxilla, the amount depending to a large extent on the patient's age; (2) forward movement of the maxillary teeth relative to the maxilla; and (3) downward and backward rotation of the mandible because of the reciprocal force placed against the chin.

ficiency should be referred for complete evaluation as early as possible. The chance of successful forward movement is essentially zero by the time sexual maturity is achieved.

Even in young patients, two side effects of treatment are almost inevitable when reverse headgear is used (see Figure 8-33): forward movement of maxillary teeth relative to the maxilla and downward and backward rotation of the mandible. For this reason, in addition to being preadolescent, the ideal patients for treatment with this method would have both:

- Normally positioned or retrusive, but not protrusive, maxillary teeth
- Normal or short, but not long, anterior facial vertical dimensions

The Delaire face mask design (Figure 8-34) is best described as "deceptively simple," in that it is remarkably unobtrusive and consequently is well accepted by children, who will wear it about as well as the standard headgear. The attachment is to a maxillary splint incorporating all the teeth. This can be removable, if enough retention can be gained, or bonded. If a three-dimensional deficiency exists,

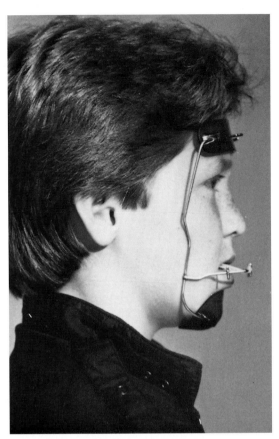

FIGURE 8-34 Delaire-type facemask or reverse headgear used to place forward traction against the maxilla.

so that the maxilla is narrow as well as deficient anteroposterior and vertically, slow expansion can be done simultaneously with protraction. A banded or bonded expansion appliance provides a convenient attachment for the face mask. It is doubtful, however, that the expansion itself offers any net gain in forward movement of the maxilla.

Mandibular Excess. Extraoral force applied via a chin cup (Figure 8-35) is not completely analogous to the use of extraoral force against the maxilla because there are no sutures to influence. If the cartilage of the mandibular condyle were a growth center with the capacity to grow independently, one would not expect chin cup therapy to be particularly successful. From the opposite and more contemporary view that condylar growth is largely a response to translation as surrounding tissues grow, a more optimistic view of the possibilities for growth restraint would be warranted. Research in recent years (see Chapter 2) indicates that the second view of mandibular growth is more correct. Nevertheless, results from chin cup therapy are usually discouraging.

There are two major ways to direct force against the mandible (Figure 8-36). The first is to apply it on a line directly through the mandibular condyle, with the intent of impeding mandibular growth in exactly the same way that extraoral force against the maxilla impedes its growth. This works in experimental animals,[37] but in humans the changes are considerably less impressive. Perhaps the difficulty can be attributed to the nature of the temporomandibular joint, which makes it difficult to create a

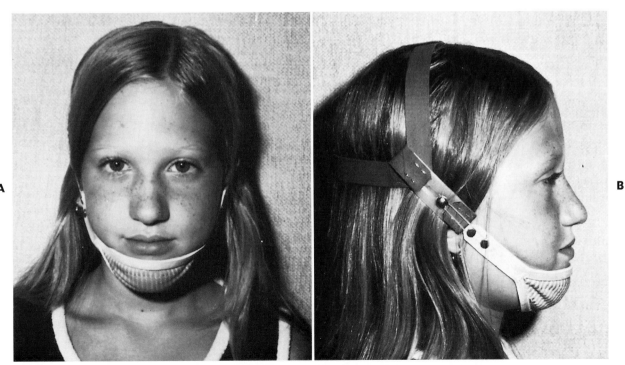

FIGURE 8-35 Chin cup appliance with a soft cup in clinical use. **A,** Anterior view; **B,** lateral view. Note that the force direction is slightly below the head of the condyle.

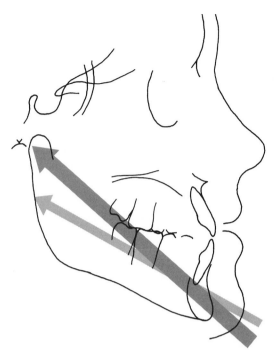

FIGURE 8-36 There are two main approaches to chin cup therapy, as shown diagrammatically here: heavy force aimed directly at the condylar area, or lighter force aimed below the condyle to produce downward rotation of the mandible.

restraining force against the condyle, or it may reflect a more fundamental difference between maxillary and mandibular growth (see Chapter 9).

A second approach to chin cup therapy is to orient the line of force application below the mandibular condyle, so that the chin is deliberately rotated downward and backward. Less force is applied than when direct growth restriction is the objective. In essence, an increase in facial height is traded for a decrease in the prominence of the chin. This can be quite effective within the limits established by excessive face height. Obviously, it would work best in individuals who had short facial vertical dimensions initially (Figure 8-37).

When extraoral force is applied against the chin, it is difficult to avoid tipping the lower incisors lingually. An elastic type of chin cup (the sort worn by football players, adapted for orthodontic use) transfers a significant amount of force to the base of the alveolar process and causes uprighting of the lower incisors. Even when a more rigid chin cup is used, a component of dental displacement in addition to the desired skeletal change is usually observed.[35] If the mandibular dentition was protrusive initially, of course, uprighting of the incisors is desirable. In most cases, however, the incisor uprighting is an undesirable side effect and can cause crowding.

Functional appliances for mandibular prognathism work in exactly the same way as the second approach to chin cup therapy: they rotate the mandible downward and backward. The construction bite for Class III functional

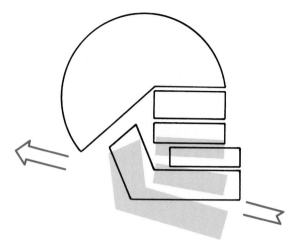

FIGURE 8-37 Diagrammatic representation of a typical response to chin cup therapy, showing the downward and backward rotation of the mandible accompanied by an increase in facial height.

appliances is based on opening the mandible on a hinge, creating additional vertical space into which eruption of the teeth is guided. Just the reverse of the eruption pattern in Class II treatment is desired: the upper molars should erupt more than the lower. Although there are several types of Class III functional appliances, none of these create any direct force to restrain the mandible.

The ideal patient for chin cup or functional appliance treatment of excessive mandibular growth has:
- A mild skeletal problem, with the ability to bring the incisors end-to-end or nearly so
- Short vertical face height
- Normally positioned or protrusive, but not retrusive, lower incisors

It is possible to combine maxillary protraction and chin cup force against the mandible, which accentuates downward-backward rotation of the mandible,[38] but patients with severe Class III problems, especially those with mandibular prognathism, will eventually require surgical correction (see Chapter 22). Modification of excessive mandibular growth can be successful only within narrow limits, whatever the appliance system. Maxillary deficiency is somewhat more treatable, but bringing the maxilla forward more than a few millimeters is unlikely. As a guideline, more than 4 mm reverse overjet in a preadolescent child indicates that surgery eventually will be needed.

CLASS II PROBLEMS IN ADOLESCENTS

The goal of treatment for Class II problems in adolescents (in addition to correcting any other problems that are present) is to establish the correct overjet and buccal segment occlusion. Exactly how this was expected to occur has been viewed differently at different times. Edward Angle was confident that if Class II elastics were used, differential

"Pitchfork" Analysis

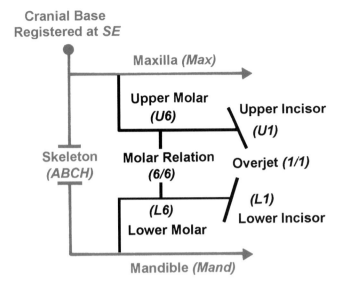

$$Max + Mand = ABCH$$
$$ABCH + U6 + L6 = 6/6$$
$$ABCH + U1 + L1 = 1/1$$

FIGURE 8-38 The "pitchfork analysis," which projects changes related to Class II correction to the occlusal plane, is a convenient way to show how dental and skeletal changes in both arches sum to produce the total change in occlusal relationships. As one might expect, a mix of dental and skeletal changes occur during treatment of almost any type, but apparently similar total changes can be produced in a variety of ways. (Redrawn from Johnston LE, *Brit J Orthod* 23:93, 1996.)

growth of the mandible would produce most if not all the correction. When early cephalometric data showed that this rarely occurred and that most of the correction was produced by tooth movement, skeletal changes were discounted and it was expected that most of the correction would have to be produced by moving the teeth. More recently, the demonstration of growth modification by headgear and functional appliances led to renewed optimism about growth in adolescents contributing to the correction. The questions now are whether enough growth to make a difference can be expected in this age group and what mix of treatment responses can be expected.

There are no data from clinical trials of adolescent Class II treatment. The outcomes of treatment with different methods, however, have been evaluated by many investigators, so that a reasonable body of data exists for comparison of alternatives. Lysle Johnston has proposed a method of cephalometric analysis designed to specifically address the question of exactly what does happen in Class II treatment.[39] His "pitchfork analysis" (Figure 8-38) sums the skeletal and dental components of Class II correction along the occlusal plane so that it is easy to see how the end result was obtained. To the extent possible, this thinking is used in the following discussion of the relative merits of various treatment plans for adolescent Class II problems.

There are four major approaches to Class II problems in adolescents: growth modification with headgear or functional appliance and three variations of tooth movement: (1) distal movement of maxillary molars, and eventually the entire upper dental arch, (2) retraction of maxillary incisors into a premolar extraction space, and (3) a combination of retraction of the upper teeth and forward movement of the lower teeth.

Growth Modification in Adolescents

The guiding principle is that growth can only be modified when it is occurring. Because dental and skeletal development are not tightly linked (see Chapter 2), treatment starting with the eruption of the permanent teeth could come almost anywhere from the beginning to the end of the adolescent growth spurt. Obviously, growth modification would be more successful when more growth remains.

As a general guideline, even in the most favorable circumstances it is unlikely that more than half of the changes needed to correct Class II malocclusion in an adolescent would be gained by differential jaw growth (i.e., a 3-4 mm contribution from growth to the total Class II correction would be as much as one could hope for).[40] The more mature the patient, the less growth change should be expected. Both the phase 2 results from the UNC clinical trial and data from retrospective analyses show that favorable growth often occurs in adolescents and that early (preadolescent) treatment is not routinely superior in guiding growth. Because growth can be so unpredictable, often it is necessary to plan adolescent treatment so that the amount of tooth movement can be adjusted in compensation for whatever growth did occur.

An additional factor in the selection of a growth modification appliance comes into play with adolescents, its compatibility with a fixed appliance on the teeth. A complete fixed appliance cannot be used in the mixed dentition, so this does not affect the choice of headgear vs. a functional appliance for early treatment. In adolescents there is no reason to delay aligning the teeth, and a growth modification appliance that makes this difficult or impossible is a disadvantage. Headgear is compatible with fixed appliances but most functional appliances are not. If a functional appliance is desired for adolescent treatment, often a fixed functional that allows brackets on the incisor teeth is the best choice.

To be successful, a functional appliance must displace the condyles (or stimulate the patient to displace them) a critical distance for a critical amount of time. The distance of condylar displacement rarely is considered, simply because almost any functional appliance repositions the condyles enough to be effective if it is worn enough. This becomes important, however, when we examine the growth modification effect of Class II elastics or flexible fixed units (like those in the "Jasper jumper" or similar devices—see Chapter 17). Both elastics and flexible fixed units have little growth effect and mostly move teeth, probably because they do not displace the condyles far enough. Neither elastics nor flexible fixed units should be considered a substitute for headgear or a functional appliance.

Correction by Tooth Movement

Distal Movement of the Upper Teeth.   If the upper molars could be moved posteriorly, this would correct a Class II molar relationship and provide space into which the other maxillary teeth could be retracted. If the maxillary first molars are rotated mesio-lingually, as they often are when a Class II molar relationship exists, correcting the rotation moves the buccal cusps posteriorly and provides at least a small space mesial to the molar (Figure 8-39). Tipping the crowns distally to gain space is more difficult, and bodily distal movement is more difficult still. The problem is that the second and third molars are in the way, and there is little or no space in the maxillary tuberosity to move all the molars back. Vertical growth helps: it is much easier to tip a molar distally if it can extrude at the same time.

From this perspective it is easy to understand that the most successful way to move a first molar distally is to extract the second molar, which creates space for the tooth movement. In the absence of vertical growth this is the only way to create significant distal movement. Extraction of maxillary second molars and distal movement of the remaining upper teeth can successfully correct moderate Class II malocclusion in mature adolescents with limited growth potential.[41] Even with second molar extraction,

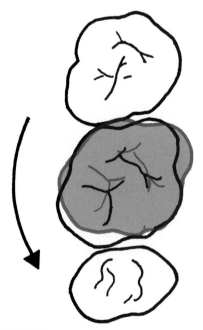

FIGURE 8-39   In a patient with Class II malocclusion, the upper first molar usually is rotated mesio-lingually. Correcting this rotation, which is necessary to obtain proper occlusion with the lower first molar, moves the buccal cusps distally. This improves the buccal occlusal relationship and creates at least a modest amount of space for retraction of other maxillary teeth.

however, one should not expect more than 4 mm distal movement. The ideal patient for this plan, therefore, is one who has less than a full cusp Class II molar relationship. Either extra-oral force or Class II elastics can be used to produce the tooth movement. Each has advantages and disadvantages. Headgear provides heavy intermittent rather than light continuous force and is ineffective unless patients wear it most of the time, but it concentrates the force where it is needed and may contribute to growth modification. It is easier to get patients to wear Class II elastics full-time or nearly so, and the force magnitude is appropriate for tooth movement, but the elastics tend to bring the lower arch forward.

Distal movement of upper molars is difficult when second molars are present. Both molars can be tipped back, especially if they also elongate. Creating the force system is a problem. One possibility is Class II elastics against a maxillary arch arranged so the force is concentrated against the upper first molars (see Chapter 17). This creates some distal movement of the upper teeth, but the molar relationship is corrected mostly by the lower molar coming forward. Palatal anchorage for the molar movement can be created by splinting the maxillary premolars and including an acrylic pad in the splint so that it contacts the palatal mucosa. In theory, the palatal mucosa resists displacement; in clinical use, tissue irritation is likely. Force to move the molars back can be derived from nickel-titanium springs, magnets, or other spring arrangements (Figure 8-40).[42,43] Even with the more elaborate appliances of this type, not more than half the total Class II correction can be expected from distal movement of the molars. Even if they are tipped back further than that initially, they come forward again when the other maxillary teeth are retracted.

Retraction of the Upper Incisors into a Premolar Extraction Space.   A straightforward way to correct excessive overjet is to retract the protruding incisors into space created by extracting the maxillary first premolars. If mandibular first or second premolars also are extracted, Class II elastics can be used to bring the lower molars forward and retract the upper incisors, correcting both the molar relationship and the overjet. Without lower extractions, Class II elastic use would have to be minimal, and extra-oral force might be needed. The patient would have a Class II molar relationship, but normal overjet, at the end of treatment.

It is important to remember that extraction space must be available after the teeth are aligned to be useful for Class II correction. As we have pointed out previously, there are two reasons for extraction: to provide space to align crowded/protrusive incisors or to allow differential anteroposterior movement of the upper and lower teeth. The same extraction space cannot be used for both purposes.

Premolar extraction for Class II correction can produce excellent occlusion, but there are potential problems with this approach. If the patient's Class II malocclusion is primarily due to mandibular deficiency, retracting the maxillary incisors would create a maxillary deformity to go with the mandibular one—which is difficult to justify as correct treatment (see the discussion of Class II camouflage in adults, on p. 281). Extractions in the lower arch allow the molars to come forward into a Class I relationship, but it would be important to close the lower space without retracting the lower incisors. For facial esthetics, usually it is better not to retract upper incisors the entire width of the extraction space, but then the lower arch would have to come forward. If Class II elastics are used, the upper incisors are elongated as well as retracted, which can produce an undesirable "gummy smile."

Combined Retraction of the Upper Teeth and Forward Movement of the Lower Teeth. If some forward movement of the lower arch can be accepted, there would be no need to extract in the lower arch and perhaps no need to extract in the upper arch. Correction could be achieved just with the use of Class II elastics (or their equivalent). It is possible to correct most Class II malocclusions by prolonged use of Class II elastics without extractions. The correction is achieved, however, much more by forward movement of the lower arch than by moving the upper teeth back. Rarely, excess overjet and Class II buccal segments are due to a distally positioned lower arch, and then moving it forward is exactly what is needed. Vertical growth is needed when inter-arch elastics are used, to prevent rotat-

ing the mandible down and back as the lower molars are elongated, and even then, the elastics may produce an unesthetic elongation of the upper incisors.

Almost always, however, moving the lower incisors anteriorly more than 2 mm leads to instability and relapse. Lip pressure that moves the lower incisors lingually leads to incisor crowding, return of overjet, and return of overbite (because the incisors tend to erupt back into occlusal contact from their lingual position). If non-extraction treatment of adolescent Class II problems is accomplished primarily with prolonged use of Class II elastics, the result is likely to be a convex profile with protrusive lower incisors and a prominent lower lip. This is best described as relapse waiting to occur.

Adolescent Class II Treatment: Summary

In the absence of favorable growth, the review above makes it apparent that treating a Class II relationship in adolescents is difficult and that compromises may have to be accepted in order to correct the occlusion. Fortunately, even though growth modification cannot be expected to totally correct an adolescent Class II problem, some forward movement of the mandible relative to the maxilla does contribute to successful treatment of the average patient. Mandibular growth is important even if differential anteroposterior growth does not occur, because vertical growth allows the use of elastics or other extrusive mechanics.

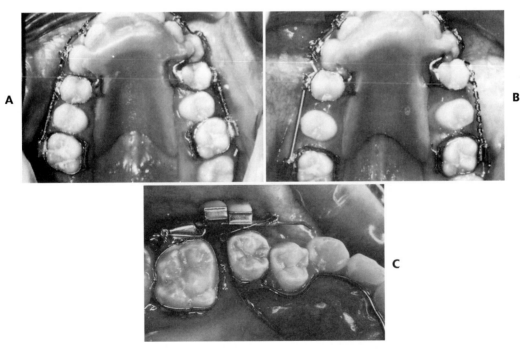

FIGURE 8-40 Distal movement of maxillary molars can be produced during Class II treatment by a variety of methods. The most effective at present are NiTi coil springs (**A, B**), magnets in repulsion (**C**), or an active lingual arch, as in the pendulum appliance (see Figure 17-4). Note that a stabilizing lingual arch with a button against the anterior palate is used for anchorage with all these approaches. The distal movement is primarily tipping, and this type of treatment is most effective when vertical growth allows the molar to extrude as it moves distally. (**A, B,** Courtesy Dr. Anthony Gianelly; **C,** Courtesy Dr. Wick Alexander.)

Only a small amount of net distal movement of upper molars, beyond what is gained by de-rotating them, can be expected unless second molars are extracted. Major retraction of upper incisors requires extraction, and moving the incisors back more than 4 mm requires premolar extraction. Moving the mandibular teeth forward on their base more than 2 mm or so produces an unstable situation that is likely also to be unesthetic. Unless there is some favorable mandibular growth, therefore, premolar extraction appears to be necessary to produce a stable orthodontic correction of many adolescent Class II problems.

Extraction of premolars in adolescent Class II treatment has been criticized in recent years on two grounds: that it leads to TM joint problems because the incisors are likely to be retracted too much and that it compromises facial esthetics.

The relationship, if any, between TM dysfunction and premolar extraction is difficult to assess because data from well-controlled studies are not available. No relationships between symptoms of TMD and the type of orthodontic treatment were noted in any of a considerable series of reports in the early 1990s. The best data come from a study in which a careful compilation of retrospective data was used to create two groups of patients whose "borderline" Class II malocclusions could have been treated equally plausibly with or without premolar extraction. One group had extractions, the other did not. Both groups had low scores for signs or symptoms of dysfunction, and there was no difference between them in any aspect of TM joint function.[44] There is simply no evidence to support the allegation that premolar extraction causes TMD.

The effect of premolar extraction on facial esthetics is even more difficult to assess, because extraction is only one determinant of where the incisors end up. The extraction decision in Class II adolescents often is influenced by the degree of crowding or protrusion, not just by considerations of anteroposterior movement of teeth. For example, a Class II patient with incisor crowding that might not be an indication for extraction in a Class I patient, might need extraction to tolerate even a modest amount of Class II elastics. When discriminant analysis based on consideration of crowding and protrusion was used to create clear-cut extraction and non-extraction groups within a large retrospective sample of adolescent Class II patients, extraction did reduce lip prominence more than non-extraction, but the non-extraction patients had less prominent lips on long-term recall.[45] One cannot automatically assume, therefore, that premolar extraction flattens the profile too much in adolescent Class II patients—but clearly it has the potential to do so, if the incisors are retracted too much.

Because the primary indication for premolar extraction in adolescent Class II patients is a lack of mandibular growth, this leads directly to further consideration of treatment in late adolescence and adult life, when little or no growth can be expected.

SKELETAL PROBLEMS IN OLDER PATIENTS: CAMOUFLAGE VS. SURGERY

Beyond the adolescent growth spurt, even though some facial growth continues, too little remains to correct skeletal problems. The possibilities for treatment, therefore, are either displacement of the teeth relative to their supporting bone, to compensate for the underlying jaw discrepancy, or surgical repositioning of the jaws (Figure 8-41). Displacement of the teeth, as in retraction of protruding incisors, often is termed *camouflage*. The name is well chosen, because the objective of the treatment is to correct the malocclusion while making the underlying skeletal problem less apparent. Because skeletal Class II problems often can be camouflaged rather well, most camouflage treatment is for Class II patients. Class III and long face problems, in contrast, do not camouflage well, in the sense that correcting the occlusion does not conceal the skeletal problem and may make it worse.

Camouflage Treatment

With extraction of teeth to provide space for the necessary tooth movement, often it is possible to obtain correct molar and incisor relationships despite an underlying skeletal Class II or Class III jaw relationship (see Figure 8-41). The method was developed as extraction treatment was reintroduced into orthodontics in the 1930s and 1940s. In that era, it was the major approach to treating skeletal problems. At the time that extraction for camouflage became popular, growth modification as a treatment approach had been largely rejected as ineffective, and surgical techniques to correct skeletal problems had barely begun to be developed. It seemed appropriate, therefore, for the orthodontist to accept the limitations in skeletal relationships and concentrate on the dental occlusion.

Camouflage also implies that repositioning the teeth will have a favorable, or at least not a detrimental, effect on facial esthetics. For patients with mild to moderate skeletal Class II problems, displacement of the teeth relative to their bony bases to achieve good occlusion is compatible with reasonable facial esthetics, and the camouflage can be quite successful (Figure 8-42). In more severe Class II problems, it may be possible to obtain good occlusion only at considerable expense to facial esthetics. If the upper incisors must be displaced far distally to compensate for mandibular deficiency, the esthetic result is increased prominence of the nose and an overall appearance of mid- and lower face deficiency (Figure 8-43).

Camouflage also can be used in patients with mild skeletal Class III problems, in whom adjustment of incisor position can achieve acceptable occlusion and reasonable facial esthetics (Figure 8-44). Unfortunately, in even moderately severe skeletal Class III problems, camouflage is much less successful. Extraction of lower premolars combined with Class III elastics and extraoral force can im-

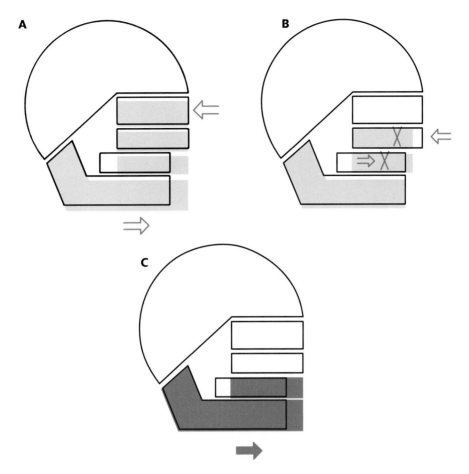

FIGURE 8-41   There are three major possibilities for correction of skeletal mandibular deficiency; **A,** differential growth of the lower jaw, bringing the dentition forward with it; **B,** camouflage, achieved in most cases by extracting premolars and then closing the space by retracting the maxillary anterior teeth while bringing the mandibular posterior teeth forward (at least a small amount of vertical growth is needed because most aspects of the orthodontic mechanotherapy tend to extrude the teeth); **C,** surgical advancement of the mandible. Growth modification is most successful in preadolescent patients; camouflage is most useful for adolescents with moderately severe problems; jaw surgery is most useful for patients with no remaining growth potential and severe problems.

prove the dental occlusion for many Class III patients, but the treatment rarely produces successful camouflage and frequently makes esthetics worse. Even minimal retraction of the lower incisors often magnifies the chin prominence that was a major reason for seeking treatment initially (Figure 8-45).

Because extractions provide space to displace the remaining teeth only in the anteroposterior plane of space, camouflage rarely succeeds with skeletal vertical problems. The force systems used to reposition dental segments tend to extrude posterior teeth and are likely to make both the occlusion and the facial appearance worse.

Camouflage as a treatment plan implies that growth modification to overcome the basic problem is not feasible. Because of the extrusive nature of most orthodontic mechanics, however, it helps to have some vertical growth during treatment to avoid downward and backward rotation of the mandible. For that reason, camouflage works

best in late adolescents who are past the pubertal growth spurt but still have some growth remaining. Although this type of treatment is possible for nongrowing adults, it is more difficult because the potentially extrusive components of any mechanical system must be much more carefully controlled (see Chapter 21).

The characteristics of a patient who would be a good candidate for camouflage treatment are:
- Too old for successful growth modification
- Mild to moderate skeletal Class II or mild skeletal Class III
- Reasonably good alignment of teeth (so that the extraction spaces would be available for controlled anteroposterior displacement and not used to relieve crowding)
- Good vertical facial proportions, neither extreme short face (skeletal deep bite) nor long face (skeletal open bite)

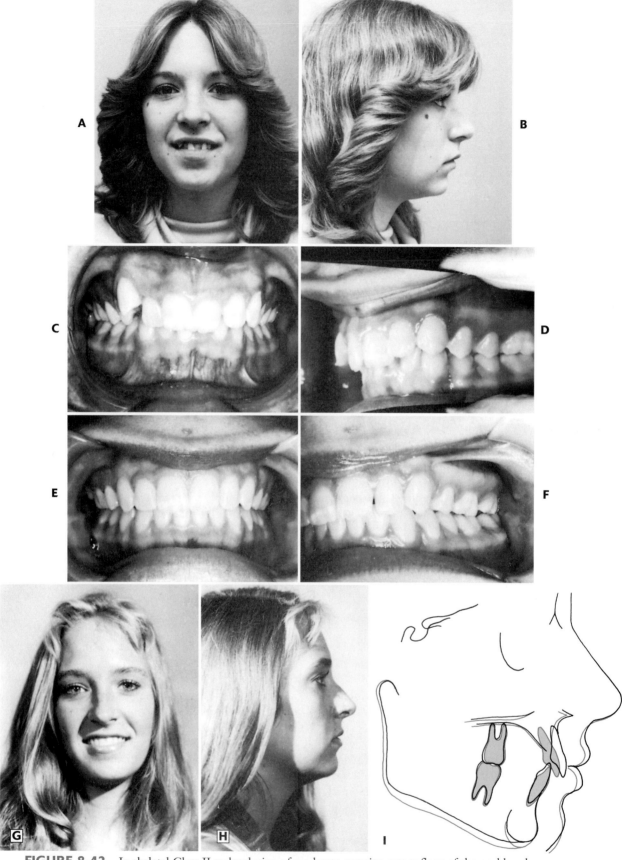

FIGURE 8-42 In skeletal Class II malocclusion of moderate severity, camouflage of the problem by displacement of the incisor teeth can be quite successful, as in this girl who was age 16 at the beginning of treatment. **A** and **B,** Facial appearance before treatment; occlusal relationships before (**C** and **D**) and after (**E** and **F**) treatment with extraction of maxillary first premolars; **G** and **H,** facial appearance at age 18, after treatment; **I,** cephalometric superimposition showing the retraction of the upper incisors.

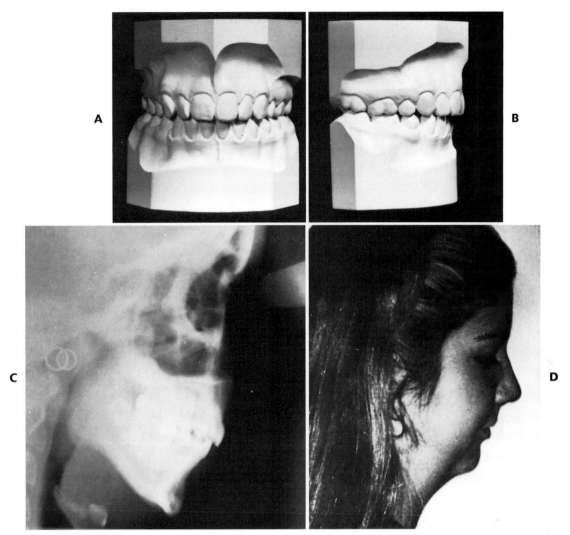

FIGURE 8-43 If mandibular deficiency is severe, orthodontic treatment for Class II malocclusion may result in reasonably satisfactory occlusal relationships but poor facial esthetics (i.e., a failure of camouflage). **A** and **B,** Occlusal relationships after premolar extractions and 4 years of orthodontic treatment; **C** and **D,** profile relationships after treatment. The term *camouflage* is chosen to emphasize that successful treatment must produce acceptable facial esthetics as well as acceptable dental occlusion.

Conversely, camouflage treatment designed to correct the occlusion despite jaw relationship problems should be avoided in:

- Severe Class II, moderate or severe Class III, and vertical skeletal discrepancies
- Patients with severe crowding or protrusion of incisors, in whom the extraction spaces will be required to achieve proper alignment of the incisors
- Patients with excellent remaining growth potential (in whom growth modification treatment should be used) or non-growing adults with more than mild discrepancies (in whom orthognathic surgery usually offers better long-term results)

Surgical Correction

Although surgical procedures to correct mandibular prognathism date back to the beginning of the 20th century, much progress in orthognathic surgery has occurred quite recently, in the 1980s and 1990s. At this point, surgical techniques have been developed that allow severe problems of any type to be corrected. Excellent results require careful coordination of the orthodontic and surgical phases of treatment. The principles of combined surgical and orthodontic treatment are discussed in some detail in Chapter 22.

The characteristics of a patient who would be treated best by surgically repositioning the jaws are:

- Severe skeletal discrepancy or extremely severe dentoalveolar problem
- Adult patient (little if any remaining growth), or younger patient with extremely severe or progressive deformity
- Good general health status (mild, controlled systemic disease acceptable)

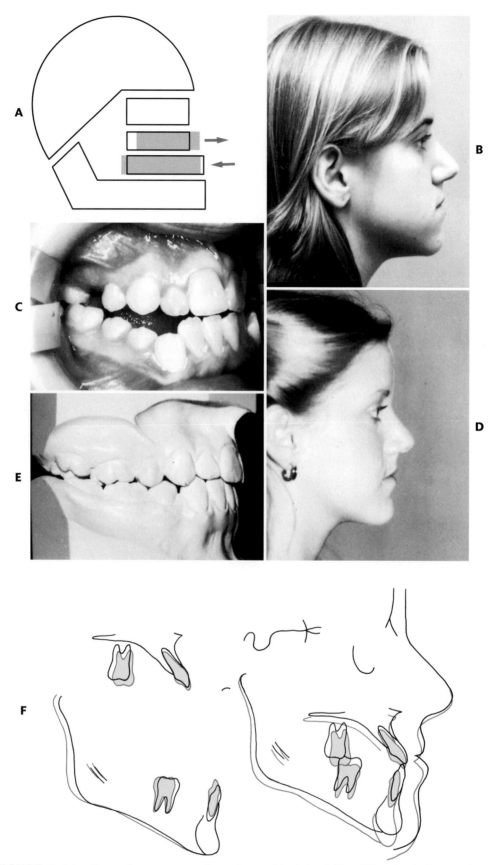

FIGURE 8-44 Camouflage treatment for patients with skeletal Class III malocclusion can be successful if the skeletal discrepancy is mild. **A,** Diagrammatic representation of Class III camouflage with moderate forward movement of maxillary teeth and retraction of mandibular teeth; **B** and **C,** profile and dental relationships in a 14-year-old girl; **D** and **E,** profile and dental relationships at age 16, after treatment with extraction of upper and lower first premolars; **F,** cephalometric superimposition showing changes in treatment. For this patient, as for many Class III patients, downward and backward rotation of the mandible in addition to displacement of the teeth was an important component of the treatment.

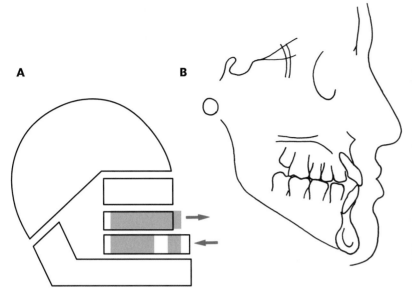

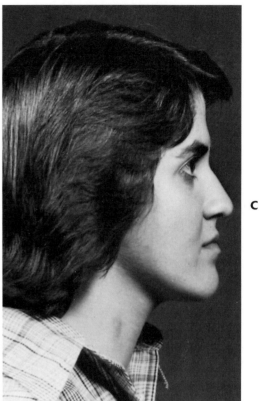

FIGURE 8-45   A, Diagrammatic representation of attempted camouflage for a more severe skeletal Class III problem, showing the obvious chin prominence created by retracting mandibular incisor teeth; **B,** cephalometric tracing, and **C,** profile relationships for a patient after treatment in which lower but not upper premolars were retracted, lower incisors were retracted and upper incisors were tipped forward. She was unhappy with the prominence of her chin and sought further surgical treatment to correct it.

An important principle of treatment planning is that orthodontic camouflage and orthodontic preparation for surgery often require exactly opposite tooth movements. The reason is found in the concept of "dental compensation for skeletal discrepancy." This can occur naturally as well as being created by orthodontic camouflage treatment. In mandibular prognathism, for instance, as the individual grows the upper incisors tend to protrude while the lower incisors incline lingually. By the time growth is completed, the dental discrepancy usually is smaller than the jaw discrepancy. Tooth position has compensated at least partially for the jaw discrepancy. Some degree of dental compensation accompanies most skeletal jaw discrepancies, even without treatment.

If the jaws are to be repositioned surgically, this dental compensation must be removed. Otherwise, when the jaws fit, the teeth will not. Orthodontic preparation for surgery usually involves removing, not creating, dental compensation and therefore is just the opposite of conventional orthodontic treatment. The result is that vigorous orthodontic treatment to correct the malocclusion in a patient with a difficult skeletal problem may eventually make surgical correction all but impossible without another session of orthodontic treatment to undo the original orthodontics. The patient, of course, is not likely to be pleased by this news. It is appropriate to attempt growth modification in younger patients with severe problems. As a general rule, however, an attempt at camouflage in a patient who may well need surgery should be avoided unless a successful outcome can be clearly predicted. Therapeutic diagnosis is a good way to evaluate the response to conservative orthodontic treatment but is not applicable to treatment based on extreme tooth movements for attempted camouflage.

Camouflage vs. Surgery in Postadolescent Class II Patients. The boundary between orthodontic and surgical treatment is particularly troublesome for teenagers with Class II problems. Given the risk of camouflage failure vs. the greater cost and morbidity of orthognathic surgery, what do you do with the rather mature 14 year old with a full cusp Class II malocclusion, 10 mm overjet, and an obvious mandibular deficiency? The choices are maxillary premolar extraction to provide space to retract the upper incisors or surgical mandibular advancement. Although no clinical trial has occurred (and probably never will, given the problems in randomly assigning patients to surgery), some data now are available to more clearly indicate the limits of camouflage and therefore the indications for surgery for postadolescent Class II patients.

In an individual who is past the adolescent growth spurt, the best single indicator of a problem too severe for likely success with camouflage is >10 mm overjet. That is particularly true if the mandible is short, the lower teeth already protrude relative to the mandible so that the chin is well behind the teeth, and/or the face is long (Figure 8-46).[46]

Two other factors to consider in the decision for orthodontics vs. surgery are the possible role of augmentation genioplasty as an adjunct to Class II camouflage and the risk of root resorption with camouflage treatment. A limiting factor in orthodontic Class II treatment is the extent to

ADOLESCENT CLASS II
Indications for Surgery

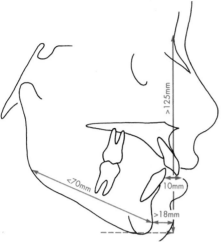

FIGURE 8-46 For adolescent Class II patients, the best indicator of the limits of satisfactory orthodontic correction is the simplest thing one can measure—overjet. More than 10 mm overjet in a patient who is past the peak of the adolescent growth spurt suggests that surgical correction probably would be needed, especially if the lower incisors are protrusive relative to a deficient mandible (Pg-Nperp >18 mm), the mandible is short (mandibular body length < 70 mm), and/or face height is long (> 125 mm). Mandibular body length (GoPg) is a more reliable indicator than total length (CoPg), probably because of the difficulty in accurately locating condylion and variations in chin morphology.

which the lower teeth can be moved forward relative to the mandible. Moving the lower incisors forward more than 2 mm is highly unstable unless they were severely tipped lingually, but this is likely to occur during camouflage treatment when Class II elastics are used unless lower premolars were extracted. Often it is undesirable esthetically to retract the upper incisors to the extent that would be necessary if the lower incisors were not advanced significantly. If orthodontic treatment would otherwise move the lower incisors too far forward for reasonable esthetics or stability, a lower border osteotomy to reposition the chin can both improve facial balance and decrease lip pressure against the lower incisors, improving their stability (Figure 8-47). The lower border osteotomy is no more extensive a surgical procedure than premolar extraction would be, and it can be done as an outpatient or day-op procedure at much less cost than mandibular advancement.

The relationship between root resorption and camouflage treatment also should be kept in mind. A major risk factor for severe resorption of maxillary incisor roots during orthodontic treatment is contact of the roots with the lingual cortical plate (Figure 8-48). The best data (see Chapter 9) suggest that the risk of resorption increases twenty-fold when lingual plate contact occurs. What causes the roots to contact the lingual cortical plate? Two circumstances, primarily: torquing the upper incisors back during Class II camouflage and tipping them facially in Class III

BOX 8-3

SEQUENCE OF TREATMENT IN PATIENTS WITH MULTIPLE PROBLEMS

1. Disease control
   Caries control
   Endodontics
   Initial periodontics (no osseous surgery)
   Initial restorative (no case restoration)
2. Establishment of occlusion
   Orthodontics
   Orthognathic surgery
   Periodontal maintenance
3. Definitive periodontics (including osseous surgery)
4. Definitive restorative
   Cast restorations
   Splints, partial dentures

camouflage (because the roots go lingually as the crowns go facially). Camouflage failure, in both Class II and Class III patients, often is accompanied by incisor root resorption that can complicate surgical retreatment—but fortunately, further orthodontic tooth movement without additional resorption is possible if lingual contact is avoided during retreatment (see Chapter 22).

TREATMENT PLANNING IN SPECIAL CIRCUMSTANCES

Sequence of Treatment for Patients with Multiple Dental Problems

For patients with multiple dental problems including malocclusion, the appropriate sequencing of treatment is important (Box 8-3). Although these patients usually are adults, the principles are the same for adults or children:

- Dental disease should be brought under control initially
- Orthodontic treatment, including skeletal as well as dental changes, should be carried out next
- Definitive restorative and periodontal treatment should be completed after the orthodontic phase of treatment

Control of dental disease includes a number of treatment procedures: tooth extractions if necessary, endodontic treatment if required, periodontal treatment procedures necessary to bring the patient to a point of satisfactory maintenance, and restorative treatment to eliminate the progression of dental caries.

At one time there was concern that endodontically treated teeth could not be moved. It is now clear that as long as the periodontal ligament is normal, endodontically treated teeth respond to orthodontic force in the same way as teeth with vital pulps. Although some investigators have

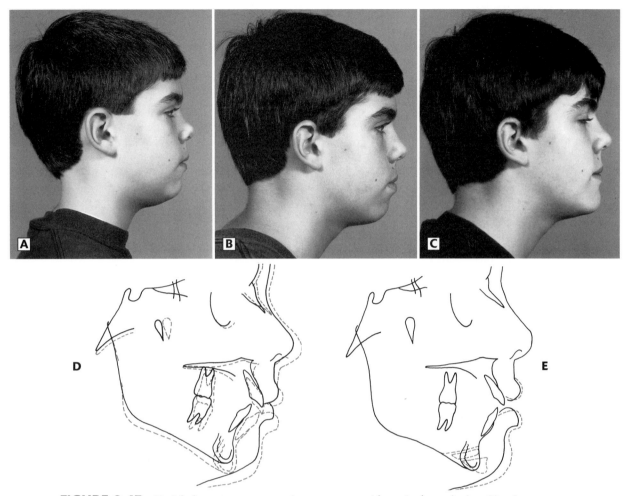

FIGURE 8-47   Facial changes, non-extraction treatment with genioplasty. **A,** Age 13 prior to treatment; **B,** age 15, with protrusion of lower incisors (that would be neither stable nor acceptably esthetic; **C,** age 15, after lower border osteotomy to slide the chin forward; **D,** superimposition of changes during orthodontic treatment. Note the forward movement of the lower incisors in the absence of favorable growth; **E,** superimposition of changes produced by lower border osteotomy and repositioning of the chin. This procedure decreases both lip separation at rest and lip pressure against the lower incisors.

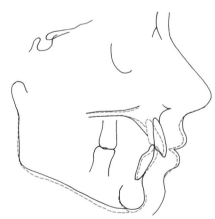

FIGURE 8-48   Contact of the roots of upper incisors with the lingual cortical plate, as in this patient, greatly increases the risk of root resorption during orthodontic treatment. This occurs most frequently when the incisor roots are torqued lingually during Class II camouflage, or when these teeth are tipped facially during Class III camouflage (the root apex moves lingually when the crown is tipped facially).

suggested that root-filled teeth are more subject to root resorption, the current consensus is that this is not a major concern.[47] Occasionally hemisection of a posterior tooth, with removal of one root and endodontic treatment of the remaining root, is desirable. It is perfectly feasible to orthodontically reposition the remaining root of a posterior tooth, should this be necessary, after the endodontics is completed. In general, prior endodontic treatment does not contraindicate orthodontic tooth movement.

Essentially all periodontal treatment procedures may be used in bringing a pre-orthodontic patient to the point of satisfactory maintenance, with the exception of osseous surgery. Scaling, curettage, flap procedures, and gingival grafts should be employed as appropriate before orthodontic treatment, so that progression of periodontal problems during orthodontic treatment can be avoided. Children or adults with mucogingival problems, most commonly a lack of adequate attached gingiva, should have free gingival grafts to create attached gingiva before the beginning of orthodontics. Since research findings indicate that 5% to 10% of children and 20% to 25% of adults who need orthodontic treatment have mucogingival problems,[48] periodontal treatment to deal with this before orthodontic therapy is needed relatively frequently (see Figure 7-25).

Further details in the sequencing of treatment for adults with multiple problems are provided in Chapters 20 and 21.

Patients with Systemic Disease Problems

Patients who are suffering from systemic disease are at greater risk for complications during orthodontic treatment but can have successful orthodontic treatment as long as the systemic problems are under control.[49]

In adults or children, the most common systemic problem that may complicate orthodontic treatment is diabetes or a prediabetic state. The rapid progression of periodontal disease in patients with diabetes is well recognized, and the indication for orthodontic treatment in these individuals is often a series of occlusal problems related to previous periodontal breakdown and loss of teeth.

If the diabetes is under good control, periodontal responses to orthodontic force are essentially normal and successful orthodontic treatment, particularly the adjunctive procedures most often desired for adult diabetics, can be carried out successfully. If the diabetic condition is not under good control, however, there is a real risk of accelerated periodontal breakdown (Figure 8-49). For this reason, careful monitoring of a diabetic patient's compliance with medical therapy is essential during any phase of orthodontic treatment. Prolonged comprehensive orthodontic treatment should be avoided in these patients if at all possible.

Arthritic degeneration may also be a factor in orthodontic planning. Juvenile rheumatoid arthritis frequently produces severe skeletal mandibular deficiency, and adult onset rheumatoid arthritis can destroy the condylar process and create a deformity (Figure 8-50). Long-term administration of steroids as part of the medical treatment may increase the possibility of periodontal problems during orthodontics. In adults, degenerative changes in the temporomandibular joint accompanying osteoarthritis may be related to occlusal problems in some instances, but this is not always or even usually the case. Orthodontic treatment is unlikely to improve degenerative temporomandibular joint problems, but if it is needed for other reasons, it will not accelerate the joint degeneration (see Chapter 21).

Comprehensive orthodontic treatment for children with other systemic diseases is also possible if the disease is controlled, but requires careful judgment about whether the benefit to the patient warrants the orthodontic treatment. It is not uncommon for the parents of a child with a severe systemic problem (e.g., cystic fibrosis) to seek orthodontic consultation in their bid to do everything possible for the unfortunate child. With the increasing long-term survival after childhood leukemia, children with this medical background also are now being seen as potential orthodontic patients. Although treatment for patients with a poor long-term prognosis is technically feasible, it is usually good judgment to limit the scope of treatment plans, accepting some compromise in occlusion to limit treatment time and intensity. Orthodontic tooth movement should be avoided in patients who have received significant radiation to the jaws.

Anomalies and Injuries

Maxillary Injuries.   Fortunately, because they are difficult to manage, injuries to the maxilla in children are rare. If the maxilla is displaced by trauma, it should be repositioned immediately if this is possible. When immediate attention to a displaced maxilla is impossible because of other injuries, protraction force from a face mask before complete healing of fractures has occurred can successfully reposition the jaw.

Asymmetric Mandibular Deficiency.   If the mandibular condyles are affected by either a congenital condition or an injury at birth or later, facial asymmetry is likely to result. Since the appropriate treatment can be quite differ-

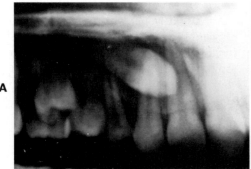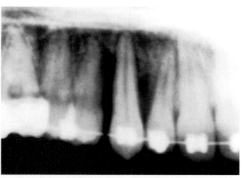

FIGURE 8-49   Patients with uncontrolled diabetes may experience rapid bone loss during orthodontic tooth movement. **A,** Impacted canine in a 13-year-old girl; **B,** 1 year later. Note the extent of bone loss around the tooth as it was being moved. During the year of active treatment, the patient had great difficulty in controlling her diabetes and was hospitalized for related problems on two occasions. (Courtesy Dr. G Jacobs.)

ent if the restriction of mandibular growth is from an injury rather than a congenital anomaly, this is an important diagnostic decision.

In the congenital syndrome of hemifacial microsomia, there is an absence of tissue in the region of the mandibular condyle. In more severe cases, the entire distal portion of the mandible may be missing, along with associated soft tissues (see Chapter 3). In less severe cases, the size of the affected area simply may be diminished, with slower growth on that side and a resulting asymmetry. An apparently similar situation of reduced growth on one side can also result from an injury to the mandibular condyle, and this is the most frequent cause of mandibular asymmetry. In hemifacial microsomia, the problem is a lack of tissue, so growth potential is reduced. In postinjury problems, there is potential for normal growth, but restriction from scarring and fibrosis of the area may prevent expression of this growth.

In planning treatment, it is important to evaluate whether the affected condyle can translate normally. If it can, as one would expect in a mild to moderate form of hemifacial microsomia or post-traumatic injury, a functional appliance could be helpful and should be tried first. If translation of the condyle is severely restricted by posttraumatic scarring, a functional appliance will be ineffective and should not be attempted until the restriction on growth has been removed.

Asymmetry with deficient growth on one side but some translation on the affected side is a particular indication for custom-designed "hybrid" functional appliances (Figure 8-51) because requirements for the deficient side will be different from those for the normal or more normal side. Often it is desirable to incorporate a bite block between the teeth on the normal side while providing space for eruption on the deficient side, so that the vertical component of the asymmetry can be addressed. In the construction bite, the mandible would be advanced more on the deficient side than on the normal side. Further details on fabrication of hybrid functional appliances are presented in Chapter 15.

The restriction of growth that accompanies little or no translation of the condyle often leads to a progressively more severe deformity as growth of other parts of the face continues. Progressive deformity of this type is an indication for early surgical intervention. There is nothing to be gained by waiting for such a deformity to become worse. The goal of surgery is to create an environment in which growth is possible, and orthodontic treatment with a hybrid functional usually is needed after surgery to release ankylosis, to guide the subsequent growth.

Hemimandibular Hypertrophy. Mandibular and facial asymmetry can also be caused by excessive growth of the mandibular condyle on one side. Growth problems of this type are almost never symmetric. They appear to be

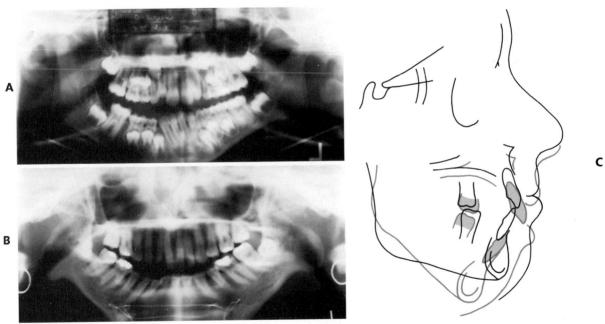

FIGURE 8-50 Rheumatoid arthritis can affect the condylar process and in the worst case can lead to loss of the entire condylar process. **A,** Panoramic radiograph of a child with rheumatoid arthritis. Note the early degenerative changes in the condyle on the left side (compare the left with the as yet unaffected right side); **B,** panoramic radiograph of a young adult with complete destruction of the condylar processes; **C,** cephalometric superimpositions for a patient with severe degeneration of the condylar process of the mandible because of rheumatoid arthritis. Age 18, after uneventful orthodontic treatment (*black*); age 29 (*red*), by which time the condylar processes had been destroyed. Note the downward-backward rotation of the mandible. (**B,** Courtesy Dr. M. Goonewardene; **C,** courtesy Dr. J.R. Greer.)

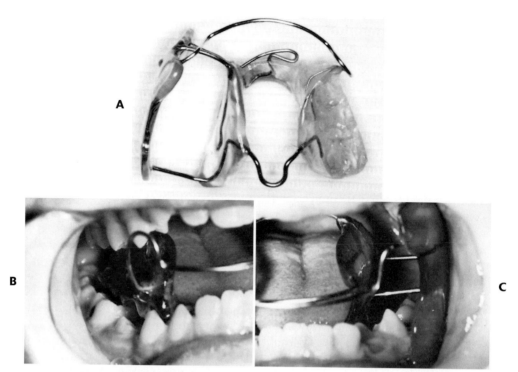

FIGURE 8-51   A "hybrid" functional appliance can be used to correct vertical and transverse jaw asymmetries. **A,** Extraoral view; **B** and **C,** intraoral views. For this patient, the appliance consists of a bite block on the right side and buccal and lingual shields on the left that allow free eruption of teeth. The construction bite, swinging the jaw to one side, is designed to correct the transverse asymmetry by producing more growth on the deficient side, while differential eruption corrects the vertical asymmetry.

caused by an escape of the growing tissues on one side from normal regulatory control, the exact mechanism of which is not understood. The condition typically appears in the late teens, most frequently in girls, but may begin at an earlier age. Because the body of the mandible is distorted by the excessive growth (usually by bowing downward on the affected side), the condition is appropriately described as hemimandibular hypertrophy—but since excessive growth at the condyle is the cause, the old name for this condition, condylar hyperplasia, was not wrong.

There are two possible modes of treatment, both surgical: (1) a ramus osteotomy to correct the asymmetry resulting from unilateral overgrowth, after the excessive growth has ceased; and (2) condylectomy to remove the excessively growing condyle and reconstruct the joint. The reconstruction usually is done with a section of rib incorporating the costochondral junction area but occasionally can be accomplished just by recontouring the condylar head ("condylar shave"). Since surgical involvement of the temporomandibular joint should be avoided if possible, the first treatment plan is preferable. This implies, however, that the abnormal growth has stopped or, in a younger patient, will stop within reasonable limits. As a practical matter, removal of the condyle is likely to be necessary in the more severe and more rapidly growing cases, while a ramus osteotomy is preferred for the less severe problems.

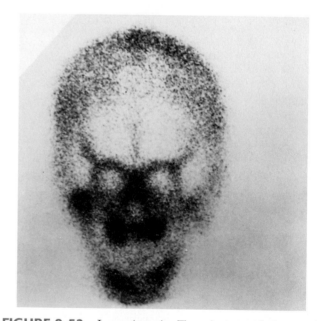

FIGURE 8-52   Image (anterior Towne's view with the mouth open) from bone scan with ^{99m}Tc in a 10-year-old boy with suspected hyperplasia of the right mandibular condyle. Note the "hot spot" in the area of the right condyle and the difference in uptake of the isotope between the right and left sides. Eruption of teeth and apposition of bone at the alveolar processes normally create heavy imaging along the dental arches.

The bone seeking isotope ^{99m}Tc can be used to distinguish an active rapidly growing condyle from an enlarged condyle that has ceased growing.[50] This short-lived gamma-emitting isotope is concentrated in areas of active bone deposition. [99m]Tc imaging of the oral structures typically shows high activity in areas around the alveolar ridge, particularly in areas where teeth are erupting. The condyles are not normally areas of intense imaging. A "hot" condyle is evidence of active growth at that site (Figure 8-52).

Unfortunately, though false positive images are rare, false negatives are not, so a negative bone scan of the condyles cannot be taken as evidence that hyperplastic growth of one condyle is not occurring. A positive unilateral condylar response on a bone scan indicates that condylectomy will probably be required, whereas a negative response means that further observation for continuing growth is indicated before the surgical procedure is selected.

Treatment Planning for Cleft Lip and Palate Patients

Patients with cleft lip and palate routinely require extensive and prolonged orthodontic treatment. Orthodontic treatment may be required at any or all of four separate stages: (1) in infancy before the initial surgical repair of the lip, (2) during the late primary and early mixed dentition, (3) during the late mixed and early permanent dentition, and (4) in the late teens after the completion of facial growth, in conjunction with orthognathic surgery.

Infant Orthopedics. An infant with a cleft lip and palate will have a distorted maxillary arch at birth in nearly every instance. In patients with a bilateral cleft, the premaxillary segment is often displaced anteriorly while the posterior maxillary segments are lingually collapsed behind it (Figure 8-53). Less severe distortions occur in infants with unilateral palatal clefts. If the distortion of arch form is extremely severe, surgical closure of the lip, which is normally carried out in the early weeks of life, can be extremely difficult. Orthodontic intervention to reposition the segments and to bring the protruding premaxillary segment back into the arch may be needed to obtain a good surgical repair of the lip. This "infant orthopedics" is one of the few instances in which orthodontic treatment for a newborn infant, before eruption of any teeth, may be indicated.

Infant orthopedics of this type was pioneered by Burston in Liverpool in the late 1950s and was carried out on a large scale at many cleft palate centers in the 1960s. In a child with a bilateral cleft, two types of movement of the maxillary segments may be needed (Figure 8-54). First, the collapsed maxillary posterior segments must be expanded laterally; then pressure against the premaxilla can reposition it posteriorly into its approximately correct position in the arch. This movement can be accomplished by a light elastic strap across the anterior segment, by an orthodontic appliance pinned to the segments that applies a contraction force, or even by pressure from the repaired lip if lip repair

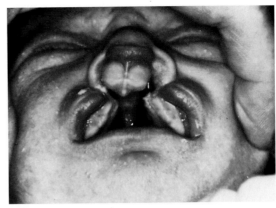

FIGURE 8-53 A forward displacement of the premaxillary segment and medial collapse of the lateral maxillary segments can be seen clearly in this photograph of a newborn infant with a bilateral cleft of the lip and palate.

is done after the lateral expansion. In patients with extremely severe protrusion, an appliance held to the maxillary segments by pins might be required, while an elastic strap or the pressure of the lip itself would be adequate with less severe problems.

In infants, the segments can be repositioned surprisingly quickly and easily, so that the period of active treatment is a few weeks at most. If presurgical movement of maxillary segments is indicated, this typically would be done beginning at 3 to 6 weeks of age, so that the lip closure could be carried out at approximately 10 weeks. A passive plate, similar to an orthodontic retainer, is then used for a few months after lip closure.

Even in children with unilateral clefts and relatively slight distortion of the arch, an improvement in the position of the premaxillary segment can be noted if a passive plate is placed, because there is a molding effect on the arch after lip closure. For these patients, the passive appliance would be placed before lip closure, then maintained for perhaps 3 months after the lip closure. Acceptance of such an appliance by the infant is surprisingly good. It serves as a "feeding plate," apparently making it easier for the infant to swallow normally. A passive plate can be left in position for most of the first year of life if desired.

After 40 years of experience with presurgical infant orthopedics, the present consensus is that these procedures offer less long-term benefit than was originally expected.[51] Soon after this treatment, the infants who have had presurgical orthopedics look much better than those who have not had it. With each passing year, however, it becomes more difficult to tell which patients had segments repositioned in infancy and which did not. The short-term benefit is more impressive than the long-term benefit. For this reason, the method is used less frequently now than when enthusiasm was at a peak.

For a few infants with extremely malpositioned segments, which occur almost exclusively in bilateral cleft lip

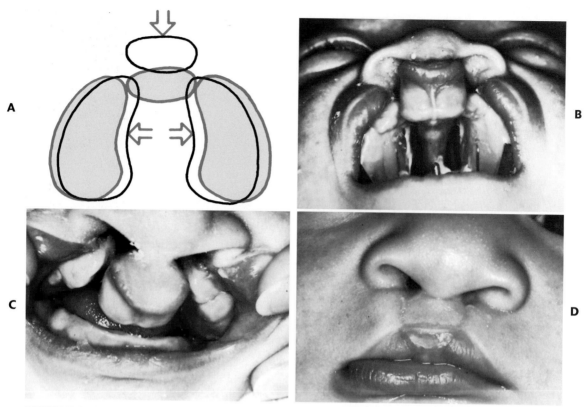

FIGURE 8-54   A, Diagrammatic representation of the movements needed to place maxillary segments in their proper position. The posterior segments must be moved laterally so that the premaxillary segment can move lingually. **B,** Infant with bilateral cleft and appliance in place to widen the posterior segments. **C,** Same infant after an elastic strap has been used to reposition the premaxillary segment lingually. **D,** Same infant after surgical repair of the cleft lip.

and palate, presurgical infant orthopedics remains useful. For the majority of patients with cleft lip or palate, however, the orthodontist is no longer called to reposition segments in infants. Instead, if the segments protrude, the lip repair may be carried out in two stages, first with a lip adhesion to provide an elastic force from the lip itself, followed at a somewhat later stage by definitive lip repair. Rather than presurgical orthopedics being recommended for nearly all infants with cleft lip or palate, at present a minority are treated with presurgical orthopedics.

At some centers, bone grafts were placed across the cleft alveolus soon after the infant orthopedics to stabilize the position of the segments. Although a few clinicians still advocate this procedure, the consensus is that early grafting of the alveolar process is contraindicated because it tends to interfere with later growth.[52] Alveolar bone grafts are better deferred until the early mixed dentition.

Late Primary and Early Mixed Dentition Treatment.   Many of the orthodontic problems of cleft palate children in the late and early mixed dentition result not from the cleft itself, but from the effects of surgical repair. Although the techniques for repair of cleft lip and palate have improved tremendously in recent years, closure of the lip inevitably creates some constriction across the anterior part of the maxillary arch, and closure of a cleft palate causes at least some degree of lateral constriction. As a result, surgically treated cleft palate patients have a tendency toward both anterior and lateral crossbite, which is not seen in patients with untreated clefts. This result is not an argument against surgical repair of the lip and palate, which is necessary for esthetic and functional (speech) reasons. It simply means that orthodontic treatment must be considered a necessary part of the habilitation of such patients.

Orthodontic intervention is often unnecessary until the permanent incisor teeth begin to erupt but is usually imperative at that point. As the permanent teeth come in, there is a strong tendency for the maxillary incisors to erupt rotated and often in crossbite (Figure 8-55). The major goal of orthodontic treatment at this time is to correct incisor position, and prepare the patient for an alveolar bone graft. Although alveolar bone grafts in infancy appear to be contraindicated, placing a bone graft in the alveolar cleft area before the permanent lateral incisors (if present) or permanent canines erupt, is advantageous. This stabilizes the cleft area and creates a healthy environment for the permanent teeth.[53] Ideally, the permanent laterals or canines should erupt through the graft (see Figure 8-55), which means that the best time to place such a graft is

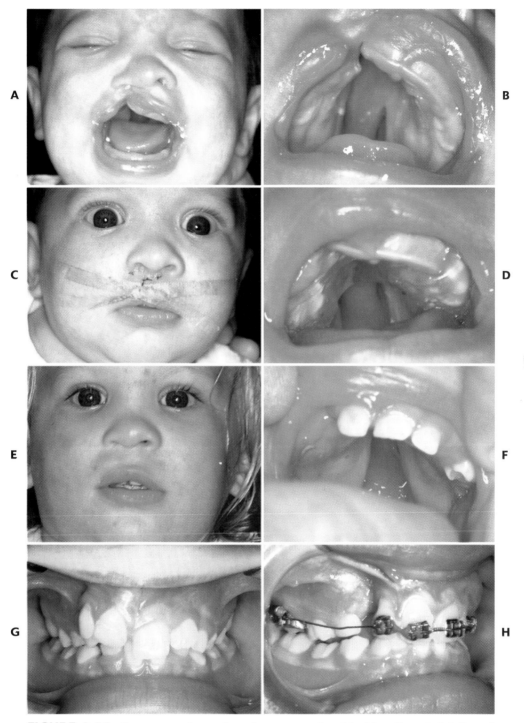

FIGURE 8-55 Long-term observation of treatment of a girl with unilateral cleft lip and palate. **A,B,** Age 8 weeks prior to lip repair. Note the displacement of the alveolar segments at the cleft site. **C,D,** Age 9 weeks after lip closure. A palatal plate has been pinned into position to control the alveolar segments while lip pressure molds them into position. This type of infant orthopedics, popular in the 1970s, is used less now than previously because its long-term efficacy is questionable. **E,F,** Age 2, prior to palate closure. **G,** Age 8, after eruption of maxillary incisors; **H,** Age 9, incisor alignment in preparation for alveolar bone graft. *continued*

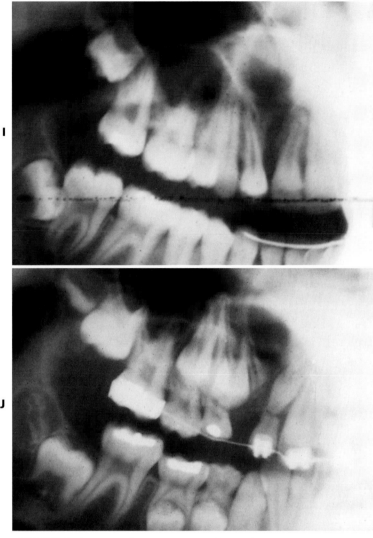

FIGURE 8-55, cont'd **I,** Panoramic radiograph, age 9, just prior to bone graft; **J,** Panoramic radiograph age 12, at completion of orthodontic treatment, showing bone fill-in at the cleft site.   *continued*

between 7 and 10 years. Any necessary alignment of incisors or expansion of posterior segments should be completed before the alveolar grafting. This now should be considered a routine part of contemporary treatment.

Early Permanent Dentition Treatment. As the canine and premolar teeth erupt, there is a tendency for posterior crossbite to develop problems, particularly on the cleft side in a unilateral situation, and the teeth are likely to be malaligned. The more successful the surgery, the fewer the problems, but in essentially every instance, fixed appliance orthodontic treatment is necessary at this time. With contemporary treatment that includes grafting of alveolar clefts, it is possible to close spaces due to missing teeth, and this now is a major objective of this phase of treatment (see Figure 8-55). If space closure is not possible, orthodontic tooth movement may be needed to position teeth as abutments for eventual fixed prosthodontics. In that circumstance, a resin-bonded bridge to provide a semipermanent replacement for missing teeth can be ex-

tremely helpful. Orthodontic treatment is often completed at age 14, but a permanent bridge in many instances cannot be placed until age 17 or 18. The semipermanent fixed bridge is preferable to prolonged use of a removable retainer with a replacement tooth. Dental implants are not appropriate for cleft areas.

Orthognathic Surgery for Patients with Cleft Lip and Palate. In some patients with cleft lip and palate, more often in males than females, continued mandibular growth after the completion of active orthodontic treatment leads to the return of anterior and lateral crossbites. This result is not so much from excessive mandibular growth as from deficient maxillary growth, both anteroposteriorly and vertically, and it is seen less frequently now because of the improvements in cleft lip/palate surgery in recent years. Orthognathic surgery to bring the deficient maxilla downward and forward may be a necessary last stage in treatment of a patient with cleft lip or palate, typically at about age 18 if required. Occasionally, surgical mandibular setback also may

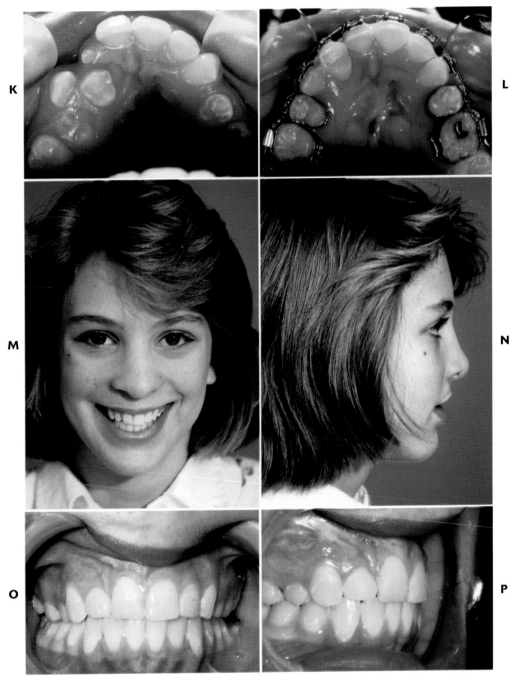

FIGURE 8-55, cont'd K, Age 11, transposed first premolar erupting in the grafted area; **L,** First premolar in lateral incisor position toward the end of active orthodontics, age 12. A tooth that erupts in a grafted area or that is moved orthodontically into the area stimulates formation of new bone that eliminates the cleft. Because teeth bring alveolar bone with them and this bone is lost in the absence of teeth, this is the only way to completely repair an alveolar cleft. **M,N,** Facial and, **O,P,** intraoral photos, age 12.

continued

be needed. After this, the definitive restorative work to replace any missing teeth can be carried out.

The decrease in the number of cleft patients needing prosthodontic replacement of missing teeth or orthognathic surgery because of problems with maxillary growth is striking. The standard of care now is closure of the space where teeth are missing, made possible by alveolar grafts at age 6-8, and atraumatic palatal surgery that minimizes interferences with growth. At one leading center, in the 1970s up to one half of all cleft patients needed fixed prosthodontics to replace missing teeth, and 10% to 15% needed orthognathic surgery. By the end of the 1980s, fewer than 10% of the cleft patients needed prosthodontic treatment and orthognathic surgery was rarely required.[54]

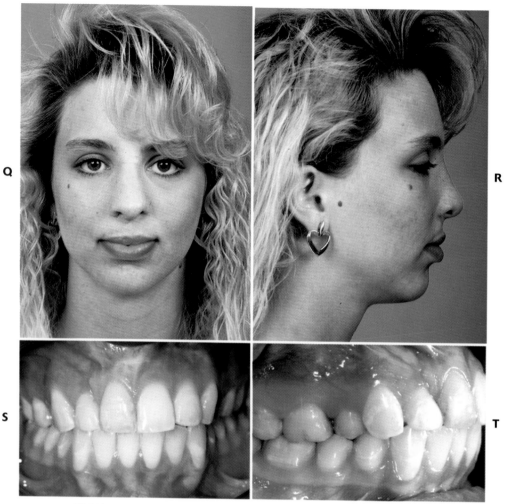

FIGURE 8-55, cont'd **Q,R,** Facial and, **S,T,** intraoral photos, age 21.

REFERENCES

1. Mosteller F, Colditz GA: Understanding research synthesis (meta-analysis), Ann Rev Public Health 17:1-23, 1996.
2. Popovich FP, et al: Burlington growth study templates, Toronto, 1981, University of Toronto Department of Orthodontics.
3. Johnston LE: A simplified approach to prediction, Am J Orthod 67:253-257, 1975.
4. Broadbent BH, Sr, Broadbent BJ, Jr, Golden WH: Bolton standards of dentofacial developmental growth, St Louis, 1975, Mosby.
5. Ackerman JL, Proffit WR: Communication in orthodontic treatment planning: bioethical and informed consent issues, Angle Orthod 65:253-262, 1995.
6. Phillips C, Hill BJ, Cannac C: The influence of video imaging on patients' perceptions and expectations, Angle Orthod 65:263-270, 1995.
7. Angle EH: Treatment of malocclusion of the teeth, ed 7, Philadelphia, 1907, SS White Manufacturing Co.
8. Case CS: The question of extraction in orthodontics, reprinted in Am J Orthod 50:658-691, 1964.
9. Little RM, Wallen TR, Riedel RA: Stability and relapse of mandibular anterior alignment: first premolar extraction cases treated by traditional edgewise orthodontics, Am J Orthod 80:349-364, 1981.
10. McReynolds DC, Little RM: Mandibular second premolar extraction—postretention evaluation of stability and relapse, Angle Orthod 61:133-144, 1991.
11. Burke SP, Silveira AM, Goldsmith LJ et al: A meta-analysis of mandibular intercanine width in treatment and postretention, Angle Orthod 68:53-60, 1998.
12. Betts NJ, Vanarsdall RL, Barber HD et al: Diagnosis and treatment of transverse maxillary deficiency, Int J Adult Orthod Orthogn Surg 10:75-96, 1995.
13. Nimkarn Y, Miles PG, O'Reilly MT, Weyant RJ: The validity of maxillary expansion indices, Angle Orthod 65:321-326, 1995.
14. Haas AJ: Rapid expansion of the maxillary dental arch and nasal cavity by opening the midpalatal suture, Angle Orthod 31:73-90, 1961.
15. Wertz R, Dreskin M: Midpalatal suture opening: a normative study, Am J Orthod 71:367-381, 1977.
16. Isaacson RJ, Wood JL, Ingram AH: Forces produced by rapid maxillary expansion, Angle Orthod 34:256-270, 1964.
17. Hicks EP: Slow maxillary expansion: a clinical study of the skeletal versus dental response to low-magnitude force, Am J Orthod 73:121-141, 1978.

18. Sarver DM, Johnston MW: Skeletal changes in vertical and anterior displacement of the maxilla with bonded rapid palatal expansion appliances, Am J Orthod Dentofacial Orthop 95:462-466, 1989.

19. Weislander L: The effect of orthodontic treatment on the concurrent development of the craniofacial complex, Am J Orthod 49:15-27, 1963.

20. Graber TM, Neumann B: Removable orthodontic appliances, ed 2, Philadelphia, 1984, W.B. Saunders.

21. McNamara JA, Howe RP, Dischinger TG: A comparison of the Herbst and Frankel appliances in the treatment of Class II malocclusion, Am J Orthod Dentofacial Orthop 98:138-144, 1990.

22. Pancherz H, Fackel U: The skeletofacial growth pattern pre- and post-dentofacial orthopedics, Eur J Orthod 12:209-218, 1990.

23. Tulloch JFC, Phillips C, Koch G, Proffit WR: The effect of early intervention on skeletal pattern in Class II malocclusion: a randomized clinical trial, Am J Orthod Dentofac Orthop 111:391-400, 1997.

24. Tulloch JFC, Proffit WR, Phillips C: Influences on the outcome of early treatment for Class II malocclusion, Am J Orthod Dentofac Orthop 111:533-542, 1997.

25. Tulloch JFC, Phillips C, Proffit WR: Benefit of early Class II treatment: progress report of a two-phase randomized clinical trial, Am J Orthod Dentofac Orthop 113:62-72, 1998.

26. Keeling SD, Wheeler TT, King GJ et al: Anteroposterior skeletal and dental changes after early Class II treatment with bionators and headgear, Am J Orthod Dentofac Orthop 113:40-50, 1998.

27. Keeling SD, Garvan CW, King GJ et al: Temporomandibular disorders after early Class II treatment with bionators and headgear: results from a randomized clinical trial, Sem Orthod 1:149-164, 1995.

28. Ghafari J, Shofer FS, Jacobsson-Hunt U et al: Headgear versus function regulator in the early treatment of Class II, division 1 malocclusion: a randomized clinical trial, Am J Orthod Dentofac Orthop 113:51-61, 1998.

29. Baumrind S, Korn EL, Molthen R, West EE: Changes in facial dimensions associated with the use of forces to retract the maxilla, Am J Orthod 80:17-30, 1981.

30. Baumrind S, Molthen R, West EE, Miller DM: Mandibular plane changes during maxillary retraction, part 2, Am J Orthod 74:603-620, 1978.

31. Orton HS, Slattery DA, Orton S: The treatment of severe 'gummy' Class II division 1 malocclusion using the maxillary intrusion splint, Eur J Orthod 14:216-23, 1992.

32. Stockli PW, Teuscher UM: Combined activator headgear orthopedics. In Graber TM, Vanarsdall RL (editors): Current orthodontic principles and techniques, ed 2, St Louis, 1994, Mosby.

33. Barbre RE, Sinclair PM: A cephalometric evaluation of anterior open bite correction with the magnetic active vertical corrector, Angle Orthod 61:93-102, 1991.

34. Verdon P: Professor Delaire's facial orthopedic mask, Denver, 1982, Rocky Mountain Orthodontic Products.

35. Merwin D, Ngan P, Hagg U et al: Timing for effective application of anteriorly directed orthopedic force to the maxilla, Am J Orthod Dentofac Orthop 112:292-299, 1997.

36. Baccetti T, McGill JS, Franchi L, McNamara JA: Skeletal effects of early treatment of Class III malocclusion with maxillary expansion and face-mask therapy, Am J Orthod Dentofac Orthop 113:333-343, 1998.

37. Janzen EK, Bluher JA: The cephalometric, anatomic and histologic changes in *Macaca mulatta*, after application of a continuous-acting retraction force on the mandible, Am J Orthod 51:823-855, 1965.

38. Takada K, Petdachai S, Sakuda M: Changes in dentofacial morphology in skeletal Class III children treated by a modified maxillary protraction headgear and a chin cup: a longitudinal cephalometric appraisal, Eur J Orthod 15:211-221, 1993.

39. Johnston LE: Balancing the books on orthodontic treatment: an integrated analysis of change, Brit J Orthod 23:93-102, 1996.

40. Konik M, Pancherz H, Hansen K: The mechanism of Class II correction in late Herbst treatment, Am J Orthod Dentofac Orthop 112:87-91, 1997.

41. Basdra EK, Stellzig A, Komposch G: Extraction of maxillary second molars in the treatment of Class II malocclusion, Angle Orthod 66:287-292, 1996.

42. Gianelly AA: Distal movement of the maxillary molars, Am J Orthod Dentofac Orthop 114:166-72, 1998.

43. Gianelly AA, Bednar J, Dietz VS: Japanese NiTi coils used to move molars distally, Am J Orthod Dentofac Orthop 99:564-566, 1991.

44. Beattie JR, Paquette DE, Johnston LE: The functional impact of extraction and non-extraction treatments: a long-term comparison in patients with "borderline", equally susceptible Class II malocclusions, Am J Orthod Dentofac Orthop 105:444-449, 1994.

45. Luppapornlap S, Johnston LE: The effects of premolar extraction: a long-term comparison of outcomes in "clear-cut" extraction and nonextraction Class II patients, Angle Orthod 63:257-272, 1993.

46. Proffit WR, Phillips C, Tulloch JFC, Medland PH: Orthognathic vs orthodontic correction of skeletal Class II malocclusion in adolescents: effects and indications, Int J Adult Orthod Orthogn Surg 7:209-220, 1992.

47. Drysdale C, Gibbs SL, Ford TR: Orthodontic management of root-filled teeth, Brit J Orthod 23:255-260, 1996.

48. Wennstrom JL: Mucogingival considerations in orthodontic treatment, Sem Orthod 2:46-54, 1996.

49. van Venrooy JR, Proffit WR: Orthondontic care for medically compromised patients, J Am Dent Assoc 111:262-266, 1985.

50. Gray RJ, Horner K, Testa HJ et al: Condylar hyperplasia: correlation of histological and clinical features, Dento-Maxillo-Facial Radiol 23:103-107, 1994.

51. Berkowitz S (editor): Cleft lip and palate: perspectives in management, San Diego, 1996, Singular Publishing Group.

52. Semb G, Shaw W: Influence of alveolar bone grafting on facial growth. In Bardach J, Morris HL (editors): Multidisciplinary management of cleft lip and palate, Philadelphia, 1990, W.B. Saunders.

53. Waite PD, Waite DE: Bone grafting for the alveolar cleft defect, Sem Orthod 2:192-196, 1996.

54. Semb G, Borchgrevink H, Saether IL et al: Multidisciplinary management of cleft lip and palate in Oslo, Norway. In Bardach J, Morris HL (editors): Multidisciplinary management of cleft lip and palate, Philadelphia, 1990, W.B. Saunders.

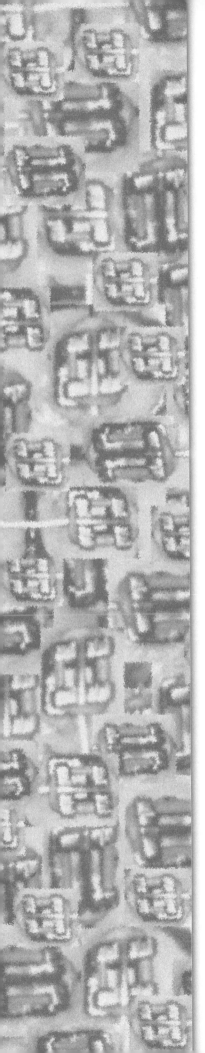

SECTION
IV

BIOMECHANICS AND MECHANICS

Orthodontic therapy depends on the reaction of the teeth, and more generally the facial structures, to gentle but persistent force. In an orthodontic context, *biomechanics* is commonly used in discussions of the reaction of the dental and facial structures to orthodontic force, whereas *mechanics* is reserved for the properties of the strictly mechanical components of the appliance system. In this section, the biologic responses to orthodontic force that underlie biomechanics are discussed in Chapter 9. Chapter 10, which is concerned with the design and application of orthodontic appliances, is largely devoted to mechanics, but includes some biomechanical considerations as well.

CHAPTER

9

The Biological Basis of Orthodontic Therapy

Orthodontic treatment is based on the principle that if prolonged pressure is applied to a tooth, tooth movement will occur as the bone around the tooth remodels. Bone is selectively removed in some areas and added in others. In essence, the tooth moves through the bone carrying its attachment apparatus with it, as the socket of the tooth migrates. Because the bony response is mediated by the periodontal ligament, tooth movement is primarily a periodontal ligament phenomenon.

Forces applied to the teeth can also affect the pattern of bone apposition and resorption at sites distant from the teeth, particularly the sutures of the maxilla and bony surfaces on both sides of the temporomandibular joint. Thus the biologic response to orthodontic therapy includes not only the response of the periodontal ligament but also the response of growing areas distant from the dentition. In this chapter, the response of periodontal structures to orthodontic force is discussed first, and then the response of skeletal areas distant from the dentition is considered briefly, drawing on the background of normal growth provided in Chapters 2 through 4.

PERIODONTAL AND BONE RESPONSE TO NORMAL FUNCTION

Periodontal Ligament Structure and Function

Each tooth is attached to and separated from the adjacent alveolar bone by a heavy collagenous supporting structure, the periodontal ligament (PDL). Under normal circumstances, the PDL occupies a space approximately 0.5 mm in width around all parts of the root. By far the major component of the ligament is a network of parallel collagenous fibers, inserting into cementum of the root surface on one side and into a relatively dense bony plate, the lamina dura, on the other side. These supporting fibers run at an angle, attaching farther apically on the tooth than on the adjacent alveolar bone. This arrangement, of course, resists the displacement of the tooth expected during normal function (Figure 9-1).

Although most of the PDL space is taken up with the collagenous fiber bundles that constitute the ligamentous attachment, two other major components of the ligament must be considered. These are (1) the cellular elements, including mesenchymal cells of various types along with vascular and neural elements; and (2) the tissue fluids. Both play an important role in normal function and in making orthodontic tooth movement possible.

The principal cellular elements in the PDL are undifferentiated mesenchymal cells and their progeny in the form of fibroblasts and osteoblasts. The collagen of the ligament is constantly being remodeled and renewed during normal function.[1] The same cells can serve as both fibroblasts, producing new collagenous matrix materials, and fibroclasts, destroying previously produced collagen. Remodeling and recontouring of the bony socket and the cementum of the root is also constantly being carried out, though on a smaller scale, as a response to normal function. Fibroblasts in the PDL have properties similar to osteoblasts, and new bone probably is formed by osteoblasts that differentiated from the local cellular population.[2] Bone and cementum are removed by specialized osteoclasts and cementoclasts, respectively. These multinucleated giant cells are quite different from the osteoblasts and cementoblasts that produce bone and cementum. Despite years of investigation, their origin remains controversial. Most are of hematogenous origin; some may be derived from stem cells found in the local area.[3]

Although the PDL is not highly vascular, it does contain blood vessels and cells from the vascular system. Nerve endings are also found within the ligament, both the unmyelinated free endings associated with perception of pain and the more complex receptors associated with pressure and positional information (proprioception).

Finally, it is important to recognize that the PDL space is filled with fluid; this fluid is the same as that found in all other tissues, ultimately derived from the vascular system. A fluid-filled chamber with retentive but porous walls could be a description of a shock absorber, and in normal function, the fluid allows the PDL space to play just this role.

Response to Normal Function

During masticatory function, the teeth and periodontal structures are subjected to intermittent heavy forces. Tooth contacts last for 1 second or less; forces are quite heavy, ranging from 1 or 2 kg while soft substances are chewed up to as much as 50 kg against a more resistant object. When a tooth is subjected to heavy loads of this type, quick displacement of the tooth within the PDL space is prevented by the incompressible tissue fluid. Instead, the force is transmitted to the alveolar bone, which bends in response.

The extent of bone bending during normal function of the jaws (and other skeletal elements of the body) is often not appreciated. The body of the mandible bends as the mouth is opened and closed, even without heavy masticatory loads. Upon wide opening, the distance between the mandibular molars decreases by 2 to 3 mm. In heavy function, individual teeth are slightly displaced as the bone of the alveolar process bends to allow this to occur, and bending stresses are transmitted over considerable distances. Bone bending in response to normal function generates piezoelectric currents (see p. 299) that appear to be an important stimulus to skeletal regeneration and repair. This is the mechanism by which bony architecture is adapted to functional demands.

Very little of the fluid within the PDL space is squeezed out during the first second of pressure application. If pressure against a tooth is maintained, however, the fluid is rapidly expressed, and the tooth displaces within the PDL space, compressing the ligament itself against adjacent bone. Not surprisingly, this hurts. Pain is normally felt after 3 to 5 seconds of heavy force application, indicating that the fluids are expressed and crushing pressure is applied against the PDL in this amount of time (Table 9-1). The resistance

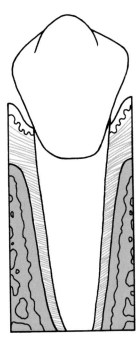

FIGURE 9-1 Diagrammatic representation of periodontal structures (bone in *pale red*). Note the angulation of the PDL fibers.

TABLE 9-1 *Physiologic Response to Heavy Pressure Against a Tooth*

Time (seconds)	Event
<1	PDL* fluid incompressible, alveolar bone bends, piezoelectric signal generated
1-2	PDL fluid expressed, tooth moves within PDL space
3-5	PDL fluid squeezed out, tissues compressed; immediate pain if pressure is heavy

*PDL, periodontal ligament.

provided by tissue fluids allows normal mastication, with its force applications of 1 second or less, to occur without pain.

Although the PDL is beautifully adapted to resist forces of short duration, it rapidly loses its adaptive capability as the tissue fluids are squeezed out of its confined area. Prolonged force, even of low magnitude, produces a different physiologic response—remodeling of the adjacent bone. Orthodontic tooth movement is made possible by the application of prolonged forces. In addition, light prolonged forces in the natural environment—forces from the lips, cheeks, or tongue resting against the teeth—have the same potential as orthodontic forces to cause the teeth to move to a different location (see the discussion of equilibrium factors in Chapter 5).

Role of the Periodontal Ligament in Eruption and Stabilization of the Teeth

The phenomenon of tooth eruption makes it plain that forces generated within the PDL itself can produce tooth movement. The eruption mechanism appears to depend on metabolic events within the PDL, including but perhaps not limited to formation, cross-linkage and maturational shortening of collagen fibers (see Marks[4] for a recent comprehensive review). This process continues, although at a reduced rate, into adult life. A tooth whose antagonist has been extracted will often begin to erupt again after many years of apparent quiescence.

The continuing presence of this mechanism indicates that it may produce not only eruption of the teeth under appropriate circumstances but also active stabilization of the teeth against prolonged forces of light magnitude. It is commonly observed that light prolonged pressures against the teeth are not in perfect balance, as would seem to be re-

quired if tooth movement were not to occur (Figure 9-2). The ability of the PDL to generate a force and thereby contribute to the set of forces that determine the equilibrium situation, probably explains this (see the discussion of equilibrium in Chapter 5).

Active stabilization also implies a threshold for orthodontic force, since forces below the stabilization level would be expected to be ineffective. The threshold for outside force, of course, would vary depending on the extent to which existing soft tissue pressures were already being resisted by the stabilization mechanism. In some experiments, the threshold for orthodontic force, if one existed at all, appeared extremely low. In other circumstances, a somewhat higher threshold, but still one of only a few grams, seemed to exist.[5] The current concept is that active stabilization can overcome prolonged forces of a few grams at most, perhaps up to the 5 to 10 gm/cm^2 often observed as the magnitude of unbalanced soft tissue resting pressures.

PERIODONTAL LIGAMENT AND BONE RESPONSE TO SUSTAINED ORTHODONTIC FORCE

The response to sustained force against the teeth is a function of force magnitude: heavy forces lead to rapidly developing pain, necrosis of cellular elements within the PDL, and the phenomenon (discussed in more detail later) of "undermining resorption" of alveolar bone near the affected tooth. Lighter forces are compatible with survival of cells within the PDL and a remodeling of the tooth socket by a relatively painless "frontal resorption" of the tooth socket. In orthodontic practice, the objective is to produce tooth movement as much as possible by frontal resorption, recognizing that some areas of PDL necrosis and undermining resorption will probably occur despite efforts to prevent this.

Biologic Control of Tooth Movement

Before discussing in detail the response to orthodontic force, it is necessary to consider the biologic control mechanisms that lead from the stimulus of sustained force application to the response of orthodontic tooth movement. Two possible control elements, biologic electricity and pressure-tension in the PDL that affects blood flow, are contrasted in the two major theories of orthodontic tooth movement. The bioelectric theory relates tooth movement at least in part to changes in bone metabolism controlled by the electric signals that are produced when alveolar bone flexes and bends. The pressure-tension theory relates tooth movement to cellular changes produced by chemical messengers, traditionally thought to be generated by alterations in blood flow through the PDL. Pressure and tension within the PDL, by reducing (pressure) or increasing (tension) the diameter of blood vessels in the ligament space, could certainly alter blood flow. The two theories are neither incom-

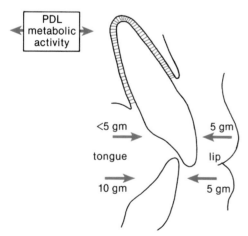

FIGURE 9-2 Resting pressures from the lips or cheeks and tongue are usually not balanced. In some areas, as in the mandibular anterior, tongue pressure is greater than lip pressure. In other areas, as in the maxillary incisor region, lip pressure is greater. Active stabilization produced by metabolic effects in the PDL probably explains why teeth are stable in the presence of imbalanced pressures that would otherwise cause tooth movement.

patible nor mutually exclusive. From a contemporary perspective, it appears that both mechanisms may play a part in the biologic control of tooth movement.

Electric signals that might initiate tooth movement initially were thought to be piezoelectric. Piezoelectricity is a phenomenon observed in many crystalline materials in which a deformation of the crystal structure produces a flow of electric current as electrons are displaced from one part of the crystal lattice to another. The piezoelectricity of many inorganic crystals has been recognized for many years and has been used in everyday technology (e.g., the crystal pickup found in inexpensive phonographic systems). Organic crystals can also have piezoelectric properties. Not only is bone mineral a crystal structure with piezoelectric properties, collagen itself is piezoelectric, and stress-generated potentials in dried bone specimens can be attributed to piezoelectricity.

Piezoelectric signals have two unusual characteristics: (1) a quick decay rate (i.e., when a force is applied, a piezoelectric signal is created in response that quickly dies away to zero even though the force is maintained) and (2) the production of an equivalent signal, opposite in direction, when the force is released (Figure 9-3).

Both these characteristics are explained by the migration of electrons within the crystal lattice as it is distorted by pressure. When the crystal structure is deformed, electrons migrate from one location to another and an electric charge is observed. As long as the force is maintained, the crystal structure is stable and no further electric events are observed. When the force is released, however, the crystal returns to its original shape, and a reverse flow of electrons is seen. With this arrangement, rhythmic activity would produce a constant interplay of electric signals, whereas

occasional application and release of force would produce only occasional electric signals.

Ions in the fluids that bathe living bone interact with the complex electric field generated when the bone bends, causing temperature changes as well as electric signals. As a result, both convection and conduction currents can be detected in the extracellular fluids, and the currents are affected by the nature of the fluids. The small voltages that are observed are called the "streaming potential." These voltages, though different from piezoelectric signals in dry material, have in common their rapid onset and alteration, as changing stresses are placed on the bone. There is also a reverse piezoelectric effect. Not only will the application of force cause distortion of crystalline structure and with it an electric signal, application of an electric field can cause a crystal to deform and produce force in doing so. Reverse piezoelectricity has no place in natural control systems, at least as far as is presently known, but there are intriguing possibilities for using external electric fields to promote bone healing and regeneration after injury.[6]

There is no longer any doubt that stress-generated signals are important in the general maintenance of the skeleton. Without such signals, bone mineral is lost and general skeletal atrophy ensues—a situation that has proved troublesome for astronauts whose bones no longer flex in a weightless environment as they would under normal gravity. Signals generated by the bending of alveolar bone during normal chewing almost surely are important for maintenance of the bone around the teeth. On the other hand, sustained force of the type used to induce orthodontic tooth movement does not produce prominent stress-generated signals. When the force is applied, a brief signal is created; when it is removed, the reverse signal appears. As long as the force is sustained, however, nothing happens. If stress-generated signals were important in producing the bone remodeling associated with orthodontic tooth movement, a vibrating application of pressure would be advantageous. Experiments indicate little or no advantage in vibrating over sustained force for the movement of teeth[7]; in fact, there may be disadvantages. It appears that stress-generated signals, important as they may be for normal skeletal function, probably have little if anything to do with the response to orthodontic tooth movement.

One should not conclude from this that all types of electric signals are unimportant in the control of tooth movement. A second type of endogenous electric signal, which is called the "bioelectric potential," can be observed in bone that is not being stressed. Metabolically active bone or connective tissue cells (in areas of active growth or remodeling) produce electronegative charges that are generally proportional to how active they are; inactive cells and areas are nearly electrically neutral. Although the purpose of this bioelectric potential is not known, cellular activity can be modified by adding exogenous electric signals. The effects, presumably, are felt at cell membranes.

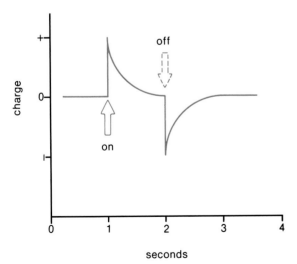

FIGURE 9-3 When a force is applied to a crystalline structure (like bone or collagen), a flow of current is produced that quickly dies away. When the force is released, an opposite current flow is observed. The piezoelectric effect results from migration of electrons within the crystal lattice.

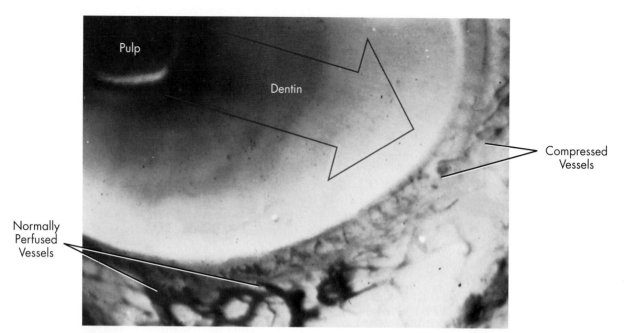

FIGURE 9-4 In experimental animals, changes in blood flow in the PDL can be observed by perfusing India ink into the vascular system while the animal is being sacrificed. The vessels are filled with India ink, so that their size can be seen easily. This specimen is seen in horizontal section, with the tooth root on the left and the pulp chamber just visible in the upper left. The PDL is below and to the right. Note that vessels have been compressed in the area of the PDL toward which the tooth is being moved. Cells disappear in the compressed areas, and the area is sometimes said to be hyalinized because of its resemblance by hyaline connective area. (Courtesy Dr. F.E. Khouw.)

Membrane depolarization triggers nerve impulses and muscle contraction, but changes in membrane potentials accompany other cellular responses as well. The external electric signals probably affect cell membrane receptors, membrane permeability, or both.[8] Both animal and human experiments indicate that when low voltage direct current is applied to the alveolar bone, modifying the bioelectric potential, a tooth moves faster than its control in response to an identical spring.[9] Electromagnetic fields also can affect cell membrane potentials and permeability, and thereby trigger changes in cellular activity. In animal experiments, a pulsed electromagnetic field increased the role of tooth movement, apparently by shortening the initial "lag phase" before tooth movement begins.[10] Electromagnetic fields can be induced within tissues by adjacent magnets, without the contact required by electrodes, and bone healing has been shown to be enhanced by certain types of fields. It is possible that this effect can be utilized in the future to enhance orthodontic tooth movement and/or alter jaw growth. Perhaps a fair conclusion is that even though stress-generated electrical signals do not explain tooth movement, electric and electromagnetic influences can modify the bony remodeling on which tooth movement depends and may yet prove useful therapeutically. It seems highly unlikely, however, that the fields generated by small magnets attached to the teeth to generate tooth-moving forces (see Chapter 10) could change the basic biology of the response to force. Recent claims that magnetic force generation reduces pain and mobility are not supported by evidence.

Pressure-Tension Theory. The pressure-tension theory, the classic theory of tooth movement, relies on chemical rather than electric signals as the stimulus for cellular differentiation and ultimately tooth movement. There is no doubt that chemical messengers are important in the cascade of events that lead to remodeling of alveolar bone and tooth movement. Because this theory does explain the course of events reasonably well, it remains the basis of the following discussion.

In this theory, an alteration in blood flow within the PDL is produced by the sustained pressure that causes the tooth to shift position within the PDL space, compressing the ligament in some areas while stretching it in others. Blood flow is decreased where the PDL is compressed (Figure 9-4), while it usually is maintained or increased where the PDL is under tension (Figure 9-5). If regions of the PDL are overstretched, blood flow may be decreased transiently. Alterations in blood flow quickly create changes in the chemical environment. For instance, oxygen levels certainly would fall in the compressed area, but might increase on the tension side, and the relative proportions of other metabolites would also change in a matter of minutes. These chemical changes, acting either directly or by stimulating the release of other biologically

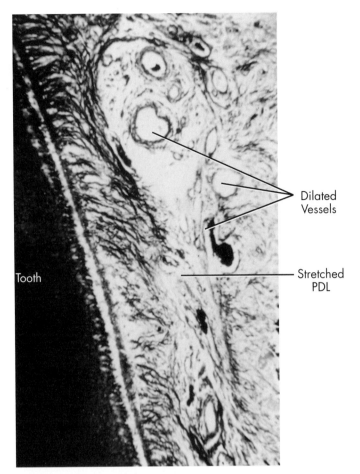

FIGURE 9-5   On the side away from the direction of tooth movement, the PDL space is enlarged and blood vessels dilate. In this vertical section from an animal perfused with India ink at the time of death, the tooth is on the left. Expanded vessels that are only partially filled can be seen on the tension side of the PDL. (Courtesy Dr. F.E. Khouw.)

TABLE 9-2   *Physiologic Response to Sustained Pressure Against a Tooth*

Time		Event
Light pressure	**Heavy pressure**	
< 1 sec		PDL* fluid incompressible, alveolar bone bends, piezoelectric signal generated
1-2 sec		PDL fluid expressed, tooth moves within PDL space
3-5 sec		Blood vessels within PDL partially compressed on pressure side, dilated on tension side; PDL fibers and cells mechanically distorted
Minutes		Blood flow altered, oxygen tension begins to change; prostaglandins and cytokines released
Hours		Metabolic changes occurring: chemical messengers affect cellular activity, enzyme levels change
~4 hours		Increased cAMP levels detectable, cellular differentiation begins within PDL
~2 days		Tooth movement beginning as osteoclasts/osteoblasts remodel bony socket
	3-5 sec	Blood vessels within PDL occluded on pressure side
	Minutes	Blood flow cut off to compressed PDL area
	Hours	Cell death in compressed area
	3-5 days	Cell differentiation in adjacent narrow spaces, undermining resorption begins
	7-14 days	Undermining resorption removes lamina dura adjacent to compressed PDL, tooth movement occurs

*PDL, periodontal ligament.

active agents, then would stimulate cellular differentiation and activity. In essence, this view of tooth movement shows three stages: (1) alterations in blood flow associated with pressure within the PDL, (2) the formation and/or release of chemical messengers, and (3) activation of cells (Table 9-2).

Effects of Force Magnitude

The heavier the sustained pressure, the greater should be the reduction in blood flow through compressed areas of the PDL, up to the point that the vessels are totally collapsed and no further blood flows (Figure 9-6). That this theoretic sequence actually occurs has been demonstrated in animal experiments, in which increasing the force against a tooth causes decreasing perfusion of the PDL on the compression side (see Figures 9-4 and 9-5).[11] Let us consider the time course of events after application of orthodontic force, contrasting what happens with heavy vs. light force (see Table 9-2).

When light but prolonged force is applied to a tooth, blood flow through the partially compressed PDL decreases as soon as fluids are expressed from the PDL space and the tooth moves in its socket (i.e., in a few seconds). Within a few hours at most, the resulting change in the chemical environment produces a different pattern of cellular activity. Animal experiments indicate that increased levels of cyclic adenosine monophosphate (AMP), the "second messenger" for many important cellular functions including differentiation, appear after about 4 hours of sustained pressure.[12] This amount of time to produce a response correlates rather well with the human response to removable appliances. If a removable appliance is worn

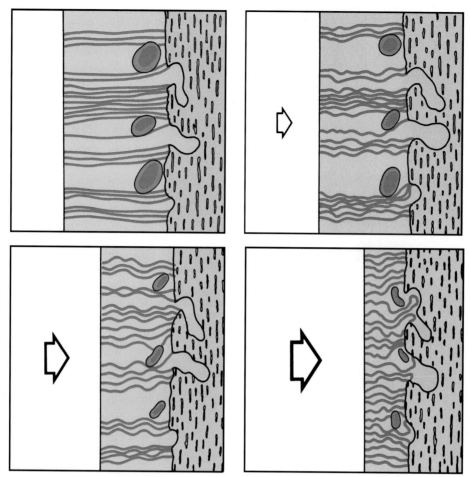

FIGURE 9-6 Diagrammatic representation of the increasing compression of blood vessels as pressure increases in the PDL. At a certain magnitude of continuous pressure, blood vessels are totally occluded and a sterile necrosis of PDL tissue ensues.

less than 4 to 6 hours per day, it will produce no orthodontic effects. Above this duration threshold, tooth movement does occur.

Until recently, very little was known about what happened in the first hours after sustained force was placed against a tooth, between the onset of pressure and tension in the PDL and the appearance of second messengers a few hours later. Experiments have shown that prostaglandin and interleukin-1 beta levels increase within the PDL within a short time after the application of pressure, and it now seems clear that prostaglandin E is an important mediator of the cellular response.[13] Changes in cell shape probably play a role. There is some evidence that prostaglandins are released when cells are mechanically deformed (i.e., prostaglandin release may be a primary rather than a secondary response to pressure).[14] It is likely that mobilization of membrane phospholipids, which leads to the formation of inositol phosphates, is another pathway toward the eventual cellular response.[15] Other chemical messengers, particularly members of the cytokine family but also nitric oxide (NO) and other regulators of cellular activity, also are involved.[16] Since drugs of various types

can affect both prostaglandin levels and other potential chemical messengers, it is clear that pharmacologic modification of the response to orthodontic force is more than just a theoretic possibility (see the discussion on p. 306 of drug interactions with orthodontic treatment).

For a tooth to move, osteoclasts must be formed so that they can remove bone from the area adjacent to the compressed part of the PDL. Osteoblasts also are needed to form new bone on the tension side and remodel resorbed areas on the pressure side. Prostaglandin E has the interesting property of stimulating both osteoclastic and osteoblastic activity, making it particularly suitable as a mediator of tooth movement. If parathyroid hormone is injected, osteoclasts can be induced in only a few hours, but the response is much slower when mechanical deformation of the PDL is the stimulus, and it can be up to 48 hours before the first osteoclasts appear within and adjacent to the compressed PDL. Studies of cellular kinetics indicate that they arrive in two waves, implying that some (the first wave) may be derived from a local cell population, while others (the larger second wave) are brought in from distant areas via blood flow.[17] These cells attack the adjacent lamina dura, remov-

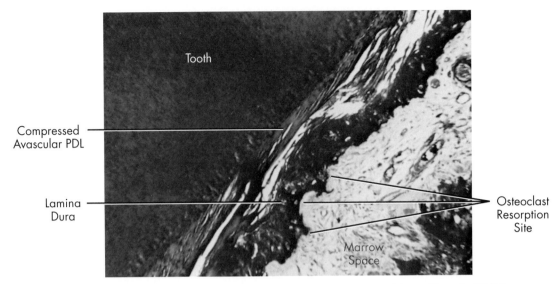

FIGURE 9-7   Histologic specimen of compressed PDL area after several days. When the PDL is compressed to the point that blood flow is totally cut off, differentiation of osteoclasts within the PDL space is not possible. After a delay of several days, osteoclasts within adjacent marrow spaces attack the underside of the lamina dura in the process called *undermining resorption*. (Courtesy Dr. F.E. Khouw.)

ing bone in the process of "frontal resorption," and tooth movement begins soon thereafter. At the same time, but lagging somewhat behind so that the PDL space becomes enlarged, osteoblasts (recruited locally from progenitor cells in the PDL) form bone on the tension side and begin remodeling activity on the pressure side.

The course of events is different if the sustained force against the tooth is great enough to totally occlude blood vessels and cut off the blood supply to an area within the PDL. When this happens, rather than cells within the compressed area of the PDL being stimulated to develop into osteoclasts, a sterile necrosis ensues within the compressed area. In clinical orthodontics it is difficult to avoid pressure that produces at least some avascular areas in the PDL, and it has been suggested that releasing pressure against a tooth at intervals, while maintaining the pressure for enough hours to produce the biologic response, could help in maintaining tissue vitality. Animal experiments support this hypothesis.[18] At present, however, there is no practical way to implement this approach. It is possible in the future that interrupted force of this type will become clinically useful, if methods for activating and de-activating springs can be worked out.

Because of its histologic appearance as the cells disappear, an avascular area in the PDL traditionally has been referred to as *hyalinized* (see Figure 9-4). Despite the name, the process has nothing to do with the formation of hyaline connective tissue but represents the inevitable loss of all cells when the blood supply is totally cut off. When this happens, remodeling of bone bordering the necrotic area of the PDL must be accomplished by cells derived from adjacent undamaged areas.

After a delay of several days, cellular elements begin to invade the necrotic (hyalinized) area. More importantly, os-

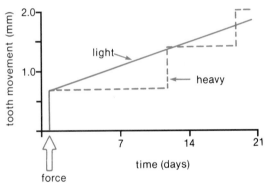

FIGURE 9-8   Diagrammatic representation of the time course of tooth movement with frontal resorption vs. undermining resorption. With frontal resorption, a steady attack on the outer surface of the lamina dura results in smooth continuous tooth movement. With undermining resorption, there is a delay until the bone adjacent to the tooth can be removed. At that point, the tooth "jumps" to a new position, and if heavy force is maintained, there will again be a delay until a second round of undermining resorption can occur.

teoclasts appear within the adjacent bone marrow spaces and begin an attack on the underside of the bone immediately adjacent to the necrotic PDL area (Figure 9-7). This process is appropriately described as *undermining resorption*, since the attack is from the underside of the lamina dura. When hyalinization and undermining resorption occur, an inevitable delay in tooth movement results. This is caused first by a delay in stimulating differentiation of cells within the marrow spaces, and second, because a considerable thickness of bone must be removed from the underside before any tooth movement can take place. The different time course of tooth movement when frontal resorption is compared with undermining resorption is shown graphically in Figure 9-8.

Not only is tooth movement more efficient when areas of PDL necrosis are avoided but pain is also lessened. However, even with light forces, small avascular areas are likely to develop in the PDL and tooth movement will be delayed until these can be removed by undermining resorption. The smooth progression of tooth movement with light force shown in Figure 9-8 may be an unattainable ideal when continuous force is used. In clinical practice, tooth movement usually proceeds in a more stepwise fashion because of the inevitable areas of undermining resorption. Nevertheless, too much force is not helpful.

Effects of Force Distribution and Types of Tooth Movement

From the previous discussion, it is apparent that the optimum force levels for orthodontic tooth movement should be just high enough to stimulate cellular activity without completely occluding blood vessels in the PDL. Both the amount of force delivered to a tooth and also the area of the PDL over which that force is distributed are important in determining the biologic effect. The PDL response is determined not by force alone, but by force per unit area, or pressure. Since the distribution of force within the PDL, and therefore the pressure, differs with different types of tooth movement, it is necessary to specify the type of tooth movement as well as the amount of force in discussing optimum force levels for orthodontic purposes.

The simplest form of orthodontic movement is tipping. Tipping movements are produced when a single force (e.g., a spring extending from a removable appliance) is applied against the crown of a tooth. When this is done, the tooth rotates around its "center of resistance," a point located about halfway down the root. (A further discussion of the center of resistance and its control follows in Chapter 10.) When the tooth rotates in this fashion, the PDL is compressed near the root apex on the same side as the spring and at the crest of the alveolar bone on the opposite side from the spring (Figure 9-9). Maximum pressure in the PDL is created at the alveolar crest and at the root apex. Progressively less pressure is created as the center of resistance is approached, and there is minimum pressure at that point.

In tipping, only one-half the PDL area that could be loaded actually is. As shown in Figure 9-9, the "loading diagram" consists of two triangles, covering half the total PDL area. On the other hand, pressure in the two areas where it is concentrated is high in relation to the force applied to the crown. For this reason, forces used to tip teeth must be kept quite low. Both experiments with animals and clinical experience with humans suggest that tipping forces should not exceed approximately 50 gm.

If two forces are applied simultaneously to the crown of a tooth, the tooth can be moved bodily (translated) (i.e., the root apex and crown move in the same direction the same amount). In this case, the total PDL area is loaded uniformly (Figure 9-10). It is apparent that to produce the same pressure in the PDL and therefore the same biologic response, twice as much force would be required for bodily movement as for tipping. To move a tooth so that it is partially tipped and partially translated would require forces intermediate between those needed for pure tipping and bodily movement (Table 9-3).

TABLE 9-3   *Optimum Forces for Orthodontic Tooth Movement*

Type of movement	Force* (gm)
Tipping	35-60
Bodily movement (translation)	70-120
Root uprighting	50-100
Rotation	35-60
Extrusion	35-60
Intrusion	10-20

*Values depend in part on the size of the tooth; smaller values appropriate for incisors, higher values for multirooted posterior teeth.

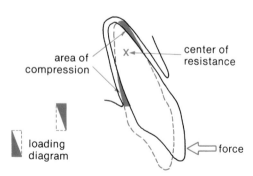

FIGURE 9-9   Application of a single force to the crown of a tooth creates rotation around a point approximately halfway down the root. Heavy pressure is felt at the root apex and at the crest of the alveolar bone, but pressure decreases to zero at the center of resistance. The loading diagram, therefore, consists of two triangles as shown.

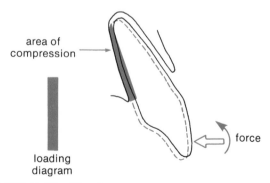

FIGURE 9-10   Translation or bodily movement of a tooth requires that the PDL space be loaded uniformly from alveolar crest to apex, creating a rectangular loading diagram. Twice as much force applied to the crown of the tooth would be required to produce the same pressure within the PDL for bodily movement as compared with tipping.

In theory, forces to produce rotation of a tooth around its long axis could be much larger than those to produce other tooth movements, since the force could be distributed over the entire PDL rather than over a narrow vertical strip. In fact, however, it is essentially impossible to apply a rotational force so that the tooth does not also tip in its socket, and when this happens, an area of compression is created just as in any other tipping movement. For this reason, appropriate forces for rotation are similar to those for tipping.

Extrusion and intrusion are also special cases. Extrusive movements ideally would produce no areas of compression within the PDL, only tension. Like rotation, this is probably more a theoretic than a practical possibility, since if the tooth tipped at all while being extruded, areas of compression would be created. Even if compressed areas could be avoided, heavy forces in pure tension would be undesirable unless the goal was to extract the tooth rather than to bring alveolar bone along with the tooth. Extrusive forces, like rotation, should be of about the same magnitude as those for tipping.

For many years it was considered essentially impossible to produce orthodontic intrusion of teeth. Clinically successful intrusion has been demonstrated in recent years, and it has become clear that doing this requires careful control of force magnitude so that very light forces are applied to the teeth. Light force is required for intrusion because the force will be concentrated in a small area at the tooth apex (Figure 9-11). As with extrusion, the tooth probably will tip somewhat as it is intruded, but the loading diagram nevertheless will show high force concentration at the apex. Only if the force is kept very light can intrusion be expected.

Effects of Force Duration and Force Decay

The key to producing orthodontic tooth movement is the application of sustained force, which does not mean that the force must be absolutely continuous. It does mean that the force must be present for a considerable percentage of the time, certainly hours rather than minutes per day. As we have noted previously, animal experiments suggest that only after force is maintained for approximately 4 hours do cyclic nucleotide levels in the PDL increase, indicating that this duration of pressure is required to produce the "second messengers" needed to stimulate cellular differentiation.

Clinical experience suggests that there is a threshold for force duration in humans in the 4-8 hour range, and that increasingly effective tooth movement is produced if force is maintained for longer durations. Although no firm experimental data are available, a plot of efficiency of tooth movement as a function of force duration would probably look like Figure 9-12. Continuous forces, produced by fixed appliances that are not affected by what the patient does, produce more tooth movement than removable appliances unless the removable appliance is present almost all the time. Removable appliances worn for decreasing fractions of time produce decreasing amounts of tooth movement. If the idea of providing brief intervals of no pressure and resumed blood flow (to improve the vitality of PDL tissues) is ever to be used clinically, it will be necessary to modify fixed appliances to do this. With removable appliances, not only are patients too unreliably compliant, the two-point contacts on teeth that are needed to control tooth movement (see Chapter 10) are too difficult to produce.

Duration of force has another aspect, related to how force magnitude changes as the tooth responds by moving. Only in theory is it possible to make a perfect spring, one that would deliver the same force day after day, no matter how much or how little the tooth moved in response to that force. In reality, some decline in force magnitude (i.e., force decay) is noted with even the springiest device after the tooth has moved a short distance (though with the new nickel-titanium materials discussed in Chapter 10, the decrease is amazingly small). With many orthodontic devices,

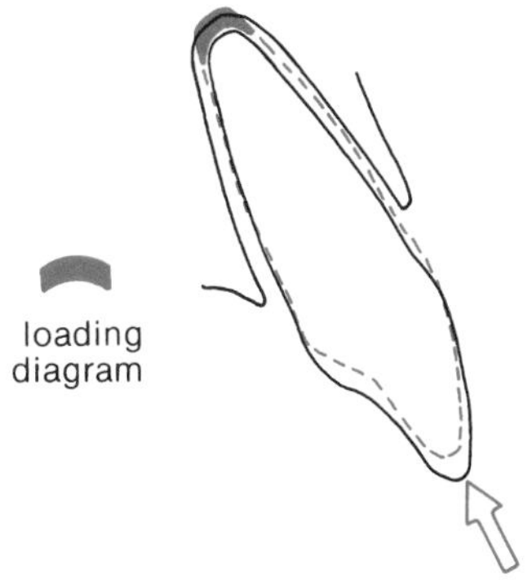

FIGURE 9-11 When a tooth is intruded, the force is concentrated over a small area at the apex. For this reason, extremely light forces are needed to produce appropriate pressure within the PDL during intrusion.

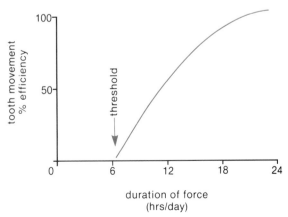

FIGURE 9-12 Theoretic plot of tooth movement efficiency versus duration of force in hours per day. Continuous force, 24 hours per day, produces the most efficient tooth movement, but successful tooth movement can be produced by shorter durations, with a threshold at about 6 hours.

the force may drop all the way to zero. From this perspective, orthodontic force duration is classified (Figure 9-13) by the rate of decay as:

- Continuous—force maintained at some appreciable fraction of the original from one patient visit to the next
- Interrupted—force levels decline to zero between activations

Both continuous and interrupted forces can be produced by fixed appliances that are constantly present.

- Intermittent—force levels decline abruptly to zero intermittently, when the orthodontic appliance is removed by the patient or perhaps when a fixed appliance is temporarily deactivated, and then return to the original level some time later. When tooth movement occurs, force levels will decrease as they would with a fixed appliance (i.e., the intermittent force can also become interrupted between adjustments of the appliance).

Intermittent forces are produced by all patient-activated appliances, such as removable plates, headgear, and elastics. Forces generated during normal function (chewing, swallowing, speaking, etc.) can be viewed as a special case of intermittently applied forces, most of which are not maintained for enough hours per day to have significant effects on the position of the teeth.

There is an important interaction between force magnitude and how rapidly the force declines as the tooth responds. Consider first the effect of a nearly continuous force. If this force is quite light, a relatively smooth progression of tooth movement will result from frontal resorption. If the continuous force is heavy, however, tooth movement will be delayed until undermining resorption can remove the bone necessary to allow the tooth movement. At that time, the tooth will change its position rapidly, and the constant force will again compress the tissues, preventing repair of the PDL and creating the need for further undermining resorption, and so on. Such a heavy continuous force can be quite destructive to both the periodontal structures and the tooth itself (as we discuss in more detail below).

Consider now the effect of forces that decay fairly rapidly, so that the force declines to zero after the tooth moves only a short distance. If the initial force level is relatively light, the tooth will move a small amount by frontal resorption and then will remain in that position until the appliance is activated again. If the force level is heavy enough to produce undermining resorption, the tooth will move when the undermining resorption is complete. Then, since the force has dropped to zero at that point, it will remain in that position until the next activation. Although the original force is heavy, after the tooth moves there is a period for regeneration and repair of the PDL before force is applied again.

Theoretically, there is no doubt that light continuous forces produce the most efficient tooth movement. Despite the clinician's best efforts to keep forces light enough to produce only frontal resorption, some areas of undermining resorption are probably produced in every clinical patient. The heavier forces that produce this response are physiologically acceptable, only if force levels decline so that there is a period of repair and regeneration before the next activation, or if the force decreases at least to the point that no second and third rounds of undermining resorption occur.

Heavy continuous forces are to be avoided; heavy intermittent forces, though less efficient, can be clinically acceptable. To say it another way: the more perfect the spring in the sense of its ability to provide continuous force, the more careful the clinician must be that only light force is applied. Some of the cruder springs used in orthodontic treatment have the paradoxic virtue of producing forces that rapidly decline to zero and are thus incapable of inflicting the biologic damage that can occur from heavy continuous forces. Several clinical studies have indicated that heavy force applications may produce more tooth movement than lighter ones, an apparently paradoxic result that can be understood from consideration of force decay characteristics.

Experience has shown that orthodontic appliances should not be reactivated more frequently than at 3-week intervals. A 4-week appointment cycle is more typical in clinical practice. Undermining resorption requires 7 to 14 days (longer on the initial application of force, shorter thereafter). When this is the mode of tooth movement and when force levels decline rapidly, tooth movement is essentially complete in this length of time. The wisdom of the interval between adjustments now becomes clear. If the appliance is springy and light forces produce continuous frontal resorption, there is no need for further activation. If the appliance is stiffer and undermining resorption occurs, but then the force drops to zero, the tooth movement occurs in the first 10 days or so, and there is an equal or longer period for PDL regeneration and repair before force is applied again. This repair phase is highly desirable and needed with many appliances. Activating an appliance too frequently, short circuiting the repair process, can produce damage to the teeth or bone that a longer appointment cycle would have prevented or at least minimized.

Drug Effects on the Response to Orthodontic Force

It is quite possible that pharmacologic agents to manipulate tooth movement in both directions will come into common use. At present, agents that stimulate tooth movement are unlikely to be encountered, although under some circumstances vitamin D administration can enhance the response to orthodontic force. Direct injection of prostaglandin into the periodontal ligament has been shown to increase the rate of tooth movement, but this is quite painful (a bee sting is essentially an injection of prostaglandin) and not very practical. Drugs that inhibit tooth movement, however, already are encountered frequently, though not yet prescribed for their tooth-stabilizing effect.

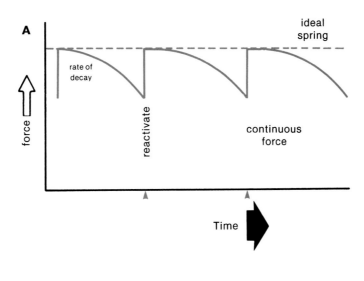

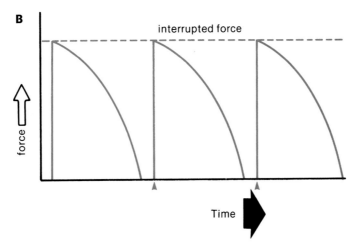

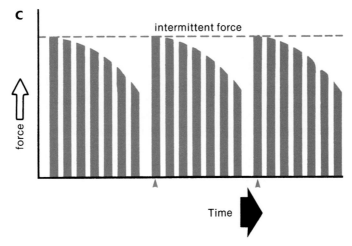

FIGURE 9-13   Diagrammatic representation of force decay. **A,** An ideal spring would maintain the same amount of force regardless of distance a tooth had moved, but with real springs the force decays at least somewhat as tooth movement occurs. Forces that are maintained between activations of an orthodontic appliance, even though the force declines, are defined as continuous. In contrast, **B,** interrupted forces drop to zero between activations. **C,** Intermittent forces fall to zero when a removable appliance is taken out, only to resume when the appliance is reinserted into the mouth. These forces also decay as tooth movement occurs.

Two types of drugs are known to depress the response to orthodontic force and may influence current treatment: the bisphosphonates used in treatment of osteoporosis (e.g., alendronate [Fosamax]), and prostaglandin inhibitors (e.g., especially the more potent members of this group that are used in treatment of arthritis, like indomethacin).

Osteoporosis is a problem particularly in postmenopausal females but is associated with aging in both sexes. Medication for this purpose, therefore, is encountered almost entirely in older adult orthodontic patients. Estrogen therapy, which is used frequently to prevent loss of bone in older women, has little or no impact on orthodontic treatment, but pharmacologic agents that inhibit bone resorption are a potential problem. At present bisphosphonates, synthetic analogues of pyrophosphate that bind to hydroxyapatite in bone, are the major class of drugs of this type. They act as specific inhibitors of osteoclast-mediated bone resorption,[19] so it is not surprising that the bone remodeling necessary for tooth movement is slower in patients on this medication. If orthodontic treatment were necessary in an older woman taking one of these agents, it would be worthwhile to explore with her physician the possibility of switching to estrogen, at least temporarily.

If prostaglandin E plays an important role in the cascade of signals that leads to tooth movement, one would expect inhibitors of its activity to affect tooth movement. Drugs that affect prostaglandin activity fall into two categories: (1) corticosteroids and nonsteroidal antiinflammatory drugs (NSAID) that interfere with prostaglandin synthesis, and (2) other agents that have mixed agonistic and antagonistic effects on various prostaglandins. In the body, prostaglandins are formed from arachidonic acid, which in turn is derived from phospholipids. Corticosteroids reduce prostaglandin synthesis by inhibiting the formation of arachidonic acid; NSAIDs inhibit the conversion of arachidonic acid to prostaglandins.

Both children and adults on chronic steroid therapy may be encountered, and the possibility of difficult tooth movement in these patients must be kept in mind. The fact that analgesics often are prostaglandin inhibitors raises the interesting possibility that the medication used by many patients to control pain after orthodontic appointments could interfere with tooth movement. Fortunately, although potent prostaglandin inhibitors like indomethacin can inhibit tooth movement,[20] the common analgesics seem to have little or no inhibiting effect on tooth movement at the dose levels used with orthodontic patients.

Several other classes of drugs can affect prostaglandin levels, and therefore could affect the response to orthodontic force. Tricyclic antidepressants (doxepin, amitriptyline, imipramine), anti-arrhythmic agents (procaine), antimalarial drugs (quinine, quinidine, chloroquine), and methyl xanthines fall into this category. In addition, the anticonvulsant drug phenytoin has been reported to decrease tooth movement in rats, and some tetracyclines (e.g., doxycycline) inhibit osteoclast recruitment, an effect similar to bisphosphonates. It is possible that unusual responses to orthodontic force could be encountered in patients taking any of these medications.

ANCHORAGE AND ITS CONTROL

Anchorage: Resistance to Unwanted Tooth Movement

The term *anchorage*, in its orthodontic application, is defined in an unusual way: the definition as "resistance to unwanted tooth movement" includes a statement of what the dentist desires. The usage, though unusual, is clearest when presented this way. The dentist or orthodontist always constructs an appliance to produce certain desired tooth movements. For every (desired) action there is an equal and opposite reaction. Inevitably, reaction forces can move other teeth as well if the appliance contacts them. Anchorage, then, is the resistance to reaction forces that is provided (usually) by other teeth, or (sometimes) by the palate, head or neck (via extraoral force), or implants in bone. At this point, let us focus on controlling unwanted tooth movement. In planning orthodontic therapy, it is simply not possible to consider only the teeth whose movement is desired. Reciprocal effects throughout the dental arches must be carefully analyzed, evaluated, and controlled. An important aspect of treatment is maximizing the tooth movement that is desired, while minimizing undesirable side effects.

Relationship of Tooth Movement to Force

An obvious strategy for anchorage control would be to concentrate the force needed to produce tooth movement where it was desired, and then to dissipate the reaction force over as many other teeth as possible, keeping the pressure in the PDL of anchor teeth as low as possible. A threshold, below which pressure would produce no reaction, could provide perfect anchorage control, since it would only be necessary to be certain that the threshold for tooth movement was not reached for teeth in the anchorage unit. A differential response to pressure, so that heavier pressure produced more tooth movement than lighter pressure, would make it possible to move some teeth more than others even though some undesired tooth movement occurred.

In fact, the threshold for tooth movement appears to be quite low, but there is a differential response to pressure, and so this strategy of "divide and conquer" is reasonably effective. As Figure 9-14 indicates, teeth behave as if orthodontic movement is proportional to the magnitude of the pressure, up to a point. When that point is reached, the amount of tooth movement becomes more or less independent of the magnitude of the pressure, so that a broad plateau of orthodontically effective pressure is created.[21]

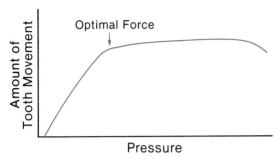

FIGURE 9-14 Theoretic representation of the relationship of pressure within the periodontal ligament to the amount of tooth movement. Pressure in the PDL is determined by the force applied to a tooth divided by the area of the PDL over which that force is distributed. The threshold for tooth movement is very small. Tooth movement increases as pressure increases up to a point, remains at about the same level over a broad range, and then may actually decline with extremely heavy pressure. The best definition of the optimum force for orthodontic purposes is the lightest force that produces a maximum or near-maximum response (i.e., that brings pressure in the PDL to the edge of the nearly-constant portion of the response curve). The magnitude of the optimum force will vary depending on the way it is distributed in the PDL (i.e., is different for different types of tooth movement [tipping, bodily movement, intrusion, etc.]).

The optimum force level for orthodontic movement is the lightest force and resulting pressure that produces a near-maximum response (i.e., at the edge of the plateau). Forces greater than that, though equally effective in producing tooth movement, would be unnecessarily traumatic and, as we will see, unnecessarily stressful to anchorage.

Anchorage Situations

From this background, we can now define several anchorage situations:

Reciprocal Tooth Movement. In a reciprocal situation, the forces applied to teeth and to arch segments are equal, and so is the force distribution in the PDL. A simple example is what would occur if two maxillary central incisors separated by a diastema were connected by an active spring (Figure 9-15). The essentially identical teeth would feel the same force distributed in the same way through the PDL and would move toward each other by the same amount.

A somewhat similar situation would arise if a spring were placed across a first premolar extraction site, pitting the central incisor, lateral incisor, and canine in the anterior arch segment against the second premolar and first molar posteriorly. Whether this technique would really produce reciprocal tooth movement requires some thought. Certainly the same force would be felt by the three anterior teeth and the two posterior teeth, since the action of the spring on one segment has an equal and opposite reaction on the other. Reciprocal movement would require the same total PDL area over which the force was distributed.

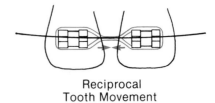
Reciprocal
Tooth Movement

FIGURE 9-15 Reciprocal tooth movement is produced when two teeth or resistance units of equal size pull against each other, as in this example of the reciprocal closure of a maxillary midline diastema.

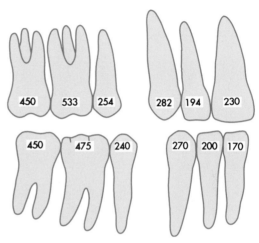

FIGURE 9-16 The "anchorage value" of any tooth is roughly equivalent to its root surface area. As this diagram shows, the first molar and second premolar in each arch are approximately equal in surface area to the canine and two incisors. (Modified from Freeman DC: *Root surface area related to anchorage in the Begg technique*, Memphis, 1965, University of Tennessee Dept. of Orthodontics, M.S. Thesis.)

Conceptually, the "anchorage value" of a tooth, that is, its resistance to movement, can be thought of as a function of its root surface area, which is the same as its PDL area. The larger the root, the greater the area over which a force can be distributed, and vice versa. As Figure 9-16 shows, the PDL area for the two posterior teeth in this example is slightly larger than the total anterior PDL area. Therefore with a simple spring connecting the segments, the anterior teeth would move slightly more than the posterior teeth. The movement would not be truly reciprocal but would be close to it.

Reinforced Anchorage. Continuing with the extraction site example: if it was desired to differentially retract the anterior teeth, the anchorage of the posterior teeth could be reinforced by adding the second molar to the posterior unit (see Figure 9-16). This would change the ratio of the root surface areas so that there would be relatively more pressure in the PDL of the anterior teeth, and therefore relatively more retraction of the anterior segment than forward movement of the posterior segment.

Note that reinforcing anchorage by adding more resistance units is effective because with more teeth (or extraoral

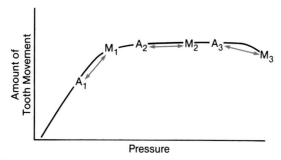

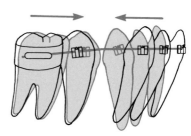

FIGURE 9-17 Consider the response of anchor teeth (A on the chart) and teeth to be moved (M) in three circumstances. In each case, the pressure in the PDL of the anchor teeth is less than the pressure in the PDL of the teeth to be moved because there are more teeth in the anchor unit. In the first case (A1-M1), the pressure for the teeth to be moved is optimal, whereas the pressure in the anchor unit is suboptimal, and the anchor teeth move less (anchorage is preserved). In the second case (A2-M2), although the pressure for the anchor teeth is less than for the teeth to be moved, both are on the plateau of the pressure-response curve, and the anchor teeth can be expected to move as much as the teeth that are desired to move (anchorage is lost). With extremely high force (A3-M3), the anchor teeth might move more than the teeth it was desired to move. Although the third possibility is theoretic and may not be encountered clinically, both the first and second situations are seen in clinical orthodontics. This principle explains the efficacy of light forces in controlling anchorage, and why heavy force destroys anchorage.

FIGURE 9-18 Displacement of anchor teeth can be minimized by arranging the force system so that the anchor teeth must move bodily if they move at all, while movement teeth are allowed to tip, as in this example of retracting incisors by tipping them posteriorly. The approach is called "stationary anchorage." In this example, treatment is not complete because the roots of the lingually tipped incisors will have to be uprighted at a later stage, but two-stage treatment with tipping followed by uprighting can be used as a means of controlling anchorage. Distributing the force over a larger PDL area of the anchor teeth reduces pressure there.

structures) in the anchorage, the reaction force is distributed over a larger PDL area. This reduces the pressure on the anchor units, moving them down the slope of the pressure-response curve. Now the shape of the pressure-response curve becomes important. Keeping the force light has two virtues. Not only does it minimize trauma and pain (see p. 312), but also it makes it possible to create anchorage by taking advantage of different PDL areas in the anchor segments. As Figure 9-17 illustrates, too much force destroys the effectiveness of reinforced anchorage by pulling the anchor teeth up onto the flatter portion of the pressure-response curve. Then the clinician is said to have slipped, burned or blown the anchorage by moving the anchor teeth too much.

Stationary Anchorage. The term *stationary anchorage*, traditionally used though inherently less descriptive than the term *reinforced anchorage*, refers to the advantage that can be obtained by pitting bodily movement of one group of teeth against tipping of another (Figure 9-18). Using our same example of a premolar extraction site, if the appliance were arranged so that the anterior teeth could tip lingually while the posterior teeth could only move bodily, the optimum pressure for the anterior segment would be produced by about half as much force as if the anterior teeth were to be retracted bodily. This would mean that the reaction force distributed over the posterior teeth would be reduced by half, and as a consequence, these teeth would move half as much.

If PDL areas were equal, tipping the anterior segment while holding the posterior segment for bodily movement would have the effect of doubling the amount of anterior retraction compared with posterior forward movement. It is important to note again, however, that successful implementation of this strategy requires light force. If the force were large enough to bring the posterior teeth into their optimum movement range, it would no longer matter whether the anterior segment tipped or was moved bodily. Using too much force would disastrously undermine this method of anchorage control.

Differential Effect of Very Large Forces. If tooth movement were actually impeded by very high levels of pressure, it might be possible to structure an anchorage situation so that there was more movement of the arch segment with the larger PDL area. This result could happen, of course, if such high force were used that the smaller segment was placed beyond the greatest tooth movement range, while the larger segment was still in it (see Figure 9-17). Because the effect would be highly traumatic, it would be an undesirable way to deliberately manage anchorage.

In fact, it is not certain that the amount of tooth movement in response to applied force really decreases with very high force levels in any circumstance, and so this type of differential movement may not really exist. By using too much force, however, it is certainly possible to produce more movement of the anchor segment than was expected, even if the mechanism is merely a differential movement of the anchor segment up the slope of the pressure-response curve rather than a decline in the response of the movement segment. Differential force is understood best in terms of the plateau portion of the curve in Figures 9-14 and 9-17, not the questionable decline at the far right.

Cortical Anchorage. A final consideration in anchorage control is the different response of cortical compared with medullary bone. Cortical bone is more resistant

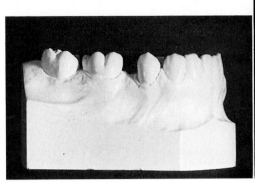
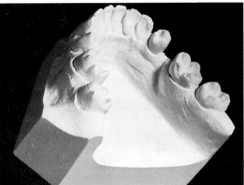

FIGURE 9-19 Loss of alveolar bone at an old extraction site can create an area of cortical bone between adjacent teeth, as the alveolar process narrows. This is one situation in which "cortical anchorage" definitely can be a factor. Closing such an extraction site is extremely difficult because of the resistance of cortical bone to remodeling.

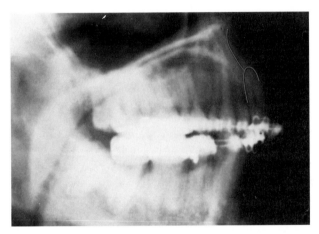

FIGURE 9-20 Extreme tipping of maxillary incisor teeth from excessive and poorly controlled orthodontic forces. In this patient, the apices of all four maxillary incisors were carried through the labial cortical plate, and pulp vitality was lost.

to resorption, and tooth movement is slowed when a root contacts it. Some authors have advocated torquing the roots of posterior teeth outward against the cortical plate as a way to inhibit their mesial movement when extraction spaces are to be closed.[22] Since the mesial movement would be along rather than against the cortical plate, it is doubtful that this technique greatly augments anchorage (although it has the potential to create root resorption—see p. 314). However, a layer of dense cortical bone that has formed within the alveolar process can certainly affect tooth movement. This situation may be encountered at an old extraction site, for example, in an adult in whom a molar or premolar was lost many years previously (Figure 9-19). It can be very difficult to close such an extraction site, because tooth movement is slowed to a minimum as the roots encounter cortical bone along the resorbed alveolar ridge.[23]

As a general rule, torquing movements are limited by the facial and lingual cortical plates. If a root is persistently

forced against either of these cortical plates, tooth movement is greatly slowed and root resorption is likely (see p. 314), but penetration of the cortical bone may occur. Although it is possible to torque the root of a tooth labially or lingually out of the bone (Figure 9-20), fortunately, it is difficult to do so.

DELETERIOUS EFFECTS OF ORTHODONTIC FORCE

Mobility and Pain Related to Orthodontic Treatment

Orthodontic tooth movement requires not only a remodeling of bone adjacent to the teeth, but also a reorganization of the PDL itself. Fibers become detached from the bone and cementum, then reattach at a later time. Radiographically, it can be observed that the PDL space widens during orthodontic tooth movement. The combination of a wider ligament space and a somewhat disorganized ligament means that some increase in mobility will be observed in every patient.

A moderate increase in mobility is an expected response to orthodontic treatment. The heavier the force, however, the greater the amount of undermining resorption expected, and the greater the mobility that will develop. Excessive mobility is an indication that excessive forces are being encountered. This may occur because the patient is clenching or grinding against a tooth that has moved into a position of traumatic occlusion. If a tooth becomes extremely mobile during orthodontic treatment, it should be taken out of occlusion and all force should be discontinued until the mobility decreases to moderate levels. Unlike root resorption (see p.314), excessive mobility will usually correct itself without permanent damage.

If heavy pressure is applied to a tooth, pain develops almost immediately as the PDL is literally crushed. There is no excuse for using force levels for orthodontic tooth movement that produce immediate pain of this type. If appropriate orthodontic force is applied, the patient feels little or nothing immediately. Several hours later, however, pain usually appears. The patient feels a mild aching sensation, and the teeth are quite sensitive to pressure, so that biting a hard object hurts. The pain typically lasts for 2 to 4 days, then disappears until the orthodontic appliance is reactivated. At that point, a similar cycle may recur, but for almost all patients, the pain associated with the initial activation of the appliance is the most severe. It is commonly noted that there is a great deal of individual variation in any pain experience, and this is certainly true of orthodontic pain. Some patients report little or no pain even with relatively heavy forces, whereas others experience considerable discomfort with quite light forces.

The pain associated with orthodontic treatment is related to the development of ischemic areas in the PDL that will undergo sterile necrosis (hyalinization). The increased tenderness to pressure suggests inflammation at the apex, and the mild pulpitis that usually appears soon after orthodontic force is applied probably also contributes to the pain. There does seem to be a relationship between the amount of force used and the amount of pain: the greater the force, the greater the pain, all other factors being equal. This is consistent with the concept that ischemic areas in the PDL are the major pain source, since greater force would produce larger areas of ischemia.

If the source of pain is the development of ischemic areas, strategies to temporarily relieve pressure and allow blood flow through compressed areas should help. In fact, if light forces are used, the amount of pain experienced by patients can be decreased by having them engage in repetitive chewing (of gum, a plastic wafer placed between the teeth, or whatever) during the first 8 hours after the orthodontic appliance is activated. Presumably this works by temporarily displacing the teeth enough to allow some blood flow through compressed areas, thereby preventing build-up of metabolic products that stimulate pain receptors. Light forces, however, are the key to minimizing pain as a concomitant of orthodontic treatment.

As we have noted above, many drugs used to control pain have the potential to affect tooth movement because of their effects on prostaglandins. It has been suggested that acetaminophen (Tylenol) should be a better analgesic for orthodontic patients than aspirin or ibuprofen because it acts centrally rather than as a prostaglandin inhibitor,[24] but with any of these agents, no evidence of inhibition of tooth movement in humans has been observed. Nonpharmacologic methods for pain control, including but by no means limited to magnets in the vicinity, would be expected to be effective with some but not all patients with orthodontic pain, just as they are for other types of pain.

It is rare but not impossible for orthodontic patients to develop pain and inflammation of soft tissues, not because of the orthodontic force, but because of an allergic reaction. There are two major culprits when this occurs: a reaction to the latex in gloves or elastics and a reaction to the nickel in stainless steel bands, brackets, and wires. Latex allergies can become so severe as to be life threatening. Extreme care should be taken to avoid using latex products in patients reporting a latex allergy. Nickel is allergenic, and nearly 20% of the U.S. population show some skin reaction to nickel-containing materials (cheap jewelry and earrings).[25] Fortunately, most children with a skin allergy to nickel have no mucosal response to orthodontic appliances and tolerate treatment perfectly well, but some do not. The typical symptoms of nickel allergy in an orthodontic patient are widespread erythema and swelling of oral tissues, developing 1-2 days after treatment is started. For such patients, titanium brackets and tubes can be substituted for stainless steel (see Chapter 12).

Effects on the Pulp

In theory, the application of light sustained force to the crown of a tooth should produce a PDL reaction but should have little if any effect on the pulp. In fact, although pulpal reactions to orthodontic treatment are minimal, there is probably a modest and transient inflammatory response within the pulp, at least at the beginning of treatment.[26] This may contribute to the discomfort that patients often experience for a few days after appliances are activated, but the mild pulpitis has no long-term significance.

There are occasional reports of loss of tooth vitality during orthodontic treatment. Usually there is a history of previous trauma to the tooth, but poor control of orthodontic force also can be the culprit. If a tooth is subjected to heavy continuous force, a sequence of abrupt movements occurs, as undermining resorption allows increasingly large increments of change. A large enough abrupt movement of the root apex could sever the blood vessels as they enter. Loss of vitality has also been observed when incisor teeth were tipped distally to such an extent that the root apex, moving in the opposite direction, was actually moved outside the alveolar process (see Figure 9-20). Again, such movements probably would sever the blood vessels entering the pulp canal.

Since the response of the PDL, not the pulp, is the key element in orthodontic tooth movement, moving endodontically treated teeth is perfectly feasible. Especially in adults receiving adjunctive orthodontic treatment (see Chapter 20), it may be necessary to treat some teeth endodontically, and then reposition them orthodontically. There is no contraindication to this practice. Although some evidence has indicated that endodontically treated teeth are more prone to root resorption during orthodontics than are teeth with normal vitality, the most recent studies suggest that this is not the case.[27] Severe root resorption should not be expected as a consequence of moving a nonvital tooth that has had proper endodontic therapy. One special circumstance is a tooth that experienced severe intrusive trauma and required pulp therapy for that reason. If such a tooth must be repositioned orthodontically, resorption seems less likely if a calcium hydroxide fill is maintained until the tooth movement is completed, and then the definitive root canal filling is placed.[28]

Effects on Root Structure

Orthodontic treatment requires resorption and apposition of bone adjacent to the root structure of teeth. For many years it was thought that the root structure of the teeth was not remodeled in the same way as bone. More recent research has made it plain that when orthodontic forces are applied, there is usually an attack on the cementum of the root, just as there is an attack on adjacent bone, but repair of cementum also occurs.

Rygh and co-workers have shown that cementum adjacent to hyalinized (necrotic) areas of the PDL is "marked" by this contact and that clast cells attack this marked cementum when the PDL area is repaired.[29] This observation helps explain why heavy continuous orthodontic force can lead to severe root resorption. Even with the most careful control of orthodontic force, however, it is difficult to avoid creating some hyalinized areas in the PDL. It is not surprising, therefore, that careful examination of the root surfaces of teeth that have been moved reveals repaired areas of resorption of both cementum and dentin of the root (Figure 9-21). It appears that cementum (and dentin, if resorption penetrates through the cementum) is

removed from the root surface, then cementum is restored in the same way that alveolar bone is removed and then replaced. Root remodeling, in other words, is a constant feature of orthodontic tooth movement, but permanent loss of root structure would occur only if repair did not replace the initially resorbed cementum.

Repair of the damaged root restores its original contours, unless the attack on the root surface produces large defects at the apex that eventually become separated from the root surface (Figure 9-22). Once an island of cementum or dentin has been cut totally free from the root surface, it will be resorbed and will not be replaced. On the other hand, even deep defects in the form of craters into the root surface will be filled in again with cementum once orthodontic movement stops. Therefore permanent loss of root structure related to orthodontic treatment occurs primarily at the apex. Sometimes there is a reduction in the lateral aspect of the root in the apical region.

Shortening of tooth roots during orthodontic treatment occurs in three distinct forms that must be distinguished when the etiology of resorption is considered.

Moderate Generalized Resorption. Despite the potential for repair, careful radiographic examination of individuals who have undergone comprehensive orthodontic treatment shows that most of the teeth show some loss of root length, and this is greater in patients whose treatment duration was longer (Table 9-4). The average shortening of root length of maxillary incisors is somewhat greater than

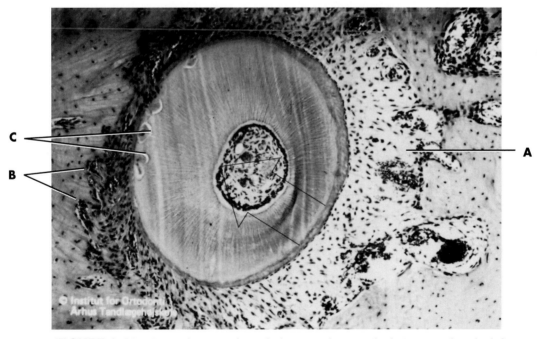

FIGURE 9-21 Coronal section through the root of a premolar being moved to the left (*arrow*). Note the zone of PDL compression to the left and tension to the right. Dilation of blood vessels and osteoblastic activity (**A**) can be seen on the right. Osteoclasts removing bone are present on the left (**B**). Areas of beginning root resorption that will be repaired by later deposition of cementum also can be seen on the left (**C**). (Courtesy Prof. B. Melsen.)

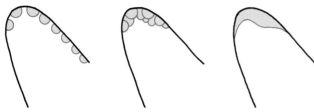

FIGURE 9-22   During tooth movement, clast cells attack cementum as well as bone, creating defects in surface of the roots. During the repair phase, these defects fill back in with cementum. Shortening of the root occurs when cavities coalesce at the apex, so that peninsulas of root structure are cut off as islands. Then the repair process smooths over the new root surface, and a net loss of root length occurs. This is why, although both the sides and the apex of the root experience resorption, roots become shorter but not thinner as a result of orthodontic tooth movement.

TABLE 9-4   *Average Root Length Change*

	Maxillary		Mandibular	
	Serial ext plus	Late ext	Serial ext plus	Late ext
Central Incisor	−1.5	−2.0	−1.0	−1.5
Lateral incisor	−2.0	−2.5	−1.0	−1.0
Canine	−1.0	−1.5	−0.5	−1.0
Second Premolar	−0.5	−1.5	−0.5	−1.5
First molar (mesial)	−0.5	−1.0	−0.5	−1.5

Data from Kennedy OB et al, *Am J Orthod* 84:183, 1983.

for other teeth, but all teeth included in the typical fixed orthodontic appliance show slight average shortening. In the Seattle study from which the data of Table 9-4 were derived, all teeth except upper second molars were banded. Note that these were the only unaffected teeth. Although 90% of maxillary incisors and over half of all teeth show some loss of root length during treatment, for the great majority of the patients, this modest shortening is almost imperceptible and is clinically insignificant.

Occasionally, however, loss of one-third or one-half or more of the root structure is observed in patients who received what seemed to be only routine orthodontic therapy (Figure 9-23). Again, it is important to distinguish between two forms of severe resorption:

Severe Generalized Resorption.   Severe root resorption of all the teeth, fortunately, is rare. Some individuals are prone to root resorption, even without orthodontic treatment—severe generalized resorption has been observed many times in individuals who never were orthodontic patients. If there is evidence of root resorption before orthodontic treatment, the patient is at considerable risk of further resorption during orthodontic treatment, much more so than a patient with no pretreatment resorption. Although hormonal imbalances and other metabolic derangements have been suspected in these susceptible patients, little evidence supports these theories. It was reported in the 1940s that a deficiency of thyroid hormone could lead to generalized root resorption, and occasionally thyroid supplements

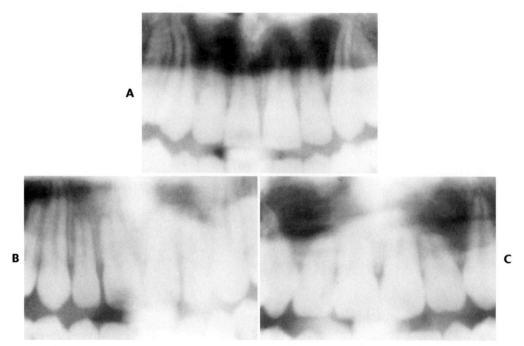

FIGURE 9-23   Root resorption accompanying orthodontic treatment can be placed into three categories as illustrated here for maxillary central and lateral incisors: **A,** category 1, slight blunting; **B,** category 2, moderate resorption, up to ¼ of root length; **C,** category 3, severe resorption, greater than ¼ of root length. See Table 9-5 for date for prevalence of these levels of resorption. (From Kaley JD, Phillips C: *Angle Orthod* 61:125-131, 1991.)

and soft tissue forms in the area.[35] If a tooth is intruded, bone height tends to be lost at the alveolar crest, so that about the same percentage of the root remains embedded in bone as before, even if the intrusion was over a considerable distance.

In most circumstances, this tendency for alveolar bone height to stay at the same level along the root is a therapeutic plus. Occasionally, it would be desirable to change the amount of tooth embedded in bone. For instance, the bone support around periodontally involved teeth could be improved by intruding the teeth and forcing the roots deeper into the bone, if the alveolar bone did not follow the intruding tooth. There are reports of therapeutic benefit from intruding periodontally involved teeth,[36] but the reduced pocketing relates to the formation of a long junctional epithelium, not to reattachment of the PDL or more extensive bony support. On occasion, it is desirable to elongate the root of a fractured tooth, to enable its use as a prosthetic abutment without crown-lengthening surgery (see Chapter 20). If heavy forces are used to extrude a tooth quickly, a relative loss of attachment may occur, but this deliberately nonphysiologic extrusion is at best traumatic and at worst can lead to ankylosis and/or resorption. Physiologic extrusion or intrusion that brings the alveolar bone along with the tooth, followed by surgical recontouring of gingiva and bone, is preferable.[37]

SKELETAL EFFECTS OF ORTHODONTIC FORCE: GROWTH MODIFICATION

Principles in Growth Modification

Orthodontic force applied to the teeth has the potential to radiate outward and affect distant skeletal locations. Orthodontic tooth movement can correct dental malocclusions; if the distant effects could change the pattern of jaw growth, there also would be the possibility of correcting skeletal malocclusions.

Our current knowledge of how and why the jaws grow is covered in some detail in Chapters 2 through 4. In brief summary, the maxilla grows by apposition of new bone at its posterior and superior sutures, in response to being pushed forward by the lengthening cranial base and pulled downward and forward by the growth of the adjacent soft tissues. Tension at the sutures as the maxilla is displaced from its supporting structures appears to be the stimulus for new bone formation. Somewhat similarly, the mandible is pulled downward and forward by the soft tissues in which it is embedded. In response, the condylar process grows upward and backward to maintain the temporomandibular articulation. If this is so, it seems entirely reasonable that pressures resisting the downward and forward movement of either jaw should decrease the amount of growth, while adding to the forces that pull them downward and forward should increase their growth.

The possibility of modifying the growth of the jaws and face in this way has been accepted, rejected, and then accepted again during the past century. Although the extent to which treatment can produce skeletal change remains controversial, the clinical effectiveness of procedures aimed at modifying growth has been demonstrated in recent years. The possibilities for growth modification treatment and the characteristics of patients who would be good candidates for it are described in Chapter 8. Here, the focus is on how the effects on growth are produced.

Effects of Orthodontic Force on the Maxilla and Midface

Teeth erupt and bring alveolar bone with them, a contribution to growth of both jaws that is of great importance in orthodontic treatment. Manipulation and control of tooth eruption is properly considered an aspect of orthodontic tooth movement and therefore has been reviewed in some detail in the section above, but growth of the alveolar process has a major effect on anteroposterior and vertical jaw relationships. The discussion below focuses on skeletal (i.e., non-dentoalveolar) growth and how orthodontic force can affect distant sites. It is important to keep in mind, however, that in treatment of patients, the dentoalveolar and skeletal effects cannot be divorced so readily.

Modification of Maxillary Growth. Besides the dentoalveolar process, the important sites of growth of the maxilla, where it might be possible to alter the expression of growth, are the sutures that attach the maxilla to the zygoma, pterygoid plates, and frontonasal area and separate the middle of the palate. These sutures are similar in some respects to the PDL, but are neither as complex in their structure nor nearly as densely collagenous (Figure 9-25). For modification of excessive maxillary growth, the concept of treatment would be to add a force to oppose the natural force that separates the sutures, preventing the amount of separation that would have occurred (Figure 9-26). For deficient growth, the concept would be to add additional force to the natural force, separating the sutures more than otherwise would have occurred.

It is difficult to measure compression or tension within sutures, and there is no way to know theoretically what is required to alter growth. Clinical experience suggests that moderate amounts of force against the maxillary teeth can impede forward growth of the maxilla, but heavier force is needed for separation of sutures and growth stimulation. When force is applied to the teeth, only a small fraction of the pressure in the PDL is experienced at the sutures, because the area of the sutures is so much larger. For this reason, even the moderate forces recommended for restraint of forward maxillary growth tend to be heavier than those recommended for tooth movement alone. For instance, a force of 250 gm per side (500 gm total) probably is about the minimum for impeding forward movement of the maxilla, and often this force or more is applied only to the first molar teeth via a facebow. Heavier force (up to 1000 gm), usually

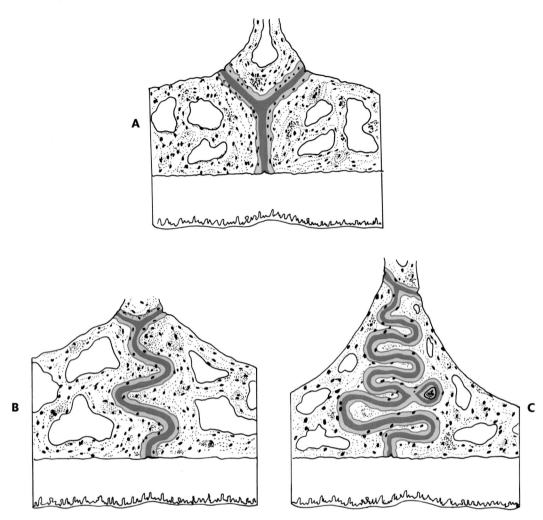

FIGURE 9-25   Like the other sutures of the facial skeleton, the mid-palatal suture becomes increasingly tortuous and interdigitated with increasing age. These diagrams show the typical histologic appearance of the mid-palatal suture in (**A**) infancy, when the suture is almost a straight line; (**B**) childhood (early mixed dentition); and (**C**) early adolescence. In childhood sutural expansion can be accomplished with almost any type of expansion device (e.g., a lingual arch). By early adolescence interdigitation of spicules in the suture has reached the point that a jackscrew with considerable force is required to create micro-fractures before the suture can open. By the late teens, interdigitation and areas of bony bridging across the suture develop to the point that skeletal maxillary expansion becomes impossible. (Redrawn from Melsen B: *Am J Orthod* 668:42-54, 1975.)

applied to a splint that distributes it over most or all the teeth, appears to be needed to bring the maxilla forward.

The effect of this much force on the dentition is a justifiable matter for concern. During growth modification treatment, tooth movement is undesirable—the objective is to correct the jaw discrepancy, not move teeth to camouflage it. As we have noted in the first part of this chapter, heavy continuous force can damage the roots of the teeth and the periodontium. Heavy intermittent force is less likely to produce damage, and intermittent force is a less effective way to induce tooth movement, probably because the stimulus for undermining resorption is diluted during the times that the heavy force is removed. It follows logically that to minimize damage to the teeth, full-time application of heavy force to the maxilla is unwise.

Because tooth movement is an undesirable side effect, it would be convenient if part-time application of heavy force produced relatively more skeletal than dental effect. At one time, it was thought that the skeletal effect of headgear was about the same with 12 to 16 or 24 hours of wear per day, while much more tooth movement occurred with solid 24-hour wear. This would be another argument for part-time rather than full-time headgear wear. However, very little data exist to support this hypothesis, and intermittent headgear wear cannot be relied on to produce a differential between tooth movement and skeletal change.

For tooth movement, there is a definite threshold for the duration of force: unless force is applied to a tooth for at least 6 hours per day, no bone remodeling occurs.

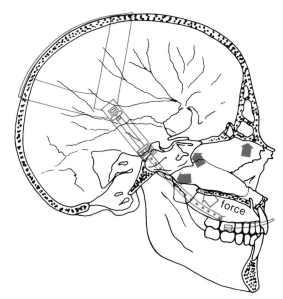

FIGURE 9-26 Extraoral force applied to the maxillary teeth radiates to the sutures of the maxilla, where it can affect the pattern of skeletal maxillary growth.

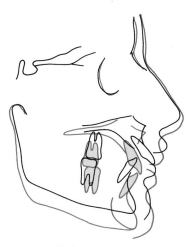

FIGURE 9-27 Cephalometric superimposition showing growth modification produced by extraoral force to the maxilla. Note that the maxilla has moved downward and backward, not in the expected downward and forward direction shown by the mandible.

Whether a similar duration threshold applies to sutures is unknown, but clinical experience suggests that it may.

Until recently the time of day when force was applied to the jaws was not considered important. It seems clear that in both experimental animals and humans, short-term growth is characterized by fluctuations in growth rates, even within a single day.[38] It has been known for some time that in growing children, growth hormone is released primarily during the evening, so it is not surprising that addition of new bone at the epiphyseal plates of the long bones occurs mostly—perhaps entirely—at night.[39] We do not know whether facial growth follows this pattern, but it is entirely possible that it does. It also is possible that tooth movement is more likely to occur during the times of active growth, since eruption occurs then and recent animal experiments have detected differences in the rate of tooth movement at different times of the day.[40] Since orthodontic patients are more likely to wear headgear at night than during the day, perhaps it is fortunate that its effect may be greatest at this time. Growth hormone release begins in the early evening, however, so it probably is important to stress that a patient should begin wearing headgear (or a functional appliance) immediately after dinner rather than waiting until bedtime.

Based on these considerations, the following "force prescription" for headgear to restrain maxillary growth in patients with Class II problems now is considered optimal:

- Force of 500 to 1000 gm total (half that per side)
- Force direction slightly above the occlusal plane (through the center of resistance of the molar teeth, if the force application is to the molars by a facebow)
- Force duration at least 12 hours per day, every day, with emphasis on wearing it from early evening (right after dinner) until the next morning

- Typical treatment duration 12 to 18 months, depending on rapidity of growth and patient cooperation (Figure 9-27)

It must be kept in mind that both orthopedic (skeletal) and orthodontic (dental) effects will be produced from use of this force prescription. The changes to be expected are outlined in Chapter 8 and have been reviewed in detail by Baumrind et al.[41] Sometimes extraoral force is used with the aim of promoting tooth movement, and then, of course, the force levels should be lighter and the duration of wear longer.

As we have discussed in Chapter 8, although modest changes can be produced by a face mask (reverse headgear), augmenting forward growth of the maxilla by producing tension in the sutures has not been as successful clinically as restraining growth. The difficulty in stimulating the entire maxilla to grow forward probably reflects our inability to produce enough force at the posterior and superior sutures to separate them in older children, but that is not the whole story. Part of the problem also is the extent of interdigitation of bony spicules across the sutural lines (see Figure 9-25).[42] As the sutures become more and more highly interdigitated with increasing age, it becomes more and more difficult to separate them. In an adolescent, enough force can be applied across the palate with a jackscrew to open a moderately interdigitated midpalatal suture, but reverse headgear cannot produce that much force in the much more extensive suture system above and behind the maxilla, once even a moderate level of interdigitation has been reached.

Tooth movement is undesirable when any type of growth modification is being attempted, but it is a particular problem

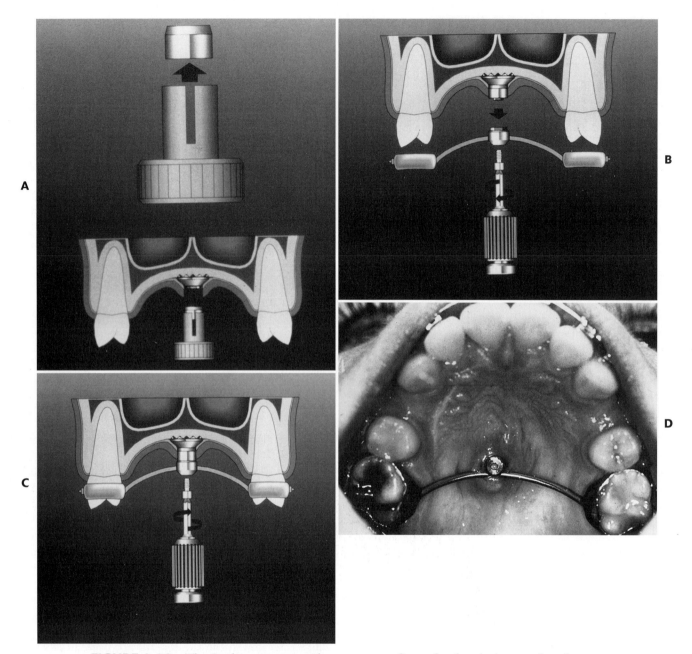

FIGURE 9-28   The Onplant system provides a temporary fixture fused to the bone surface that can be used for orthodontic anchorage. In one application of this approach, maximum anchorage for retraction of maxillary incisors could be obtained by placing an onplant in the center of the palate and using it to stabilize the maxillary posterior teeth as the anterior teeth were retracted into a first premolar extraction space. **A,** After the onplant, which is a titanium fixture coated on its base with hydroxylapatite, is placed via a lateral incision and submucosal dissection and has become integrated, it is exposed and a protective cap is placed; **B,** A transpalatal lingual arch from first molar bands is placed through a cap that fits onto the integrated fixture and **C,** is screwed into place; **D,** an onplant-stabilized lingual arch in position in a patient. The onplant is removed after treatment through the same type of incision through which it was placed—it pops loose with a tap of a chisel. (Courtesy Dr. B. Kvarnstrom, Nobel BioCare.)

in efforts to displace the maxilla forward. One way to overcome this might be to apply the reverse headgear to an implant in the maxilla. An ankylosed primary tooth, which has become fused to the bone and is no longer capable of responding to orthodontic force but will eventually be lost because of root resorption, can be considered a temporary implant. It is possible to deliberately induce ankylosis of primary canines during the mixed dentition by extracting and replanting them. Animal experiments and experience with a few human subjects[43] have shown that ankylosed primary teeth can be used to deliver force to the maxilla. Eventually, the ankylosed tooth resorbs or must be extracted, but there is little or no effect on its permanent successor. This approach may offer a way to treat maxillary deficiency patients who are at least somewhat older than the current age limits.

Adolescent patients who are losing their last primary teeth pose an even greater problem in overcoming maxillary deficiency. Inducing ankylosis of a permanent tooth to provide a point for application of force is not feasible because vertical growth, and with it further eruption of the teeth, continues into the late teens. If ankylosis of a permanent tooth occurred before vertical growth was completed, the tooth would end up out of occlusion in adult life. After healing is complete, osseointegrated implants seem to withstand orthodontic force nicely. The newly-developed onplant approach (Figure 9-28), using a post that integrates with the surface of the bone but can be removed later,[44] has considerable promise as a way of delivering force where it is needed for skeletal effects. In the future it may be possible to place onplants, perhaps in the lateral buttress of the maxilla above the dentition, and apply extraoral force against them to bring the maxilla forward. Whether this will become a practical clinical procedure remains to be seen; there is still the question of how well an adolescent would tolerate the large amount of force that probably would be needed at that age.

An ankylosed tooth or implant/onplant would provide perfect anchorage in the sense that there would be no unwanted tooth movement, but this should not be taken to mean that there would then be no constraints on the amount of possible skeletal change. Forward growth, after all, seems to be largely controlled by the soft tissue matrix in which the maxilla is embedded. Clinical experience to date suggests that more than 3 mm forward displacement of the maxilla is unlikely, probably because of soft tissue limitations.

Effects of Orthodontic Force on the Mandible

If the mandible, like the maxilla, grows largely in response to growth of the surrounding soft tissues, it should be possible to alter its growth in somewhat the same way maxillary growth can be altered, by pushing back against it or pulling it forward. To some extent, that is true, but the attachment of the mandible to the rest of the facial skeleton via the temporomandibular joint is very different from the sutural attachment of the maxilla. Not surprisingly, the response of the mandible to force transmitted to the temporomandibular joint also is quite different.

As we have discussed in Chapter 8, efforts to restrain mandibular growth by applying a compressive force to the mandibular condyle have never been very successful. Animal experiments, in which quite heavy and prolonged forces can be used, suggest that restraining forces can stop mandibular growth and cause remodeling within the temporal fossa.[45] Tooth movement is not a major problem, because the force is applied to the chin rather than the mandibular teeth. The difficulty in getting this to work with human children may be related to their willingness to cooperate with the duration and magnitude of force necessary, or may be the result of inappropriate force levels within the joint.

The duration of the chin cup force (hours/day) may be an important difference between children and experimental animals. In the animal experiments in which a force against the chin has been shown to impede mandibular growth, the force was present essentially all the time. The effect of functional ankylosis in children (see Chapter 5) demonstrates that when there is a constant interference with translation of the condyles out of the glenoid fossa, growth is inhibited, in the absence of force against the chin. An experimental animal has no choice but to wear a restraining device full-time (and tolerate heavy force levels). Children will wear a growth-modifying appliance for some hours per day, but are quite unlikely to wear it all the time even if they promise to do so. Headgear against the maxilla works well with 12 to 14 hours per day, or even less, but the mandible may be different. It is possible, though no one knows for sure, that restraint of mandibular growth may require prevention of translation on a full-time or nearly full-time basis.

It also is possible that if appropriate pressure could be created within the joint, growth could be restrained with part-time application of force. The presence of the articular disk complicates the situation, making it difficult to determine exactly what areas in and around the temporomandibular joint are being loaded by pressure against the chin. In addition, the geometry of the rounded joint surfaces makes it difficult to load the entire area (Figure 9-29).

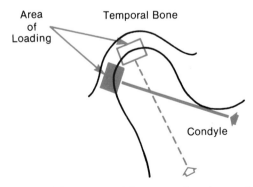

FIGURE 9-29 Extraoral force aimed at the condyle of the mandible tends to load only a small portion of the rounded surface, which is one explanation for the relative ineffectiveness of this type of attempted growth modification.

A force aimed at the top of the condyle might well restrain growth there, but growth only a few millimeters away would be unaffected, since that area would experience little or no force. If the force were aimed at the back of the condyle, the top would be minimally affected. Extremely heavy force, more than most children will tolerate, may be needed to achieve adequate force levels throughout the growing area.

It is possible to use a chin cup to deliberately rotate the mandible down and back, redirecting rather than directly restraining mandibular growth (see Chapter 8). This reduces the prominence of the chin, at the expense of increasing anterior face height. Much of the clinical success that has been obtained with restraints against the mandible can be attributed to this type of rotation.[46] Class III functional appliances produce exactly the same type of downward and backward rotation. The problem, of course, is that a patient who had excessive face height and mandibular prognathism would not be a good candidate for this type of treatment—and two thirds of the prognathic patients have a long face as well.[47]

It is fair to say that controlling excessive mandibular growth is an important unsolved problem in contemporary orthodontics. At this point, we simply cannot restrain mandibular growth with anything like the effectiveness of similar treatment for the maxilla.

On the other hand, the condyle translates forward away from the temporal bone during normal function, and the mandible can be pulled into a protruded position and held there for long durations with moderate and entirely tolerable force. If the current theory is correct, that should stimulate growth. Arguments have raged for many years over whether it really does. If growth stimulation is defined as an acceleration of growth, so that the mandible grows faster while it is being protruded, growth stimulation can be shown to occur for many (but not all) patients (see Figure 8-36). If stimulation is defined as producing a larger mandible at the end of the total growth period than would have existed without treatment, it is much harder to demonstrate a positive effect. The ultimate size of mandibles in treated and untreated patients is remarkably similar.[48]

It is possible that exactly how the mandible is held forward out of the fossa is important in determining the response. There are two mechanisms for protrusion. One is passive, that is, the mandible is held forward by the orthodontic appliance. The other is active, that is, the patient responds to the appliance by using his or her muscles, especially the lateral pterygoid, to hold the mandible forward. Stimulating (activating) the muscles was thought to be important from the beginning of functional appliance therapy, hence both the generic *functional* name and the specific term *activator.*

Up to a certain point, posturing the mandible forward does activate the mandibular musculature—both the elevators and the less powerful muscles involved in protrusion.

Some clinicians argue that it is important in taking the construction bite for a functional appliance to advance the mandible only a few millimeters, because this gives maximum activation of the muscles. If the mandible is brought forward a considerable distance, 1 cm or more, the muscles tend to be electrically silenced rather than activated. But appliances made with such extreme construction bites can be quite effective clinically, and may be just as potent in modifying mandibular (and maxillary) growth as appliances made with smaller advancements. Muscle activation, in short, is not necessary to obtain growth modification. The argument is about whether muscle activation makes these appliances work better, not whether it is necessary for them to work at all.

When the mandible is protruded (or restrained), changes can occur on the temporal as well as the mandibular side of the temporomandibular joint. Sometimes lengthening of the mandible has much less than the expected effect on a skeletal Class II malocclusion, because the temporomandibular joint remodels posteriorly at the same time the mandible is growing longer (see Figure 4-9), and occasionally forward displacement of the joint contributes noticeably to Class II correction. In experiments with monkeys, full-time mandibular protrusion leads to remodeling of the glenoid fossa and forward relocation of the temporomandibular joint,[49] and radiographs of the joint in children wearing similar appliances suggest that bone is being added to its posterior area. There are no data to suggest, however, that forward relocation of the temporomandibular joint area is a major factor in the usual clinical response to functional appliances.

Holding the mandible forward passively requires a force of a few hundred grams. If the musculature relaxes, the reaction force is distributed to the maxilla and, to the extent that the appliance contacts them, to the maxillary and mandibular teeth. The restraint of forward maxillary growth that often accompanies functional appliance treatment is another indication that extremely heavy force is not required to affect the maxilla. On the other hand, headgear usually produces a greater effect on the maxilla than a functional appliance. This implies that the reactive forces from posturing the mandible forward are below the optimum level for altering maxillary growth. When a functional appliance contacts the teeth, as most do, a force system identical to Class II elastics is created, which would move the upper teeth backward and the lower teeth forward. To maximize skeletal effects and minimize dental effects, it is clear that the reactive forces should be kept away from the teeth, in so far as possible.

From this perspective, whether the patient actively uses his musculature to posture the mandible forward or passively rests against the appliance may or may not affect the amount of mandibular growth, but it definitely affects how much tooth movement occurs and may determine the effect on the maxilla. The difference between active and passive protrusion shows up most clearly when the Herbst

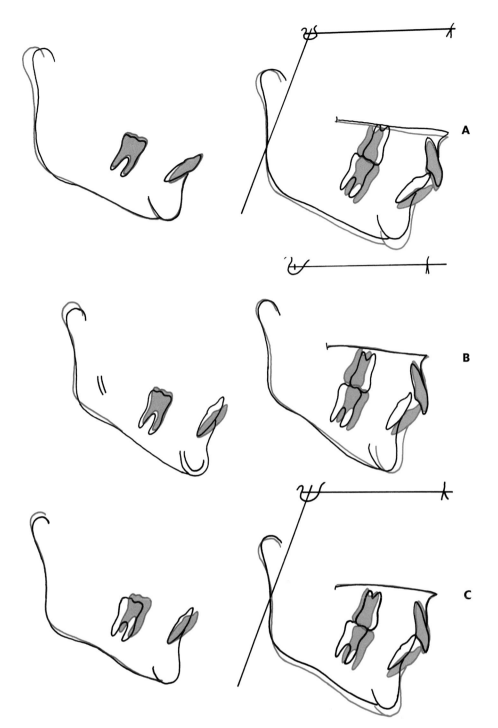

FIGURE 9-30 Functional appliance treatment can result in any combination of differential mandibular growth relative to the maxilla and cranial base (skeletal effect) and displacement of the mandibular and maxillary teeth (dental effect). Note in these tracings of the response to Herbst appliance treatment the almost total skeletal response in **A,** the combination of skeletal and dental changes in **B,** and the almost totally dentally response in **C.** Although the changes in B are typical, it is important to keep in mind that responses like A and C can occur. (Redrawn from Pancherz H: *Am J Orthod* 82:104-113, 1982). *Continued*

appliance (see Figure 11-6), the only fixed functional appliance, is used. With the Herbst appliance, the condyle is displaced anteriorly at all times, but the amount of force against the teeth is very much under the patient's control. The patient can use his or her own muscles to hold the mandible forward, with the Herbst appliance serving only as a stimulus to do so; or the appliance can passively hold the jaw forward, with no contribution from the musculature. If the muscles hold the jaw forward, there is little or no reactive force against the teeth and minimal tooth movement; if the jaw repositioning is entirely passive, force against the teeth can displace them quite significantly.

All of the possible outcomes can be seen in cephalometric tracings of patients treated with the Herbst appliance (Figure 9-30).[50] This device is potentially the most effective of the functional appliances in altering jaw growth, probably because of its full-time action, but it is also rather unpredictable in terms of the amount of skeletal vs. dental change likely to be produced. At first glance, an advantage of the Herbst appliance would appear to be that it removes cooperation and compliance as a factor in treatment. On closer examination, cooperation in terms of active versus passive posturing of the jaw is extremely important in determining the result. The Frankel appliance (see Figure 11-9), which is supported mostly by the soft tissues rather than the teeth, should be and probably is the functional appliance least likely to displace the teeth, but a Class II elastics effect can be seen even with this appliance.

The various types of functional appliances and their use in clinical treatment are reviewed in detail, along with other growth-modifying appliances, in Chapters 11 and 15.

REFERENCES

1. Bumann A, Carvalho RS, Schwarzer CL, Yen EH: Collagen synthesis from human PDL cells following orthodontic tooth movement, Eur J Orthod 19:29-37, 1997.
2. Basdra EK, Komposch G: Osteoblast-like properties of human periodontal ligament cells: an in vitro analysis, Eur J Orthod 19:615-621, 1997.
3. Yokoya K, Sasaki T, Shibasaki Y: Distributional changes of osteoclasts and pre-osteoclastic cells in periodontal tissues during experimental tooth movement, J Dent Res 76:580-587, 1997.
4. Marks SC Jr.: The basic and applied biology of tooth eruption, Connective Tissue Res 32:149-157, 1995.
5. Proffit WR: Equilibrium theory revisited: factors influencing position of the teeth, Angle Orthod 48:175-186, 1978.
6. Bassett CA: Bioelectromagnetics in the service of medicine, Electromagnetic Fields 250: 261-275, 1995 (in *Advances in Chemistry Series*).
7. Shapiro E: Orthodontic movement using pulsating force-induced piezoelectricity, Am J Orthod 73:59-66, 1979.
8. Norton LA: Stress-generated potentials and bioelectric effects: their possible relationship to tooth movement. In Norton LA, Burstone CJ (editors): The biology of orthodontic tooth movement, Boca Raton, Fla, 1989, CRC Press.
9. Giovanelli S, Festa F: Effect of electric stimulation on tooth movement in clinical application. In Davidovitch Z, Norton LA (editors): Biological mechanisms of tooth movement and craniofacial adaptation, Boston, 1996, Harvard Society for Advancement of Orthodontics.
10. Stark TM, Sinclair PM: The effect of pulsed electromagnetic fields on orthodontic tooth movement, Am J Orthod 91: 91-104, 1987.
11. Khouw FE, Goldhaber P: Changes in vasculature of the periodontium associated with tooth movement in the rhesus monkey and dog, Arch Oral Biol 15:1125-1132, 1970.
12. Davidovitch Z, Shamfield JL: Cyclic nucleotide levels in alveolar bone of orthodontically treated cats, Arch Oral Biol 20:567-574, 1975.
13. Grieve WG, Johnson GK, Moore RN et al: Prostaglandin-E and interleukin-1 beta levels in gingival crevicular fluid during human orthodontic tooth movement, Am J Orthod Dentofac Orthop 105:369-374, 1994.
14. Rodan GA, Yeh CK, Thompson DT: Prostaglandins and bone. In Norton LA, Burstone CJ (editors): The biology of orthodontic tooth movement, Boca Raton, Fla, 1989, CRC Press.
15. Sandy JR, Farndale RW, Meikle MC: Recent advances in understanding mechanically induced bone remodeling and their relevance to orthodontic theory and practice, Am J Orthod Dentofac Orthop 103:212-222, 1993.
16. Collin-Osdoby P, Nickols GA, Osdoby P: Bone cell function, regulation and communication—a role for nitric oxide, J Cellular Biochem 57:399-408, 1995.
17. Roberts WE, Ferguson DJ: Cell kinetics of the periodontal ligament. In Norton LA, Burstone CJ (editors): The biology of orthodontic tooth movement, Boca Raton, Fla, 1989, CRC Press.
18. King GJ, Keeling SD, Wronski TJ: Histomorphometric study of alveolar bone turnover in orthodontic tooth movement, Bone 12:401-409, 1991.
19. Kanis JA, Gertz BJ, Singer F, Ortolani S: Rationale for the use of alendronate in osteoporosis, Osteoporosis Int 5:1-13, 1995.
20. Zhou D, Hughes B, King GJ: Histomorphometric and biochemical study of osteoclasts at orthodontic compression sites in the rat during indomethacin inhibition, Arch Oral Biol 42:717-726, 1997.
21. Quinn RS, Yoshikawa DK: A reassessment of force magnitude in orthodontics, Am J Orthod 88:252-260, 1985.
22. Ricketts RM et al: Bioprogressive therapy, Denver, 1979, Rocky Mountain Orthodontics.
23. Goldberg D, Turley PK: Orthodontic space closure of the edentulous maxillary first molar area in adults, Int J Adult Orthod Orthognath Surg 4:255-266, 1989.
24. Roche JJ, Cisneros GJ, Acs G: The effect of acetaminophen on tooth movement in rabbits, Angle Orthod 67:231-236, 1997.
25. Janson GRP, Dainesi EA, Consolaro A et al: Nickel hypersensitivity reaction before, during and after orthodontic therapy, Am J Orthod Dentofac Orthop 113:655-660, 1998.
26. Anstendig H, Kronman J: A histologic study of pulpal reaction to orthodontic tooth movement in dogs, Angle Orthod 42:50-55, 1972.
27. Spurrier SW, Hall SH, Joondeph DR et al: A comparison of apical root resorption during orthodontic treatment in endodontically treated and vital teeth, Am J Orthod Dentofac Orthop 97:130-134, 1990.
28. Spaulding PM, Fields HW, Torney D et al: The changing role of endodontics and orthodontics in the management of traumatically intruded permanent incisors, Pediatr Dent 7:104-110, 1985.
29. Brudvik P, Pygh P: Transition and determinants of orthodontic root resorption-repair sequence, Eur J Orthod 17:177-188, 1995.
30. Mirabella AD, Artun J: Risk factors for apical root resorption of maxillary anterior teeth in adult orthodontic patients, Am J Orthod Dentofac Orthop 108:48-55, 1995.

31. Kaley JD, Phillips C: Factors related to root resorption in edgewise practice, Angle Orthod 61:125-131, 1991.

32. Kennedy DB, Joondeph DR, Osterburg SK, Little RM: The effect of extraction and orthodontic treatment on dentoalveolar support, Am J Orthod 84:183-190, 1983.

33. Sharpe W, Reed B, Subtelny JD, Polson A: Orthodontic relapse, apical root resorption and crestal alveolar bone levels, Am J Orthod Dentofacial Orthop 91:252-258, 1987.

34. Kokich VG: Interdisciplinary management of single-tooth implants, Sem Orthod 3:45-72, 1997.

35. Mantzikos T, Shamus I: Forced eruption and implant site development: soft tissue response, Am J Orthod Dentofac Orthop 112:596-606, 1997.

36. Melsen B, Agerbaek N, Markenstam G: Intrusion of incisors in adult patients with marginal bone loss, Am J Orthod Dentofac Orthop 96:232-241, 1989.

37. Ingber JS: Forced eruption: alterations of soft tissue cosmetic deformities, Int J Periodontol Rest Dent 9:417-428, 1989.

38. Hermanussen M: The analysis of short-term growth, Hormone Res 49:53-64, 1998.

39. Stevenson S, Hunziker EB, Hermann W, Schenk RK: Is longitudinal bone growth influenced by diurnal variation in the mitotic activity of chondrocytes of the growth plates? J Orthop Res 8:132-135, 1990.

40. Igarashi K, Miyoshi K, Shinoda H, Saeki S, Mitani H: Diurnal variation in tooth movement in response to an orthodontic force in rats, Am J Orthod Dentofac Orthop 114:8-14, 1998.

41. Baumrind S, Korn EL, Isaacson RJ et al: Quantitative analysis of the orthodontic and orthopedic effects of maxillary traction, Am J Orthod 83:384-398, 1983.

42. Melsen B: Palatal growth studied on human autopsy material, Am J Orthod 68:42-54, 1975.

43. Omnell ML, Sheller B: Maxillary protraction to intentionally ankylosed deciduous canines in a patient with cleft palate, Am J Orthod Dentofac Orthop 106:201-205, 1994.

44. Block MS, Hoffman DR: A new device for absolute anchorage for orthodontics, Am J Orthod Dentofac Orthop 107:251-258, 1995.

45. Janzen EK, Bluher JA: The cephalometric, anatomic and histologic changes in *Macaca mulatta* after application of a continuous-acting retraction force on the mandible, Am J Orthod 51:832-855, 1965.

46. Allen RA, Connolly IH, Richardson A: Early treatment of Class III incisor relationship using the chincap appliance, Eur J Orthod 15:371-376, 1993.

47. Proffit WR, White RP Jr: Who seeks surgical-orthodontic treatment? Int J Adult Orthod Dentofac Orthop 5:153-160, 1990.

48. Baumrind S, Korn EL, Isaacson RJ et al: Superimpositional assessment of treatment-associated changes in the temporomandibular joint and the mandibular symphysis, Am J Orthod 84:443-465, 1983.

49. Woodside DG, Metakas A, Altuna G: The influence of functional appliance therapy on glenoid fossa remodeling, Am J Orthod Dentofac Orthop 92:181-198, 1987.

50. Pancherz H: The mechanism of Class II correction in Herbst appliance treatment, Am J Orthod 82:104-113, 1982.

CHAPTER
10
Mechanical Principles in Orthodontic Force Control

Optimum orthodontic tooth movement is produced by light, continuous force. The challenge in designing and using an orthodontic appliance is to produce a force system with these characteristics, creating forces that are neither too great nor too variable over time. It is particularly important that the light forces do not decrease rapidly, decaying away either because the material itself loses its elasticity or because a small amount of tooth movement causes a larger change in the amount of force delivered. Both the behavior of elastic materials and mechanical factors in the response of the teeth must be considered in the design of an orthodontic appliance system through which mechanotherapy is delivered.

ELASTIC MATERIALS AND THE PRODUCTION OF ORTHODONTIC FORCE

The Basic Properties of Elastic Materials
The elastic behavior of any material is defined in terms of its stress-strain response to an external load. Both stress and strain refer to the internal state of the material being studied: stress is the internal distribution of the load, defined as force per unit area, whereas strain is the internal distortion produced by the load, defined as deflection per unit length.

For analysis purposes, orthodontic arch wires and springs can be considered as beams, supported either only on one end (e.g., a spring projecting from a removable appliance) or on both ends (the segment of an arch wire spanning between attachments on adjacent teeth) (Figure 10-1). If a force is applied to such a beam, its response can be measured as the deflection (bending or twisting) produced by the force (Figure 10-2). Force and deflection are external measurements. In tension, internal stress and strain can be calculated from force and deflection by considering the area and length of the beam.

For orthodontic purposes, three major properties of beam materials are critical in defining their clinical usefulness: strength, stiffness (or its inverse, springiness), and range. Each can be defined by appropriate reference to a force-deflection or stress-strain diagram (Figures 10-2 and 10-3).

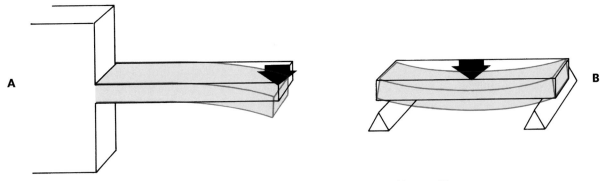

FIGURE 10-1   Cantilever (**A**) and supported beams (**B**).

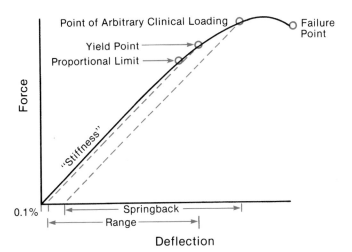

FIGURE 10-2   A typical force-deflection curve for an elastic material like an orthodontic arch wire. The stiffness of the material is given by the slope of the linear portion of the curve. The range is the distance along the X-axis to the point at which permanent deformation occurs (usually taken as the yield point, at which 0.1% permanent deformation has occurred). Clinically useful springback occurs if the wire is deflected beyond the yield point (as to the point indicated here as "arbitrary clinical loading"), but it no longer returns to its original shape. At the failure point, the wire breaks.

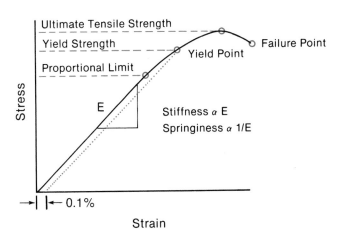

FIGURE 10-3   Stress and strain are internal characteristics that can be calculated from measurements of force and deflection, so the general shapes of force-deflection and stress-strain curves are similar. Three different points on a stress-strain diagram can be taken as representing the strength. The slope of the stress-strain curve, *E*, is the modulus of elasticity, to which stiffness and springiness are proportional.

Three different points on a stress-strain diagram can be taken as representative of the strength of a material (see Figure 10-3). Each represents, in a somewhat different way, the maximum load that the material can resist. The most conservative measure is the proportional limit, the point at which any permanent deformation is first observed. (Although there is a slight difference in the engineering definition of the term *elastic limit*, it is essentially the same point, and elastic and proportional limit may be used interchangeably.) A more practical indicator is the point at which a deformation of 0.1% is measured; this is defined as the yield strength. The maximum load the wire can sustain—the ultimate tensile strength—is reached after some permanent deformation and is greater than the yield strength. Since this ultimate strength determines the max-

imum force the wire can deliver if used as a spring, it is important clinically, especially since yield strength and ultimate strength differ much more for the newer titanium alloys than for steel wires. Strength is measured in stress units (gm/cm^2).

Stiffness and springiness are reciprocal properties:

$$Springiness = 1/Stiffness$$

Each is proportional to the slope of the elastic portion of the force-deflection curve (see Figure 10-2). The more horizontal the slope, the springier the wire; the more vertical the slope, the stiffer the wire.

Range is defined as the distance that the wire will bend elastically before permanent deformation occurs. This distance is measured in millimeters (or other length units) (see Figure 10-2). If the wire is deflected beyond its yield strength, it will not return to its original shape, but clinically useful springback will occur unless the failure point is reached. This springback is measured along the horizontal axis as shown in Figure 10-2. In many clinical situations, orthodontic wires are deformed beyond their elastic limit. Their springback properties in the portion of the load-deflection curve between the elastic limit and the ultimate strength, therefore, are important in determining clinical performance.

These three major properties have an important relationship:

$$\text{Strength} = \text{Stiffness} \times \text{Range}$$

Two other characteristics of some clinical importance also can be illustrated with a stress-strain diagram: resilience and formability (Figure 10-4). Resilience is the area under the stress-strain curve out to the proportional limit. It represents the energy storage capacity of the wire, which is a combination of strength and springiness. Formability is the amount of permanent deformation that a wire can withstand before failing. It represents the amount of permanent bending the wire will tolerate (while being formed into a clinically useful spring, for instance) before it breaks.

The properties of an ideal wire material for orthodontic purposes can be described largely in terms of these criteria: it should possess (1) high strength, (2) low stiffness (in most applications), (3) high range, and (4) high formability. In addition, the material should be weldable or solderable, so that hooks or stops can be attached to the wire. It should also be reasonable in cost. In contemporary practice, no one arch wire material meets all these requirements, and the best results are obtained by using specific arch wire materials for specific purposes.

In the United States, orthodontic appliance dimensions, including wire sizes, are specified in thousandths of an inch. For simplicity in this text, they are given in mils (i.e., .016 inch = 16 mils). In Europe and many other areas of the world, appliance dimensions are specified in millimeters. For the range of orthodontic sizes, a close approximation of sizes in millimeters can be obtained by dividing the dimensions in mils by 4 and placing a decimal point in front (i.e., 16 mils = 0.4 mm).

Orthodontic Arch wire Materials

Precious Metal Alloys.   Before the 1950s, precious metal alloys were used routinely for orthodontic purposes, primarily because nothing else would tolerate intraoral conditions. Gold itself is too soft for nearly all dental purposes, but alloys (which often included platinum and palladium along with gold and copper) could be useful orthodontically. The introduction of stainless steel made precious metal alloys obsolete for orthodontic purposes before the price increases of the 1970s also made them prohibitively expensive. Only the Crozat appliance is still occasionally made from gold, following the original design of the early 1900s (see Chapter 11).

Stainless Steel and Cobalt-Chromium Alloys. Stainless steel, or on a cobalt-chromium alloy (Elgiloy; Rocky Mountain Co.) with similar properties, replaced precious metal in orthodontics because of considerably better strength and springiness with equivalent corrosion resistance. Stainless steel's rust resistance results from a relatively high chromium content. A typical formulation for orthodontic use has 18% chromium and 8% nickel (thus the material is often referred to as an 18-8 stainless steel).

The properties of these steel wires can be controlled over a reasonably wide range by varying the amount of cold working and annealing during manufacture. Steel is softened by annealing and hardened by cold working. Fully annealed stainless steel wires are soft and highly formable. The ligatures used to tie orthodontic arch wires into brackets on the teeth are made from such "dead soft" wire. Steel arch wire materials are offered in a range of partially annealed states, in which yield strength is progressively enhanced at the cost of formability. The steel wires with the most impressive yield strength ("super" grades) are almost brittle and will break if bent sharply. The "regular" grade of orthodontic steel wire can be bent to almost any desired shape without breaking. If sharp bends are not needed, the super wires can be useful, but it is difficult to show improved clinical performance that justifies either their higher cost or limited formability.[1]

Elgiloy, the cobalt-chromium alloy, has the advantage that it can be supplied in a softer and therefore more formable state, and then can be hardened by heat treatment after being shaped. The heat treatment increases strength significantly. After heat treatment, the softest Elgiloy becomes equivalent to regular stainless steel, while harder initial grades are equivalent to the "super" steels.

Nickel-Titanium (NiTi) Alloys.   The first of the titanium alloys introduced into orthodontics in recent years, a nickel-titanium alloy marketed as Nitinol (Unitek Corp.), was developed for the space program (Ni, nickel; Ti, titanium; NOL, Naval Ordnance Laboratory) but has proved very useful in clinical orthodontics because of its exceptional springiness. In this book, the term *NiTi* is used sub-

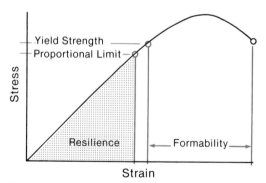

FIGURE 10-4   Resilience and formability are defined as an area under the stress-strain curve and a distance along the X-axis respectively, as shown here. Because the plastic deformation that makes a material formable also may be thought of as cold work, formability alternatively can be interpreted as the area under that part of the stress-strain curve.

sequently to refer to the family of nickel-titanium wire materials (nitinol, with the word not capitalized, also is used in this way in some other publications). Reference to a specific material is by its trademark (capitalized) name.

NiTi alloys have two remarkable properties that are unique in dentistry—shape memory and superelasticity. Like stainless steel and many other metal alloys, NiTi can exist in more than one form or crystal structure. The martensite form exists at lower temperatures, the austenite form at higher temperatures. For steel and almost all other metals, the phase change occurs at a transition temperature of hundreds of degrees. Both shape memory and superelasticity are related to phase transitions within the NiTi alloy between the martensitic and austenitic forms that occur at a relatively low transition temperature.

Shape memory refers to the ability of the material to "remember" its original shape after being plastically deformed while in the martensitic form. In a typical application, a certain shape is set while the alloy is maintained at an elevated temperature, above the martensite-austenite transition temperature. When the alloy is cooled below the transition temperature, it can be plastically deformed, but when it is heated again the original shape is restored. This property, called *thermoelasticity*, was important to the original nitinol's use in the space program but proved difficult to exploit in orthodontic applications.

After considerable experimentation, Nitinol was marketed in the late 1970s for orthodontic use in a stabilized martensitic form, with no application of phase transition effects (although efforts to take advantage of shape memory continued). As provided for orthodontic use, Nitinol is exceptionally springy and quite strong but has poor formability (Table 10-1). Other martensitic alloys marketed later (Titanal, Lancer Pacific; Orthonol, Rocky Mountain) have similar strength and springiness to Nitinol but better formability. In the following discussion, the family of stabilized martensitic alloys now commercially available are referred to as *M-NiTi*.

In the late 1980s, new nickel-titanium wires with an active austenitic grain structure appeared. These wires exhibit the other remarkable property of NiTi alloys—superelasticity—which is manifested by very large reversible strains and a non-elastic stress-strain or force-deflection curve. Burstone et al reported that such a NiTi alloy developed in China has the type of force-deflection curve shown in Figure 10-5.[2] Miura et al have described similar properties in austenitic NiTi (Sentinol) prepared in Japan,[3] and presumably equivalent properties are found in other austenitic wires now marketed (Ni-Ti and Cu-NiTi, Ormco/Sybron; Nitinol-SE, Unitek; and several others). This group subsequently is referred to as *A-NiTi*. Note in Figure 10-5 that over a considerable range of deflection, the force produced by A-NiTi hardly varies. This means that an initial arch wire would exert about the same force whether it were deflected a relatively small or a large distance, which is a unique and extremely desirable characteristic.

The unique force-deflection curve for A-NiTi wire occurs because of a phase transition in grain structure from austenite to martensite, in response not to a temperature

TABLE 10-1 *Comparative Properties of Orthodontic Wires*

	Modulus of elasticity (10^6 psi)	Material stiffness relative to steel	Set angle (degrees)*
Gold (heat-treated)	12	0.41	NA
Stainless steel	29	1.00	12
Truchrome—Rocky Mtn			
Aust. stainless steel	28	0.97	NA
Wallaby—Ormco			
Cobalt-chromium	28	0.97	12
Elgiloy—Rocky Mtn			
Cobalt-chromium (heat treated)	29	1.00	16
Elgiloy—Rocky Mtn			
Beta-titanium	10.5	0.36	35
TMA—Ormco			
A-NiTi	12[a]	0.41	87
Nitinol SE-Unitek			
M-NiTi	4.8	0.17	NA
Nitinol—Unitek			
Triple strand 9 mil	3.9[b]	0.13	42
Triple-flex—Ormco			
Coaxial 6 strand	1.25[b]	0.04	62
Respond—Ormco			
Braided rect. 9 strand	1.50[b]	0.05	49
Force 9—Ormco			
Braided rect. 8 strand	1.25[b]	0.04	56
D-Rect—Ormco			
Braided rect. A-NiTi	0.50[b]	0.02	88
Turbo—Ormco			
Optical glass	0.25	0.01	88
Optiflex—Ormco			

*Degrees of bending around ¼-inch radius before permanent deformation.
a-From initial elastic part of force-deflection; b-apparent modulus, calculated.

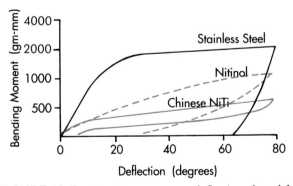

FIGURE 10-5 Bending moment vs. deflection plotted for 16 mil orthodontic wires (black, stainless steel; dashed red, stabilized martensitic NiTi [M-NiTi]; red, austenitic NiTi [A-NiTi]). Note that after an initial force level is reached, A-NiTi has a considerably flatter load-deflection curve and greater springback than M-NiTi, which in turn has much more springback than steel. (From Burstone CJ et al: *Am J Orthod* 87:445-452, 1985.)

change but to applied force. The transformation is a mechanical analogue to the thermally-induced shape memory effect. In other words, the austenitic alloy undergoes a transition in internal structure in response to stress, without requiring a significant temperature change (which is possible because for these materials, the transition temperature is very close to room temperature). Some currently-marketed wires are almost dead soft at room temperature, and become elastic at mouth temperatures, which can make them easier to place initially but the exceptional range that goes with superelasticity is obtainable only if a stress-induced transformation also occurs. This stress-induced martensitic transformation manifests itself in the almost flat section of the load-deflection curve. For a change, superelasticity is not just an advertising term (Figure 10-6).

Part of the unusual nature of a superelastic material like A-NiTi is that its unloading curve differs from its loading curve (i.e., the reversibility has an energy loss associated with it [hysteresis]) (Figure 10-7). This means the force

that it delivers is not the same as the force applied to activate it. The different loading and unloading curves produce the even more remarkable effect that the force delivered by an A-NiTi wire can be changed during clinical use merely by releasing and retying it (Figure 10-8).

For the orthodontist, wire bending in the classic sense is all but impossible with A-NiTi wires because they do not undergo plastic deformation until remarkably high force is applied (see Figure 10-6). The wires can be shaped and their properties can be altered, however, by heat-treatment. This can be done in the orthodontic office by passing an electric current between electrodes attached to the wire or a segment of it.[4] Miura et al have shown that it is possible to reposition the teeth on a dental cast to the desired posttreatment occlusion, bond brackets to the setup, force an A-NiTi wire into the brackets, and then heat-treat the wire so that it "memorizes" its shape with the teeth in the desired position.[5] The wire then incorporates all of what would otherwise be the "finishing bends" usually required in the last stages of treatment. In theory at least, this allows certain types of treatment to be accomplished with a single wire, progressively bringing the teeth toward their predetermined position. The concept is exactly the same as Edward Angle's original approach to arch expansion, which implies that the same limitations would be encountered.

The properties of A-NiTi have quickly made it the preferred material for orthodontic applications in which a long range of activation with relatively constant force is needed (i.e., for initial arch wires and coil springs). M-NiTi remains useful, primarily in the later stages of treatment when flexible but larger and somewhat stiffer wires are needed. At this point, small round nickel-titanium wires usually should be A-NiTi, while larger rectangular ones often perform better if made from M-NiTi.

Clinicians should not take it for granted that wires advertised as being superelastic all perform the same. Re-

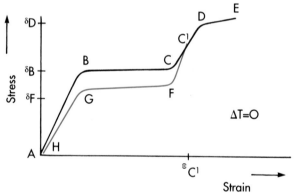

FIGURE 10-6   A stress-strain curve illustrating superelasticity due to the stress-induced transformation from the austenitic to the martensitic phase, as in A-NiTi. Section A-B represents purely elastic deformation of the austenitic phase (note in Figure 10-5 that in this phase A-NiTi is stiffer than M-NiTi). The stress corresponding to point B is the minimum stress at which transformation to the martensitic phase starts to occur. At point C, the transformation is completed. The difference between the slopes of A-B and B-C indicates the ease with which transformation occurs. After the transformation is completed, the martensitic structure deforms elastically, represented by section C-D (but orthodontic arch wires are almost never stressed into this region, and this part of the graph usually is not seen in illustrations of the response of orthodontic archwires). At point D the yield stress of the martensitic phase is reached, and the material deforms plastically until failure occurs at E. If the stress is released before reaching point D (as at point C^1 in the diagram), elastic unloading of the martensitic structure occurs along the line C^1-F. Point F indicates the maximum stress on which the stress-induced martensitic structure on unloading can exist, and at that point the reverse transformation to austenite begins, continuing to point G, where the austenitic structure is completely restored. G-H represents the elastic unloading of the austenite phase. A small portion of the total strain may not be recovered because of irreversible changes during loading or unloading.

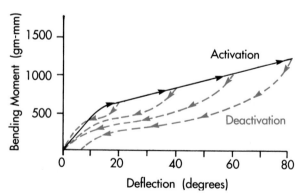

FIGURE 10-7   Activation (*solid*) and deactivation (*dashed*) curves for A-NiTi wire. Note that the unloading curves change at different activations (i.e., the unloading stiffness is affected by the degree of activation). In contrast, the unloading stiffness for steel, beta-Ti, and M-NiTi wires is the same for all activations. (From Burstone CJ et al: *Am J Orthod* 87:445-452, 1985.)

search data have shown remarkable differences in the force-deflection curves and the force delivered by ostensibly similar wires from different manufacturers (Figure 10-9).[6] Data for performance under controlled conditions, not testimonials from prominent clinicians, should be the basis for choosing a specific wire.

Beta-Titanium.   In the early 1980s, after Nitinol but before A-NiTi, a quite different titanium alloy, beta-titanium, was introduced into orthodontics. This beta-Ti material (TMA, Ormco/Sybron [the name is an acronym for titanium-molybdenum alloy]), was developed primarily for orthodontic use. It offers a highly desirable combination of strength and springiness (i.e., excellent resilience), as well as reasonably good formability. This makes it an excellent choice for auxiliary springs and for intermediate and finishing arch wires, especially rectangular wires for the late stages of edgewise treatment. As Table 10-1 shows, in many ways its properties are intermediate between stainless steel and M-NiTi.

Composite Plastics.   Additional progress in orthodontic elastic materials can be anticipated in the early 21st century. The new orthodontic materials of recent years have been adapted from those used in aerospace technology. The high-performance aircraft of the 1970s and 1980s were titanium-based, but their replacements are built of composite plastics, and there is every reason to believe that orthodontic "wires" of this type will move into clinical use in the future. It is already possible to produce fibers with better strength and springiness than non-superelastic wires, and the recently patented process of pultrusion allows both round and rectangular fibers to be produced.[7] The properties of the plastic materials can be manipulated to such an extent that another potential product is a ligature that would adapt around a wire and bracket so that it produced no additional force. This would be

highly advantageous in reducing friction (see below). An additional advantage is that the plastic fibers can be tooth-colored, and so they should have an esthetic advantage as well as a performance advantage. Like the advanced metal wires, their shape is very difficult to change once the manufacturing process is completed, which leads to a number of practical problems for clinical application. It was more than a decade before the first NiTi wires went from clinical curiosity to regular use, and a similar time period may be needed to bring the composite plastics into routine clinical orthodontics.

Comparison of Contemporary Arch wires

As we have noted previously, stainless steel, beta-Ti and NiTi arch wires all have an important place in contemporary orthodontic practice. Their comparative properties explain why specific wires are preferred for specific clinical applications (see Chapters 16 through 18). Hooke's law, which defines the elastic behavior of materials, applies to all orthodontic wires except superelastic A-NiTi. For everything else, a useful method for comparing two arch wires of various materials, sizes and dimensions is the

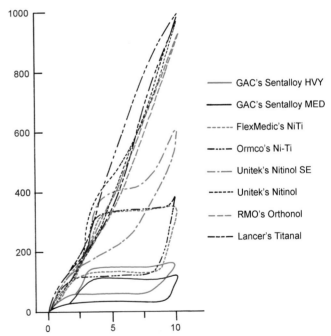

FIGURE 10-9 Force-deflection curves for commercially-available NiTi wires. RMO's Orthonol and Lancer's Titanal are martensitic, so the elastic rather than superelastic curves are expected. Note that the GAC Sentalloy wires show classic superelastic curves and low force values, while the other A-NiTi wires demonstrate partial to almost no superelasticity and force values that would be higher than optimal. In the absence of data, advertising claims for orthodontic wires must be viewed with considerable suspicion. Unlike other medical devices, no proof of performance is required before an orthodontic wire can be marketed. (From Thayer et al: *Am J Orthod Dentofac Orthop* 107:604-612, 1995).

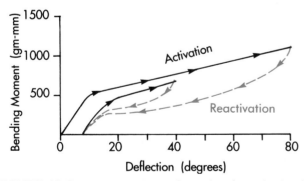

FIGURE 10-8 Activation (to 80 degrees) and reactivation (to 40 degrees) curves for austenitic NiTi wire. In each case, the loading curve is solid and the unloading curve dashed. The unloading curve indicates the force that would be delivered to a tooth. Note that the amount of force exerted by a piece of A-NiTi wire that had previously been activated to 80 degrees could be considerably increased by untying it from a bracket and then retying it—again, a unique property of this alloy. (From Burstone CJ et al: *Am J Orthod* 87:445-452, 1985.)

use of ratios of the major properties (strength, stiffness, and range):

$$\text{Strength A/Strength B} = \text{Strength ratio}$$
$$\text{Stiffness A/Stiffness B} = \text{Stiffness ratio}$$
$$\text{Range A/Range B} = \text{Range ratio}$$

These ratios have been calculated for many different wires by Kusy,[8] and the data presented here are taken from his work.

Three points must be kept in mind when these ratios are compared:

1. The ratios are functions of both physical properties and geometric factors, hence the importance of specifying both in the comparison. Geometric factors relate to both the size of the wire and its shape, whether it is round, rectangular, or square. These are discussed in more detail later in this chapter.
2. Bending describes round wires reasonably completely in orthodontic applications, but both bending and torsional stresses are encountered when rectangular wires are placed into rectangular attachments on teeth. The fundamental relationships for torsion are analogous to those in bending but are not the same. Appropriate use of the equations for torsion, however, allows torsion ratios to be computed in the same way as bending ratios.
3. The ratios apply to the linear portion of the load-deflection curve and thus do not accurately describe the behavior of wires that are stressed beyond their elastic limit but still have useful springback. This is an increasingly significant limitation as consideration passes from steel or chromium-cobalt to beta-Ti to M-NiTi. The nonlinear response of A-NiTi makes calculation of ratios for it all but impossible. Nevertheless, the ratios offer an initial understanding of the properties of traditional steel wires as compared with the newer titanium alloys, and they can be quite helpful in appreciating the effects of changing wire geometry.

In the beginning, tabulated comparative data are easiest to understand. Note in Tables 10-2 and 10-3 the comparative properties of 16, 18, and 19 × 25 mil wires in stainless steel (or chromium-cobalt), M-NiTi, and beta-Ti. In each case, the steel wire has been given an arbitrary value of 1. Note that the titanium wires in each case provide a gain in springiness and range that is greater than the loss in strength.

From Table 10-2, it can be seen that:

1. The strength of 16 and 18 M-NiTi and beta-Ti wires are the same: both are 60% as strong as steel.
2. Stiffness of the small round titanium wires is also similar, less than one-third that of steel.
3. TMA has nearly twice the range of steel, and M-NiTi has twice the range of TMA and nearly four times the range of steel. The A-NiTi alloys quickly move into the nonlinear portion of the force-

TABLE 10-2   *Elastic Property Ratios: 16 and 18 mil Wire in Bending*

	Strength		Stiffness		Range	
	.016	.018	.016	.018	.016	.018
Stainless steel	1.0		1.0		1.0	
TMA	0.6	0.6	0.3	0.3	1.8	1.8
M-NiTi	0.6	0.6	0.2	0.2	3.9	3.9

TABLE 10-3   *Elastic Property Ratios: 19× 25 Wire in Bending (B) and Torsion (T)*

	Strength		Stiffness		Range	
	B	T	B	T	B	T
Stainless steel	1.0		1.0		1.0	
TMA	0.6	0.6	0.3	0.3	1.8	2.0
M-NiTi	0.6	0.8	0.2	0.1	4.0	5.4

deflection curve and so in the strict definition of the term do not have much range, but as Figure 10-5 shows, they have tremendous springback and behave clinically as if they have very large range.

Table 10-3 shows that properties of rectangular wire in bending and torsion are quite different. Note that at this common wire size, both beta-Ti and M-NiTi have greater springiness and range than steel. M-NiTi in torsion must bend more than twice as far as TMA to deliver the same load (because of its great springiness), and thus is at a disadvantage when small precise adjustments are needed. A-NiTi would be at an even greater disadvantage in this application. Beta-Ti or steel (depending on wire size) would be a better choice for making final adjustments in tooth inclination (torque).

Table 10-4 shows wires of equivalent stiffness, with 16 mil stainless steel as the index value. Table 10-5 illustrates a sequence of rectangular wires that are increasingly stiff in torsion. The application of this information to the selection of arch wires at various stages of fixed appliance treatment is covered in detail in Chapters 16 to 18.

A more graphic and efficient method for comparing different wire materials and sizes (within the limitations described above) is the use of nomograms—fixed charts that display mathematical relationships via appropriately adjusted scales. In the preparation of a nomogram, a reference wire is given a value of 1, and many other wires can then be located appropriately in reference to it. Nomograms developed by Kusy to provide generalized comparisons of stainless steel, M-NiTi, and beta-Ti in bending and torsion are shown in Figures 10-10 and 10-11.[9] Note that because the nomograms of each set are all drawn to the same base, any

TABLE 10-4   *Wires of Equivalent Stiffness—Bending*

Wire type			
M-NiTi	Beta-Ti	Stainless steel	Relative springiness
16		17.5 (3 × 8)	6.6
19	16	12	3.3
	18	14	1.9
17 × 25		16	1.0
21 × 25		18	0.70
	19 × 25		0.37
		19 × 26	0.12

TABLE 10-5   *A Sequence of Increasingly Stiff Wires in Torsion*

Wire	Stiffness index
18 × 18 M-NiTi	1.0
17 × 25 M-NiTi	1.7
21 × 25 M-NiTi	2.8
17 × 25 beta-Ti	3.5
19 × 25 beta-Ti	4.6
21 × 25 beta-Ti	5.7
16 × 22 steel	8.0
17 × 25 steel	12
19 × 25 steel	16
21 × 25 steel	21

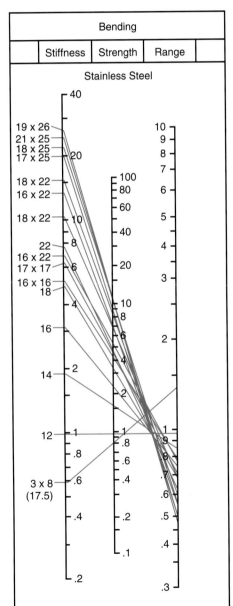
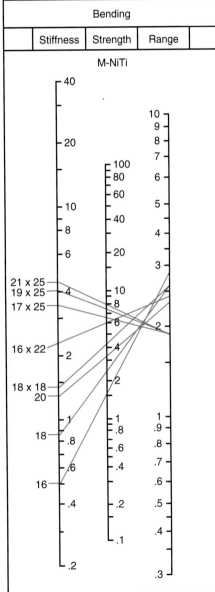
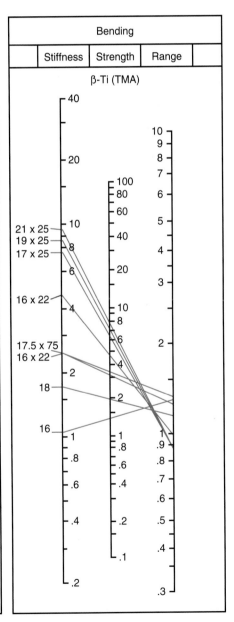

FIGURE 10-10   Bending nomograms for stainless steel, M-NiTi (Nitinol), and beta-titanium (TMA) wires. The index for all three nomograms, with an assigned value of 1, is 12 mil steel, so all values on the three nomograms are comparable. (From Kusy RP: *Am J Orthod* 83:374-381, 1983.)

wire on any one of the three nomograms can be compared with any other wire.

The nomograms are particularly helpful in allowing one to assess at a glance a whole set of relationships that would require pages of tables. For example, using Figure 10-11 to compare 21 × 25 M-NiTi to 21 × 25 beta-Ti in torsion (the appropriate comparison if the wires would be used to produce a torquing movement of the root of a tooth): 21 × 25 beta-Ti has a stiffness value of 6, while 21 × 25 M-NiTi has a value of 3, so the beta-Ti would deliver twice the force at a given deflection; the strength value for 21 × 25 beta-Ti wire is 4, while the value for this size M-NiTi wire is 6, so the NiTi wire is less likely to become per-

manently distorted if twisted into a bracket; the range value for 21 × 25 beta-Ti is 0.7, while the same size M-NiTi has a range value of 1.9, so the NiTi could be twisted nearly three times as far. The nomograms contain the information to allow a similar comparison of any one of the wire sizes listed to any other wire shown on the chart, in bending (see Figure 10-10) or torsion (see Figure 10-11).

Effects of Size and Shape on Elastic Properties

Each of the major elastic properties—strength, stiffness, and range—is substantially affected by a change in the geometry of a beam. Both the cross-section (whether the beam is circular, rectangular, or square) and the length of a

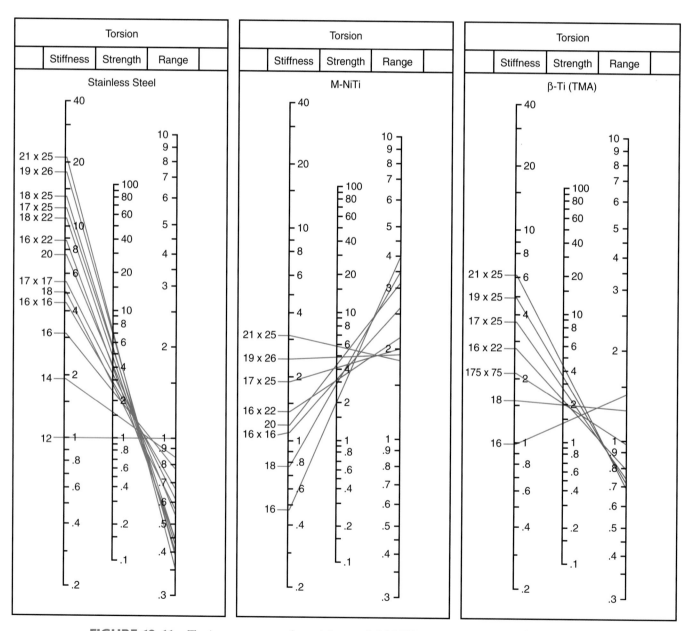

FIGURE 10-11   Torsion nomograms for stainless steel, M-NiTi (Nitinol), and beta-titanium (TMA) wires. For all three nomograms, the index wire is the same, making all values comparable. (From Kusy RP: *Am J Orthod* 83:374-381, 1983.)

beam are of great significance in determining its properties. Changes related to size and shape are independent of the material. In other words, decreasing the diameter of a steel beam by 50% would reduce its strength to a specific percentage of what it had been previously (the exact reduction would depend on how the beam was supported, as we discuss below). Decreasing the diameter of a TMA beam by 50% would reduce its strength by exactly the same percentage. But keep in mind that the performance of a beam, whether beneath a highway bridge or between two teeth in an orthodontic appliance, is determined by the combination of material properties and geometric factors.

Effects of Diameter or Cross-section. Let us begin by considering a cantilever beam, supported on only one end. In orthodontic applications, this is the type of spring often used in removable appliances, in which a wire extends from the plastic body of the removable appliance as a fingerspring. When a round wire is used as a fingerspring, doubling the diameter of the wire increases its strength eight times (i.e., the larger wire can resist eight times as much force before permanently deforming, or can deliver eight times as much force). Doubling the diameter, however, decreases springiness by a factor of 16 and decreases range by a factor of two.

More generally, for a round cantilever beam, the strength of the beam changes as the third power of the ratio of the larger to the smaller beam; springiness changes as the fourth power of the ratio of the smaller to the larger; and range changes directly as the ratio of the smaller to the larger (Figure 10-12).

The situation is somewhat more complex for a beam supported on both ends, as is the case for a segment of arch wire between two teeth. Supporting both ends makes the

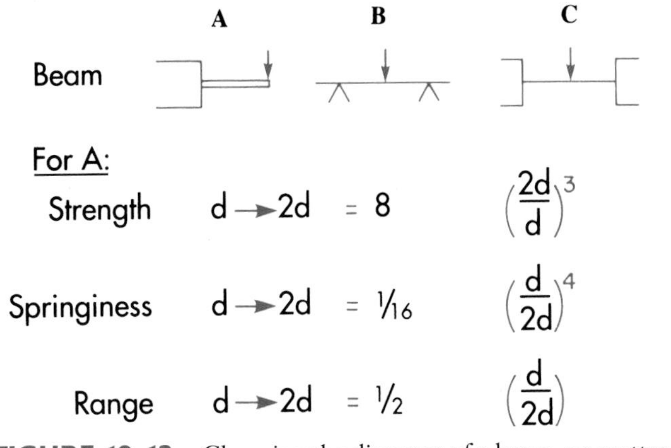

beam stronger and less flexible, particularly if the ends are tightly anchored as opposed to being free to slide. If a rectangular beam is evaluated, its dimension in the direction of bending is the primary determinant of its properties. The principle with any supported beam, however, is the same as with a cantilever beam: as the beam size increases, strength increases as a cubic function, while springiness decreases as a fourth power function and range decreases proportionately, not exponentially.

Although round beams can be placed in torsion in engineering applications, torsion is of practical importance in orthodontics only for rectangular wires that can be twisted into rectangular slots. In torsion, the analytic approach is basically similar to that in bending, but shear stress rather than bending stress is encountered, and the appropriate equations are all different. The overall effect is the same, however: decreasing the size of a wire decreases its strength in torsion while increasing its springiness and range, just as in bending.

As the diameter of a wire decreases, its strength decreases so rapidly that a point is reached at which the strength is no longer adequate for orthodontic purposes. As the diameter increases, its stiffness increases so rapidly that a point is reached at which the wire is simply too stiff to be useful. These upper and lower limits establish the wire sizes useful in orthodontics. The phenomenon is the same for any material, but the useful sizes vary considerably from one material to another. As Table 10-6 indicates, useful steel wires are considerably smaller than the gold wires they replaced. The titanium wires are much springier than steel wires of equal sizes, but not as strong. Their useful sizes therefore are larger than steel and quite close to the sizes for gold.

Effects of Length and Attachment. Changing the length of a beam, whatever its size or the material from which it is made, also dramatically affects its properties (Figure 10-13). If the length of a cantilever beam is doubled, its bending strength is cut in half, but its springiness increases eight times and its range four times. More generally, when the length of a cantilever beam increases, its strength decreases proportionately, while its springiness increases as the cubic function of the ratio of the length and its range increases as the square of the ratio of the length. Length changes affect torsion quite differently from bending: springiness and range in torsion increase proportionally with length, while torsional strength is not affected by length.

Changing from a cantilever to a supported beam, though it complicates the mathematics, does not affect the big picture: as beam length increases, there are proportional decreases in strength but exponential increases in springiness and range.

The way in which a beam is attached also affects its properties. An arch wire can be tied tightly or loosely, and the point of loading can be any point along the span. As Figure 10-12 shows, a supported beam like an arch wire is

	A	**B**	**C**
Beam			

For A:

Strength $d \rightarrow 2d$ $= 8$ $\left(\dfrac{2d}{d}\right)^3$

Springiness $d \rightarrow 2d$ $= \dfrac{1}{16}$ $\left(\dfrac{d}{2d}\right)^4$

Range $d \rightarrow 2d$ $= \dfrac{1}{2}$ $\left(\dfrac{d}{2d}\right)$

FIGURE 10-12 Changing the diameter of a beam, no matter how it is supported, greatly affects its properties. As the figures below the drawing indicate, doubling the diameter of a cantilever beam makes it 8 times as strong, but it is then only 1/16 as springy and has half the range. More generally, when beams of any type made from two sizes of wire are compared, strength changes as a cubic function of the ratio of the two cross-sections; springiness changes as the fourth power of the ratios; range changes as a direct proportion (but the precise ratios are different from those for cantilever beams).

TABLE 10-6   *Useful Wire Sizes in Various Materials (Dimensions in mils)*

	Gold	Steel	Cobalt-chromium	Beta-Ti	M-NiTi	A-NiTi
Stranded arch wire		6 to 9				
Arch wire						
Round	20 to 22	12 to 20	12 to 20	16 to 20	16 to 20	16 to 20
Rectangular	22 × 28	16 × 16 to 19 × 25	16 × 16 to 19 × 25	18 × 18 to 21 × 25	17 × 25 to 21 × 25	17 × 25 to 21 × 25
Removable appliance	30 to 40	22 to 30	22 to 30			
Lingual arch	40	30, 36, 32 × 32	30, 36	32 × 32		
Headgear		45, 51				
Auxiliary expansion arch		36, 40				

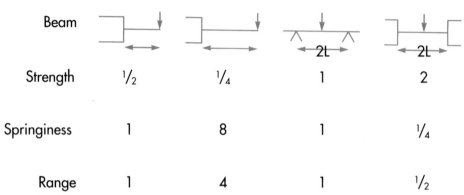

Beam				
Strength	½	¼	1	2
Springiness	1	8	1	¼
Range	1	4	1	½

FIGURE 10-13   Changing either the length of a beam or the way in which it is attached dramatically affects its properties. Doubling the length of a cantilever beam cuts its strength in half, but makes it 8 times as springy and gives it 4 times the range. More generally, strength varies inversely with length, whereas springiness varies as a cubic function of the length ratios, and range as a second power function. Supporting a beam on both ends makes it much stronger but also much less springy than supporting it on only one end. Note that if a beam is rigidly attached on both ends, it is twice as strong but only one fourth as springy as a beam of the same material and length that can slide over the abutments. For this reason, the elastic properties of an orthodontic arch wire are affected by whether it is tied tightly or held loosely in a bracket.

four times as springy if it can slide over the abutments (in clinical use, through a bracket into which it is loosely tied) rather than if the beam is firmly attached (tied tightly). With multiple attachments, as with an arch wire tied to several teeth, the gain in springiness from loose ties of an initial arch wire is less dramatic but still significant.[10]

Controlling Orthodontic Force by Varying Materials and Size-Shape. Obtaining enough orthodontic force is never a problem. The difficulty is in obtaining light but sustained force. A spring or arch wire strong enough to resist permanent deformation may be too stiff, which creates two problems: the force is likely to be too heavy initially and then decay rapidly when the tooth begins to move. A wire with excellent springiness and range may nevertheless fail to provide a sustained force if it distorts from inadequate strength the first time the patient has lunch. The best balance of strength, springiness, and range must be sought among the almost innumerable possible combinations of beam materials, diameters, and lengths.

The first consideration in spring design is adequate strength: the wire size selected must not deform permanently in use. As a general rule, fingersprings for removable appliances are best constructed using steel wire. Great advantage can be taken of the fact that fingersprings behave like cantilever beams: springiness increases as a cubic function of the increase in length of the beam, while strength decreases only in direct proportion. Thus a relatively large wire, selected for its strength, can be given the desired spring qualities by increasing its length.

In practice, this lengthening often means doubling the wire back on itself or winding a helix into it to gain length while keeping the spring within a confined intraoral area (Figure 10-14). The same technique can be used with arch wires, of course; the effective length of a beam is measured along the wire from one support to the other, and this does not have to be in a straight line (Figure 10-15). Bending loops in arch wires can be a time-consuming chairside procedure, which is the major disadvantage.

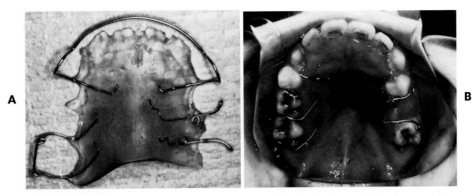

FIGURE 10-14 **A** and **B,** A removable appliance incorporating cantilever springs to reposition an upper molar and upper first premolar. Note that a helix has been bent into the base of the cantilever springs, effectively increasing their length to obtain more desirable mechanical properties.

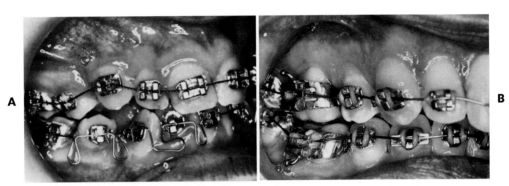

FIGURE 10-15 **A,** Improved springiness and range with steel arch wires can be obtained by either of two strategies: bending loops into the arch wire, as shown in the lower arch here, to increase the length of the beam segments between adjacent teeth; or using multiple strands of small diameter wires, as shown in the upper arch. **B,** The exceptional range and flat force-deflection curve of modern superelastic A-NiTi archwires makes it possible to use a single strand of 14 or 16 mil wire for initial alignment.

Another way to obtain a better combination of springiness and strength is to combine two or more strands of a small, and therefore springy, wire. Two 10 mil steel wires in tandem, for instance, could withstand twice the load as a single strand before permanently deforming, but if each strand could bend without being restrained by the other, springiness would not be affected. The genesis of the "twin wire" appliance system (see Chapter 12) was just this observation, that a pair of 10 mil steel wires offered excellent springiness and range for aligning teeth, and that two wires gave adequate strength although one did not. More recently, three or more strands of smaller steel wires, twisted into a cable, have come into common use (see Figure 10-15). The properties of the multistrand wire depend both on the characteristics of the individual wire strands and on how tightly they have been woven together. Current multistrand wires offer an impressive combination of strength and spring qualities.

The exceptional springiness of A-NiTi makes it a particularly attractive alternative to steel wires in the initial phases of treatment when the teeth are severely malaligned. A continuous NiTi arch wire of either type will have better properties than multistrand steel wires and properties similar to a steel arch wire with loops. TMA, as an intermediate between NiTi and steel, is less useful than either in the first stage of full-appliance treatment. Its excellent overall properties, however, make it quite useful in the later stages of treatment. It is possible, and frequently desirable, to carry out orthodontic treatment with a series of wires of approximately the same size, using a sequence from NiTi to TMA to steel. Arch wire selection in varying circumstances is discussed in more detail later in this chapter and in Chapters 16 through 18.

Rubber and Plastic Sources of Elastic Force

From the beginning, rubber bands were used in orthodontics to transmit force from the upper arch to the lower. Rubber has the particularly valuable quality of a great elastic range, so that the extreme stretching produced when a patient opens the mouth while wearing rubber bands can be tolerated without destroying the appliance. Rubber bands are also easier for a patient to remove and replace than, for instance, a heavy coil spring would be. More recently, rubber and plastic elastomers also have been used to close spaces within the arches.

From a materials point of view, the greatest problem with all types of rubber is that they absorb water and deteriorate under intraoral conditions.[11] Gum rubber, which is used to make the rubber bands commonly used in households and offices, begins to deteriorate in the mouth within a couple of hours, and much of its elasticity is lost in 12 to 24 hours. Although orthodontic elastics once were made from this material, they have been largely superseded by latex elastics, which have a useful performance life 4 to 6 times as long. In contemporary orthodontics, only latex rubber elastics should be used.

Elastomeric plastics developed in the 1960s became available for orthodontic purposes during the 1970s and are marketed under a variety of trade names. Small elastomeric modules replace wire ligature ties to hold archwires in the brackets in many applications (Figure 10-16), and also can be used to apply a force to close spaces within the arches. Like rubber, however, these elastomers tend to deteriorate in elastic performance after a relatively short period in the mouth.[12] This feature does not prevent them from performing quite well in holding arch wires in place, nor does it contraindicate their use to close small spaces. It simply must be kept in mind that when elastomers are used, the forces decay rapidly, and so can be characterized better as interrupted rather than continuous. Although larger spaces within the dental arch can be closed by sliding teeth with rubber bands or elastomeric chains, the same tooth movement can be done much more efficiently with A-NiTi springs that provide a nearly constant force over quite a large range.

Magnets as a Source of Orthodontic Force

Magnets in attraction or repulsion could generate forces of the magnitude needed to move teeth and would have the advantage of providing predictable force levels without direct contact or friction. Until rare earth magnets were developed in the 1980s, magnetic devices with enough force at reasonable separation distances were simply too bulky for orthodontic purposes. In recent years, with smaller and more powerful magnets available, there has been considerable interest in the possibility of using magnetic force in orthodontics.

The two key questions with magnets as a source of force are their biological implications and their clinical effectiveness.[13] Although the rare earth materials are potentially toxic, magnets must be in sealed cases when used intraorally to prevent corrosion, and direct cytotoxic effects have not been observed. Indirect effects of the magnetic fields on cellular activity are possible and could be helpful or harmful. There is some evidence from animal

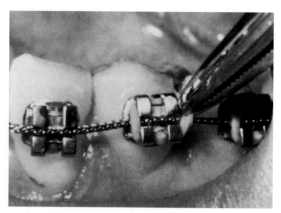

FIGURE 10-16   Elastomeric module used to hold an arch wire in a bracket.

experiments that static as well as pulsed magnetic fields increase the rate of bone formation and can accelerate the rate of tooth movement.[14] In other experiments, with magnets in close contact with skin and bone surfaces, a reduction in the number of epithelial cells and resorption of the cortical bone surface was reported.[15] With the small magnets used to generate orthodontic force, it appears that safety is not a problem. On the other hand, the weak magnetic fields they produce are quite different from those that have been shown to affect bone formation, so indirect effects on bone remodeling and tooth movement are doubtful.

There is no doubt that magnets can be clinically effective. They produce appropriate force for orthodontic tooth movement, and can be arranged to open or close spaces within the dental arches, simulate the effect of Class II or III elastics, or change jaw posture (Figure 10-17). A particularly attractive potential application is bringing impacted teeth into the arch, because if a magnet were attached to an impacted tooth when it was exposed, it would not be necessary to maintain a physical connection. There are two major problems with magnets for general orthodontic use. First, even the smallest magnets still are quite bulky compared with, for instance, a NiTi spring. Second, the force follows the inverse square law (i.e., the force changes as the square of the distance between the magnets). Force decay (or increase) as teeth move can be a problem if the magnets were close together initially.

The extent to which magnets will be used in the future in orthodontics almost surely will be a function of their biologic effects. If magnets are just another source of force, they are likely to be used only for special applications where their relative bulkiness and force characteristics are not a problem. But it turns out that even small magnetic fields change the biologic response in a favorable way, magnets could become an important part of orthodontic treatment.

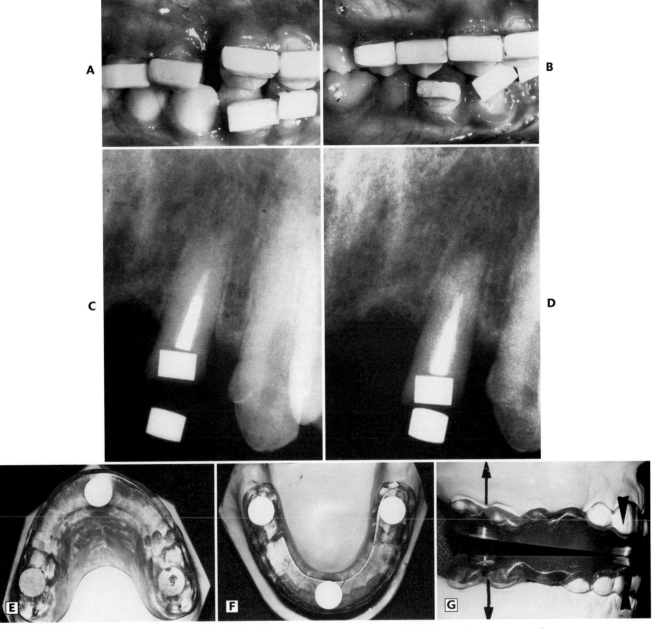

FIGURE 10-17   Magnets can be used successfully to produce either tooth movement of almost any type or jaw position changes that lead to growth effects. **A,B,** Magnets bonded to individual teeth as used for space closure; **C,D,** Use of an attractive magnet for extrusion of a damaged premolar; **E-G,** Use of magnets in a functional appliance, here arranged to exert an intrusive force posteriorly and an attractive force anteriorly, to close an anterior open bite and produce upward-forward rotation of the mandible. (Courtesy Dr. M.A. Darendeliler.)

DESIGN FACTORS IN ORTHODONTIC APPLIANCES

Two Point Contact and Control of Root Position

Definition of Terms. Before beginning to discuss control of root position, it is necessary to understand some basic physical terms that must be used in the discussion:

- *Force*—a load applied to an object that will tend to move it to a different position in space. Force, though rigidly defined in units of Newtons (mass times the acceleration of gravity), is usually measured in weight units of grams or ounces.
- *Center of resistance*—a point at which resistance to movement can be concentrated for mathematical analysis. For an object in free space, the center of resistance is the same as the center of mass. If the object is partially restrained, as is the case for a fence post extending into the earth or a tooth root embedded in bone, the center of resistance will be determined by the nature of the external constraints. The center of resistance for a tooth is at the approximate midpoint of the embedded portion of the root (i.e., about halfway between the root apex and the crest of the alveolar bone) (Figure 10-18).
- *Moment*—a force acting at a distance. A moment is defined as the product of the force times the perpendicular distance from the point of force application to the center of resistance, and thus is measured in units of gm-mm (or equivalent). If the line of action of an applied force does not pass through the center of resistance, a moment is necessarily created. Not only will the force tend to translate the object, moving it to a different position, it also will tend to rotate the object around the center of resistance.

This, of course, is precisely the situation when a force is applied to the crown of a tooth (see Figure 10-18). Not only is the tooth displaced in the direction of the force, it also rotates around the center of resistance—thus the tooth tips as it moves.

- *Couple*—two forces equal in magnitude and opposite in direction. The result of applying two forces in this way is a pure moment, since the translatory effect of the forces cancels out. A couple will produce pure rotation, spinning the object around its center of resistance, while the combination of a force and a couple can change the way an object rotates while it is being moved (Figure 10-19).
- *Center of rotation*—the point around which rotation actually occurs when an object is being moved. If a force and a couple are applied to an object, the center of rotation can be controlled and made to have any desired location. The application of a force and a couple to the crown of a tooth, in fact, is the mechanism by which bodily movement of a tooth, or even greater movement of the root than the crown, can be produced (see Figure 10-19).

Forces, Moments, and Couples in Tooth Movement. Consider the clinical problem posed by a protrud-

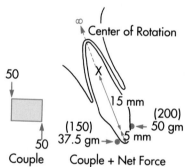

FIGURE 10-19 A couple, as shown on the left, is defined as two forces equal in magnitude and opposite in direction. The application of a couple produces pure rotation. In clinical application, two unequal forces applied to the crown of a tooth to control root position can be resolved into a couple and a net force to move the tooth. If a 50 gm force were applied to a point on the labial surface of an incisor tooth 15 mm from the center of resistance, a 750 gm-mm moment (the moment of the force, or M_F) would be produced, tipping the tooth. To obtain bodily movement, it is necessary to apply a couple, to create a moment (the moment of the couple, or M_C) equal in magnitude and opposite in direction to the original movement. One way to do this would be to apply a force of 37.5 gm pushing the incisal edge labially at a point 22 mm from the center of resistance. This creates a 750 gm-mm moment in the opposite direction, so the force system is equivalent to a couple with a 12.5 gm net force to move the tooth lingually. With this force system, the tooth would not tip, but with so light a net force, there would be only a small amount of movement. To achieve a net 50 gm for effective movement, it would be necessary to use 200 gm against the labial surface and 150 gm in the opposite direction against the incisal edge. Controlling forces of this magnitude without a fixed appliance is difficult.

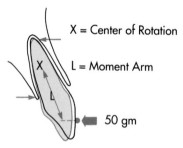

FIGURE 10-18 The center of resistance (C_R) for any tooth is at the approximate midpoint of the embedded portion of the root. If a single force is applied to the crown of a tooth, the tooth will not only translate but also rotate around C_R (i.e., the center of rotation and center of resistance are identical), because a moment is created by applying a force at a distance from C_R. The perpendicular distance from the point of force application to the center of resistance is the moment arm. Pressure in the periodontal ligament will be greatest at the alveolar crest and opposite the root apex (see Figure 9-9).

ing maxillary central incisor. If a single force of 50 gm is applied against the crown of this tooth, as might happen with a spring on a maxillary removable appliance, a force system will be created that includes a 750 gm-mm moment (see Figure 10-19). The result will be that the crown will be retracted more than the root apex, which might actually move slightly in the opposite direction. (Remember that a force will tend to displace the entire object, despite the fact that its orientation will change via simultaneous rotation around the center of resistance.) If it is desired to maintain the inclination of the tooth while retracting it, it will be necessary to overcome the moment inadvertently created when the force was applied to the crown.

One way to decrease the magnitude of the moment is to apply the force closer to the center of resistance. In orthodontics, it is impractical to apply the force directly to the root, but a similar effect could be achieved by constructing a rigid attachment that projected upward from the crown. Then the force could be applied to the attachment such that its line of action passed near or through the center of resistance. If the attachment were perfectly rigid, the effect would be to reduce or eliminate the moment arm and thereby the tipping (Figure 10-20). Since it is difficult to make the arms long enough to totally eliminate tipping, this procedure is only a partial solution at best, and it creates problems with oral hygiene.

Another way to control or eliminate tipping is to create a second moment opposite in direction to the first one. If a second counterbalancing moment could be created

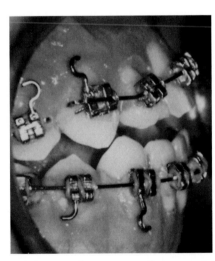

FIGURE 10-20 Attachments extending toward the center of resistance, seen here as hooks integrated into the brackets, can be used to shorten the moment arm and thereby decrease the amount of tipping when elastics or springs are used to slide teeth mesiodistally along an arch wire. This idea from the 1920s was reintroduced as part of the early straight-wire appliance. Unfortunately, the longer the hook the more effective it is mechanically but the greater the chance of oral hygiene problems leading to gingival irritation and/or decalcification. Other methods for controlling tipping are more practical.

equal in magnitude to the moment produced by the first force application, the tooth would remain upright and move bodily. A moment can be created only by application of a force at a distance, however, so this would require that a second force be applied to the crown of the tooth.

In our example of the protruding central incisor, the tendency for the incisor to tip when it was being retracted could be controlled by applying a second force to the lingual surface of this tooth, perhaps with a spring in a removable appliance pushing outward from the lingual edge near the incisal edge (see Figure 10-19). As a practical matter, it can be difficult to maintain removable appliances in place against the displacing effects of a pair of springs with heavy activation. The usual orthodontic solution is a fixed attachment on the tooth, constructed so that forces can be applied at two points. With round wires, an auxiliary spring is needed (Figure 10-21). A rectangular arch wire fitting into a rectangular bracket slot on the tooth is most widely used because the entire force system can be produced with a single wire (Figure 10-22).

It should be noted that with this approach, the two points of contact are the opposite edges of the rectangular wire. The moment arms of the couple therefore are quite small, which means that the forces at the bracket necessary to create a countervailing moment are quite large. If a rectangular arch wire is to be used to retract a central incisor bodily, the net retraction force should be small, but the twisting forces on the bracket must be large in order to generate the moment.

Moment-to-Force Ratios and Control of Root Position. The previous analysis demonstrates that control of root position during movement requires both a force to move the tooth in the desired direction, and a couple to produce the necessary counterbalancing moment for control of root position. The heavier the force, the larger the counterbalancing moment must be to prevent tipping, and vice-versa.[16]

Perhaps the simplest way to determine how a tooth will move is to consider the ratio between the moment created when a force is applied to the crown of a tooth (the moment of the force, or M_F), and the counterbalancing moment generated by a couple within the bracket (the moment of the couple, or M_C). Then it can be seen (Figure 10-23) that the following possibilities exist:

$M_C/M_F = 0$	Pure tipping (no control of rotation)
$0 < M_C/M_F < 1$	Controlled tipping (inclination of tooth changes but the center of rotation is displaced away from the center of resistance, and the root and crown move in the same direction)
$M_C/M_F = 1$	Bodily movement (equal movement of crown and root)
$M_C/M_F > 1$	Torque (root apex moves further than crown)

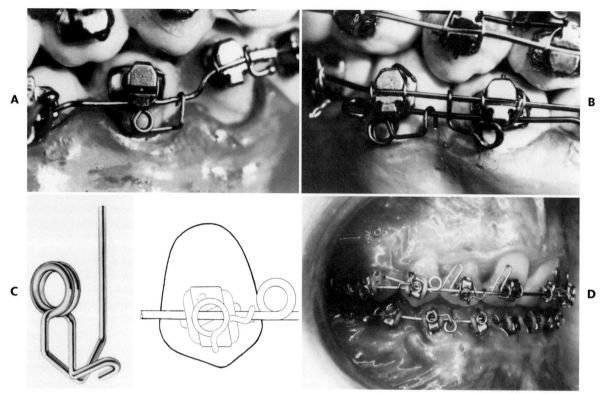

FIGURE 10-21 Auxiliary uprighting springs are used for root positioning with the Begg appliance and its modifications. **A** and **B**, Begg-style uprighting springs (which fit into a vertical slot beneath the bracket) used for root paralleling at extraction sites with the Combination-Anchorage appliance; **C**, modified uprighting springs (Sidewinder springs) that wrap around the bracket, for use with the Tip-Edge appliance; **D**, auxiliary uprighting springs and a maxillary auxiliary torquing arch wire, during treatment with the Tip-Edge appliance. (**A** and **B**, Courtesy Dr. WJ Thompson; **D**, courtesy Dr. P.C. Kesling.)

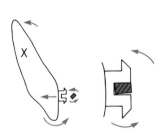

FIGURE 10-22 A rectangular arch wire fitting into a rectangular slot can generate the moment of a couple necessary to control root position. The wire is twisted (placed into torsion) as it is put into the bracket slot. The two points of contact are at the edge of the wire, where it contacts the bracket. The moment arm therefore is quite small, and forces must be large to generate the necessary M_C. Using the same tooth dimensions indicated in Figure 10-18, a 50 gm net lingual force would generate a 750 gm-mm moment. To balance it by creating an opposite 750 gm-mm moment within a 0.5 mm bracket, a torsional force of 1500 gm is required.

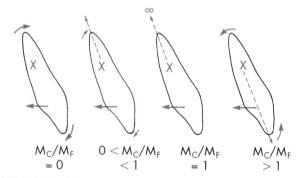

FIGURE 10-23 The ratio between the moment produced by the force applied to move a tooth (M_F) and the counterbalancing moment produced by the couple used to control root position (M_C) determines the type of tooth movement. With no M_C, ($M_C/M_F = 0$), the tooth rotates around a point near the center of resistance (pure tipping). As the moment-to-force ratio increases ($0 < M_C/M_F < 1$), the center of rotation is displaced further and further away from the center of resistance, producing what is called controlled tipping. When $M_C/M_F = 1$, the center of rotation is displaced to infinity and bodily movement (translation) occurs. If $M_C/M_F > 1$, the center of rotation is displaced incisally and the root apex will move more than the crown, producing root torque.

The moment of the force is determined by the magnitude of the force and the distance from the point of force application to the center of resistance. For most teeth, this is 8 to 10 mm, so M_F will be 8 to 10 times the force. In other words, if a 100 gm net force were used to move a tooth, a balancing moment of 800 to 1000 gm-mm (depending on root length and alveolar bone support) would be needed to obtain bodily movement. In the orthodontic literature, the relationship between the force and the counterbalancing couple often has been expressed in this way, as the "moment-to-force" ratio. In those terms, moment-to-force ratios of 1 to 7 would produce controlled tipping, ratios of 8 to 10 (depending on the length of the root) would produce bodily movement, and ratios greater than 10 would produce torque. Because the distance from the point of force application to the center of resistance can and does vary, moment-to-force ratios must be adjusted if root length, amount of alveolar bone support or point of force application differs from the usual condition. M_C/M_F ratios more precisely describe how a tooth will respond.

Remember that when a force is applied to a bracket to slide it along an arch wire, as often is the case in clinical orthodontics, the force felt by the tooth will be less than the force applied to the bracket because of frictional resistance (see further discussion on p. 344). The *net* force, after frictional resistance is subtracted, and the moment associated with the net force, are what is important. In contrast, when a couple is created within a bracket, friction rarely is a factor.

It is easy to underestimate the magnitude of the forces needed to create the balancing couple. In the example presented previously, if a 50 gm net force was used to retract a central incisor, a 500 gm-mm moment would be needed to keep it from tipping the crown moved lingually. To produce a moment of this magnitude within the confines of an 18 mil (0.45 mm) bracket would require opposite forces of 1100 gm, derived from twisting the arch wire. These forces within the bracket produce only a pure moment, so the periodontal ligament does not feel heavy force, but the necessary magnitude can come as a considerable surprise. The wire must literally snap into the bracket.

Narrow vs. Wide Brackets in Fixed Appliance Systems

Control of root position with an orthodontic appliance is especially needed in two circumstances: when the root of a tooth needs to be torqued faciolingually (as in the previous example), and when mesiodistal root movement is needed for proper paralleling of teeth at extraction sites. In the former instance, the necessary moment is generated within the bracket, and the key dimensions are those of the arch wire; in the latter circumstance, the moment is generated across the bracket, and bracket width determines the length of the moment arm.

The wider the bracket, all other things being equal, the easier it will be to generate the moments needed to bring

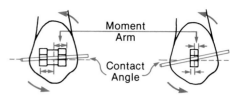

FIGURE 10-24 The width of the bracket on a tooth determines the length of the moment arm for control of mesiodistal root position. Bracket width also influences the contact angle at which the corner of the bracket meets the arch wire. The wider the bracket, the smaller the contact angle.

roots together at extraction sites or to control mesiodistal position of roots in general. Consider retracting the root of a canine tooth into a first premolar extraction site (Figure 10-24). With a retraction force of 100 gm and a 10 mm distance from the bracket to the center of resistance, a 1000 gm-mm moment will be needed. If the bracket on this tooth is 1 mm wide, 1000 gm of force will be needed at each corner of the bracket, but if the bracket is 4 mm wide, only 250 gm of force at each corner will be necessary.

This assumes even greater practical significance when the extraction site is to be closed by sliding teeth along an arch wire, and friction between the wire and bracket is encountered. Frictional resistance to sliding (discussed more fully following) is affected by the force with which the bracket contacts the arch wire and the contact angle between the wire and the bracket (see Figure 10-24). The wider bracket reduces both the force needed to generate the moment and the contact angle and is thus advantageous for space closure by sliding.

Despite their advantage when spaces are to be closed by sliding teeth on an arch wire, wide brackets have a partially offsetting disadvantage. The wider the bracket on a tooth, the smaller the interbracket span between adjacent teeth, and therefore the shorter the effective length of the arch wire segments between supports. Reducing the span of the wire segments in this way (reducing the length of the beam, in the terminology of our previous discussion) greatly decreases both the springiness of the arch wire and its range of action. For this reason, the use of extremely wide brackets is contraindicated. The maximum practical width of a wide bracket is about half the width of a tooth, and even narrower brackets have an advantage when teeth are malaligned, because the greater interbracket span gives more springiness.

Effect of Bracket Slot Size in the Edgewise System

The use of rectangular arch wires in rectangular bracket slots was introduced by Edward Angle in the late 1920s with his edgewise arch mechanism (see Chapter 12). The original appliance was designed for use with gold arch wires, and the 22 × 28 mil bracket slot size was designed to accommodate rectangular arch wires of approximately the same dimension. In Angle's concept of treatment, sliding teeth along arch wires to close extraction sites was unnecessary, because extractions for orthodontic purposes simply were not done. Torquing movements, on the other hand, were important, and a major goal of the appliance design was efficient torque. The appliance was engineered to produce appropriate force and a reasonable range of action in torsion when gold arch wires of 22 × 28 dimension were used with narrow brackets.

When steel arch wires replaced gold, Angle's original engineering calculations were no longer valid because steel wire of the same size was so much stiffer. An alternative was to redesign the edgewise appliance, optimizing the bracket slot size for steel. A reduction in slot size from 22 to 18 mil was advocated for this purpose. Even with this smaller slot size, full dimension steel wires still produce slightly greater forces than the original edgewise system did, but the properties of the appliance system are close to the original. Good torque is possible with steel wires and 18 mil edgewise brackets.

On the other hand, using undersized arch wires in edgewise brackets is a way to reduce friction if teeth are to slide along the arch wire, which was an important consideration by the time steel wire replaced gold. As a practical matter, sliding teeth along an arch wire requires at least 2 mil of clearance, and even more clearance may be desirable. The greater strength of an 18 mil arch wire compared with a 16 mil wire can be an advantage in sliding teeth. The 18 mil wire would, of course, offer excellent clearance in a 22-slot bracket, but fits too tightly for sliding space closure in an 18-slot bracket. The original 22-slot bracket therefore would have some advantage during space closure but would be a definite disadvantage when torque was needed later. With steel arch wires of 21 mil as the smaller dimension (close enough to the original 22 mil bracket slot size to give a good fit), springiness and range in torsion are so limited that effective torque with the arch wire is essentially impossible. Using wide brackets to help with space closure would make the torque problem worse. Exaggerated inclinations of smaller rectangular wires, for example, 19 × 25, are one alternative, but torquing auxiliaries (see Figure 10-21) are often necessary with undersized steel wires in 22-slot edgewise brackets.

In this situation, a role for the new titanium arch wires becomes clearer. If only steel wires are to be used, the 18 mil slot system has considerable advantage over the larger bracket slot size. With their excellent springback and resistance to permanent deformation, NiTi alloys overcome some of the alignment limitations of steel wires in wide 22 mil slot brackets, while rectangular NiTi and beta-Ti wires offer advantages over steel for the finishing phases of treatment and torque control. In short, the new titanium arch wires greatly help overcome the major problems associated with continued use of the original edgewise slot size.

MECHANICAL ASPECTS OF ANCHORAGE CONTROL

When teeth slide along an arch wire, force is needed for two purposes: to overcome frictional resistance, and to create the bone remodeling needed for tooth movement. As we have pointed out in Chapter 9, controlling the position of anchor teeth is accomplished best by minimizing the reaction force that reaches them. Use of unnecessarily heavy force to move teeth creates problems in controlling anchorage. Unfortunately, anchor teeth usually feel the reaction to both frictional resistance and tooth movement forces, so controlling and minimizing friction is an important aspect of anchorage control.

Frictional Effects on Anchorage

When one moving object contacts another, friction at their interface produces resistance to the direction of movement. The frictional force is proportional to the force with which the contacting surfaces are pressed together and is affected by the nature of the surface at the interface (rough or smooth, chemically reactive or passive, modified by lubricants, etc.). Interestingly, friction is independent of the apparent area of contact. This is because all surfaces, no matter how smooth, have irregularities that are large on a molecular scale, and real contact occurs only at a limited number of small spots at the peaks of the surface irregularities (Figure 10-25). These spots, called *asperities*, carry all

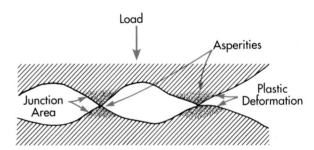

FIGURE 10-25 When two solid surfaces are pressed together or one slides over the other, real contact occurs only at a limited number of small spots, called *asperities*, that represent the peaks of surface irregularities. Even under light loads, as when an orthodontic arch wire is tied into a bracket, local pressure at the asperities is likely to form junctions between the two surfaces. These junctions shear as sliding occurs. If two materials of different hardness slide past each other (for instance, a metal wire in a ceramic bracket), the coefficient of friction is mainly determined by the shear strength and yield pressure of the softer material. When a soft material slides past a harder one (again, a metal wire in a ceramic bracket), small fragments of the soft material adhere to the hard one (see Figure 12-42), but "plowing" of asperities, which can contribute to total friction, is not observed. Although interlocking of asperities can contribute to friction, this also is negligible in most orthodontic applications because the surfaces have been ground relatively smooth. (Redrawn from Jastrzebski Z: *The nature and properties of engineering materials,* ed 2, New York, 1976, John Wiley & Sons.)

the load between the two surfaces. Even under light loads, local pressure at the asperities may cause appreciable plastic deformation of those small areas. Because of this, the true contact area is to a considerable extent determined by the applied load and is directly proportional to it.

When a tangential force is applied to cause one material to slide past the other, the junctions begin to shear. The coefficient of friction then is proportional to the shear strength of the junctions and is inversely proportional to the yield strength of the materials (because this determines the extent of plastic deformation at the asperities). At low sliding speeds, a "stick-slip" phenomenon may occur as enough force builds up to shear the junctions and a jump occurs, then the surfaces stick again until enough force again builds to break them.

Two other factors can affect the resistance to sliding: the interlocking of surface irregularities, which obviously becomes more important when the asperities are large or pointed; and the extent to which asperities on a harder material plow into the surface of a softer one. Thus the total frictional resistance will be the sum of three components: (1) the force necessary to shear all junctions, (2) the resistance caused by the interlocking of roughness, and (3) the plowing component of the total friction force.[17] In practice, if the two materials are relatively smooth and not greatly dissimilar in hardness, friction is largely determined by the shearing component.

To a surprisingly large extent, friction is a factor in orthodontic anchorage control, particularly for space closure with fixed appliances. Frictional resistance to sliding arch wires against brackets can be reduced by modifying any or all of the major factors discussed above, but it cannot be totally eliminated. It is possible in the laboratory to measure the actual friction between various wires and brackets and then to compare the magnitude of frictional resistance with the force levels needed to produce tooth movement.

Significant influences on friction in orthodontic appliances include:

Surfaces of Wires and Brackets. The concept that surface qualities are an important variable in determining friction has been emphasized by experiences in the late 1980s with both titanium wires and ceramic or plastic brackets. Stainless steel brackets slide reasonably well on steel wires, but the situation is not so fortunate with some other possible combinations.

Surface Qualities of Wires. When NiTi wires were first introduced, manufacturers claimed that they had an inherently slick surface compared with stainless steel, so that all other factors being equal, there would be less interlocking of asperities and thereby less frictional resistance to sliding a tooth along a NiTi wire than a stainless steel one. This is erroneous—the surface of NiTi is rougher (because of surface defects, not the quality of polishing) than that of beta-Ti, which in turn is rougher than steel. More importantly, however, there is little or no correlation for orthodontic wires between the coefficients of friction and surface roughness[18] (i.e., interlocking and plowing are not significant components of the total frictional resistance). Although NiTi has greater surface roughness, beta-Ti has greater frictional resistance. It turns out that as the titanium content of an alloy increases, its surface reactivity increases, and the surface chemistry is a major influence on frictional behavior. Thus beta-Ti, at 80% titanium, has a higher coefficient of friction than NiTi at 50% titanium, and there is greater frictional resistance to sliding with either than with steel. With beta-Ti, there is enough titanium reactivity for the wire to "cold-weld" itself to a steel bracket under some circumstances, making sliding all but impossible.[19]

A possible solution to this problem is alteration of the surface of the titanium wires by implantation of ions into the surface. Ion implantation (with nitrogen, carbon, and other materials) has been done successfully with beta-Ti, and has been shown to improve the characteristics of beta-Ti hip implants. In clinical orthodontics, however, implanted NiTi and beta-Ti wires have failed to show improved performance in initial alignment or sliding space closure respectively, perhaps because friction is released when teeth move as bone bends during mastication.[20,21]

Surface Qualities of Brackets. Bracket surfaces also are important in friction. Most modern orthodontic brackets are either cast or milled from stainless steel, and if properly polished have relatively smooth surfaces comparable with steel wires. Titanium brackets now are coming into use, primarily because of their better biocompatibility—some patients have an allergic response to the nickel in stainless steel and do not tolerate steel appliances. Fortunately, many individuals who show cutaneous sensitivity to nickel do not have a mucosal reaction, but the increasing number of allergic patients is becoming a problem. At best, the surface properties of titanium brackets are like those of titanium wires, and polishing the interior of bracket slots is difficult enough that these critical areas may be rougher than wires. Sliding with titanium brackets, therefore, may be problematic, particularly if titanium archwires also are used.

Ceramic brackets became quite popular in the 1980s because of their improved esthetics, but problems related to frictional resistance to sliding have limited their use. The ones made from polycrystalline ceramics have considerably rougher surfaces than steel brackets. The rough but hard ceramic material is likely to penetrate the surface of even a steel wire during sliding, creating considerable resistance, and of course this is worse with titanium wires.[22] Although single crystal brackets are quite smooth, these brackets also can damage wires during sliding, and so they also have increased frictional resistance to sliding.[23] Recently, ceramic brackets with metal slots have been introduced, a rather explicit recognition of the problems created by friction against ceramic surfaces (see further discussion of esthetic appliances in Chapter 12).

It is quite likely that composite plastic brackets will come into routine use early in the new century. They have the advantages of being tooth colored and non-allergenic, and at least in theory, should have surface properties that would not be as troublesome as ceramics. Based on laboratory data, one of the few couples that improves the coefficient of friction beyond that of an all-stainless steel couple, is the esthetic wire-bracket-ligature couple comprised of all composite materials. The polycarbonate plastic brackets that have been offered commercially to date, however, have surfaces that are too soft and have required metal slots to provide even semi-satisfactory performance.

Force of Contact. The amount of force between the wire and the bracket strongly influences the amount of friction. This is determined by two things. First, if a tooth is pulled along an arch wire, it will tip until the corners of the bracket contact the wire and a moment is generated that prevents further tipping (see Figure 10-24). If the initial tipping is to be prevented and true bodily movement produced, any wire that is smaller than the bracket initially must cross the bracket at an angle. The greater the angle, the greater the initial moment and the greater the force between the wire and the bracket. As can be seen from Figure 10-26, friction goes up rapidly as the angle between the bracket and the wire increases. Because of this, the elastic properties of the wire influence friction, especially as bracket angulation increases.[24] A more flexible wire bends and reduces the angle between wire and bracket. As noted earlier, when teeth slide along an arch wire, it is easier to generate the moments needed to control root position with a wide bracket because the wider the bracket, the smaller the force needed at its edges to generate any necessary moment. The smaller force also should reduce the frictional force proportionally.

A second force, however, is the one that largely determines friction: the force that pulls the wire into the bracket, which would be produced by the ligature holding the wire in place.[25] Perhaps this explains why laboratory data indicate that bracket width has surprisingly little effect on friction. More importantly, it illustrates why sliding along arch wires works much better when the system that holds the arch wire in the bracket does not hold the wire tightly the bracket. Modern edgewise appliances with a rigid cap that locks over the top of the bracket (see Chapter 12 for a more detailed discussion) can have several advantages, but clearly the most important one is the reduced friction that allows more effective sliding—and therefore better anchorage control as well.

Magnitude of Friction. Perhaps the most important information to be gained from a consideration of friction is an appreciation of its magnitude, even under the best of circumstances. Note in Figure 10-27 that in the passive configuration, even with a 14 wire in a 22 slot bracket, there is measurable friction. The minimum frictional resistance to sliding a single bracket along an arch wire is about 100 gm.[26] In other words, if a canine tooth is to slide along an arch wire as part of the closure of an extraction space, and

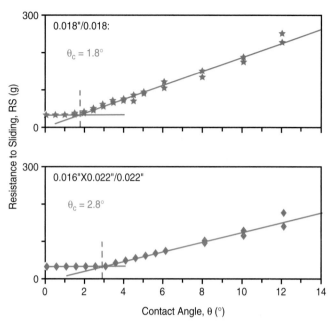

FIGURE 10-26 The amount of friction produced as a wire slides through a bracket increases as the angulation of the wire across the bracket slot increases. With a steel wire held loosely in a steel bracket, about 35 gm frictional resistance is measured under laboratory conditions, below a critical angle at which friction begins to increase (note the similarity of the initial data for the two wire/slot combinations shown here; also see Figure 10-27). Resistance to sliding can be minimized but not eliminated—this is close to the achievable minimum for steel on steel in orthodontic applications. As the upper curve shows, for a nominal 18 mil wire in an 18 slot bracket, the critical angle is 1.8°. Resistance to sliding increases linearly as the angulation increases, and for this wire/bracket combination, exceeds 200 gm at 12°. For a 16 × 22 wire in a 22 slot bracket, the critical angle is 2.8°, and resistance at 12° is about 150 gm. (Redrawn from Kusy and Whitley: *Angle Orthod* 69:71-80, 1999.)

a 100 gm net force is needed for tooth movement, approximately another 100 gm will be needed to overcome friction (Figure 10-28). The total force needed to slide the tooth therefore is twice as great as might have been expected. The frictional resistance can be reduced, but not eliminated, by replacing the ligature tie with a bracket cap so that the wire is held in place loosely.

In terms of the effect on orthodontic anchorage, the problem created by friction is not so much its presence as the difficulty of knowing its magnitude. To slide a tooth or teeth along an arch wire, the clinician must apply enough force to overcome the friction and produce the biologic response. It is difficult to avoid the temptation to estimate friction generously and add enough force to be certain that tooth movement will occur. The effect of any force beyond what was really needed to overcome friction is to bring the anchor teeth up onto the plateau of the tooth movement curve (see Figure 9-17). Then either unnecessary movement of the anchor teeth occurs, or additional steps to maintain anchorage are necessary (e.g., headgear).

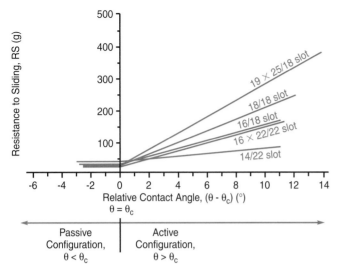

FIGURE 10-27   Laboratory data for sliding of five steel wire/bracket combinations, superimposed on the critical contact angle at which frictional resistance begins to increase (see Figure 10-26). Note the similarity of friction for all the wire-bracket combinations in the passive configuration, below the critical angle. It is possible to fit a nominal 19 × 25 wire into an 18 slot bracket because the wire typically is slightly undersized and the bracket slot is slightly oversized, but the fit is tight. The increase of friction with increasing contact angles is greatest for tightly fitting wires and least with the loosest fit. In the absence of notching phenomena, arch wire-bracket combinations with less second-order clearance ultimately bind worse than those with more clearance. (Redrawn from Kusy and Whitley: *Angle Orthod* 69: 71-80, 1999.)

Friction in the appliance system can be avoided if a spring loop is bent into the arch wire, so that arch wire segments move, taking the teeth with them instead of the teeth moving relative to the wire. Springs of this type are called *retraction springs* if they attach to only one tooth, or *closing loops* if they connect two arch wire segments (Figure 10-29). Incorporating springs into the arch wire makes the appliance more complex to fabricate and to use clinically but eliminates the difficulty in anchorage control caused by frictional resistance.

Methods to Control Anchorage

From the previous discussion, of both the biologic aspects of anchorage in Chapter 9 and the review above of frictional effects, it is apparent that several potential strategies can be used to control anchorage. Nearly all the possible approaches are actually used in clinical orthodontics, and each method is affected by whether friction will be encountered. Considering them in more detail:

   Reinforcement.   The extent to which anchorage should be reinforced depends on the tooth movement that is desired. In practice, this means that anchorage requirements must be established individually in each clinical situation. Once it has been determined that reinforcement is desirable, however, this typically involves including as many teeth as possible in the anchorage unit. For significant differential

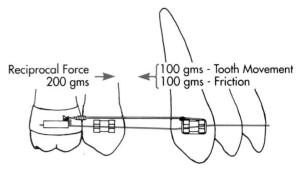

FIGURE 10-28   To retract a canine tooth by sliding it along an arch wire, an unknown amount of frictional resistance (from laboratory results, approximately equal to the force necessary to move the tooth) must be overcome. Clinically, problems in controlling anchorage because of friction arise largely because the true friction is unknown. A generous amount of force beyond what is necessary to move the tooth usually is added to ensure clinical effectiveness, but the excess force affects the anchor teeth.

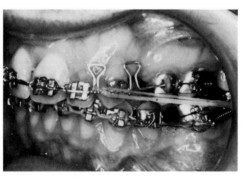

FIGURE 10-29   A closing loop is being used to retract the maxillary incisors, while a spring to slide the arch wire through the molar tube is used for space closure in the lower arch. In contemporary use, closing loops are bent into steel archwires, and teeth slide along steel wires, but the coil spring is A-NiTi. The Class II elastic from lower posterior to upper anterior also provides force to close both upper and lower spaces.

tooth movement, the ratio of PDL area in the anchorage unit to PDL area in the tooth movement unit should be at least 2 to 1 without friction, 4 to 1 with it. Anything less produces something close to reciprocal movement. Obviously, larger ratios are desirable if they can be obtained.

   Satisfactory reinforcement of anchorage may require the addition of teeth from the opposite dental arch to the anchor unit. Reinforcement may also include forces derived from structures outside the mouth. For example, to close a mandibular premolar extraction site, it would be possible to stabilize all the teeth in the maxillary arch so that they could only move bodily as a group, and then to run an elastic from the upper posterior to the lower anterior, thus pitting forward movement of the entire upper arch against distal movement of the lower anterior segment (Figure 10-30). This addition of the entire upper arch would greatly alter the balance between retraction of the lower anteriors and forward slippage of the lower posteriors.

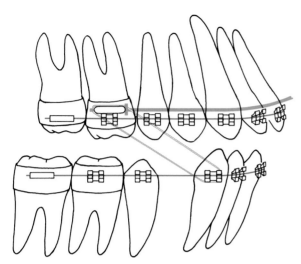

FIGURE 10-30   Reinforcement of anchorage can be produced by adding additional teeth within the same arch to the anchor unit, or by using elastics from the opposite arch to help produce desired tooth movement, as with the interarch elastic shown here. Additional reinforcement can be obtained with extraoral force, as with addition of a facebow to the upper molar to resist the forward pull of the elastic.

This anchorage could be reinforced even further by having the patient wear an extraoral appliance (headgear) placing backward force against the upper arch. The reaction force from the headgear is dissipated against the bones of the cranial vault, thus adding the resistance of these structures to the anchorage unit. The only problem with reinforcement outside the dental arch is that springs within an arch provide constant forces, whereas elastics from one arch to the other tend to be intermittent, and extra-oral force is likely to be even more intermittent. Although this time factor can significantly decrease the value of cross-arch and extraoral reinforcement, both can be quite useful clinically.

Subdivision of Desired Movement.   A common way to improve anchorage control is to pit the resistance of a group of teeth against the movement of a single tooth, rather than dividing the arch into more or less equal segments. In our same extraction site example, it would be perfectly possible to reduce the strain on posterior anchorage by retracting the canine individually, pitting its distal movement against mesial movement of all other teeth within the arch (Figure 10-31). After the canine tooth had been retracted, one could then add it to the posterior anchorage unit and retract the incisors. This approach would have the advantage that the reaction force would always be dissipated over a large PDL area in the anchor unit. Its disadvantage is that closing the space in two steps rather than one would take nearly twice as long.

Subdivision of tooth movement improves the anchorage situation regardless of whether friction is involved and where a space in the arch is located. If it is desired to slip all the posterior teeth forward (in which case the anterior teeth are the anchor unit), bringing them forward one at a time is the most conservative way to proceed. Moving them

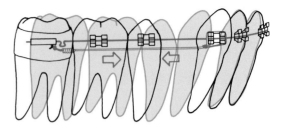

FIGURE 10-31   Retraction of the canine by itself, as the first step in a two-stage space closure, often is used to conserve anchorage, particularly when sliding teeth along an arch wire.

one at a time without friction, of course, will put less strain on anchorage than sliding them one at a time.

Tipping/Uprighting.   Another possible strategy for anchorage control is to tip the teeth and then upright them, rather than moving them bodily. In our familiar extraction site example, this would again require two steps in treatment. First, the anterior teeth would be tipped distally by being pitted against mesial bodily movement of the posterior segment (see Figure 9-18). As a second step, the tipped teeth would be uprighted, moving the canine roots distally and torquing the incisor roots lingually, again with stationary anchorage in the posterior segments. It would be extremely important to keep forces as light as possible during both steps, so that the teeth in the posterior segment were always below the optimum force range while the anterior teeth received optimum force.

Friction and Anchorage Control Strategies.   Anchorage control is particularly important when protruding incisors are to be retracted. The goal is to end up with the teeth in the correct position, not necessarily to retract them as much as possible. The desired amount of incisor retraction for any patient should be carefully planned, and the mechanotherapy should be selected to produce the desired outcome. This subject is discussed in considerably more detail in Chapter 17.

At this point, however, it is interesting to consider a relatively typical extraction situation, in which it is desired to close the extraction space 60% by retraction of the anterior teeth and 40% by forward movement of the posterior segments (Figure 10-32). This outcome would be expected from any of three possible approaches: (1) one-step space closure with a frictionless appliance; (2) a two-step closure sliding the canine along the arch wire, then retracting the incisors (as in the original Tweed technique); or (3) two-step space closure, tipping the anterior segment with some friction, then uprighting the tipped teeth (as in the Begg technique). (See Chapters 12 and 16 through 18 for a detailed discussion of these techniques.) The example makes the cost of friction in a clinical setting more apparent: the greater strain on anchorage when brackets slide along an arch wire must be compensated by a more conservative approach to anchorage control. The price is usually paid therefore in increased treatment time. The frictionless appliance, though more difficult to fabricate and manipulate, will result in the same space closure significantly faster.

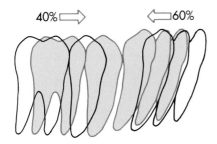

FIGURE 10-32   Closure of a premolar extraction site often is desired in a ratio of 60% retraction of incisors, 40% forward movement of molar and second premolar. This result can be obtained straightforwardly in three ways: (1) one-step space closure with a frictionless (closing loop) mechanism; (2) two-step space closure with sliding mechanics, retracting the canine individually, and then retracting the four incisors in a second step (the classic Tweed approach); or (3) two-step sliding space closure with distal tipping of the canine and incisors initially, followed by uprighting of these teeth (the classic Begg approach). Good clinical results can be obtained with all three methods. The cost of friction in space closure, with well-managed orthodontic appliances, is paid more in increased treatment time than in decreased quality of result.

Note that strategies for anchorage control are associated with particular orthodontic appliances, indeed are literally built into the appliance in many instances. The mechanical design principles discussed in this chapter have shaped the development of contemporary fixed appliances, but appliance designers have also had to consider anchorage as a design factor of considerable importance. The approach to anchorage control that is implicit in the appliance design is sometimes called the *appliance philosophy*, not quite so strange a term when viewed in this way.

DETERMINATE VS. INDETERMINATE FORCE SYSTEMS

The laws of equilibrium require not only that for every force there is an equal and opposite reactive force but also that the sum of the moments in any plane are equal to zero. In other words, the moments as well as the forces generated by an orthodontic appliance system must be balanced, in all three planes of space. It can be very difficult to visualize the total force system in orthodontics. Unexpected and unwanted tooth movement easily can result when an important component of the system is overlooked.

Force systems can be defined as statically *determinate*, meaning that the moments and forces can readily be discerned, measured and evaluated, or as *indeterminate*. Statically indeterminate systems are too complex for precisely measuring all forces and moments involved in the equilibrium. Typically, only the direction of net moments and approximate net force levels can be determined. This is more of a problem in orthodontics than in many engineering situations, because the eventual action of the system is determined by the biologic response. For instance, the amount

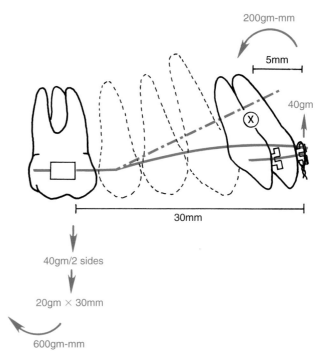

FIGURE 10-33   An intrusion arch made from rectangular wire, which fits into a rectangular tube on the molars and is tied to one point of contact on the incisor segment, is an example of a determinate one-couple system. If the arch wire is activated by pulling it down and tying it to the incisor segment so that it delivers 40 gm intrusion force (10 gm per tooth, 20 gm per side), and if the distance from the molar tube to the point of attachment is 30 mm, each molar will feel a 20 gm extrusive force in reaction and a 600 gm-mm moment to tip the crown distally. At the incisor segment, the force will create a 200 gm-mm moment to rotate the incisor crowns facially. At each molar, the extrusive force also would create a moment to roll the crown lingually. If the buccal tube were 4 mm buccal to the center of resistance, its magnitude would be 80 gm-mm.

of tooth movement will be determined to a large extent by the magnitude of the forces felt by anchor teeth and teeth whose movement is intended, not just by the differential between those forces. If the force applied to the anchor teeth is high enough to pull them up onto the plateau of the pressure-response curve, reciprocal tooth movement will occur despite a difference in PDL pressures (see Figure 9-17). Similarly, whether intrusion of incisor teeth or extrusion of posterior teeth occurs is almost totally a function of the magnitude of intrusive vs. extrusive forces, not their direction or the difference between them. Determinate force systems, therefore, are advantageous in orthodontics because they provide much better control of the magnitude of forces and couples.

For all practical purposes, determinate systems in orthodontics are those in which a couple is created at one end of an attachment, with only a force (no couple) at the other. This means that a wire that will serve as a spring can be inserted into a tube or bracket at one end, but must be tied so that there is only one point of contact on the other (Figure 10-33). When the wire is tied into a bracket on both ends, a statically indeterminate two-couple system has been created.

One-couple Systems

In orthodontic applications, one-couple systems are found when two conditions are met: (1) a cantilever spring or auxiliary arch wire is placed into a bracket or tube(s). It typically attaches to a tooth or teeth that is part of a stabilized segment (i.e., reinforced anchorage is being used); and (2) the other end of the cantilever spring or auxiliary arch wire is tied to a tooth or group of teeth that are to be moved, with a single point of force application.[27]

For analysis, the teeth in the anchor unit are considered as if stabilization had created a single large multirooted tooth, with a single center of resistance. It is important to tie teeth in an anchor unit tightly together with as rigid a stabilizing wire segment as possible. Often the posterior teeth on both sides are tied together with a rigid lingual arch, so that a single posterior stabilizing segment is created. If the goal is to move more than one tooth, the tooth movement segment similarly must be tied so the teeth become a single unit.

Cantilever Spring Applications. Cantilever springs are used most frequently to bring severely displaced (impacted) teeth into the arch (Figure 10-34). These springs have the advantage of a long range of action, with minimal decrease in force as tooth movement proceeds and excellent control of force magnitude. There are two disadvantages: (1) as with most devices with a long range of action, cantilever springs do not fail safe. If they are distorted by the patient, significant tooth movement in the wrong direction is quite possible; (2) the moment of the force on an unerupted tooth rotates the crown lingually as the tooth is brought toward the occlusal plane, which is likely to be undesirable. Although an additional force can be added to overcome this, the system rapidly can become complex. If the cantilever spring is tied into a bracket on the unerupted

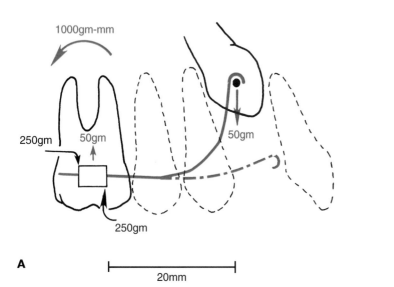

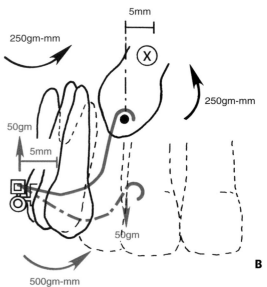

FIGURE 10-34 A cantilever spring, made from a rectangular wire that fits into a rectangular tube (or bracket) on one end and is tied to one point of contact on the other, produces a determinate one-couple system in which the forces and moments can be known precisely. **A,** Lateral view of the force system created by a cantilever spring to extrude an impacted maxillary canine. If the distance between the molar tube and a button on the canine to which the spring is tied is 20 mm, placing a 50 gm extrusive force on the canine creates a 50 gm intrusive force on the molar and also a 1000 gm-mm moment to rotate the molar crown forward around its center of resistance. If the molar tube is 4 mm in length, the moment would be created by a couple with 250 gm force upward on the mesial end of the tube and 250 gm downward on the distal end. **B,** Frontal view of the same force system. Consider the bucco-lingual (torque) moments created by the force on the molar and canine. If the center of resistance of the canine is 5 mm lingual to the button on its crown, a 50 gm extrusive force creates a 250 gm-mm moment to rotate the crown lingually (which usually is not desired). At the molar, if the center of resistance is 4 mm lingual to the tube on the buccal surface, the 50 gm intrusive force creates a 200 gm-mm moment to rotate the crown facially. But if the impacted canine is 10 mm lingual to the buccal surface of the molar, activating the spring also twists it, creating a 500 gm-mm torquing moment to rotate the molar crown lingually. The result at the molar is a net 300 gm-mm moment to torque the molar crown lingually and roots buccally. If the rectangular spring were tied into a bracket on the canine, a moment to torque its root facially could be generated, but the resulting two-couple system would be indeterminate—it would no longer be possible to know the forces and moments with certainty.

tooth so that a couple can be created for better control, the force system becomes statically indeterminate and force magnitudes are no longer known with certainty.

Auxiliary Intrusion/Extrusion Arches. The major use of one couple systems is for intrusion, typically of incisors that have erupted too much. For this purpose, light force against the teeth to be intruded is critical. An intrusion arch typically employs posterior (molar) anchorage against two or four incisors (Figure 10-35). Because the intrusive force must be light, the reaction force against the anchor teeth also is light, well below the force levels needed for extrusion and tipping that would be the reactive movements of the anchor teeth. Tying the molar teeth together with a rigid lingual arch prevents lingual tipping of the molars. In adults, usually the premolar teeth also are added to the anchor unit.

It would be easy enough to activate an auxiliary arch wire to produce extrusion of incisors rather than intrusion. This is rarely done clinically, however. The force needed for extrusion is 4 to 5 times higher than intrusion, however, so the reactive force against the anchor teeth also would be higher and the anchor teeth would not be as stable. Perhaps more importantly, the precise control of force magnitude that is the major advantage of a one-couple system, is less critical when extrusion is desired. The additional complexity of stabilizing segments and an auxiliary arch wire may not be cost effective if extrusion is the goal.

Two-couple Systems

An easy way to see the effect of changing from a determinate one-couple to an indeterminate two-couple system is to observe the effect of tying an intrusion arch into brackets on incisor teeth, rather than tying it with one-point contact.[28] The utility arch, popularized by Ricketts and used most frequently for incisor intrusion, makes just this change. Like a one-couple intrusion arch, it is formed from rectangular wire so that it will not roll in the molar tubes. Also like a one-couple intrusion arch, it bypasses the canine and premolar teeth, i.e., it is a 2 × 4 arch wire (attached to 2 molars and 4 incisors). The resulting long span provides excellent load deflection properties so that the light force necessary for intrusion can be created. The difference comes when the utility arch is tied into the incisor brackets, creating a two-couple system.

When the utility arch is activated for intrusion, the moment of the intrusive force tips the crowns facially (Figure 10-36). One way to prevent the facial tipping is to apply a force to retract the incisors, which would create a moment in the opposite direction. This could be done by cinching or tying back the intrusion utility arch. Although the retraction force could be light, any force to bring the anchor teeth mesially is likely to be undesirable.

Another strategy to control the facial tipping is immediately apparent: place a twist in the anterior segment

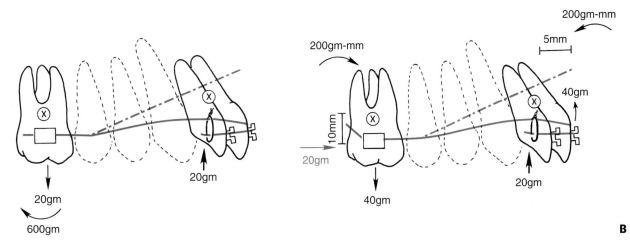

A   **B**

FIGURE 10-35 Two factors in the action of an intrusion arch are the relationship of the point of force application relative to the center of resistance of the incisor segment, and whether the incisor teeth are free to tip facially as they intrude or whether the arch is cinched back to produce lingual root torque. **A,** An intrusion arch can be tied at any point along the incisor segment. If it is tied behind the lateral incisor bracket, the force is applied in line with the center of resistance, and there is no moment to rotate the incisors facio-lingually. The effect on the anchor molar would be the same as if the intrusion arch were tied in the midline (see Figure 10-33). **B,** If the intrusion arch were tied in the midline and cinched back so it could not slide forward in the molar tube, the effect would be lingual root torque on the incisors as they intruded. Equilibrium requires that both moments and forces be balanced, so the moment on the incisors would be balanced by a similar moment on the anchor molars. Each would receive a 100 gm-mm moment to bring the crown mesially, which would require a 10 gm force at the distal of the molar tube if the distance from the tube to the molar's center of resistance is 10 mm.

of the utility arch, to torque the incisors lingually.[29] Let us examine the effect of doing this (see Figure 10-36, *B*). An effect of the couple within the bracket is to increase the intrusive force on the incisors, and also the reactive extrusive force on the molars. Although one can be sure that the magnitude of the intrusive force would increase, it is impossible to know how much—but any increase would shift the balance of tooth movement away from the desired intrusion of the incisor, for which highly controlled light force is critical, toward extrusion of the anchor teeth.

Note that the "torque bend" in the utility arch wire produces two problems. The first is the reactive force generated by the couple within the bracket. An increase in the magnitude of the intrusive force often is not anticipated from such an apparently unrelated change in the arch wire. The second problem is that the magnitude of the reactive forces is not known with certainty, which makes it impossible to accurately adjust the arch wire even if you do anticipate the increase. Both effects help explain why utility arches often produce disappointing amounts of incisor intrusion relative to molar extrusion.

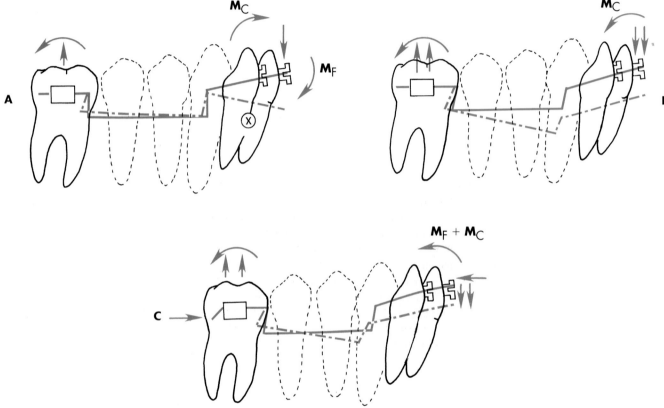

FIGURE 10-36 A utility arch often is an intrusion arch in a two-couple configuration, created by tying the rectangular intrusion arch into the brackets on the incisors. When this is done, the precise magnitude of forces and couples cannot be known, but the initial activation of the arch should be to provide about 40 grams to the incisor segment for intrusion. **A,** Activating the utility arch by placing it in the brackets creates the intrusion force, with a reactive force of the same magnitude on the anchor molar and a couple to tip its crown distally. At the incisors, a moment to tip the crowns facially (M_F) is created by distance of the brackets forward from the center of resistance, and an additional moment in the same direction is created by the couple within the bracket (M_C) as the inclination of the wire is changed when it is brought to the brackets. The moment of this couple cannot be known, but it is clinically important because it affects the magnitude of the intrusion force. **B,** Placing a torque bend in the utility arch creates a moment to bring the crown lingually, controlling the tendency for the teeth to tip facially as they intrude, but it also increases the magnitude of the intrusive force on the incisor segment and the extrusive force and couple on the molar. **C,** Cinching back the utility arch creates a force to bring the incisors lingually, and a moment of this force opposes the moment of the intrusion force. At the molar, a force to bring the molar mesially is created, along with a moment to tip the molar mesially. Especially if a torque bend still is present, it is difficult to be certain which of the moments will prevail, or whether the intrusion force is appropriate. With this two-couple system, the vertical forces easily can be heavier than desired, changing the balance between intrusion of the incisors and extrusion of the molars. (Redrawn from Davidovitch M, Rebellato J: Utility arches: a two-couple intrusion system, *Sem Orthod* 1: 25-30, 1995.)

APPLICATIONS OF COMPLEX (TWO-COUPLE) FORCE SYSTEMS

Symmetric and Asymmetric Bends

When a wire is placed into two brackets, the forces of the equilibrium always act at both brackets. There are three possibilities for placing a bend in the wire to activate it:[30]

- Symmetric V-bend, which creates equal and opposite couples at the brackets (Figure 10-37). The associated equilibrium forces at each bracket also are equal and opposite, and therefore cancel each other out. A symmetrical V-bend is not necessarily halfway between two teeth or two groups of teeth. If two teeth are involved but one is bigger than the other (e.g., a canine and lateral incisor), equal and opposite moments would require placing the bend closer to the large tooth, to compensate for the longer distance from the bracket to its center of resistance. The same would be true if two groups of teeth had been created by tying them into the equivalent of a single large multi-rooted tooth, as when posterior teeth are grouped into a stabilizing segment and used for anchorage to move a group of four incisors. A symmetrical V-bend would have to be offset, to compensate for the greater resistance of one segment.

- Asymmetric V-bend, which creates unequal and opposite couples, and net equilibrium forces that would intrude one unit and extrude the other (Figure 10-38). Although the absolute magnitude of the forces involved cannot be known with certainty (this is, after all, an indeterminate system), the relative magnitude of the moments and the direction of the associated equilibrium forces can be determined. The bracket with the larger moment will have a

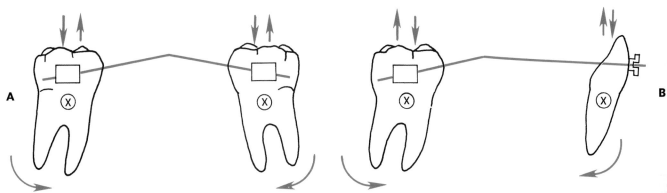

FIGURE 10-37 **A,** A symmetric V-bend is placed halfway between two units with equal resistance to movement. It creates equal and opposite moments, and the intrusive/extrusive forces cancel each other. **B,** To create equal and opposite couples, a V-bend must be displaced toward the unit with greater resistance to movement, so a symmetric V-bend between an incisor and molar would be offset toward the molar. One must know the approximate anchorage value of teeth or units of the dental arch to calculate the appropriate location of symmetric or asymmetric V-bends.

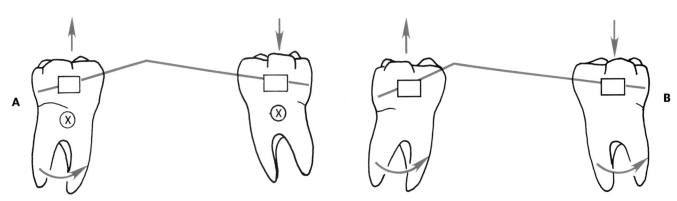

FIGURE 10-38 **A,** An asymmetric V-bend creates a greater moment on one tooth or unit than the other. As the bend moves toward one tooth, the moment on it increases and the moment on the distant tooth decreases. When the bend is one-third of the way along the interbracket span, the distant tooth receives only a force, with no moment. **B,** If the V-bend moves closer than the one-third point to one of the teeth, a moment in the same direction is created on both teeth, instead of opposite moments. A V-bend placed to parallel the roots of the adjacent teeth would not do so if the bend were too close to one of the teeth.

greater tendency to rotate than the bracket with the smaller moment, and this will indicate the direction of the equilibrium forces. As the bend moves closer to one of two equal units, the moment increases on the closer unit and decreases on the distant one, while equilibrium forces increase. When the bend is located one-third of the distance along the wire between two equal units, no moment is felt at the distant bracket, only a single force. When the bend moves closer than that to one bracket, moments at both brackets are in the same direction, and equilibrium forces increase further.

- Step bend, which creates two couples in the same direction regardless of its location between the brackets (Figure 10-39). The location of a V-bend is a critical variable in determining its effect, but the location of a step bend has little or no effect on either the magnitude of the moments or the equilibrium forces.

The general relationship between bend location and the forces and moments that are produced is shown in Table 10-7. Note that for V-bends, the force increases steadily as the beam moves off-center. For step bends, since both couples are in the same direction, the force is increased over what a symmetrical V-bend would produce.

Under laboratory conditions, the forces and couples created in a two-couple system can be evaluated experimentally.[31] With a 16 mil steel wire and an interbracket distance of 7 mm (about what would be found between central incisors with twin brackets or between narrow canine and premolar brackets), a step bend of only 0.35 mm would produce intrusive/extrusive forces of 347 grams and 1210 gm-mm couples in the same direction (see Table 10-7). Permanent distortion of the wire would occur with

a step bend of 0.8 mm. Since this force magnitude is far too great for intrusion, it is clear that extrusion would prevail. The heavy vertical forces produced by what orthodontists would consider modest bends in a light arch wire explain why extrusion is the response to step bends in continuous arch wires. With 16 mil steel wire and a 7 mm span between adjacent brackets, an asymmetric V-bend that places the apex of the wire only 0.35 mm above the bracket alos produces intrusive/extrusive forces that are far too great for intrusion (see Table 10-7), so the result here also would be extrusion.

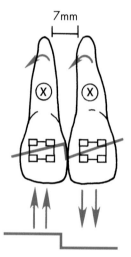

FIGURE 10-39 A step bend between two teeth produces intrusive force on one tooth, extrusive force on the other, and creates couples in the same direction. In contrast to V-bends, there is little effect on either the force or the couples when the step bend is moved off-center.

TABLE 10-7 *Force Systems From Step and V-Bends*

	Percent of total span to closest bracket	Moment far tooth/ Moment near tooth	Force general condition	Data from experiment 16 steel, 7 mm span, 0.35 mm bend	
				Force (gm)	Moment (gm-mm)
Step bend					
	All	1.0	XX	347	1210/1210
V-Bend					
	0.5	−1.0	None	0	803/803
	0.4	−0.3	X		
	0.33	0	XX		
	0.29			353	2210/262
	0.2	0.3	XXX		
	0.14			937	4840/1720
	0.1	0.4	XXXX		

(From Burstone CJ, Koening HA: Am J Orthod Dentofac Orthop 93: 59-67, 1988.)

The moments and forces are greatly reduced as inter-bracket distances increase. For instance, the same 0.35 mm step bend that produced 347 grams with a 7 mm inter-bracket span, produces only 43 grams with a 14 mm span (which is still too high for intrusion). Even with flexible arch wires, an interbracket span equivalent to the distance from the first molar to the lateral incisor is needed to obtain the light force necessary for intrusion. Longer spans also make the location of V-bends less critical. With a 7 mm interbracket span, moving a V-bend only 1.2 mm from a centered position would put it at the one-third position that totally eliminates the moment on the distant bracket. With a 21 mm span, the same error would be almost negligible. It is much easier, therefore, to control two-couple systems when the distances between attachments are relatively large, as they are when wires connect only to molars and incisors in a 2 × 4 arrangement, or to anterior and posterior segments.

Still another level of complexity exists for a 2 × 4 two-couple wire, because three-dimensional effects are produced when the wire goes around the arch from the molars to the incisors. This makes the analysis of torque bends particularly difficult. Using finite analysis modeling, Isaacson et al have shown that the general principles of 2-D analysis remain valid when 3-D analysis is done.[32] In a long-span wire like a utility arch, however, a V-bend at the molar produces significantly less moment and associated equilibrium forces than the same V-bend located at the same distance from the incisor segment. In addition, the reversal of moments so that the moment is in the same direction on the molar and the incisor, does not occur in the 3-D analysis when the V-bend moves closer than one-third of the distance to the molar or incisors. The effect is to make the effect of utility arches with complex bends even less predictable.

Utility and 2 × 4 Arches to Change Incisor Positions

The use of a two-couple utility arch to change the vertical position of incisors, and the problems that arise in controlling intrusion with this method, have been briefly outlined above. Two-couple systems work better for other types of tooth movement in which force magnitudes do not have to be controlled so precisely.

A two-couple system to change the inclination of incisors can be arranged to produce either tipping or torque. If a wire spanning from the molars to the incisors is activated to rotate incisors around their center of resistance, the crowns will move facially when the wire is free to slide through the molar tube (Figure 10-40).[33] Occasionally, this provides a convenient way to tip maxillary incisors facially to correct anterior crossbite in the mixed dentition (see Chapter 14).

If the wire is cinched back, the effect will be to torque the incisor roots lingually, and a reaction force to bring the molar mesially is created. The incisors also will extrude, while the molars will intrude and roll buccally. For incisor root torque, the long range of action provided by a 2 × 4 two-couple system is not necessarily an advantage, particularly when there is nothing to control the vertical side effects on the incisors. In patients with lingually tipped maxillary central incisors (as in Class II division 2 malocclusion), a one-couple torquing arch can be used to advantage (Figure 10-41).

Transverse Movement of Posterior Teeth

Dental posterior crossbite, requiring expansion or constriction of molars, can be approached with two-couple arch wires.[34] Then the anterior segment becomes the anchorage and movement of one or both first molars is desired (Figure 10-42). Incorporating the canines into the

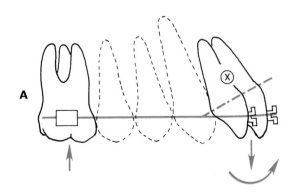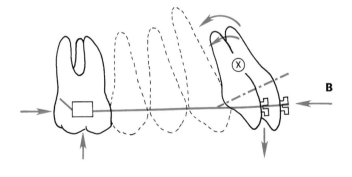

FIGURE 10-40   An asymmetric V-bend in a rectangular wire spanning from the first molars to the incisor segment produces a moment to rotate the incisors facio-lingually, with an intrusive force but no moment on the molars and an extrusive force on the incisors. **A,** If the arch wire is free to slide forward through the molar tube, the result is anterior tipping and extrusion of the incisors. Occasionally, this is desirable in the correction of anterior crossbite in the mixed dentition. **B,** If the arch wire is cinched behind the molar so that it cannot slide, the effect is lingual root torque and extrusion for the incisors and a mesial force on the molars.

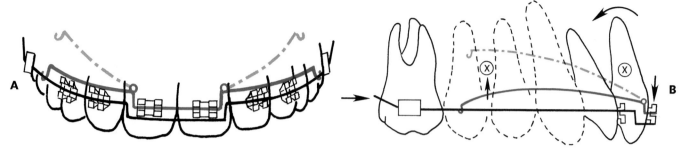

FIGURE 10-41   For torque of very upright maxillary central incisors (as in Class II division 2 malocclusion), a one-couple torquing arch designed by Burstone can be very effective. **A,** A heavy stabilizing arch is placed in all the teeth but the central incisors, contoured so that it steps below the brackets on the central incisors and contacts the facial surface of these teeth, is tied back against the molars. A wire tied into the central incisor brackets and activated by bending it down and hooking it between the first molar and second premolar, then produces the desired moment. **B,** Because the stabilizing arch wire prevents facial tipping and extrusion of the central incisors, the result is lingual root torque with optimum force over a long range. The reaction force to intrude the remaining teeth and bring them anteriorly is distributed over all the other teeth, minimizing the reaction.

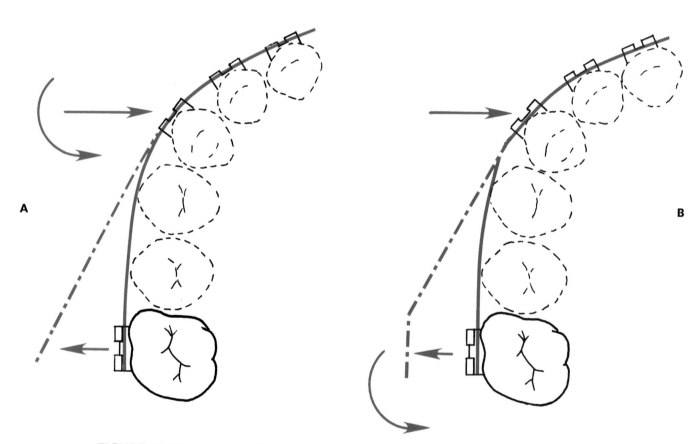

FIGURE 10-42   A 2 × 6 appliance can be used to produce transverse movement of first permanent molars. In this circumstance, the anterior segment becomes the segment, and it is important to add the canines to the anchor unit, but the premolars cannot be tied to the arch wire without destroying its effectiveness. The long span between the canine and molar is needed to produce the desired forces and moments in this two-couple system. **A,** An outward bend a few mm behind the canine bracket results primarily in expansion of the molar, with little or no rotation (with the unequal segments, this approximates the one-third position between the units of the two-couple system). **B,** An outward bend behind the canine combined with a toe-in bend at the molar results in expansion and mesial-out rotation of the molar. (Redrawn from Isaacson RJ, Rebellato J: Sem Orthod 1: 31-36, 1995.)

anchor segment is a necessity (i.e., this requires a 2 × 6 rather than a 2 × 4 appliance). A long span bypassing the premolars still is needed for appropriate force levels and control of moments. Asymmetric expansion or constriction to correct unilateral crossbite is quite feasible and often is the indication for using this method. As with other applications of two-couple systems, the large range of the appliance means that teeth can be moved a considerable distance with a single activation of the appliance. The corresponding disadvantage, of course, is that the system has poor fail-safe properties.

Lingual Arches as Two-Couple Systems

Still another example of a two-couple appliance system is a transpalatal lingual arch (or a mandibular lingual arch that does not contact the anterior teeth).[35] Lingual arches often are employed to prevent tooth movement rather than create it. The need for a lingual arch to stabilize posterior segments in many situations has been noted above. When a lingual arch is used to move teeth, spring properties are required—which means that either a different wire size or different material is needed for an active rather than a stabilizing lingual arch. Often when a flexible lingual arch is used to reposition molars, a rigid one then is needed to stabilize them while other tooth movement occurs. Steel lingual arches usually are 30 mil when tooth movement is desired, 36 mil when stabilization is needed. Replacing one with the other would require changing the tube on the molar band. To prevent this, the most practical approach is

to use a 32 × 32 TMA wire for active movement and 32 × 32 steel for stabilization, both of which will fit into the same rectangular lingual tube.[36,37] Lingual arches in general, and this approach in particular, are discussed in some detail in Chapter 12.

Whatever a lingual arch is made of, and however it is attached, its two-couple design predicts the effect of symmetric V, asymmetric V and step bends. Often it is desirable to rotate maxillary first molars so that the mesio-buccal cusp moves facially. This can be accomplished bilaterally with symmetric bends, or unilaterally with an asymmetric bend (Figure 10-43). An asymmetric activation tends to rotate the molar on the side closest to the bend and move it mesially, while the molar on the other side is displaced distally. It is tempting to think that net distal movement of upper molars can be accomplished routinely with this type of activation of lingual arches, and it has been suggested that a clinician can distalize one molar while rotating the other, then reverse the process, moving both of them back. However, the evidence indicates that significant distal movement beyond rotation of the buccal cusps is unlikely—mesial movement of the anchor molar is entirely possible.[38]

A lingual arch also can be activated to torque roots facially or lingually (Figure 10-44). Symmetric torque when molars are expanded provides bodily movement rather than tipping. An interesting approach to unilateral crossbite is the use of a lingual arch with buccal root torque (lingual crown torque) on one side pitted against buccal tipping on the other side. As Ingervall and co-workers have

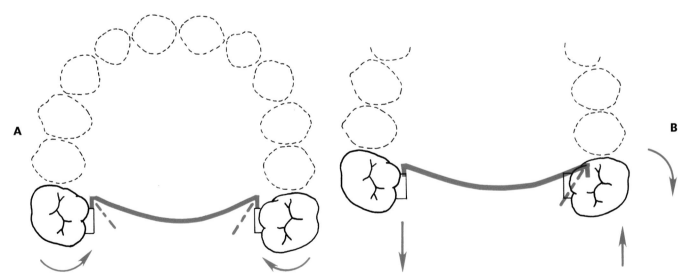

FIGURE 10-43 **A,** Bilateral toe-in bends at the first molars create equal and opposite couples, so the mesio-distal forces cancel and the teeth are rotated to bring the mesio-buccal cusp facially. When space has been lost in the maxillary arch or when a Class II molar relationship exists, this type of rotation often is desired, but a flexible rather than a rigid lingual arch is needed to obtain it. **B,** A unilateral toe-in bend rotates the molar on the side of the bend, and creates a force to move the other molar distally. Although mesial movement of the molar on the side of the bend is limited by contact with the other teeth, mesial movement may occur. Although net distalization of both molars has been claimed by bends of this type on first one side, then the other, significant distal movement of both teeth is unlikely.

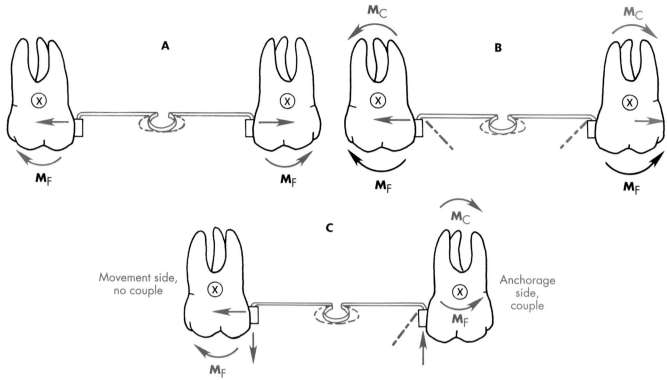

FIGURE 10-44   A, Bilateral expansion of molars can be created by expansion of a transpalatal arch, which typically is achieved by opening a loop in the mid-palate area. The moment of the expansion force tips the crowns facially. **B,** Placing a twist in the wire creates a moment to torque the roots facially. The moment of the couple must be greater than the moment of the force for this to occur. Unless a flexible wire is used for the lingual arch, it can be difficult to insert the activated lingual arch with enough twist to produce the desired torque. **C,** A twist in the wire on one side can be used to create stationary anchorage to tip the opposite molar facially. This is particularly effective if the wire is rounded on the movement side, so that a one-couple rather than two-couple system exists in the facio-lingual plane of space. (**A, B** redrawn from Rebellato. J: Two-couple orthodontic appliance systems: activations in the transverse dimension, *Sem Orthod* 1:37-43, 1995; see Ingerrall B et al: Am J Orthod Dentofac Orthop 107:418-425, 1995.)

shown quite convincingly, significant expansion on the tipping side can be produced, perhaps more effectively if the appliance is converted to a one-couple device by placing a round rather than rectangular wire in the bracket on the tipping side.[39]

A somewhat unusual application of a lingual arch would be to tip one molar distally, uprighting it. The reciprocal, of course, would be mesial tipping of the opposite molar. This activation would require a twist in the lingual wire. The location of this twist bend is not critical. The relative moments on the molar teeth will be equal and opposite, wherever the twist bend is placed.

Segmented Arch Mechanics

What is often called segmented arch mechanics is best considered an organized approach to using one-couple and two-couple systems for most tooth movements, so as to obtain both more favorable force levels and better control.[40] The essence of the segmented arch system is the establishment of well-defined units of teeth, so that anchorage and movement segments are clearly defined. The desired tooth movement is accomplished with cantilever springs where possible, so that the precision of the one-couple approach

is available, or with the use of two-couple systems through which at least net moments and the direction of equilibrium forces can be known.

An excellent example of the segmented arch approach is the design of an appliance to simultaneously retract and intrude protruding maxillary central incisors. This is difficult to accomplish because lingual tipping of the incisors tends to move the crown downward as the tooth rotates around its center of resistance. Intrusion of the root apex is necessary to keep the crown at the same vertical level relative to the lip and other teeth. This problem can be solved by creating anterior and posterior segments, using a rigid bar to move the point of force application distal to the center of resistance of the incisor segment, and applying separate intrusion and retraction forces (Figure 10-45).[41]

In segmented arch treatment, lingual arches are used for stabilization in a majority of the patients, and stabilizing wire segments in the brackets of teeth in anchor units also are used routinely. The requirements for stabilization, of course, are just the opposite of those for tooth movement: the heaviest and most rigid available wires are desired. For this reason, the 22 slot edgewise appliance is favored for segmented arch treatment. The wires used for stabilizing seg-

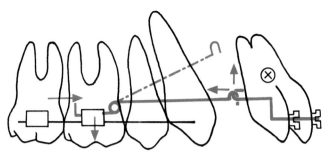

FIGURE 10-45 A segmented arch approach allows simultaneous retraction and intrusion of an anterior segment. A rigid bar in the anterior segment can be extended posteriorly so that the point of application of an intrusive force is at or distal to the center of resistance of the incisor segment. If a cantilever spring is used to apply an intrusive force at that point, the tendency of a retraction force to elongate the anterior segment can be overcome. (Redrawn from Shroff B, Yoon WM, Lindauer SJ, Burstone CJ: Simultaneous intrusion and retraction using a three-piece base arch, *Angle Orthod* 67:455-462, 1997.)

ments usually are 21 × 25 steel, which is far too stiff for tooth movement. Until 32 × 32 steel wires became available, the stabilizing lingual arches usually were 36 steel, with doubled-over ends that fit into rectangular sheaths.

Typical segmented arch treatment would call for initial alignment within anterior and posterior segments, the creation of appropriate anchorage and tooth movement segments, vertical leveling using intrusion or extrusion as needed, space closure with differential movement of anterior and posterior segments, and perhaps the use of auxiliary torquing arches. Friction as wires slide through brackets is almost always avoided, because it hampers efforts to control anchorage and introduces almost intolerable uncertainties into the calculation of appropriate force levels. Continuous archwires, particularly rectangular wires, would be reserved for the final stages of treatment when quite small but precise movements are required.

The advantages of the segmented arch approach are the control that is available, and the possibility of tooth movements that would be impossible with continuous archwires. The disadvantage is the greater complexity of the orthodontic appliance, and the greater amount of the doctor's time needed to install, adjust and maintain it. It is an interesting paradox that simplifying the engineering analysis of the appliance, by dealing insofar as possible with identifiable one- and two-couple systems, complicates the appliance rather than making it simpler.

The more complex segmented approach carries with it two other potential disadvantages that must be kept in mind. First, even with the most careful engineering analysis, it can turn out that something was overlooked in the determination of the likely outcome. Obviously, that is more likely when two-couple rather than one-couple devices are employed, but occasionally the simplifications that are part of normal engineering practice (e.g., neglecting the torque that may be created within a lingual arch bracket as tooth movement starts) can lead to surprising outcomes. It remains true that the more often something has been attempted, the more predictable the outcome is likely to be. The application of engineering theory to orthodontics is imperfect enough that a unique force system for an individual patient may not produce the expected outcome.

Second, most segmented arch mechanisms contain little or nothing to control the distance that teeth can be displaced if something goes wrong. If precisely calibrated springs with a long range of action encounter something that distorts them (e.g., a sticky candy bar) major problems can occur. The mechanical efficiency of a segmented appliance can be both an advantage and a disadvantage.

Continuous Arch Mechanics

Analysis of the effects of a continuous arch wire, one that is tied into the brackets on all the teeth, is essentially impossible. All that can be said is that an extremely complex multicouple force system is established when the wire is tied into place. The initial result is a small movement of one tooth. As soon as that occurs, the force system is changed, and the new system causes a small movement of another tooth (or a different movement of the first tooth). Either way, the result is still another complex force system, which causes another movement, leading to another change in the system, and so forth.[42] Sometimes orthodontic tooth movement is conceived as a slow, smooth transition of the teeth from one arrangement to another. Some thought about the force systems involved, particularly those with continuous arch mechanics, make it plain that this is far from the case. If it were possible to take time-lapse photographs of teeth being moved into position, we undoubtedly would see "the dance of the teeth," as the complex force systems formed and changed, producing varied effects in sequence. It is a saving grace that a continuous arch wire usually does not allow the teeth to move very far from the desired end point. In general, the mechanical efficiency of a continuous arch wire system is less than that of a segmented arch system, but its fail-safe properties are better.

Even with continuous arch mechanics, major tooth movements often are undertaken after the establishment of identifiable segments. In adults who require intrusion of incisors, there is no alternative to the use of a long-span auxiliary arch wire from stabilized posterior segments, and a one-couple intrusion arch clearly is preferable. For closure of extraction spaces, even if a continuous closing loop wire is used, posterior stabilizing and anterior tooth movement segments need to be established. Teeth may or may not slide along an arch wire during closure of extraction spaces, but especially when the 22 slot appliance is used with continuous arch wires, sliding often is a major component of the treatment mechanics.

The advantages and disadvantages of the continuous arch approach are just the reverse of those with the segmented arch approach. Continuous arch treatment is not as well defined in terms of the forces and moments that will be generated at any one time, and certainly is less elegant from an engineering perspective. But continuous arch wires often take less chair time because they are simpler to make and install, and because they have excellent fail-safe properties in most applications. In modern orthodontics, often the clinician must evaluate the trade-off between segmented and continuous arch approaches to specific problems. For those who use primarily the segmented approach, some use of continuous arch wires simplifies life. For those who use primarily continuous arch wires, some use of the segmented approach is necessary to meet specific objectives. Quite literally, you consider the benefits vs. the cost (time) and risks, and take your choice.

The development of contemporary fixed appliances and their characteristics are discussed in Chapter 12. Clinical applications of the mechanical principles reviewed in this chapter, and further information about the use of specific treatment methods, are provided in some detail in Chapters 16 to 18.

REFERENCES

1. Kusy RP, Dilley GJ, Whitley JQ: Mechanical properties of stainless steel orthodontic archwires, Clin Materials 3:41-59, 1988.
2. Burstone CJ, Qin B, Morton JY: Chinese NiTi wire: a new orthodontic alloy, Am J Orthod 87:445-452, 1985.
3. Miura F, Mogi M, Yoshiaki O et al: The super-elastic property of the Japanese NiTi alloy wire for use in orthodontics, Am J Orthod 90:1-10, 1986.
4. Miura F, Mogi M, Ohura Y: Japanese NiTi alloy wire: use of the direct electric resistance heat treatment method, Eur J Orthod 10:187-191, 1988.
5. Miura F, Mogi M, Okamoto Y: New application of super-elastic NiTi rectangular wire, J Clin Orthod 24:544-548, 1990.
6. Thayer TA, Bagby MD, Moore RN, DeAngelis RJ: X-ray diffraction of nitinol orthodontic archwires, Am J Orthod Dentofac Orthop 107:604-612, 1995.
7. Kusy RP: The future of orthodontic materials: the long view, Am J Orthod Dentofac Orthop 113:91-95, 1998.
8. Kusy RP: Comparison of nickel-titanium and beta-titanium wire sizes to conventional orthodontic arch wire materials, Am J Orthod 79:625-629, 1981.
9. Kusy RP: On the use of nomograms to determine the elastic property ratios of orthodontic archwires, Am J Orthod 83:374-381, 1983.
10. Adams DM, Powers JM, Asgar K: Effects of brackets and ties on stiffness of an arch wire, Am J Orthod Dentofac Orthop 91:131-136, 1987.
11. Bertl W, Droschl H: Forces produced by orthodontic elastics as a function of time and distance extended, Eur J Orthod 8:198-201, 1986.
12. Josell SD, Leiss JB, Rekow ED: Force degradation in elastomeric chains, Sem Orthod 3:189-197, 1997.
13. Darendeliler MA, Darendeliler A, Mandurino M: Clinical application of magnets in orthodontics and biological implications: a review, Eur J Orthod 19:431-442, 1997.
14. Darendeliler MA, Sinclair PM, Kusy RP: Effects of static and pulsed electromagnetic fields on orthodontic tooth movement, Am J Orthod Dentofac Orthop 107:578-588, 1995.
15. Linder-Aronson A, Lindskog S, Rygh P: Orthodontic magnets: effects on gingival epithelium and alveolar bone in monkeys, Eur J Orthod 14:255-263, 1992.
16. Smith RJ, Burstone CJ: Mechanics of tooth movement, Am J Orthod 85:294-307, 1984.
17. Jastrzebski ZD: The nature and properties of engineering materials, ed 2, New York, 1976, John Wiley & Sons.
18. Kusy RP, Whitley JQ: Effects of surface roughness on the coefficients of friction in model orthodontic systems, J Biomech 23:913-925, 1990.
19. Kusy RP, Whitley JQ: Friction between different wire-bracket configurations and materials, Sem Orthod 3:166-177, 1997.
20. Cobb NW III, Kula KS, Phillips C, Proffit WR: Efficiency of multistrand steel, superelastic NiTi and ion-implanted NiTi archwires in initial alignment, Clin Orthod Res, in press.
21. Kula K, Phillips C, Gibilaro A, Proffit WR: The effect of ion implantation of TMA archwires on the rate of orthodontic sliding space closure, Am J Orthod Dentofac Orthop 114:577-580, 1998.
22. Kusy RP, Whitley JQ, Prewitt MJ: Comparison of the frictional coefficients for selected arch wire-bracket slot combinations in the dry and wet states, Angle Orthod 61:293-302, 1991.
23. Saunders CR, Kusy RP: Surface topography and frictional characteristics of ceramic brackets, Am J Orthod Dentofac Orthop 106:76-87, 1994.
24. Drescher D, Bourauel C, Schumacher HA: Frictional forces between bracket and arch wire, Am J Orthod Dentofac Orthop 96:397-404, 1989.
25. Yamaguchi K, Nanda RS, Morimoto N, Oda Y: A study of force application, amount of retarding force and bracket width in sliding mechanics, Am J Orthod Dentofac Orthop 109:50-57, 1996.
26. Kusy RP, Whitley JQ: Friction between different wire-bracket configurations and materials, Sem Orthod 3:166-177, 1997.
27. Lindauer SJ, Isaacson RJ: One-couple systems, Sem Orthod 1:12-24, 1995.
28. Davidovitch M, Rebellato J: Utility arches: a two-couple intrusion system, Sem Orthod 1:25-30, 1995.
29. Ricketts RM: Bioprogressive therapy as an answer to orthodontic treatment needs, part 2, Am J Orthod 70:241-268, 1976.
30. Isaacson RJ, Lindauer SJ, Davidovitch M: The ground rules for arch wire design, Sem Orthod 1:3-11, 1995.
31. Burstone CJ, Koenig HA: Creative wire bending—the force system from step and V bends, Am J Orthod Dentofac Orthop 93:59-67, 1988.
32. Isaacson RJ, Lindauer SJ, Conley P: Responses of 3-dimensional archwires to vertical V-bends: comnparisons with existing 2-dimensional data in the lateral view, Sem Orthod 1:57-63, 1995.

33. Isaacson RJ, Rebellato J: Two-couple orthodontic appliance systems: torquing arches, Sem Orthod 1:31-36, 1995.
34. Rebellato J: Two-couple orthodontic appliance systems: activations in the transverse dimension, Sem Orthod 1:37-43, 1995.
35. Rebellato J: Two-couple orthodontic appliance systems: transpalatal arches, Sem Orthod 1:44-54, 1995.
36. Burstone CJ, Manhartsberger C: Precision lingual arches: passive applications, J Clin Orthod 22:444-452, 1988.
37. Burstone CJ: Precision lingual arches: active applications, J Clin Orthod 23:101-109, 1989.
38. Dahlquist A, Gebauer U, Ingervall B: The effect of a transpalatal arch for correction of first molar rotation, Eur J Orthod 18:257-267, 1996.
39. Ingervall B, Gollner P, Gebauer U, Frolich K: A clinical investigation of the correction of unilateral molar crossbite with a transpalatal arch, Am J Orthod Dentofac Orthop 107:418-425, 1995.
40. Burstone CJ: The segmented arch approach to space closure, Am J Orthod 82:361-378, 1982.
41. Shroff B, Yoon WM, Lindauer SJ, Burstone CJ: Simultaneous intrusion and retraction using a three-piece base arch, Angle Orthod 67:455-462, 1997.
42. Smith RJ, Burstone CJ: Mechanics of tooth movement, Am J Orthod 85:294-307, 1984.

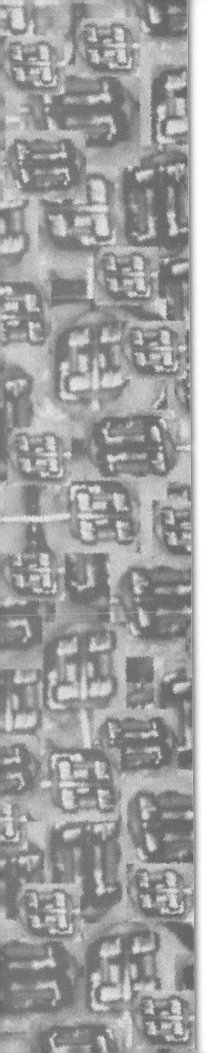

SECTION

V

FIXED AND REMOVABLE APPLIANCES

Contemporary orthodontic treatment involves the use of both fixed and removable appliances. Although removable appliances play only a supporting role in comprehensive treatment now, they are an important part of preliminary treatment for preadolescents, adjunctive treatment for adults, and retention for all types of patients. The indications for functional appliances for growth modification are discussed in Chapter 8; Chapter 11 describes all types of removables useful at present, with emphasis on the components approach to designing functional appliances for individual patients.

Comprehensive treatment now is done with fixed attachments for all teeth, almost always using a modern edgewise appliance with offset, angulated, and torqued bracket slots to reduce the need for routine first, second, and third order bends in arch wires. In Chapter 12, banding and bonding as methods for attaching fixed appliances are described and illustrated, and the characteristics of current edgewise appliances are discussed in detail.

CHAPTER

11

Removable Appliances

Removable orthodontic appliances have two immediately apparent advantages: they can be removed on socially sensitive occasions, which makes them (at least initially) more acceptable to patients, and they are fabricated in the laboratory rather than directly in the patient's mouth, reducing the dentist's chair time during the initial part of treatment. In addition, they allow some types of growth guidance treatment to be carried out more readily than is possible with fixed appliances. These advantages for both the patient and the dentist have ensured a continuing interest in removable appliances.

There are also obvious disadvantages: the response to treatment is heavily dependent on patient compliance, since the appliance can be effective only when the patient chooses to wear it; and it is difficult to obtain the two-point contacts on teeth necessary to produce complex tooth movements, which means that the appliance itself may limit the possibilities for treatment. Because of these limitations, removable appliances are most useful for the first of two phases of treatment, and contemporary comprehensive treatment is dominated by fixed, non-removable appliances.

THE DEVELOPMENT OF REMOVABLE APPLIANCES

In the United States, Victor Hugo Jackson was the chief proponent of removable appliances among the pioneer orthodontists of the early 20th century. At that time, neither the modern plastics for baseplate materials nor stainless steel wires for clasps and springs were available, and the appliances were rather clumsy combinations of vulcanite bases and precious metal or nickel-silver wires.

In the early 1900s, George Crozat developed a removable appliance fabricated entirely of precious metal that is still used occasionally. The appliance consisted of an effective clasp for first molar teeth modified from Jackson's designs, heavy gold wires as a framework, and lighter gold fingersprings to produce the desired tooth movement (Figure 11-1). At the time the Crozat appliance was developed, a typical fixed appliance consisted of bands only on first molars, with wire ligatures tied to a heavy labial or lingual archwire to align malposed teeth by expanding the dental arch. The Crozat appliance was a removable but more flexible version of the same device. Its metal framework and improved clasps made it greatly superior to alternative removables of that time. The clasping was good enough to allow the use of light interarch elastics, and Class II elastics were employed with Crozat appliances to treat Class II malocclusions.

The Crozat appliance attracted a small but devoted following, primarily in the area around New Orleans. It is still used by some practitioners but had little impact on the mainstream of American orthodontic thought and practice. From the beginning, the emphasis in American orthodontics has been on fixed appliances, and the steady progression of fixed appliance techniques in the United States is described and illustrated in Chapter 12.

For a variety of reasons, development of removable appliances continued in Europe despite their neglect in

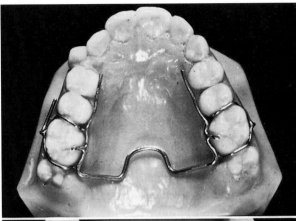

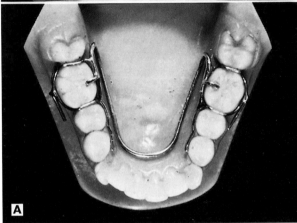

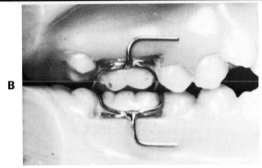

FIGURE 11-1 Crozat appliances for the upper and lower arch. **A,** Occlusal view, showing the transverse connectors that allow lateral expansion; **B,** close-up of the Crozat clasps, which utilize fingers extending into the mesio-buccal and disto-buccal undercuts.

orthodontists to emphasize removable appliances that could be made with available materials. (Precision steel attachments were not available until long after World War II; fixed appliances required precious metal.)

The interesting result was that in the 1925 to 1965 era, American orthodontics was based almost exclusively on the use of fixed appliances, while fixed appliances were essentially unknown in Europe and all treatment was done with removables, not only for growth guidance but also for tooth movement of all types.

A major part of European removable appliance orthodontics of this period was functional appliances for guidance of growth. A functional appliance by definition is one that changes the posture of the mandible, holding it open or open and forward. Pressures created by stretch of the muscles and soft tissues are transmitted to the dental and skeletal structures, moving teeth and modifying growth. The monobloc developed by Robin in the early 1900s is generally considered the forerunner of all functional appliances, but the activator developed in Norway by Andresen in the 1920s (Figure 11-2) was the first functional appliance to be widely accepted.

Andresen's activator became the basis of the "Norwegian system" of treatment. Both the appliance system and its theoretic underpinnings were improved and extended elsewhere in Europe, particularly by the German school led by Haupl, who believed that the only stable tooth movement was produced by natural forces and that alterations in function produced by these appliances would give stable corrections of malocclusion.

This philosophic approach was diametrically opposite to that espoused by Angle and his followers in the United States, who emphasized fixed appliances to precisely position the teeth. These opposing beliefs contributed to the great differences between European and American orthodontics at mid-20th century.

Functional appliances were introduced into American orthodontics in the 1960s, largely in the beginning through the influence of Egil Harvold after he joined the faculty at the University of Toronto, and later from personal contact by a number of American orthodontists with their European counterparts. (Fixed appliances spread to Europe at the same time through similar personal contacts.) A major boost to functional appliance treatment in the United States came from the publication of animal experiment results in the 1970s showing that skeletal changes really could be produced by posturing the mandible to a new position and holding out the possibility that true stimulation of mandibular growth could be achieved (see Chapter 9). Although some of the enthusiasm for functional appliance treatment caused by the favorable animal experiments has faded in the light of less impressive results from clinical trials and retrospective clinical studies (see Chapter 8), functional appliances have achieved a major place in contemporary growth modification treatment.

the United States. There were three major reasons for this trend: (1) Angle's dogmatic approach to occlusion, with its emphasis on precise positioning of each tooth, had less impact in Europe than in the United States; (2) social welfare systems developed much more rapidly in Europe, which meant that the emphasis tended to be on limited orthodontic treatment for large numbers of people, often delivered by general practitioners rather than orthodontic specialists; and (3) precious metal for fixed appliances was less available in Europe, both as a consequence of the social systems and because the use of precious metal in dentistry was banned in Nazi Germany, forcing German

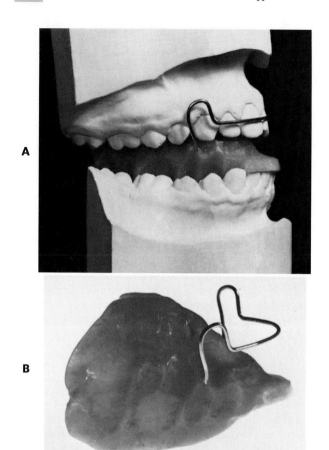

FIGURE 11-2 The Andresen-type activator is a tooth-borne passive appliance that was the first widely used functional appliance. The appliance opens the bite, and the mandible is advanced for Class II correction. **A,** The design incorporates a labial bow for control of maxillary anterior teeth and an acrylic cap over the lower incisors to control both eruption and mesial movement. **B,** The facets cut in the acrylic help direct eruption of the posterior teeth, mesially in the lower arch and distally and buccally in the upper arch. The lingual flange is the primary mechanism to position the mandible.

In the European approach of the mid-20th century, removable appliances often were differentiated into "activators," or functional appliances aimed at modifying growth, and "active plates" aimed at moving teeth. In addition to the functional appliance pioneers, two European orthodontists deserve special mention for their contributions to removable appliance techniques for moving teeth. Martin Schwartz in Vienna developed and publicized a variety of "split plate" appliances (Figure 11-3, *A*), which could produce most types of tooth movements. Philip Adams in Belfast modified the arrowhead clasp favored by Schwartz into the Adams crib, which became the basis for English removable appliances and is still the most effective clasp for orthodontic purposes (see Figure 11-3, *B*).

Within the past 20 years, the dichotomy between European and American orthodontics has largely disappeared. European-style removable appliances, particularly

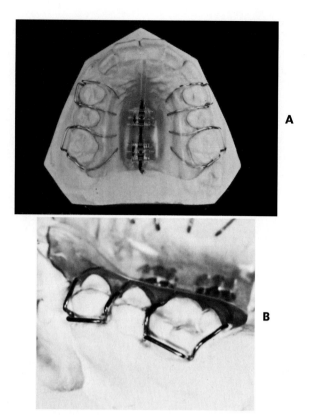

FIGURE 11-3 **A,** A split-plate maxillary expansion appliance of the type popularized by Martin Schwartz in Vienna. **B,** This appliance is retained by Adams clasps, which have replaced the arrowhead clasps favored by Schwartz.

for growth modification during first-stage mixed dentition treatment, have become widely used in the United States, while fixed appliances have largely replaced removables for comprehensive treatment in Europe and elsewhere throughout the world. This trend has been accelerated by the replacement of orthodontic bands with bonded attachments, which makes the placement of fixed appliances easier for both the dentist and the patient (see Chapter 12).

At present, removable appliances are indicated primarily for three major uses:
- Growth modification during the mixed dentition
- Limited (tipping) tooth movements, especially for arch expansion or correction of individual tooth malposition
- Retention after comprehensive treatment

The focus of this chapter is on the fabrication and adjustment of functional appliances and active plates. The indications for use of functional appliances in growth modification and considerations in planning arch expansion treatment are discussed in some detail in Chapter 8, and the biologic responses that underlie growth modification are described in Chapter 9. The clinical use of removable appliances in contemporary mixed dentition treatment is covered in Chapters 13 through 15, and retention is discussed in Chapter 19.

FUNCTIONAL APPLIANCES FOR GROWTH MODIFICATION

Because the design and fabrication of many types of functional appliances are covered in detail in a recent text devoted to the subject,[1] the goal here is to put these devices in perspective. They are understood best when viewed as falling into one of three broad categories, and as made up from a set of possible components that can be combined as needed in the design of an appliance for any individual patient.

Categories of Functional Appliances

Passive Tooth-borne Appliances.   These appliances have no intrinsic force-generating capacity from springs or screws and depend only on soft tissue stretch and muscular activity to produce treatment effects.

Activator.   The original functional appliance design (see Figure 11-2) was a block of plastic covering the teeth of both arches and the palate, made to fit loosely, advance the mandible several millimeters for Class II correction, and open the bite 3-4 mm. In addition to their effects on jaw growth, these essentially passive appliances can tip anterior teeth and control eruption of teeth to alter vertical dental relationships. The original design had facets or flutes (see below) trimmed into the body of the appliance to direct erupting posterior teeth mesially or distally, so despite the simple design, dental relationships in all three planes of space could be changed. In current activator designs, flutes are replaced by a plastic shelf to impede eruption of upper posterior teeth while allowing eruption of lower posterior teeth, and lower incisors are capped to control forward displacement of the lower arch (Figure 11-4).

Bionator.   Originated by Balters and sometimes still bearing his name, the bionator (Figure 11-5) is best described briefly as a cut-down activator. Palatal coverage is eliminated. As with the activator, lingual flanges stimulate forward posturing of the mandible and shelves or blocks between the teeth provide vertical control.

Herbst Appliance.   This device (Figure11-6), developed in the early 1900s and reintroduced in the 1970s by Pancherz, can be either a fixed or removable appliance. The maxillary and mandibular arches are splinted with frameworks that usually are cemented or bonded but can be removable, and connected with a pin-and-tube device that holds the mandible forward. Occasionally a modification of this appliance is superimposed on traditional fixed appliances (see Chapter 17). Jaw position is controlled by a pin and tube apparatus that runs between the arches. Pressure against the teeth can produce significant tooth movement in addition to any skeletal effects and, even if the appliance is fixed in place, the amount of skeletal vs. dental change is affected by patient compliance (see Chapter 9).

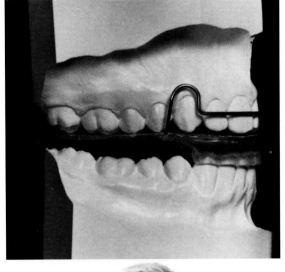

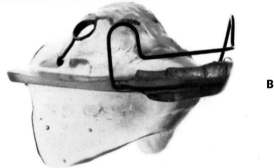

FIGURE 11-4   A, This Woodside-type activator has a modest vertical opening and the mandible is advanced so that the incisors are in an edge-to-edge relationship for Class II Correction. The maxillary posterior teeth are prevented from erupting by the acrylic shelf, while the mandibular posterior teeth are free to erupt; thus the appliance will induce a rotation of the occlusal plane, which usually is desirable in functional appliance treatment because it makes it easier to change a Class II to a Class I molar relationship. **B,** This appliance also has a deep lingual flange extension and a displacement spring on the upper first molars, which requires the patient to actively maintain the appliance in the proper position. It was once thought that a loosely-fitting appliance contributed to activation of the mandibular musculature, but research has not supported this concept, so modern activators are more likely to incorporate clasps than displacing springs.

Twin Block.   This appliance (Figure 11-7), recently popularized by Clark, is a modification of the Schwartz double plate mechanism. Like the Herbst, although it can be used as either a removable or cemented device, it is most effective when fixed in place. Its maxillary and mandibular portions are configured so the interaction of the two parts controls how much the mandible is postured forward and how much the jaws are separated vertically. This is similar to the Herbst appliance in that pressure against the teeth rather than the mucosa is employed to bring the jaw forward. Relief or presence of the plastic blocks can control eruption of the anterior and posterior

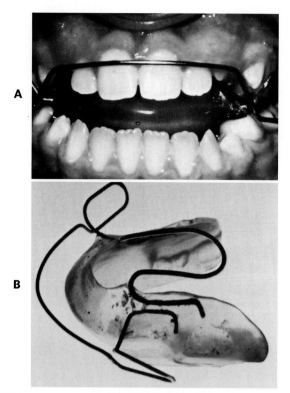

FIGURE 11-5 The Balters-type bionator is another of the tooth-borne passive appliances. **A,** This appliance uses a lingual flange to regulate the posture of the mandible and usually incorporates a buccinator wraparound as an extension of the labial bow. **B,** The design, which removes much of the bulk of the activator, can include posterior facets or acrylic occlusal stops to control the amount and direction of eruption.

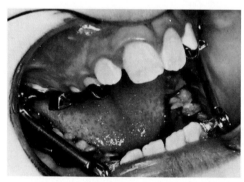

FIGURE 11-6 The Herbst appliance is the only fixed functional appliance. The maxillary and mandibular splints usually are cemented or bonded to the teeth (but can be removable and clasp-retained). The upper and lower splints are joined by the pin and tube apparatus that dictates the mandibular position.

teeth, and extraoral force can be applied to the maxillary portion of the appliance. The appliance has the advantage of allowing nearly a full range of mandibular movement, easy acclimation and reasonable speech, so that it can be worn most of the time. The greatest disadvantage is that

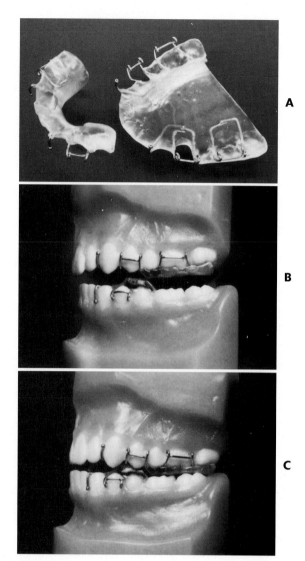

FIGURE 11-7 The twin-block appliance consists of individual maxillary and mandibular plates with ramps that guide the mandible forward when the patient closes down. **A,** Maxillary and mandibular appliances outside the mouth; **B,** arch relationships when the plates first contact; **C,** arch relationships as the ramps force the mandible forward as the patient closes down.

displacement of incisors can occur freely despite the absence of active springs or screws.

Active Tooth-borne Appliances. These are largely modifications of activator and bionator designs that include expansion screws or springs to move teeth (expansion activator, orthopedic corrector, sagittal appliance, any number of activators carrying the developer's name, and many others) (Figure 11-8).

In the correction of a Class II malocclusion, some transverse expansion of the upper arch is nearly always needed, as can be seen by having the patient hold the lower jaw forward in a Class I position; a crossbite tendency is usually apparent. The springs or screws in active functional appliances were added to the basic design in some instances

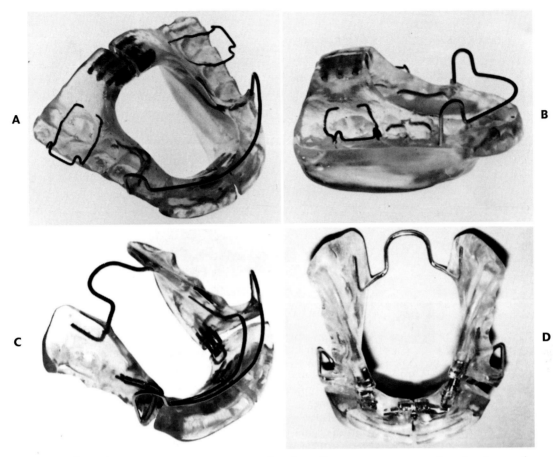

FIGURE 11-8 The expansion activator and orthopedic corrector are examples of active tooth-borne appliances. **A** and **B,** The expansion activator resembles the classic activator design with the addition of anterior and posterior screws to facilitate transverse expansion. This modification also requires posterior clasps to aid in retention. Note the minimal lingual flanges. The posterior occlusal stops can be modified to direct eruption. **C** and **D,** The orthopedic corrector is closer in design to the bionator but it incorporates a wire bow for transverse expansion and screws for intra-arch expansion. The sagittal appliance is similar in that it also contains screws in the canine-premolar region to increase arch length. These screws produce much more forward tipping of incisors than posterior movement of molars and also create unphysiologic force levels. Although appliances of this type were frequently used in Europe a generation ago, they have little or no place in contemporary orthodontics and are not recommended.

to provide this expansion, but in many appliances an additional goal was further expansion of the upper and lower arches to correct crowding.

In functional appliance treatment of preadolescent children, anteroposterior movement of upper and lower incisors to camouflage jaw discrepancies almost always is undesirable. Every millimeter of incisor tipping (camouflage) is a millimeter of potential skeletal correction that has been lost. This means that active springs for camouflage are likely to detract from the overall effectiveness of growth modification treatment. Springs and screws for transverse expansion to correct crowding also can produce unstable results and should be used cautiously (see Chapter 8 and the discussion of combined functional-active plate treatment at the end of this chapter).

Tissue-borne Appliances. The functional regulator of Frankel is the only tissue-borne functional appliance (Figure 11-9). A small pad against the lingual mucosa beneath the lower incisors stimulates mandibular repositioning. Much of the appliance is located in the vestibule, however, and it alters both mandibular posture and the contour of facial soft tissue. It serves as an arch expansion appliance in addition to its effects on jaw growth because the arches tend to expand when lip and cheek pressure is removed.

Components Approach to Functional Appliances

Each functional appliance, no matter what name it carries, is simply a melding of wire and plastic components. If one understands the different component parts of these

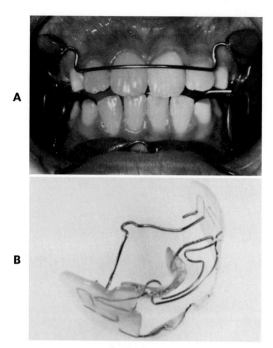

FIGURE 11-9 The Frankel appliance is the only tissue-borne functional appliance. **A,** With the mandible postured forward for Class II correction, there usually is less vertical opening than with other functional appliances. **B,** The large buccal shields and lip pads reduce soft tissue pressure on the dentition; the lingual pad dictates the mandibular position. The appliance looks bulky, but for the most part it is restricted to the buccal vestibule, and therefore it interferes less with speech and is more compatible with 24-hour wear than most other functional designs.

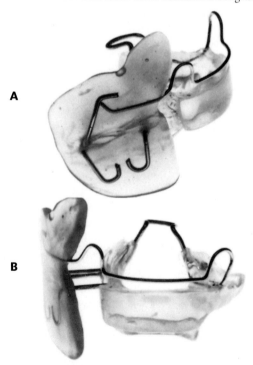

FIGURE 11-10 The components approach to functional appliance design is particularly apparent in an appliance for treatment of asymmetric growth. This appliance uses buccal and lingual shields on the right side, with the teeth free to erupt on that side, and a bite block anteriorly and on the left.

appliances and how the components translate into treatment effects, it is possible to plan functional appliance treatment by combining the appropriate components to deal with specific aspects of the patient's problems. This approach demands more knowledge and thought during treatment planning and appliance design, but should lead to more appropriate treatment for the patients. This can be described as the components approach to functional appliance therapy.

The components approach leads to custom-designed appliances for individual patients, so that the therapy is focused on that patient's specific problems. Appliance designs for asymmetry problems are particularly likely to end up quite different from any conventional design (Figure 11-10), but subtle variations in the appliance for common Class II problems can enhance treatment.

Functional and tooth-controlling components are listed and briefly annotated in Table 11-1. The functional components generate forces by altering posture of the mandible, changing soft tissue pressures against the teeth, or both. Although the functional components are the heart of the device, often they are only a small portion of the total appliance, the bulk of which is devoted to controlling the position of the teeth.

TABLE 11-1   *Functional Appliance Components*

Component	Comment
Functional Components	
Lingual flanges	Contact with mucosa; most effective
Lingual pad	Contact with mucosa; less effective
Sliding pin and tube	Contact with teeth; variable tooth displacement
Tooth-supported ramps	Contact with teeth; tooth displacement likely
Lip pads	Secondary effect only on mandibular position
Tooth-Controlling Components	
Arch expansion	
Buccal shields	Passive, effective
Buccinator bow, other wire shield	Passive, less effective
Expansion screws and/or springs	Must activate slowly; questionable stability
Vertical control	
Occlusal or incisal stops	Prevent eruption in discrete area
Bite blocks	Prevent eruption of all posterior teeth
Lingual shield	Facilitate eruption
Stabilizing Components	
Clasps	No effect on growth modification
Labial bow	Keep away from incisors, lingual tipping undesirable
Anterior torquing springs	Needed to control lingual tipping, especially with headgear-activator combination

Functional Components. In most functional appliances, flanges against the alveolar mucosa below the mandibular molars or lingual pads contacting the tissue behind the lower incisors provide the stimulus to posture the mandible to a new position (Figure 11-11). Growth modification is most effective if the patient uses his or her own musculature to posture the mandible forward, as opposed to the mandible being held forward by external pressure while the patient relaxes. Note that contact of the pad or flange with soft tissue, not the teeth, is the key to mandibular repositioning. If the lingual component of the appliance contacts the mandibular incisors, it also can produce a labially directed force against these teeth as the mandible attempts to return to normal resting posture. For this reason, activators and bionators usually are relieved behind the lower incisors.

Ramps supported by the teeth are another mechanism for posturing the mandible forward. It is much better to have two ramps in contact, as in the twin block appliance (see Figure 11-7), than to have the lower anterior teeth contact a ramp only on the upper appliance. Even so, an undesirable amount of tooth movement is likely to occur because of direct pressure against the teeth.

The sliding pin and tube components of the Herbst appliance also force the mandible to be positioned forward by holding the teeth (see Figure 11-6). If the appliance is bonded or cemented, this approach has the advantage that the postural change is permanent (at least until the dentist removes the appliance) and the disadvantage that pressure against the teeth, which produces compensatory incisor movements, cannot be avoided.

If a vertical and/or distal extraoral force is desired, a facebow can be fitted into headgear tubes attached to almost any type of tooth-borne functional appliance (i.e., almost anything except a Frankel appliance) (see Figure 11-16). This application of extra-oral force is especially useful for patients with a combination of mandibular deficiency and vertical maxillary excess who have a growth pattern in which the mandible tends to rotate downward and backward.

Lip pads positioned low in the vestibule (Figure 11-12) force the lip musculature to stretch during function, presumably improving the tonicity of the lips and perhaps

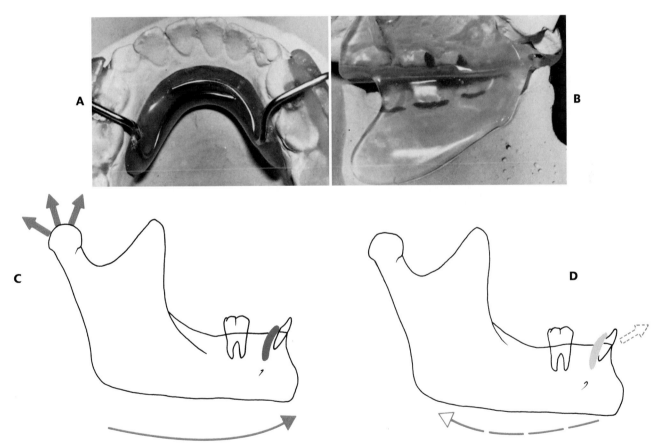

FIGURE 11-11 The lingual pad or flange determines the anteroposterior and vertical mandibular posture for most functional appliances. **A,** The small lingual pad from a Frankel appliance; **B,** the extensive lingual flange from a modified activator; **C,** the lingual components not only position the mandible forward but, **D,** also exert a protrusive effect on the mandibular incisors when the mandible attempts to return to its original position, especially if some component of the appliance contacts these teeth.

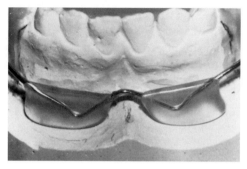

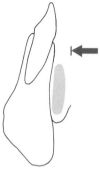

FIGURE 11-12   Lip pads hold the lips away from the teeth and force the lips to stretch to form an oral seal. The lip pad is positioned low in the vestibule and must have the proper inclination to avoid soft tissue irritation.

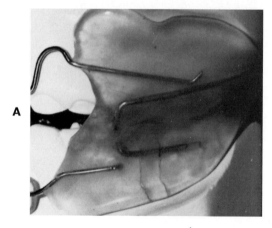

FIGURE 11-13   **A,** A buccal shield holds the cheek away from the dentition and, **B,** facilitates posterior dental expansion by disrupting the tongue-cheek equilibrium. The shield is placed away from the teeth in areas where arch expansion is desired. If the shield is extended to the depth of the vestibule, there is the potential for periosteal stretching that facilitates deposition of bone (*dashed arrows*).

promoting some soft tissue remodeling that would contribute to stability of changes in incisor position. As functional components, they are best considered an adjunct to the mandibular repositioning mechanism rather than a primary component of it.

Tooth-Controlling Components.

Arch Expansion Components.   Plastic buccal shields (Figure 11-13) and wires to hold the soft tissues away from the teeth like the buccinator bow shown in Figure 11-14, *A,* are used to remove the buccal soft tissue from contact with the dentition. The effect is to disrupt the tongue-cheek equilibrium, and this in turn leads to facial movement of the teeth and arch expansion. A combination of lip pads and buccal shields will result in an increase in arch circumference as well. The plastic buccal shield is more effective in producing buccal expansion than wires to hold the cheeks away from the teeth.

Expansion screws and springs can be used to actively increase the transverse dimension of the arches or to modify the anteroposterior dimension of the appliance (see Figure 11-8). They generate tooth-moving forces within the appliance, beyond those generated by the patient's soft tissues and function, and are discussed in more detail in the section on active plates at the end of this chapter. As a general guideline, passive expansion achieved from changing soft tissue pressures is preferred over active expansion during functional appliance treatment whose primary aim is to modify growth.

Vertical Control Components.   When acrylic or wire is placed in contact with a tooth and the vertical dimension is opened past the normal postural position, the stretch of the soft tissue will exert an intrusive force on the teeth (Figure 11-15). Intrusion usually does not occur, probably because the force is not constant, but if the patient wears the appliance most of the time, eruption is impeded. Thus the presence or absence of occlusal or incisal stops, including

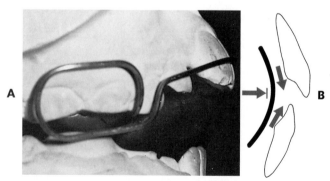

FIGURE 11-14   **A,** In this bionator, a "buccinator bow" of wire facial to the premolars provides something of the same effect as a plastic buccal shield (but is less effective for that purpose.) **B,** A lingual shield restricts the resting tongue (and thumbs, fingers, and other foreign objects) from the position between the teeth. The acrylic shield is placed behind the anterior teeth, leaving the anterior teeth free to erupt while (typically) the posterior teeth are blocked.

bite blocks, provides a way to control the vertical position of anterior or posterior teeth, allowing teeth to erupt where this is desired and preventing it where it is not.

Lingual shields remove the resting tongue from between the teeth (see Figures 11-10 and 11-14, *B*). This has the effect of enhancing tooth eruption. A lingual shield is particularly important if eruption of posterior teeth is desired on one side but not the other. Since teeth erupt mostly at night, if the patient can place the tongue between the teeth during sleep, eruption is likely to be impeded.

Stabilizing Components. An assortment of clasps can be used to help retain a functional appliance in position in the mouth (Figure 11-16, see also the discussion of clasps for active plates, on p. 380). Although it was thought in the early days of functional appliances that a loose fit was important and therefore clasps were contraindicated, it is clear now that growth effects with and without clasps are remarkably similar. Clasps often help the first-time wearer to adapt to the appliance. They can be used initially and then removed or deactivated, if desired, when the patient has learned to wear the appliance.

The labial bow across the maxillary incisor teeth that is included in many functional appliances should be considered and managed as a stabilizing component in almost all instances. Its purpose is to help guide the appliance into proper position, not to tip the upper incisors lingually. For this reason the labial bow is adjusted so it does not touch the teeth when the appliance is seated in position. Even

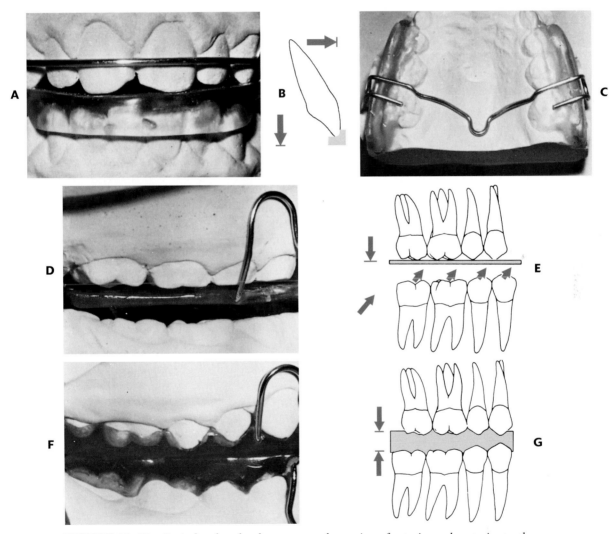

FIGURE 11-15 Incisal and occlusal stops control eruption of anterior and posterior teeth, respectively. **A,** The acrylic above and in front of the incisal edges prohibits eruption of these incisors; **B,** incisal stops can extend to the facial surface and control the anteroposterior incisor position, as shown for the upper arch in this diagram and for the lower arch in **A; C,** posterior stops can be constructed of wire or, **D,** acrylic; **E,** this positioning of the occlusal stops inhibits maxillary eruption but allows mandibular teeth to erupt; **F,** the complete acrylic posterior bite block, **G,** eliminates both maxillary and mandibular eruption and is extremely useful in controlling vertical facial dimensions.

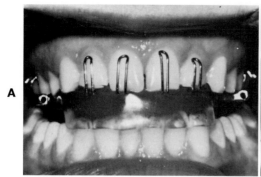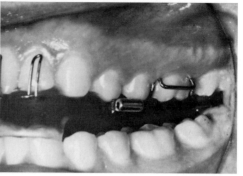

FIGURE 11-16   The Stockli-type activator is used in conjunction with high-pull headgear and incorporates torquing springs to control lingual tipping of the upper incisors. **A,** The vertically-oriented springs contact the incisors near the cervical line, while the incisal edge of these teeth is prevented from moving lingually by the acrylic. This creates the couple needed for bodily movement or torque of the incisors. **B,** A facebow placed in the tubes augments horizontal restriction of maxillary growth and controls descent of the maxilla. The clasps add retention, which is needed to help maintain the torquing springs in position. With an appliance of this type, posterior bite blocks can be used to prevent eruption in both arches in open bite patients, or the acrylic can be trimmed as illustrated here, to allow mandibular but not maxillary posterior teeth to erupt.

then it often contacts them during movement or displacement of the appliance. Undesirable lingual tipping of incisors during functional appliance wear, therefore, usually reflects a failure of the child to keep the mouth closed while wearing an appliance with a labial bow.

Torquing springs, which contact the incisors in the cervical third, are aimed at counteracting the tipping movement often produced by a labial bow (see Figure 11-16). They are considered particularly important when extraoral force is used against an activator or bionator (see Chapter 15).

Clinical Management of Functional Appliances

Impressions.   The impressions for functional appliance fabrication differ somewhat from those for orthodontic diagnostic records in two important ways:

1. Areas where appliance components will contact soft tissues must be clearly delineated. Most appliances use contact with the lingual mucosa to stimulate forward posturing, so usually this is the critical area. The impression must include the alveolar process below the lower molars if long lingual flanges are to be employed.

2. The impression must not stretch and excessively displace soft tissues in an area of contact with the appliance. This is critical when lip pads and buccal shields are planned. Too much extension of the impression will result in pads and shields that are too long and will cause soft tissue irritation and ulceration when the appliance is worn.

Bite Registration.   The construction bite for a functional appliance for Class II patients advances the mandible so that the condyles are out of the fossae and separates

the jaws by a predetermined amount. In theory, small increments of mandibular advancement should produce a greater skeletal effect relative to the dental effects by minimizing pressures against the teeth. For this reason, Frankel has been the strongest advocate of small advancements and minimal vertical separation of the jaws.[2] In clinical practice, however, how far the mandible is advanced seems to make little or no difference in the response, up to a limit of 7 to 8 mm.[3] Greater advancement than that leads to patient discomfort, which can reduce compliance. For most patients, we recommend limiting the initial advancement to 4 to 6 mm.

The vertical opening depends on the appliance design and purpose. The minimum opening, typically used with the Frankel appliance, is 3 to 4 mm. This amount of space is necessary for the connectors between the facial and lingual components of the appliance. With interocclusal stops or facets to guide eruption, 4 to 5 mm are needed, and if bite blocks to limit posterior eruption are planned, 5 to 6 mm of separation are needed.

To take the bite impression, it is better to use a wax that is relatively hard when chilled. Tongue blades embedded in the wax can be used to control the vertical separation and provide an indicator of the amount of advancement (Figure 11-17), unless even a single tongue blade would produce too much separation.

Decisions on Appliance Design.   The components approach suggests that there is no ideal appliance that can be used in all situations, nor is there necessarily a single optimum appliance design for a specific malocclusion. How the possible components should be put together is determined by two things: (1) exactly what is desired in the treatment, and (2) practical considerations of cost, complexity, and acceptability of the appliance to the patient. As a gen-

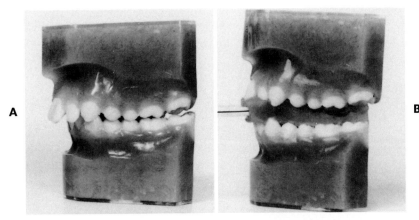

FIGURE 11-17   The construction bite for a functional appliance typically advances the patient from the initial occlusal relationship (**A**) by 4 to 6 mm, to a Class I molar relationship (**B**). One convenient way to control the vertical separation of the jaws in the construction bite is to use one or more tongue blades, so that when the patient closes as far as the tongue blades will allow, the molars are separated by the desired distance. A notch in the tongue blade also can be used to help the patient find the correct advancement. In normal clinical use, a single tongue blade would be employed for a patient with a bite as deep as this one, so that vertical separation was limited to about 4 mm.

eral rule, it is better to use contact of lingual flanges with the soft tissue to produce forward posturing of the mandible, rather than pressure against the teeth. The reason is simple: pressure against the teeth leads to camouflage-type tooth movement, which is usually undesirable. For the same reason, active elements within a functional appliance must be considered as having the potential to diminish, not augment, the growth modification desired from treatment.

As a general rule also, simple and sturdy functional appliance designs are more effective than complex and fragile ones. Preadolescent children are not known for their gentle treatment of appliances; if something can be broken easily, it will be. The original activators have a significant advantage from this perspective.

Vertical control always is a key element, and one of the advantages of functional appliances is the control of eruption they provide. Blocking the eruption of some teeth and allowing the eruption of others is the key to correcting deep bite or open bite problems. A major indication for using extraoral force with a functional appliance is a severe long-face open bite problem (see Chapters 8 and 15).

Finally, acceptability to the patient is critical. If the child cannot be persuaded to wear the appliance regularly for at least half the time, growth modification is unlikely to succeed. What one child accepts willingly, another may not; sometimes a child who reacts poorly to a tooth-borne appliance will wear a tissue-borne design, and vice versa. One important factor in acceptability is the extent of interference with speech, which can make full-time wear impossible. The original activators do interfere with speech;

removing the palatal plastic and making the appliance less bulky helps significantly (while also making the appliance more fragile, of course). From this perspective, the bionator design is better; twin blocks or Frankel appliances produce even less interference with speech and can be quite compatible with full-time wear.

Appliance Adjustments.   Clinical adjustment of a functional appliance depends on its components and purpose. Typical adjustments include (1) trimming of interocclusal elements to allow teeth to erupt where desired. Often the lower molars should erupt to level the lower arch and facilitate Class II correction, while other teeth are prevented from erupting (see Figures 11-2 and 11-4). Then a clinical adjustment to clear appliance material from their eruption path is important; (2) adjustment of the labial bow, almost always to reduce its contact with the anterior teeth, not to increase it; and (3) outward bending of buccal shields and lip pads, to facilitate arch expansion.

Clinical adjustment of the amount of mandibular advancement may or may not be practical, depending on the method for advancement that was chosen. With lingual flanges, a new construction bite and new appliance is the best way to produce a further advancement. The Frankel appliance can be sectioned so that its lingual pad slips further forward and cold-cure acrylic is added in the gap (Figure 11-18), but the fit of the appliance may be compromised and many clinicians prefer to make a new appliance when more advancement is needed. With the Herbst appliance, increments of advancement can be produced readily by adding spacers to the sliding pin and tube assembly.

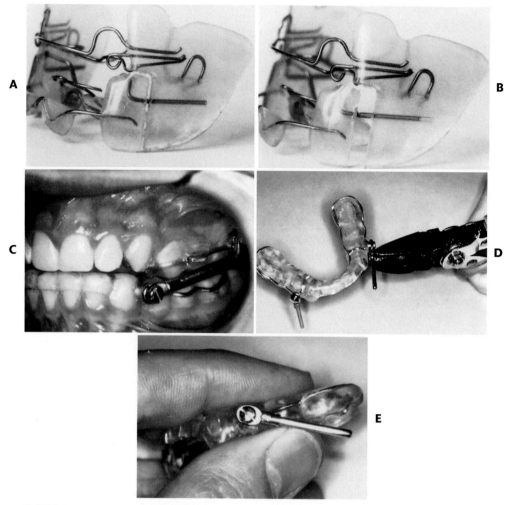

FIGURE 11-18   Both the Frankel and Herbst appliances can be adjusted to increase the amount of mandibular advancement. The Frankel appliance is cut as shown (**A**), and the lip pads and lingual pad are slipped anteriorly (**B**), guided by the wire embedded in the appliance during its construction. The Herbst appliance (**C**) is advanced further by placing a sleeve (**D** and **E**) over the rod that connects the upper and lower portions of the appliance.

REMOVABLE APPLIANCES FOR TOOTH MOVEMENT

Tooth movement with removable appliances almost always falls into one of two major categories: (1) arch expansion, in which groups of teeth are moved to expand the arch perimeter; and (2) repositioning of individual teeth within the arch.

Active Plates for Arch Expansion

The indications for arch expansion as a method of treatment for crowding and malalignment of teeth are presented in Chapters 7 and 8. Obviously, a careful diagnostic evaluation is required to summarize all the characteristics of an individual malocclusion, and the treatment plan must be calculated to achieve maximum benefit for the patient. It is neither wise nor practical to reduce the diagnosis and treatment planning to simple generalities. However, the

greater the crowding, the greater the chance of relapse after expansion treatment, and the greater the chance that reducing the amount of tooth structure would produce a better long-term result. Active plates therefore are most useful when only a few millimeters of space are needed.

The framework of an active plate is a baseplate made from acrylic or a similar (perhaps thermoplastic) material. This serves as a base in which screws or springs are embedded and to which clasps are attached. The active element of an expansion plate is almost always a jackscrew placed so that it holds the parts of the plate together. Opening the screw with a key then separates the sections of the plate. The use of a screw offers the advantage that the amount of movement can be controlled, and the baseplate remains rigid despite being cut into two parts. The disadvantage is that the force system is very different from the ideal one for moving teeth. Rather than providing a light but continuous force, activation of the screw produces a heavy force that

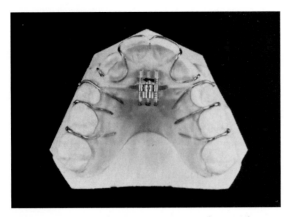

FIGURE 11-19 A Schwartz-type active plate, with a screw, is being used to move the maxillary incisors forward, to correct an anterior crossbite. An active plate of this type, though reasonably effective in tipping the incisors forward, must be activated very slowly to prevent excessive force against the teeth and displacement of the plate. From a biological perspective, the force system is just the reverse of an ideal light continuous force.

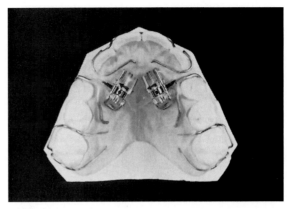

FIGURE 11-20 The "Y plate" designed by Schwartz to simultaneously expand the maxillary posterior teeth laterally and the incisors anteriorly. As with all screw-activated appliances, very slow and careful activation of the screws is required. As a general rule, appliances of this type are no longer recommended.

decays rapidly, and rapid reactivation of the appliance has the potential of damaging the teeth.

When a screw is used to apply force against a group of teeth, however, the amount of force felt by any individual tooth is reduced. In addition, even with the best clasps, if the force levels become too high, the appliance is likely to be displaced before damage can occur. This displacement is the most common problem with expansion plates: activating the screw too rapidly results in the appliance being progressively displaced away from the teeth rather than the arch being expanded as desired.

Most screws open 1 mm per complete revolution, so that a single quarter turn produces 0.25 mm of tooth movement. The rate of active tooth movement should not exceed 1 mm per month. The screw to activate a removable appliance to expand the maxillary arch should under no circumstance be activated more than twice a week, a rate that would produce movement of 1 mm per month bilaterally. With the plates of this type, it is usually preferable to place the appliance in the mouth, turn the screw with the appliance held firmly in position, and not remove it for several hours after activation. This maximizes the chance that the removable appliance will continue to fit.

Anterior Expansion of Maxillary Incisors. One of the simplest uses of an active plate for expansion is to correct a maxillary anterior crossbite when there is room to accommodate the teeth in their appropriate positions within the arch (Figure 11-19). If this is done in an adult, usually it is necessary to bring the baseplate material up over the occlusal surface of the posterior teeth, to separate the teeth vertically, and allow clearance for the upper incisors to move out of crossbite. In a child, these posterior bite blocks may not be necessary.

Retention for a plate of this type sometimes can be obtained simply by allowing the baseplate material to flow slightly into buccal and lingual undercuts. Alternatively and more typically, clasps are incorporated, which extend into buccal undercuts of posterior teeth. A screw behind the incisors completes the appliance.

Transverse Expansion of the Arches. The most common circumstance in which arch expansion is appropriate is a constricted maxillary arch, with a tendency toward crossbite. An active plate split in the midline (see Figure 11-3) will expand the arch almost totally by tipping the posterior teeth buccally, not by opening the mid-palatal suture and widening the maxilla itself. For this reason, removable plates are not indicated for skeletal crossbites or for dental expansion of more than 2 mm per side. Excellent clasping is required to prevent displacement of the plate.

Lateral expansion of the mandibular arch with a removable appliance is much more difficult than maxillary expansion, because the screw must be placed more anteriorly. Expanding the mandibular intercanine distance with an anteriorly positioned screw in a removable appliance is not recommended, because the force is concentrated against the incisor and canine teeth so that excessive forces easily can be produced, and because mandibular intercanine expansion is notoriously unstable.

Simultaneous Anterior and Posterior Expansion. It is also possible to expand, particularly in the maxillary arch, by dividing the baseplate into three rather than two segments. This design was the basis of Schwartz's original "Y plate," used to simultaneously expand the maxillary posterior teeth laterally and the incisors anteriorly (Figure 11-20). If plates of this type are activated slowly and carefully, they can be quite effective in arch expansion. The major problem with such a plate, as with any screw-activated device, is the heavy intermittent force system, which requires slow and careful tooth movement.

A variant of the Y plate divides the baseplate into only two sections, one large and one small (Figure 11-21). With an asymmetrically divided plate, activation of the screw will

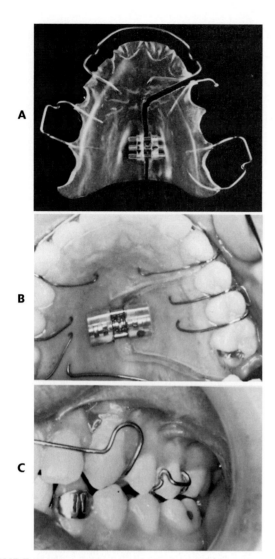

FIGURE 11-21 A variant of the Y plate, used to produce more expansion on the left than the right side in this patient with a unilateral crossbite tendency. Differential expansion occurs because the teeth on the patient's left side, adjacent to the small section of the plate, receive more force from opening the screw than teeth adjacent to the large segment. **A,** Appliance before insertion; **B,** intraoral view of a similar appliance after some expansion; **C,** crossbite partially corrected.

produce more force per unit area in the smaller baseplate segment than in the larger, and therefore there should be more movement of the teeth in the small segment. Carrying this idea to an extreme would lead to putting a single tooth in the small segment, with all other teeth contained in the large segment. This approach is not recommended, however, because too much force is produced by an activation if it is concentrated against a single tooth. The practical limit for the number of teeth in a small segment is two or three. As a general rule, springs rather than screws should be used if the movement of only one or two teeth is required.

It is also possible to use a split-plate design and a screw to expand an arch in an anteroposterior direction, as for example with an appliance to open space for a blocked out ca-

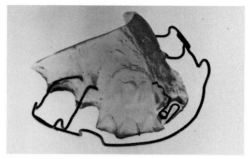

FIGURE 11-22 Maxillary removable appliance with a lingual spring to move one lateral incisor labially and a Hawley-type labial bow to control the amount of labial movement. The Hawley labial bow is characterized by the loops in the canine region; it can be attached into the baseplate distal to the canines or soldered to clasps on the molars, as illustrated here. As a design principle, an active component of a removable appliance should be restrained by the baseplate or by a restraining wire after the desired tooth movement has occurred; the labial bow here is the restraining wire.

nine or a premolar. The same objection to screws applies to this circumstance: the force is concentrated on too few teeth, and is just the opposite of what is desired for physiologic tooth movement. For this reason, screw-activated appliances cannot be recommended for intra-arch expansion. Using a screw for this purpose is at best obsolete and at worst positively dangerous.

All split-plate appliances produce only tipping tooth movement, because the edge of the plate contacts each tooth at only one point. There is no practical way to produce the couple necessary for labial or buccal root torque (see Chapter 10). Even when tipping is an acceptable result in expansion, a fixed appliance with only a few teeth banded (i.e., a lingual arch) produces similar effects and is often a better choice. Removable expansion plates, in short, have limited indications in children and adults.

Removable Appliances with Springs for Positioning Individual Teeth

In contrast to the heavy, rapidly decaying forces produced by a screw, nearly optimum light continuous forces can be produced by springs in a removable appliance. Like the edges of an active plate, however, these springs contact the tooth surface at only one point, and it is difficult to use them for anything but tipping tooth movements. The guideline for tooth movement with a spring from a removable appliance therefore is that this is acceptable for a few millimeters of tipping movement. Root control is needed for more than 3 to 4 mm of crown movement.

One possible use of a removable appliance is to retract flared incisors, and for this purpose, a long labial bow with loops for greater flexibility and adjustment is normally used. The classic labial bow with loops in the canine regions bilaterally was designed by Charles Hawley in the 1920s (Figure 11-22), and a removable appliance incorporating it is still often called a Hawley appliance or (since it

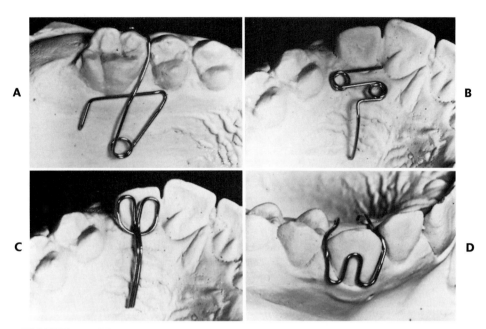

FIGURE 11-23 A variety of springs for possible use with a removable appliance: **A,** helical spring for distal tipping of a molar; **B,** double helical spring for labial tipping of a lateral incisor; **C,** paddle spring for labial movement of an incisor (note that this design provides better control over the position of the part of the spring that contacts the tooth, at the cost of greater potential occlusal interference); **D,** buccal loop spring, to tip a canine lingually. The attachment portion of a spring of this type must be contoured carefully as it extends into the baseplate so that it does not interfere with the desired tooth movement.

is frequently used as a retainer after comprehensive treatment) a Hawley retainer. A wire labial bow is usually included in removable appliances even if there is no desire to reposition the anterior teeth, because it provides some anterior stabilization for the appliance and helps control the position of incisor teeth that are not meant to be moved (see Figure 11-22).

Spring Designs for Individual Teeth. In designing springs to move a tooth facially, lingually, or mesio-distally within the arch, two important principles must be kept in mind: (1) the design must ensure adequate springiness and range while retaining acceptable strength. This usually means using recurved or looped wires for additional length; and (2) the spring must be guided so that its action is exerted only in the appropriate direction.

Because smaller wires are not strong enough, it is unwise to fabricate springs for removable appliances from steel wire smaller than 20 mil (0.5 mm); larger diameter wires usually are preferred. In general, it is better to use a larger wire for its (considerably) greater strength, and then gain springiness and range by increasing the length of the spring, than to use a smaller wire initially. Examples of springs for specific purposes are shown in Figure 11-23.

The major problem with long flexible springs is that the spring can deflect three-dimensionally even though tooth movement in only one direction is usually desired. For instance, if a spring is placed against a lingually positioned incisor, it will be ineffective if it distorts vertically,

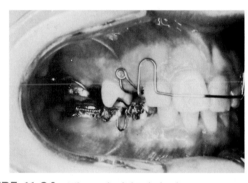

FIGURE 11-24 The end of this helical spring to tip the first premolar posteriorly is held in position because it engages the mesial undercut of the premolar. Placing the end of the spring in an undercut also aids in retention of the appliance, whereas a spring not held in position tends to displace itself and the appliance.

sliding down the lingual surface toward the incisal edge. This is a problem with any spring against any tooth surface: unless the spring remains in its planned position, its action will be unpredictable.

This difficulty can be overcome in three ways:

1. Place the spring in an undercut area of the tooth, so that it cannot slip toward the occlusal surface (Figure 11-24). The spring may then have an extrusive as well as a horizontal component of force, but this usually does not cause a practical problem. For posterior teeth, this is the preferred solution.

2. Use a guide to hold the spring in its proper position (Figure 11-25). This approach is often necessary with active springs to move canines and incisors labially, because no undercuts are available on the lingual surface. The guide can be either a rigid wire over the spring, or a shelf of baseplate material extending over the top of the spring to prevent its displacement (see Figure 11-22).

3. Bond an attachment to the tooth surface to provide a point of positive attachment for the spring. This approach is more practical now than it was before the development of modern bonding materials. On the other hand, it is no more difficult to bond a bracket for fixed appliance technique than to bond a stop against which a removable spring would rest. Tooth movements that can be accomplished with removable appliances only by bonding attachments for springs, in other words, may be an indication for using a fixed appliance technique.

The problem of controlling exactly where a spring contacts a tooth, more than any other factor, makes it difficult to control root position in removable appliance treatment. As an example, consider the problem of torquing a maxillary central incisor with a removable appliance. To move the root back while maintaining the crown in approximately the same position, it is necessary to generate a moment by applying two forces against the crown of the tooth. If a spring is applied from the lingual against the incisal edge, while a

wire bow contacts the middle or gingival portion of the labial surface, the necessary force system can be achieved (see Figure 10-19). It is almost impossible to keep the lingual spring from slipping out of position without bonding material to the lingual surface, creating a ledge toward the incisal edge into which the spring can fit securely.

Exactly the same problems arise if spaces within the arch are closed using a removable appliance. It is possible, with a removable appliance, to tip teeth together at an extraction site or large diastema but virtually impossible to generate the moments necessary for proper root paralleling. In theory, one could place a spring on each side of the teeth being moved together, one high and the other low, to create a root paralleling moment (Figure 11-26). In practice, it is difficult to keep the springs in position without either notching the teeth or bonding an attachment. Furthermore, the forces necessary to generate the moments are high enough that it is very difficult to keep them from displacing a removable appliance. Using screws instead of springs, so that a section of the baseplate contacts the teeth, slightly improves the ability to control the point of force application. This does not overcome the other disadvantages, however, and introduces the additional complication of inappropriate force magnitude and duration. This inability to control root position is a major limitation of active removable appliances. If tooth movement requirements go beyond simple tipping of teeth, a fixed rather than removable appliance is almost always indicated.

Clasps.   Retention of an active appliance is critical to its success. The best springs are ineffective if the appliance becomes displaced. It is probably fair to say that clasps are even more important than springs in determining how well a removable appliance performs clinically.

Adams Clasp.   By far the most useful and versatile clasp for contemporary removable appliances is the Adams[4] crib. This clasp, a modification of Schwartz's arrowhead clasp, is designed to engage the mesio-buccal and disto-buccal undercuts of individual posterior teeth. It has the significant advantage over the arrowhead clasp that it does not tend to separate the teeth, and it has excellent retentive properties.

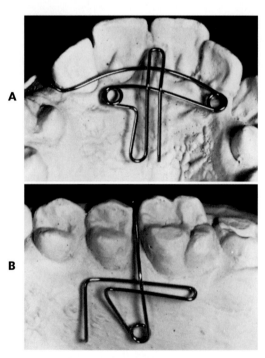

FIGURE 11-25   A long spring requires a guide to hold the spring in proper position. **A,** Wire guide for spring to tip the upper incisors forward. If a removable appliance is used to tip incisors for correction of an anterior crossbite, a spring of this type, rather than the screw arrangement shown in Figure 11-19, is preferred. **B,** Wire guide for spring to tip upper molar distally.

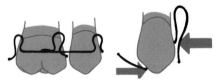

FIGURE 11-26   Diagrammatic representation of the spring assembly necessary for bodily retraction of a canine with a removable appliance. The mesial spring exerts a heavier force than the distal spring, leaving a net force to move the canine distally, while the couple necessary for control of root position is created by the opposing action of the two springs. Although bodily movement with a removable appliance is theoretically possible with spring arrangements of this type, the spring adjustments and clasp arrangements become too complex for practical clinical use. A fixed appliance is necessary if bodily tooth movement is needed.

The Adams clasp is made of 28 mil (0.7 mm) wire, except that 24 mil (0.6 mm) wire is preferred for clasps on canines. The first step in fabricating an Adams clasp, establishing the distance between the retentive points, is critically important, because there is no way to compensate for a significant error. Partially preformed clasps with varying bridge lengths and preformed retentive points are available commercially, but the clasp must be fabricated individually from that point.

The retentive points of the clasp must fit well into the undercuts for good retention. When this clasp is used for children, it may be necessary for the points to slip slightly into the gingival crevice. This step is accomplished by trimming away stone interproximally on the laboratory cast, so that the clasp can fit far enough down the tooth. Steps in the fabrication of an Adams clasp are illustrated in Figure 11-27.

When a new removable appliance is received from the laboratory, or when a patient returns for adjustments, it is often necessary for the dentist to tighten the clasps. Most of the time, this adjustment is done as illustrated in Figure 11-28, *A*, by simply bending the clasp slightly gingivally

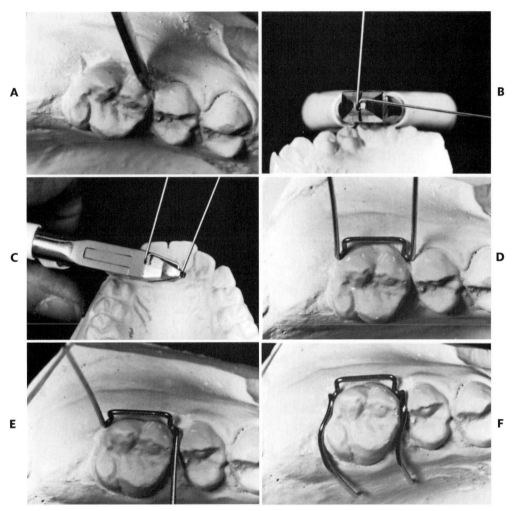

FIGURE 11-27 Steps in the fabrication of Adams crib. **A,** Carving the cast, exposing the mesio-buccal and disto-buccal undercuts into which the retentive points will insert. This is a critically important step in fabricating a clasp for a young child. **B,** Forming a retentive point from 28 mil (0.7 mm) wire. If preformed components are used, this step can be omitted. **C,** Angulation of the retentive points, which must sit at about 45 degrees to the bridge portion of the clasp that connects the retentive points. This adjustment is required if preformed components are used. **D,** The partially formed clasp, showing the retentive points in position, with the bridge portion of the clasp at least 1 mm away from the buccal surface. **E,** Contouring the attachment portion of the clasp over the top of the contacts. It is important that the wire be contoured as close to the occlusal surface of the teeth as possible to minimize occlusal interferences. **F,** Completed clasp, showing the clearance between the bridge portion and the buccal surface of the tooth, and the contouring of the attachment portion of the clasp on the lingual side of the contact point. If the clasp wire is not bent down sharply into the lingual embrasure, interference with the lower teeth is almost inevitable. Note also that the wire ends are bent toward the palate, ensuring a small space beneath the wires so that acrylic will surround the portion of the wire contained in the baseplate.

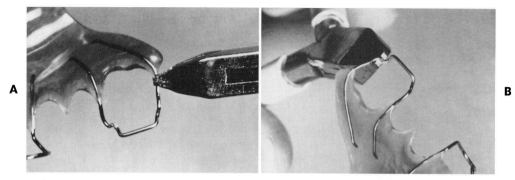

FIGURE 11-28   Clinical adjustments of an Adams clasp. **A,** Tightening the clasp by bending it gingivally at the point where the wire emerges from the baseplate. This is the usual adjustment for a clasp that has become loose after repeated insertions and removals of an appliance. **B,** Adjustment of the clasp by bending the retentive points inward. This alternative method of tightening a clasp is particularly useful during the initial fitting of an appliance.

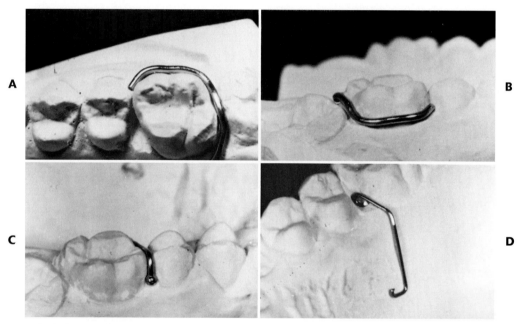

FIGURE 11-29   Other possible clasps for removable appliances. **A** and **B,** Circumferential molar clasp, extending into the mesio-buccal undercut; **C,** ball clasp, extending into the buccal embrasure; **D,** lingual extension clasp, made from fine wire (usually 16 mil) extending into the lingual embrasure.

from its point of attachment. It is also possible to bend the retentive points inward to obtain better contact in the undercut areas (Figure 11-28, *B*), which really should be necessary only if the laboratory fabrication of the clasps was imperfect.

As a general principle, the more active a removable appliance is to be and the greater the force applied during its use, the more clasping is required to hold it in place. It is possible to modify the Adams clasp by soldering an extension to the buccal bridge portion of the clasp, which allows an additional retentive point to be placed in the next embrasure. This is particularly useful in older patients as a means of gaining retention from a second molar as well as

a first molar. The same approach can be used to clasp both premolars if needed. The Adams clasp is so effective, however, that three or four retentive points on each side will support almost any practical type of movement with a removable appliance (see Figure 11-19).

Of the dozens of other clasp designs that can be used, three deserve brief mention here:

Circumferential Clasp.   The circumferential clasp (Figure 11-29, *A* and *B*) is particularly useful for second molars, and occasionally for canines. This clasp's greatest virtue is that it is easier to keep out of occlusal contact than the Adams clasp. However, it does not compare with the Adams clasp in retentive ability and should be considered only a supporting rather than a truly retentive element. For practical purposes, a circumferential clasp might be adequate for a retainer but not for an active removable appliance.

Ball Clasp. The ball clasp (see Figure 11-29, *C*), like the Adams clasp, extends across the embrasure between adjacent teeth and uses undercuts on the buccal surface. These clasps are easy to fabricate, which is their major advantage, but because of their short span they are relatively stiff and unable to extend as deeply into the undercuts as an Adams clasp. Ball clasps should be considered only when the demands on them will be limited.

Lingual Extension Clasp. Any wire that crosses the occlusal table can interfere with occlusion, so it would be ideal to have a clasp that operated only from the lingual (see Figure 11-29, *D*). In theory, extending a spring element into the lingual embrasures should provide retention, but in fact, it is difficult to develop and use clasping of this type. A short loop of 16 mil (0.4 mm) wire can be placed into the first molar-second premolar embrasure from the lingual on most patients and can provide enough retention for a maxillary removable retainer.

Offsetting the advantage of no wire crossing the occlusal surface, these clasps have several disadvantages: they are difficult or impossible to adjust, are prone to breakage, may cause tissue irritation, and can separate the teeth if too active. They can be useful for retainers but are not recommended for active removable appliances.

Clinical Adjustments

The fit of any removable appliance depends on the stability of its framework or baseplate. For this reason, maxillary removable appliances tend to be both better tolerated by patients and more successful than mandibular removables. The horseshoe-shaped mandibular appliances are inevitably somewhat flexible, making them less stable and less comfortable. This often is made worse by the presence of lingual undercuts in the mandibular molar region, so that an appliance must be extensively trimmed to make insertion possible—but it is important to adjust the appliance so that the patient can place and remove it without great difficulty.

As treatment proceeds, three adjustments are necessary when an active removable appliance is being used appropriately: tightening of clasps when they become loose, activation of the spring or springs, and removal of material from the baseplate. Adams clasps usually require a minor adjustment at each appointment, bending them as described previously (see Figure 11-28).

Activation of the springs of a removable appliance must be done carefully, and not more than approximately 1 mm at a time. The more the spring is activated, the more difficult it becomes to keep it in the proper position. Too much activation usually displaces either the spring or the whole appliance.

Often it is necessary to trim away baseplate material to complete the activation of a spring. Baseplate material must not be removed near a clasp, since this would allow that

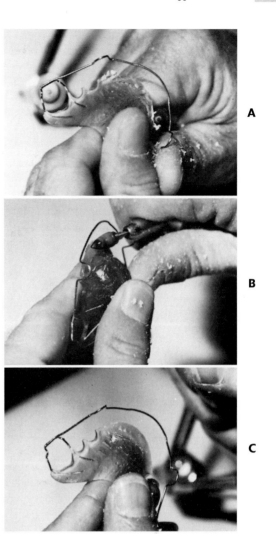

FIGURE 11-30 Removal of baseplate material is necessary to allow lingual movement of teeth, as with this maxillary removable appliance to tip the incisors lingually. **A,** Removal of acrylic at the incisal edge; **B,** removal of baseplate material above the incisal edge, to accommodate the expected tipping tooth movement; **C,** the appliance after trimming, in which 1 mm of baseplate material has been removed.

anchor tooth to move and retention of the appliance would be lost. On the other hand, baseplate material must be removed from the path of a tooth that is to be moved, which means that the baseplate must be trimmed for all lingual and most mesio-distal movements (Figure 11-30). Failure to relieve the baseplate near a spring is a common error.

A patient who is wearing an active removable appliance should be seen at 4- to 6-week intervals. Springs should be adjusted to produce approximately 1 mm of tooth movement (which may require slightly more activation of the spring than that) and the baseplate should be relieved to provide a similar amount of clearance. At the next appointment, the spring is reactivated and the baseplate is again relieved by a similar amount. Trimming the baseplate only the amount that a tooth can move in one appointment interval preserves the fit of the appliance and provides a fail-safe feature if the patient does not return for the next appointment at the expected time. An active spring, with nothing to check its action, could produce an excessive response.

Preventing an excessive response by limiting the relief of the baseplate is possible only when a tooth is being moved lingually, not labially. The same fail-safe effect, however, can be achieved by placing a labial or buccal restraining wire. For example, it may be a good idea to incorporate both a lingual spring and a labial restraining wire in an appliance to move a single tooth labially. The spring is activated to produce the tooth movement, and the restraining wire is adjusted to prevent excessive movement if the spring becomes distorted (see Figure 11-22). Split-plate appliances cannot be made fail-safe in this way, but since it is necessary for the patient to activate a screw and because the rate of activation is quite slow, these appliances have less danger of an excessive response.

COMBINED FUNCTIONAL AND ACTIVE PLATE TREATMENT

In theory, there is no reason that growth guidance with a functional removable appliance cannot be combined with active tooth movement produced by springs or screws. As noted above, the original activators did not use any springs or screws, but essentially all of the modified activators developed in Europe after World War II added the elements of active plates to an activator framework so that teeth could be moved while jaw growth was controlled.

Incorporating active elements into a functional removable appliance (see Figure 11-8) is a decidedly mixed blessing. There are three problems. The first is that correcting the occlusal relationships by actively moving teeth is not the goal of functional appliance therapy, and in fact tooth movement may prevent the modification in jaw position that is desired as a result of functional treatment. To take Class II malocclusion as an example, the more the occlusion is corrected by springs that move the lower incisors forward relative to the mandible, the less the skeletal change that will be produced (Figure 11-31). Adding springs or screws to push the teeth toward the desired occlusion does make the treatment proceed faster, but the result may be worse than that achieved by a functional appliance without active springs.

The second problem with active functional appliances is the questionable long-term stability of arch expansion. Functional appliances are less successful in correcting crowding and irregularity within the arches than in improving a Class II open bite or deep bite occlusal relationship. A major motivation for including active elements in a functional appliance is that this provides a way to correct crowding within the arches at the same time that jaw discrepancies are being treated. It does not follow logically, however, that more arch expansion can be tolerated by patients whose jaw growth is being manipulated, nor is there evidence to support that contention.

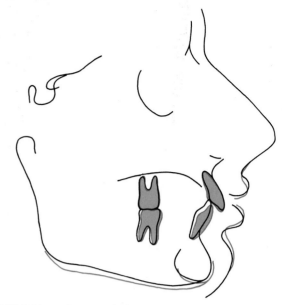

FIGURE 11-31 Cephalometric superimposition showing an unsatisfactory response to a removable functional appliance for a skeletal Class II malocclusion. Note the lack of skeletal response, but dental changes including forward movement of the lower incisors, slight retraction and elongation of the upper incisors, and downward and backward rotation of the mandible. Adding springs to a functional appliance, if it accentuates this pattern of tooth movement, makes the treatment response worse rather than better.

The third problem is that precise tooth positions cannot be achieved with springs or screws in removable appliances. The European active-functional appliances of the 1950s and 1960s were an attempt to provide comprehensive treatment within the framework of removable appliance orthodontics. For many patients, no matter how clever the design, the problems caused by limited two-point contact with the teeth become overwhelming, and either a fixed appliance must be used to finish the case, or a compromise result must be accepted.

This means that in contemporary orthodontics, there are few indications for removable appliances designed to provide all aspects of treatment like those commonly used in Europe a generation ago.

REFERENCES

1. Graber TM, Rakosi T, Petrovic AG (editors): Dentofacial orthopedics with functional appliances, St Louis, 1997, Mosby.
2. Falck F, Frankel R: Clinical relevance of step-by-step mandibular advancement in treatment of mandibular retrusion, Am J Orthod Dentofac Orthop 96:333-341, 1989.
3. DeVincenzo JP, Winn MW: Orthopedic and orthodontic effects resulting from the use of a functional appliance with different amounts of protrusive activation, Am J Orthod Dentofac Orthop 96:181-190, 1989.
4. Adams CP: The design and construction of removable appliances, ed 4, Bristol, England, 1970, John Wright & Sons.

CHAPTER
12

Contemporary Fixed Appliances

The mechanical principles underlying the use of any fixed appliance are discussed in detail in Chapter 10. This chapter is devoted to the historical development of fixed appliances, including the progression from original edgewise to the contemporary edgewise appliance; to the methods by which fixed attachments are placed (i.e., banding and bonding techniques); and to the characteristics of the modern fixed appliance.

Contemporary fixed appliances are predominantly variations of the edgewise appliance system. The only current fixed appliance system that does not incorporate the edgewise system's ability to use rectangular arch wires in a rectangular slot is the Begg appliance, and there is renewed interest in the use of rectangular arch wires at the finishing stage of Begg treatment. The focus in this and the succeeding chapters, therefore, is almost entirely on use of the contemporary edgewise appliance, with occasional reference to Begg technique.

THE DEVELOPMENT OF CONTEMPORARY FIXED APPLIANCES

Angle's Progression to the Edgewise Appliance

Edward Angle's position as the "father of modern orthodontics" is based not only on his contributions to classification and diagnosis but also on his creativity in developing new orthodontic appliances. With few exceptions, the fixed appliances used in contemporary orthodontics are based on Angle's designs from the early 20th century. Angle developed four major appliance systems:

The E-Arch. In the late 1800s, a typical orthodontic appliance depended on some sort of rigid framework to which the teeth were tied so that they could be expanded to the arch form dictated by the appliance. Angle's first appliance, the E-arch, was an improvement on this basic design (Figure 12-1). Bands were placed only on molar teeth, and a heavy labial arch wire extended around the arch. The end of the wire was threaded, and a small nut placed on the threaded portion of the arch allowed the arch wire to be advanced so that the arch perimeter increased. Individual teeth were simply ligated to this expansion arch. This appliance still could be found in the catalogs of some

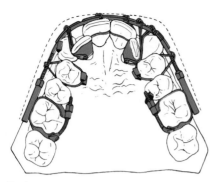

FIGURE 12-1 Edward Angle's E-arch, from the early 1900s. Ligatures from a heavy labial arch were used to bring malposed teeth to the line of occlusion.

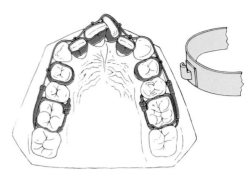

FIGURE 12-2 Angle's ribbon arch appliance, introduced about 1910, was well-adapted to bring teeth into alignment but was too flexible to allow precise positioning of roots.

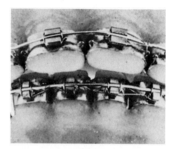

FIGURE 12-3 Angle's edgewise appliance received its name because the arch wire was inserted at a 90-degree angle to the plane of insertion of the ribbon arch. The rectangular wire was tied into a rectangular slot with wire ligatures, making excellent control of root position possible. Eyelets in the corners of the bands were tied to the arch wire as needed for rotational control, as on the distal of the upper left central incisor.

mail-order orthodontic laboratories as late as the 1980s, perhaps because of its simplicity, and despite the fact that it can deliver only heavy interrupted force.

Pin and Tube. The E-arch was capable only of tipping teeth to a new position. It was not able to precisely position any individual tooth. To overcome this difficulty, Angle began placing bands on other teeth and used a vertical tube on each tooth into which a soldered pin from a smaller arch wire was placed. With this appliance, tooth movement was accomplished by repositioning the individual pins at each appointment.

An incredible degree of craftsmanship was involved in constructing and adjusting this pin and tube appliance, and although it was theoretically capable of great precision in tooth movement, it proved impractical in clinical use. It is said that only Angle himself and one of his students ever mastered the appliance. The relatively heavy base arch meant that spring qualities were poor, and the problem therefore was compounded because many small adjustments were needed.

Ribbon Arch. Angle's next appliance modified the tube on each tooth to provide a vertically positioned rectangular slot behind the tube. A ribbon arch of 10 × 20 gold wire was placed into the slot and held with pins (Figure 12-2). The ribbon arch was an immediate success, primarily because the arch wire, unlike any of its predecessors, was small enough to have good spring qualities and was quite efficient in aligning malposed teeth. Although the ribbon arch could be twisted as it was inserted into its slot, the major weakness of the appliance was that it provided relatively poor control of root position. The resiliency of the ribbon arch wire simply did not allow generation of the moments necessary to torque roots to a new position.

Edgewise. To overcome the deficiencies of the ribbon arch, Angle reoriented the slot from vertical to horizontal and inserted a rectangular wire rotated 90 degrees to the orientation it had with the ribbon arch—thus the name "edgewise" (Figure 12-3). The dimensions of the slot were altered to 22 × 28 mils, and a 22 × 28 precious metal wire was used. These dimensions, arrived at after extensive experimentation, did allow excellent control of crown and root position in all three planes of space.

After its introduction in 1928,[1] this appliance became the mainstay of multibanded fixed appliance therapy, although the ribbon arch continued in common use for another decade.

OTHER EARLY APPLIANCE SYSTEMS

Before Angle, placing attachments on individual teeth simply had not been done, and Angle's concern about precisely positioning each tooth was not widely shared during his lifetime. In addition to a variety of removable appliances utilizing finger springs for repositioning teeth, the major competing appliance systems of the first half of the 20th century were the labiolingual appliance, which used bands on first molars and a combination of heavy lingual and labial arch wires to which fingersprings were soldered to move individual teeth, and the twin-wire appliance (Figure 12-4). This appliance used bands on incisors as well as molars and featured twin 10 mil steel arch wires for

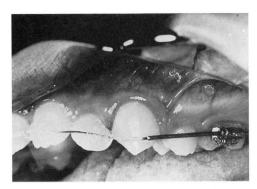

FIGURE 12-4 The twin-wire appliance used two strands of 10 mil wire for initial alignment of the incisor teeth. Incisors and first molars had fixed attachments (here, plastic brackets), but canines and premolars were not usually banded. A heavy tube extending forward from the first molar was used to protect the delicate twin wires.

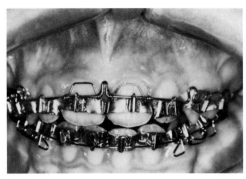

FIGURE 12-5 The Begg appliance is a modification of the ribbon arch attachment, into which round arch wires are pinned. A variety of auxiliary arch wires are used in this system to obtain control of root position.

alignment of the incisor teeth. These delicate wires were protected by long tubes that extended forward from the molars to the vicinity of the canines. None of these appliances, however, were capable of more than tipping movements except with special and unusual modifications.

Begg Appliance

Given Angle's insistence on expansion of the arches rather than extraction to deal with crowding problems, it is ironic that the edgewise appliance finally provided the control of root position necessary for successful extraction treatment. The appliance was being used for this purpose within a few years of its introduction. Charles Tweed, one of Angle's last students, was the leader in the United States in adapting the edgewise appliance for extraction treatment. In fact, little adaptation of the appliance was needed. Tweed moved the teeth bodily and used the subdivision approach for anchorage control, first sliding the canines distally along the arch wire, then retracting the incisors (see Figure 10-31).

Raymond Begg had been taught use of the ribbon arch appliance at the Angle school before his return to Australia in the 1920s. Working independently in Adelaide, Begg also concluded that extraction of teeth was often necessary, and set out to adapt the ribbon arch appliance so that it could be used for better control of root position.

Begg's adaptation took three forms: (1) he replaced the precious metal ribbon arch with high-strength 16 mil stainless steel wire as this became available in the late 1930s; (2) he retained the original ribbon arch bracket, but turned it upside down so that the bracket slot pointed gingivally rather than occlusally; and (3) he added auxiliary springs to the appliance for control of root position. In the resulting Begg appliance (Figure 12-5),[2] friction was minimized because the area of contact between the narrow ribbon arch bracket and the arch wire was very small and the force of the wire against the bracket was also small. Begg's strategy for anchorage control was tipping/uprighting (see Figure 9-18).

Although the progress records with his approach looked vastly different, it is not surprising that Begg's overall result in anchorage control was similar to Tweed's, since both used two steps to overcome some frictional problems. The Begg appliance is still seen in contemporary use though it has declined in popularity. It is a complete appliance in the sense that it allows good control of crown and root position in all three planes of space. The greatest difficulty in using the appliance comes in the final stage, where it can be difficult to precisely position the teeth.

Combinations of Begg and edgewise appliances have been proposed on many occasions. At present, there are two ways to retain some of the tipping/uprighting mechanics used with the Begg appliance while taking advantage of rectangular arch wires in a rectangular slot for the finishing stage. One is to use a bracket with both a ribbon arch (Begg) slot and an edgewise slot[3]; the other is to use a modified bracket that allows tipping in one direction, so that the rectangular slot is available for both root uprighting and torque (Figure 12-6).[4]

Contemporary Edgewise: The Modern Appliance

The Begg appliance became widely popular in the 1960s because it was more efficient than the edgewise appliance of that era, in the sense that equivalent results could be produced with less investment of the clinician's time. Developments since then have reversed the balance: the contemporary edgewise appliance has evolved far beyond the original design while retaining the basic principle of a rectangular wire in a rectangular slot, and now is more efficient than the Begg appliance—which is the reason for its almost universal use now. Major steps in the evolution of the edgewise appliance include:

Automatic Rotational Control. In the original appliance, Angle soldered eyelets to the corners of the bands, so a separate ligature tie could be used as needed to correct rotations or control the tendency for a tooth to rotate as it

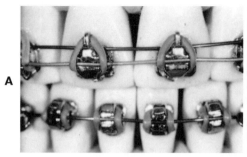
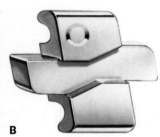
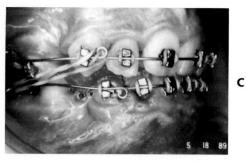

FIGURE 12-6   Modified brackets to allow a combination of Begg and edgewise mechanics. **A,** Stage-4 bracket, with 18 × 25 or 22 × 28 edgewise slots and a 22 × 32 gingival slot in which a wire can be pin-retained. For this patient in the first stage of treatment, the base (gingival) wire is 18 mil steel and the edgewise wire is 16 mil NiTi (see Chapter 15 for additional views of this bracket in use). **B,** Tip-Edge bracket, with a rectangular slot cut away on one side to allow crown tipping in that direction with no incisal deflection of the arch wire. This allows the teeth to be tipped in the initial stage of treatment, but a rectangular wire used for torque in finishing. **C,** Tip-Edge brackets in the initial stage of treatment, with small diameter steel arch wires. See Figure 10-21 for additional views of these brackets in use. (**A,** Courtesy Dr. W.J. Thompson; **B** and **C,** courtesy Dr. P.C. Kesling.)

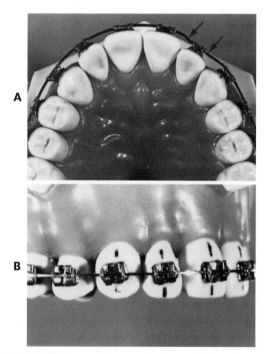

FIGURE 12-7   Typodont with contemporary straight-wire brackets on the right side and conventional twin brackets on the left. **A,** Bends in the arch wire to compensate for the lateral incisor position are required on the conventional side (*arrows*), whereas on the straight-wire side, a thicker base for the lateral bracket provides the same positioning without a bend in the wire. **B,** On the straight-wire side, each bracket slot is also angulated individually and cut at an angle, eliminating angulating and torquing bends.

was moved (see Figure 12-3). Now rotation control is achieved without the necessity for an additional ligature by using either twin brackets (Figure 12-7) or single brackets with extension wings that contact the underside of the arch wire (Lewis brackets) (see Figure 12-34) to obtain the necessary moment in the rotational plane of space.

Alteration in Bracket Slot Dimensions.   The significance of reducing Angle's original slot size from 22 to 18 mils and the implications of using the larger slot with undersize steel wires have been discussed in Chapter 10. In essence, there are now two modern edgewise appliances, because the 18 and 22 slot appliances are used rather differently. Chapters 16-18 focus on these differences. In addition, edgewise bracket slots are now routinely deeper than Angle originally proposed—usually 30 mil. The deeper bracket slot allows better engagement of large arch wires and the possibility of placing two smaller arch wires simultaneously if desired.

Straight-wire Prescriptions.   Angle used the same bracket on all teeth, as did the other appliance systems. In the 1980s Andrews developed bracket modifications for specific teeth, to eliminate the many repetitive wire bends that had been necessary up to that time to compensate for differences in tooth anatomy. The result was the "straight wire" appliance.[5] This was the key step in improving the efficiency of the edgewise appliance. The straight wire appliance included:

Variation in Bracket Thickness to Compensate for the Varying Thickness of Individual Teeth.   In the original edgewise appliance, faciolingual bends in the arch wires (*first-order,* or *in-out, bends*) were necessary to compensate for variations in the contour of labial surfaces of individual teeth. In the contemporary appliance, this compensation is built into the base of the bracket itself (Figure 12-7, *A*), reducing the need for compensating bends (but not eliminating them, because of individual variations in tooth thickness).

Angulation of Bracket Slots.   Angulation of brackets relative to the long axis of the tooth is necessary to achieve proper positioning of the roots of most teeth. Originally, this mesio-distal root positioning required angled bends in the arch wire, called *second-order,* or *tip,* bends. Angulating

TABLE 12-1   *A Generalized Angulation and/or Torque Prescription for "Straight-Wire" Edgewise Appliances*

	Maxillary		Mandibular	
	Angulation	Torque	Angulation	Torque
Central	+5°	+14°	0°	−1°
Lateral	+8°	+7°	0°	−1°
Canine	+10°	−3°	+6°	−7°
First premolar	0°	−7°	0°	−14°
Second premolar	0°	−7°	0°	−17°
First molar	+10°	−10°	0°	−25°
Second molar	+10°	−10°	0°	−30°

the bracket or bracket slot decreases or removes the necessity for these bends in arch wires (Figure 12-7, *B*).

Torque in Bracket Slots. Because the facial surface of individual teeth varies markedly in inclination to the true vertical, in the original edgewise appliance it was necessary to place a varying twist (referred to as *third-order*, or *torque*, bends) in segments of each rectangular arch wire, in order to make the wire fit passively. Torque bends were required for every patient in every arch wire, not just when roots needed to be moved facially or lingually, in order to avoid inadvertent movements of properly positioned teeth. The bracket slots in the contemporary edgewise appliance are inclined to compensate for the inclination of the facial surface, so that third-order bends are less necessary.

The angulation and torque values built into the bracket are often referred to as the *appliance prescription*.

A generalized prescription to minimize second- and third-order bends is illustrated in Table 12-1. Obviously, this would precisely position the average tooth, but would not be exactly correct for any deviations from the average—and most teeth do deviate from the average. Modern computer-assisted design methods allow custom brackets to be produced for an individual patient's teeth, based on laser scans of the surfaces of those particular tooth. For this to work, however, not only is custom fabrication required, but also the bracket must be placed on the tooth in precisely the planned position, which requires a positioning jig or template (see indirect bonding, on p. 400). Whether the total elimination of compensating bends in finishing wires is worth this degree of appliance preparation has not yet been determined.

The prescriptions of current commercially-available appliances, and a detailed discussion of the implications of their rather large differences, are presented at the end of this chapter.

Self-Ligating Brackets. Placing wire ligatures around tie wings on brackets to hold arch wires in the bracket slot can be a time-consuming procedure. The elastomeric modules introduced in the 1970s largely replaced wire ligatures for two reasons: they are quicker and easier to place, and they can be used in chains to close small spaces within the arch or prevent spaces from opening.

It also is possible to use a cap built into the bracket itself to hold wires in position, and a number of brackets of this type have been offered at various times. In the 1980s, a bracket with a latching spring clip (the SPEED bracket, Orec Corp.) was offered that now enjoys considerable use, and recently several other brackets with rigid clips to hold the arch wire in place have appeared (Figure 12-8). In comparison with ligating conventional brackets with elastomeric modules, these brackets can be latched and unlatched somewhat more quickly, but elastomeric chains still may be needed to control spaces within the arch, so the speed of placing and removing arch wires is not a compelling advantage.

It turns out, however, that the self-ligating brackets provide considerably less frictional resistance to sliding than conventionally-ligated brackets.[6,7] The force with which the wire is forced against the bracket by the ligature tie is a major determinant of friction (see Chapter 10), and the clip holds the arch wire in place without forcing it against the bottom of the bracket slot. The original spring clip design was better with steel arch wires; if superelastic arch wires are used, there is no need to obtain additional springiness from the bracket clip, and the sturdier rigid clip seems advantageous. However, what is an advantage for sliding is a disadvantage for frictionless space closure. The spring clips may not hold a wire in place well enough to deliver adequate moments to prevent tipping when closing loops are used, and with rigid clips, it can be quite difficult to fully engage full-dimension wires.

Lingual Appliances. A major objection to fixed orthodontic appliances has been their visible placement on the facial surface of the teeth. This has always been one reason for the use of removable appliances. The introduction of bonding in the 1970s made it possible to place fixed attachments on the lingual surface of teeth and produce an invisible fixed appliance, and attachments designed for placement on the lingual surface were first offered soon after bonding was introduced.

In theory, it should be possible to obtain the same three-dimensional control of crown and root position from the lingual surface as the labial, and considerable progress has been made toward this goal, but the small

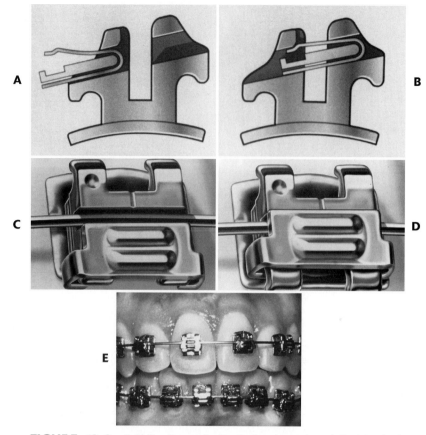

FIGURE 12-8 Self-ligating orthodontic brackets. **A** and **B,** Twinlock brackets open and closed; **C** and **D,** Damon SL brackets, open and closed; **E,** Damon SL brackets in clinical use. (Courtesy Ormco-A Company.)

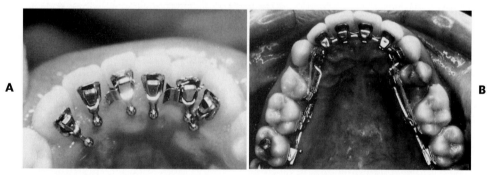

FIGURE 12-9 Adapting the edgewise appliance so that it can be placed on the lingual surface requires drastic alterations in the shape of the brackets, but the principle of a rectangular wire in a rectangular slot remains. Lingual appliances continue to evolve, and the current brackets are quite different from those used when the appliance was first introduced. **A,** Close-up of brackets for lower incisors; **B,** complete lingual appliance for the maxillary arch. (**A,** Courtesy Ormco-A Company; **B,** courtesy Dr. D. Fillion.)

interbracket span between lingual attachments is a major problem (Figure 12-9). The situation is somewhat reminiscent of Edward Angle's problems with the pin and tube appliance: the relative stiffness of wires used with the lingual appliance means that it requires more frequent adjustments, but the appliance is relatively inaccessible and quite difficult to adjust. Although comprehensive treatment of less severe malocclusions can be accomplished with current lingual appliances,[8] the difficulty, duration and cost of treatment are all significantly increased. Despite considerable progress, the initial promise of lingual appliances has not yet been fulfilled.

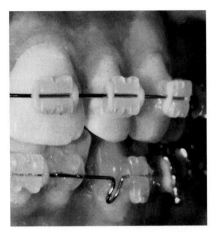

FIGURE 12-10   Ceramic brackets can be successfully bonded to the facial surface. They are esthetic, like their plastic predecessors, but both long-term appearance and dimensional stability are much improved.

Clear or Tooth-Colored Appliances.   Placing a fixed appliance out of sight on the lingual surface is one way to improve its esthetics. Another is to keep the fixed appliance on the labial surface but make it the same color as the teeth. Clear plastic brackets and plastic-coated arch wires were the first attempt to make a labial appliance almost invisible. A number of problems were encountered when these were introduced in the 1970s. The major one was that neither the brackets nor the arch wire coatings were durable enough to hold up in the mouth. The brackets discolored and broke, and the coatings came off the wires. In addition, uncoated wires did not slide freely in plastic brackets, and coated wires tended to be even worse. The initial failure of esthetic labial appliances was a major incentive toward lingual appliances.

With the development of ceramic brackets in the late 1980s (Figure 12-10), the situation changed. Although the first ceramic brackets had a number of problems, they did not discolor, and even with uncoated arch wires, patients appreciated their better esthetic qualities. Almost immediately, ceramic brackets achieved a degree of clinical utilization that their plastic predecessors had never approached, and the use of lingual appliances declined. It quickly became clear, however, that the sole advantage of ceramic brackets is their better esthetics. There are problems with bulkiness, possible enamel damage, and especially friction. On the other hand, using these brackets on the labial surface is considerably easier for doctor and patient than using a lingual appliance, and the esthetic improvement is considerable even when ceramic brackets are limited just to the maxillary anterior teeth.

The characteristics of the contemporary edgewise appliance, and the status of the materials from which it can be fabricated, are reviewed in detail in the last section of this chapter, after a discussion of banding vs. bonding as the means of fixing the appliance in place.

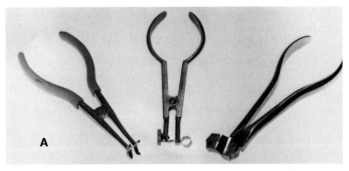

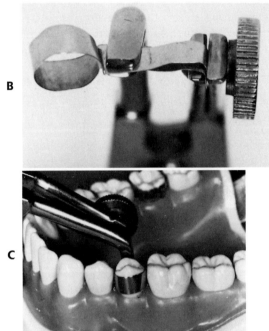

FIGURE 12-11   Forming a custom band from a strip of band material. **A,** Three types of band-forming pliers to stretch band material for a tight fit around the teeth; **B,** close-up view of band material in the pliers; **C,** band being formed on a lower premolar.

BANDS FOR ATTACHMENTS

Indications for Banding

Until recently, the only practical way to place a fixed attachment was to put it on a band that could be cemented to a tooth. The pioneer orthodontists of the early 1900s used clamp bands, which were tightened around molar teeth by screw attachments. Only with the advent of custom-fitted pinched bands was it practical to place fixed attachments on more than a few teeth. To fabricate pinched bands, a special pliers was used to stretch thin gold band material around the tooth, and the seam on the lingual surface was soldered and then ground smooth (Figure 12-11).

When steel replaced gold as the common orthodontic material, pinched bands were welded rather than soldered, with the welded seam bent over on the lingual surface and welded flat. The first preformed steel bands were a by-product of the manufacture of anatomically shaped steel crowns for restorative purposes. Preformed steel bands came into widespread use during the 1960s and are now available in anatomically correct shapes for all teeth.

There are definite advantages to bonding attachments directly to the tooth surface. Bonded attachments have no interproximal component, and therefore require no separation of teeth and are less painful. They are easier than bands both to put on and to remove, and they are also more esthetic because the highly visible metallic band material is eliminated. They make it easier to handle tooth-size problems during treatment by leaving the interproximal surfaces accessible for modification if needed. Bonded attachments are less irritating to the gingiva and less prone to produce decalcification and white spots on the teeth, although they do not totally eliminate this problem. For these reasons, it is no longer appropriate to routinely place bands on all teeth that are to receive fixed attachments. However, a number of indications still exist for use of a band rather than a bonded attachment, including:

1. Teeth that will receive heavy intermittent forces against the attachments. An excellent example is an upper first molar against which extraoral force will be placed via a headgear. The twisting and shearing forces often encountered when the facebow is placed or removed are better resisted by a steel band than by a bonded attachment.

2. Teeth that will need both labial and lingual attachments, especially if the lingual attachment will not be tied to some other part of the appliance. Although it is possible to bond on both sides of a tooth, it is usually easier for both the dentist and the patient to place a band with welded labial and lingual attachments than to go through two separate bonding procedures. More importantly, bonded lingual attachments are likely to be swallowed or aspirated if something comes loose. It is safer to have a lingual attachment attached to a band.

3. Teeth with short clinical crowns. Bands can be placed subgingivally, and as a general rule, the gingival margin of a band should either go slightly subgingival or should clear the gingival margin by at least 2 mm, so that the area of exposed enamel can be cleaned. If attached to a band, a tube or bracket can slightly displace the gingiva as it is carried into proper position. It is much more difficult to do this with bonded attachments. The decision to band rather than bond second premolars in adolescents is often based on the length of the clinical crown.

4. Tooth surfaces that are incompatible with successful bonding. It is more difficult to bond brackets or tubes to surfaces that have been restored than to enamel, but recent advances in bonding technology have largely overcome the problems of bonding to

amalgam, precious metal, and porcelain veneers.[9] Some nonrestored surfaces are also extremely difficult to prepare for bonding; teeth affected by fluorosis are the primary example. A good band initially is better than a series of unsuccessful bonds in some difficult situations.

Although there are exceptions, the rule in contemporary orthodontics is that bonded attachments are almost always preferred for anterior teeth; bonds or bands may be used on premolars, depending on the height of the clinical crown and whether lingual attachments are needed; and bands usually are preferred for molars, especially if both buccal and lingual attachments are needed.

This rule suggests that preformed molar and premolar bands should be available in a contemporary orthodontic practice. Incisor and canine bands are needed so rarely and in such unusual circumstances that pinching a band from band material, rather than relying on preformed anterior bands, may be the most appropriate approach.

Separation

Tight interproximal contacts make it impossible to properly seat a band, which means that some device to separate the teeth usually must be used before banding. Although separators are available in many varieties, the principle is the same in each case: a device to force or wedge the teeth apart is left in place long enough for initial tooth movement to occur, so that the teeth are slightly separated by the appointment at which bands are to be fitted. Separation can be painful, particularly for anterior teeth, and the necessity for separation must be considered a disadvantage of banding and its absence an advantage of bonding.

Three main methods of separation are used for posterior teeth: (1) brass wire, which is twisted tightly around the contact as shown in Figure 12-12 and left in place for 5 to 7 days; (2) separating springs (Figure 12-13), which exert a scissors action above and below the contact, typically opening enough space for banding in approximately 1 week; and (3) elastomeric separators ("doughnuts"), applied as shown in Figure 12-14, which surround the contact point and squeeze the teeth apart over a period of several days.

From the patient's perspective, steel spring separators are the easiest to tolerate, both when they are being placed and removed, and as they separate the teeth. These separators tend to come loose and may fall out as they accomplish their purpose, which is their main disadvantage and the reason for leaving them in place only a few days. Brass wire and elastomeric separators are more difficult to insert, but are usually retained well when they are around the contact, and so may be left in position for somewhat longer periods. Because elastomeric separators are radiolucent, a serious problem can arise if one is lost into the interproximal space. It is wise to use a brightly colored elastomeric material to make a displaced separator more visible, and these separators should not be left in place for more than 2 weeks.

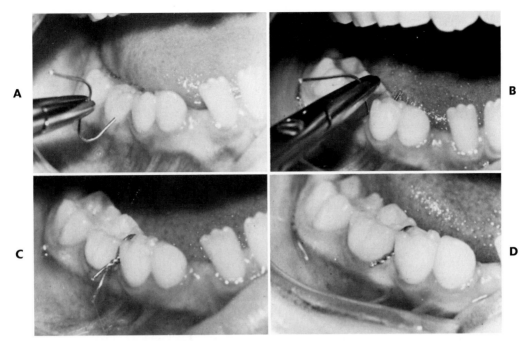

FIGURE 12-12   Separation with brass wire. **A,** 20 mil soft brass wire bent in an open hook shape; **B,** wire passed beneath the contact; **C,** wire brought back over the contact and twisted slightly; **D,** wire pigtail cut to 3 mm length and tucked in the gingival crevice. A brass wire separator of this type is normally left in place 5 to 7 days.

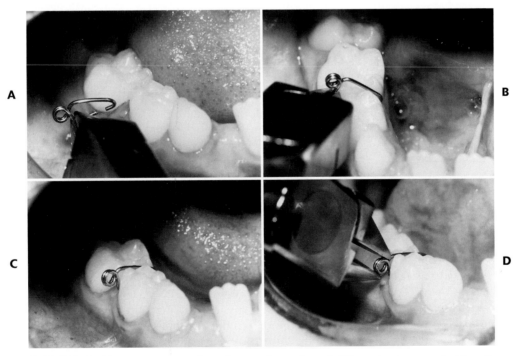

FIGURE 12-13   Separation with steel separating springs. **A,** The spring is grasped with a pliers at the base of its shorter leg; **B,** the bent-over end of the longer leg is placed in the lingual embrasure, and the spring is pulled open so the shorter leg can slip beneath the contact; **C,** the spring in place, with the helix to the buccal; **D,** the spring can be removed most easily by squeezing the helix, forcing the legs apart.

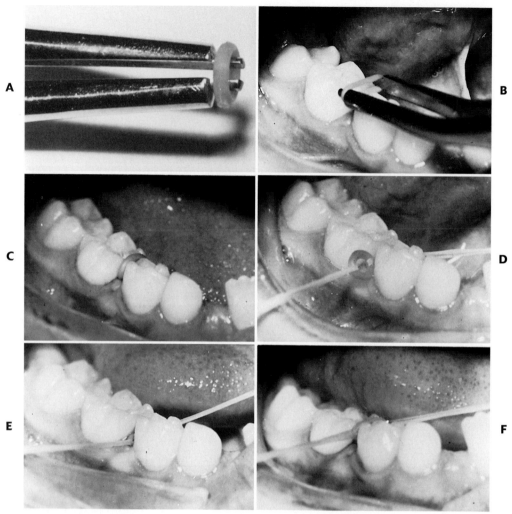

FIGURE 12-14 Separation with an elastomeric ring or "doughnut." **A,** The elastomeric ring is placed over the beaks of a special pliers; **B,** the ring is stretched, then one side is snapped through the contact; **C,** the separator in place; **D,** an alternative to the special pliers is two loops of dental floss, placed so they can be used to stretch the ring. The dental floss is snapped through the contact; **E,** the doughnut is placed underneath the contact point, then; **F,** the doughnut is snapped into position. At that point, the dental floss is removed.

Fabricating and Fitting Bands

It is possible to purchase preformed bands and to weld attachments to them in the dental office. However, it is cost-effective to obtain preformed bands with prewelded attachments, especially if a contemporary edgewise appliance with precisely angulated attachments is selected, because production jigs to assure accurate placement are needed to weld the attachments.

Fitting a preformed band involves stretching the stainless steel material over the tooth surface. This simultaneously contours and work-hardens the initially rather soft band material. It follows that heavy force is needed to seat a preformed band, stretching it to place. The necessary force should be supplied by the masticatory muscles of the patient, not by the arm strength of the dentist or dental assistant. Patients can bite harder and with much greater control, a fact best appreciated on the rare occasions when a patient is unable to bite bands to place.

Preformed bands are designed to be fitted in a certain sequence, and it is important to follow the manufacturer's instructions. A typical upper molar band, for example, is designed to be placed initially by hand pressure on the mesial and distal surfaces, bringing the band down close to the height of the marginal ridges. Then it is driven to place by pressure on the mesiobuccal and distolingual corners (Figure 12-15). Usually the final seating is with heavy biting force on the distolingual surface. Lower molar bands are designed to be seated initially with hand pressure on the proximal surfaces, and then with heavy biting force along the buccal but not the lingual margins. Maxillary premolar bands are usually seated with alter-

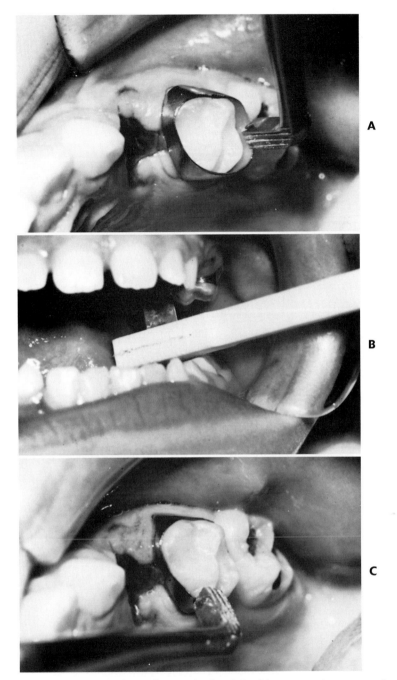

FIGURE 12-15   Fitting a preformed maxillary molar band (in this case, a primary second molar; the steps are the same for primary and permanent maxillary molars). **A,** The band is pressed over the height of contour with finger pressure or an instrument with a serrated tip; **B,** heavy biting force on the band seating instrument is used to seat the band, with the final pressure application to seat the bank on the disto-lingual corner, as shown here; **C,** open margins are burnished with a hand instrument.

nate pressure on the buccal and lingual surfaces, while mandibular premolar bands, like mandibular molars, are designed for heavy pressure on the buccal surface only.

It is easier to fabricate a pinched band for an anterior than a posterior tooth, simply because access to the lingual surface is better. The steps in pinching an incisor band are shown in Figure 12-16. In contemporary practice, this technique would rarely if ever be done—only when bonding was not possible for some specific reason.

Cementation

Cementing orthodontic bands is similar to cementing cast restorations but differs in important details. The differences relate to the fact that in restorative dentistry, most if

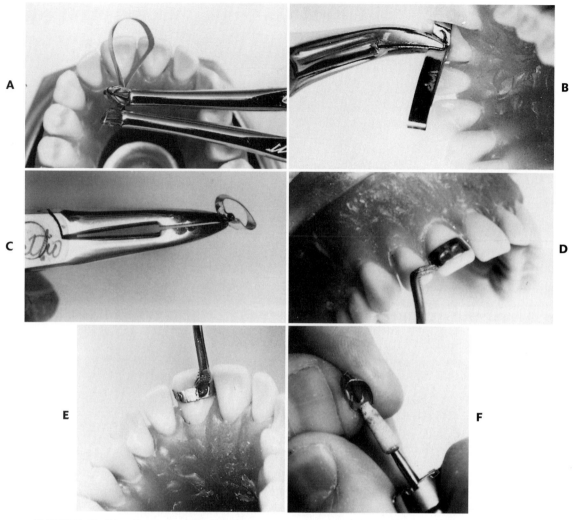

FIGURE 12-16   On rare occasions, it is not possible to bond a bracket to an incisor tooth, and because incisor bands are used so rarely now, a preformed band may not be available. Fabricating a band from strip band material may be necessary. This is done by forming a loop of band material, carrying it over the tooth and contouring it to the labial surface, and pinching it tightly against the lingual surface, using either a special band-forming pliers (**A**) or a Weingart or How pliers (**B** and **C**). The lingual tab then is welded, the band is placed back on the tooth and seated firmly (**D**), and the tab is bent flat and welded again (**E**). Often it is desirable to contour the lingual portion of the interproximal band material to avoid tissue irritation (**F**). The final step is to weld a bracket to the facial surface.

not all enamel has been removed and the cement contacts dentin, whereas in orthodontic treatment, the cementation is entirely to enamel.

Zinc phosphate cement remains useful for orthodontic purposes. The cements of this type for orthodontic use, however, differ from those used in restorative dentistry in that the liquid contains more free phosphoric acid. Relatively mild cements are needed for restorative purposes, because the open dentinal tubules allow free acid to irritate the pulp. A relatively acid cement is needed for orthodontic purposes, so that an acid-etch of the enamel surface, not unlike that created before bonding, is produced to aid in retention. In addition, orthodontic cement is mixed thicker than the cement for an inlay or a crown, because the escape

of excess cement from the margins of a band is not the same problem that escape of cement from beneath an inlay can be, and a thicker mix provides greater strength.

Recent work with glass ionomer cement has demonstrated that the retention of molar bands is better with this material than with zinc phosphate cement.[10] Glass ionomer cement also has the potential for fluoride release from the material over some months, and tends to be retained against the teeth instead of the band if the cement fractures. Both these properties provide at least some protective effect against decalcification around or under bands. The major disadvantage of glass ionomer is its slow setting time and the need to keep it isolated from moisture while it sets up. Nevertheless, it appears that this material is likely to

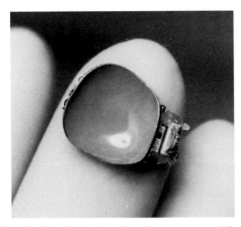

FIGURE 12-17 Molar band ready to cement. The cement must cover all the anterior surface of the band. Placing a gloved finger over the top of the band helps express cement gingivally when the band is carried to place.

displace zinc phosphate as the preferred material for cementing orthodontic bands.

With both zinc phosphate and glass ionomer materials, cementation of multiple bands is greatly facilitated by using a cold mixing slab. A cold slab also allows a greater amount of powder to be incorporated into the cement liquid, producing a stronger cement. Keeping the mixing slab in a freezer before use (the "frozen slab technique") is the preferred approach.

All interior surfaces of an orthodontic band must be coated with cement before it is placed, so that there is no bare metal. As the band is carried to place, the occlusal surface should be covered so that cement is expressed from the gingival as well as the occlusal margins of the band (Figure 12-17).

BONDED ATTACHMENTS

The Basis of Bonding
Bonding of attachments, eliminating the need for bands, was a dream for many years before rather abruptly becoming a routine clinical procedure in the 1980s. Bonding is based on the mechanical locking of an adhesive to irregularities in the enamel surface of the tooth and to mechanical locks formed in the base of the orthodontic attachment. Successful bonding in orthodontics, therefore, requires careful attention to three components of the system: the tooth surface and its preparation, the design of the attachment base, and the bonding material itself.

Preparation of the Tooth Surface. Before bonding an orthodontic attachment, it is necessary to remove the enamel pellicle and to create irregularities in the enamel surface. This is accomplished by gently cleaning and drying the enamel surface (avoiding heavy pumicing), then treating it with an etching agent, usually 35% to 50%

unbuffered phosphoric acid for 20-30 seconds. Longer etching times can be counterproductive.[11] The effect is to remove a small amount of the softer interprismatic enamel and open up pores between the enamel prisms, so the adhesive can penetrate into the enamel surface (Figure 12-18). It is convenient to apply the etching agent in a gel rather than a liquid form, simply because gels make it easier to confine the etch to a prescribed area and are as effective as liquids (Figure 12-19). The tooth surface must not be contaminated with saliva, which promotes immediate remineralization, until bonding is completed; otherwise, re-etching is required.

Rather than opening up minute irregularities extending into the enamel surface, another possible way to prepare for bonding would be to build up irregular deposits on the enamel surface and thus obtain a mechanical interlocking with the bonding agent. The loss of enamel surface when acid-etch bonds are removed is minimal, but the buildup approach would, at least in theory, eliminate any loss of enamel. Although a system to chemically attach sulfite materials to the enamel surface in preparation for bonding has been offered commercially, the bond between the sulfite and the enamel surface is relatively weak, resulting in frequent clinical bond failures.[12] Because the buildup material breaks cleanly away from the enamel surface, there is less cleanup at debanding, but this is no advantage if the bracket comes loose prematurely. Further progress is needed before acid etching can be replaced by enamel buildup.

Surface of Attachments. The base of a metal bonded attachment must be manufactured so that a mechanical interlock between the bonding material and the attachment surface can be achieved. Either chemical bonding or mechanical interlocking can be used with ceramic brackets (Figure 12-20). The strength of chemical bonds can become high enough to create problems in debonding (see p. 401), so mechanical retention now is preferred for ceramic as well as metal brackets.

Bonding Materials. A successful bonding material must meet a set of formidable criteria: it must be dimensionally stable; it must be quite fluid, so that it penetrates the enamel surface; it must have excellent inherent strength; and it must be easy to use clinically.

At present, filled acrylic (bis-GMA) resins are the preferred bonding materials. These are available in a variety of formulations that differ mainly in the composition and extent of the fillers, and in the arrangement—chemical- or light-activation—to initiate polymerization of the resin. Although several fluoride-releasing bonding materials have been offered commercially, it has not yet been possible to develop one that has any lasting protective effects.[13]

Direct Bonding Technique
Direct bonding of attachments can be used quite successfully as a routine clinical procedure, and even when most attachments are bonded indirectly, it is indicated whenever a single bracket must be changed or replaced. After

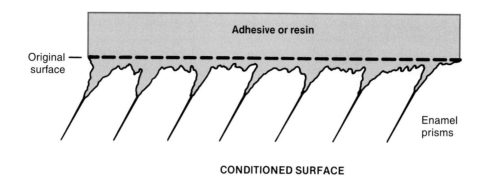

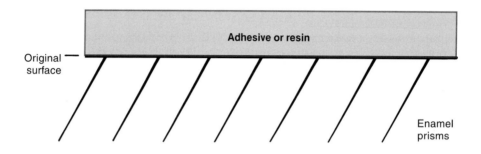

FIGURE 12-18   Diagrammatic representation of the effect of preparation of the enamel surface before bonding. Pretreatment with phosphoric acid creates minute irregularities in the enamel surface, allowing the bonding material to form penetrating "tags" that mechanically interlock with the enamel surface.

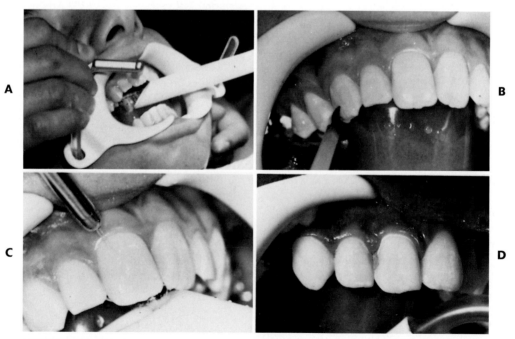

FIGURE 12-19   Steps in preparation for bonding. **A,** The tooth surface is pumiced gently if stain or plaque is present. This step can be omitted in patients with excellent oral hygiene. **B,** The etch material is applied to the area where the bracket will be placed. **C,** After approximately 30 seconds, the etching material is rinsed away, and the tooth surface is dried. **D,** The chalky or frosted appearance of the enamel surface after proper etching.

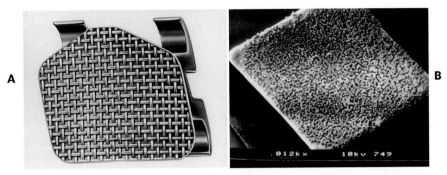

FIGURE 12-20 **A,** For steel brackets, the bonding material is attached mechanically to the bracket base by penetrating into undercuts usually provided by a fine mesh welded or brazed onto the back of a metal bracket. **B,** Ceramic brackets can be coupled chemically to the bonding material with silane coupling, or mechanical undercuts can be employed, as provided for this ceramic bracket (the back of the bracket is viewed here under magnification) by tiny balls of the ceramic material. Mechanical bonding is one way to make debonding of ceramic brackets easier and less hazardous. (Courtesy Ormco-A Company.)

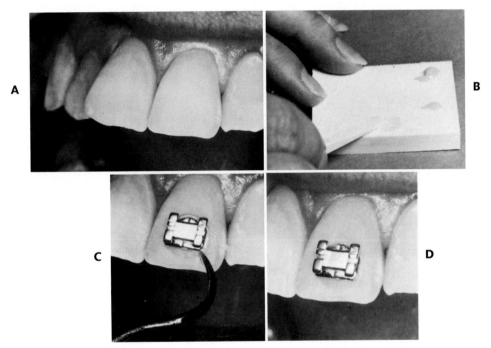

FIGURE 12-21 Steps in direct bonding. **A,** Teeth after preparation of the tooth surface. A liquid sealant (usually the monomer of the bonding agent) can be applied at this stage if desired. **B,** A small quantity of the bonding material is mixed so that it will set in 30 to 60 seconds. **C,** Bonding material is placed on the back of the bracket, and the bracket is pressed to place against the enamel surface, causing excess bonding material to be expressed around the edges. This is removed immediately with a scaler, before the material sets. **D,** The bonded bracket, immediately after cleanup. In this technique, a separate mix of bonding material is used for each tooth.

preparation of the tooth surface via an acid etch, either a chemically-activated composite resin with a very rapid setting time or a light-activated material can be used.

The major difficulty with direct bonding is that the dentist must be able to judge the proper position for the attachment and must carry it to place rapidly and accurately. There is less opportunity for precise measurements of bracket position or detailed adjustments than there would be at the laboratory bench. It is generally conceded that for

this reason, direct bonding does not provide as accurate a placement of brackets as indirect bonding. On the other hand, direct bonding is easier, faster (especially if only a few teeth are to be bonded), and less expensive (because the laboratory fabrication steps are eliminated).

Steps in the direct bonding technique, using an individual mix of chemically-activated resin for each bracket, are illustrated in Figure 12-21. Most bonding now is done by this method.

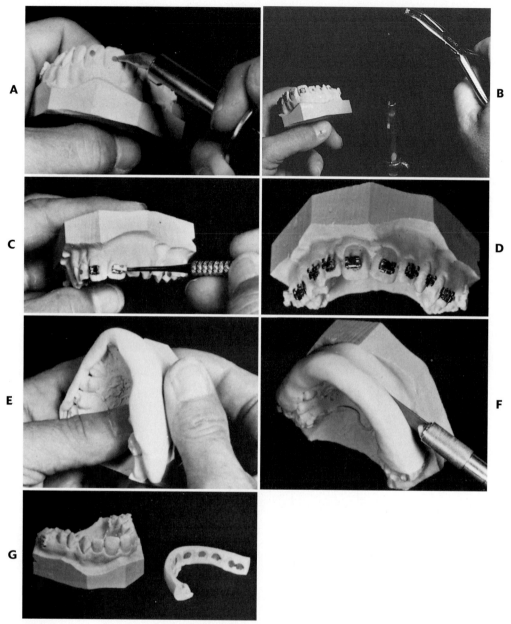

FIGURE 12-22 Laboratory steps in indirect bonding. **A,** A spot of candy adhesive is applied to the labial surface of each tooth on the working cast. **B,** Each bracket is warmed in a flame, then pressed to place against the surface of the cast. The warmth melts the candy adhesive. **C,** The position of each bracket can be precisely adjusted by warming an instrument in the flame and pressing it against the bracket until the adhesive softens, allowing the bracket to be moved slightly. **D,** Brackets positioned on the working cast. **E,** The transfer tray is formed by adapting a carrier material, usually silicone rubber, over the working cast and the adapted brackets. **F,** The tray is trimmed to remove excess material from the labial vestibule, but tray material is left extending onto the occlusal and incisal surfaces of the teeth. **G,** The completed tray is removed from the working cast by soaking in warm water, and the remaining candy adhesive is washed away from the inner surface of the brackets with hot water.

Indirect Bonding Technique

Indirect bonding is done by placing the brackets on a model in the laboratory, then using a template or tray to transfer the laboratory positioning to the teeth. The advantage is the more precise location of brackets that is possible in the laboratory. An alginate impression, poured relatively rapidly, gives an accurate enough working cast for

indirect bonding. Custom impression trays and silicone or rubber impressions are not necessary. Laboratory steps in indirect bonding are illustrated in Figure 12-22.

For indirect bonding, "no-mix" chemically-activated materials usually are employed. The composite resin is placed on the tooth surface in unpolymerized form, while the polymerization catalyst is placed on the back of the

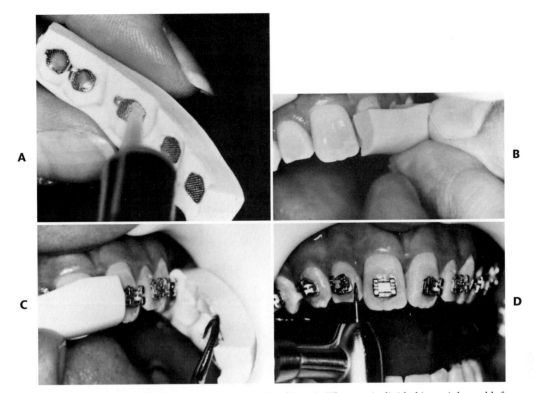

FIGURE 12-23 Clinical steps in indirect bonding. **A,** The tray is divided into right and left halves, if desired for easier handling. The adhesive material, if a third generation resin is used, or the paste portion of a fourth generation resin, is applied to the back of each bracket in the transfer tray. The catalyst portion of a fourth generation resin is placed on the tooth surface, so that mixing occurs when the two components contact each other when the tray is carried to the mouth. **B,** The tray or tray section is carried to place, and pressed firmly against the teeth. **C,** After the adhesive has set, the tray material is gently peeled away from the teeth. **D,** Excess bonding material is removed, with a carbide finishing bur if hardened third generation adhesive is encountered, or with a scaler if unset fourth generation material is present. If a light-activated material is the bonding agent, a translucent transfer tray is needed.

brackets. When the tray carrying the brackets is placed against the tooth surface, the resin immediately beneath the bracket is activated and polymerizes, but excess resin around the margins of the brackets does not polymerize and can easily be scaled away when the bracket tray is removed. This overcomes one of the greatest problems with indirect bonding, the difficulty of clean-up of excess bonding material when it has hardened. This clinical technique is illustrated in Figure 12-23.

At present, indirect bonding is used routinely by some practitioners, but is reserved for special circumstances by most. Custom brackets that were manufactured for an individual patient require the precision of indirect bonding. More generally, the poorer the visibility, the more difficult direct bonding becomes, and the greater the indication for an indirect approach. For this reason, indirect bonding is almost a necessity for lingual attachments. Bonding an isolated lingual hook or button is not difficult, but precisely positioning the attachments for a lingual appliance is, and even the placement of a fixed lingual retainer is done more easily with indirect technique and a transfer tray.

Debonding

It is as important to remove a fixed appliance safely as to place it properly. Bands are largely retained by the elasticity of the band material as it fits around the tooth. This is augmented by the cement that seals between the band and the tooth, but a band retained only by cement was not fitted tightly enough. Neither zinc phosphate nor glass ionomer cement bonds strongly to enamel or stainless steel band material. When the band is distorted by force to remove it, the cement breaks away from the band or the tooth, and there is almost no chance of damaging the enamel surface.

The greater strength of bonding adhesives becomes a potential problem in debonding. When a bonded bracket is removed, failure at one of three interfaces must occur: between the bonding material and the bracket, within the bonding material itself, or between the bonding material and the enamel surface. If a strong bond to the enamel has been achieved, which is the case with the modern materials, failure at the enamel surface is undesirable, because the bonding material may tear the enamel surface as it pulls away from it. The interface between the bonding material and the bracket is the usual, and preferred, site of failure when brackets are removed. The safest way to remove metal brackets is to distort the bracket base, which induces failure between it and the bonding adhesive. This damages the bracket so that it cannot be reused. The major reason for not recycling and reusing brackets is the possibility of enamel damage when they are removed without distorting the base. If brackets can be removed without damage they can be cleaned, sterilized and reused without risk to the patient, in exactly the same way as other medical devices.

Ceramic brackets are a particular problem for debonding, because their base cannot be distorted. They break before they bend. There are two ways to create adhesion between a ceramic bracket and the bonding adhesive: mechanical retention through undercuts on the bracket base, as is done with metal brackets; or chemical bonding between the adhesive and a treated bracket base. It is quite possible to create such a strong bond between the adhesive and a chemically treated bracket base that failure will not occur there—but then when the bracket is removed, there is a real chance of enamel surface damage. Reports of enamel damage on debonding began to appear soon after ceramic brackets were introduced, and have been a problem ever since.

Modifications to ceramic brackets to enhance the chance of debonding at the right interface, and electro-thermal and laser techniques to weaken the adhesive during debonding, are discussed in the section below on modern bracket materials.

CHARACTERISTICS OF CONTEMPORARY EDGEWISE ATTACHMENTS

Edgewise Brackets and Tubes in the Contemporary "Straight-Wire" Appliance

The contemporary edgewise appliance uses slightly different brackets or tubes that are custom-made for each tooth, with the goal of minimizing the number of bends in arch wires needed to produce an ideal arrangement of the teeth—hence the "straight-wire" name (Figure 12-24). An important concept is that unless the appliance has been modified from the original design, first-, second-, and third-order bends are necessary to provide a passive fit of an arch wire when the teeth are ideally aligned, and are *not* used just to correct malaligned teeth.

Variations in Bracket Base Thickness and Elimination of First-Order Bends. Elimination of first-order bends requires varying the thickness of the bracket base for individual teeth and placing attachments for molars at an angle to the buccal surface, so that molar rotation can be controlled automatically.

The varying thickness of anterior bracket bases is shown in Figure 12-25. Because of the prominence of the canine in each arch, its bracket base must be thin, bring-

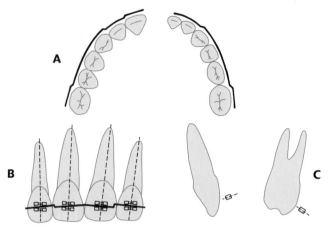

FIGURE 12-24 First-, second-, and third-order bends in edgewise wires. **A,** First-order bends in a maxillary (*left*) and mandibular (*right*) arch wire. Note the lateral inset required in the maxillary arch wire, and the canine and molar offset bends that are required in both. **B,** Second-order bends in the maxillary incisor segment to compensate for the inclination of the incisal edge of these teeth relative to the long axis of the tooth. **C,** Third-order bends for the maxillary central incisors and maxillary first molars showing the twist in the arch wire to provide a passive fit in a bracket or tube on these teeth. Twist in an arch wire provides torque in a bracket; the torque is positive for the incisor, negative for the molar.

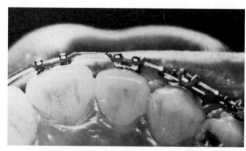

FIGURE 12-25 First-order, or in-out, bends in the anterior sector of arch wires can be minimized by varying the thickness of the bracket base. Note the thin bracket base for the canine, thick base for the lateral incisor, and intermediate thickness for the central incisor in this contemporary appliance. An elastomeric chain ties the anterior teeth together.

ing the labial surface of these teeth close to the arch wires. The difference in prominence between the maxillary lateral incisor and canine means that the bracket base for the lateral incisor, in contrast, must be quite thick, while the maxillary central incisor is intermediate. In the mandibular arch, the canine tooth is less prominent, so while a thin bracket base is used on the canine, an intermediate thickness base can be used on both lower lateral and central incisors. Bracket thickness for both maxillary and mandibular premolars is approximately equivalent to that of the canines.

Especially in the maxillary arch, control of molar rotation is important if good interdigitation of the teeth is to be achieved. Placing a tube flat along the buccal surface of an upper molar would result in rotating it as shown in Figure 12-26. For good occlusion, the buccal surface must sit at an angle to the line of occlusion, with the mesio-buccal cusp more prominent than the distobuccal cusp. For this reason, the tube or bracket specified for the upper molar should have at least a 10-degree offset (Figure 12-27), as should the tube for the upper second molar.

A similar phenomenon occurs with the lower molars, but to a lesser extent. The offset for the lower first molar tubes should be 5 to 7 degrees, about half as much as for the upper molar. The offset for the lower second molar should be at least as large as for the first molar. Offsets in some typical commercially available appliances are shown in Table 12-2 (the listed prescriptions are available in most instances from several different manufacturers).

Variations in Bracket Slot Angulation and Elimination of Second-Order Bends.   In the original edgewise appliance, second-order bends, sometimes called artistic positioning bends, were an important part of the finishing phase of treatment (see Figure 12-24, *B*). These bends were necessary because the long axis of each tooth is inclined relative to the plane of a continuous arch wire (Figure 12-28). Without adequate second-order bends, the incisor teeth are positioned too straight up and down with the roots too close together, producing an effect sometimes disparagingly called the "orthodontic look" (Figure 12-29). The contemporary edgewise brackets that have a built-in tip for maxillary incisor teeth routinely produce a more esthetically pleasing arrangement of the incisors than was achieved in many instances with the early fixed appliances.

Distal tip of the upper first molar is also needed to obtain good interdigitation of the posterior teeth. As shown in Figure 12-30, if the upper molar is too vertically upright, even though a proper Class I relationship apparently exists, good interdigitation cannot be achieved. Tipping the molar distally brings its distal cusps into occlusion and creates

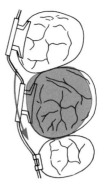

FIGURE 12-26   The rhomboidal surface of the upper, and to a lesser extent the lower, molars means that placing a springy arch wire through attachments that were flat against the facial surface would produce a mesio-lingual rotation of these teeth, causing them to take up too much space in the arch. Compensation requires a bend in the arch wire, or placing the tube at an angle offset to the facial surface.

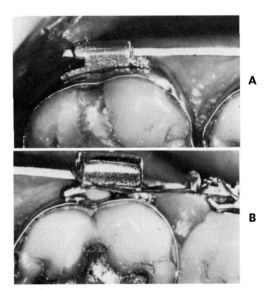

FIGURE 12-27   Tubes for the upper second molar (**A**) and upper first molar (**B**) in a contemporary appliance. Note the offset position of the tube so that a first-order bend in the wire is unnecessary.

TABLE 12-2   *Molar Tube Offset*

	Maxilla		Mandible	
	First Molar	**Second Molar**	**First Molar**	**Second Molar**
Straight wire (Andrews)	10	10	0	0
Straight wire (Roth modified)	14	14	4	4
Alexander	15	6	6	6
Burstone	10	6	5	6
Hilgers	15	12	12	12
Bioprogressive (Ricketts)	15	15	0, 12	0, 12
Bioprogressive (Bench)	0, 15	12	0, 6	6
Level anchorage (Root/Tweed)	12	12	12	12
Hasund	10	6	4	6
Cetlin	14	14	4	6
Orthos	15	15	0	5

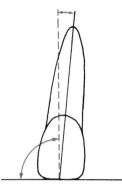

FIGURE 12-28 A second-order bend, or an inclination of the bracket slot to produce the same effect, is necessary for the maxillary incisors because the long axes of these teeth are inclined relative to the incisal edge. The smaller angle (shown above) is the bracket angulation or the tip. (Redrawn from Andrews LF: *J Clin Orthod* 12:179, 1976.)

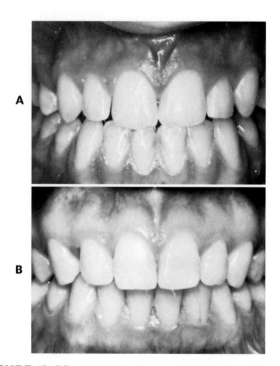

FIGURE 12-29 Achieving the proper inclination of the maxillary incisors is important for good esthetics. **A,** Dental appearance of a patient treated in the 1960s, with inadequate incisor torque and inclination. **B,** Dental appearance of a patient treated recently with a contemporary edgewise appliance, showing improved torque and inclination.

the space needed for proper relationships of the premolars. Bracket and tube inclinations (tip) in some commercially available prescriptions are shown in Table 12-3.

Little if any tip is needed in the canines and premolars when an arch wire is fitted to an ideal arch. An inclination of the bracket slot for canines and premolars may be part of a straight-wire prescription, however, for two reasons: root paralleling at extraction sites and tip of posterior teeth for anchorage.

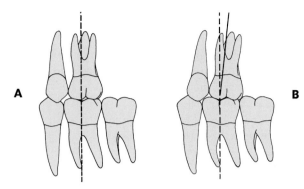

FIGURE 12-30 A distal inclination or tip of the maxillary first molar is important for proper posterior occlusal function. If the mesio-buccal cusp occludes in the mesial groove of the mandibular first molar, creating an apparently ideal Class I relationship, proper interdigitation of the premolars still cannot be obtained if the molar is positioned too upright (**A**). Tipping the molar distally (**B**) allows the premolars to interdigitate properly. (Redrawn from Andrews LF: *Am J Orthod* 62:296, 1972.)

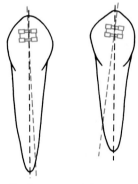

FIGURE 12-31 Inclination of the bracket slots on canines and premolars is not needed for normal positioning. Inclining the canine and second premolar brackets toward a first premolar extraction space, however, can be used to create an automatic root paralleling moment. Bracket inclinations of this type can produce too much root proximity at extraction sites and must be used with caution.

If the bracket slots on the canine and second premolar are inclined as shown in Figure 12-31, a straight arch wire will automatically produce a root-paralleling moment during the closure of a first premolar extraction site. The problem with bracket inclinations of this type is that the desired effect can easily be overdone, so that the root apices have been brought too close together at the conclusion of orthodontic treatment. Furthermore, larger slot inclinations are required on the canines and second premolars for patients who have first premolar extractions than are appropriate for nonextraction patients. Bizarre tooth positions can result if extraction brackets are used on nonextraction patients, or if the finishing phase of treatment is prolonged. Special "extraction brackets" that deviate significantly from the inclinations shown in Table 12-3 must be used with considerable caution.

TABLE 12-3 *Bracket and/or Tube Inclination (Tip)*

	Maxilla						
	Central	Lateral	Canine	1st premolar	2nd premolar	1st molar	2nd molar
Straight wire (Andrews)	5	9	11	2	2	5	5
Straight wire (Roth modified)	5	9	13	0	0	0	0
Alexander	5	8	10	0	0	0	0
Burstone	5	8	10	0	0	0	0
Hilgers	5	8	10	0	0	0	0
Bioprogressive (Ricketts)	0	8	5	0	0	0	0
Bioprogressive (Bench)	5	9	9	0	0	0	0
Level anchorage (Root/Tweed)	4	7	0	0	0	0	−15
Hasund	5	8	13	0	0	3	0
Cetlin	5	9	7	0	0	0	0
Orthos	5	9	10	0	4	0	0
Orthos AP*	4	6	8	4	6	0	0

	Mandible						
	Central	Lateral	Canine	1st premolar	2nd premolar	1st molar	2nd molar
Straight wire (Andrews)	2	2	5	2	2	2	2
Straight wire (Roth modified)	2	2	7	−1	−1	−1	−1
Alexander	0	0	6	0	0	−6	−6, 0
Burstone	0	0	6	0	0	0	0
Hilgers	0	0	6	0	0	−5	−5
Bioprogressive (Ricketts)	0	0	5	0	0	5	5
Bioprogressive (Bench)	2	2	5	0	0	−5, 0	−5
Level anchorage (Root/Tweed)	2	2	−4	−4	−6, −4	−10, −6	−15, −10
Hasund	0	0	5	0	0	0	0
Cetlin	0	0	7	0	0	0	0
Orthos	2	4	6	3	3	0	0
Orthos AP*	0	0	2	3	6	0	0

*For Asian patients.

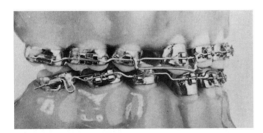

FIGURE 12-32 Distal tipping of the posterior teeth with second-order bends in rectangular wire is used in the Tweed technique to provide increased anchorage. Brackets and molar tubes angulated to produce the same distal tipping are used in one contemporary straight-wire appliance, and distal tipping of molars for anchorage purposes is included in several other appliance prescriptions. (From Tweed CH: *Clinical Orthodontics*, St Louis, 1966, Mosby.)

A second reason for incorporating tip in posterior brackets relates to anchorage control. In the Tweed technique for managing premolar extraction treatment with the original edgewise appliance, it was considered important to "prepare anchorage." This was done by deliberately tipping the molar teeth distally so that they would better resist mesial displacement during space closure (Figure 12-32). One presently available appliance (Level Anchorage, Unitek) is designed to allow the Tweed technique to be used without the necessity for the second-order bends that were an important part of the original technique. In this appliance, distal tipping of the molars and premolars is a built-in feature. Interestingly, a number of the other appliance prescriptions also include some distal tipping of the molars, which is not desired in the final position of these teeth and seems to have been incorporated as a gesture toward anchorage control.

The same inclinations that tip crowns distally also tend to bring the roots mesially, and careless use of an appliance with tip built into the posterior brackets can lead to loss of anchorage. If the molars are tipped somewhat distally at the end of orthodontic treatment and the patient has vertical growth remaining (a critical point), the molars will upright into the normal position. In non-growing patients, tipbacks in the molars do not resolve so neatly on their own. As with inclined brackets on canines and premolars, inclined attachments on molars should be used with a clear understanding of the effects that will be produced. In most circumstances, they are not recommended.

Variations in Bracket Slot Inclination (Torque) and Elimination of Third-Order Bends. If the bracket for a rectangular arch wire is placed flat against the labial or buccal surface of any tooth, the plane of the bracket slot will twist away from the horizontal, often to a considerable extent. With the original edgewise appliance, it was necessary to place a twist in each rectangular arch wire to compensate for this (see Figure 12-24). Failure to place third-order bends meant that in the anterior region, the teeth would become too upright, while posteriorly the buccal cusps of molars would be depressed and the lingual cusps elevated (Figure 12-33). Cutting the bracket slot into the bracket at an angle, which is called *placing torque in the bracket*, allows a horizontally flat rectangular arch wire to be placed into the bracket slots without incorporating twist bends.

The torque needed in many bracket slots is considerable. For incisors, the bracket slot must be at an angle so that the roots are lingually positioned relative to the crowns (positive torque). Canines stand relatively upright, whereas premolars and molars require increasing amounts of negative torque to position the roots buccally, not lingually.

The amount of torque recommended in the various appliance prescriptions varies more than any other feature of contemporary edgewise appliances (Table 12-4). Although a number of factors are important in establishing the appropriate torque, three are particularly germane to how much torque is used for any particular bracket: (1) the value that the developer of the appliance chose as the average normal inclination of the tooth surface (this varies considerably among individuals and therefore can be different in "normal" samples); (2) where on the labial surface (i.e., how far from the incisal edge) the bracket is intended to be placed (the inclination of the tooth surface varies depending on where the measurement is made, so that an appliance meant to be placed rather gingivally would have different torque values from one placed more incisally); and (3) the expected "play" in the bracket slot between the wire and the slot. As Table 12-5 demonstrates, the effective torque produced by undersized rectangular wires is far less than the bracket slot prescription might lead one to expect. Torque prescriptions for 18-slot brackets tend to be more conservative (i.e., have less torque in the brackets) than those for 22-slot appliances. This is because 17 or 18 mil rectangular steel arch wires are routinely placed in 18-slot brackets, whereas 21 or 22 mil steel wires may never be used with 22-slot brackets; thus the torque in the bracket slot tends to be more effective in the 18-slot appliance. As rectangular full-dimension titanium wires are used more and more with the 22-slot appliance, however, it is important to remember that the torque prescription may need to be adjusted to compensate for the better-fitting wires.

Variations in the shape and contour of individual teeth mean that any given inclination or torque built into a bracket will be correct for some teeth and incorrect for oth-

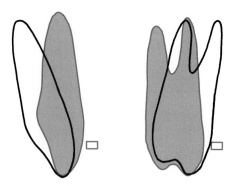

FIGURE 12-33 The plane of a flat rectangular arch wire relative to a maxillary incisor and molar is shown in red. To produce the proper facio-lingual position of both anterior and posterior teeth, either a rectangular arch wire must be twisted (torqued), or the bracket slot must be cut at an angle to produce the same torque effect. Otherwise, the improper inclination shown in red will be produced. Proper torque is necessary, not to move teeth, but to prevent undesired movement.

ers because there is so much variation in the morphology of individual teeth. Slight errors in positioning brackets and bands also contribute to deviations from the ideal appliance prescription. For these reasons, even with the contemporary appliances, some third-order bends in finishing are almost always required, and some first- and second-order bends are likely to be necessary.

Bracket Widths and Slot Sizes

Bracket Width. In the original edgewise appliance, a narrow single bracket was placed in the center of the tooth, and small eyelets were soldered near the corners of the bands to provide for control of rotations (see Figure 12-3). Even before the replacement of bands with bonded attachments made eyelets impractical for anterior teeth, two more convenient methods for obtaining rotational control had largely superceded them: the use of two brackets on the labial surface, creating a twin or Siamese bracket, and the use of wings extending from the single bracket (Figure 12-34). Both single brackets with wings or an extended base width and twin brackets remain important in contemporary use.

Biomechanical considerations in the choice of wide (twin) or narrow (single) brackets are discussed in some detail in Chapter 10. In brief summary, wider brackets allow more positive control of tooth inclination (tip) and are easier to use when teeth slide along arch wires. Wider brackets inevitably reduce interbracket span, however, which makes both initial alignment and detailed finishing (alignment and torque) more difficult because arch wires become stiffer as interbracket span decreases.

There is no reason that wide brackets cannot be used on some teeth and narrow ones on others in the same patient, and just this arrangement is incorporated into some contemporary appliances. However, one cannot evade the basic mechanical principle: the very increase in bracket width that provides better control of root position mesio-

TABLE 12-4 *Bracket and/or Tube Torque*

	Maxilla						
	Central	Lateral	Canine	1st premolar	2nd premolar	1st molar	2nd molar
Straight wire (Andrews)	7	3	−7	−7	−7	−9	−9
Straight wire (Roth modified)	12	8	−2	−7	−7	−14	−14
Alexander	14	7	−3	−7	−7	−10	−10
Burstone	7	3	−7	−7	−10	−10	0
Hilgers	22	14	7	7	−7	−10	−10
Bioprogressive (Ricketts)	22	14	7	0	0	0	0
Bioprogressive (Bench)	17	10	7	−7	−7	−10, 0	−10
Level anchorage (Root/Tweed)	15	7	0	−7	−7	−10	−10
Hasund	22	14	−2	−11	−11	−20	−25
Cetlin	12	8	−2	−7	−7	−14	−14
Orthos	15	9	−3	−6	−8	−10	−10
Orthos AP*	11	9	0	−2	−3	−10	−10

	Mandible						
	Central	Lateral	Canine	1st premolar	2nd premolar	1st molar	2nd molar
Straight wire (Andrews)	−1	−1	−11	−17	−22	−30	−33
Straight wire (Roth modified)	−1	−1	−11	−17	−22	−30	−30
Alexander	−5	−5	−7	−11	−17	−22	−27
Burstone	−1	−1	−11	−17	−22	−27	−27
Hilgers	−1	−1	7	11	−17	−27	−27
Bioprogressive (Ricketts)	0	0	7	0	−14	−22	−32
Bioprogressive (Bench)	−1	−1	7	−11	−22	−27, 0	−27
Level anchorage (Root/Tweed)	0	0	0	−11	−11	−22	−22
Hasund	0	0	−11	−11	−17	−22	−25
Cetlin	0	0	−5	−11	−17	−25	−25
Orthos	−5	−5	−6	−7	−9	−10	−10
Orthos AP*	3	3	−2	−8	−8	−10	−10

*For Asian patients.

TABLE 12-5 *Effective Torque*

Wire size	Play (degrees)	Bracket torque angle (degrees)		
		10	22	30
		Effective Torque		
18-Slot Bracket				
16 × 16	10.9	0.0	11.1	19.1
16 × 22	9.3	0.7	12.7	20.7
17 × 25	4.1	5.9	17.9	25.9
18 × 18	1.5	8.5	20.5	28.5
18 × 25	1.0	9.0	21.0	29.0
22-Slot Bracket				
16 × 22	21.9	0	0.1	8.1
17 × 25	15.5	0	6.5	13.5
19 × 25	9.6	0.4	12.4	20.4
21 × 25	4.1	5.9	17.9	25.9
21.5 × 28	1.8	8.2	20.2	28.2

Note: based on nominal wire and/or slot sizes; actual play is likely to be greater.
(From Sernetz: *Kieferorthop Mitteil* 7:13-26, 1993.)

distally also reduces the springiness of arch wires. Conversely, any modification of a twin bracket that decreases interbracket span inevitably reduces control of tooth inclination. Because of this, arch wire choices will be affected throughout treatment by the width of the brackets.

18- vs. 22-Slot. Biomechanical factors related to use of 18 as compared with 22 mil bracket slots are also discussed in some detail in Chapter 10. Briefly, the 22 mil bracket slot was originally selected to produce optimum performance with gold arch wires. It remained in use after gold was replaced by smaller stainless steel wires primarily because of its advantages in sliding teeth along the wire. With the 18 mil bracket slot, it is common to almost completely fill the slot with a rectangular steel arch wire at the finishing stage of treatment, whereas with the 22 mil bracket slot, steel full-dimension arch wires are forbiddingly stiff and either undersized steel wires or larger but more flexible titanium arch wires can be used to control this problem. Although the factors of bracket width and slot size interact strongly, slot size is even more important than bracket width in determining arch wire sizes and sequence at each stage of treatment.

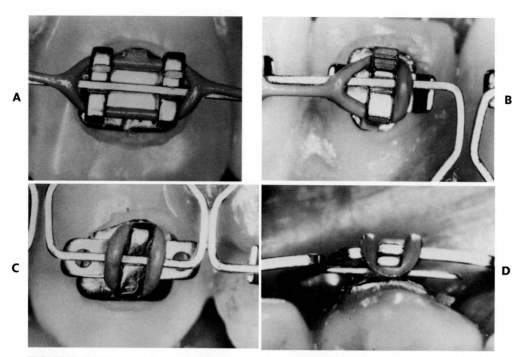

FIGURE 12-34   Either twin brackets or single brackets with wings are used in the contemporary edgewise, and it is not unusual to find a combination of bracket types within a single contemporary appliance prescription. **A,** Twin bracket for maxillary central incisor, with the bracket in a rhomboid or "diamond" configuration to provide the desired 5 degree inclination of the bracket slot; **B,** single bracket with upswept wings (Lewis bracket) for a lower incisor. Note the elastomeric chain tie, which tends to produce rotation. The bracket wing on the right side, contacting the undersurface of the arch wire, provides an antirotation couple with a moment arm from the bracket to the end of the wing. **C,** Single bracket with flat wings (Lang bracket) on a maxillary canine. **D,** Occlusal view of Lang bracket. Note that on canines, the curvature of the arch wire tends to bring it into contact with flat wings. These wings can be bent to the precisely desired position for rotational control after the bracket is placed on the tooth.

Auxiliary Attachments

Auxiliary attachments are an integral part of the contemporary edgewise appliance. They fall into four categories:

Headgear Tubes.   These 45 or 51 mil round tubes are placed routinely on maxillary first molars (Figure 12-35, *A*). They are used for the insertion of the inner bow of a facebow appliance (see Chapter 15) and can also accept a heavy auxiliary labial arch wire. Although the headgear tube can go gingivally or occlusally relative to the slot for the main arch wire, for ease of access and better hygiene, the occlusal location is preferred.

Auxiliary Edgewise Tubes.   The major purpose for auxiliary edgewise tubes is to allow the use of segmented arch technique, which is necessary to intrude teeth and also helpful in other situations. A rectangular auxiliary tube, placed gingivally to the plane of the main arch wires, should be present on both the upper and lower first molars. With this arrangement, the upper first molar typically has a convertible tube-bracket for the main arch wires, a gingivally positioned auxiliary rectangular tube, and an occlusally positioned headgear tube. The lower molar has a convertible tube-bracket for the

main arch wires and a gingivally positioned auxiliary tube (Figure 12-35, *B*).

Auxiliary rectangular tubes on the canines are also used during closure of extraction spaces in the appliance designed by Burstone for segmented arch technique (Figure 12-36). The auxiliary tube on the canine allows the use of springs connecting the anterior and posterior segments that are separate from the base arch wires in either segment. Auxiliary tubes on the canines are only needed for space closure in special circumstances and can be added to an arch wire segment (see Chapter 20). For this reason, they are not routinely used on canines in contemporary appliance prescriptions. The auxiliary tubes for the molars are a necessity for leveling by intrusion and are strongly recommended in all patients.

Auxiliary Labial Hooks.   Hooks for interarch elastics are routinely incorporated into the labial attachments for first and second molars in both arches (see Figure 12-35). These are used as needed for Class II, Class III, or cross-elastics (elastics that correct Class II, Class III, or crossbite relationships, respectively). Although integral hooks are convenient at certain stages of treatment, they

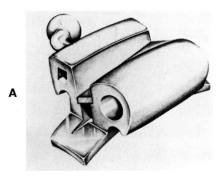
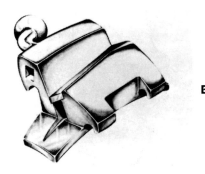

A   B

FIGURE 12-35 Contemporary edgewise tube-bracket attachments to first molars. **A,** Maxillary first molar attachment with convertible bracket slot, occlusal round headgear tube, and gingival auxiliary rectangular tube. **B,** Mandibular first molar attachment with convertible bracket slot and gingival auxiliary rectangular tube. (Courtesy Ormco-A Company.)

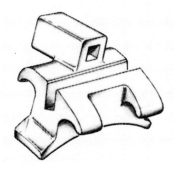
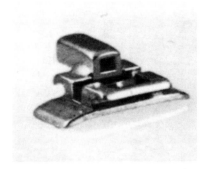

FIGURE 12-36 Burstone canine bracket, combining a rectangular bracket slot with a vertical tube that is used for attachment of retraction springs. (Courtesy Ormco-A Company.)

are full-time food traps and should be used with caution in patients with doubtful oral hygiene. Large hooks, like the "power arms" once recommended to facilitate sliding space closure (see Figure 10-20), are such a hygiene problem that they are rarely used now despite their mechanical advantage.

Lingual Arch Attachments. Heavy stabilizing lingual arches can serve as an important adjunct in anchorage control. They are an important part of segmented arch technique and are needed when auxiliary arch wires are used for leveling by intrusion. They also can be an important adjunct for anchorage control in space closure in premolar extraction cases, regardless of whether a totally segmented arch approach is used (see Chapter 10).

There are two modern lingual arch attachments. One, the standard method until the late 1980s, is the horizontal lingual sheath, made to accept a doubled-over segment of 36 or 30 mil steel wire (Figure 12-37). The other is a lingual bracket made to accept 32×32 beta-Ti or steel wire (Figure 12-38).[14] Twin vertical tubes are an acceptable but

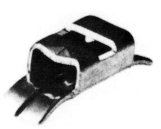

FIGURE 12-37 Horizontal lingual sheath to accept doubled-over 30 or 36 mil steel wire. (Courtesy 3M-Unitek.)

less effective alternative; the single vertical tubes used in mid-century are no longer recommended (see Chapter 13).

In modern orthodontics, lingual arches are used for two quite different purposes: stabilization of the arch, to reinforce anchorage; and tooth movement. For stabilization, the lingual arch needs to be as stiff and rigid as possible. For

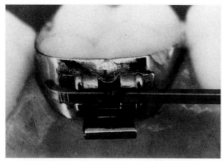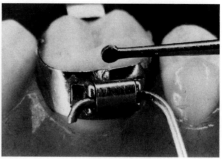

A   B

FIGURE 12-38   The most recent development in lingual arches is the use of a lingual bracket with a 32 × 32 slot and locking cap (**A,** open; **B,** closed, with opening tool shown). The rectangular wire gives excellent three-dimensional control of the molars. The lingual arch can be made from either beta-Ti or steel wire. The more resilient beta-Ti wire is used when tooth movement is desired, the more rigid steel wire when the primary purpose is stabilization for anchorage. (Courtesy Ormco-A Company).

tooth movement, it should be flexible, so that light forces and a reasonable range of action are produced.

With steel lingual arches, 36 mil wire is preferred for stabilization, while 30 mil is better for tooth movement. This produces a problem if the treatment plan calls for using a lingual arch for some tooth movement initially, then leaving it in place for stabilization. It is not practical to remove molar bands and change lingual arch brackets in the middle of treatment, but tooth movement followed by stabilization is a common treatment plan. For example, a lingual arch often is used initially to rotate maxillary molars disto-bucally, and then is left in place while these teeth serve as anchorage for other tooth movement (see Chapter 16). Despite its excessive stiffness for the tooth movement, the 36 mil version of steel lingual arches performs better clinically in these cases. The new lingual arch brackets offer the possibility of using 32 × 32 beta-Ti wire for the initial tooth movement, then replacing it with 32 × 32 steel for stabilization.[15]

Lingual Cleats or Buttons.   It is convenient to have a lingual cleat or button on at least one molar, to allow the use of cross-elastics if necessary during treatment. In addition, lingual cleats on premolars and canines can help in controlling rotations during space closure (see Chapter 17). It is common practice to place a lingual cleat or button on banded posterior teeth, but isolated bonded lingual attachments are not recommended because of the risk that they could become detached and be swallowed by the patient. If it is necessary to use a bonded lingual attachment, tying it to the labial arch wire is a way to control this risk.

Appliance Materials

Stamped vs. Cast Stainless Steel Brackets.   The brackets and tubes for an edgewise appliance must be precisely manufactured so that the internal slot dimensions are accurate to at least 1 mil. Until the recent introduction of ceramic and titanium brackets, fixed appliances had been fabricated entirely from stainless steel for many years, and steel remains the standard material for appliance components.

There are two ways to produce steel edgewise brackets and tubes: from thin metal strip material that is stamped to shape, or by casting. Although stamped brackets and tubes were used almost routinely until the prescription straight-wire appliances were introduced, cast attachments are both more accurate and more durable, and clearly are superior. Most of the brackets and tubes for contemporary appliances now are castings, but some inexpensive appliances still use stamped brackets and tubes. Effective use of the straight-wire approach all but demands the precision of castings.

Nickel Sensitivity: Titanium as an Alternative to Stainless Steel.   Nickel is a potentially allergenic material. Given the significant nickel content of stainless steel, it is fortunate for orthodontists that mucosal allergic reactions to nickel are much less prevalent than cutaneous reactions. Cutaneous sensitization to nickel often develops from skin contact with cheap jewelry, and 10% or more of the population now have some degree of sensitivity to nickel.[16] Most patients who show skin reactions tolerate stainless steel orthodontic appliances quite satisfactorily, but an increasing number do not. Some European countries are now considering a ban on steel orthodontic appliances because of the risk of allergic responses.

The metal alternatives to steel are precious metal, long since abandoned because of performance and cost considerations, and titanium, which contains no nickel and is exceptionally biocompatible. Titanium arch wires have been used since the 1980s. Titanium brackets are difficult to fabricate, but now are available and seem to perform satisfactorily. For patients with nickel allergy, the choice would be between these brackets and non-metallic ones.

Non-Metallic Appliance Materials.   Recurring efforts have been made to make fixed appliances more esthetic by eliminating their metallic appearance. A major impetus

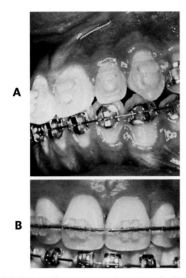

FIGURE 12-39   Clear or tooth-colored plastic brackets can be used on incisors to decrease the visibility of orthodontic appliances. **A,** Polycarbonate incisor brackets with an unconventional shape to minimize bracket failure. Frictional resistance to sliding is a particular problem with brackets of this type; **B,** plastic brackets with metal slots embedded into the body of the bracket. The metal slots reduce sliding friction but the bracket still is not rigid enough for active torque. With a metal arch wire in place, the metal slot is not obvious.

TABLE 12-6 *Ceramic Brackets*	
Material	**Manufacturer, name**
Polycrystallion alumina (PCA)	American, 20/20
	Dentarum, Fascination
	GAC, Allure
	Rocky Mtn, Signature
	Unitek, Transcend and many others
PCA with metal slot	Unitek, Clarity
Monocystalline alumina	A Co., Starfire
Polycrystalline zirconia	Yamaura, Toray

to the development of bonding for orthodontic attachments was the elimination of the unsightly metal band. Tooth-colored or clear brackets for anterior teeth became practical when successful systems for direct bonding were developed (Figure 12-39). Although they were introduced with considerable enthusiasm in the early 1980s, plastic brackets suffered from three largely unresolved problems: (1) staining and discoloration, particularly in patients who smoke or drink coffee; (2) poor dimensional stability, so that it is not possible to provide precise bracket slots or build in all the straight-wire features; and (3) friction between the plastic bracket and metal arch wires that makes it very difficult to slide teeth to a new position. Using a metal slot in the plastic bracket helps the second and third problems, but even with this modification, plastic brackets are useful only when complex tooth movements are not required.

Ceramic brackets, which were first made available commerically in the late 1980s, largely overcome the esthetic limitations of plastic brackets in that they are quite durable and resist staining. In addition, they can be custom-molded for individual teeth and are dimensionally stable, so that the precise bracket angulations and slots of the straight-wire appliance can be incorporated. Four different types of ceramic brackets currently are available (Table 12-6). The new brackets were received enthusiastically and immediately achieved widespread use, but problems with fractures of brackets, friction within bracket slots, wear on teeth contacting a bracket, and enamel damage from bracket removal soon became apparent.

Fractures of ceramic brackets are a problem in two ways: loss of part of the brackets (e.g., tie wings) during arch wire changes or eating, and cracking of the bracket when torque forces are applied. Ceramics are a form of glass, and like glass, ceramic brackets tend to be brittle. Because the fracture toughness of steel is much greater, ceramic brackets must be bulkier than stainless steel brackets, and the ceramic design is much closer to a wide single bracket than is usual in steel. Under stress in the laboratory, metal brackets begin to deform under lower loads than those at which ceramic brackets fail, but the ceramic brackets break catastrophically at the point of failure, with no plastic deformation.

Most currently-available ceramic brackets are produced from alumina, either as single-crystal or polycrystalline units. In theory, single-crystal brackets should offer greater strength, which is true until the bracket surface is scratched. At that point, the small surface crack tends to spread, and fracture resistance is reduced to or below the level of the polycrystalline materials.[17] Scratches, of course, are likely to occur during the course of treatment.

For successful torquing tooth movements, moments between 2000 and 3500 gm-mm are required. Both theoretical analysis and clinical testing suggest that under stresses of this magnitude, fracture of ceramic brackets is likely to occur.[18] For this reason, despite their straight-wire features, it may be necessary to use torquing auxiliaries to complete the final positioning of incisor teeth when ceramic brackets are employed.

Although ceramic brackets are better in this regard than plastics, frictional resistance to sliding has proved to be greater with ceramic than with steel brackets. Because of the multiple crystals, polycrystalline alumina brackets have relatively rough surfaces (Figure 12-40). Even though monocrystalline alumina is as smooth as steel, these brackets also show greater friction than steel, perhaps reflecting a chemical interaction between the wire and bracket material. With ceramic as with steel brackets, friction is worst with beta-Ti wires (Figure 12-41).[19] The bracket surface can abrade the surface of the relatively soft beta-Ti wire, so that small pieces of the wire are pulled out and adhere to the bracket (Figure 12-42). Even with steel wires, nicks and

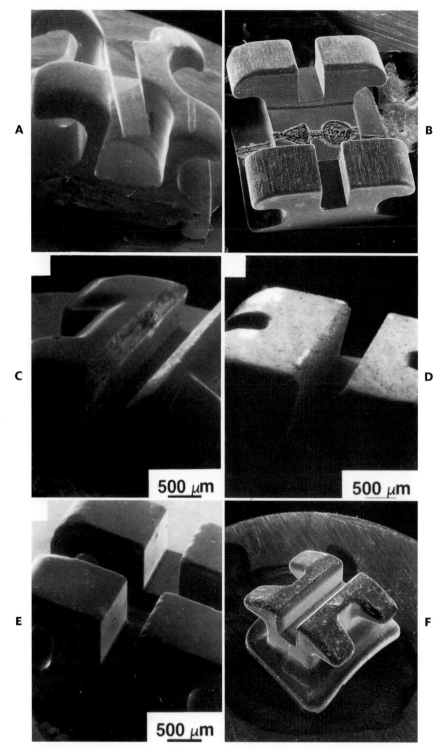

FIGURE 12-40   Scanning electron microscope views of brackets. **A,** stainless bracket (Uni-Twin, 3M-Unitek); **B,** commercially pure titanium (Rematitan, Dentarum); **C,** polycrystalline alumina (Allure, GAC); **D,** polycrystalline alumina (Transcend, 3M-Unitek); **E,** monocrystalline alumina (Starfire, A Co.); **F,** polycrystalline zirconia (Toray, Yamaura). Note the smooth surfaces of the monocrystalline alumina and steel brackets compared with the rougher surface of the polycrystalline alumina and zirconia brackets (which vary from one manufacturer to another). The titanium bracket slot is smooth but not quite as smooth as steel. (Courtesy Dr. R. Kusy.)

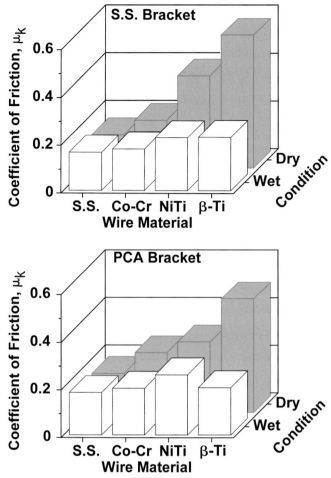

FIGURE 12-41   Coefficients of friction for the wet (human saliva) and dry states, for four arch wires sliding in stainless steel and polycrystalline alumina (PCA) brackets. Note that the NiTi and beta-Ti wires look much worse under dry than wet conditions, in comparison with steel and cobalt-chromium wires. Friction is quite similar in the steel and ceramic brackets. (Redrawn from Kusy and Whitley: *Sem Orthod* 3:166-177, 1997.)

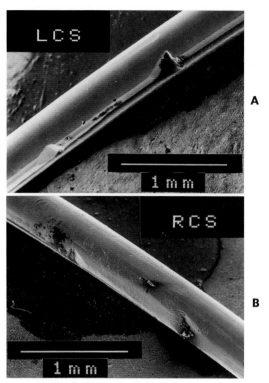

FIGURE 12-42   Scanning electron microscope view of a steel wire that was severely notched by sliding through a ceramic bracket: **A,** at the left and, **B,** at the right canine region. In general, ceramic brackets cause more damage to wires than stainless steel brackets, regardless of the opposing wire alloy. Note that the damage is greatest on the lingual aspect of the canine region. (Copyright R. Kusy; reprinted with permission.)

cuts in the surface of the wire often are observed after movement of the wire against a ceramic bracket. The importance of increased friction depends to some extent on technique: the more the orthodontist will close spaces by sliding, the more important it is, and conversely, the more loops are used for space closure, the more friction can be tolerated.

Although occlusal contacts against brackets are avoided when possible, many patients bite against a bracket or tube at some point in treatment. If the occlusion is against a steel bracket, little or no wear of enamel occurs, but ceramic brackets can abrade enamel quite rapidly (Figure 12-43). This risk is largely avoided if ceramic brackets are placed only on the upper anterior teeth, which is the location where improved esthetics is most important. Most patients will accept ceramic brackets only where they are most visible and steel or titanium brackets elsewhere, and in most circumstances this is now the preferred arrangement to prevent enamel abrasion.

As noted above in the section on debonding, ceramic brackets also can be a problem when it comes time for bracket removal. Distorting the ceramic bracket base to induce failure between the bracket and adhesive is not possible. For safe debonding, it is best to select ceramic brackets with mechanical retention between the base and the adhesive, not chemical retention. Some recently introduced brackets have an additional interface at the bracket base that is designed to be the point of failure. Ceramic brackets with a metal slot will fracture at the slot, and if a bracket of this type has mechanical retention at the bracket base, this facilitates removal.

In addition, the debonding technique is important. The current recommendation is to either:

1. use a debonding instrument that concentrates force at the bracket-adhesive interface (sharp cutter), or an instrument that induces an asymmetric shearing rather than a torquing stress,[20] or
2. use a thermal or laser instrument to weaken the adhesive (by heating it), to induce failure within the bonding agent itself. Thermal debonding of this

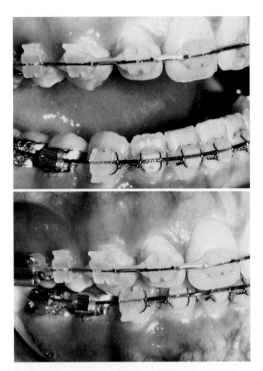

FIGURE 12-43   Ceramic brackets can cause abrasion of teeth if they are in occlusal contact. Note the abrasion of the mesial surface of the maxillary right canine in this patient, caused by contact with the mandibular canine bracket. Ceramic brackets for the mandibular arch must be used with extreme care to avoid this complication.

type is quite effective in reducing the chance of enamel damage. Unfortunately, it introduces the chance of pulpal damage unless the heat application is controlled quite precisely.[21]

Just as composite plastic fibers are likely to replace metal arch wires in clinical orthodontics (see Chapter 10), it seems highly probable that composite plastic brackets will become the standard in another few years. Composite plastics with better physical properties than metal already exist. It is just a matter of overcoming the engineering problems to produce satisfactory brackets. The better esthetic qualities of these materials compared with metal become almost a fringe benefit.

Pre-formed Arch wires and Arch Form

As another contributor to increased efficiency, preformed arch wires are an important part of the modern appliance. For all practical purposes, there is no choice but to use preformed NiTi and beta-Ti wires. What arch form should be employed?

The concept that dental arch form varies among individuals is driven home to most dentists in full denture prosthodontics, where it is taught that the dimensions and shape of the dental arches are correlated with the dimensions and shape of the face. The same variations in arch form and dimensions of course exist in the natural dentition, and it is not the goal of orthodontic treatment to produce dental arches of a single ideal size and shape for everyone.

The basic principle of arch form in orthodontic treatment is that within reason, the patient's original arch form should be preserved. Most thoughtful orthodontists have assumed that this would place the teeth in a position of maximum stability, and long-term retention studies support the view that posttreatment changes are greater when arch form is altered than when it is maintained.[22] The normal variations in arch form, however, are not reflected in the preformed arch wires presently available, and it is important to keep in mind during orthodontic treatment that if preformed arch wires are used, their shape should be considered a starting point for the adjustments necessary for proper individualization (Figure 12-44).

When a Class II malocclusion is present, there is a tendency for the maxillary arch to assume an excessively tapered form. In most Class II patients, it can be seen that when the lower arch is brought forward into a proper relationship, there is an incompatibility in arch form because the upper arch is too constricted across the canines and premolars (Figure 12-45). In this circumstance, it is necessary during orthodontic treatment to change the maxillary arch form. As a more general guideline, if the maxillary and mandibular arch forms are incompatible at the beginning of treatment, the mandibular arch form should be used as a basic guide. Obvious exceptions are encountered, however, in patients in whom the mandibular arch form has been distorted. This distortion can happen in a number of ways, the most common being lingual displacement of the mandibular incisors by habits or heavy lip pressures, and unilateral drift of teeth in response to early loss of primary canines or molars. Although some judgment is required, the arch form desired at the end of orthodontic treatment should be determined at the beginning, and the patient's occlusal relationships should be established with this in mind.

Despite wide acceptance of the idea that arch forms vary among individuals, there is a long orthodontic tradition of seeking a single ideal arch form. For many years, the Bonwill-Hawley arch form dominated orthodontic thinking. This arch form was based on establishing the anterior segment of the dental arch, from canine to canine, on a segment of the arc of a circle, and extending the posterior segments along a straight line. The radius of the arch varied depending on the size of the incisor teeth, so that arch dimensions differed as a function of tooth size, but arch form was constant for all individuals. The patient's original arch form was not considered. This approach can no longer be recommended.

An excellent mathematical description of the natural dental arch form is provided by a catenary curve, which is the shape that a loop of chain would take if it were suspended from two hooks. The length of the chain and the width between the supports determine the precise shape of the curve. When the width across the first molars is used to establish the posterior attachments, a catenary curve fits

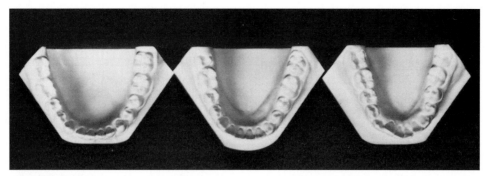

FIGURE 12-44 Lower casts of three untreated potential orthodontic patients. Note the difference in arch form.

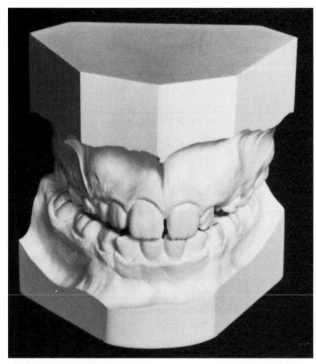

FIGURE 12-45 Frontal view of the dental casts of this boy with a typical Class II malocclusion, with the casts placed into a Class I molar relationship. Note that a crossbite results because of the relatively narrow upper arch. In treatment of Class II patients, this effect usually requires some change in upper arch form.

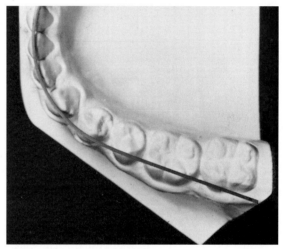

FIGURE 12-46 Preformed arch wire with catenary arch form on a lower dental cast from an untreated patient. Note the good correspondence between the arch form and the line of occlusion, except for the second molar.

the dental arch form of the premolar-canine-incisor segment of the arch very nicely for most individuals. Exceptions include patients whose arches would fall into the prosthodontists' classifications of square or tapering arch forms. For all individuals, the fit is not as good if the catenary curve is extended posteriorly, because the dental arch normally curves slightly lingually in the second and third molar region (Figure 12-46). Most of the preformed arch wires offered by contemporary manufacturers are based on a catenary curve, with average intermolar dimensions.

Although these arch wires are a good starting point, it is apparent that even if one accepts the catenary curve as ideal, their shape should be modified if the first molar widths are unusually wide or narrow. Modifications to accommodate for a generally more tapering or more square morphology are also appropriate, and the second molars must be "tucked in" slightly.

Another mathematical model of dental arch form, originally advocated by Brader and often called the *Brader arch form*, is based on a trifocal ellipse. The anterior segment of the trifocal ellipse closely approximates the anterior segment of a catenary curve, but the trifocal ellipse gradually constricts posteriorly in a way that the catenary curve does not (Figure 12-47). The Brader arch form, therefore, will more closely approximate the normal position of the second and third molars. It also differs from a catenary curve in producing somewhat greater width across the premolars.

Preformed arch wires prepared to an average Brader arch form are available commercially in a limited range of sizes, which can reduce the amount of individualization necessary. Like the catenary curve, however, the Brader arch form represents what the prosthodontists would call a mid-range arch form, which will require some alteration

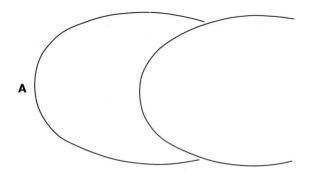

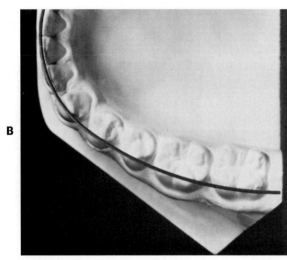

FIGURE 12-47   **A,** The Brader arch form for preformed arch wires is based on a trifocal ellipse, which slightly rounds the arch in the premolar region compared with a catenary curve and constricts it posteriorly. **B,** An arch wire formed to the Brader curve fits much better in the second molar region for this untreated patient than a catenary curve would (compare with Figure 12-46).

for either the relatively square or relatively tapering normal arch form variations. Recently, several manufacturers have offered preformed arch wires that appear to be variations of the Brader arch, with advertisements that suggest these wires are more compatible with expansion therapy than conventional arch forms; however, there are no data to support this contention. More refined mathematical descriptions of typical human arch forms have appeared recently,[23] and it is likely that better mathematical models will improve the preformed arch wires available in the near future.

It is important to keep in mind that the adjustments placed in brackets for all of the straight-wire edgewise systems have nothing to do with arch form, which is still established by the shape of the arch wires connecting the brackets. Arch form is particularly important during the finishing stage of treatment, when heavy rectangular arch wires are employed. Preformed arch wires are often listed in the catalogs as "arch blanks" and the name is appropriate, since this properly implies that a degree of individualization of the shape of the preformed arch wires will be required to accommodate the needs of patients.

REFERENCES

1. Angle EH: The latest and best in orthodontic mechanisms, Dent Cosmos 70:1143-1158, 1928.
2. Begg PR, Kesling PC: Begg orthodontic theory and technique, ed 3, Philadelphia, 1977, W.B. Saunders.
3. Zuriarrain JL, Echeverria JE, del Valle J, Thompson WJ: Our experience in combining mechanics, Am J Orthod Dentofac Orthop 110:575-589, 1996.
4. Kesling PC, Rocke RT, Kesling CK: Treatment with Tip-Edge brackets and differential tooth movement, Am J Orthod Dentofac Orthop 99:387-401, 1991.
5. Andrews LF: Straight wire: the concept and appliance, San Diego, 1989, LA Wells.
6. Berger JL: The SPEED appliance: a 14-year update on this unique self-ligating orthodontic mechanism, Am J Orthod Dentofac Orthop 105:217-223, 1994.
7. Pizzoni L, Revnholt G, Melsen B: Frictional forces related to self-ligating brackets, Eur J Orthod 20:283-291, 1998.
8. Creekmore T: Lingual orthodontics—its renaissance, Am J Orthod Dentofac Orthop 96:120-137, 1989.
9. Powers JM, Kim HB, Turner DS: Orthodontic adhesives and bond strength testing, Sem Orthod 3:147-156, 1997.
10. Stirrups DR: A comparative trial of a glass ionomer and a zinc phosphate cement for securing orthodontic bands, Brit J Orthod 18:15-20, 1991.
11. Olsen ME, Bishara SE, Boyer DB et al: Effect of varying etching times on the bond strength of ceramic brackets, Am J Orthod Dentofac Orthop 109:403-409, 1996.
12. Artun J, Bergland S: Clinical trials with crystal growth conditioning as an alternative to acid-etch enamel pretreatment, Am J Orthod 85:333-340, 1984.
13. Banks PA, Burn A, O'Brien K: A clinical evaluation of the effectiveness of including fluoride into an orthodontic bonding adhesive, Eur J Orthod 19:391-396, 1997.
14. Burstone CJ: Precision lingual arches: passive applications, J Clin Orthod 22:444-452, 1988.
15. Burstone CJ: Precision lingual arches: active applications, J Clin Orthod 23:101-109, 1989.
16. Bass JK, Fine H, Cisneros GJ: Nickel hypersensitivity in the orthodontic patient, Am J Orthod Dentofac Orthop 103: 280-285, 1993.
17. Flores DA, Caruso IM, Scott GE, Jeroudi MT: The fracture strength of ceramic brackets: a comparative study, Angle Orthod 60:269-276, 1990.
18. Holt MH, Nanda RS, Duncanson MG: Fracture resistance of ceramic brackets during arch wire torsion, Am J Orthod Dentofac Orthop 99:287-293, 1991.
19. Kusy RP, Whitley JQ: Friction between different wire-bracket configurations and materials, Sem Orthod 3:166-177, 1997.
20. Bishara SE, Fehr DE: Ceramic brackets: something old, something new, a review, Sem Orthod 3:177-188, 1997.
21. Dovgan JS, Walton RE, Bishara SE: Electrothermal debracketing: patient acceptance and the effects on the dental pulp, J Dent Res 69:300, 1990 (abst. 1531).
22. Joondeph DB, Riedel RA: Retention. In Graber TM, Vanarsdall RL (editors): Orthodontics: current principles and techniques, ed 3, St. Louis, Mosby, in press.
23. Braun S, Hnat WH, Fender WE, Legan HL: The form of the human dental arch, Angle Orthod 68:29-36, 1998.

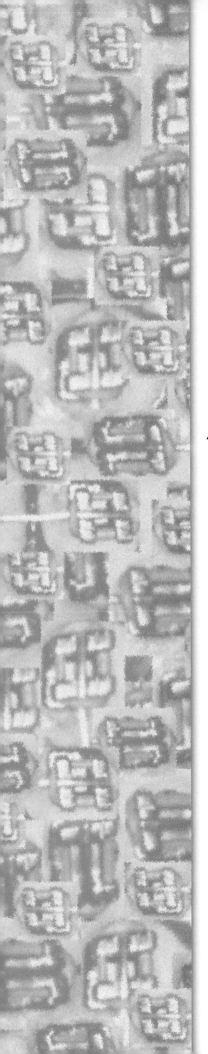

SECTION

VI

TREATMENT OF ORTHODONTIC PROBLEMS IN PREADOLESCENT CHILDREN

"Preventive and interceptive orthodontics," as a description of orthodontic treatment in children, is largely devoid of meaning in an era when treatment for a preadolescent child usually is followed by comprehensive treatment in the early permanent dentition. The problem with this description, though semantic, is not trivial: it encourages inappropriate expectations from this treatment, implying that if the right treatment were done at an early age, no further treatment would be needed. "Prevention" of malocclusion is possible only in a few special circumstances. "Interceptive" treatment can be very helpful in reducing the severity of problems but rarely is so successful that later treatment becomes unnecessary. The current concept is that most children who have orthodontic treatment in the preadolescent years will require a second stage of treatment after their succedaneous teeth erupt.

Despite this, treatment in the mixed dentition (or occasionally in the primary dentition) can be very helpful. In the discussion that follows, treatment is described in terms of appropriate responses to specific situations—without the "preventive" or "interceptive" labels.

Orthodontic problems in children can be divided conveniently into nonskeletal (dental) and skeletal problems, which are treated by tooth movement and by growth modification, respectively. Treatment of nonskeletal problems is described in Chapters 13 and 14, and skeletal problems are discussed in Chapter 15. The complexity of the treatment procedures varies. Some are definitely within the scope of the general practitioner, whereas others rarely should be attempted outside specialty practice. Even the simplest treatment in children requires continuous reevaluation to be sure that the expected response is occurring. The transition of the dentition, coupled with rapid growth, means that rapid changes can and do occur. In children, appliance therapy tends to be simpler than in adults, where all changes that occur must be caused by tooth movement, but treatment planning and monitoring are more complex. Whether treatment in children involves skeletal or nonskeletal problems, the totality of changes must be considered. Although diagnosis and treatment planning are not discussed in this section, which focuses on treatment, careful analysis and planning are imperative before any treatment begins.

Treatment of Moderate Nonskeletal Problems in Preadolescent Children

Our approach to treatment of dental problems in preadolescent children is built around the triage scheme presented in some detail in Chapter 6. The triage makes two critical distinctions: first between nonskeletal and skeletal orthodontic problems, then by severity among the nonskeletal problems. In this chapter, we presume that these distinctions have been made and using facial form analysis or (less frequently) cephalometric analysis and then space analysis as the key diagnostic procedures. This chapter focuses on treatment procedures for children who would be selected by that process. They have moderately severe orthodontic problems, or potential problems, that are within the purview of any dentist.

CROWDED AND IRREGULAR TEETH

Irregular and malaligned teeth in the early mixed dentition arise from two major causes: (1) lack of adequate space for alignment, which causes an erupting tooth to be deflected from its normal position in the arch; and (2) interferences with eruption, which prevent a permanent tooth from erupting on a normal schedule and secondarily can lead to space problems because other teeth drift to improper positions. The goal of early treatment is either to prevent teeth from drifting and reducing the space available for the permanent teeth, or to create some additional space within the dental arch so that alignment becomes possible. From this perspective, the guidelines used in the triage scheme must be kept in mind: more than 3 to 4 mm of discrepancy between the amount of space available for the teeth and the amount of space required is a severe problem, not a moderate one.

Missing Primary Teeth with Adequate Space: Space Maintenance

Early loss of a primary tooth presents a potential alignment problem because drift of permanent or other primary teeth is likely unless it is prevented by space maintenance. Space maintenance is appropriate only when adequate space is available and all unerupted teeth are present and at the proper stage of development. If there is not enough space or if succedaneous teeth are missing, space maintenance alone is inadequate. The indications and contraindications for space maintenance are discussed in Chapter 7; the discussion here focuses on the treatment procedures.

Several treatment techniques can be used successfully for space maintenance, depending on the specific situation.

Band and Loop Space Maintainers. The band and loop is a unilateral fixed appliance indicated for space maintenance in the posterior segments. It is used most frequently to maintain the space of a primary first molar before eruption of the permanent first molar, but it also can be used to maintain the space of either a primary first or second molar after the permanent first molar has erupted. The simple cantilever design makes it ideal for isolated unilateral space maintenance (Figure 13-1). Because the loop has limited strength, this appliance must be restricted to holding the space of one tooth and is not expected to accept functional forces of chewing. Although bonding a rigid or flexible wire across the edentulous space has been advocated as an alternative, this arrangement has not proved satisfactory clinically. It also is no longer considered advisable to solder the loop portion to a stainless steel crown because this precludes simple appliance removal and replacement. Teeth with stainless steel crowns should be banded like natural teeth.

If a primary second molar has been lost, the band can be placed on either the primary first molar or the permanent first molar. Some clinicians prefer to band the primary tooth in this situation because of the risk of decalcification around any band, but primary first molars are challenging to band because of their morphology, which converges occlusally and makes band retention difficult. A more important consideration is the eruption sequence of the succedaneous teeth. The primary first molar should not be banded if the first premolar is developing more rapidly than the second premolar, because loss of the banded abutment tooth would require replacement of the appliance.

Ideally, the loop portion should be wide enough faciolingually to allow eruption of the permanent premolar without removing the appliance, but this arrangement is difficult to achieve. The loop also should be in close approximation to the ridge without impinging on the soft tissue. It should not restrict any physiologic movement or adjustment of the adjacent teeth, such as the lateral adjustment of the primary canines that accompanies eruption of the permanent incisors and provides anterior space for the incisors.[1] An occlusal rest is an optional addition to the loop portion of the appliance when it is used in the posterior segments. This addition (see Figure 13-1, *D*) prevents gingival tipping of the appliance and the abutment teeth, which can result in gingival irritation and space loss. Unfortunately, the loop provides little if any functional replacement for the missing tooth and will not prevent supereruption of teeth in the opposing arch.

Before eruption of the permanent incisors, if a single primary molar has been lost bilaterally, a pair of band and loop maintainers are recommended instead of the lingual arch that would be used if the patient were older. This is

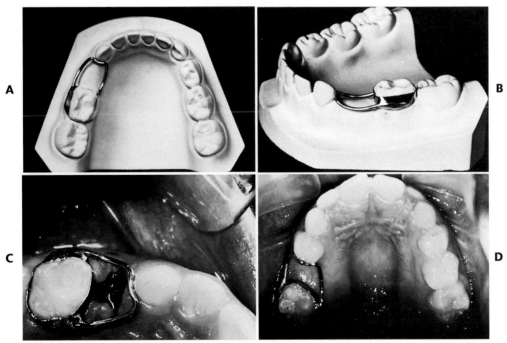

FIGURE 13-1 A band and loop space maintainer is generally used in the mixed dentition to save the space of a single prematurely lost primary molar. It consists of a band on either a primary or permanent molar and a wire loop to maintain space. **A,** The loop portion made from 36 mil wire is carefully contoured to the abutment tooth without restricting lateral movement of the primary canine and **B,** the loop is also contoured to within 1.5 mm of the alveolar ridge. The solder joints should fill the angle between the band and wire to avoid food and debris accumulation. **C,** A completed band and loop maintainer in place after extraction of a primary first molar; **D,** an occlusal rest, shown here on the primary first molar, can be added to the loop portion to prevent the banded teeth from tipping mesially.

advisable because the permanent incisor tooth buds are lingual to the primary incisors and often erupt lingual to their predecessors. The bilateral band and loops enable the permanent incisors to erupt without interference from a lingual arch wire. At a later time the two bands and loops can be replaced with a single lingual arch if necessary.

Partial Denture Space Maintainers. The partial denture is most useful for bilateral posterior space maintenance when more than one tooth has been lost per segment and the permanent incisors have not yet erupted. In these cases, because of the length of the edentulous space, band and loop space maintainers are contraindicated, and the lingual position of the unerupted permanent incisors and their likely lingual position at initial eruption make the lingual arch a poor choice. The partial denture also has the advantage of replacing occlusal function. Another indication for this appliance is posterior space maintenance in conjunction with replacement of anterior teeth for esthetics (Figure 13-2). Replacement of primary anterior teeth for esthetics is reasonable, but anterior space maintenance is unnecessary because arch circumference generally is not lost even if the teeth drift and redistribute the space.[2]

Excellent retention of a partial denture appliance is necessary for good patient compliance and usually requires several clasps. The clasps must accommodate the lateral movement of the primary canines that occurs during permanent incisor eruption. For this reason, clasps on these teeth may have to be removed or adjusted periodically. Frequently, the acrylic portion of the appliance must be modified to allow permanent teeth to erupt. Problems often encountered with partial dentures in a young child are failure to wear the appliance, which leads to space loss, or the other extreme, failure to remove it for cleaning, which can cause soft tissue irritation.

Distal Shoe Space Maintainers. The distal shoe is the appliance of choice when a primary second molar is lost before eruption of the permanent first molar. This appliance consists of a metal or plastic guide plane along which the permanent molar erupts. The guide plane is attached to a fixed or removable retaining device (Figure 13-3). When fixed, the distal shoe is usually retained with a band instead of a stainless steel crown so that it can be replaced by another type of space maintainer after the permanent first molar erupts. Unfortunately, this design limits the strength of the appliance and provides no functional replacement for the missing tooth. If primary first and second molars are missing, the appliance must be removable because of the length of the edentulous span and the guide plane is incorporated in a partial denture. This type of appliance can provide some occlusal function.

To be effective, the guide plane must extend into the alveolar process so that it contacts the permanent first molar approximately 1 mm below the mesial marginal ridge, at or before its emergence from the bone. An appliance of this

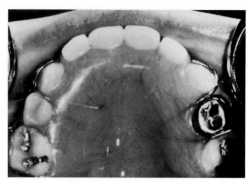

FIGURE 13-2 The removable partial denture is used to replace anterior teeth for esthetics and, at the same time, maintain the space of one or more prematurely lost primary molars. For this patient, the four incisors and the primary right first molar are replaced by the partial denture. Multiple clasps, preferably Adams' clasps, are necessary for good retention. Both the clasps and the acrylic need frequent adjustment to prevent interference with physiologic adjustment of primary teeth during eruption of permanent teeth. The C-clasps on the primary canines provide limited retention and are good examples of clasps that need continued careful attention.

type is tolerated well by most children but is contraindicated in patients who are at risk for subacute bacterial endocarditis or who are immunocompromised, because complete epithelialization around the intra-alveolar portion has not been demonstrated.[3] Careful measurement and positioning are necessary to ensure that the blade will ultimately guide the permanent molar. Faulty positioning is the most common problem with this appliance.

Lingual Arch Space Maintainers. A lingual arch is indicated for space maintenance when multiple primary posterior teeth are missing and the permanent incisors have erupted (Figure 13-4, *A* and *B*). A conventional lingual arch, attached to bands on the primary second or permanent first molars and contacting the cingula of the maxillary or mandibular incisors, prevents anterior movement of the posterior teeth and posterior movement of the anterior teeth.

A lingual arch space maintainer is usually soldered to the molar bands but can be removable, depending on the number of adjustments anticipated and the care of the appliance expected from the patient. Removable lingual arches (e.g., those that fit into attachments welded onto the bands) are more prone to breakage and loss because they use frictional retention instead of solder joints and because the lingual arch wires usually have acute bends that help to form some type of attachment or locking mechanism. The tight bends weaken the wires by introducing high stress points. Regardless of whether it is removable, the lingual arch should be positioned to rest on the cingula of the incisors, approximately 1 to 1.5 mm off the soft tissue, and should be stepped to the lingual in the canine region to remain away from the primary molars

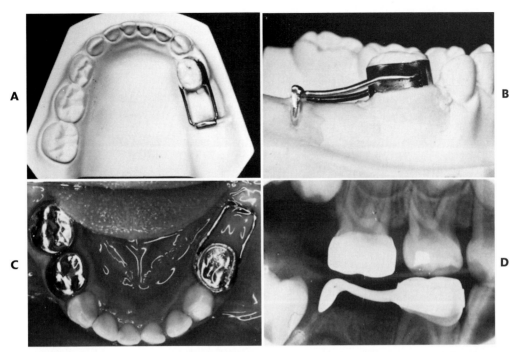

FIGURE 13-3   The distal shoe space maintainer is indicated when a primary second molar is lost before eruption of the permanent first molar and is usually placed at or very soon after the extraction of the primary molar. **A,** The loop portion, made of 36 mil stainless steel wire, and the intra-alveolar blade are soldered to a band so the whole appliance can be removed and replaced with another space maintainer after the permanent molar erupts. **B,** The loop portion must be contoured closely to the ridge since the appliance cannot resist excessive occlusal forces from the opposing teeth. **C,** This distal shoe space maintainer was placed at the time of extraction of the primary second molar. **D,** The blade portion must be positioned so that it extends approximately 1 mm below the mesial marginal ridge of the erupting permanent tooth to guide its eruption. This position can be measured from pretreatment radiographs and verified by a radiograph taken at try-in or post-cementation. An additional occlusal radiograph can be obtained if the faciolingual position is in doubt.

and the unerupted premolars (Figure 13-4, *C*). The most common problems with lingual arches are distortion, breakage, and loss. Careful instructions to parents and patients often alleviate these problems. Maxillary lingual arches of this type are not familiar to many clinicians but are contraindicated only in patients whose bite depth causes the lower incisors to contact the arch wire on the lingual of the maxillary incisors (Figure 13-4, *D*). When bite depth does not allow use of a conventional design, either the Nance lingual arch or a transpalatal arch can be used.

The Nance arch is simply a maxillary lingual arch that does not contact the anterior teeth but approximates the anterior palate (Figure 13-4, *E*). The palatal portion incorporates an acrylic button that contacts the palatal tissue, which in theory provides resistance to anterior movement of the posterior teeth. The appliance is an effective space maintainer, but soft tissue irritation can be a problem. The acrylic portion can become embedded in the soft tissue if the palatal tissue hypertrophies because of poor hygiene or if the appliance is distorted.

The transpalatal arch runs directly across the palatal vault, avoiding contact with the soft tissue (Figure 13-4, *F*). When permanent maxillary molars move anteriorly, they rotate mesiolingually around the large lingual root. The transpalatal arch reduces anterior molar movement by preventing this rotation. The best indication for a transpalatal arch is when one side of the arch is intact and several primary teeth are missing on the other side. In this situation, the rigid attachment to the intact side usually provides adequate stability for space maintenance. When primary molars have been lost bilaterally, however, both permanent molars may tip mesially despite the transpalatal arch, and a conventional lingual arch or Nance arch is preferred. The most common problems with the transpalatal arch are failure to adequately maintain space and failure of the appliance to remain passive. If the appliance is not passive, unexpected vertical and transverse movements of the permanent molars can occur.

A flowchart is provided to help guide decision making for space maintenance (Figure 13-5).

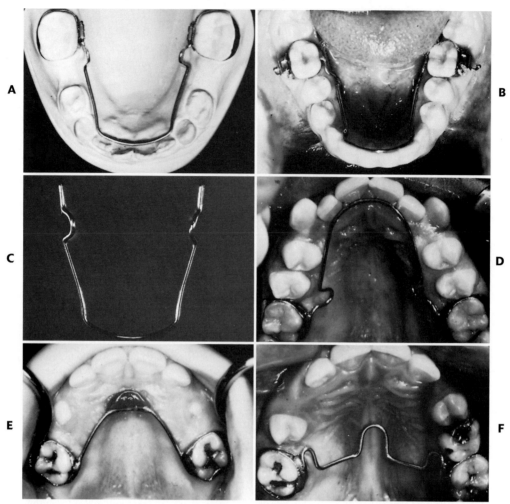

FIGURE 13-4   The lingual holding arch is generally used to maintain space for premolars after premature loss of the primary molars when the permanent incisors have erupted. **A,** The arch is made of 36 mil wire with adjustment loops mesial to the permanent first molars. **B,** This soldered lingual arch successfully maintained the space for the premolars. **C,** The ideal arch is stepped away from the premolars to allow their eruption without interference, which results in a keyhole design. The wire is also 1.5 mm away from the soft tissue at all points. **D,** A maxillary lingual arch is used when the overbite is not excessive, or **E,** a Nance arch with an acrylic button in the palatal vault is indicated if the overbite is excessive. The palatal button must be monitored because it may cause soft tissue irritation. **F,** The transpalatal arch prevents a molar from rotating mesially into a primary molar extraction space, and this largely prevents its mesial migration. Several teeth should be present on at least one side of the arch when a transpalatal design is employed as a sole space maintainer.

Irregular Incisors, No Space Discrepancy

In some children space analysis shows that enough space for all the permanent teeth ultimately will be available, but relatively large permanent incisors and primary molars cause transient crowding of the permanent incisors. This crowding is usually expressed as mild faciolingual displacement or rotation of individual anterior teeth.

Studies of children with normal occlusion indicate that when they go through the transition from the primary to the mixed dentition, up to 2 mm of incisor crowding may resolve spontaneously without treatment (see Chapter 4). From this perspective, as a general rule there

is no need for treatment when less than 2 mm of incisor crowding is observed during the mixed dentition. Not only is reduction of this small amount of crowding probably not warranted, there is no evidence that long-term stability will be greater if the child receives early treatment to improve alignment.

If exaggerated parental concern creates a problem, or if slightly more anterior irregularity is present, one could consider disking the interproximal enamel surfaces of the primary lateral incisors (Figure 13-6) or canines (Figure 13-7) as the anterior teeth erupt. When the enamel thickness at the height of contour is reduced, additional space

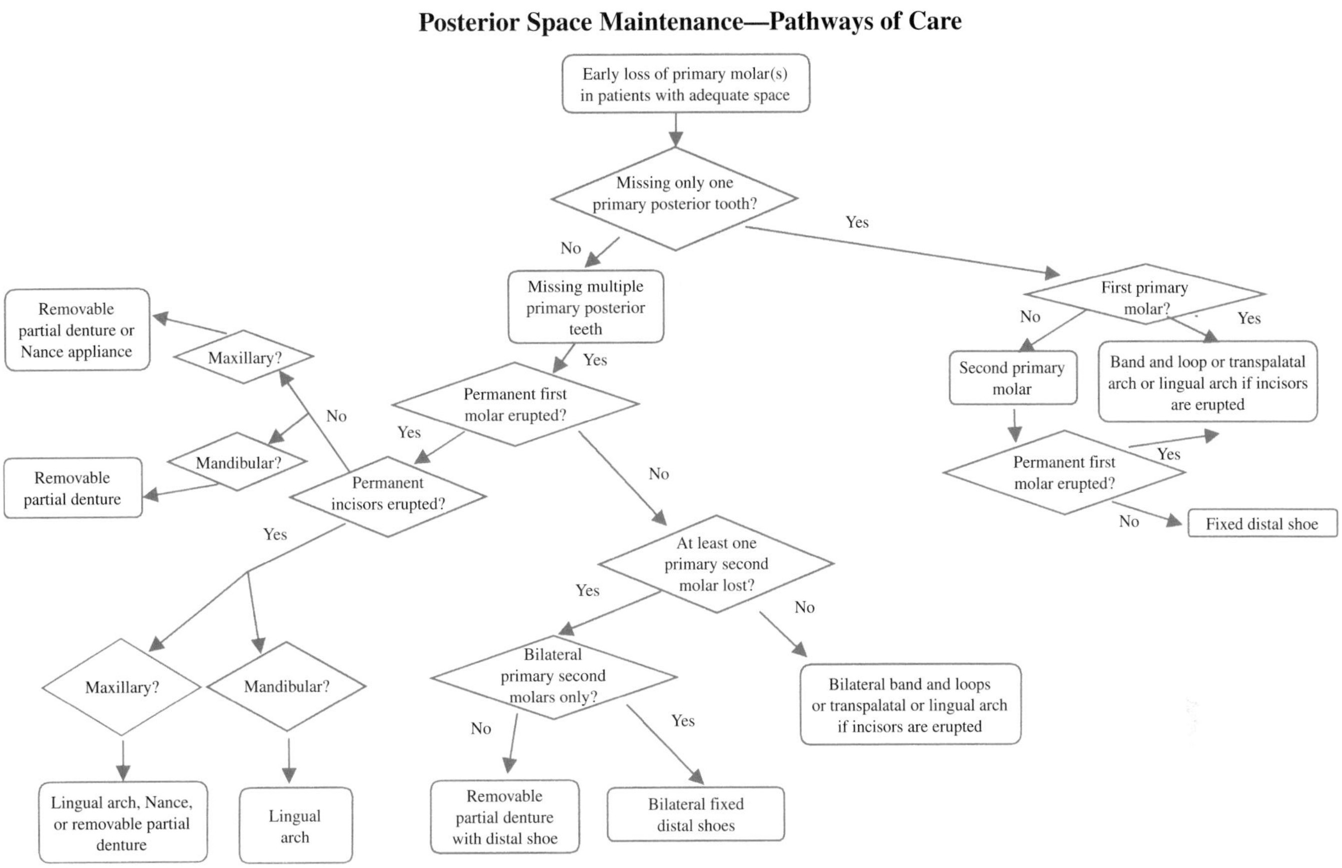

Posterior Space Maintenance—Pathways of Care

Early loss of primary molar(s) in patients with adequate space

Missing only one primary posterior tooth?

No → Missing multiple primary posterior teeth

Yes → First primary molar?

No → Second primary molar

Yes → Band and loop or transpalatal arch or lingual arch if incisors are erupted

Permanent first molar erupted?

Yes → (Band and loop or transpalatal arch or lingual arch if incisors are erupted)

No → Fixed distal shoe

Permanent first molar erupted?

Yes → Permanent incisors erupted?

No → At least one primary second molar lost?

Yes → Bilateral primary second molars only?

No → Removable partial denture with distal shoe

Yes → Bilateral fixed distal shoes

No → Bilateral band and loops or transpalatal or lingual arch if incisors are erupted

Maxillary? → No → Mandibular? → Removable partial denture

Maxillary? → Removable partial denture or Nance appliance

Permanent incisors erupted? → Yes → Maxillary? → Lingual arch, Nance, or removable partial denture

Mandibular? → Lingual arch

FIGURE 13-5 This flowchart can be used to aid decision making regarding possible options for space maintenance in the primary and mixed dentitions. Answers to the questions posed in the chart should lead to successful treatment pathways.

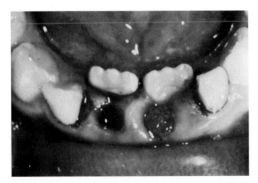

FIGURE 13-6 Disking of primary incisors is a method to reduce anterior crowding and provide space for erupting permanent incisors during the early transitional dentition years.

becomes available for spontaneous alignment. Minor amounts of disking do not cause patient discomfort, but maximum disking may require local anesthesic and produce some postoperative sensitivity. It is possible to gain as much as 3 to 4 mm of anterior space through this procedure. Because up to 2 mm of crowding may resolve spontaneously, this method should probably be reserved for situations when 3 to 4 mm of anterior crowding exist.

Correction of any incisor rotations caused by this transitional crowding requires controlled movement to align and derotate them, using an arch wire and bonded attachments on the incisors. It may be wise to defer this therapy until comprehensive treatment is begun in the early permanent dentition. If it is undertaken in the mixed dentition, the permanent first molars should be banded (and ideally reinforced with a lingual arch to serve as anchorage and to maintain posterior stability and arch dimensions). If the arch wire is not supported between the first molar and incisors, it must be relatively large for strength in the buccal segments and may have to incorporate loops for flexibility in the incisor region. If the primary first molars are also bonded, a smaller and more flexible wire can be used because the length of the molar segment arch wire span is reduced. After alignment has been achieved, if root position needs to be corrected, a rectangular wire is required to finish the tooth movement. It is rare that a child who needs this type of treatment in the mixed dentition does not require further treatment after all permanent teeth have erupted, so extensive early treatment is not often indicated.

The treatment just described is aimed at anterior irregularity only. If the transitional crowding is great enough that there is considerable crowding when the permanent

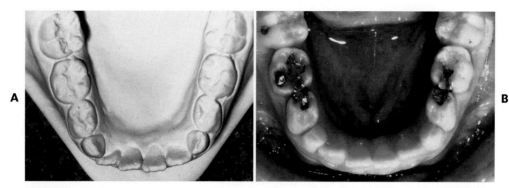

FIGURE 13-7 Disking can be used on multiple surfaces of primary teeth—especially the primary canines—when limited transitional crowding is apparent. **A,** This pretreatment cast shows minor anterior crowding. **B,** Disking of the mesial and distal surfaces of the primary canines allowed spontaneous alignment to occur without appliance therapy.

canines erupt even though there is adequate total space available, the patient really requires a more aggressive form of space supervision and treatment known as space management. This crowding occurs because the combined width of the erupting permanent canine, first premolar, and primary second molar is greater than the total width of the permanent canine and premolars. Because manipulation of the leeway space ultimately will require adjustment of molar relationships, it is considered a more complex type of treatment and is discussed in Chapter 14.

Localized Space Loss (3 mm or Less): Space Regaining

After premature loss of a primary tooth, space may be lost from drift of other teeth before a dentist is consulted. Then, repositioning the teeth to regain space rather than just space maintenance to stabilize the situation is required. Up to 3 mm of space can be reestablished in a localized area with relatively simple appliances and a good prognosis. Space loss greater than that constitutes a severe problem and is discussed in Chapter 14.

Maxillary Space Regaining. Generally, space is easier to regain in the maxillary arch than in the mandibular arch because of the increased anchorage for removable appliances afforded by the palatal vault and the possibility for use of extraoral force (headgear). Space lost from tipping can be regained when the crown of the tooth is tipped back to its original position, but space lost by bodily tooth movement requires that the tooth be bodily repositioned.

Permanent maxillary first molars can be tipped distally to regain space with either a fixed or removable appliance, but bodily movement requires a fixed appliance. Because the molars tend to tip forward and rotate mesiolingually, distal tipping for 2 to 3 mm of space regaining is often satisfactory.

A removable appliance retained with Adams' clasps and incorporating a helical fingerspring adjacent to the tooth to be moved is very effective. This appliance is the ideal design for tipping one molar (Figure 13-8). One posterior tooth can

be moved up to 3 mm distally during 3 to 4 months of full-time appliance wear. The spring is activated approximately 2 mm to produce 1 mm of movement per month. The molar generally will derotate spontaneously as it is tipped distally.

If bodily movement of one or both permanent maxillary first molars is necessary in regaining space, it sometimes can be accomplished by using headgear or an arch wire with excellent anchorage. These methods are addressed in Chapter 14.

Regardless of the method used to regain these limited amounts of space, a space maintainer is required when adequate space has been restored. A fixed space maintainer is recommended, rather than trying to maintain the space with the removable appliance that was used for space regaining.

Mandibular Space Regaining. Removable appliances can be used for space regaining in the mandibular arch just as they are in the maxillary arch, but as a rule they are less satisfactory because they are more fragile and prone to breakage, and because they do not fit as well. Problems with tissue irritation frequently are encountered, and patient acceptance tends to be poorer than with maxillary removable appliances.

If space has been lost on one side of the mandibular arch, the appliance of choice is a removable lingual arch incorporating a loop that can be opened to provide the necessary distal force (Figure 13-9). It is important to activate the lingual arch so that the molar is tipped up and back, while the reaction force is expressed largely downward on the cingulum area of the lower incisors. Nevertheless, there is an inevitable tendency to also tip the incisors forward.

An alternative for unilateral mandibular space regaining is a fixed appliance and an arch wire, which provide excellent anchorage. This method is discussed in Chapter 14.

If space has been lost bilaterally, a lingual arch also can be used, but pitting posterior movement of both molars against the anchorage offered by the incisors means that significant forward displacement of the incisors must be expected.

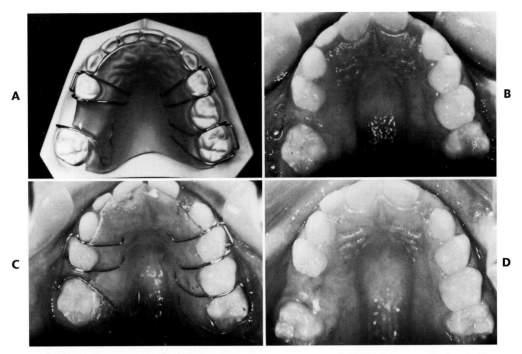

FIGURE 13-8 A removable appliance with a fingerspring is used to regain space by tipping a permanent first molar distally. **A,** The appliance incorporates multiple Adams' clasps and a 28 mil helical spring that is activated 1 to 2 mm per month. **B,** Premature loss of the primary second molar has led to mesial drift and rotation of the permanent first molar. **C,** This removable appliance can be used to regain up to 3 mm of space. **D,** After space regaining the space should be maintained with a band and loop or lingual arch if the permanent incisors have erupted.

An alternative fixed appliance for mandibular space regaining is the lip bumper, which is a labial appliance fitted to tubes on the molar teeth (Figure 13-10). The idea is that the appliance presses against the lip, which creates a distal force to tip the molars posteriorly. Although some posterior movement of the molars can be observed when a lip bumper is used, the appliance also alters the equilibrium of forces against the incisors, removing any restraint from the lip on these teeth. The result is that forward movement of lower incisors occurs with a lip bumper.[4] Depending on the type of lip bumper used and its clinical manipulation, transverse widening also may occur.[5]

On balance, the effects of the active lingual arch and the lip bumper are similar. A lingual arch can be left in place as a space maintainer after space has been regained. A lip bumper is not a good space maintainer and should be replaced with band and loop maintainers or a lingual arch for long-term maintenance of the space that was regained.

Generalized Moderate Crowding (4 mm or Less)

Children with incisor crowding and small space discrepancies can be treated with modest amounts of arch expansion during the early mixed dentition. Since further comprehensive treatment in the early permanent dentition probably will be required (because canines and premolars often

erupt in poor positions even if adequate space has been created), the cost effectiveness of mixed dentition treatment of this type must be considered carefully. One can look at this group from two perspectives: there is minimal benefit from early treatment unless there are major esthetic concerns, and therefore little or no reason to intervene; or alternatively, this group does not need much treatment, it should be relatively easy to provide, and there is always the possibility that if early treatment is done, later treatment might not be necessary.

Some practitioners have advocated arch expansion in the primary[6] and early mixed dentitions[7] on the theory that this would assure more space at a later time. To date, there is no credible evidence that early intervention to "prepare," "develop," "balance," or expand arches by any other name has any efficacy in providing a less crowded permanent dentition at a substantial post-retention time point. Unfortunately, even in children who had mild crowding initially, incisor irregularity can recur soon after early treatment if retention is not managed carefully.[8] Parents and patients should know the issues and uncertainties associated with this type of treatment.

The major reason for early intervention for incisor crowding in a child who has moderate space discrepancy, is esthetic concern because of obvious crowding. This can occur when substantial transitional crowding due to the

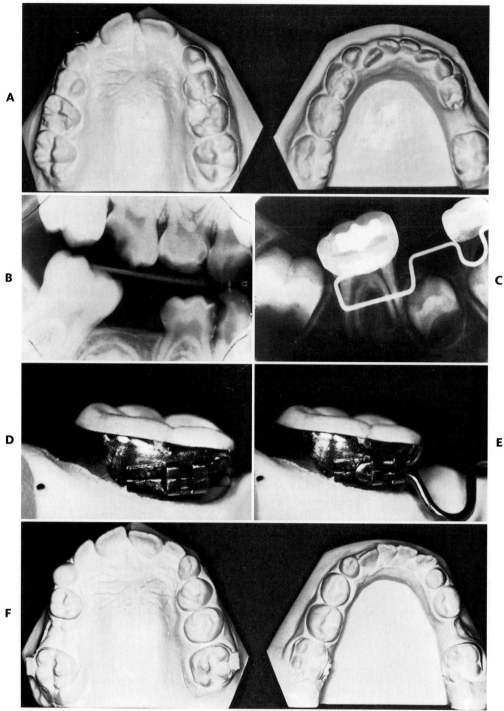

FIGURE 13-9   Space regaining in a child with space loss in the upper and lower arches. **A,** Casts demonstrating loss of space as a result of caries and early loss of a primary molar. **B,** Bitewing radiograph shows space loss caused by mesial tipping of upper and lower permanent first molars. **C,** An active lingual arch, inserted from the distal in this case, was used for mandibular space regaining. **D,** When an active lingual arch is inserted from the mesial, the welded attachment on the band should be tipped up on the mesial to allow easy placement and removal. **E,** Note that when the lingual arch is fully seated, the dimple on the distal of the sheath into which it inserts serves as a lock to retain the arch wire. **F,** Casts of this patient after treatment with a mandibular lingual arch and maxillary headgear, showing the space regaining that was achieved. At this point, space maintainers will be needed.

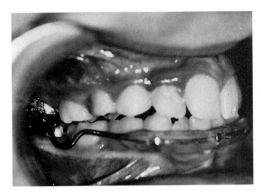

FIGURE 13-10 A lip bumper constructed of a 36 mil wire bow with an acrylic pad, which fits into tubes on the permanent first molars, is sometimes used to increase arch length by moving the molars distally and causing the incisors to move anteriorly. This occurs when the appliance stretches the lower lip and transmits force to move the molars back. The appliance also disrupts the equilibrium between the lip and tongue and allows the anterior teeth to move facially. The result is probably nearly equal molar and incisor change. (Courtesy Dr. M. Linebaugh.)

larger permanent incisors is superimposed on a real, though minor, space shortage. The amount of disking required to alleviate the crowding would expose the pulps of the primary canines or cause extreme sensitivity. The options are to (1) remove the primary canines as the crowding occurs, which allows better alignment but creates the possibility that the permanent incisors will tip lingually, reducing the arch length even more (Figure 13-11), or (2) move the teeth facially into a larger arch circumference.

A conservative approach to this dilemma is to place a lingual arch after the extraction of the primary canines and allow the incisors to align. Ultimately the lingual arch or another appliance can be used to increase the arch length. A word of caution is necessary here. Clinical experience indicates that a considerable degree of faciolingual irregularity will resolve if space is available, but rotational irregularity will not. If the incisors are rotated or severely irregular and early correction is felt to be important, a multiply bonded and banded appliance is indicated (Figure 13-12).

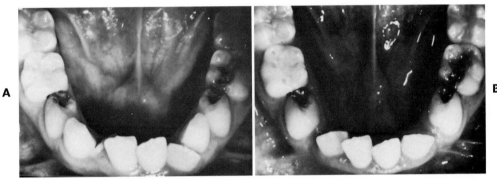

FIGURE 13-11 Extraction of primary canines as a method to reduce anterior irregularity. **A,** This patient has a sizable amount of anterior crowding and irregularity. **B,** The primary canines were extracted, which allowed some alignment, but the incisors have tipped lingually and further reduced the arch length.

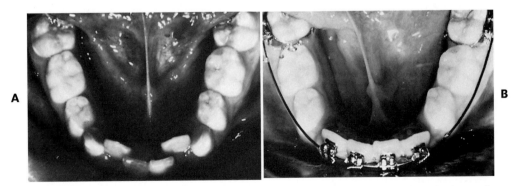

FIGURE 13-12 Alignment of anterior teeth and incisor advancement with multiple attachments and an arch wire. **A,** This patient has crowding and irregularity that (**B**) were reduced by extraction of the primary canines and alignment and advancement of the incisors using an arch wire and multiple attachments.

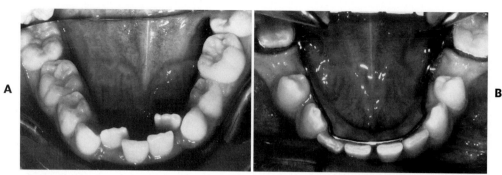

FIGURE 13-13   Arch expansion with a lingual arch in the early and late mixed dentition stages. **A,** This patient has a space shortage in the mixed dentition and anterior irregularity that were treated by (**B**) expanding the arch with an active lingual arch. These arches can be removable or soldered. The removable arches are simpler to adjust, but the soldered arches are more durable.

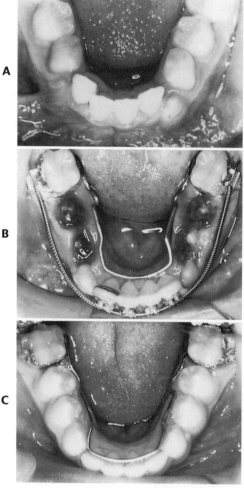

FIGURE 13-14   Moderate arch-length increases can be accomplished using a multiple bonded and banded appliance and a mechanism for expansion. **A,** This patient has moderate lower arch irregularity and space shortage. **B,** The appliance is in place with the tooth movement completed. In this case, coil springs served to generate the tooth moving force, but other methods using loops and flexible arch wires are available. Note the lingual arch used to control transverse molar dimensions. **C,** The lingual arch is adjusted by opening the loops and advancing the arch so it can serve as a retainer following arch wire and bonded attachment removal.

A more aggressive alternative is early arch expansion, moving the teeth facially. If this is to be attempted, the teeth that are to be moved, the direction, and the type of tooth movement (tipping vs. bodily) should be established. Whether primary canines should be extracted to provide additional space for alignment of the incisors is an issue that also should be addressed. Lower incisor teeth usually can be tipped 1 to 2 mm facially without much difficulty, which creates up to 4 mm of additional arch length. If the overbite is excessive and the upper and lower incisors are in contact, however, facial movement of the lower incisors will not be possible unless the upper incisors also are proclined. Finally, the status of the keratinized tissue facial to the lower incisors must be evaluated. Adequate, noninflamed issue is required for a healthy long-term supporting structure. If facial movement is anticipated and the amount and quality of tissue is questionable, a periodontal consultation is appropriate. Surgical or nonsurgical management of the tissue may be required prior to beginning the tooth movement.

When expansion by tipping the incisors facially is indicated, two methods should be considered. One is to use a removable lingual arch (Figure 13-13). The expansion can be accomplished by slightly opening the loops located mesial to the banded molars. Until the teeth have moved, the activated lingual arch will rest higher on the lingual surface of the incisors than is ideal and should exert a downward force to tip the incisors facially. Small amounts of activation are necessary since the wire is large and capable of delivering heavy forces. Two or three 1 to 1.5 mm activations at monthly intervals will achieve the desired result and the appliance can then serve as a passive retainer or be replaced with a soldered lingual arch. The other method is to band the permanent molars, bond brackets on the incisors, and use a compressed coil spring on a labial arch wire to gain the additional space (Figure 13-14). The multiple band and bond technique is usually followed with a lingual arch for retention. What distinguishes these two methods is the ability of the bonded and banded appliance to provide rotational and mesiodistal space control, while the lingual arch can only tip the teeth.

Although it is possible to tip lower incisors facially with a removable appliance incorporating several clasps and finger springs, a fixed appliance provides significantly better control of the tooth movement and fewer problems with compliance.

ANTERIOR DENTAL SPACING

Maxillary Midline Diastema

A small maxillary midline diastema, which is present in many children, is not necessarily an indication for orthodontic treatment. The unerupted permanent canines often lie superior and distal to the lateral incisor roots, which forces the lateral and central incisor roots toward the midline while their crowns diverge distally (Figure 13-15). In its extreme form, this condition of flared and spaced incisors is called the "ugly duckling" stage of development (see Chapter 4). These spaces tend to close spontaneously when the canines erupt and the incisor root and crown positions change. Until the canines erupt, it is difficult to be certain whether treatment will be necessary.

When a larger diastema is present, a midline supernumerary tooth or a midline soft tissue or intrabony lesion must always be suspected. A maxillary occlusal or periapical radiograph will reveal whether a pathologic condition exists in the area. Missing permanent lateral incisors also can lead to a large space between the central incisors because the permanent central incisors frequently move laterally and occupy the available space. Treatment for these more severe diastema problems is discussed in Chapter 14. Some digit sucking habits can lead to diastemas and spacing and are considered later in this chapter.

The major indications for closure of an uncomplicated midline diastema in the mixed dentition are: (1) an esthetic complaint, or (2) positioning of the central incisors that inhibits eruption of the lateral incisors or canines.

A small but unesthetic diastema (2 mm or less) can be closed by tipping the central incisors together. A maxillary removable appliance with clasps, fingersprings, and possibly an anterior bow will successfully complete this type of

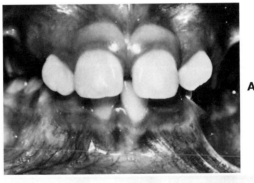

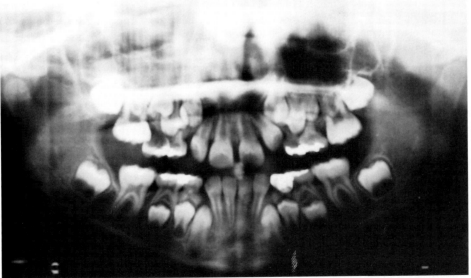

FIGURE 13-15 The "ugly duckling" phase. **A,** Spacing and mesial root position of the maxillary incisors results from the position of the unerupted permanent canines. **B,** This panoramic radiograph shows that the canines are erupting and in close proximity to the roots of the lateral incisors. The diastemas usually close when the canines erupt.

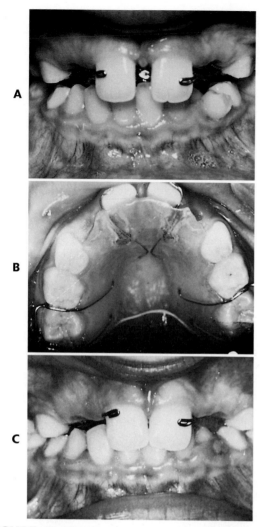

FIGURE 13-16   Closure of the midline diastema with a removable appliance. **A,** The midline diastema is closed with a removable appliance and fingersprings by tipping the teeth mesially. **B,** The 28 mil helical fingersprings are activated to move the incisors together. **C,** The final position can be maintained with the same appliance.

treatment (Figure 13-16). Use of this appliance presupposes that the incisors do not require root repositioning (bodily movement). Under no circumstances should an unsupported elastic be used around the teeth—there is a high probability that the elastic will slip apically and destroy the periodontal attachment.

The second treatment indication for a diastema is more challenging because tipping movements usually are not adequate and the diastema is likely to be larger than 2 mm. If by chance a large diastema exists and the teeth are tipped apart, they can be tipped back together and retained with a removable appliance. On the other hand, most large unesthetic diastemas will require bodily mesiodistal repositioning of the incisors. This is more challenging biomechanically and is discussed in Chapter 14.

Generalized Anterior Spacing

Excess space is not a frequent finding in the mixed dentition in the absence of incisor protrusion. It can result from either small teeth in normal-sized arches or normal-sized teeth in large arches. Unless the space presents an esthetic problem, it is reasonable to allow eruption of the remaining permanent teeth before closing the space with fixed appliances. Fixed appliances are necessary because the teeth need to be moved bodily into a smaller arch circumference. The long-term prognosis of closure of excess space is good, and the arch length does not continue to reduce drastically and result in crowding.[9]

Eruption Problems

Over-retained Primary Teeth.   A permanent tooth should replace its primary predecessor when approximately three fourths of the root of the permanent tooth has formed, whether or not resorption of the primary roots is to the point of spontaneous exfoliation. A primary tooth that is retained beyond this point can be considered overretained and should be removed. If a portion of the permanent tooth crown is visible and the primary tooth is mobile to the extent that the crown will move 1 mm in the facial and lingual direction, it is probably advisable to allow the child to "wiggle" the tooth out. If that can not be accomplished, gauze or conventional extractions are indicated. Most over-retained primary maxillary molars have either the buccal roots or the large lingual root intact. By contrast, most primary mandibular molars have either the mesial or distal root still intact.

An over-retained primary tooth leads to gingival inflammation and hyperplasia that cause pain and bleeding and sets the stage for deflected eruption paths that can result in irregularity and crossbite. Once the primary tooth is out, if space is adequate, moderately abnormal facial or lingual positioning will usually be corrected by the equilibrium forces of the lip, cheeks, and tongue. Generally, incisors will erupt lingually and then move facially when the primary tooth exfoliates (Figure 13-17). This emergence position is due to the lingual position of the developing tooth bud. In the canine and premolar areas, the permanent tooth can emerge either facially or lingually and will tend to move toward the correct position. If correction has not occurred when overbite is achieved, however, further alignment is unlikely in either the anterior or posterior quadrants, and a crossbite will result.

Ankylosed Primary Teeth.   Ankylosed primary teeth with permanent successors constitute a potential alignment problem for the permanent teeth. Although they usually resorb in the normal manner without creating long-term problems,[10] occasionally they are retained by an attachment in the cervical region and are not exfoliated on schedule. This can delay the erupting permanent tooth or deflect it from the normal eruption path. Appropriate management of an ankylosed primary tooth consists of maintain-

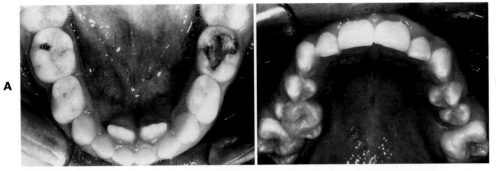

FIGURE 13-17   Permanent teeth often erupt in abnormal positions as a result of retained primary teeth. **A,** These lower central incisors erupted lingually because the permanent incisors have not been lost and their tooth buds are positioned lingual to the primary incisors. This is a common occurrence in this area and is the main reason lingual arches should not be placed until after lower incisors erupt. **B,** This maxillary premolar has been deflected facially because of the retained primary molar. Removal of teeth by the patient or extraction in both cases will allow some spontaneous alignment.

ing it until an interference with eruption or drift of other teeth begins to occur (Figure 13-18), then extracting it and placing a space maintainer or other space management appliance if needed.

When an ankylosed tooth is extracted prematurely, the space should be maintained by the techniques previously described. If occlusal discrepancies have developed from supereruption of a tooth or teeth in the opposing arch, the use of partial dentures for space maintenance may be possible only after extensive occlusal adjustments. Unless opposing permanent teeth have supererupted, the vertical irregularity will be resolved during the establishment of the occlusal plane in the permanent dentition. If tipping of adjacent teeth over the ankylosed tooth is recognized before it has progressed too far, the ankylosed primary molar can be restored with a stainless steel crown to maintain the space. This remedy is only temporary. When significant vertical facial growth and eruption occur, the ankylosed tooth again will be out of occlusion. If the tipping of adjacent teeth has progressed and space has been lost, the primary tooth should be removed and the permanent teeth repositioned to regain space. Any vertical bony discrepancies will be eradicated when the succedaneous tooth brings bone with it during eruption.

The situation is completely different when the ankylosed primary tooth has no permanent successor. Then, the ankylosed primary tooth should be extracted before a large vertical occlusal discrepancy develops to avoid long-term periodontal problems (Figure 13-19).[11] Because erupting teeth bring alveolar bone with them, in planning and executing treatment it is best to move teeth into the edentulous space so that bone is maintained and any potential or real periodontal defects eliminated. Space maintenance, therefore, may be contraindicated even if replacement of the missing tooth—rather than space closure—is the long-term plan. The longer the ankylosed primary tooth is left in place,

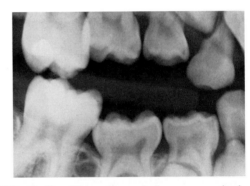

FIGURE 13-18   This radiograph demonstrates both anterior and posterior teeth tipping over adjacent ankylosed primary molars. The ankylosed teeth should be removed if significant tipping and space loss are occurring.

the greater the chance of a long-term defect because bone is not developed. It is advisable to have an experienced clinician remove these teeth. Unless the extraction is managed carefully, an even worse periodontal defect may occur.

Ectopic Eruption

Lateral Incisors.   Eruption is ectopic when a permanent tooth causes either resorption of a primary tooth other than the one it is supposed to replace or resorption of an adjacent permanent tooth. When the permanent lateral incisor erupts, resorption of the primary canine is common. Potential alignment problems result if the primary tooth is lost prematurely or if the underlying permanent tooth is blocked from erupting.

Loss of the primary canine from ectopic eruption usually indicates lack of enough space for all the permanent incisors but occasionally may result solely from an aberrant eruption path of the lateral incisor. When only one primary canine is lost prematurely, the lateral incisor will erupt into

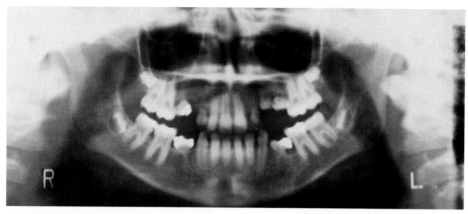

FIGURE 13-19 Ankylosed primary teeth should be carefully removed when vertical discrepancies begin to develop if they have no successors. Teeth can be allowed to erupt into the edentulous space and then repositioned prior to implant or prosthetic replacement so that large periodontal defects such as those adjacent to the primary molars in this patient do not develop. Because no permanent teeth will erupt into these spaces in this patient, the bone level will not be improved.

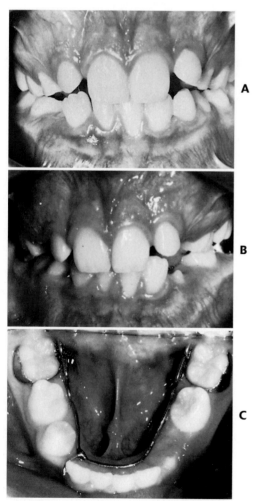

FIGURE 13-20 Midline shift resulting from tipping. **A,** These incisors tipped to the patient's right when the primary right canine was lost prematurely. **B,** The teeth have been tipped back to the left and overcorrected using a fingerspring and a removable appliance. **C,** They are currently maintained in this position with a lingual arch and a soldered spur.

the primary canine space on that side and the midline usually will shift in that direction (Figure 13-20, *A*). If both mandibular canines are lost, the permanent incisors can tip lingually, which reduces the arch circumference and increases the apparent crowding. In either case, space analysis, including an assessment of the anteroposterior incisor position and the facial profile, is needed to determine whether space maintenance, space regaining, or more complex treatment is indicated.

When one primary canine is lost, treatment is needed to prevent or correct a midline shift. Depending on the overall assessment, the dentist can either remove the contralateral canine or maintain the position of the lateral incisor on the side of the canine loss using a lingual arch with a spur. If a midline shift has occurred from tipping the appropriate treatment can be implemented with a removable or fixed appliance (Figure 13-20, *B* and *C*). If both canines are lost, an active lingual arch for expansion, a passive lingual arch for maintenance, or no treatment may be indicated. In some children, space analysis will reveal that the crowding associated with ectopic eruption of lateral incisors is so severe that complex treatment (e.g., fixed appliances, perhaps premolar extraction) is required.

Maxillary First Molars. Ectopic eruption of the permanent first molar presents an interesting problem that is usually diagnosed from routine bitewing radiographs. Some reports suggest that this painless and often unrecognized condition is related to a small and distally positioned maxilla as well as steeply angulated and large permanent molars.[12] Others have found no skeletal relationships.[13] Lack of timely intervention may cause loss of the primary molar and space loss as the permanent molar erupts mesially. Because of the frequency of self-correction of ectopic eruption, a period of watchful waiting is indicated when only small amounts of resorption are observed (Figure 13-21). If the blockage of eruption

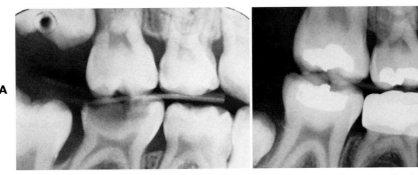

FIGURE 13-21 Ectopic eruption of the permanent first molar is usually diagnosed from routine bitewing radiographs. If the resorption is limited, the situation may be observed. **A,** The distal root of the primary maxillary second molar shows minor resorption from ectopic eruption. **B,** This radiograph taken approximately 18 months later illustrates that the permanent molar was able to erupt without treatment.

persists for 6 months or if resorption continues to increase, treatment is indicated.

Several methods can be helpful when intervention is necessary.[14] The basic approach is to move the ectopically erupting tooth away from the tooth it is resorbing. If a limited amount of movement is needed but little or none of the permanent first molar is visible clinically, a 20 mil brass wire looped and tightened around the contact between the primary second molar and the permanent molar is suggested (Figure 13-22). It may be necessary to anesthetize the soft tissue to place the brass wire, and depending on the tooth position and depth of the contact between the permanent and primary molars, it can be very difficult to successfully direct the brass wire subgingivally. The brass wire should be tightened approximately every 2 weeks. Treatment is slow but reliable.

A steel spring clip separator, available commercially, may work if only a small amount of resorption of the primary molar roots exists. These clips are difficult to place if the point of contact between the permanent and primary molars is much below the cementoenamel junction of the primary molar. Elastomeric separators wedged mesial to the first molar also can be used for this purpose but are not recommended. They have the potential to become dislodged in an apical direction and cause periodontal irritation. If this occurs, the separators can be hard to locate and retrieve, especially if the material is not radiopaque.

If resorption is more severe and more distal movement is required than can be provided by these simple appliances, the situation becomes more complex. A useful fixed appliance is a band on the second primary molar, supported by a transpalatal lingual arch when maximum control is desired, with a cantilever arm extending distally behind the unerupted permanent molar. Then a spring or elastomer is hooked from the end of the cantilever to a button bonded on the molar, generating a force to move it distally. This is not the situation for the type of space regaining discussed above. Severe resorption of the primary molar may require its extraction, and the permanent molar will erupt so far

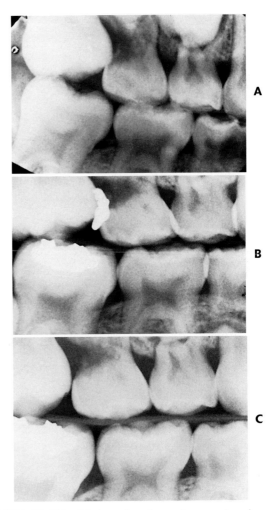

FIGURE 13-22 Moderately advanced resorption from ectopic eruption of the permanent maxillary first molar requires active intervention. **A,** This distal root of the primary maxillary second molar shows resorption and no self-correction. **B,** A 20 mil dead soft brass wire is looped around the contact between the teeth and tightened at approximately 2-week intervals; **C,** the permanent tooth is dislodged distally and erupts past the primary tooth that is retained.

Ectopic Eruption of Permanent Maxillary First Molar—Pathways of Care

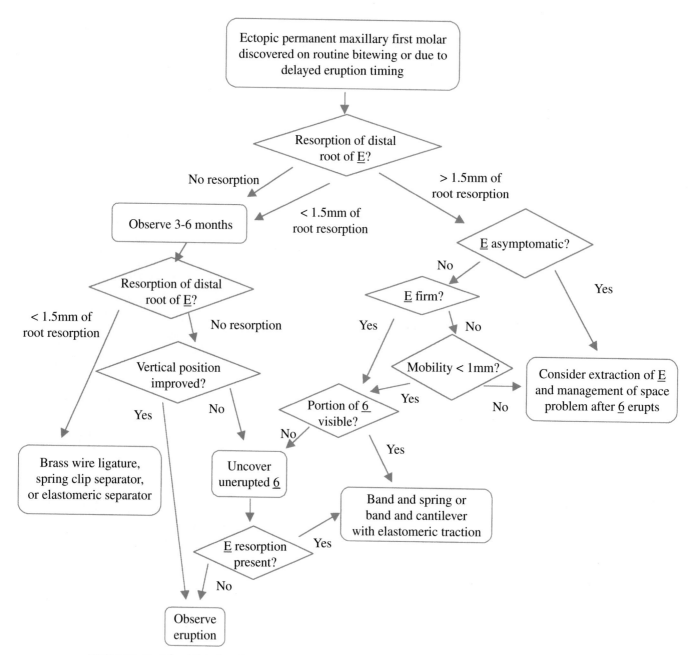

FIGURE 13-23 This flowchart can be used to aid decision making regarding possible options when a permanent molar is ectopically erupting during the mixed dentition. Answers to the questions posed in the chart should lead to successful treatment pathways. Some of the complex treatments are described in Chapter 14.

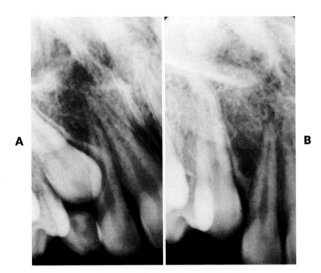

A   **B**

FIGURE 13-24   This patient demonstrates a change in position of the unerupted canine relative to the adjacent lateral incisor root that is apparently associated with extraction of the overlying primary canine. **A,** Note the overlap of the canine crown and the incisor root. **B,** Following extraction of the primary canine the permanent canine crown migrated distally and erupted in a normal position.

mesially that a major space problem is created. Treatment methods for these complex dilemmas are discussed in Chapter 14.

A flowchart (modified from Kennedy and Turley[14]) summarizes the decision making for ectopic eruption of permanent first molars (Figure 13-23).

Maxillary Canines.   Ectopic eruption of maxillary canines occurs relatively frequently and can lead to either or both of two problems: (1) impaction of the canine and/or (2) resorption of permanent lateral incisor roots. When the primary canine is not mobile, there is no observable or palpable facial canine bulge, and the patient is approximately 10 years of age, a panoramic or periapical radiograph is indicated. In this situation, the panoramic film is an excellent screening tool, but periapical radiographs have proven more helpful in localizing the teeth and delineating overlap of the unerupted teeth. Radiographs prior to this stage are not reliable for prediction of the canine path of eruption.[15]

When mesial inclination of the erupting permanent canine is detected and no incisor root resorption is noted, the treatment of choice is to extract the overlying primary canine (Figure 13-24). Ericson and Kurol found that if the permanent canine crown was overlapping less than half of the root of the lateral incisor, there was an excellent chance (91%) of normalization of the path of eruption. When more than half of the lateral incisor root was overlapped, early extraction of the primary tooth resulted in a 64% chance of normal eruption and likely improvement in the position of the canine even if it was not totally corrected.[16]

The beginning of resorption of the permanent incisor roots indicates a severe problem with canine position. In addition to extraction of the primary canine, usually it is necessary to surgically expose the permanent canine and use orthodontic force to bring it to its correct position. This comprehensive treatment will extend into the early permanent dentition period (see Chapter 16).

OCCLUSAL RELATIONSHIP PROBLEMS

Posterior Crossbite

Theoretically, treatment of posterior crossbite differs markedly, depending on the underlying cause of the crossbite situation. Skeletal crossbites, usually resulting from a narrow maxilla but occasionally from an excessively wide mandible, generally are treated by heavy forces to open the midpalatal suture and make the maxilla wider. Dental crossbites are treated by moving the teeth with lighter forces. Although this is a correct concept for adolescents in the late mixed and early permanent dentition, the lesser interdigitation of the midpalatal suture in the early mixed dentition (see Chapter 8) means that even modest forces will cause both skeletal and dental changes.[17] For this reason, palatal expansion with heavy force from a jackscrew appliance is reserved for adolescents (who may nevertheless still be in the late mixed dentition). Heavy force and rapid expansion are not indicated in the primary or early mixed dentition. There is a significant risk of distortion of the nose if this is done in younger children (see Figure 8-16).

Posterior crossbite in a child often appears to be unilateral but on close examination usually is found to result from bilateral constriction of the maxillary arch and a shift of the mandible to one side on closure. More severe constriction may result in a bilateral crossbite without mandibular shift, and occasionally, a true unilateral posterior crossbite from an intra-arch or jaw asymmetry will be noted. These more severe crossbites must be considered severe problems. Their treatment is discussed in Chapter 15.

Crossbites caused by a mandibular shift should be treated as soon as they are discovered and are among the few conditions recommended for treatment in the primary dentition. An uncorrected mandibular shift can produce, at the least, undesirable soft tissue growth modification, dental compensation, and dental abrasion of primary and permanent teeth. Further, the presence of a mandibular shift complicates the diagnostic process by making interarch relationships difficult to determine, and a constricted maxilla reduces space to accommodate the teeth.

There are three basic approaches to the treatment of moderate posterior crossbites in children: equilibration to eliminate mandibular shift, expansion of a constricted maxillary arch, and repositioning of individual teeth to deal with intra-arch asymmetries.

In a few cases, mostly observed in the primary dentition or the early mixed dentition, a shift into posterior crossbite will be due solely to interference caused by the primary canines (Figure 13-25). These patients can be diagnosed by careful positioning of the mandible. They require only limited equilibration of the primary canines to eliminate the interference and the resulting lateral shift into crossbite.

More commonly, a child with a mandibular shift has a bilateral maxillary constriction. Even a small constriction creates dental interferences that force the mandible to shift to a new position for maximum intercuspation (Figure 13-26). A greater maxillary constriction will allow the maxillary teeth to fit inside the mandibular teeth and will not be accompanied by a mandibular shift (Figure 13-27). Both of these types of crossbite should be corrected in the primary dentition if discovered then, unless the permanent first molars are expected to erupt in less than 6 months. In that situation, it is better to allow the permanent molars to erupt so that correction can include these teeth if neces-

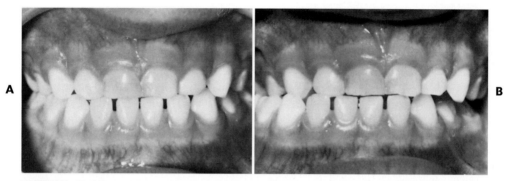

FIGURE 13-25 Minor canine interferences leading to a mandibular shift. **A,** Initial contact; **B,** Shift into centric occlusion. The slight lingual position of the primary canines can lead to occlusal interferences and an apparent posterior crossbite. This cause of posterior crossbite is infrequent and is best treated by occlusal adjustment of the primary canines.

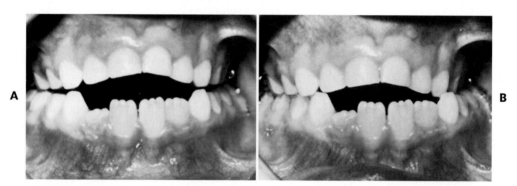

FIGURE 13-26 Moderate bilateral maxillary constriction. **A,** Initial contact; **B,** Shift into occlusion. Moderate bilateral maxillary constriction often leads to posterior interferences upon closure and a lateral shift of the mandible into an apparent posterior crossbite. This problem is best treated by bilateral maxillary expansion.

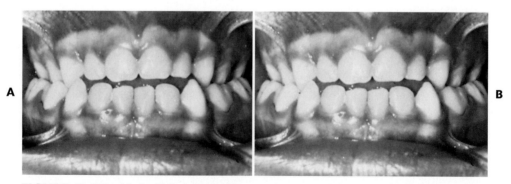

FIGURE 13-27 Marked bilateral maxillary constriction. **A,** Initial contact; **B,** Full occlusion (no shift). A marked bilateral maxillary constriction often produces no interferences upon closure, and the patient has a bilateral posterior crossbite in centric relation. This problem is best treated by bilateral maxillary expansion.

sary. Expansion of the maxillary arch will both correct the crossbite and increase the arch circumference by variable amounts depending on the site of expansion.[18] The increase in arch circumference may have benefits for crowding and irregularity.

It is possible to treat posterior crossbite with a split-plate type of removable appliance incorporating a wire spring or jackscrew for force generation (see Figure 11-21). Removable appliances rely on patient compliance for success, and the fact that the appliance is retained by clasps limits the force that can be used because the appliance can be displaced easily. This approach is less successful and less cost-effective than an expansion lingual arch.[19]

Another possibility is using a banded or bonded jackscrew appliance for maxillary expansion. These appliances deliver high forces and are usually reserved for either gross maxillary skeletal constrictions that require large amounts of correction, or for older children who have more interdigitation of the maxillary midpalatal suture and who require more force to open the suture (see Chapter 16).

The preferred appliance for correction of maxillary dental constriction in a preadolescent child is an adjustable lingual arch that requires little patient cooperation. Both the W-arch and the quad helix are reliable and easy to use. The W-arch is a fixed appliance constructed of 36 mil steel wire soldered to molar bands (Figure 13-28). To avoid soft tissue irritation, the lingual arch should

be constructed so that it rests 1 to 1.5 mm off the palatal soft tissue. This appliance will move both primary and permanent teeth and may accelerate the rate of normal expansion of the midpalatal suture, particularly in a young child. Therefore, correction will result from a combination of skeletal and dental change even if only dental or skeletal change was desired. This is of no consequence and will require no difference in either treatment or retention techniques.

The W-arch is activated simply by opening the apices of the W and is easily adjusted to provide more anterior than posterior expansion, or vice versa, if this is desired. Bending the anterior palatal portion of the wire increases the posterior arch width, and bending the wire bilaterally near the solder joint at the molar bands increases the anterior arch width (see Figure 13-28, *A*). The appliance delivers proper force levels when opened 3 to 4 mm wider than the passive width and should be adjusted to this dimension before being inserted.

Expansion should continue at the rate of 2 mm per month (1 mm tooth movement on each side) until the crossbite is slightly overcorrected. In other words, the lingual cusps of the maxillary teeth should occlude on the lingual inclines of the buccal cusps of the mandibular molars at the end of active treatment (Figure 13-29). Intraoral appliance adjustment is possible but may lead to unexpected changes. For this reason, removal and recementation are

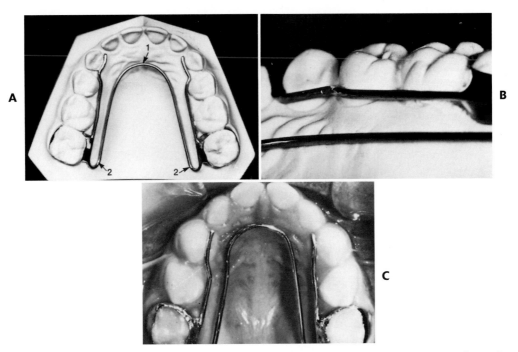

FIGURE 13-28 The W-arch appliance is ideal for bilateral maxillary expansion. **A,** The appliance is fabricated from 36 mil wire and soldered to the bands. The lingual wire should contact the teeth involved in the crossbite and extend not more than 1 to 2 mm distal to the banded molars to eliminate soft tissue irritation. Activation at point 1 produces posterior expansion and activation at point 2 produces anterior expansion. **B,** The lingual wire should remain 1 to 1.5 mm away from the marginal gingiva and the palatal tissue. **C,** This W-arch is being used to correct a bilateral constriction in the primary dentition.

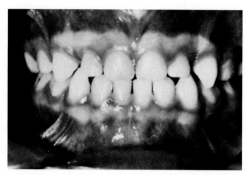

FIGURE 13-29   A posterior crossbite should be overcorrected until the maxillary posterior lingual cusps occlude with the lingual inclines of the mandibular buccal cusps, as shown here, and then retained for approximately 3 months. After retention, slight lingual movement of the maxillary teeth results in a stable result.

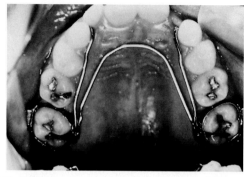

FIGURE 13-30   The W-arch can be made removable by fabricating it with attachments on the molar teeth. This appliance design is inviting but is difficult to manage and more prone to appliance breakage.

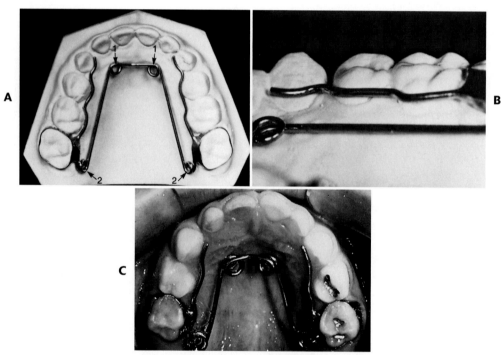

FIGURE 13-31   The quad helix used to correct bilateral maxillary constriction. **A,** The appliance is fabricated from 38 mil wire and soldered to the bands. The lingual wire should contact the teeth involved in the crossbite and extend no more than 1 to 2 mm distal to the banded molars to eliminate soft tissue irritation. Activation at point 1 produces posterior expansion, while activation at point 2 produces anterior expansion. **B,** The lingual wire should remain 1 to 1.5 mm away from the marginal gingiva and palatal tissue. **C,** This quad helix is being used to correct a bilateral maxillary constriction in the primary dentition.

recommended at each active treatment visit. Most posterior crossbites require 2 to 3 months of active treatment and 3 months of retention (during which the W-arch is left passively in place) for stability.

A variant of this appliance uses cemented bands with attachments that allow the active arch to be removed and activated without removing the bands (Figure 13-30). Although this technique is attractive in principle, it is diffi-

cult to activate the appliance in the desired direction and have it remain passive in all other dimensions. Unwanted and unexpected intrusion and extrusion of teeth are common with this technique, and it is more prone to appliance breakage.

The quad helix is a more flexible version of the W-arch. It is constructed with 38 mil steel wire and helices that increase the range and springiness of the appliance

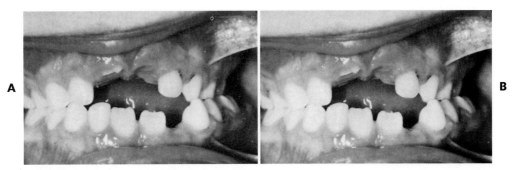

FIGURE 13-32   True unilateral maxillary posterior constriction. **A,** Initial contact. **B,** Full occlusion (no shift). True unilateral constriction has a unilateral posterior crossbite in centric relation and in centric occlusion, without a lateral shift. This problem is best treated with unilateral posterior expansion.

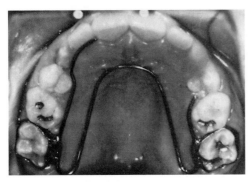

FIGURE 13-33   An unequal W-arch used to correct a true unilateral maxillary constriction. The side of the arch to be expanded has fewer teeth against the lingual wire than the anchorage unit. Even with this arrangement, both sides can be expected to show some expansion movement.

(Figure 13-31). The helices in the anterior palate are bulky, which can effectively serve as a reminder to aid in stopping a finger habit. The combination of a posterior crossbite and a finger-sucking habit is the best indication for this appliance. The extra wire incorporated in this appliance gives it slightly greater range of action than the W-arch, but the forces are equivalent. Because the anterior portion is more flexible, some children manipulate the arch and either distort or weaken the wire, which can result in soft tissue irritation or breakage. Appropriate forces are produced when the appliance is widened by 3 to 8 mm. This adjustment can be performed either intra- or extraorally, but care must be exercised with intraoral adjustments. Overcorrection, attention to soft tissue irritation, and 3 months of retention are also recommended with this appliance.

Some children do have true unilateral crossbites, usually from unilateral maxillary constriction. This condition is diagnosed by discovering a unilateral crossbite in centric relation and in maximum intercuspation without a mandibular shift (Figure 13-32). In these cases the ideal treatment is to move selected teeth on the constricted side of the upper arch. The easiest way to accomplish this

movement is to arrange an orthodontic appliance so that there are more teeth in the anchorage unit than in the unit where teeth are expected to move. To a limited extent, this goal can be achieved by using different length arms on a W-arch or quad helix (Figure 13-33), but some bilateral expansion must be expected. An alternative method is to use a mandibular lingual arch to stabilize the lower teeth and attach cross-elastics to the maxillary teeth that are at fault. This type of arrangement is more complicated and requires cooperation by the patient to be successful, but is more unilateral in its effect. A third alternative is to use a removable appliance that has been sectioned asymmetrically (see Figure 11-21). This has the effect of pitting more teeth against fewer teeth and results in asymmetric movement. Of course, this appliance has the same restrictions as all removable appliances: its success depends on both the quality of its retentive clasps and the patient's cooperation.

All of the appliances described here are aimed at correction of teeth in the maxillary arch, which is usually where the problem is located. If teeth in both arches contribute to the problem, cross-elastics between banded or bonded attachments in both arches (Figure 13-34) can reposition both upper and lower teeth. Cross-elastic treatment requires cooperation since the patient has to wear the elastics full-time and replace them at least once a day. The vector of the elastic pull moves the teeth vertically as well as faciolingually, which will extrude the posterior teeth and reduce the overbite. Therefore cross-elastics should be used with caution in children with increased lower face height or limited overbite. Crossbites treated with elastics should be overcorrected, and the bands left in place immediately after active treatment. If there is relapse, the elastics can be reinstated without rebanding or rebonding. When the occlusion is stable after several weeks without elastic force, the attachments can be removed. The most common problem with this form of crossbite correction is lack of cooperation from the child.

A flowchart is provided to help guide decision making for posterior crossbites (Figure 13-35).

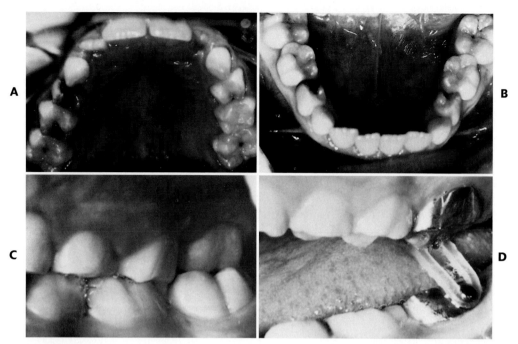

FIGURE 13-34 Cross-elastics are indicated for crossbite correction when maxillary and mandibular teeth need to be moved. **A,** This patient has the permanent maxillary left first molar displaced lingually and (**B**) the permanent mandibular left first molar displaced facially. **C,** This results in a posterior crossbite between these teeth. **D,** The cross-elastic is placed between the buttons welded on the bands. The elastic should be worn full-time and changed frequently.

Anterior Crossbites

In planning treatment for anterior crossbites, it is critically important to differentiate skeletal problems of deficient maxillary or excessive mandibular growth from crossbites due only to displacement of teeth.[20] If the etiologic factor is truly dental and space is available, the problem should be corrected when it is encountered. The most common etiologic factor of nonskeletal anterior crossbites is lack of space for the permanent incisors, and it is important that the treatment plan focus on management of the total space situation in addition to the crossbite. Since the permanent tooth buds form lingual to the primary teeth, a shortage of space may force the permanent maxillary incisor teeth to remain lingual to the line of the arch and erupt into crossbite. If the developing crossbite is discovered before eruption is complete and overbite has not been established, the adjacent primary teeth can be extracted to provide the necessary space (Figure 13-36). Primary teeth should be extracted bilaterally to prevent the midline from migrating to the side of a unilateral extraction where extra room is available.

Dental anterior crossbites diagnosed after the incisors have erupted and overbite is established require appliance therapy for correction. The first concern is adequate space for tooth movement, which usually requires bilateral disking, extraction of the adjacent primary teeth, or opening space for tooth movement. The diagnostic evaluation should determine whether tipping will provide appropriate correction (often it will, because the problem arose as eruption paths were deflected). If teeth are tipped when bodily movement is required, stability of the result is questionable.

In a young child, the best method for tipping maxillary and mandibular anterior teeth out of crossbite is a removable appliance using fingersprings for facial movement of maxillary incisors (Figure 13-37) or (less frequently) an active labial bow for lingual movement of mandibular incisors. Two maxillary anterior teeth can be moved facially with one 22 mil double helical cantilever spring. Z-springs (see Chapter 11) are another possibility, but these deliver excessively heavy forces that dislodge the appliance and lack range of action. The removable appliance should have multiple clasps for retention, but a labial bow on this appliance is usually contraindicated because it can interfere with facial movement of the incisors and would add little or no retention.

An anterior or posterior biteplate to reduce the overbite while the crossbite is being corrected is usually unnecessary in children unless the overbite is excessively deep. A reasonable approach is to place the appliance without a biteplate and attempt tooth movement. If, after 2 months, the teeth in the opposing arch are moving in the same direction as the teeth to which the force is being applied, a biteplate is indicated and can be added to the appliance. Because teeth are not in occlusion except during swallowing and parafunctional habits, a biteplate should be needed only in a child with a clenching or grinding habit. Using a biteplate risks the chance that teeth not in contact with the appliance or the opposing arch will erupt excessively.

Posterior Crossbite—Pathways of Care

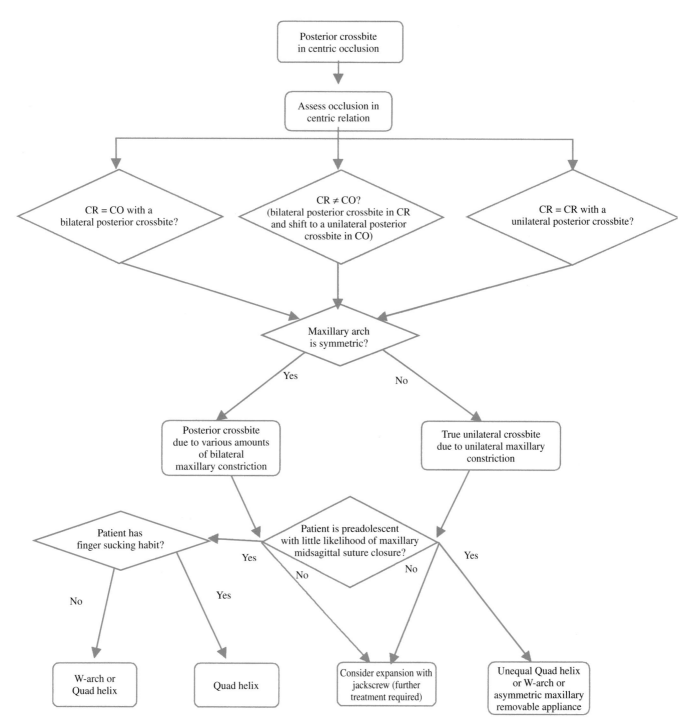

FIGURE 13-35 This flowchart can be used to aid decision making regarding possible options for posterior crossbite correction in the primary and mixed dentitions. Answers to the questions posed in the chart should lead to successful treatment pathways. Some of the complex treatments are described in Chapter 14.

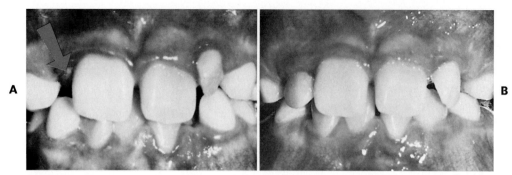

FIGURE 13-36   Developing anterior crossbites can be treated by extracting adjacent primary teeth if space is not available for the erupting permanent teeth. **A,** The permanent maxillary right lateral incisor is beginning to erupt lingual to the other anterior teeth. **B,** Extraction of both primary maxillary canines has allowed spontaneous correction of the crossbite.

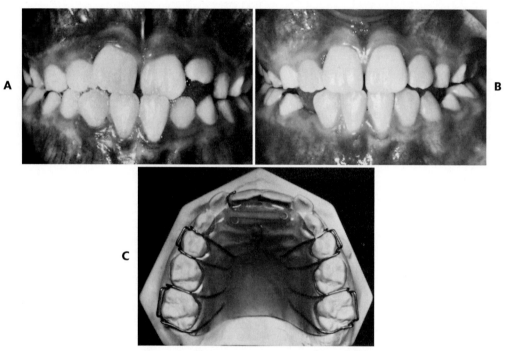

FIGURE 13-37   Anterior crossbite correction with a removable appliance to tip teeth. **A,** The permanent maxillary left central incisor has erupted into crossbite and (**B**) has been corrected with a removable appliance. **C,** This appliance is used to tip both central incisors facially with a 22 mil double helical fingerspring activated 1.5 to 2 mm per month to produce 1 mm per month of tooth movement. Note that plastic baseplate material extends over the spring to maintain its vertical position (see Chapter 11). The appliance is retained with multiple Adams' clasps.

A maxillary lingual fingerspring can be activated 1.5 to 2 mm per month and will produce approximately 1 mm of tooth movement in that time. Greater activation will slow tooth movement because of excessive force, and lesser activation will prolong treatment unnecessarily. The appliance requires nearly full-time wear to be effective and efficient. The offending teeth should be slightly overcorrected and retained until overbite is adequate to retain the corrected tooth positions. One or two months of retention with a passive appliance is usually sufficient, but if overbite is inadequate, the appliance should be continued as a passive retainer until incisor eruption has established an overbite. The most common problems associated with these simple removable appliances are lack of patient cooperation, poor design leading to lack of retention, and improper activation.

Teeth also can be tipped out of anterior crossbite using fixed appliances, either with or without attachments placed on individual teeth. Fixed appliances have a greater range of action and are more continuous in force application than removable appliances. This technique reduces some of the need for patient compliance, but will not overcome the resistance of a determined and destructive child. See Chapter 14 for the use of fixed appliances for anterior crossbite correction.

A flowchart is provided to help guide decision making for anterior crossbites (Figure 13-38).

Anterior Crossbite—Pathways of Care

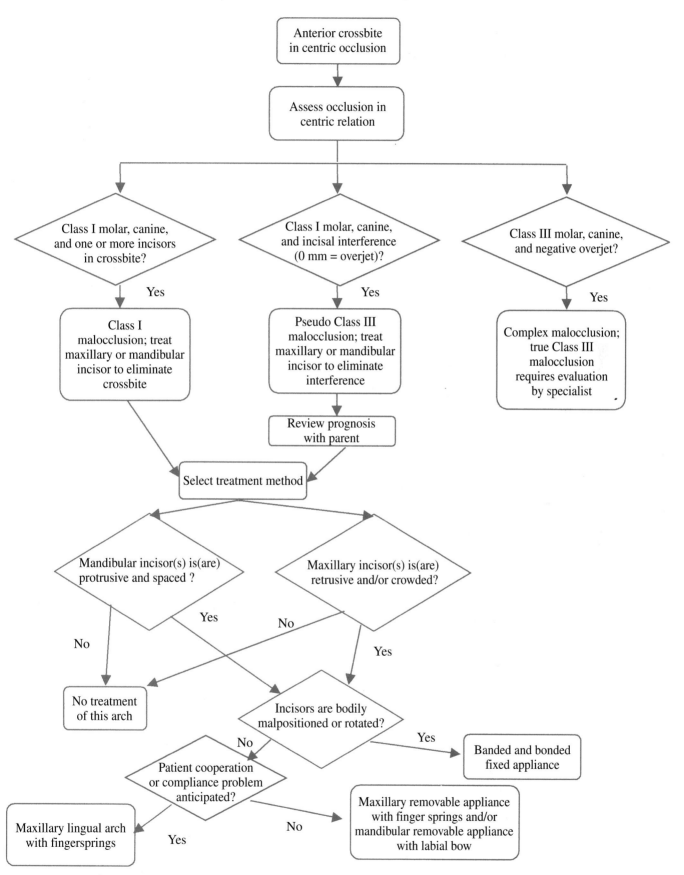

FIGURE 13-38 This flowchart can be used to aid decision making regarding possible options for anterior crossbites in the primary and mixed dentitions. Answers to the questions posed in the chart should lead to successful treatment pathways. Some of the complex treatments are described in Chapter 14.

Maxillary Dental Protrusion and Spacing.   Treatment for maxillary dental protrusion during the early mixed dentition is indicated only when the maxillary incisors protrude with spaces between them and are esthetically objectionable or in danger of traumatic injury. When this condition occurs in a child who has no skeletal discrepancies, it is often a sequela to prolonged thumbsucking. Eliminating the thumb habit prior to tooth movement is advisable (see the next section).

If there is adequate vertical clearance and space within the arch, the maxillary incisors can be tipped lingually with a removable or a fixed appliance. A Hawley-type removable appliance (see Chapter 11) utilizing multiple clasps and a 28 mil labial bow can be effective for this purpose (Figure 13-39). The labial bow is activated 1.5 to 2 mm and will achieve approximately 1 mm of retraction per month. One and one-half millimeters of plastic must be removed lingual to the maxillary incisors to allow tooth movement into this area and to accommodate the soft tissue that often piles up on the side of a tooth to which it is moving. The plastic and the labial bow should both be adjusted and evaluated at each appointment.

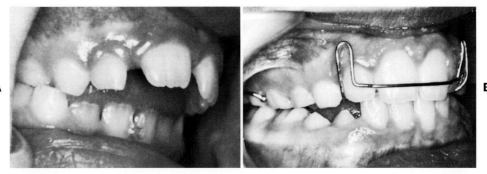

FIGURE 13-39   A removable appliance can be used to retract protrusive incisors that require lingual tipping when space and overbite permit. **A,** This patient has protrusive incisors and spacing caused by a prolonged thumb habit. **B,** A removable appliance is used to tip the incisors lingually by activating the 28 mil labial bow 1.5 to 2 mm and relieving the plastic lingual to the incisors at each appointment.

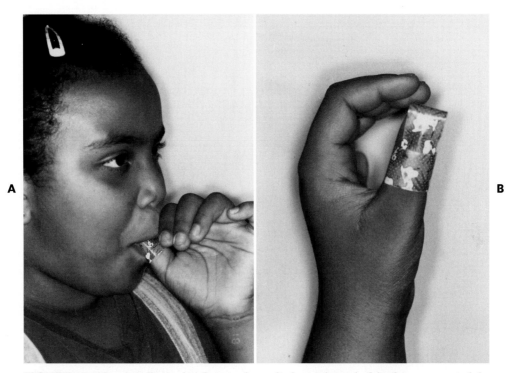

FIGURE 13-40   An adhesive bandage can be applied over the end of the finger to remind the child not to suck and to reduce the enjoyment. The bandage should be anchored at its base for retention with waterproof tape, so that it will stay in place if sucking is still attempted. (Courtesy Dr. B. Joo.)

If the overbite is enough to bring the upper and lower incisors into vertical contact, however, the upper incisors cannot be retracted until the overbite is corrected. In some properly selected patients this can be corrected with a biteplate that allows eruption of posterior teeth and reduces the overbite (see Chapter 14), but it is rare that Class II malocclusion is not part of the total picture when overjet and overbite both are present. This presents a much more complex treatment problem.

Fixed appliance therapy is recommended if the teeth require significant retraction, bodily movement or correction of rotations. This type of treatment is more complex and addressed in Chapter 14.

Oral Habits and Open Bites

Although children engage in a number of oral habits, digit and pacifier sucking are the most common, occurring at some time in the majority of children.[21] The effect of such a habit on the hard and soft tissues depends on its duration, frequency and intensity (see Chapter 5). Although it is possible to deform the alveolus and dentition during the primary dentition years with an intense habit, much of the change is related to the anterior teeth. Maxillary incisors are tipped facially, mandibular incisors are tipped lingually, and some incisors are prevented from erupting. As one would expect, overjet increases and overbite decreases. In some instances, maxillary intercanine and intermolar width may be narrowed resulting in a posterior crossbite. Girls are more likely than boys to continue finger sucking after beginning school.

When comparing digit sucking to pacifier use, there is some evidence for increased prevalence of posterior crossbites with pacifiers.[22] Pacifier shapes that are designed to produce a more physiologic sucking pattern have not been proven to be beneficial when compared with other pacifiers or to finger sucking.[23]

Most children discontinue pacifier use by age 4 or age 5 at the latest. The social pressures of school are a strong deterrent. As long as the habit stops before the eruption of the permanent incisor, most of the changes resolve spontaneously. By that time, the majority of children have stopped their sucking habit. Another group still suck but want to stop, and yet another small group do not want to stop. If a child does not want to quit sucking, habit therapy, especially appliance therapy, is not indicated.

As the time of eruption of the permanent incisors approaches, the simplest approach to habit therapy is a straightforward discussion between the child and the dentist that expresses concern and includes an explanation by the dentist. This "adult" approach (and restraint from intervention by the parents) is often enough to terminate the habit but is most effective with older children.

Another level of intervention is reminder therapy. This is for the child who wants to quit but needs help. Any one of several reminders that are introduced with explanation to the child can be useful. One of the simplest approaches is to secure an adhesive bandage with waterproof tape on the finger that is sucked (Figure 13-40). Remember that the anterior portion of the quad helix appliance can be quite useful as a reminder (see Figure 13-31).

If the reminder approach fails, a reward system can be implemented that provides a small tangible reward daily for not engaging in the habit. In some cases, a large reward must be negotiated for complete cessation of the habit.

If all the above fail and the child really wants to quit, an elastic bandage loosely wrapped around the elbow prevents the arm from flexing and the fingers from being sucked. If this is necessary, it is usually only at nights and 6 to 8 weeks of intervention should be sufficient. Once again, the child should understand that this is not punishment.

If the previous methods have not succeeded in eliminating the habit, the child who wants to stop sucking can be fitted with a cemented reminder appliance to actively impede sucking (Figure 13-41). These appliances can be deformed and removed by children who are not compliant and do not truly wish to stop the finger habit, so cooperation still is important. This appliance can also be used as a retainer following posterior crossbite correction if a finger sucking habit remains.

The appliance consists of a maxillary lingual arch and a crib constructed of soldered wire so that it is difficult to insert the thumb into the mouth. Heavy wire (38 to 40 mil) should be used to eliminate any flexibility. This appliance is bulky but not sharp, and it can be secured to either the primary second molars or the permanent first molars. A removable appliance is contraindicated because lack of compliance is part of the problem. The purpose of the therapy must be explained so the patient realizes that the appliance serves as a reminder and not as punishment. If this is understood by the child as a "helping hand," the treatment will be successful and psychological problems will not result.[24] When sucking apparently ceases, the appliance should be retained in place for approximately 6 months to

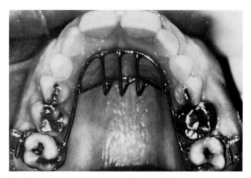

FIGURE 13-41 A cemented habit crib made of 38 to 40 mil wire can be used as a reminder along with an explanation to interrupt a fingersucking habit. The appliance can be cemented to either primary or permanent molars and should be extended anteriorly to interfere with the finger position during sucking. The amount of overbite will also help determine the appliance position.

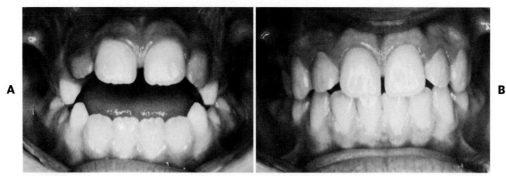

FIGURE 13-42   Open bites observed during the transitional dentition years often close spontaneously. **A,** This patient had good skeletal relationships and an open bite during the early mixed dentition years. **B,** Four years later, without appliance therapy, the open bite has spontaneously closed. (Courtesy Dr. R. Scholz.)

ensure the habit has truly stopped. Commonly these cemented reminders leave an imprint on the tongue that will resolve when the appliance is removed. The appliances also trap food and can lead to mouth odor, so excellent oral hygiene is beneficial.

The open bites associated with sucking in children with normal jaw relationships often resolve after sucking stops and the remaining permanent teeth erupt. An appliance to laterally expand a constricted maxillary arch or re-

tract flared and spaced incisors may be needed, but the open bite should require no further treatment in children with good skeletal proportions (Figure 13-42).[25]

Open bites that persist almost always have a significant skeletal component and careful diagnosis of the contributing factors is required.[26] The treatment of more severe and persistent open bites is discussed in Chapter 15.

A flowchart is provided to help guide decision making for open bite problems (Figure 13-43).

Oral Habits—Pathways of Care

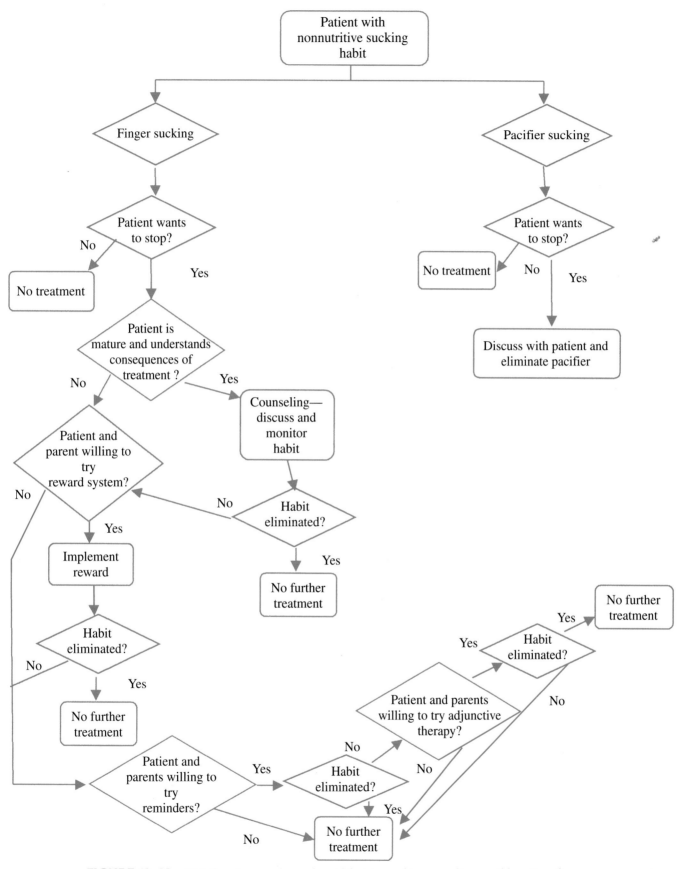

FIGURE 13-43 This flowchart can be used to aid decision making regarding possible options for nonnutritive sucking habits during the primary and mixed dentitions. Answers to the questions posed in the chart should lead to successful treatment pathways.

REFERENCES

1. Moorrees CFA: The dentition of the growing child: a longitudinal study of dental development between 3 and 18 years of age, Cambridge, Mass., 1959, Harvard University Press.
2. Christensen J, Fields HW: Space maintenance in the primary dentition. In Pinkham JR et al (editors): Pediatric dentistry: infancy through adolescence, ed 3, Philadelphia, 1999, W.B. Saunders.
3. Mayhew M, Dilley G, Dilley D et al: Tissue response to intragingival appliances in monkeys, Pediatr Dent 6:148-152, 1984.
4. O'Donnell S, Nanda RS, Ghosh J: Perioral forces and dental changes resulting from mandibular lip bumper treatment, Am J Orthod 113:247-55, 1998.
5. Nevant CT, Buschang PH, Alexander RG, Steffen JM: Lip bumper therapy for gaining arch length, Am J Orthod Dentofacial Orthop 100:330-336, 1991.
6. McInaney JB, Adams RM, Freeman M: A nonextraction approach to crowded dentitions in young children: early recognition and treatment, J Am Dent Assoc 101:252-257, 1980.
7. Spillane LM, McNamara JA: Maxillary adaptation to expansion in the mixed dentition, Seminars in Orthod 1:176-187, 1995.
8. Little RM, Riedel RA, Stein A: Mandibular arch length increase during the mixed dentition: postretention evaluation of stability and relapse, Am J Orthod Dentofacial Orthop 97:393-404, 1990.
9. Little R, Riedel R: Postretention evaluation of stability and relapse—mandibular arches with generalized spacing, Am J Orthod 95:37-41, 1989.
10. Kurol J, Thilander B: Infraocclusion of primary molars and the effect on occlusal development, a longitudinal study, Eur J Orthod 6:277-293, 1984.
11. Kurol J, Thilander B: Infraocclusion of primary molars with aplasia of the permanent successor: a longitudinal study, Angle Orthod 54:283-94, 1984.
12. Pulver F: The etiology and prevalence of ectopic eruption of the maxillary first permanent molar, J Dent Child 35:138-146, 1968.
13. Bjerklin K, Kurol J: Ectopic eruption of the maxillary first permanent molar: etiologic factors, Am J Orthod 84:147-55, 1983.
14. Kennedy DB, Turley PK: The clinical management of ectopically erupting first permanent molars, Am J Orthod Dentofacial Orthop 92:336-345, 1987.
15. Ericson S, Kurol J: Longitudinal study and analysis of clinical supervision of maxillary canine eruption, Community Dent Oral Epidemiol 14:172-176, 1986.
16. Ericson S, Kurol J: Early treatment of palatally erupting maxillary canines by extraction of the primary canines, Eur J Orthod 10:283-295, 1988.
17. Ngan P, Fields H: Orthodontic diagnosis and treatment planning in the primary dentition, J Dent Child 62:25-33, 1995.
18. Adkins MD, Nanda RS, Currier GF: Arch perimeter changes on rapid palatal expansion, Am J Orthod 97:10-19, 1990.
19. Ranta R: Treatment of unilateral posterior crossbite: comparison of the quad-helix and removable plate, J Dent Child 55:102-104, 1988.
20. Ngan P, Hu AM, Fields HW: Treatment of Class III problems begins with differential diagnosis of anterior crossbites, Pediatr Dent 19:386-95, 1997.
21. Christensen JR, Fields HW, Adair SM: Oral habits. In Pinkham JR, Casamassimo PS, Fields HW, McTigue DJ, Nowak AJ (editors): Pediatric dentistry: infancy to adolescence, ed 3, Philadelphia, 1999, W.B. Saunders.
22. Paunio P, Rautava P, Sillanpää M: The Finnish family competence study: the effects of living conditions on sucking habits in 3-year-old Finnish children and the association between these habits and dental occlusion, Acta Odontol Scand 51:23-29, 1993.
23. Adair SM, Milano M, Dushku JC: Evaluation of the effects of orthodontic pacifiers on the primary dentitions of 24-59-month-old children: preliminary study, Pediatr Dent 14:13-18, 1992.
24. Haryett R, Hansen R, Davidson P et al: Chronic thumbsucking: the psychological effects and the relative effectiveness of the various methods of treatment, Am J Orthod 53:559-585, 1967.
25. Worms F, Meskin L, Isaacson R: Openbite, Am J Orthod 59:589-595, 1971.
26. Ngan P, Fields H: Open bite: a review of etiology and management, Pediatr Dent, 19:91-98, 1997.

CHAPTER

14

Complex Nonskeletal Problems in Preadolescent Children

This chapter focuses on treatment procedures for the mixed dentition patients identified as complex nonskeletal problems during the later stages of the triage process outlined in Chapter 6. Although there is no skeletal involvement in their malocclusion, they have either severe enough crowding and malalignment that major arch expansion or extraction would be required, or other problems leading to major displacements of teeth within the arches.

In contrast to the moderately severe problems discussed in Chapter 13, these complex problems are unlikely to be solved with either simple orthodontic appliances or short duration of treatment. Before we begin a discussion of treatment approaches, it is appropriate to review some of the major differences between early (mixed dentition) and later (permanent dentition) treatment for problems of this type.

SPECIAL CONSIDERATIONS IN EARLY TREATMENT

Among the important points to consider when early treatment is considered are these:

The Goals of the Treatment Must Be Clearly Outlined and Understood

For a child with a complex problem, it is highly likely that a second stage of treatment in the early permanent dentition will be required, even if early treatment is carried out effectively and properly (Figure 14-1). There is a limit to the time and cooperation that patients and parents are willing to devote to treatment. Unless appropriate end points are set in advance, it is easy for mixed dentition treatment to extend over several years, even when skeletal growth is not a factor. Patients can be "burned out" by the time they are ready for comprehensive treatment in the early permanent dentition.

This means that the diagnosis and treatment planning are just as demanding and important as in comprehensive treatment. If the treatment goals are not clear, setting appropriate endpoints will be impossible. In early treatment, all aspects of the occlusion usually are not modified to ideal or near ideal. The original alignment, overjet, and overbite will have to be accepted if they are not treated, and the treated teeth will have to coordinate and interdigitate with the untreated teeth. Essentially, the final result is dictated by the untreated teeth and arch. For instance, if the lower arch is not ideally aligned, it will be difficult to ideally align the upper arch and have proper

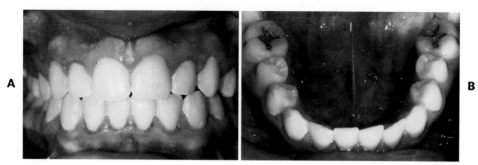

FIGURE 14-1   When limited treatment is done in the mixed dentition, it is highly likely that a second stage of treatment will be required later, or a less-than-ideal result will have to be accepted. **A,** This completed patient shows limited overbite and overjet in the maxillary left incisor region. **B,** Because only the maxillary arch had a fixed appliance, the pretreatment irregular alignment in the lower arch was accepted. It is difficult to have ideal relationships when only one arch is treated.

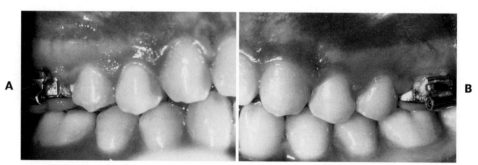

FIGURE 14-2   This patient wore headgear during the mixed dentition but was unable to obtain equal molar and canine correction on the right and left. Because only one arch was treated, interarch mechanics could not be used to remedy this problem.

coordination of the teeth without interferences. Likewise, if there is a substantial curve of Spee in the lower arch and only the upper arch is leveled, the overbite and overjet will be excessive. That is acceptable if the remainder of the total correction is to be accomplished later.

Fewer Options Are Available, and Patient Cooperation Is More Critical

In mixed dentition treatment with a partial appliance, there simply are fewer options available. For instance, if a Class II patient does not wear a headgear as prescribed in limited treatment, you are out of luck—starting over with a different approach is about the only option. In comprehensive treatment, there are the options of Class II elastics, interarch springs, Herbst attachments or guide planes. Although some of these options also require cooperation, one of the alternatives may catch the imagination of the recalcitrant patient and allow treatment to be completed in an acceptable manner. In limited treatment, the options are not there (Figure 14-2). Therefore, carefully picking the patients and working within their range of cooperation is critical.

There Are Important Biomechanical Differences Between Complete and Partial Appliances

The typical fixed appliance for mixed dentition treatment is a "2 × 4" arrangement (2 molar bands, 4 bonded incisors). When a fixed appliance includes only some of the teeth, archwire spans are longer, large moments are easy to create, and the wires themselves are more springy and less strong (see Chapter 10).

This can provide some biomechanical advantages. For example, intrusion of teeth is easier with long spans of wire that keep forces light and allow the appropriate moments to be generated. On the other hand, the wires are more prone to breakage and distortion. There is little indication for use of the newer superelastic wires when long unsupported spans exist. Simple multistranded steel wires and looped stainless steel configurations are more effective. Because the available permanent teeth are grouped in anterior (incisor) and posterior (molar) segments, a segmented arch approach to mechanics often is required. The apparently simple fixed appliances used in the mixed dentition can be

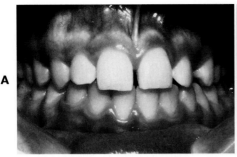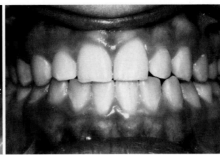

FIGURE 14-3 **A,** This patient had limited overbite on the left side where an impacted canine was located. **B,** The patient still has limited overbite after extrusion of the canine because appliances were only used on the maxillary, so no inter-arch elastics could be used.

quite complex to use appropriately (see Chapter 10). They are better described as deceptively simple.

Anchorage Control Is Both More Difficult and More Critical

With only the first molars available as anchorage in the posterior segment of the arch, there are limits to the amount of tooth movement that should be attempted in the mixed dentition. In addition, stabilizing lingual arches are more likely to be necessary as an adjunct to anchorage. In children with moderate problems, flexible lingual arches often are employed to produce tooth movement, for instance, to increase arch length. In those with severe problems, a rigid lingual arch is more likely to be used to control anchorage, while bonded brackets and labial archwires produce the desired tooth movement.

Space Closure Must Be Managed with Particular Care

Otherwise, when all teeth are not banded or bonded, the teeth without attachments will tend to be squeezed out of the arch. Unanticipated side effects of space closure that would not be encountered with a complete fixed appliance often are a problem in mixed dentition treatment.

Interarch Elastics Must Be Used Sparingly if at all

The side effects of Class II or Class III elastics make them risky in the extreme with partial fixed appliances like the typical mixed dentition 2 × 4 arrangement. They are not recommended under most circumstances unless a complete fixed appliance is present (Figure 14-3). Cross elastics can be employed in the mixed dentition, in the treatment of unilateral crossbite.

Retention Often Is Needed between Mixed Dentition Treatment and Eruption of the Permanent Teeth

After any significant tooth movement, it is important to maintain the teeth in their new position until a condition

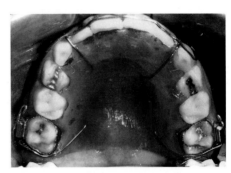

FIGURE 14-4 When retention is used between early (phase 1) and later (phase 2) treatment, creative planning of bow and clasps positions is required to avoid interference with erupting teeth and maintain the effectiveness of clasps. Note that the labial bow crosses the occlusion distal to the lateral incisors rather than in the area where the canines will erupt, and the molar clasps adapt to the bands and headgear tubes.

of stability is reached. That is as true in the mixed dentition as later. In fact, careful retention may be even more necessary after early treatment. The final stage of transition from the mixed to the permanent dentition is a particularly unstable time. For instance, mesial drift of molars that shortens arch length normally occurs then, but this can be disastrous if arch expansion was the goal of early treatment.

In mixed dentition patients, retention must be planned with two things in mind: the patient's current vs. initial condition and subsequent changes in the dentition and occlusion (Figure 14-4). With removable retainers, the location and design of clasps, wires, and labial bows should make them either modifiable or removable. Wires through edentulous areas can interfere with eruption of the permanent teeth in that area, and clasps on primary teeth will be of limited use because these teeth will be lost. Preadolescent children, even those who were quite cooperative with active treatment, tend not to be reliable patients for removable retainers, so the greater control provided by fixed rather than removable retainers must be balanced against the greater hygiene risk of fixed devices.

SPACE DEFICIENCY PROBLEMS

Space Deficiency Largely Due to Allowance for Molar Shift: Space Management

Management of Incisor Crowding.   Some children have considerable incisor irregularity in the mixed dentition due to the transitional incisor crowding, but space analysis shows that if loss of leeway space from mesial drift of first permanent molars could be prevented, there would be no space deficiency. For other patients, the large leeway space would nearly accommodate all the teeth and only a small amount of expansion would be required if mesial movement of the molars were prevented. When this strategy for treatment of crowding is adopted, intervention begins as late as possible and capitalizes most on the space differential between the primary second molar and the second premolar, sometimes known as the "E space." It is critically important to prevent either mesial movement of the first molars or lingual tipping of incisors, so appliance therapy—at least in the form of a lingual arch—will be necessary from the time any primary teeth are extracted until the end of the transition to the permanent dentition.

Usually a combination of early extraction of primary canines and disking to reduce the width of primary molars is necessary to allow the permanent incisors, canines, and premolars to erupt and align (Figure 14-5). A lingual arch that will support the incisor teeth and control the molar position by preventing any mesial shift is the minimum orthodontic appliance therapy. As in moderate space problems, the lingual arch can be activated slightly to tip molars distally and incisors facially to obtain a modest increase in arch length (Figure 14-6). A lip bumper also can be used in the lower arch to maintain the position of the molars or perhaps tip them slightly distally, while removing lip pressure and allowing the incisors to move facially. The effect of lingual arches and lip bumpers in the lower arch is remarkably similar; forward movement of the incisors is the major way in which additional space is gained.

When space is created in this way, the incisors often align spontaneously if the irregularity is from faciolingual tipping, but rotations are less likely to resolve. Correction of any incisor rotations requires controlled movement to align and derotate them, using an arch wire and bonded attachments on the incisors. It may be wise to defer this therapy until comprehensive treatment is begun in the early permanent dentition. If it is undertaken in the mixed dentition, the permanent first molars should be banded (and ideally reinforced with a lingual arch) to serve as anchorage and to maintain posterior stability and arch dimensions. If the arch wire is not supported between the first molar and incisors, it must be relatively large for strength in the buccal segments and may have to incorporate loops for flexibility in the incisor region. If the primary first molars are also bonded, a smaller and more flexible wire can be used because the length of the molar segment arch wire span is reduced. After alignment has

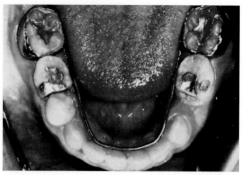

FIGURE 14-5   Disking primary posterior teeth in conjunction with space maintenance is an effective method to use the leeway space and all available arch length. Note that the disking must be completed perpendicular to the occlusal plane so that the height of contour of the tooth is reduced. Occlusally convergent slices that do not reduce the mesiodistal width of the tooth are not helpful.

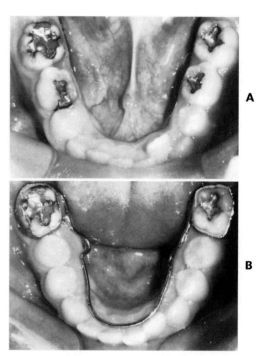

A

B

FIGURE 14-6   A lingual arch in conjunction with primary tooth extraction can be an effective way to manage the available arch length by taking advantage of the leeway space and reducing crowding. **A,** The primary second molars are in place, and there is some anterior crowding that is within the range of the leeway space. **B,** The primary second molars were extracted, and a lingual arch was placed immediately to take advantage of the leeway space. Subsequently, the second premolars erupted and the incisors aligned.

been achieved, if root position needs to be corrected, a rectangular wire is required to finish the tooth movement.

When the incisor segment is straight without anterior arch curvature, extraction of primary canines usually leads to spacing of the incisors or maintenance of essentially the same arch form. Alignment does not improve even when the space is available and a lingual arch is in place to serve

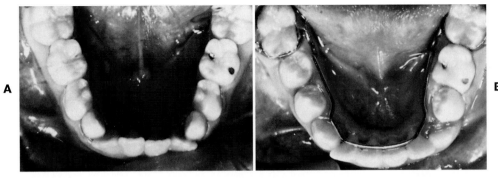

FIGURE 14-7   Anterior crowding combined with a straight anterior incisor segment. **A,** Straight incisors segments with lateral incisors that overlap the mesial of the primary canine (**B**) usually do not align into ideal arch form when the primary canines are extracted, even if a lingual arch is used.

as a template for tooth position (Figure 14-7). In most of these children, crowding will again be evident when the canines and first premolars erupt and selective disking or extraction of the primary second molars and continued space control with a lingual arch will be necessary. Deferring treatment until as late as possible—when the premolars are erupting—usually is the best judgment.[1]

Anterior Intra-arch Asymmetry.   Another problem that often needs to be addressed in the mixed dentition is anterior arch asymmetry. This is usually a shift of the dental midline to one side because of the premature loss of one primary canine caused by root resorption when the adjacent lateral incisor erupted. Loss of one primary canine often indicates a moderate space deficiency. If no permanent teeth will be extracted to provide additional space in the arch, this problem needs to be addressed before the remaining permanent teeth erupt because as more teeth erupt in asymmetric positions, overall arch perimeter will shorten and lead to a substantial space discrepancy with total arch asymmetry.

The mildest form of asymmetry is a significant but small (2 mm) midline shift. If the arch length is adequate, the incisors can be aligned and tipped back to their optimum location using a removable appliance and fingersprings. In some cases, disking or extraction of a primary canine or molar will be required to provide the necessary room for this correction even if space in the arch is predicted to be adequate. This technique is discussed in Chapter 13.

If bodily drift and rotational change has accompanied the midline change, the anterior teeth should be bonded and aligned with an arch wire. The force to move the teeth is usually generated by a coil spring placed on the arch wire (Figure 14-8). Regardless of the type of tooth movement or the appliance used for correction, retention will be needed until the remaining permanent teeth erupt (Figure 14-9).

Correction of Molar Relationship.   Because the molars have not been allowed to shift forward into the leeway space when space management is employed, they often are maintained in the end-to-end relationship that is

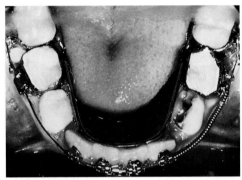

FIGURE 14-8   Bonded anterior teeth and banded posterior teeth, with a lingual arch to reinforce anchorage, are used to move the anterior teeth bodily. The coil spring generates the force to move the teeth along the arch wire.

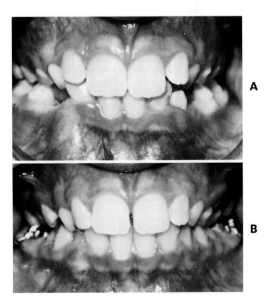

FIGURE 14-9   Midline shift requiring bodily movement. **A,** The midline of the mandibular arch has bodily shifted to the patient's right because of premature loss of a primary canine. **B,** The teeth were moved back to their proper position using a fixed appliance and are supported until eruption of the canines with a lingual holding arch.

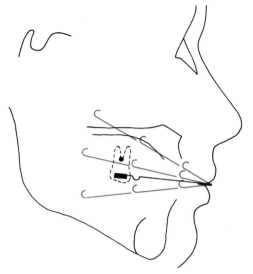

FIGURE 14-10   The effect of headgear on the molar is determined by the relationship of the outer bow of the facebow to the center of resistance of the tooth (in this figure, the dot in the midroot area) and the direction of pull (headcap, neckstrap, or combination anchorage). Facebow options for headgear are illustrated here. The vertical position of the outer bow can be high, straight, or low and its length can be short, medium, or long. Further details of the facebow and anchorage combinations and their effects are discussed in Chapter 15.

normal before the premolars erupt instead of moving into a Class I relationship. For that reason, space management also must include treatment to obtain a Class I molar relationship (i.e., if the lower molar is prevented from coming forward, the upper molar must be moved back). In the mixed dentition, the possibilities are extraoral force (headgear to the molars) or some type of molar distalizing appliance. If a second stage of treatment definitely is planned, later correction of the molar relationship (after the permanent teeth have erupted) might involve fixed appliances and interarch (Class II) elastics.

Headgear.   To change an end-to-end molar relationship to Class I by moving the upper molars distally, either by tipping both molars distally or by bodily movement, extraoral force via a facebow to the molars is the most effective and straightforward method.[2] The force is directed

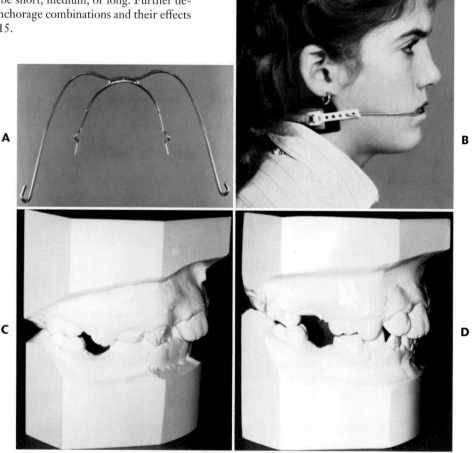

FIGURE 14-11   Extraoral force to a facebow can be used to tip molar crowns distally for space regaining. **A,** Symmetric facebow with a 45 mil inner bow is inserted into the tubes on the molar bands, and the outer bow is attached to an extraoral strap. **B,** The long, low outer bow attached to a cervical neckstrap is ideal to tip molar crowns distally for space regaining. **C,** This patient has bilateral space loss as a result of mesial tipping of the molars. **D,** Space has been regained using a headgear in the upper arch and a lingual arch in the lower. Note the increased space and improved permanent molar relationships.

specifically to the teeth that need to be moved, and reciprocal forces are not distributed on the other teeth that are in the correct positions. The force should be as nearly constant as possible to provide effective tooth movement and should be light because it is concentrated against only two teeth. The more the child wears the headgear, the better; 14 to 16 hours per day is minimal. Approximately 100 gm of force per side is appropriate. The teeth should move at the rate of 1 mm/month, so a cooperative child would need to wear the appliance for 3 months to obtain the 3 mm of correction that would be a typical requirement in this type of treatment.

If the outer bow of the headgear is positioned so that the resultant force vector passes occlusal to the center of resistance, which is near the midpoint of the root (Figure 14-10), the molar crown will tip distally. Distal crown tipping will occur if the facebow is attached to a neckstrap with either a medium length, straight or long, low outer bow (Figure 14-11). Distal tipping also would occur with a medium length, straight outer bow attached to a headcap as long as the resultant force vector passes occlusal to the center of resistance.

For bodily movement, the outer bow must be positioned so that the resultant force is through the center of resistance. Bodily movement can be attained with a medium length outer bow in combination with either a headcap or neckstrap (Figure 14-12, *A*). To move the molar roots distally most conveniently, the outer bow should be short and high so the resultant force is above the center

of resistance. This is achieved most conveniently with a headcap for force application (Figure 14-12, *B*).

A simple method to check for position of the resultant force relative to the center of resistance is to watch the portion of the headgear where the inner and outer bows meet, between the lips. If connecting the outer bow to the neckstrap or headcap raises this junction point of the inner and outer bows, the roots will move distally. If the junction moves down, the crown is going to tip distally. When the junction is stable, bodily movement will result.

It is important to remember that the direction of headgear pull relative to the crown also will determine whether the molar will be extruded, maintained at the same vertical level, or intruded as it is moved distally. A neckstrap attachment produces a downward as well as backward force on the molar and will extrude it, and adjusting the outer bow to control distal tipping when a neckstrap is used increases the extrusive force. In space management, however, the duration of extraoral force is only a few months and—even with cervical headgear extrusion of the molar—is unlikely to become a problem. Tooth movement should occur at the rate of 1 mm per month. Nevertheless, high pull headgear is an excellent option. Baumrind et al reported that this approach is particularly effective in producing distal molar movement.[3]

Asymmetric Headgear. Sometimes both molars have to be moved distally, but one requires substantially more movement than the other. To accomplish this, an asymmetric facebow with a neckstrap attachment can be used to

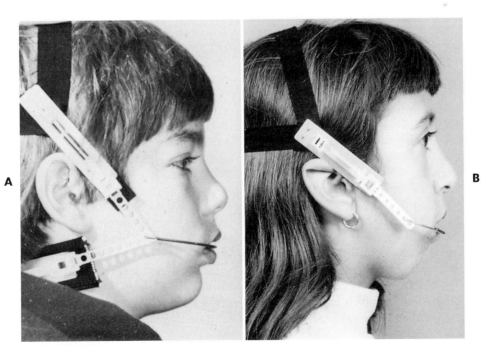

FIGURE 14-12 Bodily molar movement for space regaining is best achieved with a specific headgear-facebow configuration. **A,** A combination of a headcap and a neckstrap attached to a shorter and higher outer bow than that used for crown tipping is optimal. **B,** Using an even shorter and higher outer bow with a high pull headcap is the best way to move molar roots distally.

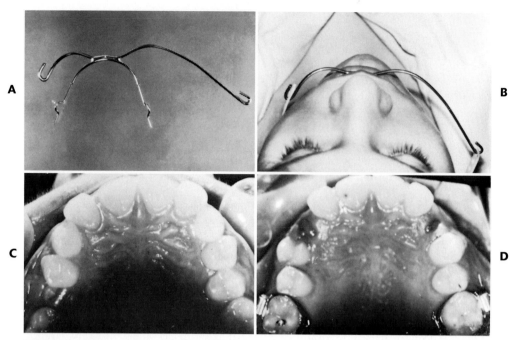

FIGURE 14-13   Asymmetric forces, achieved with a headgear by using an asymmetric outer bow, can be useful in regaining bilateral but asymmetric lost space. **A,** The outer bow is cut short on the side that needs the smaller distal movement and is left long on the side requiring the greater distal correction. **B,** When the appliance is in place, before the neckstrap is attached, the side with the long outer bow should be approximately 4 to 5 cm from the cheek. The distance is reduced when force is applied by the strap and the outer bow rotates toward the face. **C,** Intra-orally a bilateral space shortage is evident, more on the right side than the left, because of premature loss of a primary molar. **D,** Good asymmetric headgear wear resulted in space available for all succedaneous teeth.

deliver more force to one tooth than the other (Figure 14-13).[4] This will result in more movement on the side with the longer outer bow but will also move that tooth toward lingual crossbite. This approach does not work with a high pull headcap. Asymmetric cervical headgear is neither as easy to adjust nor as comfortable to wear as symmetric headgear, and it requires excellent patient compliance. For space regaining, it should be used only to deal with bilateral but asymmetric space loss—not true unilateral space loss, which is treated best with a removable appliance.

Intra-arch Appliances.

Molar Rotation.   The mildest form of maxillary space loss is mesiolingual rotation of the maxillary molars around the large lingual root (Figure 14-14, *A*). This can result from modest mesial drift into space lost because of proximal caries or minor space loss after early extraction of maxillary second primary molars. This type of space loss can be recognized by the lack of molar buccal offset (the facial surface is normally more prominent than the primary molar or premolars) and an end-to-end permanent molar relationship.

Bilateral derotation of these teeth with a soldered or removable 36 mil transpalatal arch with an adjustment loop has been advocated to improve alignment and distalize the teeth, increasing arch perimeter (Figure 14-14, *B*).[5] As

inviting as this approach appears, recent evidence indicates that although the teeth do derotate, they are just as likely to move mesially as distally,[6] so neither increased arch perimeter nor an improvement in molar relationships is guaranteed. One of the methods described below is likely to be required.

Distal Molar Movement.   If bodily distal movement of one or both permanent maxillary first molars is necessary to adjust molar relationships and space, if there are adequate anterior teeth for anchorage, and if some anterior incisor movement can be tolerated, several appliances can be considered. All are built around the use of a heavy lingual arch, usually with an acrylic pad against the anterior palate to provide anchorage (Figure 14-15). Often the anterior teeth also are bonded and stabilized with an arch wire. Then a force to move the molar distally is generated with a helical spring,[7] stainless steel or superelastic coil spring[8] or magnets[9] (see Figures 8-40 and 17-3). The amount of tooth movement needed to adjust upper molars for space management clearly could be obtained in this way. The only contraindication would be the complexity and cost of the apparatus, in contrast to the much simpler headgear approach.

No matter how a molar was moved distally, if the time prior to eruption of the premolars will be longer than a few

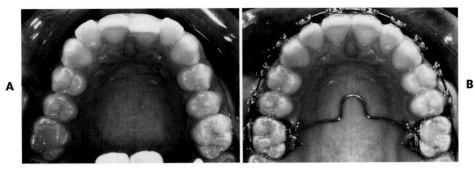

FIGURE 14-14   Molar rotation using a transpalatal arch. **A,** This patient has mesially rotated upper first molars at the beginning of treatment. **B,** During the early phases of treatment the molars were derotated using the transpalatal arch. This movement usually improves interdigitation with the lower molars but cannot be counted on to increase the available space by moving the upper molars distally.

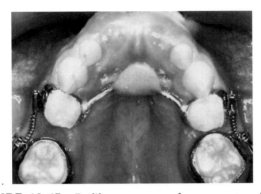

FIGURE 14-15   Bodily movement of permanent molars to regain space can be accomplished using a fixed appliance that is reinforced with a lingual arch. This method, although complex, has the capability to localize the active forces and resist unwanted reactive forces. A lingual arch incorporating a Nance-type palatal button is placed from a primary tooth adjacent to the area of space loss extending to the other side of the arch. This provides the anchorage to resist the force of repositioning the permanent molars. A compressed coil spring provides the force to reposition the molar and extends from the anchorage unit to the molar. Tooth movement should proceed at approximately 1 mm per month and be retained with a band and loop or lingual arch. (Courtesy Dr. M. Mayhew.)

months, it will be necessary to hold them back after they are repositioned. A Nance appliance is probably the best insurance to guard against repeated space loss.

It is rare that a child who receives this type of treatment in the mixed dentition does not require further treatment after all permanent teeth have erupted. If minor irregularity can be accepted until the patient is ready for comprehensive treatment, the total treatment time and appliance wear can be shortened.

Severe Localized Space Loss (>3 mm)

Space loss can progress quickly and exceed the 3 mm amount that can be dealt with using removable or simple fixed appliances. When localized space loss is 4 mm or

more, the decision must be made either to attempt to regain the space, accepting the need for major tooth movement and complex appliance therapy, or to extract a permanent tooth. Either way, a second stage of comprehensive treatment in the early permanent dentition is likely to be needed.

The treatment necessary to regain the space, especially if a second stage of treatment will be required in any event, may be more than is reasonable when one analyzes the cost/benefit ratio. Extraction with space closure often is a better choice. In that circumstance, the mixed dentition treatment can be limited to maintenance of the existing space, so that the ultimate space closure occurs under control when the complete fixed appliances are present. This should be kept in mind as the major space regaining procedures are discussed below.

Maxillary Space Regaining.   Bilateral space loss, as in bilateral drift of both first molars after early extraction of both primary second molars, creates a condition identical to the one described under space management if the drift is not too severe. Moving both molars back up to 3 mm can be accomplished with either headgear or an intra-arch appliance, exactly as described previously. The more typical space regaining situation is unilateral loss of space. Failure to maintain space after extraction of a carious maxillary second primary molar or ectopic eruption of the permanent first molar are the major causes.

For unilateral space regaining, a fixed intra-arch appliance is preferred. This would be essentially identical to the one made for bilateral use but with only one side activated. The excellent anchorage provided by the rest of the appliance can produce distal movement of the molar on only one side with good success. When a molar drifts mesially, it usually tips, and space regaining is facilitated because bodily movement is not required in most instances.

An asymmetric facebow, as mentioned previously, is also a possibility. Remember that with this appliance, teeth on both sides of the arch will move distally, not just on one side.

Mandibular Space Regaining. Space regaining in the mandibular arch is difficult to accomplish without forcing the incisors labially. A fixed appliance with multiple banded/bonded attachments, perhaps supported by interarch elastics and extraoral force, may be required to move a lower molar back after it has drifted mesially. Bodily distal movement of lower molars is almost impossible, but with excellent anchorage and careful activation of a fixed appliance, it is possible to tip a molar distally to regain space.

As an alternative for unilateral mandibular space regaining, a lingual arch can be used to support the tooth movement and provide anchorage when used in conjunction with a segmental arch wire and coil spring (see Figure 14-15). This is analogous to the method previously described for the maxilla, but a mandibular lingual arch inevitably is less stable than a maxillary one. Usually the lower lingual arch runs from one permanent first molar to the opposing primary first molar on the side where the space is to be regained. This primary molar also has a bracket on the facial surface of the band. A coil spring then can be compressed on a segmental arch wire between the primary and permanent molars. The regained space must be maintained, preferably with a passive lingual arch to bands on both permanent first molars.

Severe Generalized Arch Length Discrepancy (>4 mm)

Severe crowding usually is obvious even before a space analysis can be completed. These children have little developmental spacing between primary incisors and occasionally some crowding in the primary dentition. The two major symptoms of severe crowding in the early mixed dentition are severe irregularity of the erupting permanent incisors and early loss of primary canines caused by eruption of the permanent lateral incisors. The children with the largest arch length discrepancies often have reasonably well aligned incisors in the early mixed dentition, because the primary canines were lost when the lateral incisors erupted. After a definitive analysis of the profile and incisor position,

the decision must be made to either expand the arches or extract permanent teeth (see Chapter 8 for a review of factors influencing this decision). In the presence of severe crowding, limited treatment of the problem will not be sufficient.

A key question, which remains unanswered, is whether early expansion of the arches (before all permanent teeth erupt) gives more stable results than later expansion (in the early permanent dentition). Partly in response to the realization that recurrent crowding occurs in many patients who were treated with premolar extractions (see Chapter 8), a number of approaches to early arch expansion recently have regained some popularity in spite of a lack of data to document their effectiveness. Expansion can involve any combination of several possibilities: maxillary dental or skeletal transverse expansion by tipping teeth facially or by expanding the midpalatal suture, respectively; mandibular buccal segment expansion by facial movement of the teeth; or advancement of the incisors or distal movement of the molars in either arch.

The most aggressive approach to early expansion uses maxillary and mandibular removable lingual arches in the complete primary dentition.[10] This produces an increase in both arch perimeter and width. The expansion is maintained for variable periods during the mixed and permanent dentition years. Lutz and Poulton examined long-term results of this approach and found little change in intercanine width when control and treated patients were compared, but they did observe a small amount of buccal segment expansion and arch perimeter increase.[11] The ability of this technique to meet the challenge of anterior crowding is questionable and unsubstantiated.

A less aggressive approach, in terms of timing, is to expand the upper arch in the early mixed dentition, using a lingual arch (or perhaps a jackscrew expander—but this must be done carefully and slowly in the early mixed dentition) to produce dental and skeletal changes (Figure 14-16). The necessary mandibular incisor and buccal segment expansion, as well as molar uprighting, can be obtained with a utility arch (Figure 14-17).[12] Some authors

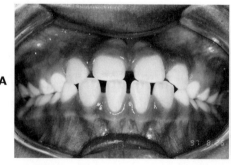
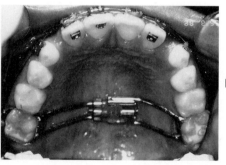

FIGURE 14-16 Some practitioners advocate early expansion by opening the midpalatal suture, usually using a jack-screw type appliance as in this patient, even in the absence of a posterior crossbite or an apparent arch length shortage, on the theory that this will improve the long-term stability of arch expansion. Little or no data exist to support this contention.

have suggested that this not only provides more space and better esthetics but can eradicate disharmonies between the arches that are present in Class II and Class III malocclusions due to inexplicable anterior and posterior skeletal adjustments.[13] Data supporting the long-term effectiveness of this technique are unavailable. It seems unlikely that the soft tissues, which establish the limits for arch expansion (see Chapter 5), would react quite differently to transverse expansion at different ages, or that jaw growth in other planes of space would be greatly affected by transverse expansion.

Another alternative is to use a functional appliance that incorporates lip and buccal shields (see Chapter 15) or a lip bumper (Figure 14-18) to reduce the resting pressure of the lips and cheeks and produce dental expansion. Lip pads and buccal shields will lead to anterior movement of the incisors and buccal movement of the primary molars or premolars, which allows the teeth to align themselves along a larger arch circumference. After additional space has been created, a retainer is needed. Although adequate evidence indicates that these appliances can create expansion, its stability has not been documented.[14] A functional appliance rarely is indicated in a child with no skeletal problem.

A combination of maxillary lingual arch appliances to rotate upper molars; headgear, sometimes supplemented by fixed or removable appliances to distalize upper molars; and a mandibular lip bumper to increase lower arch dimensions by moving incisor and buccal segments facially and lower molars distally, has been advocated as an effective way to produce major arch expansion.[15] Studies that evaluated the use of lip bumpers to increase lower arch length have yielded variable results. Most document some arch width changes, modest distal molar movement, and variable incisor proclination during treatment.[16,17]

Finally, arch expansion can be obtained by aligning the anterior teeth with bonded attachments and arch wires, and this can be combined with other types of expansion. As described previously, the teeth can be tipped facially and buccally, increasing the available arch length (Figure 14-19).

Early expansion with both functional appliance components (including the lip bumper) and/or fixed appliances has three major limitations: the long duration of treatment from the primary or early mixed dentition through the eruption of the permanent teeth; the possibility of creating unesthetic dentoalveolar protrusion; and the uncertain stability of the long-term result. Although it seems reasonable to assume that stability would be better if the initial space

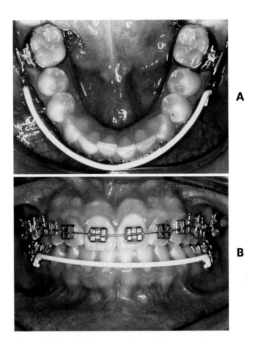

FIGURE 14-18 A lip bumper can be used to increase deficient mandibular arch length. **A,** Because of its long span, the lip bumper must be constructed from heavy wire to prevent distortion. **B,** The wire is adjusted to be 1.5 to 2 mm facial to the lower incisors, and the plastic shield that usually is added to increase contact with the lip typically is adjusted to fit at least two millimeters below the incisal edges. In theory, this increases the lip pressure that is transmitted to the molars and increases distal molar movement.

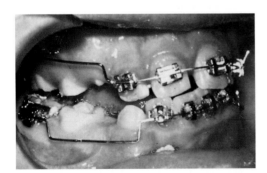

FIGURE 14-17 A utility arch can be used to intrude, tip, or reposition either maxillary or mandibular incisors, but with the limited anchorage provided by only the first molars, posterior teeth can be expected to move as well. The arch wire is stepped away from the occlusal plane to eliminate distortion from interference with food during chewing.

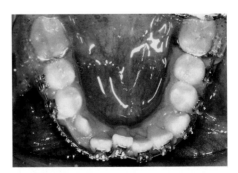

FIGURE 14-19 For mixed dentition treatment of significant lower crowding and irregularity, banded/bonded attachments and an arch wire provide the most efficient approach. This patient has a degree of crowding that indicates fixed appliance treatment; note the use of a superelastic coil spring to create space for the erupting mandibular right canine.

discrepancy were small and initial incisor protrusion were minimal, even this is not well documented at present.

Because several millimeters of space can be generated by a number of the techniques cited here, the ability to accomplish such changes is not the critical question. Rather, the question is the wisdom of major early expansion of the arches, given the questionable stability and potentially compromised esthetic results.

Very Severe Crowding: Serial Extraction? In many children with severe crowding, a decision can be made during the early mixed dentition that expansion is fruitless and that permanent teeth will have to be extracted. A planned sequence of tooth removal can reduce crowding and irreg-

ularity during the transition from the primary to the permanent dentition. It will also allow the teeth to erupt over the alveolus and through keratinized tissue, rather than being displaced buccally or lingually. This sequence, often termed *serial extraction*, simply involves the timed extraction of primary and, ultimately, permanent teeth to relieve severe crowding. It was advocated originally as a method to treat severe crowding without or with minimal use of appliance therapy but is now viewed as an adjunct to later comprehensive treatment instead of a substitute for it. Although serial extraction makes later comprehensive treatment easier and often quicker, by itself it usually does not result in ideal tooth position or closure of excess space.

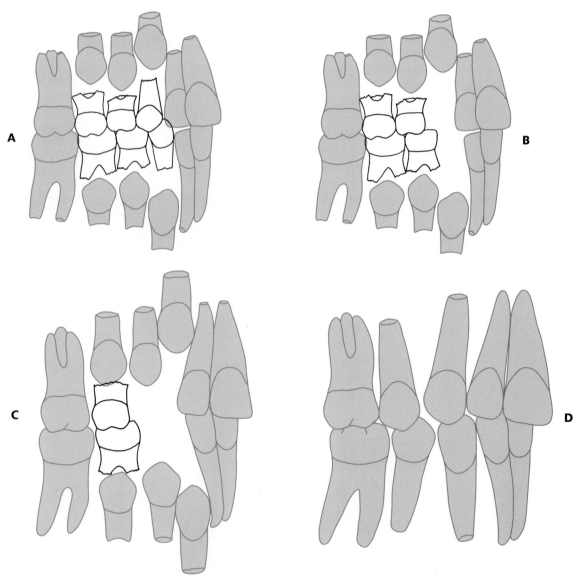

FIGURE 14-20 Serial extraction is used to relieve severe arch length discrepancies. **A,** The initial diagnosis is made when a severe space deficiency is documented and there is marked incisor crowding. **B,** The primary canines are extracted to provide space for alignment of the incisors. **C,** The primary first molars are extracted when one half to two thirds of the first premolar root is formed to speed eruption of the first premolars. **D,** When the first premolars have erupted they are extracted and the canines erupt into the remaining extraction space. The residual space is closed by drifting and tipping of the posterior teeth unless full appliance therapy is implemented.

Serial extraction is directed toward *severe* dental crowding. For this reason, it is best used when no skeletal problem exists and when the space discrepancy is large—greater than 10 mm per arch. If the crowding is severe, little space will remain, which means there will be little tipping and uncontrolled movement of the adjacent teeth into the extraction sites. If the initial discrepancy is smaller, more residual space must be anticipated.

Serial extraction treatment begins in the early mixed dentition with extraction of primary incisors if necessary, followed by extraction of the primary canines to allow eruption and alignment of the permanent incisors (Figure 14-20). As the permanent teeth align without any appli-

ances in place, there is usually some lingual tipping of the lower incisors, and overbite often increases during this stage. Labiolingual displacements resolve better than rotational irregularity. After extraction of the primary canines, crowding problems are usually under control for 1 to 2 years, but foresight is necessary. The goal is to influence the permanent first premolars to erupt ahead of the canines so that they can be extracted and the canines can move distally into this space. The maxillary premolars usually erupt before the canines, so the eruption sequence is rarely a problem in the upper arch. In the lower arch, however, the canines often erupt before the first premolars, which causes the canines to be displaced facially. To avoid this result, the

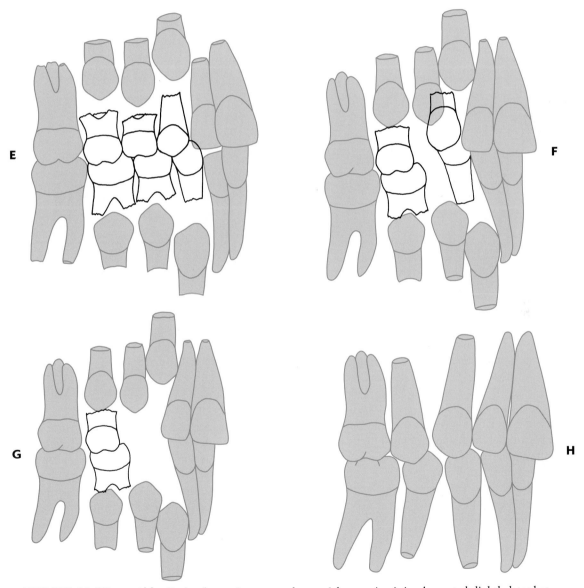

FIGURE 14-20, cont'd   **E,** An alternative approach to serial extraction is implemented slightly later but under the same conditions and **F,** begins with extraction of the primary first molars so that there is less lingual tipping of the incisors and less tendency to develop a deep bite. Extraction of the primary first molars also encourages early eruption of the first premolars. **G,** When the first premolars have erupted, they are extracted and the canines erupt into the remaining extraction space. **H,** The residual space is closed by drifting and tipping of the posterior teeth unless full appliance therapy is implemented.

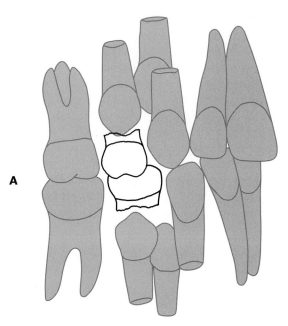

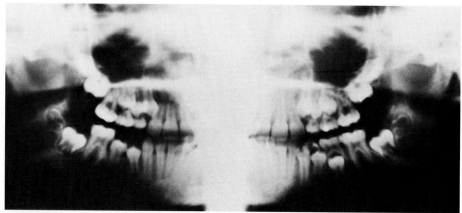

FIGURE 14-21   A complication of serial extraction is premature eruption of the permanent canines. **A,** When this occurs the first premolars are impacted between the canines and the second premolars. **B,** In this situation (note the lower right quadrant for this patient), the first premolars usually have to be surgically removed (a procedure often called enucleation).

lower primary first molar should be extracted when there is ½ to ⅔ root formation of the first premolar. This usually will speed up the premolar eruption and cause it to enter the arch before the canine (see Figure 14-20, *C*). The result is easy access for extraction of the first premolar before the canine erupts (see Figure 14-20, *D*).

A complication can occur if the primary first molar is extracted early and the first premolar still does not erupt before the canine. This can lead to impaction of the premolar that requires later surgical removal (Figure 14-21). At the time the primary first molar is removed, it may be obvious that the canine will erupt before the premolar. In this case the underlying premolar can also be extracted at the same time—a procedure termed *enucleation*. If possible, however, enucleation should be avoided because the erupting premolar brings alveolar bone with it. Early enucleation can leave a bone defect that may persist.

The increase in overbite mentioned previously can become a problem requiring later treatment. A variation in the extraction sequence has been proposed in an effort to overcome this problem.[18] The mandibular primary canines are retained and some space for anterior alignment is made available when the permanent laterals erupt by extracting the primary first molars instead. With this approach, eruption of the permanent first premolars is encouraged, and the incisors are less prone to tip lingually (see Figure 14-20, *E* through *H*). The major goal of serial extraction is prevention of incisor crowding, however, some crowding often persists if the primary canines are retained. In many patients with severe crowding, the primary canines are lost to ectopic eruption of the laterals and cannot be maintained.

After the first premolar has been extracted, the second primary molars should exfoliate normally. The premolar ex-

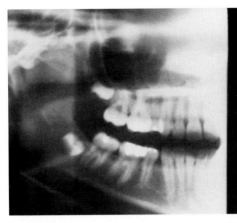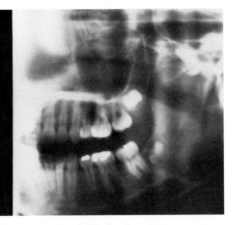

FIGURE 14-22 This patient had serial extraction not followed by fixed appliance treatment with an excellent result. Properly timed serial extraction usually results in incomplete space closure. Teeth drift together by tipping, which results in nonparallel roots between the canine and second premolar. Lack of root parallelism, residual space, and other irregularities can be addressed with subsequent fixed appliance therapy.

traction space closes partially by mesial drift of the second premolar and permanent first molar but largely by distal eruption of the canine. If serial extraction is not followed by mechanotherapy, ideal alignment, root positioning, overbite, and space closure are usually not achieved (Figure 14-22).

EXCESS SPACE

Large Maxillary Midline Diastema

As noted in Chapter 13, there are two reasons for closing a maxillary midline diastema: to improve the esthetic situation, and to provide enough space for the permanent canines to erupt when the separated central incisors have forced the lateral incisors into the canine area. In a child whose permanent canines have not yet erupted, a diastema of 2 mm or less is likely to close spontaneously and is not an indication for treatment. A diastema greater than 2 mm is unlikely to close spontaneously. If by chance a large diastema exists and the teeth are tipped apart, they can be tipped back together and retained with a removable appliance (see Figure 13-16). The second treatment indication for diastema closure is a more challenging treatment problem in most instances because most large unesthetic diastemas require bodily repositioning of the incisors.

When the situation demands bodily mesiodistal movement, an anterior segmental arch wire from central to central incisor or the classic 2 × 4 appliance can be quite satisfactory. Initial alignment of the incisors with a flexible wire is required. Then a stiffer arch wire can be employed as the teeth slide together (16 × 22 mil steel is a good choice during the space closure) (Figure 14-23). The force to move the incisors together can be provided by an elastomeric chain tying these teeth together, or by a coil spring compressed over the arch wire between the first molar and lateral incisors. The diastema closure is more predictable if

only mesiodistal movement, not retraction, is required. If the incisors are to be retracted as the space closes, careful attention to the posterior anchorage is required.

The experienced clinician's desire to close diastemas at an early age is tempered by knowledge of how difficult it can be to keep the space closed. If the lateral incisors and canines have not erupted, a Hawley-type retainer will require constant modification. An alternative approach for retention if the overbite is not prohibitively deep is to bond a 17.5 mil multistranded arch wire to the linguocervical portion of the incisors (Figure 14-24). This will provide excellent retention with less maintenance.

Another retention problem may be caused by the presence of a large or inferiorly attached labial frenum. A frenectomy after space closure and retention may be necessary in some cases, but it is difficult to determine the potential contribution of the frenum to retention problems from its morphology alone. Therefore a frenectomy before treatment is contraindicated, and a post-treatment frenectomy should be attempted only if a continued tendency of the diastema to reopen and unresolved bunching of tissue between the teeth show that it is necessary.[19]

Generalized Spacing with Protrusion

As mentioned in Chapter 13, generalized spacing of the teeth is not a frequent finding in the mixed dentition in the absence of incisor protrusion. When maxillary anterior teeth are spaced because the incisors protrude, the teeth may require tipping or bodily movement during retraction. A fixed appliance almost always is required. Large spaces, bodily displacement, and rotations are indications for fixed appliances. In these cases, an arch wire should be used with bands on posterior teeth and bonded brackets on anterior teeth. This appliance must provide a retracting and space closing force, which can be obtained from closing loops incorporated into the arch wire or from a section of elastomeric chain (Figure 14-25) (see also Chapter 17).

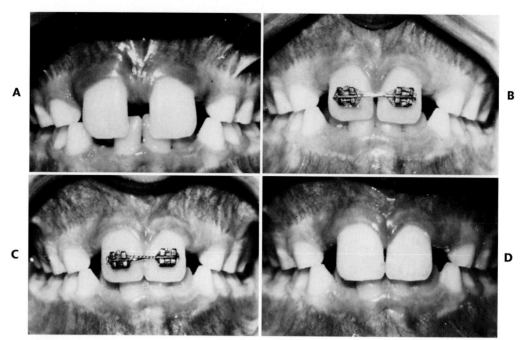

FIGURE 14-23 Closure of a diastema with a fixed appliance. **A,** This diastema requires closure by moving the crowns and roots of the central incisors. **B,** The bonded attachments and rectangular wire control the teeth in three planes of space while the elastomeric chain provides the force to slide the teeth along the wire. **C,** Immediately after space closure, the teeth are retained and (**D**) usually require a fixed lingual retainer at least until the permanent canines erupt (see Figure 14-24).

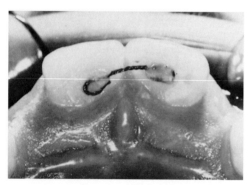

FIGURE 14-24 A fixed retainer to maintain diastema closure. A bonded 17.5 mil multistrand wire with loops bent into the ends is bonded to the lingual surfaces of anterior teeth to serve as a permanent retainer. This flexible wire allows physiologic mobility of the teeth and reduces bond failure but can be used only when the overbite is not excessive.

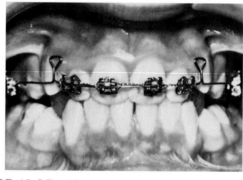

FIGURE 14-25 This closing loop arch wire was used to retract protrusive maxillary incisors and close space. Each loop was activated approximately 1 mm per month, and the posterior anchorage was reinforced with a headgear.

Bodily incisor retraction also places a large strain on the posterior teeth, which tends to pull them forward. Depending on the amount of incisor retraction and space closure, a headgear, chosen with consideration for vertical facial and dental characteristics, may be necessary for supplemental anchorage support. Again, as with expansion of arches for space, a major distinction between the use of the removable vs. fixed appliance is the type of tooth movement desired and the need to control tooth rotations. Rotations can only be efficiently managed with banded

and bonded appliances. Additionally, arch form alteration and posterior space closure can only be accomplished with fixed appliances.

Missing Permanent Teeth

When permanent teeth are congenitally missing, the patient must have a thorough evaluation to determine the correct treatment because any of the diagnostic variables of profile, incisor position, and space availability or deficiency can be crucial in treatment planning.

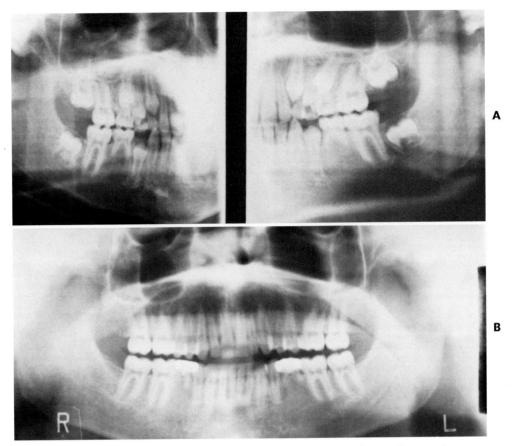

FIGURE 14-26 Primary mandibular second molars can be retained when the second premolars are missing. **A,** This patient has missing mandibular second premolars identified before orthodontic treatment. **B,** The primary mandibular second molars that have excellent root structure were reduced mesiodistally and restored with stainless steel crowns during the finishing stages of orthodontic treatment to provide good occlusion.

The most commonly missing permanent teeth are the mandibular second premolars and the maxillary lateral incisors. These two conditions pose different problems. If the patient has an ideal or an acceptable occlusion, maintaining primary second molars is a reasonable plan, since many primary molars can be retained at least until the patient reaches the early twenties if root resorption and caries have not been a problem (Figure 14-26). Many reports exist of primary posterior teeth surviving until the patient is 40 to 60 years of age. If the primary molars, which are larger than the second premolars, are retained, some reduction of their mesiodistal width is often necessary to improve the posterior interdigitation of the teeth. A limiting factor in reducing the size of primary molars and then closing space is the mesiodistal divergence of the primary molar roots. Teeth can move no closer together than their roots will allow, so a nonideal posterior occlusion may be the best that can be achieved.

When retained primary posterior teeth are lost and require prosthetic replacement, especially if this occurs before vertical growth is completed in the late teens, in many cases it is possible to use less expensive and less invasive resin-bonded bridges as an alternative to conventional bridges and preparations. Another possibility, which has become increasingly attractive in recent years and is likely to be the method of choice in the future, is the intraosseous implant. It is better to defer definitive crown and bridge treatment until the late teens, and imperative that implants not be done until growth is completed.[20]

Long-term retention of primary laterals, in contrast, is almost never an acceptable plan. When the lateral incisors are missing, one of two sequelae usually is observed. In some patients, the erupting permanent canine resorbs the primary lateral incisor and spontaneously substitutes for the missing lateral incisor, which means that the primary canine has no successor (Figure 14-27). Some of these patients are seen as adults with primary canines in place, but most primary canines are lost by the end of adolescence even if their successors have erupted mesially. Less often, the primary lateral is retained until the canine is replaced by its proper successor. The long-term prognosis of retained primary lateral incisors is poor and their small size makes them unesthetic. If adequate space exists, implants now are preferred for replacements. Leaving the permanent canine in the

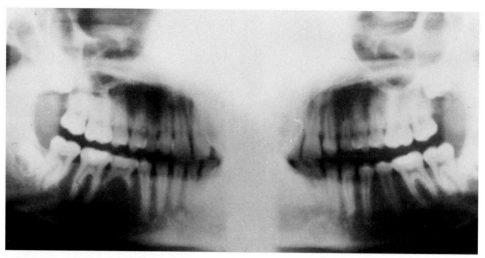

FIGURE 14-27 Missing permanent maxillary lateral incisors are often replaced spontaneously by permanent canines. This phenomenon occurs without intervention, but the resorption noted on the retained primary canines probably will continue to progress. If implants to eventually replace the missing laterals are planned, it is desirable for the canines to erupt mesially so that alveolar bone forms in the area of the future implant. The canines can be moved into their final position just prior to the implant surgery.

lateral position until near the end of the growth period, then moving it into its proper position, is the best strategy to obtain adequate alveolar bone in the future implant area (see Chapter 21). Under no circumstances should an anterior implant be placed until vertical growth is completed. The management of prosthetic replacement of missing laterals is covered in some detail in Chapter 21.

If permanent teeth are missing and there is inadequate space for the complete permanent dentition, the potential solutions include orthodontic space closure. In some of these cases, missing permanent teeth can be treated as if they had been extracted to relieve the crowding. The mandibular second premolars and the maxillary lateral incisors (the permanent teeth most often missing) generally would not be the first teeth chosen for extraction. Primary teeth should be extracted to promote drift of permanent teeth for space closure only after consultation with a specialist. These patients will require comprehensive treatment during adolescence.

The second premolars have a tendency to form late and may be thought to be missing, only to be discovered to be forming at a subsequent visit. Good premolars seldom form after the child is 8 years of age. If the space, profile, and jaw relationships are good, it is possible to extract the primary second molars at age 7 to 9 and allow the first molars to drift mesially (Figure 14-28, *A* and *B*). The mesial drift of the posterior teeth, along with some distal drift of the anterior teeth, can produce partial or even complete space closure. Unfortunately, the amount and direction of the drift vary (Figure 14-28, *C* through *H*). Early extraction can reduce the treatment time, but comprehensive orthodontic treatment is usually needed for completion of treatment.[21]

When permanent lateral incisors are missing and space closure is desired, it helps if the primary lateral incisors are replaced by the permanent canines. When this process is occurring naturally, little immediate attention is necessary at that stage. Sometimes, the absence of lateral incisors causes a large diastema to develop between the permanent central incisors. To maximize mesial drift of the erupting permanent canines, this diastema should be closed and retained as described above (Figure 14-29). Before the first premolars erupt, the primary canines should be extracted if they are not resorbing, so the premolars can migrate into the canine positions and other posterior teeth can move mesially and close space (Figure 14-30). In this situation also, comprehensive orthodontic treatment, recontouring of the anterior teeth, and resin build-ups to improve esthetics are necessary to complete the treatment (Figure 14-31), but the amount of treatment and treatment length can be greatly reduced by timely removal of primary teeth.

In patients with a congenitally missing tooth or teeth in one area but crowding in another, autotransplantation also is a possible solution. Teeth can be transplanted from one position to another in the same mouth, with a good prognosis for long-term success if done when the transplanted tooth has approximately one half of its root formed. This means that the decision for autotransplantation must be made during the mixed dentition. This technique is most commonly used to move premolars into location of missing incisors. A combination of careful surgical intervention and positioning of the transplant, followed by light orthodontic forces to achieve final tooth position, and restorative treatment to recontour the crown of the transplanted tooth, can result in long-term functional and esthetic success (Figure 14-32).[22]

Text continued on p. 470.

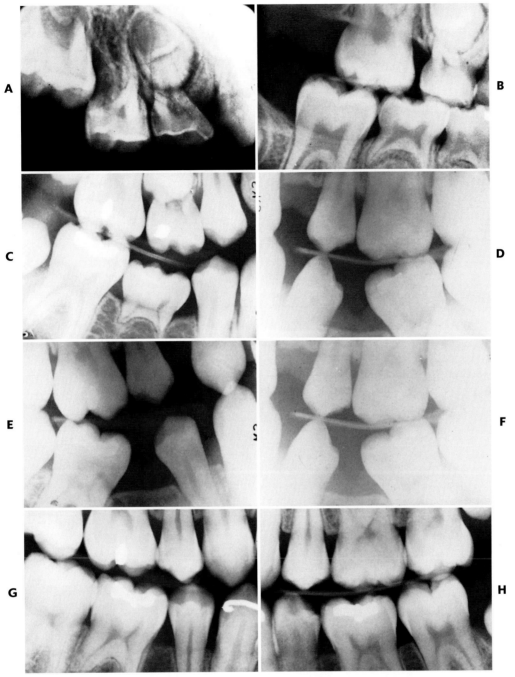

FIGURE 14-28 Missing second premolars can be treated by extraction of primary second molars to allow drifting of the permanent teeth and spontaneous space closure. **A,** This patient has ectopic eruption of the permanent maxillary first molar and a missing permanent maxillary second premolar. Since there was no other evidence of a malocclusion, the primary molar was extracted and **B,** the permanent molar drifted anteriorly and closed the space during eruption. This eliminates the need for a prosthesis at a later date. **C** and **D,** Another patient has bilaterally missing permanent mandibular second premolars, and the decision was made to extract the retained primary molars to allow as much spontaneous drift and space closure as possible before full appliance therapy. **E** and **F,** There was drift of the posterior teeth anteriorly and drift of the anterior teeth distally, but the space did not completely close. This pattern of drift is highly variable and unpredictable. **G** and **H,** The residual space was closed and the roots paralleled with full appliances.

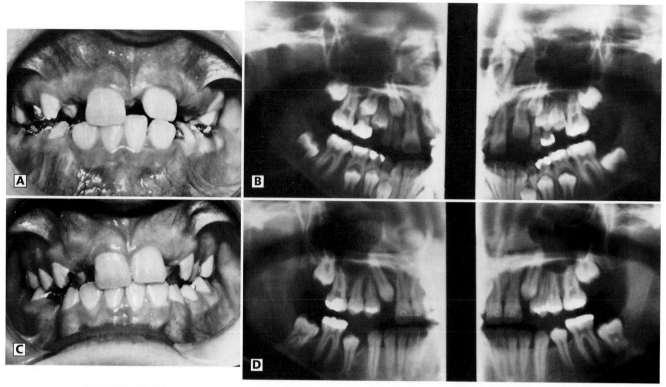

FIGURE 14-29 Missing permanent lateral incisors often allow a large diastema to develop between the permanent central incisors. **A,** This patient has that type of diastema, and the unerupted permanent canines will be substituted for the missing lateral incisors. **B,** This radiograph shows the unerupted canines in an excellent position for substitution for the lateral incisors. **C,** The diastema has been closed to obtain maximum mesial drift of the canines. **D,** This technique enables the canines to erupt closer to their final position and eliminates unnecessary tooth movement during full appliance therapy.

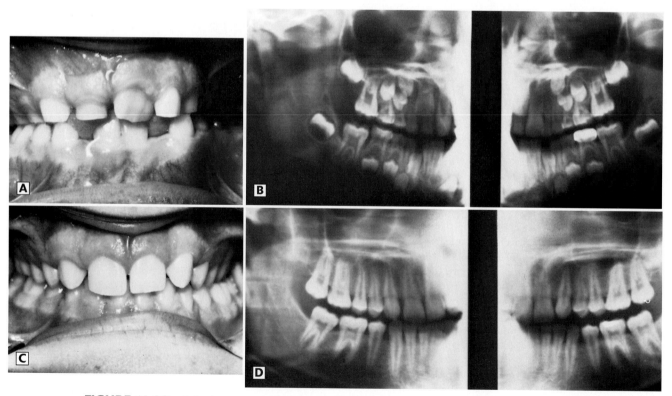

FIGURE 14-30 Selective removal of primary teeth when permanent maxillary lateral incisors are missing can lead to a shortened second phase of fully banded treatment. **A** and **B,** This patient had primary canines and first molars extracted to maximize the mesial drift of the permanent posterior teeth. **C** and **D,** This intervention resulted in good tooth position that will require little fixed appliance therapy to complete.

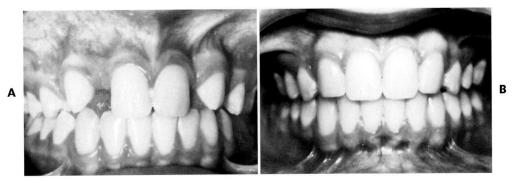

FIGURE 14-31 When permanent maxillary lateral incisors are missing, the permanent canines can be substituted for the missing incisors. **A,** This patient has missing lateral incisors and anterior irregularity. **B,** The permanent canines were substituted for the lateral incisors, the excess space closed, and resin was added to the canines to alter their morphology so they would resemble the missing lateral incisors.

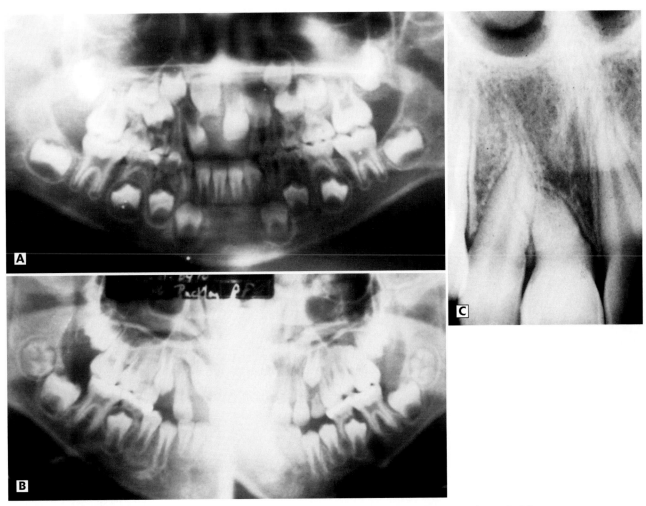

FIGURE 14-32 This patient demonstrates the utility of autotransplant procedures. **A,** The permanent maxillary right central incisor is located high in the maxilla and inverted. Conventional exposure of the tooth followed by orthodontic traction would require an extended treatment time and could result in a gingival defect if the tooth perforated the mucosa while being moved through the vestibule. **B,** The tooth has been surgically transplanted and a ligature attached so traction can begin. Note that root formation has continued. **C,** The tooth in final position after orthodontic traction with reasonable root length, good periodontal health, and physiologic mobility.

ERUPTION PROBLEMS

Supernumerary Teeth

Supernumerary teeth can disrupt both the normal eruption of other teeth and their alignment if and when they do erupt. Treatment is aimed at extraction of the supernumeraries before problems arise, or at minimizing the effect if other teeth have already been displaced.

The most common location for supernumerary teeth is the anterior maxilla. These teeth are often discovered on a panoramic or occlusal radiograph when a child is about 6 to 7 years of age, either during a routine examination or when permanent incisors fail to erupt. The simple cases are those in which a single supernumerary tooth is present and superficially located. If the tooth is not inverted, it will often erupt before the normal tooth and can be extracted before it interferes with the adjacent teeth.[23] In a few instances, multiple supernumerary teeth will be located superficially, and uncomplicated extractions can be performed without interfering appreciably with the normal teeth.

As a general rule, the more supernumeraries that are present, the more abnormal their shape and the higher their position, the harder it will be to manage the situation. Several abnormal supernumeraries are likely to have disturbed the position and eruption timing of the normal teeth before their discovery, and tubercle teeth are unlikely to erupt (Figure 14-33). Extractions should be completed as soon as the supernumerary teeth can be removed without harming the developing normal teeth. The surgeon may wish to delay intervention until continued root development has improved the access for extraction and prog-

nosis for the teeth that will remain. This is a reasonable approach, but the earlier the supernumeraries can be removed, the more likely that the normal teeth will erupt without further treatment. Conversely, the later the extraction, the more likely that the remaining normal teeth will need surgical exposure, orthodontic traction, or both to bring them into the arch.

Managing the Sequela of Delayed Eruption

Delayed Incisors. Some evidence indicates that changes in the overlying keratinized tissue occur in long-standing edentulous regions.[24] These changes contribute to slow eruption of an incisor after the supernumerary tooth blocking it and the overlying bone have been removed. If the delayed incisor is located superficially, it can be exposed with a simple soft tissue incision and usually will erupt rapidly (Figure 14-34). When the tooth is more deeply positioned, the adjacent tissue can be repositioned and the crown exposed, which usually leads to normal eruption. If there is further delay, traction can be applied to the exposed crown using a bonded attachment and fixed appliances (Figure 14-35).

If it is likely that unerupted teeth displaced by a supernumerary will have to be moved orthodontically, because of the distance they have been displaced or for other reasons, an attachment should be bonded to each unerupted tooth as it is exposed. Then a wire ligature or (better) a precious metal chain is attached to the bracket and extended out of the tissue so traction can be applied using a fixed appliance. Attachments sometimes are difficult to bond because of contamination of the tooth surface by saliva and hemorrhage, but the alternative approach of looping a wire

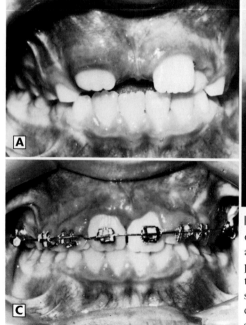
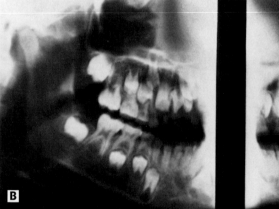
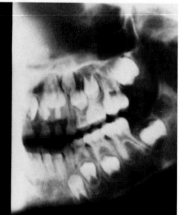

FIGURE 14-33   Multiple supernumerary teeth in the maxilla are often the cause of spacing and delayed eruption of anterior teeth. **A,** This patient has an exceptionally wide diastema and delayed eruption of the maxillary lateral incisors. **B,** The panoramic radiograph reveals three supernumeraries of various shapes and orientations. Conical and noninverted supernumeraries usually erupt, whereas tubercle shaped and inverted ones do not. **C,** The supernumeraries were removed, the diastema closed, and the remaining permanent teeth aligned with fixed appliances after they erupted.

around the cervical part of the crown requires more extensive bone removal and can compromise the ultimate health of the periodontal attachment.

A removable appliance can be used to produce the traction, but even though the appliance uses the palate as an anchorage source, tooth movement can be difficult to control and patient compliance is critical. A fixed appliance is much more efficient.

To obtain the necessary anchorage, a fixed appliance to bring an unerupted tooth into the arch should extend from molar to molar, attaching to as many other teeth as feasible, which during the mixed dentition years may mean some primary molars and canines. Before the unerupted tooth is clinically visible, the extruding force can be delivered by an elastomeric module, helical cantilever spring, or NiTi auxiliary (piggyback) wire. Any of these devices can be extended from a relatively stiff arch wire to the attachment on the unerupted tooth. Elastomeric materials produce a force that is relatively high initially but decays rapidly, so theoretically they are less desirable than springs that produce light continuous force. Despite this, because a displaced permanent tooth often is high in the vestibule, the inefficient but nonbulky elastomeric modules are often less irritating than springs and are an excellent starting point.

The best option at present often is to use the flexibility of the new superelastic arch wires (A-NiTi) while stabilizing across the edentulous area with another stiffer wire to control the reciprocal forces. This is accomplished by tying the superelastic wire over the base arch wire except in the area of the unerupted tooth, and deflecting it gingivally there to provide the traction (Figure 14-36) (see also Chapter 16). This combination of wires offers a simple and efficient method for moving unerupted teeth. Final root positioning can be achieved either in the mixed

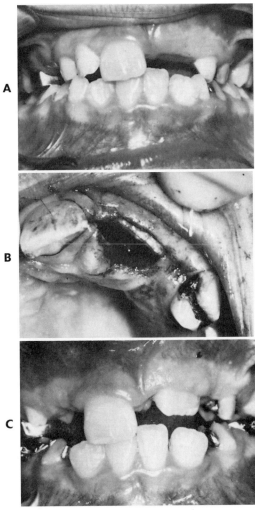

FIGURE 14-34 Overlying soft tissue may be the cause of delayed eruption after surgical intervention to remove primary or supernumerary teeth. **A,** This unerupted permanent maxillary left central incisor is covered by only soft tissue. **B,** Removal of a limited amount of the tissue while maintaining a band of keratinized tissue on the facial area (**C**) usually results in rapid eruption.

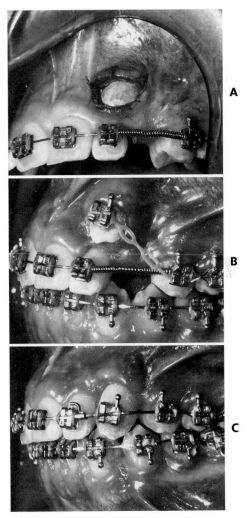

FIGURE 14-35 Unerupted canines sometimes require surgical exposure and traction to bring them into position in the dental arch. **A,** Initial traction with an elastomeric chain; **B,** tooth movement is continued using a continuous arch wire; **C,** the canine in final position.

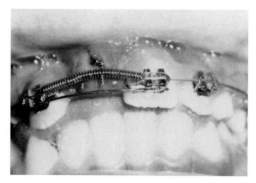

FIGURE 14-36 Traction to reposition unerupted permanent teeth can be applied by a variety of mechanisms. One of the most effective is a superelastic (A-NiTi) auxiliary wire in conjunction with a heavy stabilizing arch wire. The flexible superelastic wire is displaced apically to provide light continuous force, while the heavy arch wire tied into other brackets stabilizes the adjacent teeth as a unit and eliminates the reactive tipping movements. The coil spring to open space for the unerupted tooth can be removed after adequate space is created.

dentition or left until a second stage of treatment during the permanent dentition if one is anticipated.

Recently, it has been suggested that a magnet could be bonded to an unerupted tooth, so magnetic attraction could be used to move the tooth without the necessity of a ligature physically tying it to an appliance. The second magnet to provide the attractive force could be incorporated into a removable appliance or attached to an arch wire.[25,26] This method appears to have great promise for the future, as more powerful magnets that are safe to use intraorally are developed.

When force of any appreciable magnitude is applied, the unerupted tooth should begin to move. Failure to move indicates ankylosis. Sometimes a small bridge of bone is all that is preventing movement, and further surgical intervention (gentle luxation—see Chapter 16) can be helpful.

Delayed First Molars. Ectopic eruption, usually of a permanent maxillary first molar, also can be a cause of delayed eruption. If it is not possible to place a brass wire or separating spring (see Chapter 13), or if greater distal movement of the unerupted permanent first molar is required and access can be gained to the occlusal surface of the molar, a simple fixed appliance can be fabricated to move the molar distally. The appliance consists of a band on the primary molar (which can be further stabilized with a lingual arch) with a soldered 28 mil helical spring attached (Figure 14-37). A ledge of resin or a metal button is bonded to the permanent molar's occlusal surface for engagement of the spring. Alternatively, the spring can be bonded directly to the occlusal surface, but this makes spring adjustment difficult. Another option is to solder a heavy wire cantilever to a band on the primary second molar and extend it distally. An elastomeric chain can be stretched between the cantilever, and a button bonded to the occlusal surface of the molar. Occasionally it is difficult

to bond to the partially erupted tooth because the occlusal surface is contaminated by saliva. This may make it necessary to cut a preparation in the occlusal surface of the erupting molar so the end of the spring can lodge in the preparation and grip the tooth. The tooth is restored following tooth movement.

The technique detailed above can be extremely valuable as a means to disengage the erupting permanent tooth and retain the primary tooth. If the permanent molar has caused extensive resorption of the primary molar, there may be no choice but to extract it, and one should expect the permanent molar to continue to move mesially and shorten the arch length. Unless the second premolar is missing and the arch length is purposefully to be reduced, or unless considerable mesial molar movement is tolerable and later premolar extraction is planned, a distal shoe that guides the erupting molar should be placed after the extraction. Even if this technique is used, some space has already been lost and the permanent molar will have to be repositioned distally, using headgear[2] or another type of space regaining appliance as described above in this chapter.

CROSSBITES OF DENTAL ORIGIN

For both posterior and anterior crossbites, the distinction between skeletal and dental is important. Full-cusp bilateral posterior crossbite is quite likely to have a skeletal component. A unilateral posterior crossbite can be due to maxillary or mandibular skeletal asymmetry. If multiple teeth are in anterior crossbite, it is quite likely that the problem is a jaw discrepancy, not just displacement of teeth. Treatment procedures for these skeletal problems during the mixed dentition years are covered in Chapter 15.

Dental crossbites, in contrast, are due to displacement of teeth. They usually affect only some of the teeth in an area of the arch, as a rule are less severe so that occlusal interferences on closure often are present. Posterior dental crossbite is much more likely to be due to displacement of maxillary than mandibular teeth.

Posterior Crossbite

The apparently unilateral posterior crossbite seen frequently in young children, which usually is due to mild bilateral constriction of the maxillary arch that creates occlusal interferences and a mandibular shift on closure, is not a severe problem and has been discussed in Chapter 13.

When true unilateral posterior crossbite exists because maxillary teeth are displaced, three relatively simple methods can be applied: unequal W-arches or quad helixes, lower arches stabilized with lingual arches to support crosselastics to the maxillary teeth, or a removable appliance that has been sectioned asymmetrically. All are described in Chapter 13. A final alternative, the most elegant biomechanically, is to use a lingual arch activated as a one-couple device, so that bodily movement on the anchorage side is

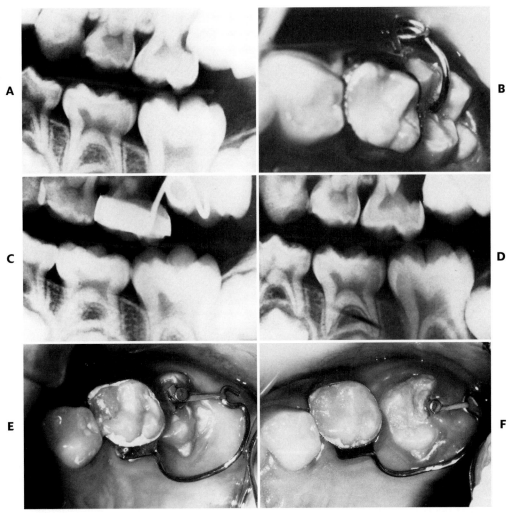

FIGURE 14-37   Ectopic eruption with severe resorption may require appliance therapy. **A,** This primary maxillary second molar shows severe resorption. **B,** If the occlusal surface of the permanent molar is accessible, the primary molar can be banded and a 20 mil spring soldered to the band. **C,** The permanent molar is tipped distally out of the resorption defect and (**D**) once disengaged, is free to erupt. **E** and **F,** Another appliance to reposition an ectopically erupting maxillary first molar is a band on the second primary molar with a soldered wire (28 mil steel) cantilever arm. An elastomeric chain is attached from the arm to a button bonded on the ectopic molar. Both the arm and the elastomeric attachment serve as sources of elastic force. Bonding the button and replacing the chain, however, can be challenging.

pitted against facial tipping on the movement side (see Figure 10-44). With any of these methods, the teeth will be tipped rather than moved bodily, which usually is satisfactory in correcting dental crossbites.

Anterior Crossbite

Dental anterior crossbite usually involves only one or two teeth that were displaced because of severe crowding. Crossbite correction becomes possible only after space for the teeth has been created by disking or, more frequently, extraction of the primary canines. Although some anterior crossbites can be treated with removable appliances as described in Chapter 13, a fixed appliance is more effective and is required to correct severely displaced incisors.

One of the simplest fixed appliances for this purpose is a maxillary lingual arch with fingersprings (sometimes referred to as whip springs). This appliance is indicated for a very young child or preadolescent with whom compliance problems are anticipated. It consists of a 36 mil maxillary lingual arch to which 22 mil springs are soldered (Figure 14-38). The springs are usually soldered on the opposite side of the arch from the tooth to be corrected, in order to increase the length of the spring and are most effective if they are approximately 15 mm long. This length provides exceptional flexibility and range, but occasionally a spur is needed to serve as a guide wire to keep the wires from slipping over the incisal edge of the incisors. When these springs are activated properly at each

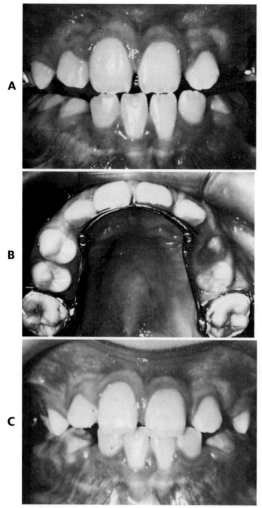

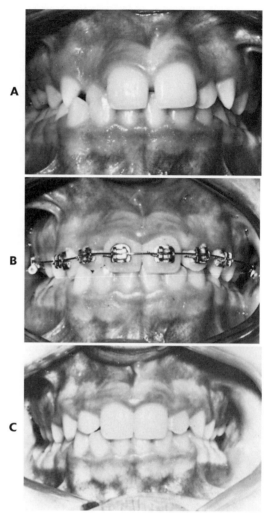

FIGURE 14-38   **A,** An anterior crossbite caused by lingual position of the maxillary incisors can be corrected using (**B**) a 36 mil lingual arch with soldered 22 mil finger springs. A guide wire can be placed between the incisors as shown here to keep the springs from moving incisally. **C,** After correction, the appliance can be modified to serve as a retainer by soldering the free ends of the springs to the lingual arch.

FIGURE 14-39   Fixed appliance treatment with bonded attachments and arch wires used to correct anterior crossbite and alignment problems. **A,** The maxillary right lateral incisor is in crossbite, and the other maxillary anterior teeth are malaligned. **B,** The anterior teeth are bonded and the permanent first molars banded so that an arch wire can be used to efficiently correct the rotation and faciolingual displacement. **C,** The patient shows a stable correction after retention and appliance removal.

monthly visit (advancing the spring about 3 mm), they produce tooth movement at the optimum rate of 1 mm per month. Overcorrection and retention are recommended with this appliance. The greatest problems with it are distortion and breakage from poor patient cooperation and poor oral hygiene, which can lead to decalcification and decay.

Another fixed appliance method to tip the maxillary incisors forward is the use of posterior bands and anterior bonded attachments with a round arch wire. This may be the best choice for a somewhat older mixed dentition patient with crowding, rotations, and more permanent teeth in crossbite (Figure 14-39). In these children, adjacent primary teeth may not be available for disking, and permanent teeth need to be moved facially or apart to provide

the space specifically where it is needed. With generalized crowding and irregularity, a flexible wire can be used to solve both problems. If only selected teeth are at fault, a stiffer arch wire with a superelastic "piggyback" overlay to provide local flexibility (see Chapter 16) would be more appropriate.

A 2 × 4 arch wire approach also can be used to provide any mix of facial tipping and lingual root torque to bring maxillary incisors out of crossbite (see Figure 10-40).[27] If the arch wire is placed with an asymmetric V-bend with a greater moment to the incisors but is free to move anteriorly and slide through the molar tube, the incisors will tip facially and increase the overjet. If the arch wire is tied back or cinched to the molars, it will provide lingual root torque to the incisors.

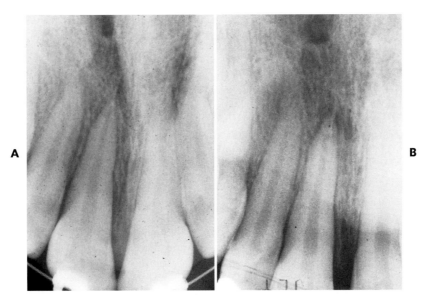

FIGURE 14-40 Multiple vertical positioned radiographs are required for an adequate diagnosis of previously traumatized teeth. **A,** This radiograph displays no periapical pathology 2 weeks after the trauma to the central incisors, but **B,** this radiograph exposed at the same time from a different vertical position shows a periapical radiolucency at the apex of the maxillary right central incisor.

Controlling the teeth in three planes of space is much more difficult than simply tipping them and requires careful planning and excellent clinical technique. As with any anterior crossbite correction, these teeth should be stabilized for 1 to 2 months after tooth movement and can then be released without further retention if the overbite is sufficient. Patient care for the appliance is the most critical factor during treatment.

DEEP BITE

Before treating a deep bite, it is necessary to establish its cause. The problem may result from reduced lower face height and lack of eruption of the posterior teeth, or from overeruption of the anterior teeth. The possible treatments attack the cause of the problem and are mutually exclusive.

Removable biteplate appliances to reduce the overbite can be used for patients who have less than normal eruption of the posterior teeth (which is usually associated with reduced face height). An anterior biteplate is incorporated into a removable appliance so that the mandibular incisors occlude with the plastic plane lingual to the maxillary incisors. This approach prevents the posterior teeth from occluding and encourages their eruption, which may take several months. The appliance must be worn on a full-time basis during this phase of treatment. The posterior eruption is hard to regulate, and once the proper vertical dimension has been established, the biteplate must continue to be worn or the anterior teeth will erupt and the deep bite will return.

A utility arch that incorporates molar and incisor teeth can be used during the mixed dentition to intrude, tip, or reposition both molars and incisors (see Figure 14-17). This appliance is versatile and effective in reducing overbite by relative intrusion but it can be difficult to control and often produces unwanted reciprocal movements (see Chapter 10 for details of the biomechanics of the utility arch). Molar extrusion should be expected with any incisor change. Molar rotation often occurs, and the arch wire may become imbedded in the buccal mucosa. A lingual arch to reinforce the anchorage usually is needed. Like many effective orthodontic appliances, the utility arch is deceptively simple and must be used with considerable care.

A more challenging approach to deep bite is necessary when the maxillary or mandibular anterior teeth have erupted excessively. For these patients the task is to stop the eruption (relatively intrude) or actually intrude the incisors. This type of tooth movement requires light continuous forces and careful management of the posterior teeth that provide anchorage. Realistically, although bite depth changes can be made in the mixed dentition by intrusion of anterior teeth, intrusion is difficult to retain—even in later phases of full appliance therapy. For this reason, intrusion as a part of early treatment is seldom required. It is often better to defer this treatment until the early permanent dentition, using an intrusion arch during the first stage of comprehensive fixed appliance therapy (see Chapter 16 for details).

TRAUMATIC DISPLACEMENT

A common problem that requires orthodontic intervention is repositioning traumatically displaced teeth. When teeth are treated immediately following a traumatic injury, they are usually repositioned with finger pressure and stabilized (with a light wire or nylon filament) for 7 to 10 days. At this point, the teeth usually exhibit physiologic mobility, and the prognosis is better if they are not splinted any longer.

For teeth that have been displaced in any direction and are consolidated in their new position, light orthodontic forces should allow successful repositioning. It is wise to counsel the patient and parents to be aware that pain, swelling, or discharge are signs of pulpal necrosis and require endodontic therapy. The larger the displacement and the more developed the root, the more likely it is that pulp therapy will be required. Nevertheless, any tooth can become nonvital following a traumatic injury. For this reason, follow-up periapical radiographs should be taken at various vertical positions at 2 to 3 weeks, 6 to 8 weeks, and 1 year post-injury to check for pathologic changes (Figure 14-40). This is a good policy if a patient has been referred for repositioning of displaced teeth, or if a patient in active orthodontic treatment sustains trauma.

If the teeth have been displaced vertically, it is best to begin traction as soon as possible (Figure 14-41). All severely intruded teeth with mature apices become nonvital.[28] Early repositioning is critical to reduce the chance of ankylosis, improve access for endodontics, and complete the diagnosis; crown and root fractures can remain undiagnosed even following extensive radiographs. Within 2 weeks of the injury, the tooth should have been moved enough to allow endodontic access—ideally, it would be at or near the pre-trauma position. Pulp therapy is best instituted within 2 weeks to reduce the possibility of resorption.[29]

The methods used to reposition teeth displaced by supernumeraries (see earlier in this chapter) are equally applicable to teeth that were intruded by trauma. The hallmarks of good treatment are tissue compatibility, good hygiene, appropriate (light) forces, and efficient use of the appliance. After the tooth has been fully erupted, it can be retained and finally positioned. If further tooth movement will be needed during a second stage of comprehensive treatment, calcium hydroxide can be retained in the pulp chamber until active tooth movement is completed as a hedge against resorption.

Teeth with extrusion luxation injuries that were not immediately reduced pose a difficult problem. These teeth have reduced bony support and a poor crown root ratio. Attempts to intrude them result in bony defects between the teeth, so orthodontic intrusion is not a good plan. When the discrepancy is minor to moderate, reshaping the tooth by crown reduction may be the best plan (Figure 14-42).

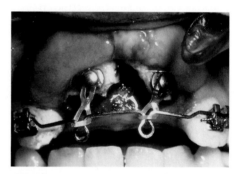

FIGURE 14-41 Early traction following intrusion of permanent teeth is critical to complete the diagnosis, prevent ankylosis, and ensure adequate endodontic access if necessary.

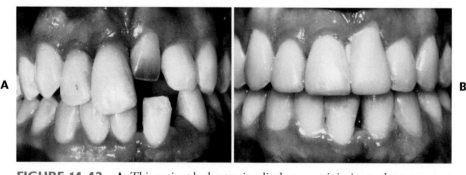

FIGURE 14-42 **A,** This patient had extrusive displacement injuries to the permanent incisors. **B,** Because it is difficult to intrude these teeth and eliminate the subsequent bony defect, the crowns of these teeth were reduced to provide a better crown-root ratio and improve the appearance.

REFERENCES

1. Gianelly AA: One-phase versus two phase treatment, Am J Orthod 108:556-9, 1995.
2. Kurol J, Bjerklin K: Treatment of children with ectopic eruption of the maxillary first permanent molar by cervical traction, Am J Orthod 86:483-492, 1984.
3. Baumrind S, Korn EL, Isaacson RJ et al: Quantitative analysis of orthodontic and orthopedic effects of maxillary traction, Am J Orthod 84:384-398, 1983.
4. Hershey H, Houghton C, Burstone C: Unilateral face-bows: a theoretical and laboratory analysis, Am J Orthod 79:229-249, 1981.
5. Cetlin NM, Ten Hoeve A: Nonextraction treatment, J Clin Orthod 17:396-413, 1983.
6. Dahlquist A, Gebauer U, Ingervall B: The effect of a transpalatal arch for correction of first molar rotation, Eur J Orthod 18:257-267, 1996.
7. Byloff FK, Darendeliler MA: Distal molar movement using the pendulum appliance, part 1: Clinical and radiographic indications, Angle Orthod 67:249-60, 1997.
8. Gianelly AA, Bednar J, Dietz VS: Japanese NiTi coils used to move molars distally, Am J Orthod 99:564-6; 1991.
9. Bondemark L, Kurol J: Molar distal movement with magnets Class II correction with magnets and superelastic coils followed by straight-wire mechanotherapy: occlusal changes during and after dental therapy, J Orofac Orthop 59:127-38,1998.
10. McInaney JB, Adams RM, Freeman M: A nonextraction approach to crowded dentitions in young children: early recognition and treatment, J Am Dent Assoc 101:252-257, 1980.
11. Lutz HD, Poulton D: Stability of dental arch expansion in the deciduous dentition, Angle Orthod 55:299-315, 1985.
12. Bench RW, Gugino CF, Hilgers JJ: Bioprogressive therapy, part VIII, J Clin Orthod 12:279-298, 1978.
13. McNamara JA, Brudon W: Orthodontic and orthopedic treatment in the mixed dentition, Ann Arbor, Mich., 1995, Needham Press.
14. Owen A: Morphologic changes in the sagittal dimension using the Frankel appliance, Am J Orthod 80:573-603, 1981.
15. Ten Hoeve A: Palatal bar and lip bumper in nonextraction treatment, J Clin Orthod 272-91, 1985.
16. Osborn WS, Nanda RS, Currier GF: Mandibular arch perimeter changes with lip bumper treatment, Am J Orthod 99:527-532, 1991.
17. O'Donnell S, Nanda RS, Ghosh J: Perioral forces and dental changes resulting from mandibular lip bumper treatment, Am J Orthod. 113:247-55,1998.
18. Dewel B: A critical analysis of serial extraction in orthodontic treatment, Am J Orthod 45:424-455, 1959.
19. Edwards J: The diastema, the frenum and the frenectomy: a clinical study, Am J Orthod 71:489-508, 1977.
20. Cronin RJ Jr, Oesterle LJ: Implant use in growing patients: Treatment planning concerns, Dent Clin North Am 42: 1-34,1998.
21. Joondeph D, McNeill R: Congenitally absent second premolars: an interceptive approach, Am J Orthod 59:50-66, 1971.
22. Paulsen HU, Andreasen JO, Schwartz O: Pulp and periodontal healing, root development and root resorption subsequent to transplantation and orthodontic rotation: a long-term study of autotransplanted premolars, Am J Orthod 108:630-40,1995.
23. Primosch R: Anterior supernumerary teeth assessment and surgical intervention in children, Pediatr Dent 3:204-215, 1981.
24. DiBase D: Mucous membrane and delayed eruption, Trans Br Soc Study Orthod 56:149-158, 1969-70.
25. Vardimon AD, Graber TM, Drescher D, Bourauel C: Rare earth magnets and impaction, Am J Orthod Dentofac Orthop 100:494-512, 1991.
26. Bondemark L, Kurol J, Hallonsten AL, Andreasen JO: Extrusion with magnets. Attractive magnets for orthodontic extrusion of crown-root fractured teeth, Am J Orthod 112:187-93, 1997.
27. Isaacson RJ, Rebellato J: Two-couple orthodontic appliance systems: torquing arches, Sem Orthod 1:31-36, 1995.
28. Andreasen JO, Andreasen FM: Textbook and color atlas of traumatic injuries to the teeth, ed 3, Copenhagen, 1994, Munksgaard.
29. Turley PK, Crawford LB, Carrington KW: Traumatically intruded teeth, Angle Orthod 57:234-44, 1987.

CHAPTER

15

Treatment of Skeletal Problems in Preadolescent Children

Whenever a jaw discrepancy exists, the ideal solution is to correct it by modifying the child's facial growth, so that the skeletal problem is corrected by more growth of one jaw than the other (Figure 15-1). Unfortunately, such an ideal solution is not always possible, but growth modification for skeletal problems can be quite successful.

Treatment planning for skeletal problems has been discussed extensively in Chapter 8. The emphasis there is on new research that both confirms the possibility of changing the way the jaws grow and emphasizes the variability of the results and the relatively modest changes that often are produced. In this chapter, we assume that an appropriate treatment plan has been developed, using the guidelines from the previous chapters. The focus is on the clinical use of growth modification methods in preadolescent children. The development of functional appliances to guide jaw growth, and the various components that can be incorporated into these appliances, are covered in detail in Chapter 11. The development of headgear—the other major method for Class II treatment—is reviewed in this chapter, along with other fixed appliances for growth modification.

Growth modification, through either a functional appliance or extraoral force, is aimed at the maxillary sutures and/or the mandibular condyles. Usually this is accomplished by applying forces directly to the teeth and secondarily and indirectly to the skeletal structures, instead of applying direct pressure to the bones. Tooth movement, in addition to any changes in skeletal relationships, is inevitable. It is possible now to apply force directly against the bone by using natural implants (ankylosed teeth) that can be removed later or temporary osseointegrated implants (see Chapter 9). This approach is likely to be used more and more in the future because the dental changes that accompany growth modification often (but not always) are undesirable. Excessive tooth movement, whether it results from a weakness in the treatment plan, poor biomechanical control, or poor compliance, can cause growth modification to be incomplete and unsuccessful. Successful growth modification must consider and account for treatment effects on the dentition, as well as the skeletal structures.

The material in this chapter is organized in the context of the child's major skeletal problem, because that is the most logical way to do it. In some cases that provides a precise description—the upper or lower jaw is clearly at fault because of its position and size, and the malocclusion is almost totally due to the jaw discrepancy. More frequently, Class II or Class III malocclusions are caused by several subtle deviations from the normal, some skeletal and some dental. In such cases, the therapy must be based on the solutions to that specific patient's set of problems. In particular, dental changes that would be unwanted side effects in some patients can be quite helpful in others—and vice versa. For this reason, the secondary as well as the primary effects of the various appliances are reviewed in detail in this chapter.

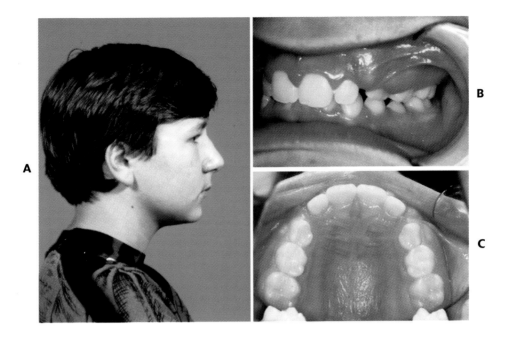

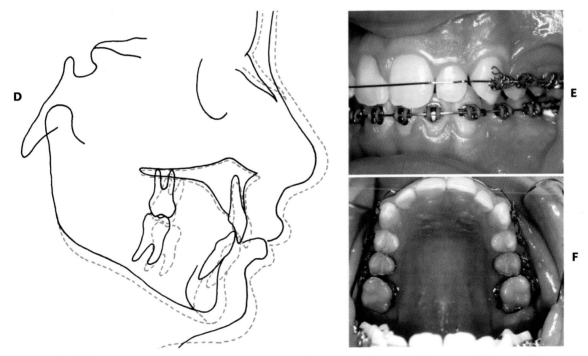

FIGURE 15-1 **A-C,** At age 11-10, this boy sought treatment because of trauma to his protruding front teeth and for correction of the crowding that was developing in the upper arch, where there was no room for the permanent canines. Skeletal Class II malocclusion, due primarily to mandibular deficiency, was apparent. Because of the damaged maxillary central incisors (one of which had a root fracture), the treatment plan called for cervical headgear to promote differential mandibular growth and create space in the maxillary arch. **D,** Fifteen months of headgear during the adolescent growth spurt produced significant improvement in the jaw relationship with differential forward growth of the mandible and created nearly enough space to bring the maxillary canines into the arch. **E-F,** A partial fixed appliance was placed, staying off the traumatized maxillary incisors until the very end of treatment, and light Class II elastics off a stabilized lower arch were used. *continued*

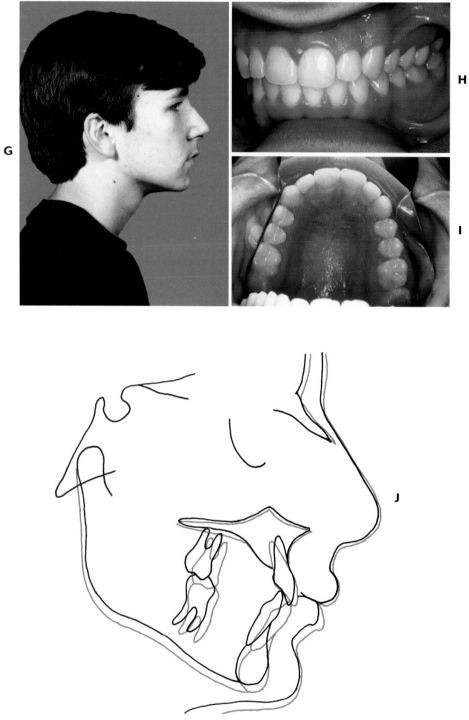

FIGURE 15-1, cont'd G-I, The 15-month second stage of treatment produced excellent dental relationships, but note in the cephalometric superimposition of changes in phase 2 (**J**) that minimal further anteroposterior growth occurred. This illustrates the importance of starting growth modification treatment in the mixed dentition prior to eruption of all permanent teeth.

THE TIMING OF GROWTH MODIFICATION

Whatever the type of appliance that is used or the kind of growth effect that is desired, if growth is to be modified, the patient has to be growing. Growth modification must be done before the adolescent growth spurt ends. In theory, it could be done at any point up to that time. The ideal timing remains somewhat controversial, but recent research has clarified the indications for treatment at various ages. This material is discussed in detail in Chapter 8 and is briefly reviewed and summarized here.

Because of the rapid growth exhibited by children during the primary dentition years, it would seem that treatment of jaw discrepancies by growth modification should be successful at a very early age. The rationale for treatment at ages 4 to 6 would be that because of the rapid rate of growth, significant amounts of skeletal discrepancy could be overcome in a short time. This implies that once discrepancies in jaw relationships are corrected, proper function will cause harmonious growth thereafter without further treatment.

If this were the case, very early treatment would be advocated for many skeletal discrepancies. Unfortunately, although most anteroposterior and vertical problems can be treated during the primary dentition years, relapse occurs because of continued growth in the original disproportionate pattern. If children are treated very early, they usually need further treatment during the mixed dentition and again in the early permanent dentition to maintain the correction.[1]

The opposite point of view would be that, since treatment in the permanent dentition will be required anyway, there is no point in starting treatment until then. Delaying treatment that long has two potential problems: (1) by the time the canines, premolars and second molars erupt there may not be enough growth remaining for effective modification, especially in girls; and (2) the child would be denied the psychosocial and functional benefits of treatment during an important period of development. It now is clear that a child can benefit from treatment during the preadolescent years if esthetic and the resultant social problems are substantial, if he or she is trauma prone, or if other specific indications exist (e.g., extreme severity, combined vertical and anteroposterior problems, asymmetry, history of trauma, etc.)—see Chapter 8. On the other hand, it seems to be neither necessary nor desirable to routinely begin treatment for moderately severe skeletal problems until the adolescent growth spurt, which often coincides with the eruption of the remaining permanent teeth. Beginning treatment too soon merely prolongs it unnecessarily. For each patient, the benefits of early treatment must be considered against the risk and cost of prolonging the total treatment period.

TREATMENT OF MANDIBULAR DEFICIENCY

Possible Approaches to Treatment

In theory, functional appliances stimulate and enhance mandibular growth, while headgear retards maxillary growth—so functional appliances would seem to be an obvious choice for treatment of mandibular deficiency, and headgear an equally obvious choice for maxillary excess. As a general rule this is correct, but the distinction between the two appliance systems and the indications for their use, are not as clear-cut as the first sentence would imply.

In functional appliance treatment, additional growth is supposed to occur in response to the movement of the mandibular condyle out of the fossa, mediated by reduced pressure on the condylar tissues or by altered muscle tension on the condyle (Figure 15-2). Although an acceleration of mandibular growth often occurs, a long-term increase in size is difficult to demonstrate (see Figure 8-24). An effect on the maxilla, although small, is almost always observed along with any mandibular effects. When the

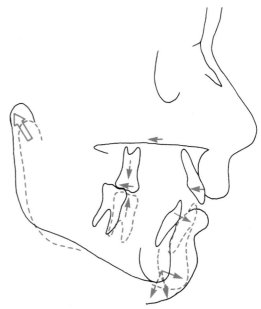

FIGURE 15-2 The side effects of functional appliance therapy for correction of a Class II skeletal malocclusion are illustrated here. The most desirable and variable effect is for the mandible to increase in length as shown by the open arrow, possibly repositioning the TM fossa by apposition. The "headgear effect" restrains the maxilla and the maxillary teeth, and mandibular repositioning often creates forces against the lower teeth that cause anterior movement of the mandibular dentition. The direction in which mandibular growth is expressed, forward and/or inferiorly, is most related to the eruption of the molars. If the molars erupt more than the ramus grows in height (*dashed arrows*), the forward mandibular change will be negated and the Class II malocclusion will not improve.

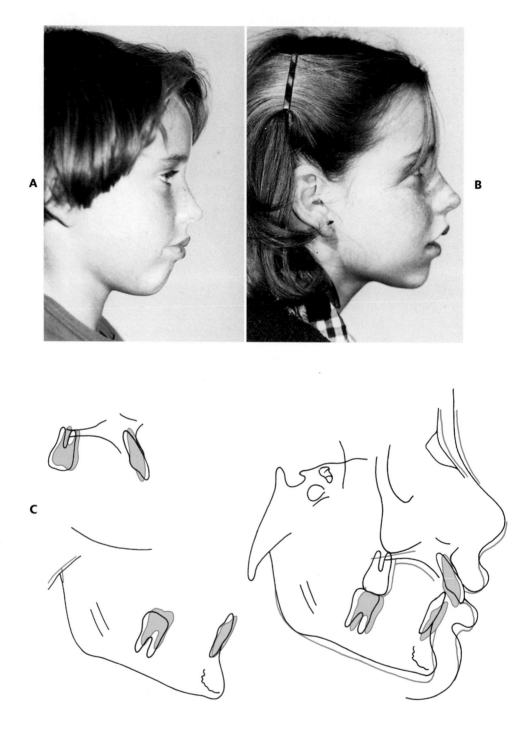

FIGURE 15-3   This child was treated with a functional appliance in an effort to correct the Class II malocclusion by changing the skeletal relationships. **A,** Pre-treatment profile; **B,** post-treatment profile; **C,** cephalometric superimposition. Note that the major skeletal change seen in the cranial base superimposition is the restriction of forward change of the maxilla. This "headgear effect" is observed in most functional appliance treatment that anteriorly positions the mandible. Note also the differential eruption of the lower molars and forward movement of the lower teeth.

mandible is held forward, the elasticity of the soft tissues produces a reactive force against the maxilla, and restraint of maxillary growth often occurs (Figure 15-3). In the Florida clinical trial (see Chapter 8), where the effects of a bionator were compared with headgear with a biteplate, the anteroposterior effects on the maxilla were similar.[2] More generally, functional appliances show a greater effect on the mandible,[3] especially in the short term, but produce some restraint of maxillary growth as well.

Functional appliances and headgear do differ in their effects on the dentition. Headgear force against the molar teeth often tips them distally but usually has little effect on other teeth. Functional appliances, especially the tooth-borne ones, often place a distal force against the upper incisors that tends to tip them lingually. This can be substantial. For removable appliances, it depends on how the relationship between the labial bow and the anterior teeth is handled and, for fixed functionals, on which anterior and posterior teeth are included in the anchorage units through supplementary bonding or banding. In addition, most functional appliances exert a protrusive effect on the mandibular dentition because the appliance contacts the lower teeth, and some of the reaction force from forward posturing of the mandible is transmitted to them. With the fixed functional appliances (e.g., Herbst, bonded twin block), usually there is greater dental change due to the continuous forces. These appliances create more protrusion of mandibular incisors than removable functionals and, in the case of the Herbst, maxillary posterior dental intrusion and more maxillary dental retrusion.[4,5,6]

The combination of maxillary dental retraction and mandibular dental protrusion that all functional appliances create is similar to the effect of interarch elastics. This "Class II elastics effect" can be quite helpful in children who have maxillary dental protrusion and mandibular dental retrusion in conjunction with a Class II skeletal problem, but the same effect is deleterious in patients who exhibit maxillary dental retrusion or mandibular dental protrusion. Mandibular dental protrusion usually contraindicates functional appliance treatment.

Functional appliances also can influence eruption of posterior and anterior teeth. It is possible to level an excessive curve of Spee in the lower arch by blocking eruption of the lower incisors while leaving the lower posterior teeth free to erupt. If upper posterior teeth are prohibited from erupting and moving forward while lower posterior teeth are erupting up and forward, the resulting rotation of the occlusal plane and forward movement of the dentition will contribute to correction of the Class II dental relationship. This is another effect of most functional appliance treatment for Class II problems (Figure 15-4).[7]

It is important to keep in mind that eruption of posterior teeth in a mandibular deficient patient is beneficial only when good vertical growth is occurring. More erup-

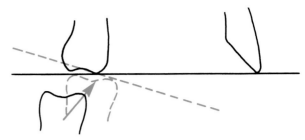

FIGURE 15-4 To facilitate Class II correction, the mesial and vertical eruption of the mandibular molar can be used advantageously. The upward and forward movement will improve the molar relationship and establish the posterior occlusal plane at the higher level.

tion of posterior teeth than growth of the ramus causes mandibular growth to be projected more downward than forward. In patients who have a tendency toward vertical rather than anteroposterior growth even without treatment, further posterior eruption must be prevented to avoid growth being expressed entirely vertically (Figure 15-5). The special problems created by excessive vertical growth are discussed later in this chapter.

The other possible treatment for a mandibular deficiency is to restrain growth of the maxilla with extraoral force (Figure 15-6) and let the mandible, continuing to grow more or less normally, catch up (Figure 15-7). Some evidence indicates that patients who wear headgear to the maxilla exhibit more mandibular growth than untreated Class II children, but generally the findings have indicated that mandibular change measured against controls is not significant.

On balance, despite the maxillary skeletal and dental effects that go along with any enhancement of mandibular growth, functional appliances usually are preferred for mixed dentition treatment of mandibular deficiency. The types of functional appliances and their components are described in Chapter 11. In the sections below, we discuss treatment procedures in using them clinically.

Treatment Procedures with Functional Appliances

Pretreatment Alignment. After treatment goals have been established and the decision has been made to use a functional appliance, the incisor position and relationships should be carefully examined. Because functional appliances for the treatment of mandibular deficiency require the mandible to be held in a protruded position to have a treatment effect, the patient's ability to posture forward at least 4 to 6 mm (i.e., to a reasonably normal mandibular position) is critical. Most mandibularly deficient children have a large overjet and can do this readily, but in some cases incisor interferences prevent the mandible from being advanced to the correct position for the bite registration. The problem can be either lingual

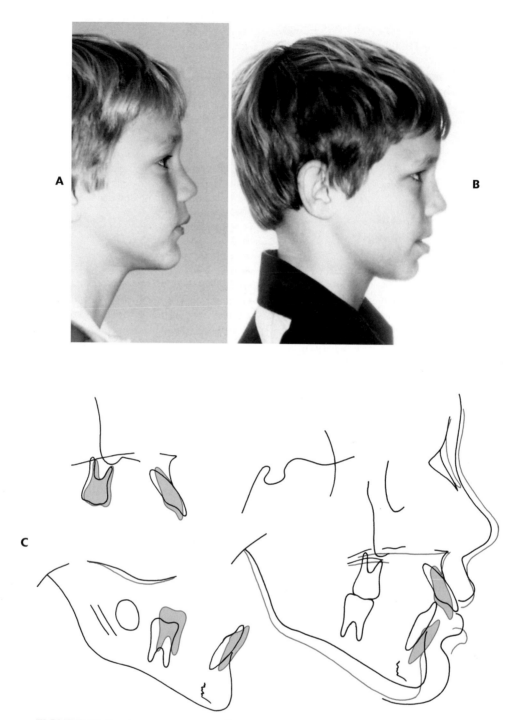

FIGURE 15-5   A poor response to Class II functional appliance treatment. **A,** Pre-treatment profile; **B,** post-treatment profile; **C,** cephalometric superimpositions. Note that before treatment the child had a tendency toward increased lower face height and a convex profile. The cranial base superimposition indicates that the mandible rotated inferiorly and backward because of excessive eruption of the lower molar, which further increased the lower face height and facial convexity. Note in the mandibular and maxillary superimpositions the anterior movement of the lower incisors, and the retraction of the upper incisors, neither of which was desirable.

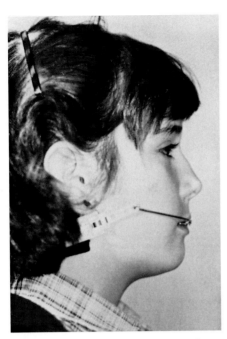

FIGURE 15-6 A Kloehn-type headgear appliance. This appliance uses a cervical neckstrap and a facebow to produce distal force on the maxillary teeth and maxilla, is aimed at altering maxillary size and position.

displacement of the upper incisors (a Class II, division 2 incisor pattern) or irregular and crowded incisors in either arch. (It must be kept in mind that facial displacement of the lower incisors, which would be produced by aligning crowded lower incisors, contraindicates functional appliance treatment).

For both the Class II, division 2 patient with limited overjet and the Class II, division 1 patient with crowded and irregular incisors, the first step in treatment is to tip the upper incisors forward and/or align them (Figure 15-8). Either fixed or removable appliances can be used for this purpose, depending on the type and magnitude of tooth movement required. This creates overjet so that an appropriate working bite can be obtained with the mandible positioned anteriorly and inferiorly to correct the horizontal and vertical deficiency. To control their tendency to relapse lingually, the repositioned incisors should be held in place for several months before the active functional appliance therapy begins.

Impressions and Working Bite. The next step in the use of a removable functional appliance is to make impressions of the upper and lower arches and register the desired mandibular position, the "working bite." The impression technique depends on the appliance components that will be used (see Chapter 11). Good reproduction of the teeth and an accurate representation of the area where the lingual pads or flanges will be placed are mandatory. If buccal shields or lip pads are to be used, it is important not to overextend the impressions so that tissue is displaced,

because this makes it difficult or impossible to accurately locate the appliance components in the vestibule. Improper location of the components leads to long-term soft tissue irritation, discomfort, difficulty in appliance adjustment, and poor patient compliance (Figure 15-9).

The working bite is obtained with multiple layers of a wax hard enough to maintain its integrity after cooling to room temperature. The patient's preliminary record casts can be used to trim the wax to a size that will register all posterior teeth, while not covering the anterior teeth (Figure 15-10). With the anterior teeth exposed, the position of the mandible easily can be judged while the bite is being taken. Care must be exercised to avoid any soft tissue interference with the wax, which will deflect the mandible or interfere with closure. This is most likely to occur in the retromolar pad region. If such an interference is not detected, the finished appliance will not seat correctly. At best, this will require reduction of the posterior plastic stops if they were integrated into the design. At worst, a new bite registration and appliance will be necessary.

The working bite for a Class II patient is obtained by advancing the mandible forward to move the condyles out of the fossa. Unless an asymmetry is to be corrected, the mandible should be advanced symmetrically so that the midline relationships do not change appreciably. We recommend a 4 to 6 mm advancement, but always one that is comfortable for the patient and does not move the incisors past an edge-to-edge incisor relationship. From a scientific perspective it appears that quite large, modest, or relatively small advancements all can produce growth modification, and that there is little difference between the results.[8]

The practical reason for recommending this modest advancement is greater patient comfort than with large advancements, which leads to better patient compliance without the need for as many appliance adjustments as smaller advancements would require.

When the mandible is advanced, the bite also must be opened. There must be enough space for the laboratory technician to place wire and plastic between the teeth to connect major components of the appliance and construct occlusal and incisor stops. The minimal posterior opening to achieve the vertical space is about 3 to 4 mm. If dental changes from differential eruption are not a major part of the desired treatment response, wire occlusal stops (as in the Frankel appliance) can be used at this minimal opening. Interocclusal stops or facets to guide eruption, as in most activators and bionators, usually require 4 to 5 mm of posterior separation to be effective. If eruption of upper and lower posterior teeth is to be limited, as in a child with excessive vertical face height (see further discussion later in this chapter), the working bite should be taken with the patient open 2 to 3 mm past the resting vertical dimension (i.e., 5 to 6 mm total opening in the molar region), so that

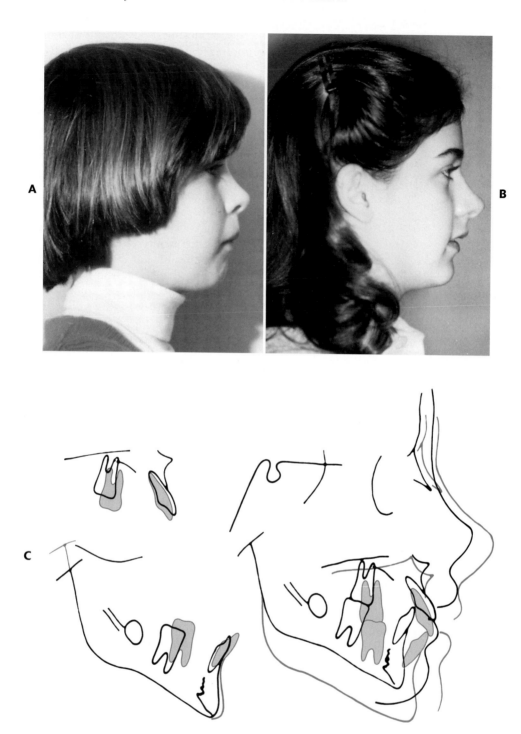

FIGURE 15-7   Headgear is sometimes used for patients with mandibular deficiencies. Facial appearance before (**A**) and after (**B**) treatment using headgear and Class II elastics; (**C**) cephalometric superimpositions of the treatment effects. This patient showed restriction of maxillary growth and some impressive mandibular growth, combined with distal movement of the upper teeth and mesial movement of the lower teeth, which were accompanied by posterior eruption.

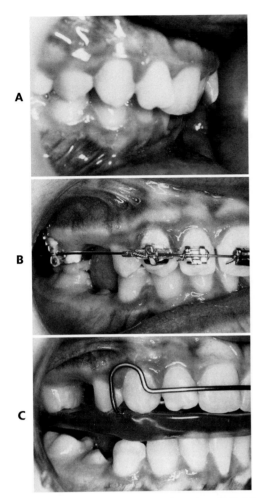

FIGURE 15-8 **A,** For this girl with a Class II division 2 malocclusion, it was impossible to take the bite registration for a functional appliance until the maxillary incisors were tipped facially; **B,** Although this change was made with a removable maxillary appliance with finger springs until recently, the prefunctional alignment now often can be accomplished more efficiently with a partial fixed appliance, as here; **C,** Same patient four months later, with a deep bite bionator in place after repositioning of the maxillary incisors was completed. It is no longer unusual to use a period of fixed appliance treatment in preparation for removable appliance treatment, the reverse of what might have been done not so long ago.

the soft tissue stretch against the bite blocks will produce a continuous force opposing eruption.

In preparation for obtaining the working bite, the wax is softened in hot water, while the child is directed to practice the working bite position. Some children can easily reproduce working bites after only a few practice tries, but others need more opportunities and perhaps some help. It is possible to aid these patients by constructing an index to guide them. This is most easily accomplished by using a stack of tongue blades with notches carved into the top and bottom blade (see Figure 15-10, *D*). This guide will stop

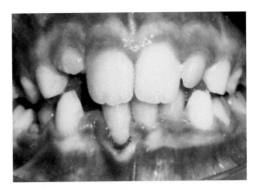

FIGURE 15-9 Patient with stripping of gingival tissue facial to the mandibular right central incisor, caused by improper placement and adjustment of a lip pad on a Frankel appliance.

the bite closure at the predetermined jaw separation and determine the anteroposterior mandibular position at the same time. Other children can be directed very simply with the use of a Boley gauge held near the teeth and "coaching" (see Figure 15-10, *E*).

To produce the working bite, the technique follows the steps illustrated in Figure 15-10. First, firmly seat the softened wax on the maxillary arch so all teeth are indexed. Next, have the child position the mandible forward to the correct position and close to the desired position, paying careful attention to reproducing the previous midline relationship. If a vertical stop made of tongue blades is used, it must remain in the proper orientation. Otherwise, as the tongue blades are inclined either inferiorly or superiorly, the mandible will either be closed and retrude or opened, respectively. When the correct bite has been obtained, the wax should be cooled and removed from the mouth. The bite should be examined for adequate dental registration and soft tissue interferences and rechecked for accuracy.

For the fixed (cemented, bonded, or partially fixed) functional appliance, accurate impressions of the teeth are essential, but extension of the impressions into the vestibules is not important.[9] If bands or steel crowns are used to retain a Herbst appliance (Figure 15-11), they are usually best adapted and retained by fitting them, making impressions over them, and then transferring them to the laboratory casts by placing them in the impressions before pouring the casts. Bands or crowns can be fabricated indirectly by a laboratory, but some accuracy is sacrificed. Most clinicians have deserted bands for retention of fixed functional appliances because they have proved to be easily distorted and broken. Metal crowns, which are fit without reducing the teeth; cast splints that can be bonded; or bonded acrylic splints are more satisfactory. The bonded splints eliminate the need to separate teeth and therefore reduce both laboratory and clinical time. The working bite for a Herbst appliance is similar to the one for a removable functional appliance, typically with

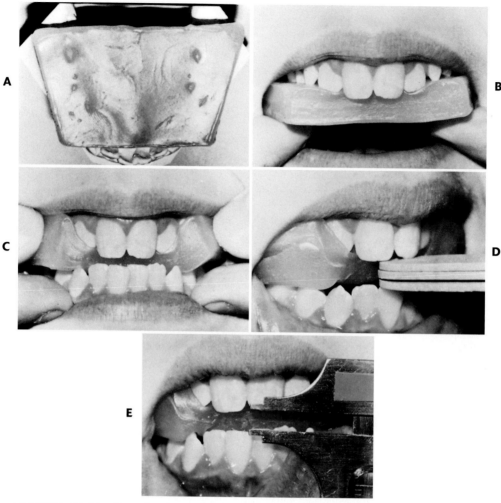

FIGURE 15-10 Steps for obtaining a "working bite" for functional appliance construction. **A,** Multiple layers of hard wax are luted together and cut to the size of the mandibular arch. Care must be taken not to cover the anterior teeth or extend the wax to areas of soft tissue interference. **B,** The softened wax is seated on the maxillary posterior teeth and pressed into place to ensure good indexing of the teeth. **C,** The mandible is guided to the correct anteroposterior and vertical position on observation of the midline relationships and the incisal separation. **D,** Either stacked tongue blades or, **E,** a Boley gauge can be used to control the amount of closure and help the patient reproduce the correct bite. The wax is then cooled with air and removed for inspection. Definite registration of both maxillary and mandibular teeth is required for proper appliance construction.

4 to 6 mm advancement, but remember that pretreatment incisor positioning is just as important for these appliances.

Appliance Components and Prescriptions. The design of a functional appliance according to the components approach is discussed and illustrated in Chapter 11. An appropriate appliance prescription specifies the appliance components that would be most effective in solving the patient's specific problems. Most laboratories have incorporated the components into a checklist format that simplifies precise communication. It is important to have the appliance design in mind prior to the impressions, because the impression technique is affected by what appliance components are selected and where they will be placed.

For most mandibular deficient patients, a bionator or activator-type appliance (see Figures 11-4 and 11-5) is the simplest, most durable, and most readily accepted appliance (if designed without excessively long lingual flanges, which tend to irritate the soft tissue). Either a bionator or an activator can include headgear tubes or bite blocks, which provide versatility when vertical problems are encountered. A tongue shield is applicable in some cases but often limits the patient's acceptance of the appliance because speaking can be difficult.

If transverse expansion of the arches is required, some form of buccal shield, either attached to an activator or bionator or as part of a Frankel appliance (see Figure 11-9), is best. When buccal shields are needed, the Frankel is less

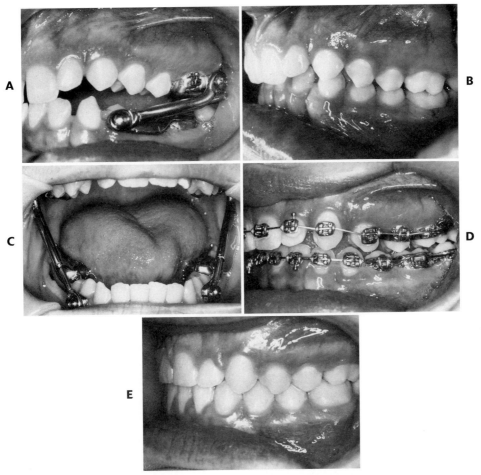

FIGURE 15-11 Clinical photos of Class II correction with a Herbst appliance. **A,** Initial malocclusion; **B** and **C,** Cantilever type Herbst appliance, attached to steel crowns on maxillary and mandibular first molars; **D,** Fixed appliance in place after 9 months of Herbst treatment. Note the molar correction and spacing within the maxillary arch; **E,** Completion of treatment.

formidable because the acrylic part is smaller, and it is easier to speak while wearing it, making it more acceptable for wear during school. It is also more delicate and easily broken, and has the potential for more soft tissue irritation. With any type of appliance, buccal shields make simultaneous use of headgear quite difficult.

The Herbst appliance, if cemented or bonded into place, has the advantage of full-time wear and circumvents some compliance problems. In spite of the fixed nature of the appliance, breakage can still be a problem with aggressive patients. Although some investigators recommend the Herbst appliance for the mixed dentition,[10] In long-term studies Pancherz noted substantial rebound in the immediate post-treatment period and recommends the Herbst appliance for the early permanent dentition, where he finds the changes more localized to the protrusion of the mandible.[4] He attributes more stability to the permanent canine intercuspation that can only be achieved in the permanent dentition.

Clinical Management of Functional Appliances

Removable Functional Appliances. When the functional appliance is returned from the laboratory, it should be checked for correct construction and fit on the working cast. The best technique for delivery is to adjust the appliance and work with the child to master insertion and removal before any discussion with the parent. This enables the child to be the full focus of attention initially and forestalls the effect of comments by the parents, such as, "How could he possibly get that thing in his mouth?"

With any functional appliance, a break-in period is helpful. This is especially important with tissue-borne appliances like the Frankel appliance. Having the child wear the appliance only a short time per day to begin with and increasing this time gradually over the first few weeks improves compliance later. To be effective, functional appliances should be worn when growth is occurring and when teeth are erupting. If the appliance is in place during these hours, theoretically, one can take advantage of the skeletal growth and either use or inhibit the tooth eruption that is occurring. Studies indicate that skeletal growth has a circadian rhythm. Most growth occurs during the evening hours when growth hormone is being secreted;[11] active eruption of teeth occurs during the same time period, typically between 8 PM and midnight or 1 AM.[12] To take practical advantage of this time period, it is suggested that children wear functional appliances from after the evening meal until they awake in the morning, which should be approximately 12 hours per day. Waiting until bed time to insert the appliance misses part of the period of active growth.

Wearing the appliance during the day may be advantageous, but this is difficult to achieve because it begins to impinge on school hours. The child should be informed that speaking may be difficult for a while, but that comfort and speaking facility will increase. Problems with speech are greatest when there is a bulk of acrylic behind or between the anterior teeth.

A good appointment schedule is to see the child at 2 weeks after insertion for inspection of the tissues and the appliance. If problems are reported, the child should be recalled at 1 week. Charts for children to record their "wearing time" are helpful, both for the data they provide and because the chart serves as a reinforcement for the desired behavior. Unfortunately, the wear time reported by patients and actual compliance often do not coincide.[13]

If a sore spot develops, the child should be encouraged to wear the appliance a few hours each day for 2 days before the appointment, so the source of the problem can be determined accurately. Usually smoothing the plastic components can be accomplished quickly. Gross adjustments should be avoided, because appliance fit and purpose can be greatly altered. For example, heavy reduction of the lingual flanges will allow the patient to position the mandible in a more posterior position.

Most components that occupy the vestibular area have a high potential for irritation if overextended or oriented improperly to the soft and hard tissues. It is not unusual to have to trim back buccal shields at their most anterior and posterior extent, but this should not be overdone. Lip pads facial to the lower incisors may have to be adjusted and contoured during treatment to eliminate gingival irritation.

Because the initial mandibular advancement is limited to a modest 4 to 6 mm and many children require more anteroposterior correction, a new appliance may be needed after 6 to 12 months of wear and a favorable response. Although a Frankel appliance can be sectioned and adjusted to change the amount of advancement (see Figure 11-18), the fit deteriorates, and better compliance is obtained by just making a new appliance. It is a good idea to reevaluate progress at 8 to 10 months after delivery with new records or at least a progress cephalometric radiograph. If little or no change has occurred in that time, then compliance is poor, the design is improper, or the patient is not responding to the appliance. In any case, a new treatment plan is needed.

Fixed Functional Appliances. At insertion of the Herbst appliance or a cemented twin block (Figure 15-12), discussion should focus on care of the appliance and acceptable mandibular movements. Because these appliances are fixed, a wear schedule is not required, but some patients initially have problems adapting to the appliance and the forward mandibular position. It is good to warn the patient and parents of this and assure them that accommodation increases rapidly after several days. Soft tissue irritation is not a major problem with the Herbst or twin block, but the teeth may be more sensitive than with removable functional appliances. Patients should be instructed that the appliance is meant to remind them to posture the mandible forward, not to force the mandible

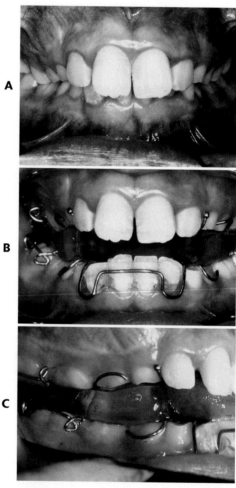

FIGURE 15-12   The twin block appliance can be used as a cemented (fixed) or removable appliance. This patient had a Class II deep bite malocclusion (**A**) treated with a twin block appliance that clearly (**B**) opened the bite and (**C**) advanced the mandible. The separate upper and lower units interdigitate via a ramp that can be seen extending forward from the maxillary primary canine area. The appliance often is cemented at insertion and later made removable, as was the case here. Adjustments can be made to the occlusal coverage and the inclines to modify eruption and the amount of advancement.

forward with heavy pressure on the teeth. In this sense, sore teeth for an extended amount of time may indicate poor cooperation.

The Herbst appliance must be carefully inspected for breakage at each visit. After a positive treatment response is noted, changes in the pin and tube length can be made during treatment to increase the amount of advancement simply by adding washer-type sleeves to the pin to restrict insertion of the pin into the tube (see Figure 11-18). The twin block appliance can have plastic resin added to the inclines to increase the advancement without totally remaking the appliance. Plastic also can be removed adjacent to the teeth to allow drift, and especially on the occlusal surfaces to encourage eruption when that is desirable.

It is possible to make a Herbst appliance partially fixed and partially removable. Typically, this involves a fixed upper and removable lower splint. In this case, the fixed and removable parts should be carefully explained, so that the child does not remove or loosen the appliance due to a misunderstanding. Likewise, the twin block can be made removable after an initial wear period.

A fixed Herbst appliance usually is worn for 6 to 8 months, at which point the desired correction should have been obtained. If the patient is still in the mixed dentition at that point, it is important to use a removable functional appliance of the activator or bionator type, which should be worn approximately 12 hours per day for a number of months as a retainer. In the early permanent dentition, a fixed appliance can serve to retain the changes produced during the functional treatment.[14] The twin block can serve as its own retainer after a 6 to 8 month fixed period, when it can be uncemented or debonded and changed to a removable appliance.

Treatment of Vertical Deficiency (Short Face)

Some children exhibit a skeletal vertical deficiency (short face), almost always in conjunction with an anterior deep bite and some degree of mandibular deficiency and often with a Class II, division 2 malocclusion. Skeletally, the condition often can be described as Class II rotated to Class I. The reduced face height is often accompanied by everted and prominent lips that would be appropriate if the face height were normal. Children with vertical deficiency can be identified at an early age.[15] They usually have a normal maxilla but have decreased eruption of maxillary and mandibular teeth. Many tend to have a low mandibular plane angle (skeletal deep bite) and a long mandibular ramus. Growth is expressed in an anterior direction, with a tendency toward upward and forward rotation of the mandible. The challenge in correcting these problems is to increase eruption of posterior teeth and influence the mandible to rotate downward without decreasing chin prominence too much.

In a patient with Class II malocclusion, one way to correct such problems is with cervical headgear, taking advantage of the extrusive tendency of extraoral force directed

below the center of resistance of the teeth and the maxilla (Figure 15-13). The other way is to use a functional appliance (with or without mandibular advancement, depending on the anteroposterior jaw relationship) that allows free eruption of the posterior teeth.

Because most short face children also have a Class II malocclusion, it is important whether the eruption that occurs during treatment is primarily of the upper or the lower molars. Cervical headgear produces more eruption of the upper molars, while eruption can be manipulated with a functional appliance so that either the upper or lower molars erupt more. Class II correction, however, is easier if the lower molar erupts more than the upper, which means that—all other factors being equal—the functional appliance would be preferred (Figure 15-14).

The ability of functional appliances to control eruption of posterior teeth can be used during treatment of children with a significant anteroposterior mandibular deficiency *and* reduced face height in an effort to take maximal advantage of mandibular growth by having it expressed in an anterior direction. First, all vertical eruption is blocked. Then, after the anteroposterior correction is complete, a child treated in this manner may exhibit a posterior open bite when the appliance is not in place (Figure 15-15). At that point, the posterior bite block gradually is cut away while correct overbite is maintained anteriorly, so that slow eruption of posterior teeth back into occlusion can occur. This type of treatment places into sharp focus the interaction between the anteroposterior and vertical planes of space that must be addressed during growth modification treatment. The priority is placed on the most severe problem. It is remedied, and then the accompanying problems are addressed.

The fixed functional appliances tend not to be good choices in the mixed dentition treatment of short face problems. Certainly, the Herbst, with its propensity to intrude the upper molars, is not an attractive option for younger patients needing increased vertical dimensions, even though the mandibular plane angle usually does not change very much in Herbst treatment.[16] The twin block does offer some options to manage posterior eruption when the acrylic is modified during treatment.

It is appropriate to remember that eruption occurs more rapidly in some patients than others and probably is affected by resting mandibular posture and freeway space, as well as the amount of appliance wear. Some short face children show extremely rapid mandibular growth when the bite is opened and incisor overlap is removed, even with so simple an appliance as a bite plate. Unfortunately, this phenomenon does not always occur, and except for the rare patients in whom there is no mandibular deficiency, posturing the mandible forward to allow the construction of a functional appliance is the better approach. Delivery and adjustment of a functional appliance for a vertically deficient patient is similar to that already discussed under mandibular deficiency.

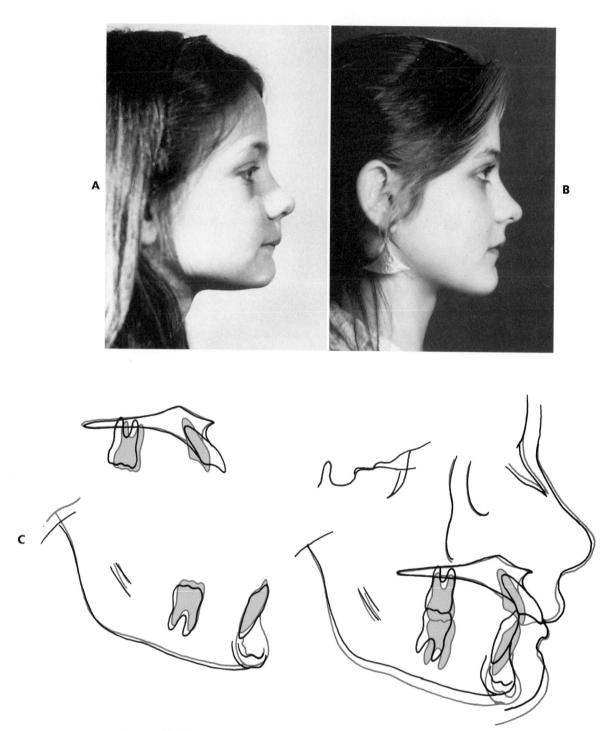

FIGURE 15-13   Increased vertical development in a child who initially had decreased lower anterior face height. **A,** Pre-treatment profile; **B,** post-treatment profile; **C,** cephalometric superimpositions. This result was accomplished by increasing the maxillary molar eruption with a cervical pull headgear, which resulted in downward movement of the mandible and improved facial esthetics.

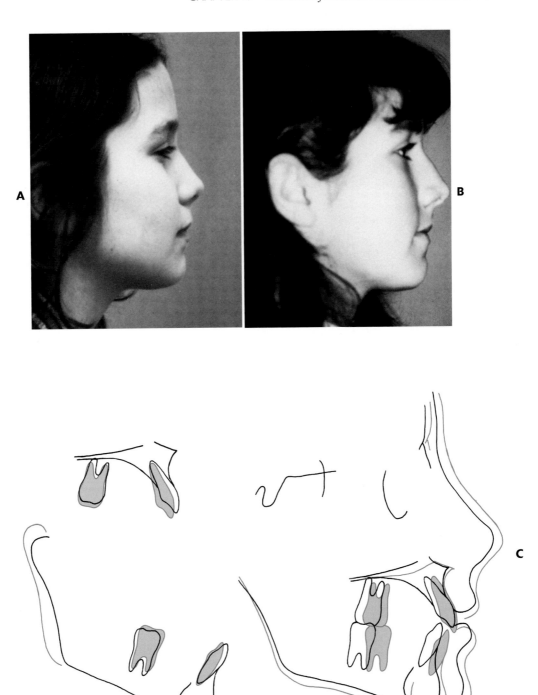

FIGURE 15-14 Functional appliance treatment to increase vertical development in a child who initially had a Class II malocclusion and slightly decreased lower anterior face height. **A,** Pre-treatment profile. Note the convexity, with equal contributions of maxillary protrusion and mandibular retrusion, and somewhat decreased lower face height; **B,** Post-treatment profile, with reduced convexity and well-balanced vertical facial proportions; **C,** cephalometric superimpositions. The tracings indicate that the correction was accomplished by limiting anterior movement of the maxilla while the mandible grew downward and forward. The maxillary and mandibular superimpositions show little incisor change, in conjunction with eruption of the lower molar, which increased the vertical facial development and aided in the Class II dental correction.

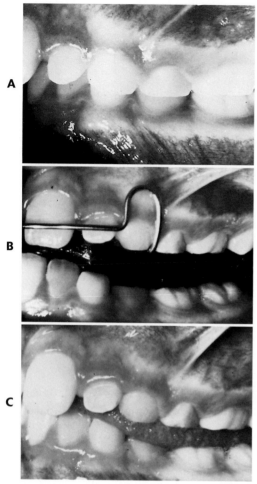

FIGURE 15-15 Posterior bite blocks can be used with any appliance that advances the mandible, in an effort to limit posterior eruption and take maximum advantage of growth in an anteroposterior direction, but the desirable skeletal changes may be accompanied by undesirable dental effects. **A,** The pre-treatment occlusal relationships; **B,** when the mandible is advanced, bite blocks are incorporated to prevent posterior eruption. **C,** After a phase of appliance therapy that resulted in anteroposterior changes, there is a posterior open bite, which can be closed at that point by reducing the plastic bite blocks.

MAXILLARY EXCESS

Excessive growth of the maxilla in children with Class II malocclusion often has a vertical as well as an anteroposterior component (i.e., there is too much downward as well as forward growth). Both components can contribute to skeletal Class II malocclusion, because if the maxilla moves downward, the mandible rotates downward and backward. The effect is to prevent mandibular growth from being expressed anteriorly. The goal of treatment is to restrict growth of the maxilla while the mandible grows into a more prominent and normal relationship with it (Figure 15-16). Although the application of extraoral force

is the obvious approach, functional appliance treatment also can be helpful, particularly in the treatment of excessive vertical growth.

Principles in the Use of Extraoral Force

The Development of Extraoral Appliances. Extraoral force, in the form of headgear appliances very similar to those used today, was used by the pioneer orthodontists of the late 1800s. Both Kingsley and Angle described and used astonishingly modern-appearing appliances of this sort, apparently with reasonable success. As orthodontics progressed in the early twentieth century, however, extraoral appliances and mixed dentition treatment were abandoned, not because they were ineffective, but because they were considered an unnecessary complication. By 1920, Angle and his followers were convinced that Class II and Class III elastics not only moved teeth but also caused significant skeletal changes, stimulating the growth of one jaw while restraining the other. If intraoral elastics could produce a true stimulation of mandibular growth while simultaneously restraining the maxilla, there would be no need to ask a patient to wear an extraoral appliance, nor would there be any reason to begin treatment until the permanent teeth were available.

The first cephalometric evaluations of the effects of orthodontic treatment, which became available in the 1940s, did not support the concept that significant skeletal changes occurred in response to intraoral forces. A 1936 paper by Oppenheim revived the idea that headgear would serve as a valuable adjunct to treatment.[17] However, it was not until after World War II, when Silas Kloehn's impressive results with headgear treatment of Class II malocclusion became widely known, that extraoral force to the maxilla again became an important part of American orthodontics.[18] Cephalometric studies of patients treated with Kloehn-type headgear (see Figure 15-16), which utilized a neckstrap and relatively light (300 to 400 gm) force, showed that skeletal change in the form of a reorientation of jaw relationships did occur.[19] Experience soon revealed that although greater skeletal effects might be produced by higher levels of force than Kloehn had advocated, this required an upward direction of pull from a headcap to prevent excessive downward movement of the maxilla and a consequent downward and backward rotation of the mandible.[20]

Effects of Headgear to the Maxilla. Extraoral force against the maxilla has been documented in numerous studies, including the recent clinical trials that are described in Chapter 8, to decrease the amount of forward and/or downward growth by changing the pattern of apposition of bone at the sutures. Class II correction is obtained as the mandible grows forward normally while similar forward growth of the maxilla is restrained, so mandibular growth is a necessary part of the treatment response.

In a preadolescent child, extraoral force is almost always applied to the first molars via a facebow with a head-

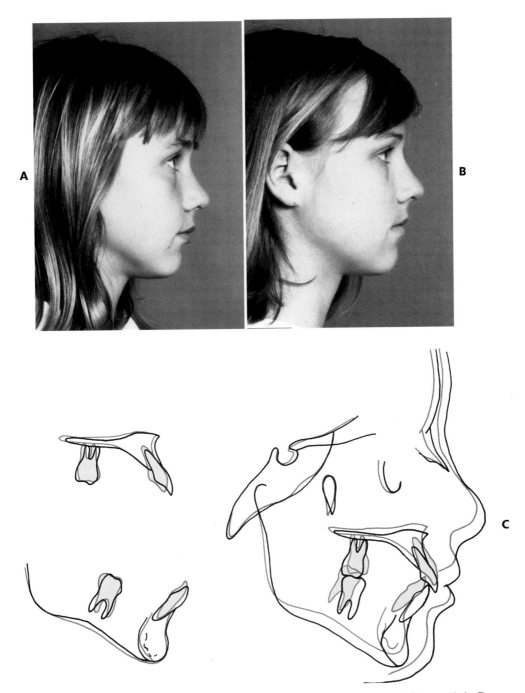

FIGURE 15-16   A good response to headgear treatment. **A,** Age 11-6; **B,** age 13-0; **C,** cephalometric superimpositions. Note the favorable downward-forward mandibular growth. For this patient, the somewhat protrusive lower incisors were part of the reason to favor headgear, because functional appliance treatment tends to move lower incisors forward but headgear treatment does not.

cap or a neckstrap for anchorage. To be effective in controlling growth, headgear should be worn regularly for at least 10 to 12 hours per day. The growth hormone release that occurs in the early evening strongly suggests that, as with functional appliances, putting the headgear on right after dinner and wearing it until the next morning—not waiting until bed time to put it on—is an ideal schedule.

The current recommendation is a force of 12 to 16 ounces (350 to 450 gm) per side. When teeth are used as the point of force application, some dental as well as skeletal effects must be expected. Extremely heavy forces (greater than 1000 gm total) are unnecessarily traumatic to the teeth and their supporting structures, while lighter forces may produce dental but not skeletal changes.

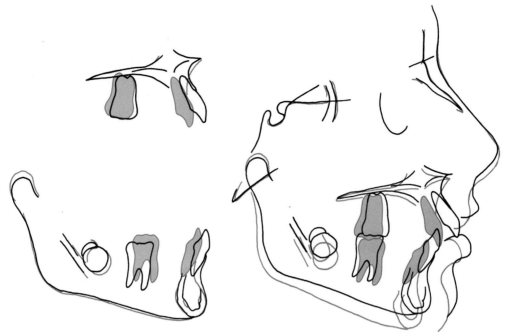

FIGURE 15-17 This child had a poor response to headgear treatment for a Class II malocclusion. The cranial base superimposition indicates that the lips were retracted and the maxilla did not grow anteriorly. The maxillary superimposition shows that the incisors were retracted and the molar movement and eruption were limited. All these effects were beneficial for Class II correction, but the mandible rotated inferiorly and backward because of the inferior movement of the maxilla and eruption of the lower molar. As a result, the profile is more convex than when treatment began and the Class II malocclusion is uncorrected.

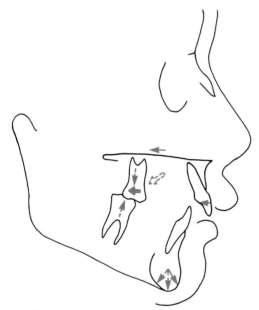

FIGURE 15-18 Headgear treatment can have several side effects that complicate correction of Class II malocclusion. If the child wears the appliance, maxillary skeletal and dental forward movement will be restricted. Although this helps in correction of the Class II malocclusion, vertical control of the maxilla and maxillary teeth is important, because this determines the extent to which the mandible is directed forward and/or inferiorly. Downward maxillary skeletal movement or maxillary and mandibular molar eruption (all shown in dashed arrows) can reduce or totally negate forward growth of the mandible.

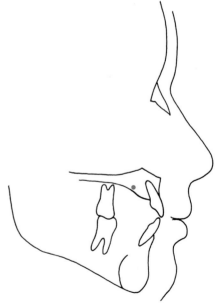

FIGURE 15-19 Although the center of resistance of the maxilla is difficult to estimate, a location above the roots of the premolar teeth, at about the location of the red dot, has been proposed. If this is true, it is difficulty to direct forces through the center of resistance by traditional force delivery systems.

To correct a Class II malocclusion, the mandible needs to grow forward relative to the maxilla. For this reason it is important to control the vertical position of the maxilla and the maxillary posterior teeth. Downward movement of either the jaw or the teeth tends to project mandibular growth more vertically, which nullifies most of the forward mandibular growth that reduces the Class II relationship (Figure 15-17). Baumrind et al have demonstrated that distal molar movement is a significant contributing factor to downward projection of mandibular growth during headgear treatment.[21] The molars should not be elongated, and distal tipping of these teeth should be minimized when the objective is a change in skeletal relationships (Figure 15-18). In addition, it is necessary to try to control the vertical growth of the maxilla.

In theory, the movement of the maxilla can be controlled in the same way as a single tooth is controlled: by managing forces and moments relative to the center of resistance of the jaw (Figure 15-19). In practice, it is difficult to analyze exactly where the center of resistance and center of rotation of the maxilla might be, but it is above the teeth. Directing the line of force closer to the center of resistance is a major reason for including an upward direction of pull for most children who have headgear force to the maxilla.

Selection of Headgear Type.   There are three major decisions to be made in the selection of headgear. First, the headgear anchorage location must be chosen to provide a preferred vertical component of force to the skeletal and dental structures. A high pull headcap (Figure 15-20, *A*) will place a superior and distal force on the teeth and maxilla. A cervical neckstrap (Figure 15-20, *B*) will place an inferior and distal force on the teeth and skeletal structures. When the headcap and neckstrap are combined (Figure 15-20, *C*), the force direction can be varied by altering the proportion of the total force provided by each component. If each delivers equal forces, the resultant force is slightly upward and distal for both the teeth and the maxilla. The initial choice of headgear configuration should be based on the original facial pattern: the more vertically excessive growth is present, the higher the direction of pull and vice versa, but it must be kept in mind that considerable variation in growth response can occur.[22]

The second decision is how the headgear is to be attached to the dentition. The usual arrangement is a facebow to tubes on the permanent first molars. Alternatively, a removable appliance can be fitted to the maxillary teeth and the facebow attached to this appliance. This appliance can take the form of a maxillary splint or a functional appliance. This alternative approach is particularly indicated for children with vertically excessive growth (see later in this chapter). Attaching headgear to an archwire anteriorly is possible but rarely practical in mixed dentition children.

Finally, a decision must be made as to whether bodily movement or tipping of the teeth or maxilla is desired. Since the center of resistance for a molar is estimated to be

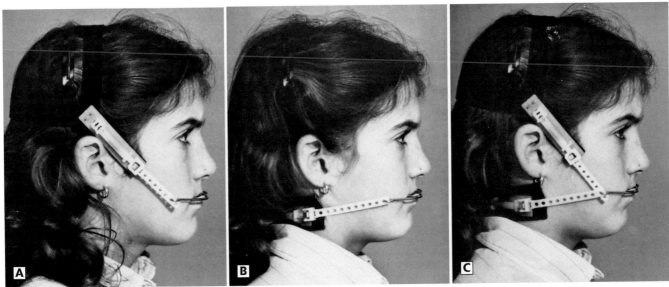

FIGURE 15-20   Various types of headgear provide different directions of force for different clinical situations. **A,** High-pull headgear consists of a headcap connected to a facebow. The appliance places a distal and upward force on the maxillary teeth and maxilla. **B,** Cervical headgear is made up of a neckstrap connected to a facebow. This appliance produces a distal and downward force against the maxillary teeth and the maxilla. **C,** The combination headgear is a marriage of the high-pull and cervical headgears, with both connected to a facebow. When the force is equal from each headgear, a distal and slightly upward force is placed on the maxillary teeth and maxilla. Varying the proportions of the total force derived from the headcap and neckstrap allows the result force vector to be altered.

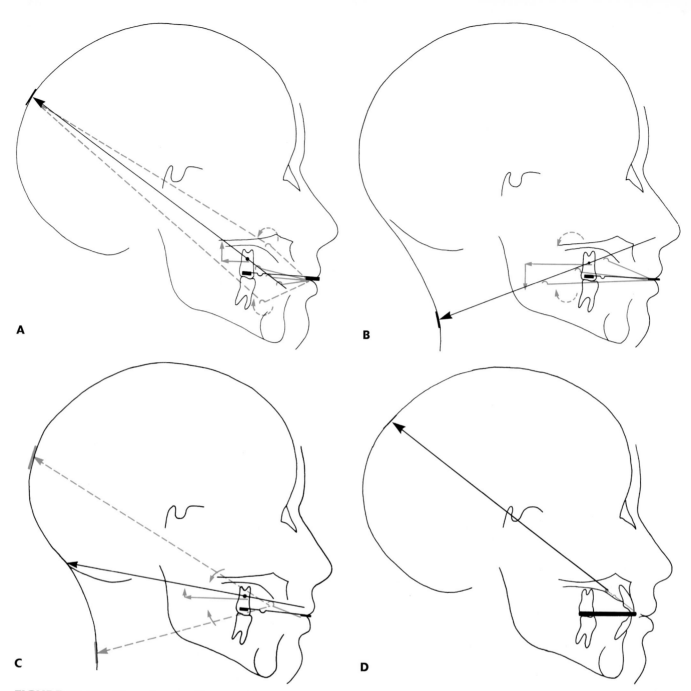

FIGURE 15-21 These diagrams illustrate effects of four commonly used types of facebow and extraoral anchorage attachments. In each diagram, the inner bow is shown in black, and the various outer bow possibilities in red or dotted red. **A,** High-pull headgear (head-cap) to the first molar. To produce bodily movement of the molar (no tipping), the line of force (*black arrow*) must pass through the center of resistance of the molar tooth. This will produce both backward and upward movement of the molar. Note that the line of force is affected by the length and position of the outer bow, so that a longer outer bow bent up or a shorter one bent down could produce the same line of force. If bow length or position produces a line of force above or below the center of resistance (*dotted red*), the tooth will tip with the root or the crown, respectively, going distally because of the moment that is produced. **B,** Cervical headgear (neckstrap) to the first molar. Again, bodily movement is produced by an outer bow length and position that places the line of force through the center of resistance of the molar; but with a lower direction of pull, the tooth is extruded as well as moved backward. Note that the outer bow of a facebow used with cervical traction nearly always is longer than the outer bow used with a high-pull headcap. If the line of force is above or below its center of resistance, the tooth will tip with the root or crown, respectively, going distally as indicated by the dotted arrows. **C,** Combination headgear to the first molar, using both a headcap and a neckstrap. The resultant force vector (*black*) determines the movement of the molar, which in this example will be back and slightly up. With the resultant line through the center of resistance, the moments created by the headcap and neckstrap cancel. Again, if the resultant force vector is above or below the center of resistance, the tooth will tip. **D,** High-pull headgear to a short facebow inserted into a maxillary splint. With all the teeth splinted, it is possible to consider the maxilla as a unit and to relate the line of force to the center of resistance of the maxilla. As with headgear force against the first molar, the relationship of the line of force to the center of resistance of the maxilla determines the rotational effect on the maxilla.

in the midroot region, force vectors above this point should result in distal root movement. Forces through the center of resistance of the molar should cause bodily movement, and vectors below this point should cause distal crown tipping. The length and position of the outer headgear bow and the form of anchorage (i.e., headcap, neckstrap, or combination) determine the vector of force and its relationship to the center of resistance of the tooth. These factors determine the molar movement.

The various combinations of force direction (anchorage), length of outer bow, and position of outer bow are diagrammatically illustrated in Figure 15-21. For example, if a cervical neckstrap is to be used, either a medium-length high or long straight outer bow will provide distal root movement along with extrusion. With a cervical neckstrap, a high short or low medium-length outer bow will produce distal crown tipping along with distal and extrusive molar movement.

As in any growth modification treatment, tooth movement generally is an undesirable side effect, and with headgear, tooth movement is minimized by causing the teeth to move bodily if they move at all.

Similar considerations apply to the maxilla: unless the line of force is through its center of resistance, rotation of the jaw (the skeletal equivalent of dental tipping) will occur.

Control of the line of force relative to the maxilla is easier when a splint covering all the teeth is used to apply the headgear force. The facebow is usually attached to the splint in the premolar region, so that the force can be directed through the center of resistance of the maxilla that is estimated to be located above the premolar roots (see Figure 15-21, *D*). Distal tipping of the maxillary incisors is likely to occur, however, because of the distal component of the force delivered to these teeth.

Clinical Procedures in Headgear Use

For headgear treatment in a preadolescent child, molar bands with headgear tubes (and any other attachments that might be needed later in treatment) are fitted and cemented (see Chapter 12 for details of appliance components). Preformed facebows are supplied in a variety of inner bow sizes and usually also have an adjustment loop as part of the inner bow. The inner bow should fit closely around the upper arch without contacting the teeth except at the molar tubes (within 3 to 4 mm of the teeth at all points) (Figure 15-22). The correct size can be selected by fitting the bow against the maxillary cast. It is then placed into the tube on one side for an examination of how it fits relative to the other tube and the teeth. By adjusting the loops to expand or contract the inner bow and by bending

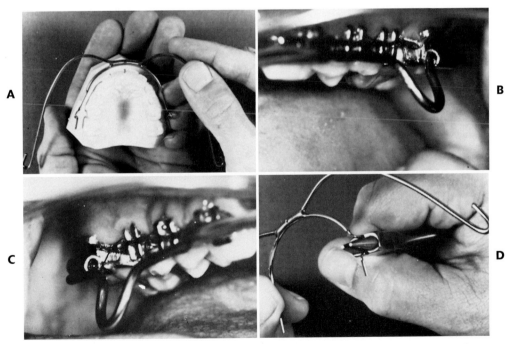

FIGURE 15-22 The steps for fitting a facebow for a headgear. **A,** Facebow inner bows come in graduated sizes. A simple method for selecting the appropriate size is to fit the bow to the pretreatment maxillary cast. **B,** After the bow is placed in one molar headgear tube, **C,** it is adjusted to be passive and aligned with the tube on the other molar band. It should be easy to insert and remove at this point. Often the adjustment loops mesial to the maxillary first molar need to be opened or closed to move the inner bow farther from or closer to the anterior teeth. **D,** Similarly, the inner bow must often be stepped away from the teeth in the buccal segments. This can be accomplished by bending the adjustment loop lingually and, *Continued*

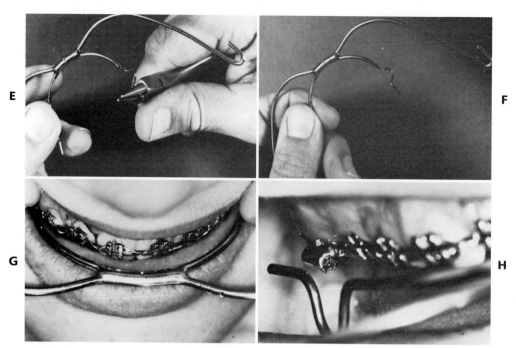

FIGURE 15-22, cont'd E, bending the portion of the bow that inserts in the molar tube back to its original position. **F,** When the inner bow is then expanded, there is no interference with the buccal teeth. The inner bow must be expanded by 1 to 2 mm to keep the posterior teeth out of crossbite as anteroposterior changes are made. **G,** These adjustments should result in the inner bow being several millimeters from the teeth and resting passively between the lips. Vertical adjustments can be made at the molar adjustment loops. **H,** The inner bow must be expanded by 1 to 2 mm to keep the posterior teeth out of crossbite as anterposterior changes are made.

the short portion of the bow that fits into the molar tubes, it is possible to make the bow passive, allow clearance from the teeth, and have the bow rest comfortably between the lips (Figure 15-23, *A*). The extension of the inner bow out the end of the headgear tubes should be evaluated. Ideally the end of the inner bow would be flush with the tube, but certainly there is no need for it to extend more than 1 mm past the end of the tube. This limited extension will reduce tissue irritation in the back of the mouth and friction during application and removal.

As a Class II molar relationship is corrected, the relative forward movement of the lower arch will produce a crossbite tendency unless the upper arch width is expanded. This must be taken into account from the beginning of treatment. The inner bow should be expanded by 2 mm symmetrically so that when it is placed in one tube, it rests just outside the other tube. The patient will need to squeeze the inner bow as it is inserted to make it fit the tubes, thus providing the appropriate molar expansion.

The outer bow should rest several millimeters from the cheeks (Figure 15-23, *B*). It must be cut to the proper length and have a hook formed at the end (Figure 15-24). The length and the vertical position of the outer bow are selected to achieve the correct force direction relative to the center of resistance (see Figure 15-21).

This can actually be accomplished quite simply after the inner and outer bow relationships to the teeth and face have been adjusted. With the bow in place, by placing your fingers on the outer bow and simulating the direction of force application at different points bilaterally, the reaction of the teeth can be determined. If the force you place with your fingers lifts the junction of the inner and outer bows between the lips, the headgear will move the roots distally. Conversely, if the force drops the bow between the lips, the molar crowns will be tipping distally. If neither occurs, the teeth will be moving bodily.

The appropriate headcap, neckstrap or combination of the two is fit by selecting the appropriate size. A spring mechanism—not elastic bands or straps—is strongly recommended to provide the force. The springs deliver consistent forces that can be documented and easily adjusted. The spring attachment is adjusted to provide the correct force with the patient sitting up or standing—not reclining in the dental chair (Figure 15-25, *A* and *B*). It is usually a good idea to start with a low force level to acclimate the patient to the headgear and then gradually increase the force at subsequent appointments. Even if the correct force level is set at the first appointment, the forces will drop when the strap stretches slightly and contours to the patient's neck. Once the forces are correct,

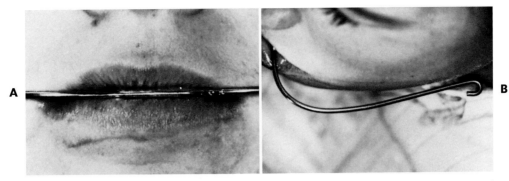

FIGURE 15-23 A, The facebow should be adjusted so that the junction of the inner and outer bows rests passively between the lips. **B,** The outer bow should rest several millimeters from the soft tissue of the cheek. This adjustment must be checked both before and after the straps for the headcap or neckstrap are attached.

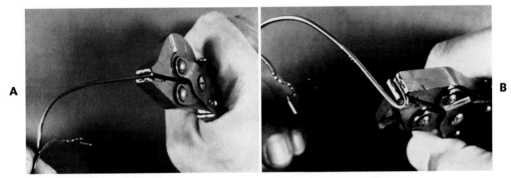

FIGURE 15-24 The length of the outer bow is critical to the desired dental changes. **A,** After the correct length is chosen and the outer bow cut with a pliers, **B,** a hook is bent at the end with a heavy pliers.

the bow position must be rechecked since the pull of the straps often alters the previous bow position so that it needs adjustment.

The child should place and remove the headgear under supervision several times to be certain that he or she understands how to manipulate it and to ensure proper adjustment. Most headgear is worn after school, during relaxed evening hours and during sleep. It is definitely not indicated for vigorous activity, bicycle riding, or general roughhousing. Children should be instructed that if anyone grabs the outer bow, they should also grab the bow with their hands. This will prevent breakage and injury. The headgear straps must be equipped with a safety-release mechanism (Figure 15-25, *C* to *E*) to prevent the bow from springing back at the child and injuring him or her if it is grabbed and pulled by a playmate. Severe injuries, including loss of sight, have occurred from headgear accidents of this type.[23] In a recent review of commercially available headgear release mechanisms that included 18 different designs, Stafford et al noted that almost all released at 10 to 20 pounds of force and concluded that the amount of extension before release occurred and the consistency of release were the most important variables from a safety perspective.[24]

Vertical Excess

Children with excessive face height (e.g., with a skeletal open bite or long face syndrome) generally have a normal upper face and elongation of maxillary and mandibular posterior teeth,[25] which accounts for the steep mandibular plane and the large discrepancy between posterior and anterior face height. The ideal treatment for these patients would be to control all subsequent vertical growth so that the mandible would rotate in an upward and forward direction (Figure 15-26).

Unfortunately, vertical facial growth extends into the adolescent and postadolescent years, which means that even if growth can be modified successfully in the mixed dentition, active retention is likely to be necessary for a number of years.

There are several possible approaches to this long face pattern of growth. In the order of their clinical effectiveness, the possible approaches are:

High Pull Headgear to the Molars. One approach to vertical excess problems is to maintain the vertical position of the maxilla and inhibit eruption of the maxillary posterior teeth. This can be attempted with high-pull headgear to the posterior teeth, that is worn 14 hours a day

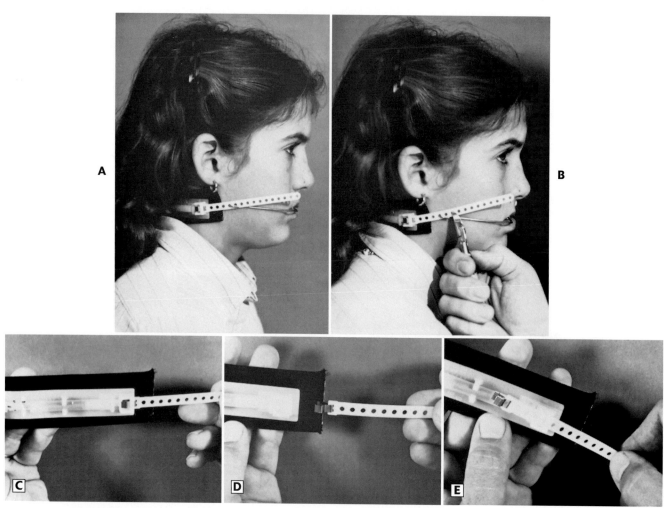

FIGURE 15-25   Adjustment of the neckstrap. **A,** The neckstrap is attached to the facebow and the proper force obtained from the spring mechanism by moving the hook to adjacent holes on the neckstrap. **B,** When the force is correct, the plastic connector is cut so that one extra hole is present in front of the correct hole. This provides a tab for the patient to grasp when placing the headgear. **C,** The spring mechanism delivers a predetermined force when the plastic connector is moved forward and aligned with a calibration mark. **D,** If the connector is stretched farther, such as it might be if someone grabbed the facebow and pulled on it, the plastic connector strap will release, preventing the bow from springing back into the patient's face and causing injury. **E,** The connector can be threaded through the back of the mechanism to reassemble it after operation of the safety release.

with a force greater than 12 ounces per side (Figure 15-27). If the headgear involves a conventional facebow to the first molar, delivery and adjustment of the headgear are identical to the high-pull headgear described previously for Class II problems. When comparisons are made using varied vertical and horizontal vectors of force, those with the greatest high-pull vector demonstrated the most vertical control of the upper molars.[26,27]

High-Pull Headgear to a Maxillary Splint.   A more effective headgear approach for children with excessive vertical development is the use of a plastic occlusal splint (Figure 15-28) to which the facebow is attached.[28] This allows vertical force to be directed against all the maxillary

teeth—not just the molars—and appears to have a substantial maxillary dental and skeletal effect with good vertical control. An appliance of this type would be most useful in a child with excessive vertical development of the entire maxillary arch and too much exposure of the maxillary incisors from beneath the lip (i.e., a long face child who does not have anterior open bite). To achieve both skeletal and dental correction, the patient must be compliant throughout what can be a very long treatment period.

Unfortunately, this type of appliance allows mandibular posterior teeth to erupt freely, and if this occurs, there may be neither redirection of growth nor favorable upward and forward rotation of the mandible.

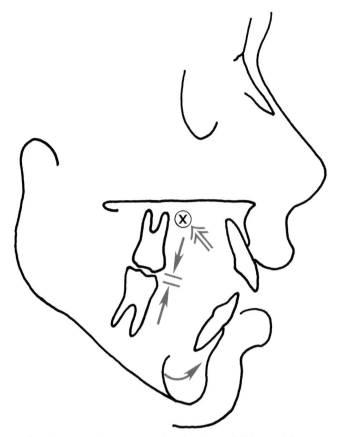

FIGURE 15-26   Mandibular-deficient children with excessive lower face height need treatment with an appliance that restricts posterior eruption and limits decent of the maxilla. This allows mandibular growth to be expressed anteriorly rather than vertically.

Functional Appliance with Bite Blocks.   A more effective alternative is the use of a functional appliance that includes posterior bite blocks (Figure 15-29). The retraction force of the headgear is replaced by the somewhat lesser "headgear effect" of the functional appliance. The primary purpose of the appliance is to inhibit eruption of posterior teeth and vertical descent of the maxilla. The appliance can be designed with or without positioning the mandible anteriorly, depending on how much mandibular deficiency is present.

Regardless of whether the mandible is brought forward in the working bite, the bite must be opened past the normal resting vertical dimension if molar eruption is to be affected. When the mandible is held in this position by the appliance, the stretch of the soft tissues (including but not limited to the muscles) exerts a vertical intrusive force on the posterior teeth. In children with anterior open bites the anterior teeth are allowed to erupt, which reduces the open bite, while in the less common long face problems without open bite, all teeth are held by the bite blocks. Because there is no compensatory posterior eruption, all mandibular growth should be directed more anteriorly.

In the short term, this type of functional appliance treatment is effective in controlling maxillary vertical skeletal and dental growth.[29] This tends to project mandibular growth anteriorly and helps to close anterior open bites (Figure 15-30). Because of the long period of continued vertical growth, if a functional appliance is used for the first phase of treatment, posterior bite blocks or other components to control vertical growth and eruption will be

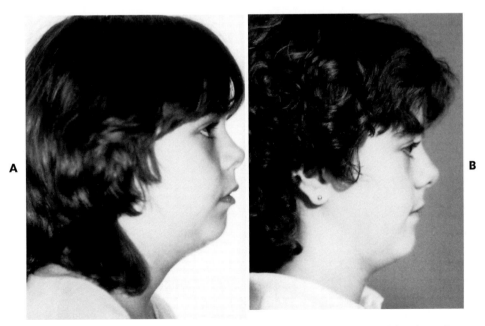

FIGURE 15-27   These photos show an excellent response to high-pull headgear for a child with excessive lower face height. **A,** Pre-treatment profile; **B,** post-treatment profile;

Continued

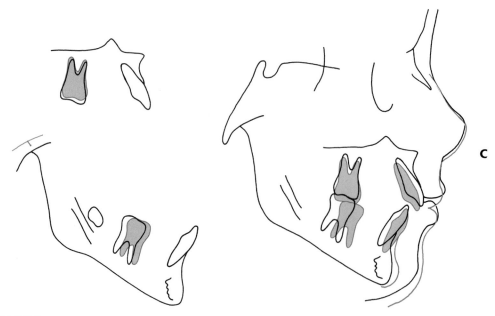

FIGURE 15-27, cont'd C, cephalometric superimposition. The cranial base superimposition shows that the maxilla and the maxillary teeth did not move inferiorly; as a result the mandible grew forward and not downward. The mandibular superimposition shows that the lower molar drifted forward into the leeway space. The incisor positions relative to the maxilla and mandible did not change.

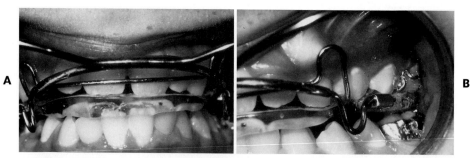

FIGURE 15-28 A and **B,** A plastic maxillary splint can be connected to a small conventional inner headgear bow and a high-pull headgear cap to deliver an upward and backward force to the entire maxilla. The splint limits dental eruption better than headgear just to the first molars.

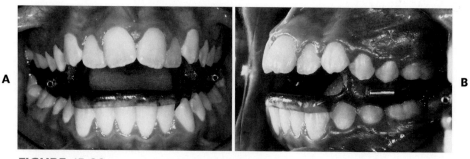

FIGURE 15-29 A and **B,** Bite blocks between the posterior teeth can be added to a functional appliance, as shown here, to provide more complete control of the eruption of posterior teeth. High pull headgear can be worn with an appliance of this type if headgear tubes are included.

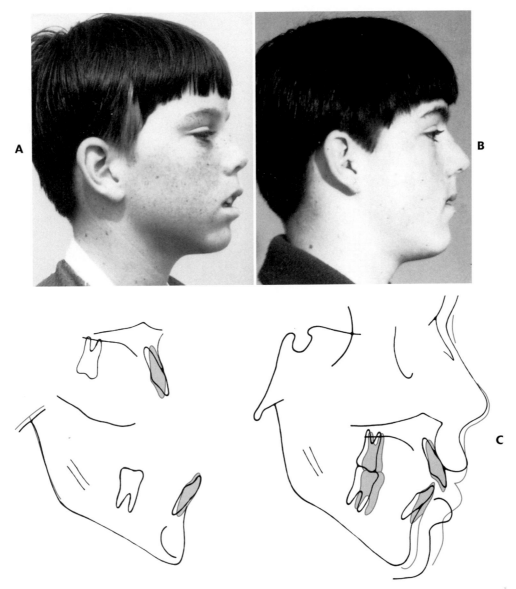

FIGURE 15-30 These tracings demonstrate a good response to functional appliance treatment designed to control vertical development with posterior bite blocks in a child with excessive lower face height. **A,** Pre-treatment profile; **B,** post-treatment profile. **C,** Cephalometric superimpositions indicate that no posterior eruption occurred, and all mandibular growth was directed anteriorly. Face height was maintained and anterior eruption closed the open bite. Maxillary and mandibular molar positions relative to their supporting bone were maintained.

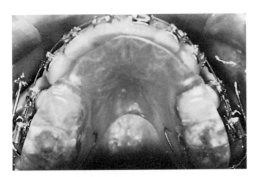

FIGURE 15-31 During fixed appliance treatment, posterior eruption can be controlled by using removable posterior bite blocks to separate the posterior teeth beyond the resting vertical dimension. This creates an intrusive force on teeth in contact with the blocks, which is generated by the stretch of the facial soft tissues. The appliance is retained by clasps over the headgear tubes.

needed during fixed appliance therapy (Figure 15-31) and probably into retention. This is necessary because fixed appliances do not control eruption well.

High-Pull Headgear to a Functional Appliance with Bite Blocks. The most effective approach to growth modification involving vertical excess and a Class II relationship and the preferred method for children with severe problems is a combination of extraoral force in the form of high-pull headgear and a functional appliance with posterior bite blocks to anteriorly reposition the mandible and control eruption.[30] The extraoral force increases the control of maxillary growth and allows the force to be delivered to the whole maxilla rather than to simply the permanent first molars (Figure 15-32). The high-pull headgear improves retention of the functional appliance and produces a force direction near the estimated center of resistance of

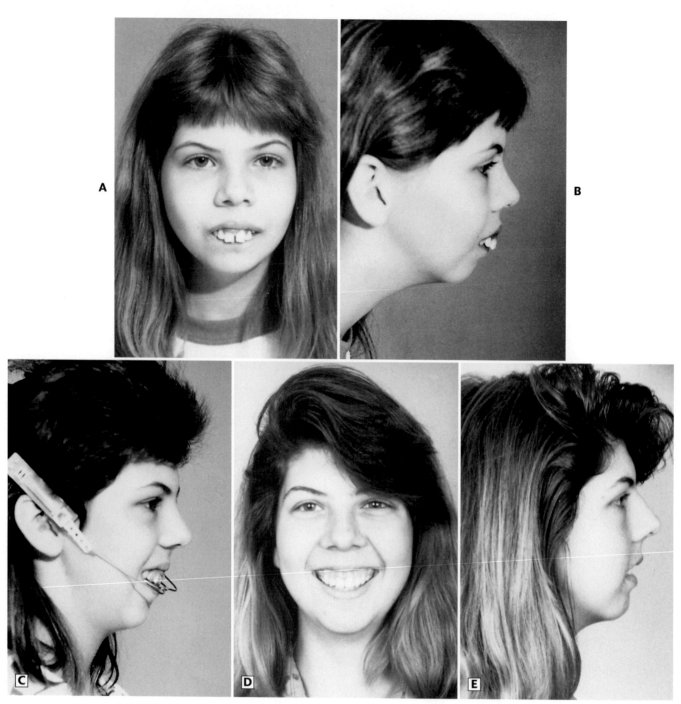

FIGURE 15-32 A severe long face mandibular deficient condition is treated best with high-pull headgear attached to a functional appliance with posterior bite blocks. **A** and **B,** Facial appearance before treatment; **C,** headgear with attachment to functional appliance. **D** and **E,** Post-treatment facial appearance; *continued*

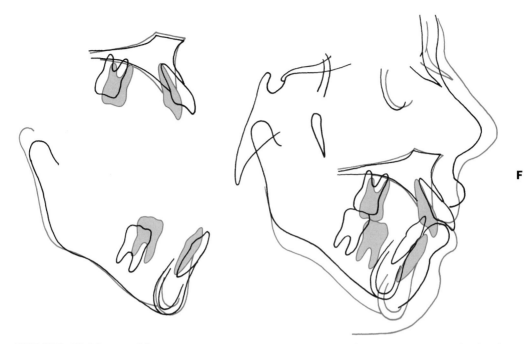

FIGURE 15-32, cont'd **F,** cephalometric superimpositions. Before treatment, note the facial convexity, increased lower face height, lip incompetence, and exposure of the maxillary incisors. The superimpositions show an overall downward and forward growth of the mandible, with no increase in the mandibular plane angle and good control of the vertical position of the teeth.

the maxilla (see Figure 15-21, *D*). The functional appliance provides the possibility of enhancing mandibular growth while controlling the eruption of the posterior and anterior teeth.

Modifications of the activator or bionator can be constructed using various functional appliance components to enhance or diminish the active dental changes. When a headgear-activator combination is used, it is a good idea to add torquing springs to the activator (Figure 15-33) to reduce the tipping effect on maxillary anterior teeth. In this case, which is a notable exception among the active functional appliances, the active components are designed to decrease dental and increase skeletal effects.[31]

Clinical management of the headgear-functional appliance is an amalgamation of techniques used for each of these appliances individually but with some interesting modifications. First, the impressions for the functional appliance are made and the working bite obtained as with any functional appliance. The headgear tubes are incorporated into the bite blocks in the premolar region (Figure 15-34). At the time of functional appliance delivery, a headcap is made for the patient and a small, if not the smallest, facebow is adjusted to fit the headgear tubes. Usually the adjustment loops need to be closed so the bow is not placed too far anteriorly.

The facebow-functional appliance combination is taken to the mouth and adjusted so the outer bow is consistent with a resultant force through the estimated center of resistance of the maxilla. With the inner bow resting passively between the lips as it should, the short or moderate

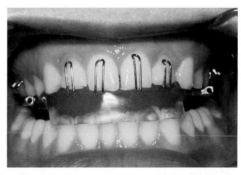

FIGURE 15-33 Torquing springs used with headgear-functional appliance combinations are designed to apply a moment to the incisor crowns and produce bodily incisor movement, or at least overcome some of the lingual incisor tipping common with functional appliances.

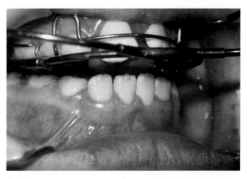

FIGURE 15-34 Headgear tubes can be incorporated into any tooth-borne functional appliance so that additional distal and vertical force can be applied with a facebow and headcap.

length outer bow must be bent upward. The headcap is connected to the facebow and the force adjusted to approximately 400 gm per side. After the facebow is attached, its position may require additional adjustment.

As with any appliance, the patient should demonstrate competence in placement before leaving the initial appointment. The child is instructed to attach the facebow extraorally, place the facebow-functional appliance combination in the mouth, and then attach the headcap. It usually is better for the child to build up wearing time incrementally for the functional appliance during waking hours. Use of the headgear during sleeping hours can begin immediately.

MAXILLARY DEFICIENCY

Transverse Maxillary Constriction

Skeletal maxillary constriction, which is distinguished by a narrow palatal vault, usually produces a posterior crossbite, and posterior crossbite due to a narrow maxilla is an indication for treatment at the time it is discovered. It can be corrected by opening the midpalatal suture, which widens the roof of the mouth and the floor of the nose at any time prior to the end of the adolescent growth spurt.

Several methods of arch expansion are possible, but to obtain skeletal effects, it is necessary to place force directly across the suture. In preadolescent children, three methods can be used for palatal expansion: a split removable plate with a jackscrew or heavy midline spring; a lingual arch, often of the quad-helix design; or a fixed palatal expander with a jackscrew that is either banded or bonded. The rapid palatal expander can be activated for either rapid (0.5 mm or more per day), semirapid (0.25 mm/day), or slow (1 mm/week) expansion. Removable plates and lingual arches produce slow expansion. For each of the possible methods, appropriate questions are: Does it achieve the expansion? Does it have iatrogenic side effects? and, Is the expansion stable?

Palatal Expansion in the Primary and Early Mixed Dentition. Because less force is needed to open the suture in younger children, it is relatively easy to obtain palatal expansion. All three types of appliances can produce both skeletal and dental expansion in the early mixed dentition.[32] Although some studies have reported increases in vertical facial relationships with maxillary expansion,[33] long-term evidence indicates this change is transitory.[34] It has also been demonstrated that it is possible to control vertical growth and posterior eruption with posterior occlusal coverage.[35]

With a removable appliance, the rate of expansion must be quite slow, and the force employed during the process must be low because of problems with retention. Multiple clasps that are well adjusted are mandatory. Because of the instability of the teeth during the expansion process, failure to wear the appliance even for 1 day requires adjustment of the jackscrew, usually by the practi-

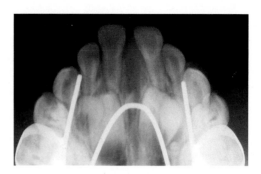

FIGURE 15-35 Prior to adolescence, the midpalatal suture can be opened during maxillary expansion using a number of methods. This occlusal radiograph taken during the primary dentition years illustrates sutural opening in response to the W-arch appliance.

tioner, to constrict the appliance until it again fits and expansion can be resumed. Compliance in activation and wear time are always issues with these appliances. Successful expansion with a removable appliance can take so much time that it is not cost-effective.

Lingual arches of the W-arch and quad helix designs (see Chapter 11) have been demonstrated to open the midpalatal suture in young patients (Figure 15-35). These appliances generally deliver a few hundred grams of force and provide slow expansion. They are relatively clean and reasonably effective, producing a mix of skeletal and dental change.

Fixed jackscrew appliances attached to bands or bonded splints also can be used in the early treatment of maxillary constriction. Banding permanent molars and primary second molars is relatively simple, but banding primary first molars can be challenging. Using a bonded appliance in the mixed dentition is relatively straightforward. This appliance can deliver a variety of forces and can extinguish habits by virtue of its bulk. In young children, in comparison with a lingual arch, there are two major disadvantages. First, the fixed jackscrew appliance is more bulky than an expansion lingual arch and more difficult to place and remove. The patient inevitably has cleaning problems, and either the patient or parent must activate the appliance. Second, a fixed appliance of this type can be activated rapidly, which in young children is a disadvantage—not an advantage. Rapid expansion should not be done in a young child. There is a risk of distortion of facial structures with rapid expansion (see Figure 8-16), and there is no evidence that rapid movement and high forces produce better or more stable expansion.

Many functional appliances incorporate some components to expand the maxillary arch either intrinsic force-generating mechanisms like springs and jackscrews or buccal shields to relieve buccal soft tissue pressure. When arch expansion occurs during functional appliance treatment (Figure 15-36), it is possible that some opening of the midpalatal suture contributes to it, but the mix of skeletal and dental change is not well-documented.

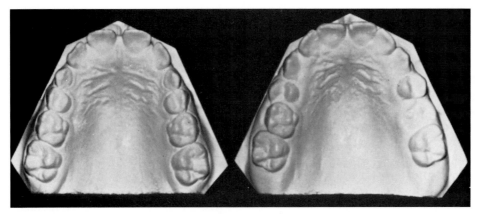

FIGURE 15-36 The pre-treatment cast on the left and the progress cast on the right demonstrate the increase in transverse dimension that usually occurs in response to Frankel appliance therapy as a result of the alteration of the cheek-tongue equilibrium.

A 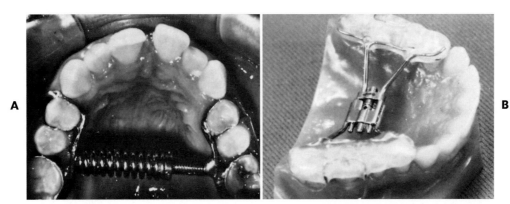 **B**

FIGURE 15-37 **A,** This banded palatal expander uses a screw device together with a spring to deliver the forces to the maxilla. The spring produces more constant force levels than are obtained with a nonflexible system. **B,** This expander is retained by bonding the acrylic resin to the teeth (with the facial and lingual but not the occlusal surfaces etched). It incorporates bite blocks to control the tendency for dental extrusion and downward mandibular rotation as a consequence of the lateral expansion. The wire loop on the facial facilitates debonding (see Figure 16-15). (Courtesy Dr. David Sarver.)

On balance, therefore, slow expansion with an active lingual arch is the preferred approach to maxillary constriction in young children in the primary and early mixed dentitions. A fixed jackscrew appliance is an acceptable alternative if activated carefully and slowly.

Palatal Expansion in the Late Mixed Dentition. With increasing age, the midpalatal suture becomes more and more tightly interdigitated, but in most individuals, it remains possible to obtain significant increments in maxillary width up to age 15 to 18. Expansion in adolescents is discussed in some detail in Chapter 16.

Even in the late mixed dentition, sutural expansion requires placing a relatively heavy force directed across the suture to move the halves of the maxilla apart. A fixed jackscrew appliance (either banded or bonded) is required (Figure 15-37). As many teeth as possible should be included in the anchorage unit. In the late mixed dentition, root resorption of primary molars may have reached the point that these teeth offer little resistance, and it may be wise to wait for eruption of the first premolars before beginning expansion.

Rapid or Slow Expansion? In the late mixed dentition, either rapid or slow expansion is clinically acceptable. As we have reviewed in some detail in Chapter 8, it now appears that slower activation of the expansion appliance (i.e., at the rate of about 1 mm/week) provides approximately the same ultimate result over a 10 to 12 week period as rapid expansion, with less trauma to the teeth and bones (see Figure 8-18).

Rapid expansion typically is done with two turns daily of the jackscrew (0.5 mm activation). This creates 10 to 20 pounds of pressure across the suture—enough to create microfractures of interdigitating bone spicules. When a screw is the activating device, the force is transmitted immediately to the teeth and then to the suture. Sometimes a large coil spring is incorporated along with the screw, which modulates the amount of force, depending on the length and stiffness of the spring (see Figure 15-37, *A*). The suture opens wider and faster anteriorly because of the buttressing effect of the other maxillary structures in the posterior regions. A diastema usually appears between the central incisors as the bones separate in this area (Figure 15-38). Expansion usually is continued until the maxillary lingual cusps occlude with the lingual inclines of the buccal cusps of the mandibular molars. When expansion has been completed, a 3-month period of retention with the appliance in place is recommended. After the 3-month retention period, the fixed appliance can be removed, but a removable retainer that covers the palate is often needed as further insurance against early relapse (Figure 15-39).

The theory behind rapid activation was that force on the teeth would be transmitted to the bone, and the two halves of the maxilla would separate before significant tooth movement could occur. In other words, rapid activa-

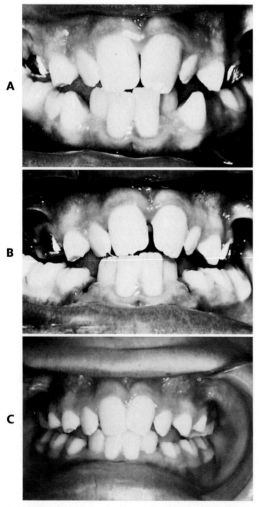

FIGURE 15-38   Spacing of the maxillary central incisors during rapid palatal expansion. **A,** When the appliance is placed and treatment begins, there is only a tiny diastema; **B,** after 1 week of expansion, the teeth have moved laterally with the skeletal structures; **C,** after retention, a combination of skeletal relapse and pull of the gingival fibers has brought the incisors together and closed the diastema.

tion was a way to maximize skeletal change and minimize dental change. It was not realized initially that during the time it takes for bone to fill in the space that was created between the left and right halves of the maxilla, skeletal relapse begins to occur almost immediately, even though the teeth are held in position. The central diastema closes from a combination of skeletal relapse and tooth movement created by stretched gingival fibers. The net treatment effect therefore is approximately equal skeletal and dental expansion (see Chapter 8).

Slower activation of the expansion appliance at the rate of 1 mm/week, which produces about 2 pounds of pressure in a mixed dentition child, opens the suture at a rate that is close to the maximum speed of bone formation.[36] The suture is not obviously pulled apart on radiographs, and no midline diastema appears, but both skeletal and dental changes occur. After 10 to 12 weeks, approximately the same roughly equal amounts of skeletal and dental expansion are present that were seen at the same time with rapid expansion. When bonded slow and rapid palatal expanders in early adolescents were compared in a recent study, the major difference was greater expansion across the canines in the rapid expansion group. This translated into a predicted greater arch perimeter change but similar opening of the suture posteriorly.[37] It appears that simply turning the screw more slowly (e.g., one turn every other day) in a typical fixed expansion appliance is effective. Alternatively, a spring to produce 2 pounds of force can be used.[36]

Clinical Management of Palatal Expansion Devices. Most traditional palate expansion devices use bands for retention on first premolars and permanent first molars if possible. During the late mixed dentition years the first premolars often are not fully erupted and are difficult to band. If the primary second molars are firm, they can be banded along with the permanent first molars. Alternatively but less desirably, only the permanent first molars can be banded. With this approach, the appliance is generally extended anteriorly, contacting the other posterior primary and erupting permanent teeth near their gingival margins.

The bands are stabilized in an impression while it is poured, so they are retained in the completed working

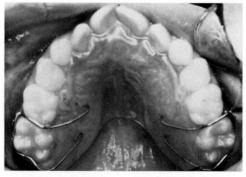

FIGURE 15-39   Following palatal expansion, an acrylic retainer that covers the palate is needed to control relapse.

model. A soldered wire framework and plastic palatal portions, if desired, are added during appliance fabrication. After crossbite correction is completed, band removal can be difficult because the teeth are mobile and sensitive. In those cases, sectioning the bands is appropriate.

An alternative approach is to use a bonded palatal expander (see Figure 15-37, *B* and *C*). During fabrication of the working casts, plastic is generally extended over the occlusal and facial and lingual surfaces of the posterior teeth. When the appliance is returned from the laboratory, because of poor dimensional stability and distortion of the plastic portion, it may be necessary to relieve the acrylic where it seats on the maxillary teeth, reline this area with additional plastic, and refit the appliance in the mouth. By removing the appliance before final polymerization, it can be trimmed and further adjusted without complication. Generally, a composite resin is used to retain the appliance, with only the facial and lingual surfaces of the posterior teeth etched. Etching the occlusal surface is not recommended—bonding there is unnecessary for retention and can greatly complicate appliance removal.

Removal of the appliance is accomplished with a band remover engaged under a facial or lingual plastic margin, and is facilitated by including loops of wire extending from the facial surfaces (see Figure 16-15). The appliance can be sectioned, but this is time-consuming and usually unnecessary. Complete resin removal can be laborious, so using only an adequate amount of resin is crucial. There is a delicate balance. Inadequate resin will lead to excessive leakage onto the unbonded surfaces, which can result in decalcification, or appliance loss. Too much resin, on the other hand, can make tooth and appliance cleaning, as well as appliance removal, difficult. For these reasons, some clinicians use glass ionomer cement for retention. The strength of the material usually is adequate but bonding failure may occur. Fluoride release from these cements may prove advantageous in the short term.

Anteroposterior and Vertical Maxillary Deficiency

Both anteroposterior and vertical maxillary deficiency can contribute to Class III malocclusion. If the maxilla is small or positioned posteriorly, the effect is direct. If it does not grow vertically, the mandible rotates upward and forward, producing an appearance of mandibular prognathism that may be due more to the position of the mandible than its size.

For children with a-p and vertical maxillary deficiency, the preferred treatment is to move the maxilla into a more anterior and inferior position, which also increases its size as bone is added at the posterior and superior sutures. A wide range of treatment timing has been reported,[38] but careful evaluation and meta-analysis[39] indicate treatment is most effective when combined with maxillary expansion before age 10. When force is applied to the teeth for transmission to the sutures, tooth movement in addition to skeletal change is inevitable.

Clinical Management of Facemask Treatment. Generally, it is better to defer maxillary protraction until the permanent first molars have erupted and can be incorporated into the anchorage unit. Following palatal expansion or in conjunction with it, a facemask that obtains anchorage from the forehead and chin (Figure 15-40) is

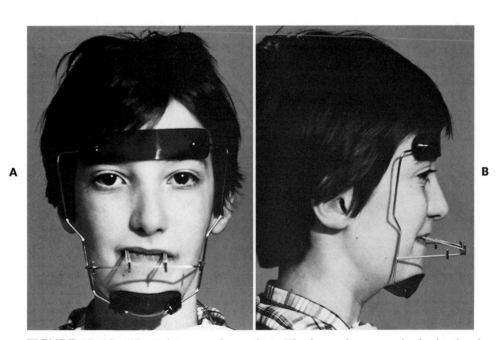

FIGURE 15-40 The Delaire-type facemask. **A,** The facemask contacts the forehead and chin for anchorage and should be adjusted several millimeters away from the other soft tissues. **B,** Adjustment of the wire framework will produce the desired fit and direction of pull on the maxilla (usually downward for increased vertical facial development and patient comfort) when the elastics are placed from the mask to splint.

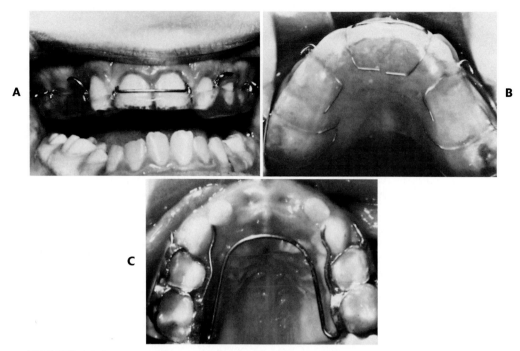

FIGURE 15-41   A maxillary removable splint is often used to make the upper arch a single unit for maxillary protraction. **A,** The splint incorporates hooks in the canine-premolar region for attachment of elastics and, **B,** should cover the anterior and posterior teeth and occlusal surfaces for best retention. Note that the hooks extend gingivally, so that the line of force comes closer to the center of resistance of the maxilla. Multiple clasps also aid in retention. A bonded expander or wire splint, **C,** also can be used and consists of four bands on primary teeth connected by a palatal wire and having hooks on the facial. A splint of this type allows simultaneous expansion if desired.

used to exert a forward force on the maxilla via elastics that attach to a maxillary appliance. To resist tooth movement as much as possible, the maxillary teeth should be splinted together as a single unit. The maxillary appliance can be banded, bonded, or removable (Figure 15-41). A removable plastic splint that covers the occlusal surfaces of the teeth often is satisfactory. Multiple clasps combined with plastic that extends over the incisal edges usually provide adequate retention. If necessary, the splint can be bonded in place, but this causes hygiene problems and should be avoided if possible for long-term use. It also is possible to use a heavy wire splint that incorporates a lingual arch (for arch expansion) cemented to the primary and molars and whatever permanent teeth are available (see Figure 15-41, *C*). Whatever the method of attachment, the appliance must have hooks for attachment to the face mask that are located in the canine-primary molar area above the occlusal plane. This places the force vector nearer the center of resistance of the maxilla and limits maxillary rotation (Figure 15-42).

For most young children, a facemask is as well-accepted as conventional headgear. Contouring an adjustable facemask for a comfortable fit on the forehead is not difficult for most children. There are a variety of designs that accommodate mandibular movement and eyeglasses if necessary.

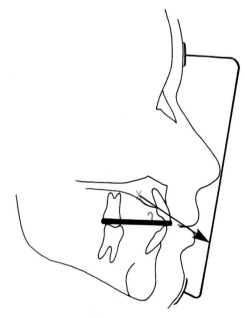

FIGURE 15-42   With the splint over the maxillary teeth and forward pull from the facemask, the hooks on the splint should be elevated. Even so, the line of force is likely to be below the center of resistance of the maxilla, so some downward rotation of the posterior maxilla and opening of the bite anteriorly can be anticipated.

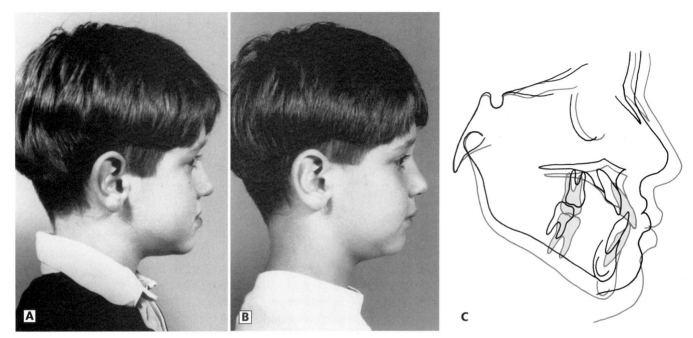

FIGURE 15-43   In a young child, facemask treatment can produce some forward displacement of the maxilla. **A,** Before facemask treatment, age 7; **B,** post-treatment, age 8-6, at the point the facemask was stopped. He wore it 12 hours per day for 14 months; **C,** cephalometric superimposition age 7 to 10, showing the amount of change maintained over 18 months. Note that three things occurred during the treatment: (1) forward movement of the maxilla, almost surely more than would have occurred without treatment; (2) forward displacement of the maxillary teeth; and (3) downward-backward rotation of the mandible. All three effects are typical responses to facemask treatment; often, as here, the downward rotation of the mandible is the major element in improving the Class III relationship. In young children, the magnitude of the skeletal change is usually greater than the dental change. In adolescents, the change is almost entirely tooth movement.

The plastic forehead and chin pads occasionally require re-lining with plastic for an ideal fit or with an adhesive-backed protective pad to reduce soft tissue irritation.

Approximately 12 ounces of force per side is applied for 14 hours per day. Most children with maxillary deficiency are deficient vertically as well as anteroposteriorly, which means that a slight downward direction of elastic traction between the intraoral attachment and the facemask frame usually is desirable. Moving the maxilla down as well as forward rotates the mandible downward and backward, which contributes to correction of a skeletal Class III relationship. A downward pull would be contraindicated, however, if lower face height were already large.

Although the goal of facemask therapy is forward displacement of the maxilla, both downward-backward rotation of the mandible, backward displacement of the mandibular teeth, and forward displacement of the maxillary teeth typically occur in response to this type of treatment (Figure 15-43).[40] Often mandibular rotation and displacement of maxillary teeth— not forward movement of the maxilla—are the major components of the treatment result.

Controlling Tooth Movement by Applying Force to Implants.
Clearly, a major negative side effect of the maxillary protraction procedure is maxillary dental movement that detracts from the skeletal change. Shapiro and Kokich deliberately ankylosed primary canines so they could be used as "natural implants." With traction against a maxillary arch stabilized by these teeth, they were able to demonstrate approximately 3 mm of maxillary protraction in one year, with minimal dental change.[41] If a child with maxillary retrusion has spontaneous ankylosis of primary molars, a splint can be fabricated to use these teeth as implants and gain the same biomechanical advantage (Figure 15-44). It also would be possible to use temporary implants or onplants[42] as a point of attachment, avoiding pressure against the teeth (see Chapter 9), and it is likely that this method will come into regular clinical use in the near future.

Functional Appliances for Maxillary Protraction.
Another possible treatment for correction of maxillary deficiency is a functional appliance made with the mandible positioned posteriorly and rotated open and with pads to stretch the upper lip forward (Figure 15-45). In theory, the lip pads, as used in Frankel's FR-III appliance, stretch the periosteum in a way that stimulates forward growth of the maxilla. The available data, however, indicate little true forward movement of the upper jaw.[43] Instead, most of the improvement is from dental changes. The appliance, which allows the maxillary molars to erupt and move mesially

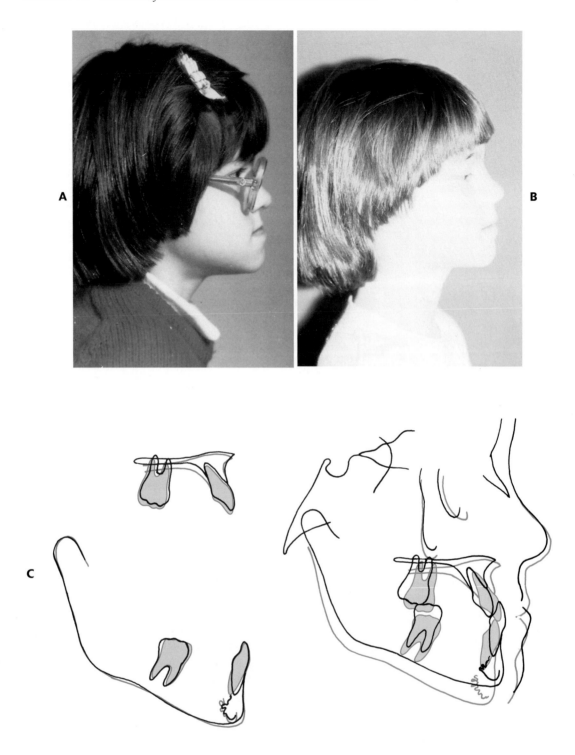

FIGURE 15-44   When ankylosed primary teeth are available for attachment of a facemask, an improved skeletal response can be obtained, as in this patient. **A,** Pre-treatment profile; **B,** post-treatment profile; **C,** cephalometric superimpositions. Note the improvement in the facial concavity, and downward-backward rotation of the mandible, with almost totally skeletal and no dental change. The maxilla rotated down posteriorly, as would be predicted from the relationship of the line of force to its center of resistance.

while holding the lower molars in place vertically and anteroposteriorly, tips the maxillary anterior teeth facially and retracts the mandibular anterior teeth (Figure 15-46). This tooth movement helps in the development of a normal overbite and overjet but has little effect on the skeletal malocclusion. Rotation of the occlusal plane also contributes to the change from a Class III to a Class I molar relationship (Figure 15-47). If the functional appliance rotates the chin down and back (see the following section), the Class III relationship will improve, but again with no effect on the maxilla. In short, functional appliance treatment, even with the use of upper lip pads, has little or no effect on maxillary retrusion.

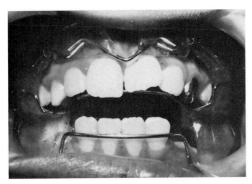

FIGURE 15-45 The Frankel III appliance stretches the soft tissue adjacent to the maxilla, attempting to stimulate forward growth of the maxilla by stretching the periosteum, and does not advance the mandible. The vertical opening is used to enhance downward and forward eruption of maxillary posterior teeth.

MANDIBULAR EXCESS

Children who have Class III malocclusion because of excessive growth of the mandible are extremely difficult to treat. The treatment of choice would appear to be a restraining device (e.g., chin cup/chin cap) to inhibit the growth of the mandible, at least preventing it from projecting forward as much as otherwise would have occurred. Functional appliances also have been advocated for mandibular excess patients. Inhibiting mandibular growth has proven to be almost impossible (see Chapter 8), so with both types of appliances, the major effect is downward and backward rotation of the mandible, which decreases anteroposterior projection of the chin by making the face longer. There is some evidence that a chin cup is more effective in young children under age 7 than the same treatment used later.[44] Unfortunately, despite efforts to modify excessive mandibular growth, many of these children ultimately need surgery, and the chin cup treatment is essentially camouflage.

Extraoral Force to the Mandible: Chin Cup Treatment

In theory, extraoral force directed against the mandibular condyle would restrain growth at that location. Despite success in animal experiments, most human studies have found little difference in mandibular dimensions between treated and untreated subjects (see Chapter 8).[45,46] What chin cup therapy does accomplish is a change in the direction of mandibular growth, rotating the chin down and back. In addition, lingual tipping of the lower incisors oc-

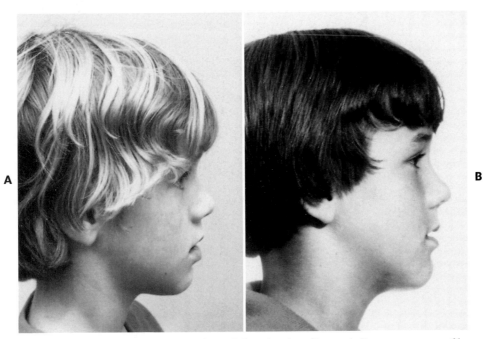

FIGURE 15-46 Response to a Class III functional appliance. **A,** Pre-treatment profile; **B,** post-treatment profile; *Continued*

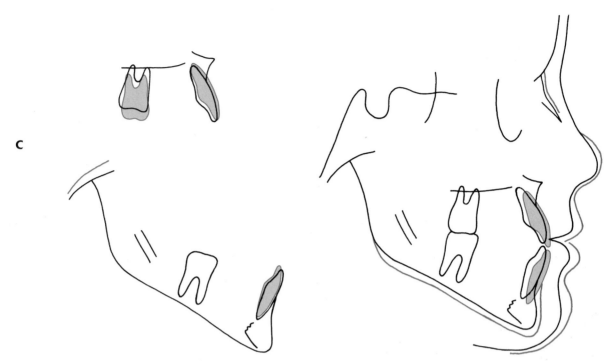

C

FIGURE 15-46, cont'd C, cephalometric superimpositions. Note in the cranial base superimposition that the mandible rotated inferiorly and posteriorly to a less prominent position. The maxillary incisors moved facially and the mandibular incisors tipped lingually. Note the differential eruption of the upper molar, which also contributes to correction of the occlusal relationships. In essence, this method trades increased face height for decreased chin prominence.

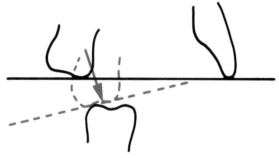

FIGURE 15-47   To facilitate Class III correction, the mesial and vertical eruption of the maxillary molar can be emphasized. This will improve the molar relationships and establish the posterior occlusal plane at a lower level. Rotation of the occlusal plane in this direction facilitates normal interdigitation of the molars in a Class III patient.

curs as a result of the pressure of the appliance on the lower lip and dentition (Figure 15-48).[44]

This type of treatment is appropriate with normal or reduced lower anterior face height but is contraindicated for a child who has excessive lower face height. In essence, the treatment becomes a trade-off between decreasing the anteroposterior prominence of the chin and increasing face height. From this perspective, more Asian than white children can benefit from chin cup treatment because of their generally shorter face heights, not because of a difference in the treatment response. Unfortunately, the majority of white children with excessive mandibular growth have normal or excessive face height, so that only small amounts of mandibular rotation are possible without producing a long-face deformity.

A hard chin cup can be custom fitted from plastic, using an impression of the chin; a commercial metal or plastic cup can be used if it fits well enough; or a soft cup can be made from a football helmet chin strap. Any of these can irritate the soft tissue of the chin and may require a protective liner or talcum powder for comfort. The more the chin cup or strap migrates up toward the lower lip during appliance wear, the more lingual movement of the lower incisors will be produced. Soft cups may produce more tooth movement in this manner than hard ones.

The headcap that includes the spring mechanism can be the same one used for high-pull headgear. It is adjusted in the same manner as the headgear to direct a force of approximately 16 to 24 ounces per side through the head of the condyle or a somewhat lighter force below the condyle. Once it is accepted that mandibular rotation is the major treatment effect, lighter force oriented to produce greater rotation makes more sense.

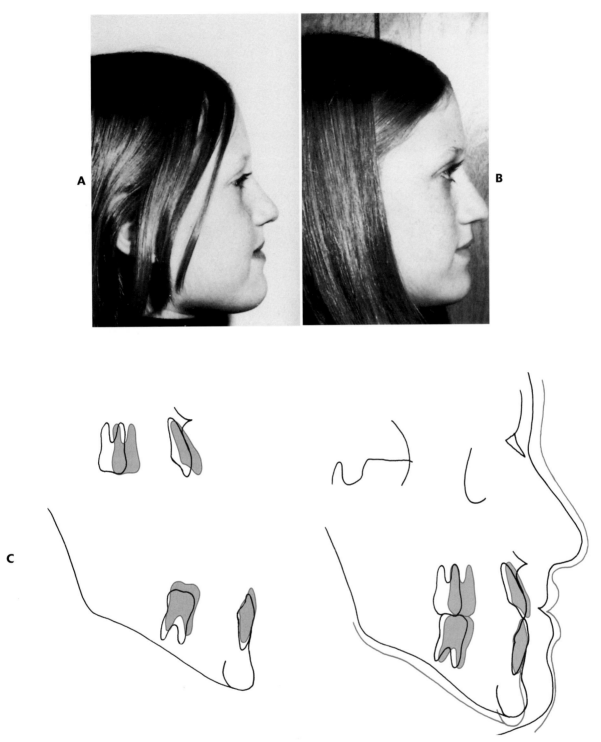

FIGURE 15-48   A typical response to chin-cup treatment. **A,** Pre-treatment profile; **B,** post-treatment profile; **C,** cephalometric superimpositions. The mandible rotated inferiorly and posteriorly to a less prominent position and the maxillary incisors moved labially as the mandibular incisors tipped lingually in response to the pressure of the chin cup. This treatment reduces mandibular protrusion by increasing anterior face height, very similarly to the effect of Class III functional appliances.

Class III Functional Appliances

Class III functional appliances for excessive mandibular growth make no pretense of restraining mandibular growth. They are designed to rotate the mandible down and back and to guide the eruption of the teeth so that the upper posterior teeth erupt down and forward while eruption of lower teeth is restrained. This rotates the occlusal plane in the direction that favors correction of a Class III molar relationship (see Figure 15-47). These appliances also tip the mandibular incisors lingually and the maxillary incisors facially, introducing an element of dental camouflage for the skeletal discrepancy. The only difference from a functional appliance for a maxillary deficiency patient is the absence of lip pads.

Although the theory of the functional appliance is quite different from that of the chin cup, the treatment effects are very similar, and the two approaches are approximately equally effective (or, in severe cases, equally ineffective).

To produce the working bite for a Class III functional appliance, the steps in preparation of the wax, practice for the patient, and the use of a guide to determine the correct vertical position are identical to the procedure for Class II patients. However, the working bite itself is significantly different: the mandible is rotated open on its hinge axis but is not advanced. This type of bite is easier for the dentist to direct because light force can be placed on the chin point to retrude the mandible.

How far the mandible is rotated open depends on the type of appliance and the need to interpose bite blocks and occlusal stops between the teeth to limit eruption. Less vertical opening would be needed for an appliance with lip pads to try to encourage forward movement of the maxilla than for one that encourages eruption and deliberately rotates the mandible significantly back. Appliance adjustments and instructions are similar to those for Class II appliances except that maxillary anterior lip pads (which are not recommended in most cases) often cause soft tissue irritation and must be observed carefully.

Modifying true mandibular prognathism is a difficult task regardless of the chosen method. This problem often leads to irrational choices by practitioners and parents in attempts to control crossbite and poor facial esthetics as the child grows and to avoid surgical treatment when the child has matured. The limited success of early intervention is a reality that must be recognized. For a child with severe prognathism, no treatment until orthognathic surgery can be done at the end of the growth period may be the best treatment.

FACIAL ASYMMETRY IN CHILDREN

Although most people have some facial asymmetry, asymmetric development of the jaws severe enough to cause a problem is relatively rare. Asymmetry in a child can be due to congenital anomalies (e.g., hemifacial microsomia or to hemimandibular hypertrophy) beginning at an early age but usually arises as a result of a fracture of the condylar process of the mandible. The asymmetry in such cases is due to a restriction on growth after the injury—not the displacement of fragments that occurred at the time of injury (see Chapter 5).[47]

When a condylar fracture is diagnosed in a child, maintaining function is the key to normal growth. Function does not mean simple opening and closing hinge movements, but must also include translation of the mandibular condyles. Translation is necessary for normal growth in the long term and for regeneration and stretch of the associated soft tissues in the short term. Fortunately, most jaw fractures in preadolescent children can be treated with little or no surgical manipulation of the segments and little immobilization of the jaws, because the bony segments are self-retentive and the healing process is rapid. Treatment should involve short fixation times (usually maintained with intraoral intermaxillary elastics) and rapid return to function.[48] Open reduction of the fracture should be avoided. A functional appliance during the post-injury period can be used to minimize any growth restriction. The appliance is a conventional activator or bionator-type appliance that symmetrically advances the mandible to nearly an edge-to-edge incisor position. Using this appliance, the patient is forced to translate the mandible, and any remodeling can occur with the mandible in the unloaded and forward position.

Many condylar fractures are not diagnosed at the time of injury, so when a child with asymmetric mandibular deficiency is seen, trauma is the most likely cause even if an injury is not reported. The key to establishing the prognosis for growth modification is the extent to which the affected side can translate. Even if the mandible deviates to the affected side on opening, reasonably normal growth is possible if some degree of translation occurs. Hybrid functional appliances (i.e., those that blend several components designed to address specific problems) can be a powerful treatment tool in these situations (Figure 15-49). Although they may appear confusing, these appliances are simply various components logically combined to achieve specific purposes.

Surgical intervention in an asymmetry situation (or other facial growth problem) prior to adolescence has only one goal: to create an environment in which growth is possible. Therefore surgery is indicated only when abnormal growth is progressively making a problem worse, as in ankylosis that keeps one side from growing or active growth at one condyle—even when significant asymmetry is present. Treatment with a hybrid functional appliance will be needed, possibly before surgery to decompensate the dental arches and certainly after surgery to correct the primary growth problem and guide function. Because of the complexity of treatment planning and the probability that surgery will also be needed, children with progressive deformities usually are better managed through a major medical center.

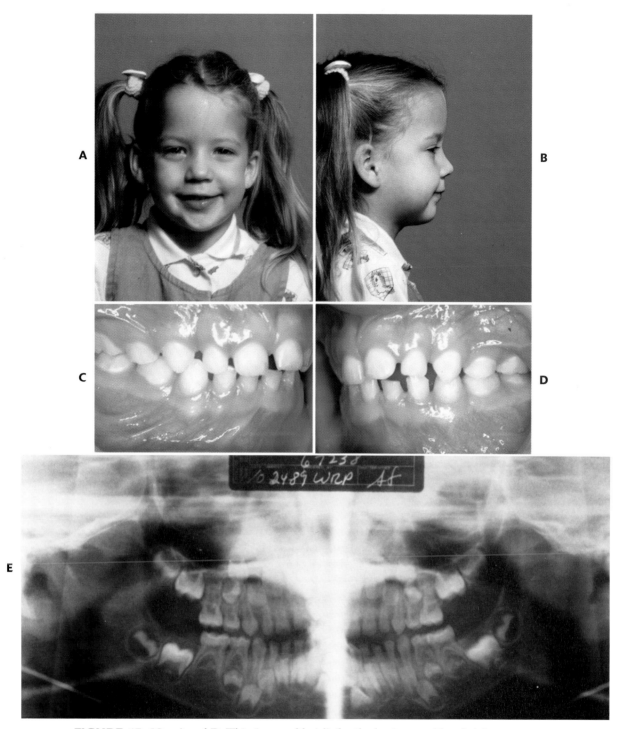

FIGURE 15-49 **A** and **B,** This 5-year-old girl's family dentist noted her facial asymmetry, with the chin off to the left (she deviated even more on opening) and referred her for further evaluation. **C** and **D,** Her buccal occlusion was normal (Class I) on the right and Class II on the left. **E,** The panoramic radiograph showed the classic appearance of a unilateral condylar fracture. Note the normal condyle on the right and only a condylar stub on the left. The injury almost surely occurred at age 2 when she fell but was not diagnosed at the time.

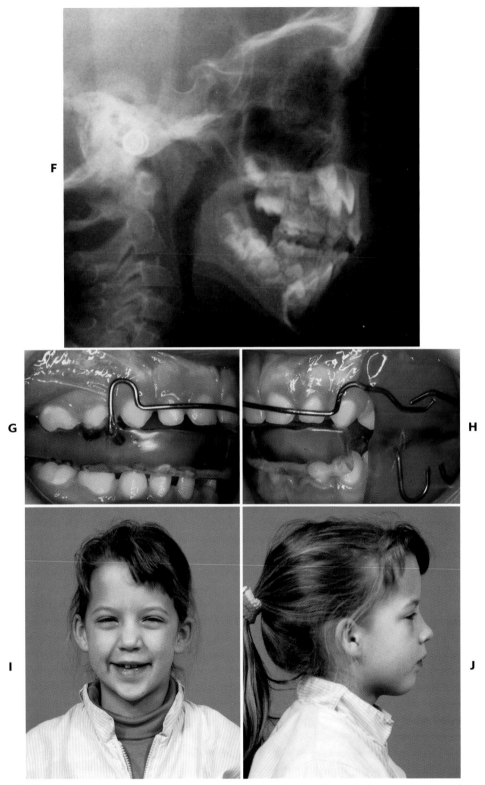

FIGURE 15-49, cont'd F, Note the two mandibular borders on the cephalometric radiograph due to the shorter ramus on the left. **G** and **H,** She was treated with a series of hybrid functional appliances, with buccal and lingual shields on the left, and a bite block anteriorly and on the right. The objective was to encourage mandibular growth and tooth eruption on the deficient left side and restrain eruption on the right. It is important to keep the tongue from between the teeth on the side where eruption is desired, thus the lingual shield on the left side (cannot be seen in the photos) was a critically important part of the appliance. **I** and **J,** Facial views 2 years later. *Continued*

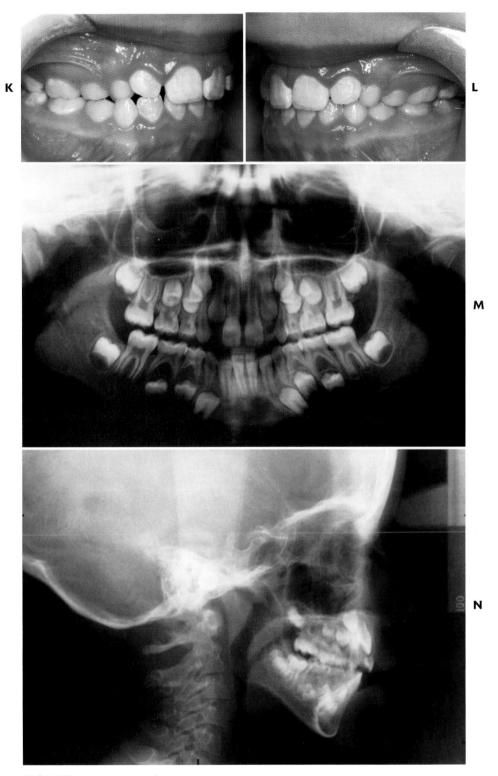

FIGURE 15-49, cont'd K and **L,** Intraoral views 2 years later. Note the improvement in both facial symmetry and occlusion. Treatment with hybrid functional appliances was continued. **M,** Panoramic and **N,** cephalometric progress views. Note the regeneration of the left condyle and reduction in the difference in height of the two mandibular rami.

Continued

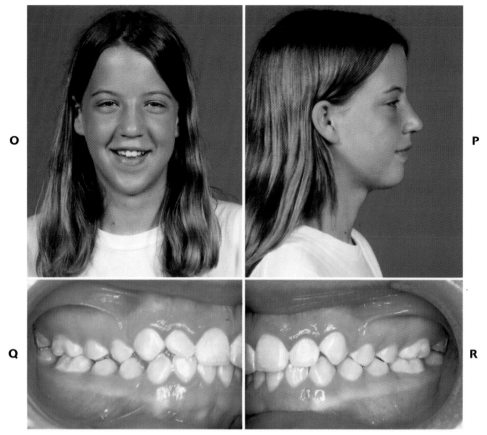

FIGURE 15-49, cont'd   **O** and **P,** Facial and **Q** and **R,** intraoral views at age 13, with nearly complete resolution of the facial asymmetry although the mandible still deviates to the left on wide opening. Functional appliance treatment was discontinued at age 10, and there has been no further orthodontic therapy.

REFERENCES

1. Wieslander L: Long-term effect of treatment with the head-gear-Herbst appliance in the early mixed dentition: stability or relapse?, Am J Orthod Dentofac Orthop 104:319-29, 1993.
2. Keeling SD, Wheeler TT, King GJ et al: Anteroposterior skeletal and dental changes after early Class II treatment with bionators and headgear, Am J Orthod Dentofac Orthop 113:40-50, 1998.
3. Tulloch JFC, Phillips C, Proffit WR: Benefit of early Class II treatment: Progress report of a two-phase randomized clinical trial, Am J Orthod Dentofac Orthop 113:62-72, 1998.
4. Pancherz H: The effects, limitations, and long-term dento-facial adaptations to treatment with the Herbst appliance, Sem Orthod 3:232-243, 1997.
5. Lund DI, Sandler PJ: The effects of twin blocks: a prospective controlled study, Am J Orthod Dentofac Orthop 113:104-10, 1998.
6. Mills CM, McCulloch KJ: Treatment effects of the twin block appliance: a cephalometric study, Am J Orthod Dentofac Orthop 114:15-24, 1998.
7. Pancherz H, Malmgren O, Hagg U et al: Class II correction in Herbst and Bass therapy, Eur J Orthod 11:17-30, 1989.

8. DeVincenzo JP, Winn MW: Orthopedic and orthodontic effects resulting from the use of a functional appliance with different amounts of protrusive activation, Am J Orthod Dentofac Orthop 96:181-90,1989.
9. McNamara JA, Howe RP: Clinical management of the acrylic splint Herbst appliance, Am J Orthod Dentofac Orthop 94:142-149, 1988.
10. Lai M, McNamara JA Jr: An evaluation of two-phase treatment with the Herbst appliance and preadjusted edgewise therapy, Sem Orthod 4:46-58, 1998.
11. Stevenson S, Hunziker EB, Hermann W, Schenk RK: Is longitudinal bone growth influenced by diurnal variation in the mitotic activity of chondrocytes of the growth plates? J Orthop Res 8:132-135, 1990.
12. Risinger RK, Proffit WR: Continuous overnight observation of human premolar eruption, Arch Oral Biol 41:779-89, 1996.
13. Sahm G, Bartsch A, Witt E: Micro-electronic monitoring of functional appliance wear, Eur J Orthod 12:297-301, 1990.
14. Pancherz H, Fackel U: The skeletofacial growth pattern pre- and post-dentofacial orthopedics: a long-term study of Class II malocclusions treated with the Herbst appliance, Eur J Orthod 12:209-218, 1990.
15. Nanda SK: Patterns of vertical growth of the face, Am J Orthod Dentofac Orthop 93:103-116, 1988.

16. Ruf S, Pancherz H: The effect of Herbst appliance treatment on the mandibular plane angle: a cephalometric roentgenographic study, Am J Orthod Dentofac Orthop 110:225-9, 1996.
17. Oppenheim A: Biologic orthodontic therapy and reality, Angle Orthod 6:69-79, 1936.
18. Kloehn S: Guiding alveolar growth and eruption of the teeth to reduce treatment time and produce a more balanced denture and face, Am J Orthod 17:10-33, 1947.
19. Wieslander L: The effects of orthodontic treatment on the concurrent development of the craniofacial complex, Am J Orthod 49:15-27, 1963.
20. Armstrong MM: Controlling the magnitude, direction and duration of extraoral force, Am J Orthod 59:217-243, 1971.
21. Baumrind S, Molthen R, West, EE, Miller D: Mandibular plane changes during maxillary retraction, part 2, Am J Orthod 74:603-621, 1978.
22. Boecler PR, Riolo ML, Keeling SD, TenHave TR: Skeletal changes associated with extraoral appliance therapy: an evaluation of 200 consecutively treated cases, Angle Orthod 59:263-70, 1989.
23. Chaushu G et al: Infraorbital abscess from orthodontic headgear, Am J Orthod Dentofac Orthop 112:364-366, 1997.
24. Stafford GD, Caputo AA, Turley PK: Characteristics of headgear release mechanisms: safety implications, Angle Orthod 68:319-326, 1998.
25. Fields H, Proffit W, Nixon W et al: Facial pattern differences in long-faced children and adults, Am J Orthod 85:217-223, 1984.
26. Ucem TT, Yuksel S: Effects of different vectors of forces applied by combined headgear, Am J Orthod Dentofac Orthop 113:316-23, 1998.
27. Baumrind S, Korn EL, Isaacson RJ et al: Quantitative analysis of orthodontic and orthopedic effects of maxillary traction, Am J Orthod 84:384-398, 1983.
28. Orton HS, Slattery DA, Orton S: The treatment of severe 'gummy' Class II division 1 malocclusion using the maxillary intrusion splint, Eur J Orthod 14:216-23, 1992.
29. Weinbach JR, Smith RJ: Cephalometric changes during treatment with the open bite bionator, Am J Orthod Dentofac Orthop 101:367-74, 1992.
30. Lagerstrom LO, Nielsen IL, Lee R, Isaacson RJ: Dental and skeletal contributions to occlusal correction in patients treated with the high-pull headgear—activator combination, Am J Orthod Dentofac Orthop 97:495-504, 1990.
31. Stockli PW, Teuscher UM: Combined activator headgear orthopedics. In (Graber TM and Vanarsdall RL, editors) Orthodontics: current principles and techniques, St Louis, 1994, Mosby.
32. Sandikcioglu M, Hazar S: Skeletal and dental changes after maxillary expansion in the mixed dentition, Am J Orthod Dentofac Orthop 111:321-7, 1997.
33. daSilva Filho OG, Villas Boas M, Capelozza Filho L: Rapid palatal expansion in the deciduous and mixed dentitions: a cephalometric evaluation, Am J Orthod Dentofac Orthop 100:171-81, 1991.
34. Chang JY, McNamara JA Jr, Herberger TA: A longitudinal study of skeletal side effects induced by rapid maxillary expansion, Am J Orthod Dentofac Orthop 112:330-337, 1997.
35. Asanza S, Cisneros GJ, Nieberg LG: Comparison of Hyrax and bonded expansion appliances, Angle Orthod 67:15-22, 1997.
36. Hicks E: Slow maxillary expansion: a clinical study of the skeletal versus the dental response to low magnitude force, Am J Orthod 73:121-141, 1978.
37. Akkaya S, Lorenzon S, Ucem TT: Comparison of dental arch and arch perimeter changes between bonded rapid and slow maxillary expansion procedures, Eur J Orthod 20:255-61, 1998.
38. Merwin D, Ngan P, Hagg U et al: Timing for effective application of anteriorly directed orthopedic force to the maxilla, Am J Orthod Dentofac Orthop 112:292-299, 1997.
39. Kim J, Marlos A, Graber T. Metal: The effectiveness of protraction face mask therapy: a meta-analysis. Am J Orthod Dentofac Orthop 115:675–685, 1999.
40. da Silva Filho OG, Magro AC, Capelozza Filho L: Early treatment of the Class III malocclusion with rapid maxillary expansion and maxillary protraction, Am J Orthod Dentofac Orthop 113:196-203, 1998.
41. Shapiro PA, Kokich VG: Treatment alternatives for children with severe maxillary hypoplasia, Eur J Orthod 6:141-147, 1984.
42. Block MS, Huffman DR: A new device for absolute anchorage for orthodontics, Am J Orthod Dentofac Orthop 107:251-258, 1995.
43. Ulgen M, Firatli S: The effects of the Frankel's function regulator on the Class III malocclusion, Am J Orthod Dentofac Orthop 105:561-567, 1994.
44. Sugawara J, Mitani H: Facial growth of skeletal Class III malocclusion and the effects, limitations, and long-term dentofacial adaptations to chin cap therapy, Sem Orthod 3:244-254, 1997.
45. Sakamoto T, Iwase I, Uka A et al: A roentgenocephalometric study of skeletal changes during and after chin cap treatment, Am J Orthod 85:341-350, 1984.
46. Sugawara J, Asano T, Endo N, Matani H: Long-term effects of chincup therapy on skeletal profile in mandibular prognathism, Am J Orthod Dentofac Orthop 98:127-33, 1990.
47. Proffit WR, Turvey TA, Vig KW: Early fracture of the mandibular condyles: frequently an unsuspected cause of growth disturbances, Am J Orthod 78:1-24, 1980.
48. Blakey GH, Ruiz R, Turvey TA: Management of facial fractures in the growing patient. In Fonseca RJ, Walker RV, Betts NJ, Barker HD (editors): Oral and maxillofacial trauma Philadelphia, 1997, W.B. Saunders.

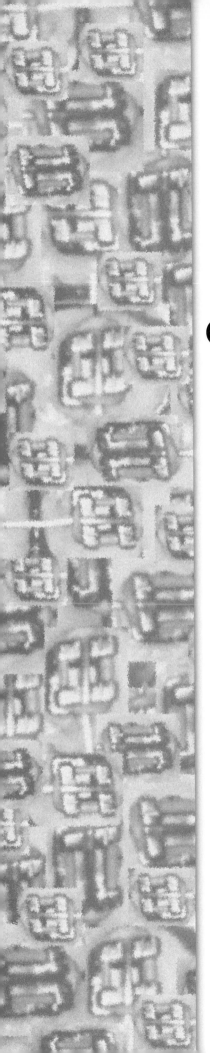

SECTION

VII

COMPREHENSIVE ORTHODONTIC TREATMENT IN THE EARLY PERMANENT DENTITION

Comprehensive orthodontic treatment implies an effort to make the patient's occlusion as ideal as possible, repositioning all or nearly all the teeth in the process. From this perspective, the mixed dentition treatment described in Chapters 13 through 15 is not comprehensive, despite its importance, because the final position of all the permanent teeth is not affected. A second phase of comprehensive treatment after the permanent teeth erupt, during which the details of occlusal relationships are established, is usually needed for children with moderate or severe malocclusion even if significant improvement occurred during a first phase of treatment in the mixed dentition.

The ideal time for comprehensive treatment is during adolescence, when the succedaneous teeth have just erupted, some vertical and anteroposterior growth of the jaws remains, and the social adjustment to orthodontic treatment is no great problem. Not all adolescent patients require comprehensive treatment, of course, and limited treatment to overcome specific problems can certainly be done at any age. Comprehensive treatment is also possible for adults, but it poses some special problems. These are discussed in Chapter 21.

Comprehensive orthodontic treatment usually requires a complete fixed appliance. In the chapters that follow, the use of a contemporary edgewise appliance that incorporates offsets, angulation, and torque in the brackets (i.e., a "straight wire" appliance) is assumed during much of the discussion. Three major stages of treatment are used to conveniently divide comprehensive treatment into sequential steps for discussion in Chapters 16 through 18. In each of these chapters, the different arch wires and arch wire sequences for sliding vs. loop mechanics and 22 versus 18 slots are emphasized. A brief description of treatment with the Begg appliance is included at appropriate points.

Whatever the orthodontic technique, treatment must be discontinued gradually, using some sort of retention appliance for a time, and this important subject is covered in the last chapter of this section.

CHAPTER

16

The First Stage of Comprehensive Treatment: Alignment and Leveling

The idea of dividing treatment into stages, which makes it easier to discuss technique, is particularly associated with the Begg technique. The three major stages discussed in this and the following two chapters are those traditionally used to describe the stages of Begg treatment,[1] but the division is reasonably applicable to edgewise treatment as well. These major stages of comprehensive treatment are: (1) alignment and leveling, (2) correction of molar relationship and space closure, and (3) finishing. The latter two stages are covered in Chapters 17 and 18, respectively. Not every patient will require the steps of each treatment stage, but whatever the technique, it is likely that both the arch wires and the way they are utilized will be changed at the various stages. In theory at least, there is more to be done in the finishing stage with the Begg appliance, particularly torquing of incisors and root uprighting of canines and premolars, than if a contemporary edgewise appliance is used. Nevertheless, the considerations are the same, and at least some appliance adjustment is needed to finish comprehensive treatment with even the most cleverly preadjusted edgewise appliance.

GOALS OF THE FIRST STAGE OF TREATMENT

Treatment for any patient should be undertaken only after a thorough analysis of the patient's problems, the preparation of a treatment plan to maximize benefit for that patient, and the development of a sequence of orthodontic treatment steps (arch wires and their activation, i.e., mechanotherapy) to produce the desired result. The diagnostic and treatment planning procedure outlined in Chapters 6 and 7, which culminates in an outline of the steps in treatment, is recommended.

In almost all patients with malocclusion, at least some teeth are initially malaligned. The great majority also have either excessive overbite, resulting from some combination of an excessive curve of Spee in the lower arch and an absent or reverse curve of Spee in the upper arch, or (less frequently) anterior open bite with excessive curve of Spee in the upper arch and little or none in the lower arch. The goals of the first phase of treatment are to bring the teeth into alignment and correct vertical discrepancies by leveling out the arches. In this form, however, neither goal is stated clearly enough. For proper alignment, it is necessary not only to bring malposed teeth into the arch, but also to specify and control the anteroposterior position of incisors, the width of the arches posteriorly, and the form of the dental arches. Similarly, in leveling the arch, it is necessary to determine and control whether the leveling occurs by elongation of posterior teeth, intrusion of incisors, or some specific combination of the two (see Chapter 7 for treatment planning details).

The form of the dental arches obviously varies between individuals. Although the orthodontist has some latitude in changing arch form, and indeed must do so in at least one arch if the upper and lower arch are not compatible initially, more stable results are achieved when the patient's original arch form is preserved during orthodontic treatment (see Chapter 12 for a discussion of arch form and arch wire shape). The light resilient arch wires used in the first stage of treatment need not be shaped to the patient's arch form as carefully as the heavier arch wires used later in treatment, but from the beginning, the arch wires should reflect each individual's arch form. If preformed arch wires are used, from the beginning the appropriate large, medium or small arch form should be selected.

Because the orthodontic mechanotherapy will be different depending on exactly how alignment and leveling are to be accomplished, it is extremely important that the desired position of the teeth at the end of each stage of treatment be clearly visualized before that stage is begun (Figure 16-1). The best alignment procedures will result in incisors that are far too protrusive, for instance, if the extractions necessary to prevent protrusion were not part of the plan. Similarly, unless leveling by intrusion is planned when it is needed, the appropriate mechanics are not likely to be selected.

In this and the subsequent chapters, it is expected that the appropriate goals for an individual patient have been clearly stated, and the discussion here concerns only the treatment techniques necessary to achieve those goals. Orthodontic treatment without specific goals can be an excellent illustration of the old adage, "If you don't know where you're going, it doesn't matter which road you take."

ALIGNMENT

Principles in the Choice of Alignment Arches

In nearly every patient with malaligned teeth, the root apices are closer to the normal position than the crowns, because malalignment almost always develops as the eruption paths of teeth are deflected. Putting it another way, a tooth bud occasionally develops in the wrong place, but (barring surgery that displaces all tissues in the area, as sometimes happens in cleft palate repairs, or the severe tipping from lip pressure that displaces maxillary central incisors in Class II, division 2 cases) the root apices are likely to be reasonably close to their correct positions even though the crowns have been displaced as the teeth erupted. To bring teeth into alignment, a combination of labiolingual and mesiodistal tipping guided by an arch wire is needed, but root movement usually is not. Several important consequences for orthodontic mechanotherapy follow from this:

1. Initial arch wires for alignment should provide light, continuous force of approximately 50 grams, to produce the most efficient tipping tooth movement. Heavy force, in contrast, is to be avoided.
2. The archwires should be able to move freely within the brackets. For mesiodistal sliding along an arch wire, at least 2 mil clearance between the arch wire and the bracket is needed, and 4 mil clearance is desirable. This means that the largest initial arch wire that should be used with an 18-slot edgewise bracket is 16 mil, whereas 14 mil would be more satisfactory. With the 22-slot bracket, an 18 mil arch wire would be close to ideal from a bracket clearance point of view. Whatever the arch wire, it should

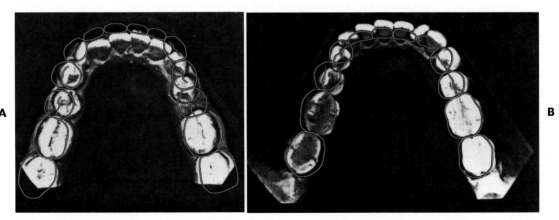

FIGURE 16-1   Goals of the first stage of treatment can be visualized on a print (from an ordinary office copy machine) of the dental arches. **A,** Expansion of the arch in a 12-year-old girl, to provide space for a blocked-out second premolar. Some anterior movement of the incisors will occur, but this can be partially prevented by including a component of lateral expansion. **B,** Alignment of crowded incisors with premolar extraction in a young adult. With the incisors aligned in the same anteroposterior position, about half the extraction space on each side will remain. This view does not show space required for leveling, which must not be overlooked in planning (see Chapter 6).

be ligated loosely in the bracket (indeed, this is probably the critical factor in determining frictional resistance to sliding).

3. Rectangular arch wires, particularly those with a tight fit within the bracket slot so that the position of the root apex could be affected, normally should be

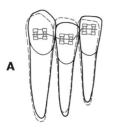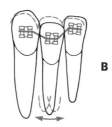

FIGURE 16-2 A tightly fitting resilient rectangular arch wire for initial alignment is almost always undesirable because it produces back-and-forth movement of the root apices as the teeth move into alignment. This occurs because the moments generated by the arch wire change as the geometry of the system changes with alterations in tooth position. **A,** Diagrammatic representation of the alignment of a malposed lateral incisor with a round wire and clearance in the bracket slot. With minimal moments created within the bracket slot, there is little displacement of the root apex. **B,** With a resilient rectangular arch wire, back-and-forth movement of the apex occurs before the tooth ends up in essentially the same place as with a round wire. This has two disadvantages: it increases the possibility of root resorption, and it slows the alignment process.

avoided. The principle is that it is better to tip crowns to position during initial alignment, rather than displacing the root apices; the corollary is that although a highly resilient rectangular arch wire such as 17 × 25 NiTi could be used in the alignment stage, this is not advantageous because the rectangular arch wire will create unnecessary and undesirable root movement during alignment (Figure 16-2). Round wires for alignment are preferred. There is no reason to pay extra for a high-performance rectangular wire for initial alignment, when alignment with it predictably will be slower and potentially more damaging to the roots than with a smaller round wire.

4. The springier the alignment arch wire, the more important it is that the crowding be at least reasonably symmetric. Otherwise, there is a danger that arch form will be lost as asymmetrically irregular teeth are brought into alignment. If only one tooth is crowded out of line (or if an impacted tooth has to be brought into alignment—see below), a rigid wire is needed that maintains arch form except where springiness is required, and an auxiliary wire should be used to reach the malaligned tooth (Figure 16-3).

Properties of Alignment Arch Wires

The wires for initial alignment require a combination of excellent strength, excellent springiness, and a long range of action. Ideally, there would be an almost flat load-

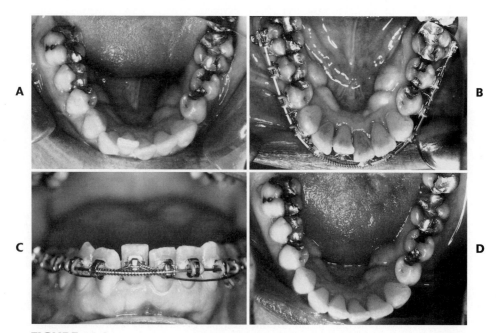

FIGURE 16-3 Use of an auxiliary superelastic wire for incisor alignment. **A,** Irregular incisors in an adult with periodontal bone loss; **B** and **C,** After space was opened for the right lateral incisor, a superelastic wire segment tied beneath the brackets was used to bring the lateral incisor into position, while arch form was maintained by a heavier arch wire in the bracket slots; **D,** alignment completed. This approach allows use of optimal force on the tooth to be moved and distributes the reaction force over the rest of the teeth in the arch.

deflection curve, with the wire delivering about 50 gm (the optimum force for tipping) at almost any degree of deflection. The variables in selecting appropriate arch wires for alignment are the arch wire material, its size (diameter or cross-section), and the distance between attachments (interbracket span). These factors have been discussed in Chapter 10 but are briefly reviewed here. Considering them in turn:

Arch wire Material.   The titanium-based arch wires, both nickel-titanium (any of the NiTi wires) and beta-titanium (TMA), offer a better combination of strength and springiness than do steel wires (see Chapter 10). The NiTi wires, however, are both springier and stronger in small cross-section than beta-Ti. For this reason, NiTi wires are particularly useful in the first stage of treatment, and the remarkably flat load-deflection curve for superelastic NiTi (austenitic NiTi, A-NiTi) makes it the preferred material. It is important to keep in mind that not all ostensibly superelastic wires offer the same performance, however (see Figure 10-9). The choice of a superelastic wire should be based on performance data—and a product with advertising claims but no data should be regarded with considerable suspicion. If steel is used at this stage, either multistranded wires or loops to increase springiness (see following) are needed. Beta-Ti rarely is the best choice for an initial arch wire.

Size of Wire.   For the superelastic A-NiTi wires, the manufacturer's preparation of the material determines the clinical performance (Figure 16-4), so wire size is a concern primarily with respect to clearance in the bracket slot. For M-NiTi, beta-Ti or steel wires, wire size is an important criterion. As wire size increases, strength increases rapidly, while springiness decreases even more rapidly. For alignment, the smallest diameter (and therefore the springiest) wire that has adequate strength would be preferred. When multiple strands of the same diameter wire are used, strength is added while springiness is relatively unaffected. This method of combining steel strands that individually would not be strong enough, makes steel wires without loops practical at the initial stage of treatment.

Distance Between Attachments.   As the distance increases between the points of attachment of a beam, strength decreases rapidly while springiness increases even more rapidly. The width of brackets determines beam length when continuous arch wires are used (unless brackets are bypassed): the wider the individual brackets, the smaller the interbracket span. For this reason, elastic arch wires become very much stiffer when wide brackets reduce interbracket span. This is a particularly important consideration when non-superelastic wires are used initially.

As we have discussed in Chapter 10, it is logical to use narrow brackets with 18-slot edgewise, for two reasons: (1) in the latter stages of treatment the rectangular steel arch wires that fill the slot are more effective with larger interbracket spans, and (2) sliding teeth along the arch wire to close extraction spaces is relatively unimportant. With 22-slot edgewise, since the larger slot provides the clearance needed for sliding but makes it difficult to obtain close engagement of rectangular arch wires with loops in closing extraction spaces, wider brackets are preferred. Prior to almost routine use of superelastic wires, bracket slot size and interbracket span were such strong influences on arch wire choice that different wires often were used with the 18 and 22 slot appliances. This is no longer the case. But with superelastic wires it is necessary to pay more attention to maintaining arch form during alignment, to the point that now alignment when crowding is reasonably symmetric must be viewed differently from alignment in highly asymmetric situations.

Alignment of Symmetric Crowding with the Edgewise Appliance

Arch wire Choices.   The flat load-deflection curve of superelastic NiTi (see Figure 16-4) makes it ideal for initial alignment when the degree of crowding is similar on the two sides of the arch. The superelastic wire provides remarkable range over which a tooth can be moved without generating excessive force. Under most circumstances initial alignment can be accomplished simply by tying 14 or 16 mil A-NiTi that delivers about 50 gm into the brackets of all the teeth, being careful not to tie too tightly, and observing the patient without the necessity of other changes (Figure 16-5). The size of the superelastic wire is not a critical variable, except that 18 mil wires should not be used in the 18 slot appliance.

It is possible now to obtain superelastic wires that are almost totally passive when cold, but deliver the desired force when at mouth temperature. Placing a chilled wire is much easier than placing a springy one, and this can be significant advantage under some circumstances. On the other hand, once mouth temperature has been reached, there is no reason to expect such a thermally-sensitive wire to perform better than one without this feature.

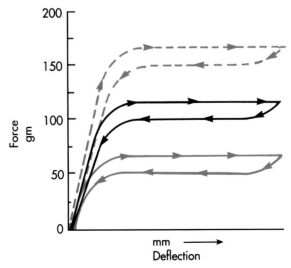

FIGURE 16-4   Force-deflection curves for 16 mil A-NiTi wires (Sentinol) prepared by the manufacturer to have different force delivery characteristics of 50, 100, and 150 gm.

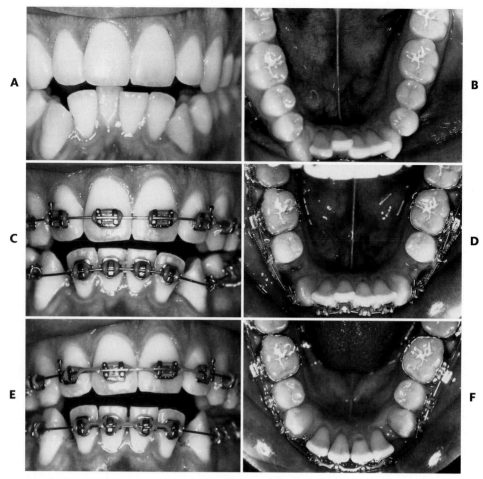

FIGURE 16-5   Alignment of lower incisors with the superelastic equivalent of the original "drag loop." **A** and **B**, initial; **C** and **D**, simultaneous retraction of canines with superelastic coil springs that provide 75 grams of force, and alignment of incisors with a superelastic NiTi wire that provides 50 grams; **E** and **F**, completion of alignment after 5 months of treatment.

The major objection to superelastic NiTi is that it is expensive. If a large range is not necessary, a triple-stranded 17.5 mil multistranded steel wire (3 × 8 mil) offers good properties at a fraction of the cost (Figure 16-6). In theory, this size would be too large for effective use in 18-slot brackets. Clinical research has shown, however, that in both the 18 and 22 appliance, if these wires are recontoured monthly and retied with elastomeric ligatures, the time to alignment is equivalent to A-NiTi.[2] Force levels certainly are more variable and patient discomfort probably is greater than with superelastic wires, but it is difficult to demonstrate this clinically.

The reason for this surprisingly good clinical performance probably is that flexible arch wires allow the teeth to move relative to each other during chewing, as alveolar bone bends under masticatory loads (see Chapter 9). This releases frictional binding and allows the bracket to slide along the arch wire to the next point at which friction stops it. But the lower cost of the steel arch wire is quickly overbalanced by the additional clinical time necessary to retie it,

especially if it must be taken out, adjusted to remove any areas of permanent distortion, and then re-ligated.

Laboratory data and clinical experience suggest that similar performance to the multistrand steel wire could be obtained with M-NiTi, a variety of more elaborate multistrand wires (coaxial wires, for instance, that have several smaller wires wound over a larger core wire), or with loops in small diameter steel wires. Both M-NiTi and coaxial multistrand wires are expensive, and the time to bend loops in 14 or 16 steel wires also is expensive. These wires, though they were the standard of treatment for initial alignment only a few years ago, have little or no place in current therapy.

As one might expect, the extreme springiness of superelastic wires is not a totally unmixed blessing. When these wires are tied into a malocclusion, they have a tendency to "travel" around the arch as the patient chews, especially if function is mostly on one side. Then the wire sticks out the back of the molar tube on one side, and may come out of the tube on the other side. Occasionally this can be extreme enough to produce the kind of situation Mark Twain called

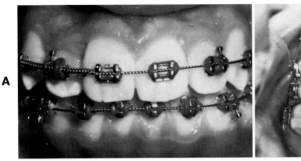
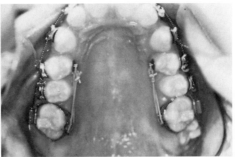

FIGURE 16-6   17.5 mil twist wire remains a good choice for initial alignment in the 22 slot edgewise appliance, if the teeth are not severely irregular. **A,** Note that the twist wire in the mandibular arch is not fully engaged in all the brackets at this point; replacement of the wire and elastomeric ligatures will be needed to complete the alignment. **B,** Occlusal view of the maxillary arch of a different patient. Elastomeric ties to lingual attachments are being used to facilitate correction of rotations. It is important to tie isolated lingual attachments so they will remain attached to the appliance if they come loose from the tooth, so they will not be swallowed.

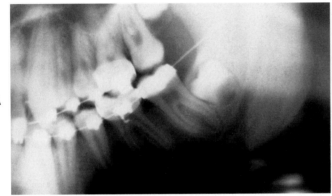
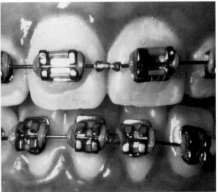

FIGURE 16-7   One problem with superelastic wires for initial alignment is their tendency to "travel" so that the wire slips around to one side, protruding distally from the molar tube on one side and slipping out of the tube on the other. **A,** Panoramic radiograph of a patient in whom the wire traveled distally on one side to the point that it penetrated into the ramus, almost to the depth of an inferior alveolar block injection (interestingly, the patient reported only mild discomfort!); **B,** The most effective way to prevent travel is to tightly crimp a split tube segment onto the wire between two adjacent brackets, as done here between the central incisors. The location of the stop is not critical. Some preformed wires now have a dimple in the midline to prevent the arch wire from sliding excessively.

"marvelous and dismaying" (Figure 16-7, *A*). Arch wire travel can be prevented by crimping a stop tightly onto the arch wire between any two brackets that are reasonably close together (see Figure 16-7, *B*). A stop of this type should be used routinely on initial superelastic wires.

Alignment in Premolar Extraction Situations.   In patients with severe crowding of anterior teeth, it is necessary to retract the canines into premolar extraction sites to gain enough space to align the incisors. In extremely severe crowding, it is better to retract the canines independently before placing attachments on the incisors. This can be done either with segmental retraction loops (Figure 16-8), or by sliding the canines along a relatively rigid wire (16 steel, for instance) that does not contact the incisors. Sliding the canines produces more stress on the posterior anchorage, so critical anchorage is an indication for the retraction loops.

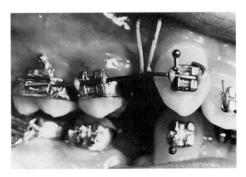

FIGURE 16-8   In this severely crowded child, initial retraction of the maxillary right canine is being done with a loop in 19 × 25 beta-Ti wire. The loop can be adjusted to tip the crown distally or produce bodily retraction. Independent retraction of the canine in this way is most applicable when the canine is severely displaced mesially or when the anchorage control strategy (see Chapter 17) calls for canine retraction as a first stage procedure.

In more typical and less extreme crowding, it is possible to simultaneously tip the canines distally and align the incisors. Until recently, the best way to do this was to use a loop arch wire of the design shown in Figure 16-9, *A*. The principle is that described by Stoner[3] as a "drag loop." The loop in the extraction site is gabled sharply and activated slightly, producing a gentle space-closing force with an

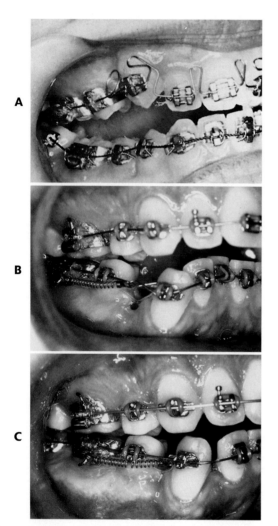

FIGURE 16-9 **A,** For this patient a rolled or drag loop in 14 mil steel wire is being used in the maxillary arch to tip the canine distally into the extraction site while the incisors are being aligned independently. If the loop in the extraction site is gently activated by pulling the posterior end of the wire 1 to 1.5 mm through the molar tube and bending it up, a force is generated to tip the canine distally, as the wire segment passing through the canine is prevented from sliding distally by the loop configuration to the mesial. As the canine tips distally, however, the mesial loop opens up, and the canine retraction provides space for alignment of the incisors without either proclining or retracting them. **B,** The modern equivalent of the drag loop uses superelastic coil springs in conjunction with a superelastic arch wire, to tip the canines distally while the incisors align. These views show the initial arch wire and spring assembly to retract the mandibular right canine, and **C,** 5 months later, with the canine upright, after being tipped distally.

anti-tip moment on the posterior teeth. As the activated distal loop closes, the loop mesial to the canine opens, allowing the canine to tip back independently while the incisors are being aligned.

The same independent distal movement of the canines now can be obtained with an A-NiTi arch wire without loops, and A-NiTi coil springs from the first molars to tip the canines distally (Figure 16-9, *B* and *C*). When this is done, the spring should be chosen to deliver only 50 gm, and an arch wire preformed by the manufacturer to have an exaggerated reverse curve of Spee should be chosen, to limit forward tipping of the molars. As with the drag loop, the idea is to pit distal tipping of the canines against forward bodily movement of the molars.

Alignment in Nonextraction Situations. Alignment in nonextraction cases requires increasing arch length, moving the incisors further from the molars. In this circumstance, just tying a superelastic wire into the bracket slots is ineffective. Two objects cannot occupy the same space at the same time, so alignment cannot occur until space to allow it is created.

With multistrand wires, the easiest way to increase arch length during alignment is to bend a loop mesial to the molars so that the wire is held just anterior to the incisors before it is tied in. At subsequent appointments the adjustment loop is opened, again advancing the wire slightly, until the teeth come into alignment.

The superelastic equivalent of this procedure is to crimp a stop on the wire at the molar tube, so that it holds the wire just in front of the incisors (Figure 16-10). The greater range of the superelastic wire means that the activation can be somewhat greater. At subsequent appointments, if more arch length is needed, an additional stop or stops can be quickly slipped into position, without even removing the wire or religating it. Obviously, this type of arch expansion will carry the incisors facially, and so it is not indicated in the presence of severe crowding unless incisor protrusion is desired.

Alignment of Asymmetric Crowding with the Edgewise Appliance

When all or nearly all the crowding is in one place, what is needed is an arch wire that is rigid where the teeth are already aligned, and quite springy where they are not. Nothing in this world is an unmixed blessing, and the extreme springiness of a superelastic wire means that if it is tied into an asymmetrically maligned arch, teeth distant to the site of malalignment will be moved. An impacted canine is the prime example of asymmetric malalignment. This situation is discussed more specifically below, but it is easy to understand that if a continuous superelastic wire were tied to the impacted tooth and to the lateral incisor and premolar adjacent to it, the incisor and premolar would be tipped into the canine space the same amount that the canine was pulled toward proper position. If one lateral incisor is blocked out of the arch and must be brought into position, the same guideline applies: a superelastic wire to bring it into alignment would move the adjacent canine and central incisor much more than would be desired.

Until recently, asymmetric crowding usually was treated by bending loops into 14 or 16 mil steel wire, as a way of gaining greater springiness in the area where it was most needed. A box loop (Figure 16-11, *A*) often was employed. The same side effects that any continuous wire would produce occurred with this type of loop, but the movement of the teeth adjacent to the displaced one was minimized by the relative stiffness of the wire in that area compared to its stiffness within the loop.

It is easy to add a small diameter superelastic wire as an auxiliary spring, so that a stiff main arch (16 or 18 steel) can be tied into all the teeth except the displaced one (or two—the same system works with small segments of two teeth). A segment of superelastic NiTi can be laid in the brackets on top of the main arch wire, or tied below the brackets of the anchor teeth, and tied to the bracket on the displaced tooth (see Figure 16-11, *B* and *C*). With this arrangement, the correct light force to bring the displaced tooth into alignment is provided by the NiTi wire, and the reciprocal force is distributed over all the rest of the teeth. The result is efficient movement of the displaced tooth, with excellent preservation of arch form.

Note that there are two advantages of the superelastic auxiliary wire: control of the tendency to distort arch form, and light force against the tooth to be moved. Although auxiliaries of this type are recommended routinely in modern orthodontics, it would be particularly important to use this method rather than bending loops in steel wire for adult patients with a reduced periodontal ligament area (see Chapter 21).

Alignment with Begg Technique

The narrow brackets used in Begg technique provide the maximum possible interbracket span without placing loops in arch wires. It was originally common practice with this appliance to use loops in 16 mil steel archwires to facilitate initial alignment (Figure 16-12, *A*). Indeed, loops for alignment were introduced into American edgewise orthodontics from the early Begg appliance. In Begg technique the initial alignment wires bypass the premolars and span from

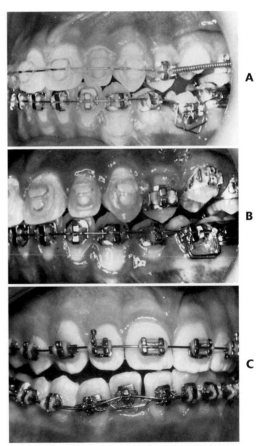

FIGURE 16-11   Box loop in 14 mil steel wire to elevate a mandibular second premolar into occlusion. **A,** Loop at initial placement; **B,** 8 weeks later. Use of a highly resilient wire like A-NiTi in this situation risks distortion of arch form if the superelastic wire is tied into all the brackets, and if only a single wire is employed, a loop remains the preferred approach when only a single tooth is badly malaligned. **C,** The most efficient way to align a single tooth is to use a superelastic wire to bring the displaced tooth into position, while a heavier steel wire maintains arch form. The superelastic auxiliary can be tied on top of the heavier arch wire in the bracket slots, or tied beneath the brackets as shown in Figure 16-3.

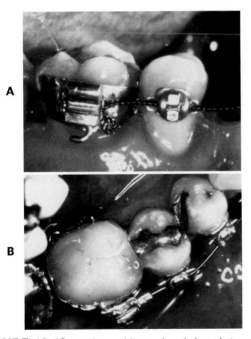

FIGURE 16-10   When additional arch length is needed, advanced stops in the flexible initial arch wire are useful. **A,** Loop stops can be formed in a multistranded steel wire; **B,** Crimped split tube segments, like those used to prevent travel, serve well as advanced stops for superelastic initial wires.

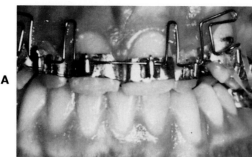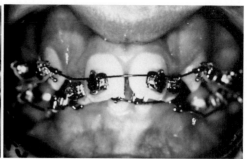

FIGURE 16-12 **A,** Alignment loops in 16 mil steel wire, in a patient wearing the Begg appliance in the upper arch. **B,** Alignment with the modern combination anchorage technique, with a dual-flex wire. The anterior section is NiTi, and the posterior section is steel. This dual-stiffness wire allows the elimination of loops in Begg technique, while retaining the needed stiffness of the posterior part of the initial arch wire. (**B,** Courtesy Dr. WJ Thompson.)

the molar to the canine. This long posterior span of wire makes it difficult to use a highly flexible titanium-based arch wire at the initial stage without losing control of molar position (see leveling, following). Although alignment loops are used less in current Begg therapy than they were previously,[4] this remains a valuable adjunct to Begg treatment. The modern alternative is a wire that is flexible in the anterior segment and stiff posteriorly, which can be produced by varying the heat treatment during manufacture of NiTi wires, or by combining steel and NiTi segments (see Figure 16-12, *B*).

SPECIAL PROBLEMS IN ALIGNMENT

Crossbite Correction

It is important to correct posterior crossbites and mild anterior crossbites (one or two displaced teeth) in the first stage of treatment. Severe anterior crossbites (all the teeth), in contrast, are usually not corrected until the second stage of conventional treatment, or might remain pending surgical correction. For both posterior and anterior crossbites, it is obviously important to make the appropriate distinctions between skeletal and dental problems, and to quantitate the severity of the problem. The appropriate diagnostic steps are discussed in Chapters 6 and 7. The assumption here is that appropriate treatment has been selected, and the discussion is solely about implementing a treatment plan based on differential diagnosis.

Individual Teeth Displaced Into Anterior Crossbite. Anterior crossbite of one or two teeth almost always is an expression of severe crowding, and is most likely to occur when maxillary lateral incisors that were somewhat lingually positioned to begin with, are forced even more lingually by lack of space. Correction of the crossbite requires first opening enough space for the displaced teeth, then bringing them into proper position in the arch (Figure 16-13).

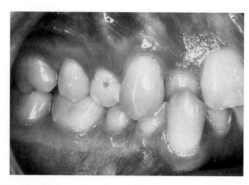

FIGURE 16-13 Correction of a dental anterior crossbite, as in this young adult, almost always requires opening enough space for the lingually displaced maxillary incisor before attempting to move it facially into arch form.

Occlusal interferences may make this difficult. The patient may tend to bite brackets off the displaced teeth, and as the teeth are moved "through the bite", occlusal force pushes them one way while the orthodontic appliance pulls them the other. It may be necessary to use a bite plate temporarily to separate the posterior teeth and create the vertical space needed to allow the teeth to move. The older the patient, the more likely it is that a bite plate will be needed. During rapid growth in early adolescence, often incisors that were locked in anterior crossbite can be corrected without a bite plate. After that, one probably will be required.

Transverse Maxillary Expansion by Opening the Midpalatal Suture. It is relatively easy to widen the maxilla by opening the midpalatal suture before and during adolescence, but this becomes progressively more difficult as patients become older. The chances of successful opening of the suture are nearly 100% before age 15, but begin to decline thereafter because of the increased interdigitation of the sutures.[5]

Patients who are candidates for opening the midpalatal suture may have such severe crowding that even with this arch expansion, premolar extraction will be required. In these patients, however, separation of the suture should be the first step in treatment, before either extraction or alignment. The first premolar teeth are useful as anchorage for the lateral expansion and can serve for that purpose even if they are to be extracted later, and the additional space provided by the lateral expansion facilitates alignment.

Sometimes, transverse maxillary expansion can provide enough additional space to make extraction unnecessary, but rarely is it wise to use sutural expansion as a means of dealing with a crowding in an individual who already has normal maxillary width (see Chapter 8). Opening the midpalatal suture should be used primarily as a means of correcting a skeletal crossbite, making a narrow maxilla normal, not a normal maxilla abnormally wide.

In the early permanent dentition, the basic mechanism for separation of the midpalatal suture is a jackscrew built into a fixed appliance that is rigidly attached to as many posterior teeth as possible. The appliance can be made so that it has plastic palate-covering shelves or can consist solely of a metal or plastic framework against the teeth, not contacting the palatal tissue (Figure 16-14). In theory, the flanges extending into the palate could cause a more bodily repositioning of the alveolar processes, but in fact, there seems to be little or no difference in the skeletal or dental response to the two types of appliances. Because the palate-covering appliance remains in contact with the soft tissue for an extended period, however, it can cause tissue irritation. For this reason, an appliance that does not contact the palate is preferred.

When the maxillary teeth move transversely, some extrusion may occur, and even if it does not, the tooth movement creates cuspal interferences that cause the mandible to rotate down and back. In deep bite patients who are still growing or in patients with a mild Class III tendency, this can be advantageous, but it is a problem in long face patients with a narrow maxilla. Adding bite blocks to a bonded expander is the best way to overcome this problem (Figure 16-15).[6]

Separation of the midpalatal suture can be produced by either rapid (Figure 16-16) or slow expansion, and the same type of palate-separating appliance can be used for either approach (see Chapter 8). Whether the expansion is done rapidly or slowly, the fixed appliance remains in place for approximately the same length of time, because a shorter period of stabilization is sufficient with slow expansion. With rapid expansion, the expansion itself is carried out in approximately 2 weeks, but the screw should then be stabilized and the appliances maintained in place for 3 to 4 months of retention. With slow expansion, approximately 2 1/2 months are needed to obtain the expansion, and the appliance can be removed in another 2 months.

Some degree of relapse can be expected after palatal expansion because of the elasticity of the palatal soft tis-

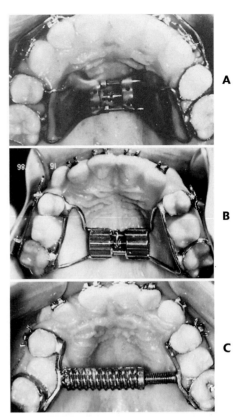

FIGURE 16-14 Palatal expansion in adolescents requires a rigid framework because of the heavy forces (2 to 4 pounds with slow expansion, 10 to 20 pounds with rapid expansion) that will be encountered. **A,** Haas-type expander with metal framework and plastic shelves contacting the palatal mucosa; **B,** Hyrax expander with metal framework only; **C,** Minn-expander, which incorporates a spring to smooth the force application but still produces heavy force if activated rapidly. Although the various expansion appliances look quite different, they produce similar results. A bonded expander, retained by bonding to the enamel rather than using bands also can be used (see Figure 16-15). With this method, the enamel is prepared for bonding only on the facial and lingual, but not the occlusal, surfaces; otherwise removing the appliance is too difficult.

sue. Therefore it is wise to overcorrect the crossbite initially (see Figure 16-16). Even if 3 to 4 months of stabilization with the palate-separating device have been provided, additional retention of the crossbite correction is needed when the fixed appliance is removed. A palate-covering removable retainer is satisfactory but may be somewhat awkward in combination with fixed appliances to align the teeth as the first stage of treatment proceeds. An alternative is a heavy labial arch wire placed in the headgear tubes, which will maintain the lateral expansion while light resilient arch wires are being used to align the teeth (Figure 16-17), or a lingual arch. The lingual arch gives better control of root position but the heavy labial arch can be fabricated much more quickly and easily.

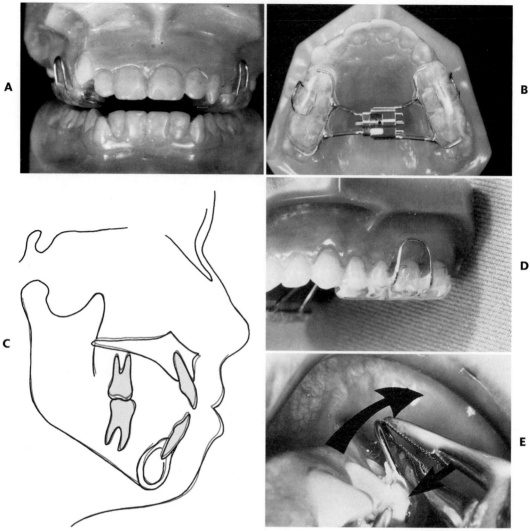

FIGURE 16-15 **A** and **B,** Palatal expander with bite blocks. With this design, intrusive pressure against the posterior teeth, created by the elastic rebound of the patient's stretched soft tissues, controls the tendency for bite opening and downward-backward rotation of the mandible that occurs with other designs of palatal expanders. **C,** Cephalometric superimposition before and after expansion, showing the very small mandibular rotation when expansion was done with a device of this type. **D** and **E,** Removal of a bonded appliance of this type is facilitated by loops extending from the appliance that can be gripped and torqued. (Courtesy Dr. David Sarver.)

Unless a direct lingual arch can be placed as soon as the expansion appliance is removed, it is wise to use the heavy labial arch at least temporarily.

Correction of Dental Posterior Crossbites. Three approaches to correction of less severe dental crossbites are feasible: a heavy labial expansion arch, as shown in Figure 16-17, an expansion lingual arch, or cross-elastics. Removable appliances, although theoretically possible, are not compatible with comprehensive treatment and should be reserved for the mixed dentition or adjunctive treatment.

The inner bow of a facebow is also, of course, a heavy labial arch, and expansion of this inner bow is a convenient way to expand the upper molars. This expansion is nearly always needed for patients with a Class II molar relationship, whose upper arch usually is too narrow to accommodate the mandibular arch when it comes forward into the correct relationship because the upper molars are tipped lingually. The inner bow is simply adjusted at each appointment to be sure that it is slightly wider than the headgear tubes and must be compressed by the patient when inserting the facebow. If the distal force of a headgear is not desired, a heavy labial auxiliary can provide the expansion effect alone. The effect of the round wire in the headgear tubes, however, is to tip the crowns outward, and so this method should be reserved for patients whose molars are tipped lingually.

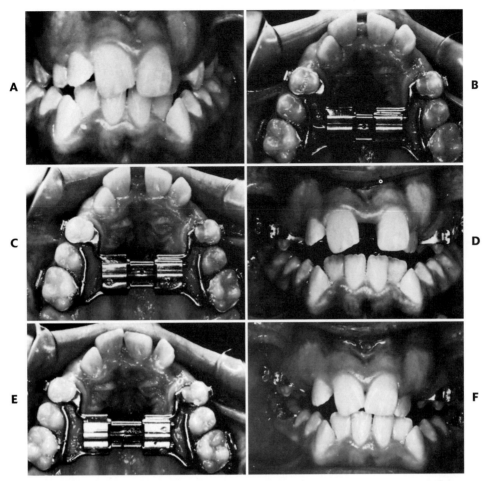

FIGURE 16-16 Rapid maxillary expansion with a jackscrew appliance to open the midpalatal suture. **A,** Maxillary constriction and crowding before treatment; **B,** jackscrew appliance in place, soldered to bands on the maxillary first molars and first premolars, with an arm contacting the second premolars. At this point, the appliance has been opened approximately 3 mm. Note the separation between the maxillary central incisors. **C,** Occlusal view after 10 days of separation. Note the wide central diastema. **D,** Labial view after 10 days of separation. A tendency toward anterior open bite is created by contact of the maxillary lingual and mandibular buccal molar cusps. **E,** Occlusal view 3 months after separation was begun and 10 weeks after the screw was stabilized by tying it with brass wire. Note the spontaneous closure of the diastema, which occurs because of a combination of elastic rebound of the gingival fibers that moves the teeth together, and skeletal relapse. **F,** Labial view at 3 months. Overcorrection of the posterior crossbite is being maintained by the stabilized appliance.

A transpalatal lingual arch for expansion must have some springiness and range of action. As a general principle, the more flexible a lingual arch is, the better it is for tooth movement but the less it adds to anchorage stability. This can be an important consideration in adolescent and adult patients. If anchorage is of no concern, a highly flexible lingual arch, like the quad helix design discussed in Chapter 13, is an excellent choice for correction of a dental crossbite. When the lingual arch is needed for both expansion and anchorage, however, the choices are 36 mil steel wire with an adjustment loop, or the new system that allows the use of 32 × 32 TMA or steel wire (Figure 16-18; see also Figure 12-38).

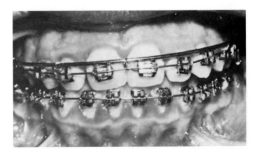

FIGURE 16-17 A heavy labial arch wire (usually 36 or 40 mil steel) placed in the headgear tubes on first molars can be used to maintain arch width after palatal suture opening while the teeth are being aligned. This is more compatible with fixed-appliance treatment than a removable retainer and does not depend on patient cooperation.

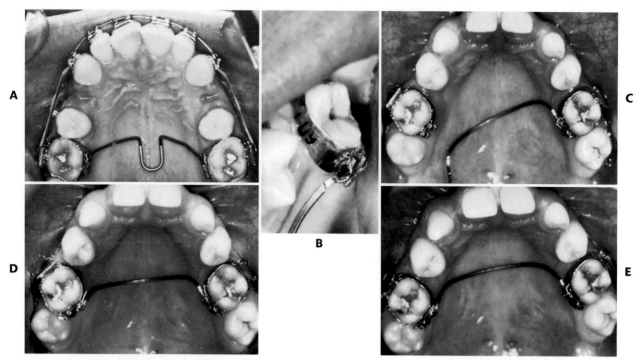

FIGURE 16-18   **A,** An expansion lingual arch of this type, using 36 mil steel wire doubled over into the horizontal lingual sheath, is often used for small amounts of expansion in the first stage of comprehensive treatment rather than the more flexible expansion arches shown in Chapter 14, because it also will contribute to stabilization of the posterior segments later, augmenting the posterior anchorage. **B,** A more efficient alternative, especially if more than a small amount of expansion is needed, is to use 32 × 32 lingual arch brackets, in which the wire is tied as shown here, or lingual cap brackets in this size (see Figure 12-38). Then a 32 × 32 TMA lingual arch can be used for the initial tooth movement, and a steel arch of the same size can be placed for the later stabilization. **C,** Activation of a TMA lingual arch (equal on the two sides); **D,** initial and, **E,** follow-up molar positions. (**B** to **E,** Courtesy Dr. C.J. Burstone.)

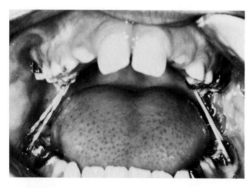

FIGURE 16-19   Cross-elastics from the lingual of the upper molars to the buccal of the lower molars. Cross-elastics are an effective way of correcting transverse dental relationships, but they also extrude teeth, and this must be kept in mind.

The third possibility for dental expansion is the use of cross-elastics, typically running from the lingual of the upper molar to the buccal of the lower molar (Figure 16-19). These elastics are effective, but their strong extrusive component must be kept in mind. As a general rule, adolescent patients can tolerate a short period of cross-elastic wear to correct a simple crossbite, because any extrusion is compensated by vertical growth of the ramus, but cross-elastics should be used with great caution, if at all, in adults. As any posterior crossbite is corrected, interference of the cusps increases posterior vertical dimension and thereby tends to rotate the mandible downward and backward, even if cross-elastics are avoided. The elastics accentuate this tendency.

If teeth are tightly locked into a posterior crossbite relationship, a bite plate to separate them vertically can make the correction easier and faster. In children and young adolescents, this is rarely needed. Use of a bite plate during transverse expansion indicates that elongation of the posterior teeth and downward-backward rotation of the mandible is an acceptable outcome.

Impacted or Unerupted Teeth

Bringing an impacted or unerupted tooth into the arch creates a set of special problems during alignment. The most frequent impaction is a maxillary canine or canines, but it is occasionally necessary to bring other unerupted teeth into the arch, and the same techniques apply for incisors, canines and premolars. Impacted lower second molars pose a different problem and are discussed separately.

The problems in dealing with an unerupted tooth fall into three categories: (1) surgical exposure, (2) attachment to the tooth, and (3) orthodontic mechanics to bring the tooth into the arch.

Surgical Exposure. It is important for a tooth to erupt through the attached gingiva, not through alveolar mucosa, and this must be considered when flaps to expose an unerupted tooth are planned. If the unerupted tooth is in the mandibular arch or on the labial side of the maxillary alveolar process, a flap should be reflected from the crest of the alveolus and sutured so that attached gingiva has been transferred to the region where the crown is exposed (Figure 16-20). If this is not done, and the tooth is brought through alveolar mucosa, it is quite likely that tissue will strip away from the crown, leaving an unsightly and periodontally compromised gingival margin.[7] If the unerupted tooth is on the palatal side, similar problems with the heavy palatal mucosa are unlikely, and flap design is less critical.

Occasionally, a tooth will obligingly erupt into its correct position after obstacles to eruption have been removed by surgical exposure, but this is rarely the case after root formation is complete. Even a tooth that is aimed in the right direction usually requires orthodontic force to bring it into position.

Method of Attachment. The least desirable way to obtain attachment is for the surgeon to place a wire ligature around the crown of the impacted tooth. This inevitably results in loss of periodontal attachment, because bone destroyed when the wire is passed around the tooth does not regenerate when it is removed. Occasionally no alternative is practical, but wire ligatures should be avoided whenever possible.

Before the availability of direct bonding, a pin was sometimes placed in a hole prepared in the crown of an unerupted tooth, and in special circumstances, this remains a possible alternative. The best contemporary approach, however, is simply to expose an area on the crown of the tooth and directly bond an attachment of some type to that surface (Figure 16-21). In many instances, a button or hook is better than a standard bracket because it is smaller. Then, a piece of fine gold chain is tied to the attachment, and before the flap is repositioned and sutured into place, this is positioned so that it extends into the mouth. The chain is much easier to tie to than a wire ligature.

Mechanical Approaches for Aligning Unerupted Teeth. Orthodontic traction to pull an unerupted tooth toward the line of the arch should begin as soon as possible after surgery. Ideally, a fixed orthodontic appliance should already be in place before the unerupted tooth is exposed, so that orthodontic force can be applied immediately. If this is not practical, active orthodontic movement should begin no later than 2 or 3 weeks postsurgically.

This means that orthodontic treatment to open space for the unerupted tooth and allow stabilization of the rest of the dental arch must begin well before the surgical ex-

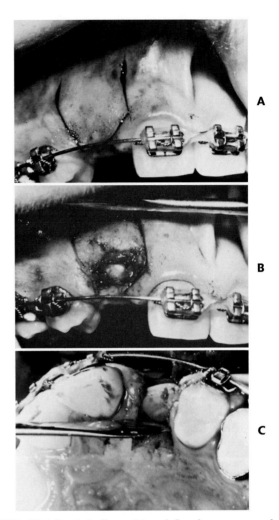

FIGURE 16-20 Apically positioned flap for exposure of an unerupted canine. **A,** Initial incision lines; **B,** crown exposed with apical repositioning of the labial tissue; **C,** lingual exposure of the same tooth.

posure. In this instance, the goals of presurgical orthodontic treatment are to create enough space if it does not exist, as often is the case; and to align the other teeth so that a heavy stabilizing arch wire (at least 18 steel, preferably a rectangular steel wire) can be in position at the time of surgery. This allows postsurgical orthodontic treatment to start immediately.

As we have noted above, an unerupted tooth is an extreme example of an asymmetric alignment problem, with one tooth far from the line of occlusion. Although a superelastic arch wire can be used if the tooth is close to the correct position (Figure 16-22, *A*), this is not recommended because of the unwanted side effects. An auxiliary NiTi wire, overlaid on the stabilizing arch in the same way as recommended above for other asymmetric alignment situations, is much better (see Figure 16-22, *B-D*), and now often is the most efficient way to bring an impacted tooth into position. The alternatives are to use a

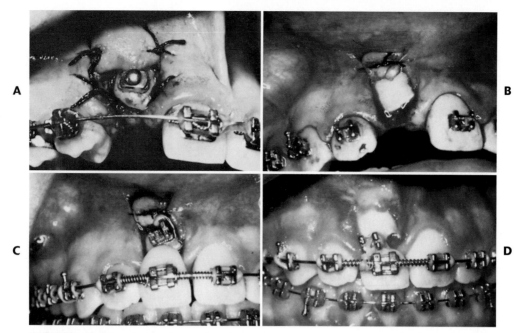

FIGURE 16-21 **A,** Attachment bonded to the labial surface of the crown of an unerupted canine (same patient as Figure 16-20), with the apically repositioned flap sutured in place. An elastomeric attachment from the arch wire to the bonded button will be used initially to bring the canine toward the line of occlusion. Later, the button will be replaced with a bonded bracket. **B,** If an unerupted incisor is labially positioned, it is important to employ an apically repositioned flap so that a gingival attachment is preserved. Then an attachment can be bonded (**C**). For this patient an elastomeric chain (**D**) looped around a rigid base arch wire is being used to bring the labially positioned incisor into the arch, which may be preferred because of its better esthetics even though mechanically this would not be as efficient as a superelastic auxiliary arch wire.

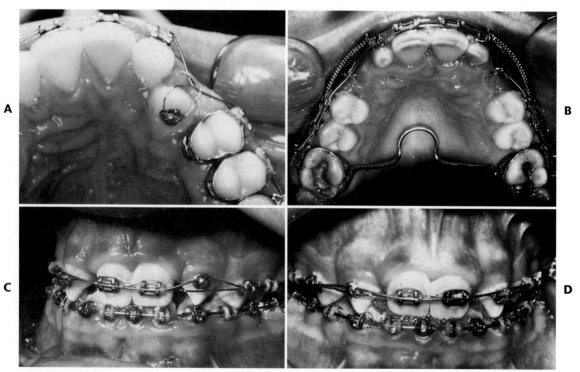

FIGURE 16-22 **A,** If an unerupted tooth is not too far out of line, a flexible arch wire like 16 A-NiTi can be tied directly to the attachment. **B,** In the more usual situation, a button is bonded to whatever portion of the tooth can be exposed, and traction (preferably by a superelastic auxiliary wire, as shown here) is applied to a ligature wire or chain that extends through the gingiva while arch form is maintained by a heavier wire in the bracket slots. **C,** Later in the same patient as in **B,** the auxiliary wire is hooked over the top of the button, bringing the tooth (**D**) down into position.

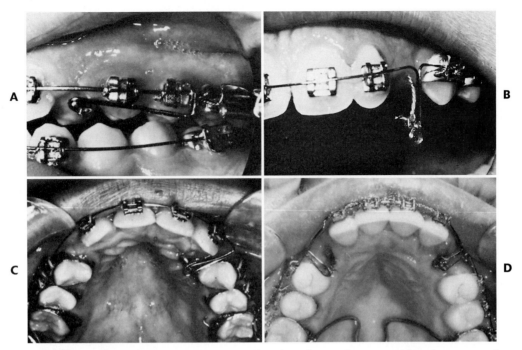

FIGURE 16-23   **A,** An auxiliary spring soldered to a base arch wire provides a long range of action to bring an unerupted canine facially and occlusally. This is more efficient than elastomeric ties. A spring bent into an arch wire also can be employed. **B,** A vertical spring bent into a 14 mil steel arch wire to bring down an impacted maxillary canine, before activation; **C,** same spring activated by rotating the loop 90 degrees. A stop against the molars, so that the wire cannot just spin in the molar tubes, is essential. **D,** If springs of this type are used bilaterally, a stabilizing lingual arch is essential. This method is also very effective, providing excellent force characteristics with a long range of action.

special alignment spring, either soldered to a heavy base arch wire or bent into a light arch wire (Figure 16-23).

Another possibility, magnetic force to initiate movement of an unerupted tooth, is especially attractive for treatment of deeply embedded teeth because no mechanical connection is required, and problems associated with premature exposure of the unerupted tooth to the oral environment can be avoided. Magnetic attraction between an attachment bonded to the tooth and an intraoral magnet would produce the tooth movement. The technique involves bonding a small magnet to an unerupted maxillary canine, and using magnetic attraction to a larger magnet contained within a palate-covering removable appliance.[8,9] The attractive force is determined by the distance between the magnets, and so can be controlled with good precision. The direction of the force depends on the orientation of the magnets, which also can be controlled, especially since the magnet within the removable appliance can be positioned almost wherever desired. Unfortunately, success depends entirely on the patient's cooperation in wearing the removable appliance with the intraoral magnet.

Ankylosis of an unerupted tooth is always a potential problem. If an area of fusion to the adjacent bone develops, orthodontic movement of the unerupted tooth becomes impossible, and displacement of the anchor teeth will occur. Occasionally, an unerupted tooth will start to move and then will become ankylosed, apparently held by only a small area of fusion. It can sometimes be freed to continue movement by anesthetizing the area and lightly luxating the tooth, breaking the area of ankylosis. If this procedure is done, it is critically important to apply orthodontic force immediately after the luxation, since it is only a matter of time until the tooth re-ankyloses. Nevertheless, this approach can sometimes allow a tooth to be brought into the arch that otherwise would have been impossible to move.

Unerupted/Impacted Lower Second Molars. Unlike impaction of most other teeth, which is an obvious problem from the beginning of treatment, impaction of lower second molars usually develops during orthodontic treatment (Figure 16-24). This occurs when the mesial marginal ridge of the second molar catches against the distal surface of the first molar, so that the second molar progressively tips mesially instead of erupting. Moving the first molar posteriorly during the mixed dentition increases the chance that the second molar will become impacted, and this possibility must be taken into account when procedures to increase mandibular arch length are employed.

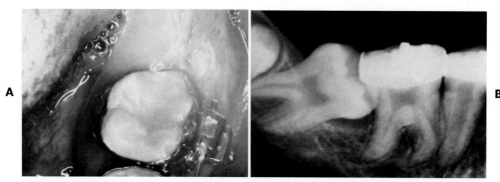

FIGURE 16-24   Impacted mandibular second molar in a 14-year-old patient. **A,** Occlusal view, **B,** radiographic view. The clinically exposed cusp is the distobuccal cusp, not the mesiobuccal cusp one would expect to see in this location. (See Figure 16-26 for treatment of this patient.)

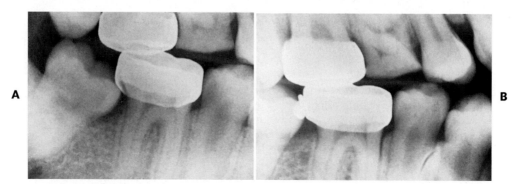

FIGURE 16-25   Brass wire separator used to de-impact a mandibular second molar. **A,** Second molar trapped beneath distal bulge of first molar; **B,** uprighting obtained with 20 mil brass wire tightened around the contact. Usually it is necessary to anesthetize the area to place a separating wire of this type. A spring clip can be used in the same way, but both brass wire and spring clips are effective only if the tooth is minimally tipped.

Correction of an impacted second molar requires that the tooth be moved posteriorly and uprighted. In most cases, if the mesial marginal ridge can be unlocked, the tooth will erupt on its own. When the second molar is not severely tipped, the simplest solution is to place a separator between the two teeth (Figure 16-25). For a more severe problem, one possibility is to solder an auxiliary spring to the arch wire mesial to the first molar and extend it posteriorly into the embrasure between the first and second molars. The long arm of such a spring gives excellent flexibility and range of action, but also makes it difficult to keep the spring in place and may lead to substantial soft tissue irritation. A better alternative is to surgically expose the second molar, bond a tube to the buccal surface, and then use an auxiliary spring inserted into this tube to upright the second molar (Figure 16-26).

An auxiliary spring often is useful to bring both upper and lower second molars into alignment when they erupt late in orthodontic treatment (Figure 16-27). The easiest way to do this is to use a segment of NiTi wire (a rectangular wire, usually 16 × 22, is preferred) from the auxiliary tube on the first molar to the tube on the second molar. This provides a light force to align the second molars while a heavier and more rigid wire remains in place anteriorly, which is much better than going back to a light round wire for the entire arch just to align the second molars.

Diastema Closure

A maxillary midline diastema is often complicated by the insertion of the labial frenum into a notch in the alveolar bone, so that a band of heavy fibrous tissue lies between the central incisors. When this is the case, a stable correction of the diastema almost always requires surgery to remove the interdental fibrous tissue and reposition the frenum. The frenectomy must be carried out in a way that will produce a good esthetic result and must be properly coordinated with orthodontic treatment.

It is an error to surgically remove the frenum and then delay orthodontic treatment in the hope that the diastema will close spontaneously. If the frenum is removed while there is still a space between the central incisors, scar tissue forms between the teeth as healing progresses, and a long

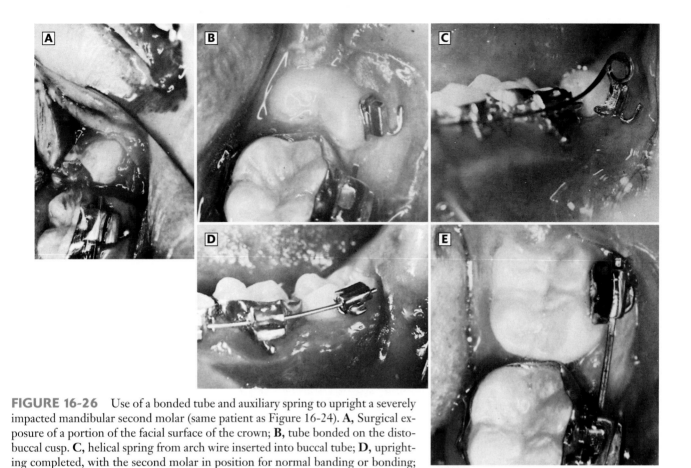

FIGURE 16-26 Use of a bonded tube and auxiliary spring to upright a severely impacted mandibular second molar (same patient as Figure 16-24). **A,** Surgical exposure of a portion of the facial surface of the crown; **B,** tube bonded on the distobuccal cusp. **C,** helical spring from arch wire inserted into buccal tube; **D,** uprighting completed, with the second molar in position for normal banding or bonding; **E,** occlusal view after uprighting.

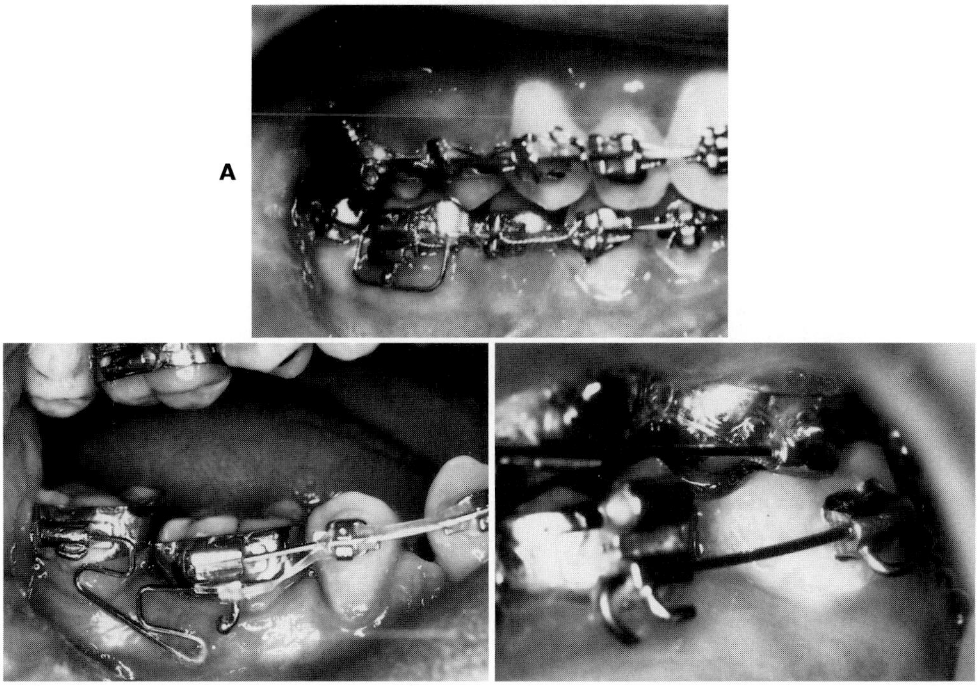

FIGURE 16-27 When a second molar is banded or bonded relatively late in treatment, often it is desirable to align it with a flexible wire while retaining a heavier arch wire in the remainder of the arch. **A,** One possibility is to solder an auxiliary spring to the main arch wire so that it extends beneath the first molar tube as shown here. **B,** If the first molar carries an auxiliary tube, an auxiliary spring can be placed into the auxiliary tube, either a steel wire with a loop as shown here, or **C,** a straight segment of rectangular A-NiTi wire, usually the most efficient procedure.

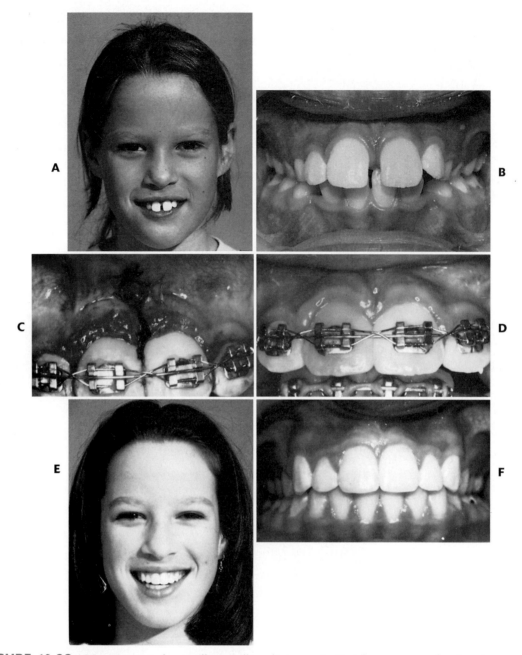

FIGURE 16-28   Management of a maxillary midline diastema. **A,** Facial appearance, showing the protruding maxillary incisors caught on the lower lip; **B,** intraoral view before treatment; **C,** teeth aligned and held tightly together with a figure-8 wire ligature, before frenectomy; **D,** appearance immediately after frenectomy, using the conservative technique advocated by Edwards in which a simple incision is used to allow access to the interdental area, the fibrous connection to the bone is removed, and the frenal attachment is sutured at a higher level; **E,** facial appearance 2 years after completion of treatment; **F,** intraoral view 2 years after treatment.

delay may result in a space that is more difficult to close than it was previously.

It is better to align the teeth before frenectomy. Sliding them together along an arch wire is usually better than using a closing loop, because a loop with any vertical height will touch and irritate the frenum. If the diastema is relatively small, it is usually possible to bring the central in-

cisors completely together before surgery (Figure 16-28). If the space is large and the frenal attachment is thick, it may not be possible to completely close the space before surgical intervention. The space should be closed at least partially, and the orthodontic movement to bring the teeth together should be resumed immediately after the frenectomy, so that the teeth are brought together quickly after the procedure. When this is done, healing occurs with the teeth together, and the inevitable postsurgical scar tissue stabilizes the teeth in their correct position instead of creating obstacles to final closure of the space.

The key to successful surgery is removal of the interdental fibrous tissue. It is unnecessary, and in fact undesirable, to excise a large portion of the frenum itself. Instead, a simple incision is used to allow access to the interdental area, the fibrous connection to the bone is removed, and the frenum is then sutured at a higher level.[10]

A maxillary midline diastema tends to recur, no matter how carefully the space was managed initially. The elastic gingival fiber network typically did not cross the midline in these patients, and the surgery interrupted any fibers that did cross. As a result, in this critical area the normal mechanism to keep teeth in contact is missing. A bonded fixed retainer is recommended (see Chapter 19).

LEVELING

The arch wire design for leveling depends on whether there is a need for absolute intrusion of incisors, or whether relative intrusion is satisfactory. This important point is discussed in detail in Chapter 7, and the biomechanical considerations in obtaining intrusion are described in Chapters 9 and 10. The discussion following assumes that an appropriate decision about the type of leveling has been made, and focuses on the rather different techniques for leveling by relative intrusion (which is really differential elongation of premolars, for the most part) as contrasted to leveling by absolute intrusion of incisors (see Figure 7-6).

Leveling by Extrusion (Relative Intrusion)

This type of leveling can be accomplished with continuous arch wires, simply by placing an exaggerated curve of Spee in the maxillary arch wire and a reverse curve of Spee in the mandibular arch wire (Figure 16-29). For most patients, it is necessary to replace the initial highly resilient alignment arch with a slightly stiffer one to complete the leveling. The choice of wires for this purpose is affected by whether the 18 or 22 slot edgewise appliance is being used.

18-Slot, Narrow Brackets.   When preliminary alignment is completed, the second arch wire is almost always 16 mil steel, with an exaggerated curve of Spee in the upper arch and a reverse curve in the lower arch. In most instances, this is sufficient to complete the leveling. An alternative is to use 16 or 18 mil M-NiTi, preformed by the manufacturer with an extremely exaggerated curve. The extreme curve is needed to generate enough force, but this can lead to problems if patients miss appointments, so these wires are not recommended for routine use.

In some patients, particularly in nonextraction treatment of older patients who have little if any remaining growth, an arch wire heavier than 16 mil steel is needed to complete the leveling of the arches. Rather than use an 18 mil arch wire, it is usually quicker and easier to add an

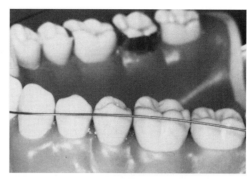

FIGURE 16-29   A reverse curve of Spee in the lower arch wire, illustrated here alongside a lower arch with which it could be used, is a satisfactory method if vertical growth will occur to compensate for the extrusion that occurs in the premolar region.

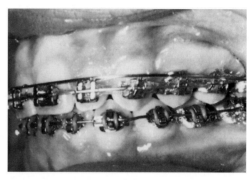

FIGURE 16-30   An auxiliary leveling arch (usually 17 × 25 steel) extending from the auxiliary tubes on the first molars and tied beneath the base arch anteriorly can be used to augment the leveling ability of continuous arch wires. With a continuous base arch wire, the effect is primarily premolar extrusion, not the incisor intrusion that a similar auxiliary arch could produce with base arch segments, but this often is what is desired in growing children. (See Figure 16-37, *D,* for an additional illustration of an auxiliary depressing arch to assist in leveling the lower arch with a continuous base arch.)

auxiliary leveling arch of 17 × 25 mil TMA or steel. This arch inserts into the auxiliary tube on the molar and is tied anteriorly beneath the 16 mil base arch (Figure 16-30). In essence, this augments the curve in the base arch and results in efficient completion of the leveling by the same mechanism as a single continuous wire. Although the auxiliary wire gives the appearance of our intrusion arch, leveling will occur almost totally by extrusion as long as a continuous rather than segmented wire is in the bracket slots.

It is sometimes said, as an argument in favor of the 22-slot appliance, that the wires available for use with the 18-slot appliance are not large enough to accomplish all necessary tooth movements. One of the few situations in which that may be true is in final leveling with continuous arch wires, which may require either a continuous 18 mil steel arch wire or the auxiliary wire suggested previously.

22-Slot, Wider Brackets. For a typical patient using the 22-slot appliance, initial alignment with a 17.5 mil twist or 16 mil A-NiTi wire is usually followed by a 16 mil steel wire with a reverse or accentuated curve, and then by an 18 mil round wire to complete the leveling. This arch wire sequence is nearly always adequate for completion of leveling, and it is rare that 20 mil wire or an auxiliary arch wire is required.

With either slot size, it is an error to place a rectangular arch wire with an exaggerated curve of Spee, because the curve creates torque to move the incisor roots lingually. Almost always that is undesirable in the lower arch. Inadvertent torque of lower incisor roots is one of the commonest mistakes with the edgewise appliance. The arch should be level before a rectangular wire is placed, and torque in any rectangular wire should be monitored carefully.

Leveling by Intrusion

Leveling by intrusion requires a mechanical arrangement other than a continuous arch wire attached to each tooth (see Chapter 10). The key to successful intrusion is light continuous force directed toward the tooth apex. It is necessary to avoid pitting intrusion of one tooth against extrusion of its neighbor, since in that circumstance, extrusion will dominate. This can be accomplished in two ways: (1) with continuous arch wires that bypass the premolar (and frequently the canine) teeth, and (2) with segmented base arch wires (so that there is no connection along the arch between the anterior and posterior segments) and an auxiliary depressing arch.

Bypass Arches. This approach to intrusion is most useful for patients who will have some growth (i.e., who are in either the mixed or early permanent dentitions). Three different mechanical arrangements are commonly used, each based on the same mechanical principle: uprighting and distal tipping of the molars, pitted against intrusion of the incisors.

A classic version of this approach to leveling is seen in the first stage of Begg technique, in which the premolar

teeth are bypassed and only a loose tie is made to the canine. A 16 mil resilient steel arch wire is fabricated as shown in Figure 16-31, using an "anchor bend" anterior to the first molar. The long span of the arch wire anterior to the anchor bend provides a gentle intrusive force on the incisors, while the reaction force on the molar tends to upright it and tip it distally. Light Class II elastic forces are used while this arch wire is in place. The result is stabilization of the lower molar against the distal tipping, at the cost of some extrusion of the molar. Hence there is a need for vertical growth while this treatment is being carried out, to prevent downward and backward rotation of the mandible. The light arch wire, however, does intrude the lower incisors. The upper incisors are being pulled downward by the Class II elastic, which counterbalances the intrusion these teeth otherwise might experience.

Exactly the same effect can be produced in exactly the same way using the edgewise appliance, if the premolars and canines are bypassed. Mulligan advocated just this approach to the fabrication of a leveling arch wire, using a 16 mil steel wire with an anchor bend similar to the initial arch wire in the Begg technique,[11] and these ideas for treatment with a "2 × 4" appliance (only 2 molars and 4 incisors included in the appliance set-up) have been presented more formally recently.[12]

A more flexible variation of the same basic idea is developed in Rickett's utility arch (Figure 16-32).[13] The utility arch is characterized by step-down bends between the first molar and the lateral incisors, so that the arch wire is less likely to be distorted by the forces of occlusion. It is fabricated of 16 × 16 mil wire, used in 18-slot brackets. In most cases, the rectangular wire is placed into the brackets with slight labial root torque to control the inclination of the teeth as the incisors move labially while they intrude. This results in a complex mechanical system, however, that becomes difficult to control (see discussion in Chapter 10).

Successful use of any of these bypass arches for leveling requires that the forces be kept light. This is accom-

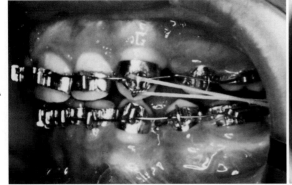
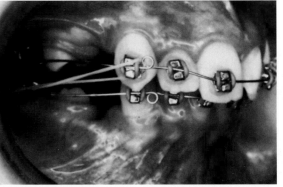

FIGURE 16-31 **A,** Illustration of 16 mil steel arch wires for leveling in the first stage of Begg technique. An "anchor bend" is placed mesial to the first molar, and the arch wire is lightly ligated or clipped as it passes the second premolar, rather than being pinned into the bracket on these teeth. **B,** Similar bends are placed in the initial wires with the modern Begg-edgewise techniques, as here with the TipEdge appliance. (**B,** Courtesy Dr. PC Kesling.)

plished in two ways: by selecting a small diameter arch wire, and by using a long span between the first molar and the incisors. Wire heavier than 16 mil steel should not be used, and Ricketts recommended a relatively soft 16 × 16 cobalt-chromium wire for utility arches to prevent heavy forces from being developed. A more modern recommendation would be 16 × 22 beta-Ti wire. Whatever the wire choice, overactivation of the vertical bends can cause loss of control of the molars in all three planes of space.

The 16 mil steel wires typically used in bypass arches, though resilient, are too stiff for efficient alignment of severely malposed incisors, even if loops are bent into the wire between adjacent teeth. Small rotations or displacements can be corrected simply by tying to a 16 mil wire and gradually bringing the wire into the bracket slot, particularly if the brackets are narrow so that interbracket span is adequate. Where significant malpositions exist, however, it is better to correct the alignment with a resilient wire, perhaps using only a resilient anterior segment, before tying a round or rectangular bypass arch into the brackets. If intrusion is desired from the beginning, an auxiliary arch for this purpose can be used along with the anterior alignment segment, as described below.

In contrast to leveling with continuous fully engaged arch wires, the size of the edgewise bracket slot is largely irrelevant when bypass arches for leveling are used. Whether the appliance is 18- or 22-slot, the bypass arch should not be stiffer than 16 mil steel wire.

Two weaknesses of the bypass arch systems limit the amount of true intrusion that can be obtained. The first is that, except for some applications of the utility arch, only the first molar is available as posterior anchorage. This means that significant extrusion of that tooth may occur. In actively growing patients with a good facial pattern, this is not a major problem, but in nongrowing patients or those with a poor facial pattern in whom molar extrusion should be avoided, the lack of posterior anchorage compromises the ability to intrude incisors. High-pull headgear to the upper molars can be added with any of the bypass arch systems to improve upper posterior anchorage, and with a

utility arch setup, the second molar and second premolar can be incorporated into the posterior segment for better anchorage control.

The second weakness is that the intrusive force against the incisors is applied anterior to the center of resistance, and therefore the incisors tend to tip forward as they intrude (Figure 16-33). Without an extraction space, forward movement of the incisors is an inevitable consequence of leveling, but often in extraction cases, this result is undesirable. The anchor bend at the molar in the Begg approach creates a space-closing effect that somewhat restrains forward incisor movement (Figure 16-34), but this also tends to bring the molar forward, straining the posterior anchorage. The same thing happens for the same reason with a Mulligan bypass arch or a utility arch. A utility arch can be activated to keep the incisors from moving forward and has the additional benefit of a rectangular cross-section anteriorly so that tipping can be controlled, but the result is still

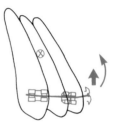

FIGURE 16-33 When the incisor segment is viewed from a lateral perspective, the center of resistance is lingual to the point at which an arch wire attaches to the crown. For this reason, the incisors tend to tip forward when an intrusive force is placed at the central incisor brackets. This tendency toward labial tipping can be controlled either by applying a force to tip the incisors distally as they are being intruded, canceling the mesial tipping, or by applying the intrusive force more posteriorly, as by attaching an intrusion arch to stabilized anterior segment more distally, in the vicinity of the lateral rather than the central incisors, for instance (see Figure 16-38).

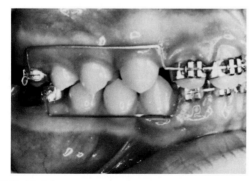

FIGURE 16-32 Utility arches for leveling, showing the long span from molars to incisors that makes it possible to produce absolute intrusion.

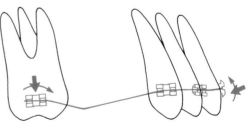

FIGURE 16-34 Diagrammatic representation of forces from a leveling arch wire that bypasses the premolars, with an anchor bend mesial to the molars. A force system is created that elongates the molars and intrudes the incisors. The wire tends to slide posteriorly through the molar tube, tipping the incisors distally at the expense of bodily mesial movement of the molars. An arch wire of this design is used in the first stage of Begg treatment but also can be used in edgewise systems. A long span from the molars to the incisors is essential.

a strain on posterior anchorage (see Chapter 10 for a detailed discussion).

The segmented arch approach to leveling developed by Burstone, which overcomes these limitations, is recommended for maximum control of the anterior and posterior segments of the dental arch.

Segmented Arch wires for Leveling. The segmented arch approach depends on establishing stabilized posterior segments and controlling the point of force application against an anterior segment. This technique requires auxiliary rectangular tubes on first molars, in addition to the regular bracket or tube. After preliminary alignment if needed, a full dimension rectangular arch wire is placed in the bracket slots of teeth in the buccal segment, which typically consists of the second premolar, first molar, and second molar. This connects these teeth into a solid unit. In addition, a heavy lingual arch (36 mil round or 32 × 32 rectangular steel wire) is used to connect the right and left posterior segments, further stabilizing them against undesired movement (Figure 16-35). A resilient anterior segmental wire is used to align the incisors, while the posterior segments are being stabilized.

For intrusion, an auxiliary depressing arch placed in the auxiliary tube on the first molar is used to apply intrusive force against the anterior segment. This arch should be made of rectangular wire that will not twist in the auxiliary tube. Burstone recommends 18 × 25 steel wire with a 2 1/2-turn helix (Figure 16-36), or 19 × 25 TMA wire without a helix.[14] More recently, preformed NiTi intrusion arches have been offered commercially, making the use of an auxiliary arch wire more convenient.[15] This depressing arch is adjusted so that it lies gingival to the incisor teeth when passive and applies a light force (10-15 gm per tooth, depending on root size) when it is brought up beneath the brackets of the incisors. It is tied underneath the incisor brackets, but not into the bracket slots, which are occupied by the anterior segment wire.

An auxiliary depressing arch can be placed while a light resilient anterior segment is being used to align malposed incisors, but it is usually better to wait to add the depressing arch until incisor alignment has been achieved and a heavier anterior segment wire has been installed. A braided rectangular steel wire or a rectangular TMA wire is usually the best choice for the anterior segment while active intrusion with an auxiliary depressing arch is being carried out.

Two strategies can be used with segmented arches to prevent forward movement of the incisors as they are intruded. The first is the same as with bypass arches: a space-closing force can be created by tying the depressing arch back against the posterior segments (see Figure 16-34). Even with stabilized posterior segments, this produces some strain on posterior anchorage.

The second and usually preferable strategy is to vary the point of force application against the incisor segment.

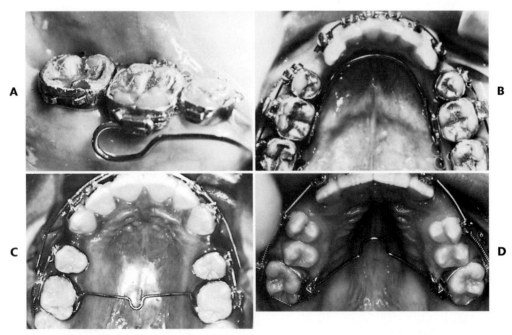

FIGURE 16-35   Mandibular stabilizing lingual arch in 36 mil steel wire, used for anchorage control in segmented arch leveling. **A,** Distal insertion into the horizontal tube on the first molar; **B,** the wire must clear the anterior segment, lying lingually and gingivally to these teeth. **C,** Maxillary transpalatal arch for anchorage control during intrusion, soldered to the first molar bands. This is effective for anchorage, but the lingual arch must be removed during finishing, and it can be awkward and difficult to cut it free. **D,** The typical removable transpalatal lingual arch uses a doubled-over segment of the wire to insert from the mesial into a horizontal tube.

If the anterior segment is considered a single unit (which is reasonable when a stiff arch wire connects the teeth within the segment), the center of resistance is located as shown in Figure 16-33. Tying the depressing arch distal to the midline, between the central and lateral incisors, or distal to the laterals (Figure 16-37), also brings the point of force application more posteriorly so that the force is applied more nearly through the center of resistance (Figure 16-38). This prevents anterior tipping of the incisor segment without causing anchorage strain.

Even with the control of posterior anchorage obtained by placing rectangular stabilizing segments and an anchorage lingual arch, the reaction to intrusion of incisors is extrusion and distal tipping of the posterior segments. With careful attention to appropriate technique with the segmented arch approach, it is possible to produce approximately four times as much incisor intrusion as molar extrusion in nongrowing adults. Although successful intrusion can be obtained with round bypass arches, the ratio of anterior intrusion to posterior extrusion is much less favorable. A utility arch can be used in conjunction with stabilized pos-

terior segments, simply by placing the utility arch into an auxiliary tube on the first molar (an arrangement recommended by Ricketts for older patients). With this alteration (Figure 16-39), the ratio of intrusion to extrusion improves. For adults, however, to control anterior tipping, it is advantageous to tie the depressing arch beneath a separate base arch wire anteriorly, rather than tying directly into the incisor brackets as is usually done with a utility arch.

At the conclusion of the first stage of treatment, the arches should be level, and teeth should be aligned to the point that rectangular steel arch wires can be placed without an exaggerated curve and without generating excessive forces. The duration of the first stage, obviously, will be determined by the severity of both the horizontal and vertical components of the initial malocclusion. For some patients, only a single initial arch wire will be required, while for others, several months may be needed for alignment, and several more months for segmental leveling, before the next stage can begin. As a principle of treatment, it is important not to move to the second stage of treatment until both leveling and alignment are adequate.

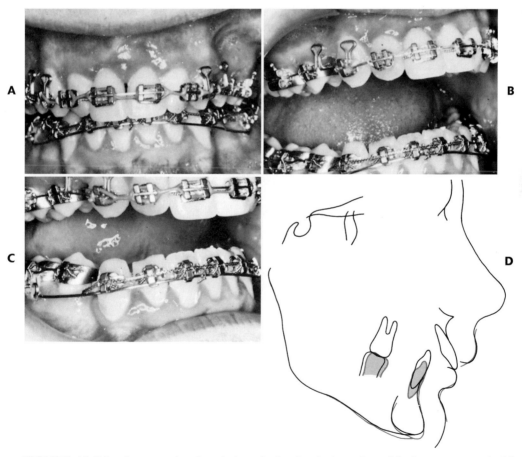

FIGURE 16-36 Segmented arch technique for leveling by intrusion of the lower incisors. **A,** After preliminary alignment, an anterior segment of 17 × 25 braided steel wire has been placed in the mandibular anterior segment. Posterior segments are stabilized, and a 17 × 25 steel depressing arch is placed in auxiliary tubes on the first molars and tied beneath the incisor brackets anteriorly; **B,** lateral view of appliance at initial activation; **C,** lateral view, 8 weeks later; **D,** cephalometric superimposition showing the amount of intrusion obtained in 3 months.

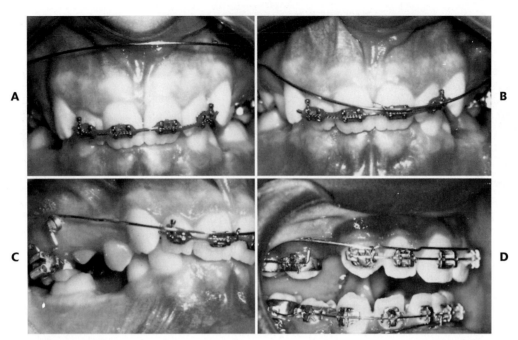

FIGURE 16-37 Segmented arch application for intrusion of maxillary incisors. **A,** The depressing arch in the vestibule, before activation. It is adjusted so that it provides about 50 gm of force, **B,** when it is deflected down to the level of the brackets. **C,** Buccal view showing the 2½ turn helix used in steel wire. For this patient, the depressing arch is tied in the midline because it is desirable for the incisors to tip forward as they depress. **D,** Buccal view of another patient. Note that the intrusion arch is tied between the lateral incisors and canines, moving the point of force appliance nearer the center of the resistance of the anterior segment to prevent labial tipping of the incisors during the intrusion. In this patient, an auxiliary wire also is being used in the lower arch, but to supplement the continuous arch that is in place. The lower leveling will occur largely by elongation of the canine and premolar, rather than by intrusion of the incisors.

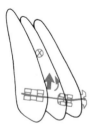

FIGURE 16-38 Tying an auxiliary depressing arch distal to the midline, as shown in Figure 16-37, moves the line of force more posteriorly and therefore closer to the center of resistance of the anterior segment, diminishing or eliminating the moment that causes tipping. Compare this figure with Figure 16-33.

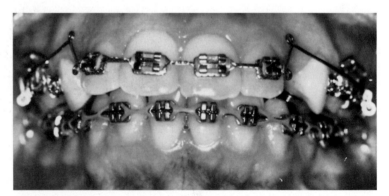

FIGURE 16-39 Utility arch inserted in auxiliary tube on molars, to intrude maxillary incisors while alignment loops are used in the buccal segments. Loops like those shown in this utility arch have two purposes: they decrease stiffness, so a larger wire than 16 × 16 steel can be used, and they can be activated to exert a distal or space-closing effect, providing a force to counteract the labial tipping of incisors that otherwise would occur.

REFERENCES

1. Begg PR, Kesling PC: Begg orthodontic theory and technique, Philadelphia, 1977, W.B. Saunders.
2. Cobb NW III, Kula KS, Phillips C, Proffit WR: Efficiency of multistrand steel, superelastic NiTi and ion-implanted NiTi arch wires for initial alignment, Clin Orthod Res, 1:12-19, 1998.
3. Stoner MM: Wire: clinical considerations. In Graber TM, Swain BF (editors): Current orthodontic concepts and techniques, ed 2, Philadelphia, 1975, W.B. Saunders.
4. Lew K: A comparison of arch wires used for initial alignment in Begg treatment, Aust Orthod J 10:180-182, 1988.
5. Melsen B: Palatal growth studied on human autopsy material, Am J Orthod 68:42-54, 1975.
6. Sarver DM, Johnston MW: Skeletal changes in vertical and anterior displacement of the maxilla with bonded rapid palatal expansion appliances, Am J Orthod Dentofac Orthop 95:462-466, 1989.
7. Vermette ME, Kokich VG, Kennedy DB: Uncovering labially impacted teeth—apically positioned flap and closed-eruption techniques, Angle Orthod 65:23-32, 1995.
8. Sandler JP: An attractive solution to unerupted teeth, Am J Orthod Dentofac Orthop 100:489-493, 1991.
9. Vardimon AD, Graber TM, Drescher D, Bourauel C: Rare earth magnets and impaction, Am J Orthod Dentofac Orthop 100:494-512, 1991.
10. Edwards JG: Soft tissue surgery to alleviate orthodontic relapse, Dent Clinics North America 37:205-225, 1993.
11. Mulligan TF: Common sense mechanics. VI. Clinical application of the diving board concept, J Clin Orthod 14: 98-103, 1980.
12. Isaacson RJ, Lindauer SJ, Rubenstein LK: Activating a 2 × 4 appliance. Angle Orthod 63:17-24, 1993.
13. Ricketts RW et al: Bioprogressive therapy, Denver, 1979, Rocky Mountain Orthodontics.
14. Burstone CJ: Deep overbite correction by intrusion, Am J Orthod 72:1-22, 1977.
15. Nanda R, Marzban R, Kuhlberg A: The Connecticut intrusion arch, J Clin Orthod 32:708-715, 1998.

CHAPTER

17

The Second Stage of Comprehensive Treatment: Correction of Molar Relationship and Space Closure

Correction of molar relationship
    Correction of molar relationship by differential growth
    Correction by distal movement of upper molars
    Differential anteroposterior tooth movement, using
        extraction spaces
    Correction with interarch elastics
Closure of extraction spaces
    Moderate anchorage situations
    Maximum incisor retraction (maximum anchorage)
    Minimum incisor retraction

At the beginning of the second stage of treatment, the teeth should be well-aligned, and any excessive or reverse curve of Spee should have been eliminated. The objectives of this stage of treatment are to correct molar and buccal segment relationships to provide normal occlusion in the anteroposterior plane of space, close extraction spaces or residual spaces in the arches, and correct excessive or negative overjet. This is possible only if the jaw relationships are reasonably correct—which means that surgery must be considered for the most severe problems. Indications for surgical treatment and the orthodontic-surgical interaction are discussed in Chapter 22.

CORRECTION OF MOLAR RELATIONSHIP

Correction of the molar relationship nearly always involves moving from a Class II or partially Class II relationship to Class I, although occasionally the treatment will be aimed at a Class III problem. Excluding surgery to reposition the jaws, there are two possibilities (1) differential growth of

the jaws, guided by extraoral force or a functional appliance, or (2) differential anteroposterior movement of the upper and lower teeth—with or without differential closure of extraction spaces. These approaches are not mutually exclusive, but growth modification is most successful in preadolescent children, so in the permanent dentition most of the correction usually has to be obtained by tooth movement intended to camouflage any skeletal contribution to the malocclusion.

Differential Growth in Adolescent Class II Treatment

The use of extraoral force or functional appliances to influence jaw growth is discussed in some detail in Chapter 15. The different timing of skeletal growth in males and females must be kept in mind when this approach is used. During adolescence, the mandible tends to grow forward more than the maxilla, providing an opportunity to improve a skeletal Class II jaw relationship. Girls mature considerably earlier than boys and are often beyond the peak of the adolescent growth spurt before the full permanent dentition is available and comprehensive orthodontic treatment can begin. Boys who mature more slowly and have a more prolonged period of adolescent growth, are much more likely to have a clinically useful amount of anteroposterior growth during comprehensive treatment.

Whether extraoral force (headgear) or a functional appliance is used to modify growth in Class II patients, a favorable response includes both restraint of maxillary growth and differential mandibular growth. Headgear is more compatible with the fixed appliances needed for comprehensive treatment, and functional appliance therapy alone is unlikely to provide a satisfactory result in the early permanent dentition. In skeletally immature patients with a permanent dentition, there is nothing wrong with a first phase of functional appliance treatment even though the permanent teeth have erupted, and then a fixed appliance to obtain detailed occlusal results, but it is likely that the functional appliance therapy will have to be modified or discontinued when the fixed appliance treatment begins. Although many clinicians would like to believe that Class II elastics (or fixed springs that have the same effect) can influence growth as well as move teeth, the evidence indicates that growth modification is unlikely with a "fixed functional" unless the rigid coupling of a Herbst appliance is used.[1]

An ideal patient for headgear in the early permanent dentition is a 12- to 14-year-old boy with a Class II problem, whose skeletal maturity is somewhat behind his stage of dental development, and who has good growth potential (Figure 17-1). Boys at age 13, it must be remembered, are on the average at the same stage of maturation as girls at 11, and significant skeletal growth is almost always continuing. On the other hand, girls at age 13 are, on the average, at the same developmental stage as boys at 15, and by this time, clinically useful changes in jaw relationship from growth guidance are unlikely.

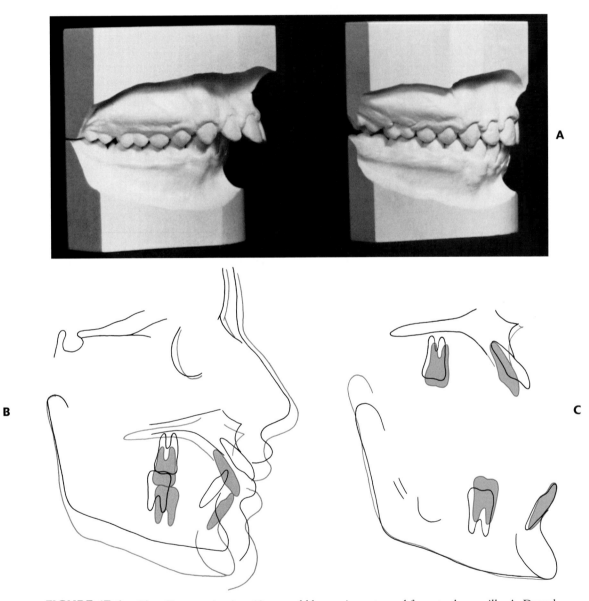

FIGURE 17-1 Class II correction in a 13-year-old boy, using extraoral force to the maxilla. **A,** Dental casts before and after treatment; **B** and **C,** cephalometric superimposition showing treatment changes. Note the large amount of vertical growth, which allowed the maxilla and maxillary dentition to be displaced distally as they moved vertically, while the mandible grew downward and forward. As the maxillary and mandibular superimpositions show, overbite was corrected by relative intrusion (i.e., the lower incisors were held at the same vertical level while the molars erupted). There was relatively more eruption of the mandibular than the maxillary molar, reflecting the upward-backward direction of headgear force, and only a small amount of distal driving of the upper molars.

Although correction of molar relationship is a major goal of the second rather than the first stage of treatment, extraoral force should be applied against the first molars from the beginning in any patient for whom molar correction by differential growth is desired. There is no reason to wait for alignment and leveling to be completed, especially since every passing day decreases the probability of a favorable growth response. The extraoral force can also help control anchorage during alignment.

Although the main purpose of extraoral force is growth modification, some tooth movement in all three planes of space inevitably accompanies it. When there is good vertical growth and the maxillary molars are allowed to elongate, the maxillary teeth erupt downward and backward, and spaces may open up in the maxillary arch. Even though the extraoral force is applied against the first molar, it is unusual for space to develop between the first molar and second premolar. Instead, the second and, to a lesser degree, the first premolars follow the molars. The result is often a space distal to the canines, along with a partial reduction of overjet as the jaw relationship improves (Figure 17-2).

When this result occurs, the preferred approach is to consolidate space within the maxillary arch at a single location, using elastomeric chains to bring the canines and incisors into an anterior segment and the molar and premolars into a posterior segment. When the molar relationship has been corrected, the residual overjet is then reduced by retracting the incisors in this nonextraction patient in exactly the same way as in a patient who had a first premolar extraction space (see the following discussion). Extraoral force should be continued until an intact maxillary arch has been achieved. Discontinuing it when only the molar relationship has been corrected is unwise, both because the maximum skeletal effect probably has not been obtained at that point, and because the retraction of the incisor teeth requires posterior anchorage, which can be reinforced by the headgear.

Correction by Distal Movement of Upper Molars

The concept of "distal driving" of the maxillary posterior teeth has a long orthodontic history. After early cephalometric studies showed that little or no distal movement of upper molars was produced by the Class II elastic treatment of that era, headgear was re-introduced as a means of moving the upper molars back. More recently, palatal anchorage has been used to create distal movement of upper molars, to create a space into which the anterior teeth can be retracted.

Although the modern methods discussed below have improved the situation, Class II correction by distal movement of upper molars has definite limits that it is important to understand and respect. With headgear, it is now clear that significant distal positioning of the upper posterior teeth relative to the maxilla occurs primarily in patients who have vertical growth and elongation of the maxillary teeth (see Figure 17-1). Without this, it is difficult to produce more than 2 to 3 mm of distal movement of the upper molars, unless the upper second molars are extracted (see p. 558). Appliances based on palatal anchorage are somewhat more successful in moving upper molars back, but complete Class II correction by this mechanism is unlikely.

Molar Rotation as a Factor in Distalization. In patients with mild to moderate skeletal Class II malocclusion, the upper molars are likely to have rotated mesially around the lingual root (see Figure 17-2, *C*), and merely correcting the rotation changes the occlusal relationship in a Class I direction. This can be done with a transpalatal lingual arch, an auxiliary labial arch, or the inner bow of a facebow. Sometimes upper molars are so mesially rotated that it is difficult or impossible to insert a facebow until the rotation has been partially corrected with a more flexible appliance.

Rotation correction is the first step in Class II treatment of almost every type.

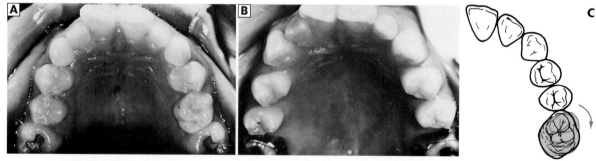

FIGURE 17-2 Space tends to open up within the maxillary arch when extraoral force to the upper first molars is used and the patient grows well. **A,** Occlusal view before treatment; **B,** same patient after 12 months of treatment with only a headgear. **C,** In patients with Class II malocclusion, the upper molars usually are rotated mesially, and part of the apparent backward movement of the first molar is a distal rotation of the buccal cusps as the tooth rotates around its lingual root. This type of rotation can be produced by a facebow or by a transpalatal lingual arch. In **B,** note the spacing in the premolar area, as gingival fibers produce distal rotation of these teeth also. When a complete fixed appliance is placed at this stage, one of the first steps is consolidation of the space distal to the canines.

Palatal Anchorage Systems for Distal Movement of Molars. Mesial movement of teeth is easier than distal movement, simply because there is much more resistance to distal movement. Successful distal movement of molars, therefore, requires more anchorage than can be supplied by just the other teeth. The relative stability of the anterior palate, both the soft tissue rugae and the cortical bone beneath them, is one possibility for obtaining this additional anchorage. Although removable appliances contact the palate, they are not effective in moving molars back, probably because they do not fit well enough. A fixed appliance that stabilizes the premolars and includes a plastic pad contacting the rugae is needed. Fortunately, most patients tolerate this with minimal problems, but contacting the palatal tissue has the potential to cause significant tissue irritation, to the point that the appliance has to be removed.

There are several possibilities for generating the molar distalizing force. A-NiTi coil springs produce an effective and nearly constant force system for the distal movement.[2] Magnets in repulsion also can be used quite effectively (Figure 17-3), but the A-NiTi springs have the additional advantage of being less bulky (see Figure 8-42) and usually are a better choice. The pendulum appliance, developed by Hilgers,[3] uses beta-Ti springs that extend from the palatal acrylic and fit into lingual sheaths on the molar tube (Figure 17-4). The effects of this appliance illustrate the potential of palatal anchorage for molar distalization.

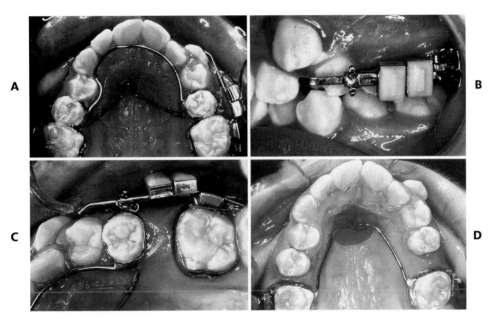

FIGURE 17-3 The use of magnets in repulsion to distalize maxillary first molars. **A,** Stabilizing lingual arch from second premolars, with one magnet attached to the premolar and the other to the first molar on the right side; **B,** Facial view of the magnet assembly. Note the arrangement for repositioning the premolar magnet as the molar moves back, to maintain the force; **C,** Progress: space opened at the rate of about 1 mm/month; **D,** Nance arch in place to maintain the molars (the left molar was distalized for 3 months, the right molar for 6 months) while distal drift of premolars occurs. A complete fixed appliance was placed a few months later to complete the treatment. (Courtesy Dr. Wick Alexander.)

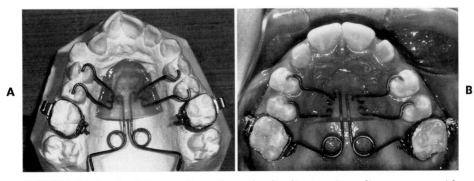

FIGURE 17-4 Pendulum appliance for molar distalization. **A,** appliance on cast, with the distalization springs not inserted into the molar tubes; **B,** Appliance in the mouth, with the springs activated. (Courtesy F. Blyloff and M.A. Darendeliler.)

In a small but well-characterized sample of patients who were treated to a super-Class I molar relationship with the pendulum appliance activated to produce 200 to 250 grams (Figure 17-5), Blyloff et al found that molar movement averaged just over 1 mm/month (1.02 ± 0.68), with a considerable degree of distal tipping of the crown and an elevation of the molar (Figure 17-6).[4] As one would expect, despite the contact of the appliance with the palate, the premolars and incisors were tipped anteriorly, but the molar moved distally 2 to 3 times as far as the anchor teeth. When the appliance was modified to minimize distal tipping of the molar, the distal movement of the molar crown was similar, but greater distal movement of the roots was obtained at the cost of increased treatment time and some additional forward movement of the incisors (Figure 17-7).[5]

However the molars were moved distally, they must be held there while the other teeth are then retracted to correct the overjet. It is one thing to move molars back, and something else to maintain them in that position. Simply leaving the distalization appliance in place for 2 to 3 months leads to distal movement of the premolars by stretched gingival fibers, but as soon as the original premolar-based lingual arch and palatal pad are removed, a new lingual arch and pad from the distalized molars must be placed (see Figure 17-6). Even so, especially if the molar tipped distally, it will tip mesially again as the space closes. Placing a tip-back in the distalizing springs will keep the molar more upright and minimize relapse, but this increases the extrusive tendency, so as with headgear, the most successful molar distalization with the pendulum appliance occurs in patients who have vertical growth during their treatment.

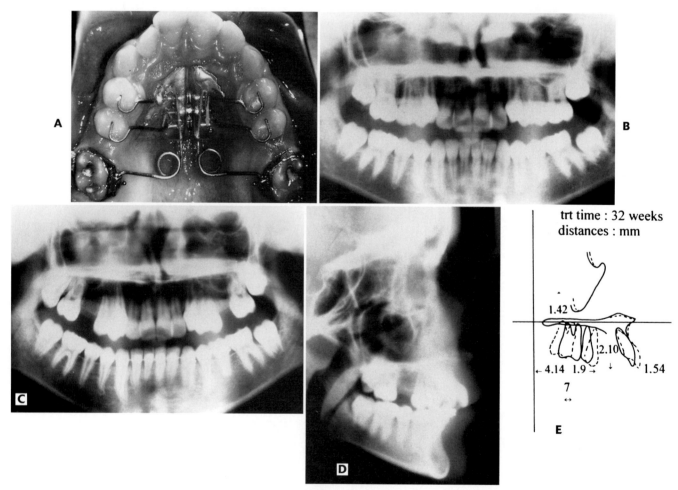

FIGURE 17-5   Correction of a Class II molar relationship by distalization of the upper molars with a pendulum appliance. **A,** Pendulum appliance with expansion screw and tip-back bends in the distalization springs, after eight months of treatment including slow expansion; **B,** panoramic radiographs before and, **C,** after distalization; **D,** cephalometric radiograph showing distalization; **E,** cephalometric superimposition showing the tooth movement achieved for this patient. Note that distal movement of the roots as well as the crowns of the molars was achieved despite modest tipping of the molars. Despite the palatal anchorage, 4 mm distal movement of the molar was accompanied by 1.5 mm mesial movement of the incisors. (Courtesy F. Blyloff and M.A. Darendeliler.)

Force from Class II elastics also can be used to push the upper molars distally, but there are two problems. First, the elastics extrude the lower molars, which means that downward-backward rotation of the mandible will occur unless the patient has some vertical growth during the period of treatment. Second, there is the risk of considerably more mesial movement of the lower teeth than distal movement of the upper teeth (Figure 17-8). If Class II elastics are used to drive upper molars distally, it is preferable at first to apply the elastic force against the first molars alone via sliding jigs, as illustrated in Figure 17-9. The upper archwire is reduced in size posteriorly to allow freer sliding, the lower arch is stabilized with a full dimension rectangular archwire, and the force of the elastics is reduced to about 100 gm (3 to 4 oz). This procedure is important not only to control forward tipping of the mandibular teeth but also to maintain transverse control of the lower arch. Class II elastics tend to widen the lower molars to the point that they can produce a molar crossbite. A heavy rectangular archwire, slightly constricted across the molars, is needed to prevent this complication.

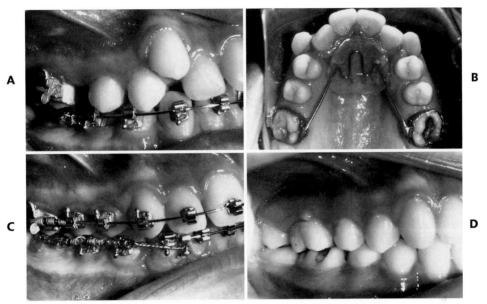

FIGURE 17-6 After molar distalization, it is important to hold the molar in position and allow distal drift of premolars to occur before placing a fixed appliance to complete the alignment of the teeth. **A,** Corrected molar relationship after distalization; **B,** lingual arch to hold distalized molars; **C,** fixed appliance in place (note the self-ligating brackets) after 6 months of premolar and canine drift with the lingual arch holding the molar largely closed the space and brought the teeth into alignment; **D,** completion of treatment. (Courtesy F. Blyloff and M.A. Darendeliler.)

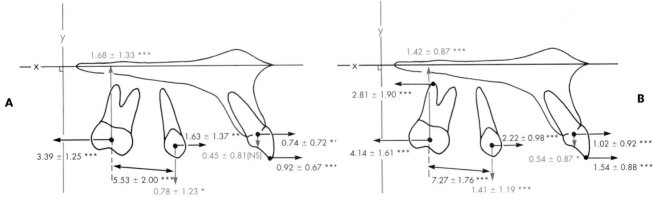

FIGURE 17-7 **A,** Mean changes in a sample of 13 patients with activation of a pendulum appliance with 250 gm force and no tipback bends; **B,** mean changes in 20 patients with a similar pendulum appliance incorporating tipback bends. The tipback bends reduced tipping of the molar as it moved distal and led to greater distal movement of the roots at the cost of increased displacement of the incisors and increased treatment time. (Redrawn from Blyloff et al: *Angle Orthod* 67:255-265, 1997.)

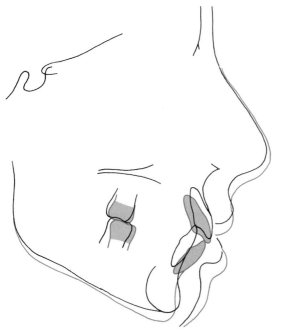

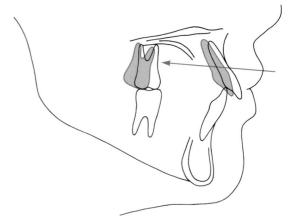

FIGURE 17-10   After extraction of maxillary second molars, extraoral force can successfully move the maxillary dentition posteriorly, as this cephalometric superimposition shows. To achieve this effect, extraoral force must be applied nearly full time, to promote efficient tooth movement. The effective limit of movement of this type is 4 to 5 mm. (Retraced from Armstrong M.M.: *Am J Orthod* 59:217-243, 1971.)

FIGURE 17-8   Cephalometric superimposition showing the response to Class II elastics in a girl in whom this was the major method for correcting a Class II malocclusion. Note that with rectangular archwires, some torque of the upper incisors was obtained. The rotational effects often associated with Class II elastics were less apparent for this patient than is sometimes the case (see also Figure 17-19), but the considerably greater forward displacement of the lower arch than retraction of the upper is typical.

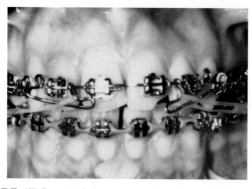

FIGURE 17-9   A "sliding jig" as illustrated here can be used to transfer Class II elastic force to the posterior segment of the maxillary arch. Rather than attaching to the maxillary archwire or anterior teeth, the elastic is hooked to the front part of the jig, which contacts the mesial surface of the first molar. In typical use, a jig later is shortened to apply the Class II force to the second premolar.

Once the upper molar has been moved into a correct relationship, the jig is altered and force applied against the second premolars. As a final step, Class II elastic force to the archwire is continued as the space between the first and second premolars is closed. With this approach, even though relatively light force is distributed over all the lower

teeth, the elastics must be worn for a long time, and mesial movement of the lower arch is an inevitable side effect.

Distalization of First Molars After Second Molar Extraction.   Moving upper first molars distally is much easier if space is created by extracting the upper second molars. Then vertical growth is not so critical in moving the first molars back, but even so, total Class II correction cannot be expected (Figure 17-10). For this reason, extraction of upper second molars to camouflage a skeletal Class II relationship should be considered only when specific indications are present (see Chapter 8). The key to success is a force system that moves the first molars and then the other teeth back without reciprocal protrusion of the anterior teeth.

For this purpose, headgear is an obvious choice. To produce tooth movement, extraoral force of moderate intensity with long duration is needed. Skeletal effects in rapidly growing patients can be achieved with fewer hours per day of headgear wear than are necessary to successfully move teeth. The patient must wear the headgear full-time or nearly so to move the maxillary teeth posteriorly. Molar extrusion should be avoided, so straight-pull or high-pull —but not cervical—headgear is indicated. The force magnitude should be large enough to simultaneously reposition all the maxillary teeth, which means that with an archwire tying the teeth together, the force should be approximately 300 gm on each side. Existing data show that with this approach, there is an excellent chance of clinical success, and that there is a 75% to 80% chance of maxillary third molars erupting into an acceptable position.[6]

Palatal anchorage is the other obvious choice and as one would expect is more successful in moving the first molar distally when the resistance of the second molar has been removed. Force levels against the first molar should be lower in second molar extraction cases. Bodily movement—not just tipping—is needed, and as with any technique that opens space mesial to the first molar, keeping the molar back while the other teeth are retracted is the key to success with this method (see Figure 17-6)

Occasionally unilateral molar distalization is indicated, typically when a unilateral Class II malocclusion is present and one side of the maxillary arch is crowded but the other is not. In patients past the adolescent growth spurt who still have at least a little vertical growth remaining, extraction of one upper second molar and asymmetric cervical headgear can produce a satisfactory treatment outcome (Figure 17-11).

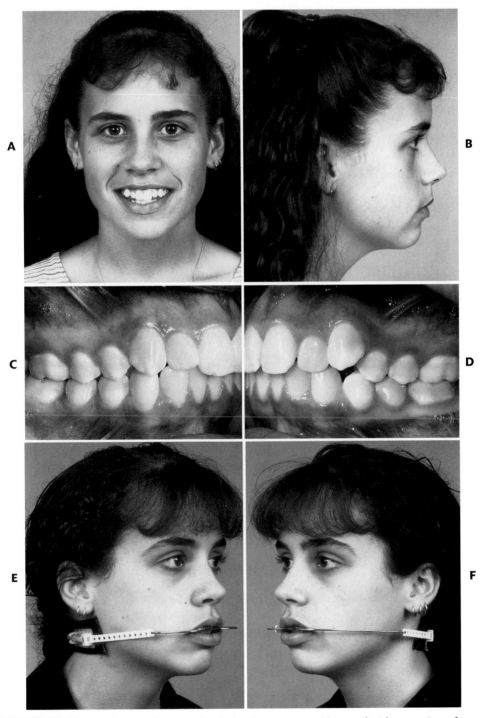

FIGURE 17-11 Unilateral Class II malocclusion in a teenage girl treated with extraction of one maxillary second molar and unilateral headgear. **A-D,** Prior to treatment. Note the maxillary midline displaced to the right and the moderate skeletal component of the malocclusion. **E** and **F,** Unilateral cervical headgear (for all practical purposes, unilateral headgear must be cervical). Note the longer outer bow on the side where greater tooth movement is desired. *continued*

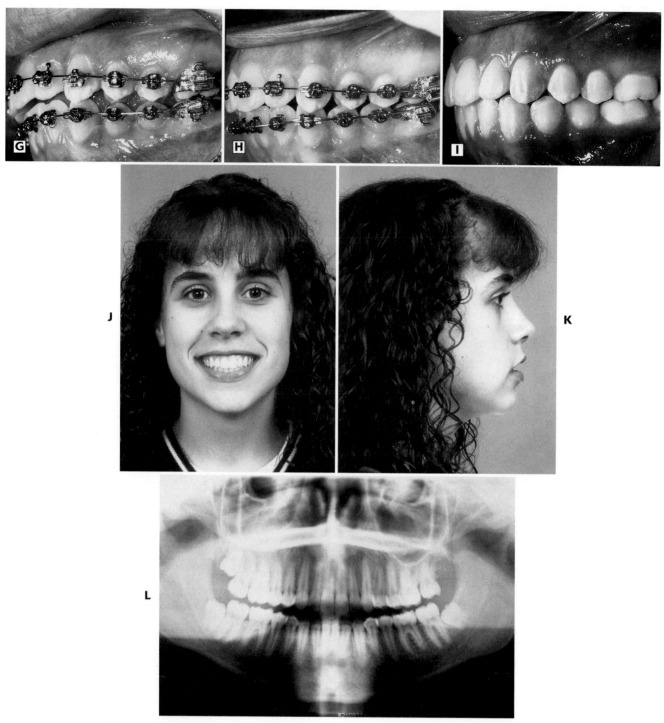

FIGURE 17-11, cont'd **G** and **H,** Progress intra-orals; **I-K,** post-treatment. Note the correction of the dental midline as well as the correction of the molar relationship. **L,** Post-treatment panoramic radiograph, showing the upper left third molar on the way to replacing the extracted second molar. There were minimal cephalometric changes, with no growth, as expected.

Differential Anteroposterior Tooth Movement Using Extraction Spaces

There are two reasons for extracting teeth in orthodontics, as discussed in detail in Chapter 7: (1) to provide space to align crowded incisors without creating excessive protrusion, and (2) to allow camouflage of moderate Class II or Class III jaw relationships when correction by growth modification is not possible. A patient who is both Class II (or III) and crowded is a particular problem because the same space cannot be used for both purposes. The more extraction space required for alignment, the less available for differential movement in camouflage, and vice versa.

An important part of treatment planning is deciding which teeth to extract and how the extraction spaces are to be closed (i.e., by retraction of incisor teeth, mesial movement of posterior teeth, or some combination). These decisions determine the orthodontic mechanics.

Class II Camouflage by Extraction of Upper First Premolars. Like upper second molar extraction, extraction of upper first premolars is a deceptively attractive

solution to Class II problems and should be adopted only when its specific indications exist (Chapter 8). With this approach, the objective during orthodontic treatment is to maintain the existing Class II molar relationship, closing the first premolar extraction space entirely by retracting the protruding incisor teeth (Figure 17-12). Anchorage must be reinforced, but one method, Class II elastics from the lower arch, is specifically contraindicated. The remaining possibilities are extraoral force to the first molars, a stabilizing lingual arch, or retraction of the maxillary anterior segment with extraoral force directly against these teeth.

Excellent reinforcement of posterior anchorage can be obtained with extraoral force if it is applied consistently and for long durations. The more constant the headgear wear, the less a stabilizing lingual arch will be needed. Conversely, a stabilizing lingual arch augments the posterior anchorage full-time, while headgear is likely to be worn a good bit less.

It seems intuitively obvious that a lingual arch with a button against the palatal tissue should be more effective than a straight transpalatal lingual arch, but when first molars

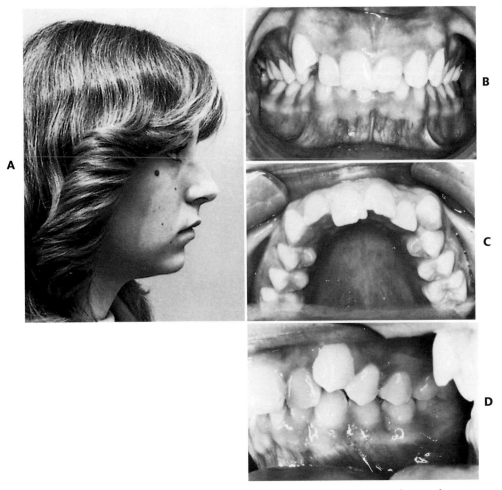

FIGURE 17-12 Records of a patient who was treated with extraction of upper first premolars for camouflage of a Class II malocclusion. **A,** Pre-treatment profile photograph; **B** to **D,** pre-treatment intraoral photographs; *continued*

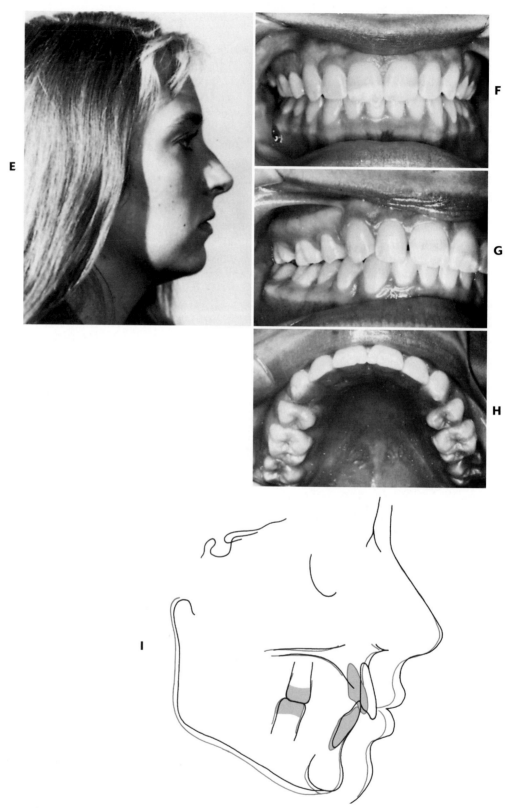

FIGURE 17-12, cont'd E, post-treatment profile; **F** to **H,** post-treatment intraoral photographs; **I,** cephalometric superimposition. For this patient, retraction of the maxillary incisors was accomplished with good anchorage control, the esthetic change was quite acceptable, and jaw function was normal.

are being stabilized in a premolar extraction case, this is not necessarily true. The effect of the lingual arch is primarily to prevent the molars from rotating mesiolingually around their palatal root, and secondarily to prevent them from tipping mesially. A straight transpalatal lingual arch (see Figure 16-35) is as effective as one with a palatal button in preventing rotation, and for most patients, the marginally better stabilization with a palatal button is not worth the cost in tissue irritation. Note that this is true when a lingual arch is used to stabilize molars, but not true when the lingual arch is to stabilize premolars, as in the molar distalization technique discussed above. When pushed mesially, premolars tip more than they rotate, and a palatal button is needed on a lingual arch to stabilize them.

In addition to headgear and/or lingual arch stabilization, all the strategies described in Chapter 10 for reducing strain on anchorage (i.e., avoiding friction, retracting canines individually, etc.) are appropriate with upper first premolar extraction and can be brought into use.

Retracting protruding maxillary anterior teeth with extraoral force (Figure 17-13) totally avoids strain on the posterior teeth and is extremely attractive from that point of view.[7] This technique has two major disadvantages: (1) The force system applied to the anterior teeth is far from ideal. When extraoral force is applied directly to the anterior segment, it is difficult to keep it from being undesirably heavy, but the force intermittently falls to zero when the headgear is removed. (2) There is significant friction not only where teeth slide along the archwire but also within the headgear mechanism itself. This makes it difficult to control the amount of force, and more friction on one side than the other may lead to an asymmetric response. In fact, it is unusual if space does not close faster on one side than the other. Excellent patient cooperation is essential. Only if the headgear is worn nearly full-time will efficient tooth movement be obtained. Although it is possible to obtain this level of cooperation, it is unwise to rely on it routinely. Patients for this approach should be selected carefully.

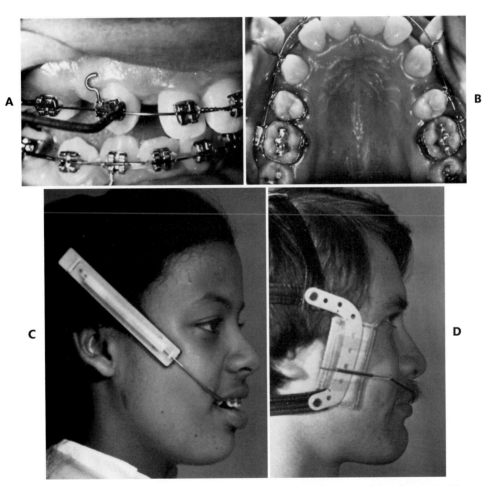

FIGURE 17-13 Retraction of the maxillary canines with a J-hook headgear. **A,** The headgear hooks over the archwire mesial to the canine bracket and pulls distally against the bracket. Approximately 200 gm of force on each side should be used; **B,** an occlusal view shows the distal translation of both canines. Note that the response at this stage is greater on one side than the other, which is not uncommon with headgear applied directly to the archwire for tooth movement; **C,** high-pull head cap with J-hooks for canine retraction; **D,** an alternative headcap, providing a more directly posterior force.

In the late 1980s, it was claimed by some dentists that extraction of upper first premolars would lead to later temporomandibular dysfunction (TD) problems. The claim was never supported by any evidence, and recent research data have refuted it.[8,9] It is important to limit first premolar extraction for camouflage of Class II malocclusion to the appropriate patients, but if this is done, it can be an excellent treatment method.

Extraction of Maxillary and Mandibular Premolars. Correction of Class II buccal segment relationships with extraction of all four first premolars implies that the mandibular posterior segments will be moved anteriorly nearly the width of the extraction space. At the same time, the protruding maxillary anterior teeth will be retracted without forward movement of the maxillary buccal segments. This, in turn, implies (though it does not absolutely require) that Class II elastics will be used to assist in closing the extraction sites.

The Begg technique is a classic illustration of the use of Class II elastics to produce differential movement of the arch segments while correcting the molar relationship. In the Begg approach, at the beginning of the second stage of treatment, light interarch elastics are added to help close space, while Class II elastics are continued (Figure 17-14). An anchor bend is placed in the upper archwire so that the maxillary anterior teeth are tipped back in part by the force system associated with the archwire itself (see Figure 16-34).

In the lower arch, the anchor bend is used to control the amount of mesial tipping of the molars. The Class II elastics reinforce and accentuate the differential tooth movements along the archwires (Figure 17-15). Friction as the archwires slide through the molar tubes during space closure is minimized by the considerable freedom between the 16 mil base arch and the 25 mil round tube through which it slides. It is extremely important that only light forces be used, so that optimum force levels are reached where tipping is desired, while forces for bodily movement remain suboptimum.

A similar mechanical arrangement, of course, can be produced with the edgewise appliance. A round wire in an edgewise bracket allows tipping of the incisors in essentially the same way as with the Begg approach, but the mesiodistal width of the canine brackets tends to keep the canine teeth more upright, thereby increasing the strain on posterior anchorage. For this reason, when a Begg-like sliding space closure in both arches is used with the edgewise appliance, reinforcement of maxillary anchorage with headgear is a good idea, and somewhat heavier Class II elastic force is needed.

It is also possible with the edgewise appliance to structure anchorage so that space closure by retraction of the maxillary anterior teeth and protraction of the mandibular posterior segments occurs without the use of Class II elastics. The best control is achieved with the segmented arch technique, using space-closing springs in each arch fabricated specifically for the type of space closure desired (see Closure of Extraction Spaces, this chapter).

When differential space closure without interarch elastics is desired, a more common approach with the edgewise appliance is to extract maxillary first and mandibular second premolars, thus altering the anchorage value of the two seg-

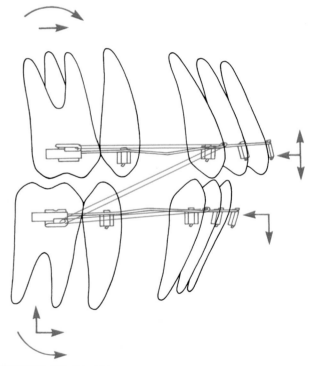

FIGURE 17-15 Diagrammatic representation of forces encountered in the second stage of Begg treatment, in which base archwires with anchor bends are combined with intra-arch and Class II elastics. The anchor bends produce bodily forward movement of the molars, but no couples are present on the incisors, so these teeth tip lingually. The anchor bends also depress the incisors and elongate the molars, which is counteracted by the Class II elastics for the upper arch but accentuated by the elastics for the lower.

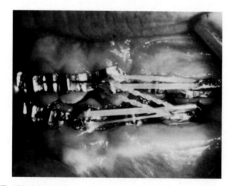

FIGURE 17-14 The second stage of Begg treatment, in which intra-arch elastics are used simultaneously with Class II elastics for space closure and correction of molar relationship. This pattern of elastic force is continued until the extraction spaces are closed. The effect is to trade forward movement of the mandibular posterior teeth for retraction of the maxillary anteriors.

ments (Figure 17-16). With this approach, routine space-closing mechanics will move the lower molars forward more than the upper, particularly if maxillary posterior anchorage is reinforced with a stabilizing lingual arch or headgear. This upper first–lower second premolar extraction pattern greatly simplifies the mechanics needed for differential space closure with continuous-arch edgewise technique.

Occasionally, however, mesial movement of the lower first molar into a second premolar extraction space is difficult to produce. This is particularly likely when the second premolar was congenitally missing and a second primary molar was extracted, because bone resorption reduces the alveolar ridge dimensions before space closure can be completed. It can be advantageous to remove only the distal root of the second primary molar, leaving the mesial part of the primary tooth in place (with a calcium hydroxide pulpotomy and temporary restoration) until the permanent tooth has been brought forward for that half of the total distance. Then the remaining half of the primary tooth is extracted, and space closure completed.

Molar Correction with Inter-arch Elastics

Without extraction spaces as previously described, Class II elastics produce molar correction largely by mesial movement of the mandibular arch, with only a small amount of distal positioning of the maxillary arch. When this pattern of tooth movement is desired, the amount of force varies with the amount of tipping allowed in the mandibular arch. With a well-fitting rectangular wire in the lower arch that is somewhat constricted posteriorly (to prevent rolling the lower molars facially and control the inclination of the lower incisors), approximately 300 gm per side is needed to displace one arch relative to the other. With a lighter round wire in the lower arch, not more than half that amount of force should be used. Incorporating the lower second molars in the appliance and attaching the elastics to a mesial hook on this tooth increase the anchorage and give a more horizontal direction of pull than hooking the elastic to the first molar.

It is important to keep in mind that with or without extraction, Class II elastics produce not only anteroposterior and transverse effects but also a vertical force (Figure 17-17). This force elongates the mandibular molars and the maxillary incisors, rotating the occlusal plane up posteriorly and down anteriorly. If the molars extrude more than the ramus grows vertically, the mandible itself will be rotated downward (Figure 17-18). Class II elastics are therefore contraindicated in nongrowing patients who cannot tolerate some downward and backward rotation of the mandible. The rotation of the occlusal plane, in and of itself, facilitates the desired correction of the posterior occlusion, but even if elongation of the lower molars can be tolerated because of good growth, the corresponding extrusion of the maxillary incisors can be unsightly.

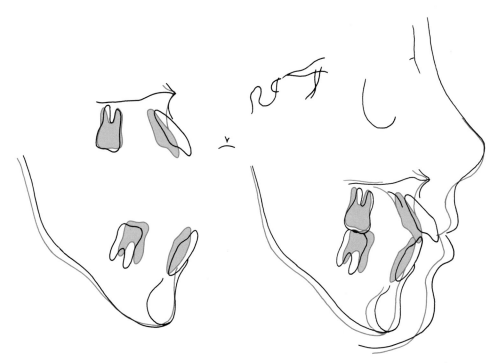

FIGURE 17-16 Cephalometric superimposition showing the result of treatment with extraction of upper first and lower second premolars. Even with second premolar extraction, some retraction of the mandibular incisors may occur, but most of the space closure will be by mesial movement of the lower molar. This adult patient experienced no growth, and a slight downward and backward rotation of the mandible occurred.

Class II elastics, in short, may produce occlusal relationships that look good on dental casts but are less satisfactory when viewed from the perspective of skeletal relationships and facial esthetics (see Figure 17-8).

Because of their vertical effects, prolonged use of Class II elastics, particularly with heavy forces, is rarely indicated. Using Class II elastics for 3 or 4 months at the completion of treatment of a Class II patient to obtain good posterior interdigitation is often acceptable. Applying heavy Class II force for 9 to 12 months as the major method for correcting a Class II malocclusion is rarely good treatment.

Class III elastics also have a significant extrusive component, tending to elongate the upper molars and the lower incisors. Elongating the molars enough to rotate the mandible downward and backward is disastrous in Class II treatment but, within limits, can help treatment of a Class III problem. If Class III elastics are used to assist in retracting mandibular incisors (see further discussion following), high-pull headgear to the upper molars worn simultaneously with the elastics can control the amount of elongation of the upper molars. Elongation of the lower incisors, however, still can be anticipated.

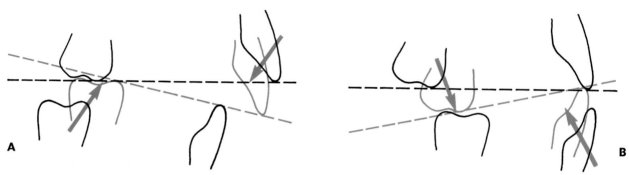

FIGURE 17-17   Rotation of the occlusal plane with Class II (**A**) and Class III (**B**) elastics. The rotation of the occlusal plane helps correct the molar relationship, and so, is helpful from that point of view, but it can be deleterious in some patients because the elongation of the molars may cause undesirable rotation of the mandible or undesirable tooth-lip relationships.

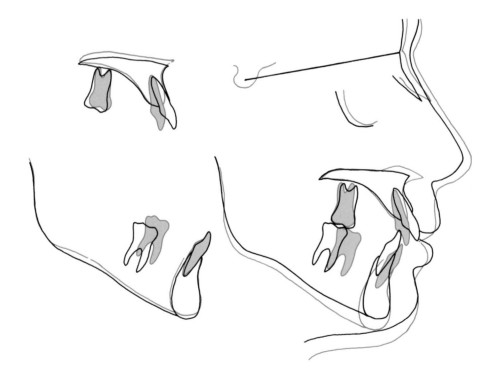

FIGURE 17-18   Cephalometric superimposition showing the vertical effects of Class II elastics in this patient, who had premolar extractions, and so, did not have forward movement of the lower incisors despite the forward movement of the lower molars. Note the elevation of the lower molar, extrusion and distal tipping of the upper incisor, rotation of the occlusal plane, and downward and backward rotation of the mandible.

CLOSURE OF EXTRACTION SPACES

To obtain the desired result of closing spaces within the arch, it is essential to control the amount of incisor retraction vs. molar-premolar protraction. Indications for extraction have been discussed in Chapters 6 and 7, and the biomechanical concepts related to control of posterior anchorage and the amount of incisor retraction are described in Chapter 10. In this section, the focus is on contemporary mechanotherapy for space closure with the 18- and 22-slot edgewise appliances.

Moderate Anchorage Situations

Most patients fall into the moderate anchorage category, meaning that after alignment of the incisors has been completed, it is desired to close the remainder of the premolar extraction space with a 50:50 or 60:40 ratio of anterior retraction to posterior protraction. The different wire sizes in 18- and 22-slot edgewise appliances require a different approach to mechanotherapy.

Moderate Anchorage Treatment with 18-Slot Edgewise: Closing Loops. Although either sliding or loop mechanics can be used, the 18-slot appliance with single or narrow twin brackets on canines and premolars is ideally suited for use of closing loops in continuous archwires. Closing loop archwires should be fabricated from rectangular wire to prevent the wire from rolling in the bracket slots. Appropriate closing loops in a continuous archwire will produce approximately 60:40 closure of the extraction space if only the second premolar and first molar are included in the anchorage unit and some uprighting of the incisors is allowed. Greater retraction will be obtained if the second molar is part of the anchorage unit, less if incisor torque is required.

The performance of a closing loop, from the perspective of engineering theory, is determined by three major characteristics: its spring properties (i.e., the amount of force it delivers and the way the force changes as the teeth move); the moment it generates, so that root position can be controlled; and its location relative to the adjacent brackets, (i.e., the extent to which it serves as a symmetric or asymmetric V-bend in a continuous wire). Clinical performance is affected not only by these characteristics but also by how well the loop conforms to additional design principles. Let us consider these in turn:

Spring Properties. The spring properties of a closing loop are determined almost totally by the wire material (at present, either steel or beta-titanium), the size of the wire, and the distance between points of attachment. This distance in turn is largely determined by the amount of wire incorporated into the loop but is affected also by the distance between brackets. Closing loops with equivalent properties can be produced from different types and sizes of wire by increasing the amount of wire incorporated into the loop as the size of the wire increases, and vice versa. Wires of greater inherent springiness or smaller cross-sectional area allow the use of simpler loop designs.

Figure 17-19, taken from the work of Booth,[10] illustrates the effects on the spring characteristics of a steel closing loop from changing wire size, the design of the loop,

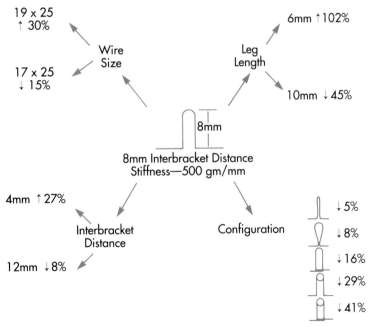

FIGURE 17-19 The effect of changing various aspects of a closing loop in an archwire. Note that an 8-mm vertical loop in 18 × 25 wire produces twice as much force as the desired 250 gm/mm. The major possibilities for producing clinically satisfactory loops are reducing wire size or incorporating additional wire by changing leg length, interbracket distance, and/or loop configuration. (Redrawn from Booth.[10])

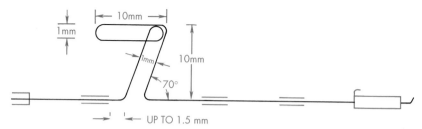

FIGURE 17-20 The Opus closing loop designed by Siatkowski offers excellent control of forces and moments, so that space can be closed under good control. The loop can be fabricated from 16 × 22 or 18 × 25 steel wire, or from 17 × 25 TMA wire. It is activated by tightening it distally behind the molar tube and can be adjusted to produce maximal, moderate, or minimal incisor retraction, but like all closing mechanisms with a long range of action, must be monitored carefully. (Redrawn from Siatkowski.[12])

and the interbracket span (the combination of these latter two parameters, of course, determines the amount of wire in the loop). Note that, as expected, changing the size of the wire produces the largest changes in characteristics, but the amount of wire incorporated in the loop is also important. The same relative effect would be observed with beta-titanium wire. For any size of wire or design of loop, beta-Ti would produce a significantly smaller force than steel.

Root-Paralleling Moments. To close an extraction space while producing bodily tooth movement, a closing loop must generate not only a closing force but also appropriate moments to bring the root apices together at the extraction site. As discussed in Chapter 10, for bodily movement the moment of the force used to move the teeth must be balanced by the moment of a couple. If its center of resistance is 10-mm from the bracket, a canine tooth being retracted with a 100-gm force must also receive a 1000 gm-mm moment if it is to move bodily. If the bracket is 1 mm wide, a vertical force of 1000 gm must be produced by the archwire at each side of the bracket (see Figures 10-28 through 10-32).

This requirement to generate a movement limits the amount of wire that can be incorporated to make a closing loop springier, because if the loop becomes too flexible, it will be unable to generate the necessary moments even though the retraction force characteristics are satisfactory. Loop design is also affected. Placing some of the wire within the closing loop in a horizontal rather than vertical direction improves its ability to deliver the moments needed to prevent tipping. Because of this and because a vertically tall loop can impinge on soft tissue, a closing loop that is only 7 to 8 mm tall while incorporating 10 to 12 mm or more of wire (e.g., a delta, L- or T-shaped loop) is preferred.

If the legs of a closing loop were parallel before activation, opening the loop would place them at an angle that in itself would generate a moment in the desired direction. Calculations show that unacceptably tall loops would be required to generate appropriate moments in this manner,[11] so additional moments must be generated by gable bends (or their equivalent) when the loop is placed in the mouth.

An elegant solution to the design of a closing loop that would provide optimum and nearly constant moment-to-force ratios at variable activations has recently been offered by Siatkowski in his Opus loop (Figure 17-20).[12]

Location of the Loop. A final engineering factor in the performance of a closing loop is its location along the span of wire between adjacent brackets. Because of its gable bends, the closing loop functions as a V-bend in the archwire, and the effect of a V-bend is quite sensitive to its position. Only if it is in the center of the span does a V-bend produce equal forces and couples on the adjacent teeth (see Figures 10-37 and 10-38). If it is one-third of the way between adjacent brackets, the tooth closer to the loop will be extruded and will feel a considerable moment to bring the root toward the V-bend, while the tooth further away will receive an intrusive force but no moment.[13] If the V-bend or loop is closer to one bracket than one third of the distance, the more distant tooth will not be intruded but will receive a moment to move the root away from the V-bend[14] (which almost never is desirable).

For routine use with fail-safe closing loops (as described later), the preferred location for a closing loop is at the spot that will be the center of the embrasure when the space is closed (Figure 17-21). This means that, in a first premolar extraction situation, the closing loop should be placed about 5 mm distal to the center of the canine tooth. The effect is to place the loop initially at the one-third position relative to the canine. The moment on the premolar increases as space closure proceeds. The design of the Opus loop calls for an off-center position with the loop 1.5 mm from the mesial (canine) bracket.

Additional Design Considerations. An important principle in closing loop design is that, to the greatest extent possible, the loop should "fail safe." This means that, although a reasonable range of action is desired from each activation, tooth movement should stop after a prescribed range of movement even if the patient does not return for a scheduled adjustment. Too long a range of action with too much flexibility could produce disastrous effects if a distorted spring were combined with a series of broken

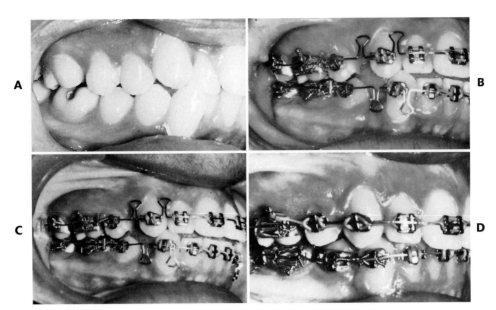

FIGURE 17-21 Stages in space closure. **A,** The original malocclusion; **B,** 16 × 22 closing loops at initial activation, after the completion of stage 1 alignment and leveling. Note the location of the closing loops and the soldered tiebacks for activation. **C,** Closing loops later during space closure; **D,** spaces closed, and finishing archwire in place.

appointments. The ideal loop design therefore would deliver a continuous, controlled force designed to produce tooth movement at a rate of approximately 1 mm per month but would not include more than 2 mm of range, so that movement would stop if the patient missed a second consecutive monthly appointment.

It also is important that the design be as simple as possible, because more complex configurations are less comfortable for patients, more difficult to fabricate clinically, and more prone to breakage or distortion. Engineering analysis, as the Opus loop demonstrates very nicely, shows that a relatively complex design is required to produce the best control of moment-force ratios. The possibilities of clinical problems from increased complexity always must be balanced against the potentially greater efficiency of the more complex design. Whether the Opus loop is simple and sturdy enough to perform well in widespread clinical use has not yet been established. Previous experience suggests that the average adolescent orthodontic patient can destroy almost any orthodontic device that is not remarkably resistant to being distorted.

A third design factor relates to whether a loop is activated by opening or closing. All else being equal, a loop is more effective when it is closed rather than opened during its activation. On the other hand, a loop designed to be opened can be made so that when it closes completely, the vertical legs come into contact, effectively preventing further movement and producing the desired fail-safe effect (Figure 17-22). A loop activated by closing, in contrast, must have its vertical legs overlap. This creates a transverse step, and the archwire does not develop the same rigidity when it is deactivated. The smaller and more flexible the

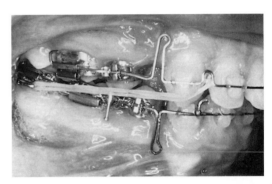

FIGURE 17-22 Closing loops in 16 × 22 wire of fail-safe design and 8-mm height used with Class II elastics in this patient. Note that the maxillary loop has been activated by pulling the wire through the molar tube and bending it up. In the mandibular arch, the loop is not active at this time, and the approximation of the legs to create a rigid archwire is apparent. The lower archwire has a tieback mesial to the first molar, so that this loop can be activated by tying a ligature from the posterior teeth to the wire rather than by bending over the end of the wire distal to the molar tube.

wire from which a closing loop arch is made, the more important it is that the wire become rigid when the loop is deactivated.

Clinical Recommendations. These design considerations indicate that an excellent closing loop for 18-slot edgewise is a delta-shaped loop in 16 × 22 wire that is activated by opening, as shown in Figures 17-21 and 17-22. Such a wire fits tightly enough in an 18 × 25 mil bracket to give good control of root position. With 10 mm of wire in the loop, the force delivery is close to the optimum, and the mechanism fails safe because contact of the vertical legs

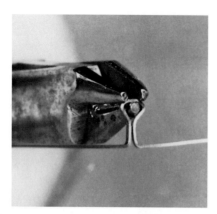

FIGURE 17-23 A three-prong pliers can be used to bring the vertical legs of a closing loop together if they are separated. The legs should touch lightly before activation of the loop by opening it.

when the loop is deactivated limits movement between adjustments and makes the archwire more rigid. It is important to activate the upper horizontal portion of a delta or T-loop so that the vertical legs are pressed lightly together when the loop is not activated (Figure 17-23). This also ensures that the loop will still be active until the legs come into contact.

With 16 × 22 wire and a loop of the delta design (so that the mechanism fails safe), with an activation of 1.0 to 1.5 mm, and with narrow 18-slot brackets, a gable bend of approximately 20 degrees on each side is needed to achieve an appropriate moment-force ratio (Figure 17-24). With wider brackets, a smaller gable bend would generate the same moment. With the same loop in stiffer wire like 17 × 25, a gable bend of any given magnitude would produce a larger moment than in 16 × 22 wire. Remember, however, that the moment-force ratio determines how teeth will move, so with a stiffer wire and the same activation a larger force would be generated and a larger moment would be needed. Optimum moment-force ratios can be achieved with several combinations of wire size, loop configuration, and gable angle and, as Siatkowski has shown, can be maintained over a variety of activations at the cost of design complexity.

A closing loop archwire is activated by pulling the posterior part of the archwire distally through the molar tubes, which activates the closing loop the desired amount (1 to 1.5 mm) and then fastening the wire in that position. The wire slides through the brackets and tubes only when it is being activated. After that, as the closing loop returns to its original configuration, and the teeth move with the archwire, not along it. There are two ways to hold the archwire in its activated position. The simplest is by bending the end of the archwire gingivally behind the last molar tube. The alternative is to place an attachment—usually a soldered tieback (see Figure 17-22)—on the posterior part of the archwire, so that a ligature can be used to tie the wire in its activated position.

With a 16 × 22 closing loop, usually it is necessary to remove the archwire and reactivate the gable bends after

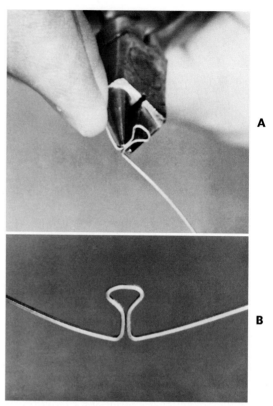

FIGURE 17-24 Gable bends for the closing loop archwire. **A,** Gable bends are placed by bending the wire at the base of the loop; **B,** appropriate gable for a 16 × 22 closing loop (40 to 45 degrees total, half that on each side).

3 to 4 mm of space closure, but a quick reactivation is all that is needed at most appointments during space closure. As a general rule, if it is anticipated that a closing loop archwire will not have to be removed for adjustment (i.e., the distance to be closed is 4 mm or less), bending the posterior end of the wire is satisfactory. It can be quite difficult to remove an archwire that has been activated by bending over the end, however, and it saves time in the long run to use tiebacks for closing loop archwires that will have to be removed and readjusted.

Specific recommendations for closing loop archwires with the 18-slot appliance and narrow brackets are:
1. 16 × 22 wire, delta or T-shaped loops, 7 mm vertical height, and additional wire incorporated in the loop to make it equivalent to 10 mm of vertical height
2. Gable bends of 40 to 45 degrees total (half on each side of the loop)
3. Loop placement 4 to 5 mm distal to the center of the canine tooth at the center of the space between the canine and second premolar with the extraction site closed

These recommendations certainly are not the only clinically effective possibilities. The principle should be that if a heavier wire (e.g., 17 × 25 mil) is used, the loop design

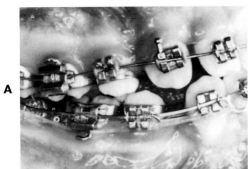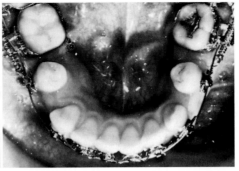

FIGURE 17-25   Sliding space closure in 22-slot edgewise. **A,** Elastomeric chain for canine retraction in the mandibular arch sliding the tooth on an undersized rectangular archwire. **B,** NiTi coil springs for retraction of first premolars in a second premolar extraction case. NiTi springs give much better control of force levels and a much greater range of action, and therefore are preferred when space is to be closed by sliding.

should be altered to incorporate additional wire for better force-deflection characteristics. Also, the gable angulations should be adjusted according to both the springiness of the loop and the width of the brackets. With wide brackets on the canines, for instance, the reduced interbracket span would make any loop somewhat stiffer, and both this and the longer moment arm across the bracket would dictate a smaller gable angle (but the range of the loop would be reduced, which is why wide brackets are not recommended).

Moderate Anchorage Space Closure with 22-Slot Edgewise.   As a general rule, space closure in moderate anchorage situations with the 22-slot edgewise appliance is done in two steps: first retracting the canines, usually sliding them along the archwire, and second, retracting the four incisors, usually with a closing loop. This two-step space closure will produce an approximately 60:40 closure of the extraction space, varying somewhat depending on whether second molars are included in posterior anchorage and incisor torque requirement.

A 19 × 25 wire is the largest on which sliding retraction of a canine should be attempted (because clearance in the bracket slot is needed), and 18 × 25 wire also can be used. An archwire with a posterior stop, usually in front of the first molar tube, is needed. This stop has the effect of incorporating all the teeth except the canine into the anchorage unit. The canine retraction can then be carried out with a coil spring, a spring soldered to the base archwire, an intra-arch latex elastic, or an elastomeric material (Figure 17-25). As a general rule, A-NiTi coil springs are preferred because they produce an almost ideal light constant force.[15] Elastics produce variable and intermittent forces, and both elastomeric chains and steel coil springs produce rapidly decaying interrupted forces.

In addition to its convenience and straightforward design, this type of sliding space closure has the important advantage that it fails safe in two ways: (1) The moments necessary for root paralleling are generated automatically by the twin brackets normally used with the 22-slot appliance. Unless the archwire itself bends, there is no danger that

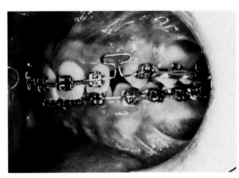

FIGURE 17-26   T-shaped loop in 18 × 25 wire, typically used with the 22-slot edgewise appliance to retract the four incisors after independent retraction of the canine.

the teeth will tip excessively. (2) The rigid attachment of the canine to the continuous ideal archwire removes the danger that this tooth will be moved far outside its intended path if the patient does not return for scheduled adjustments. For this reason, a long range of action on the retraction springs is not dangerous, as long as the force is not excessive. The ideal force to slide a canine distally is approximately 150 gm, since at least 50 gm will be used to overcome friction (see Chapter 10). A-NiTi springs can produce this level of force over a wide enough range to close an extraction space with a single activation.

The second stage in the two-stage retraction is usually accomplished with a closing loop, although it is possible to close the space now located mesial to the canines by again sliding the archwire through the posterior brackets. For this stage of incisor retraction, a rectangular wire with its smallest side at least 18 mil is needed—anything smaller rolls in the 22-slot and would allow the incisors to tip while being retracted. An 18 × 25 steel wire with a T-loop, though still too stiff, serves this purpose reasonably well while retaining the fail-safe design (Figure 17-26). Although loops in a 19 × 25 steel wire also can be used, the better force-deflection characteristics of 18 × 25 wire make it the preferred choice: the 19 × 25 loop either has to give

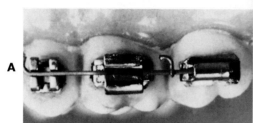
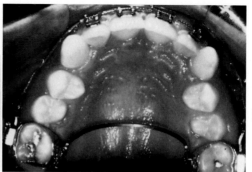

FIGURE 17-27   Stabilization of the posterior segments in Burstone's segmented arch technique requires **A,** a 21 × 25 steel wire segment in the bracket slots or tubes of the posterior teeth. Note the soldered tieback mesial to the second molar (Courtesy Dr. C.J. Burstone); and **B,** a heavy lingual arch. This current design by Burstone uses a rectangular 28 × 28 wire that is placed into a special lingual bracket on the first molars.

up the fail-safe design or is much too stiff. A third alternative, in many ways now the preferred approach, is a closing loop in 19 × 25 beta-Ti wire. This provides better properties than 18 × 25 steel (quite close to 16 × 22 steel), at the cost of more difficulty in forming the archwire.

Although the two-step procedure is predictable and has excellent fail-safe characteristics, which explains why it remains commonly used, it takes longer to close space in two steps than one.

It is possible to use a closing loop archwire for one-step (en masse) closure in the 22-slot appliance, as described previously for 18-slot edgewise. There are several possibilities, unfortunately none of them ideal. The Opus loop has excellent properties and can be used with 22-slot edgewise but is more effective in 18-slot because of the wire size. If a fail-safe design is preferred, a T-loop in 18 × 25 steel or 19 × 25 beta-Ti wire can be considered. All three of the possibilities provide less than ideal torque control of incisors during the retraction because the wire is so much smaller than the bracket slot. If en masse space closure is desired with the 22-slot appliance, a segmented arch technique offers advantages.

The segmented arch approach to space closure is based on incorporating the anterior teeth into a single segment, and both the right and left posterior teeth also into a single segment, with the two sides connected by a stabilizing lingual arch (Figure 17-27). A retraction spring is used to connect these stable bases, and the activation of the spring is varied to produce the desired pattern of space closure (Figures 17-28 and 17-29). Because the spring is separate from the wire sections that engage the bracket slots, a wire size and design that produce optimum properties can be used. An auxiliary rectangular tube, usually positioned vertically, is needed on the canine bracket or on the anterior wire segment to provide an attachment for the retraction springs (see Chapter 12). The posterior end of each spring fits into the auxiliary tube on the first molar tooth. With beta-Ti wire, the design of the retraction spring can be more simplified than the design necessary with steel wire.[16]

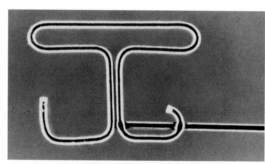

FIGURE 17-28   Composite retraction spring designed by Burstone for use with the segmented arch technique, consisting of 18 mil beta-Ti wire (the loop) welded to 17 × 25 beta-Ti. This spring can be used for either en masse retraction of incisors or canine retraction.

These springs are very effective, and with careful initial activation, an impressive range of movement can be produced before reactivation is necessary.

The greatest disadvantage of segmented arch space closure is not its increased complexity, but that it does not fail safe. Without a rigid connection between the anterior and posterior segments, there is nothing to maintain arch form and proper vertical relationships if a retraction spring is distorted or activated incorrectly. For this reason, despite the excellent results usually obtained with segmented arches and retraction springs, it is important to monitor these patients especially carefully and to avoid long intervals without observation.

Maximum Incisor Retraction (Maximum Anchorage)

It is not always desirable to retract the anterior teeth as far as possible after premolars have been extracted. In fact, over-retraction of incisors is as much of a potential problem as leaving them too prominent by not maintaining adequate posterior anchorage. When maximum retraction is needed, however, it is vital that the orthodontic mechan-

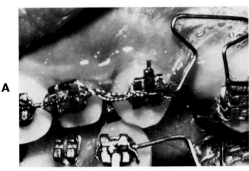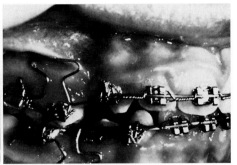

FIGURE 17-29 Space closure with the segmented arch technique. **A,** En masse retraction of the anterior maxillary segment and canine retraction in the mandibular arch (see also Figure 17-35). Note that the retraction springs fit into a vertical tube on the canine bracket. Braided wire in the maxillary anterior area will be replaced by a stabilizing anterior segment. **B,** Upper and lower en masse space closure using beta-Ti T-loops between segments in this patient with extraction of upper first and lower second premolars. (Courtesy Dr. C.J. Burstone.)

otherapy be structured to provide this. Techniques to produce maximum retraction combine two possible approaches. The first is reinforcement of posterior anchorage by appropriate means, including extraoral force, stabilizing lingual arches, and interarch elastics. The second approach involves reduction of strain on the posterior anchorage, which includes any combination of eliminating friction from the retraction system, tipping the incisors before uprighting them, or retracting the canines separately.

Maximum Retraction with the 18-Slot Appliance. With the 18-slot appliance, friction from sliding usually is avoided by employing closing loops, and tipping/uprighting is rarely part of the anchorage-control strategy. To obtain greater retraction of the anterior teeth, a sequence of steps to augment anchorage and reduce anchorage strain could be as follows:

1. Add stabilizing lingual arches and proceed with en masse space closure. The resulting increase in posterior anchorage, though modest, will change the ratio of anterior retraction to posterior protraction to approximately 2:1.

2. Reinforce maxillary posterior anchorage with extraoral force and (if needed) use Class III elastics from high-pull headgear to supplement retraction force in the lower arch, while continuing the basic en masse closure approach. Depending on how well the patient cooperates, additional improvement of retraction, perhaps to a 3:1 or 4:1 ratio, can be achieved.

3. Retract the canines independently, preferably using a segmental closing loop, and then retract the incisors with a second closing loop archwire. Used with stabilizing lingual arches (which are needed to control the posterior segments in most patients), this technique will produce a 3:1 retraction ratio. When this procedure is reinforced with headgear, even better ratios are possible.

A more detailed discussion of each of these approaches follows.

Reinforcement with Stabilizing Lingual Arches. Stabilizing lingual arches must be rigid and should be made from 36 mil or 32 × 32 steel wire. These can be soldered to the molar bands, but it is convenient to be able to remove them, and Burstone's designs (see Chapter 12) are preferred.

It is important for a lower stabilizing lingual arch to lie behind and below the lower incisors, so that it does not interfere with their retraction. If 36 mil round wire is used, the lower lingual arch is more conveniently inserted from the distal than from the mesial of the molar tube (see Figure 16-35). The maxillary stabilizing lingual arch is a straight transpalatal design. Because maximum rigidity is desired for anchorage reinforcement, an expansion loop in the palatal section of this wire is not recommended unless a specific indication exists for including it.

If lingual arches are needed for anchorage control, they should be present during the first and second stages of treatment but can and should be removed after space closure is complete. Their presence during the finishing stage of treatment, after extraction spaces have been closed, is not helpful and may interfere with final settling of the occlusion.

Reinforcement with Headgear and Interarch Elastics. Extraoral force against the maxillary posterior segments is an obvious and direct method for anchorage reinforcement. It is also possible to place extraoral force against the mandibular posterior segments, but is usually more practical to use Class III elastics to transfer the extraoral force from the upper to the lower arch.

Inter-arch elastics for anchorage reinforcement were a prominent part of the original Tweed method for maximum retraction of protruding anterior teeth. In the Tweed approach to bimaxillary protrusion, lower—but not upper—premolars are extracted initially, so that an intact upper arch is available to resist the pull of Class III elastics. This step is the first component of the anchorage

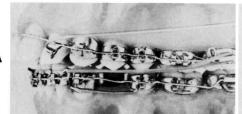 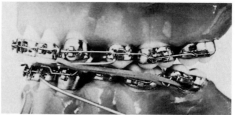

FIGURE 17-30 Anchorage preparation in Tweed technique. Class III elastics from a stabilized upper arch reinforced with headgear are being used to tip back the lower posterior teeth. Note the second order (tip-back) bends in the lower archwire. **A,** A sliding jig to the second premolar is being used to transfer the Class III elastic force to the posterior segment; **B,** anchorage preparation completed in the lingual arch. Note the distally tipped position of the lower posterior teeth and the use of Class II elastics to accomplish similar tipping of the upper posterior teeth. (From Tweed CH: *Clinical Orthodontics*, St. Louis, 1966, Mosby.)

reinforcement: pitting an intact upper arch against a segmented lower arch (and later, the reverse).

The second part of Tweed anchorage reinforcement is "anchorage preparation," achieved by tipping the molars and premolars distally (Figure 17-30). Class III elastics are used to maintain lower incisor position while this is done. The distally tipped molars then allow the incisors to be retracted further than otherwise would have occurred. Only after the lower incisors have been retracted, sliding the canine initially and then using a closing loop, are the upper premolars extracted. At that point, the lower arch is stabilized and Class II elastics are used to prepare anchorage by tipping back the upper molars, before the upper incisors are retracted (see Figure 17-30, *B*).

Although the original Tweed approach can be used with the contemporary 18-slot appliance, it is rarely indicated. Prolonged use of Class II and Class III elastics is extrusive and requires good vertical growth for acceptable results. Distally tipping the molars augments their anchorage value primarily by first moving these teeth distally, then mesially.

Segmented Retraction of the Canines. Segmented retraction of the canines with frictionless springs is an attractive method for reducing the strain on posterior anchorage and is a readily available approach with the modern 18-slot appliance. It is also possible to retract the canines by sliding them on the archwire, but the narrow brackets usually used with the 18-slot appliance and the tight clearance and relatively low strength of a 17 × 25 archwire produce less-than-optimum sliding.

For frictionless retraction of the canines, an auxiliary tube on the molar is needed. An auxiliary tube on the canine is unnecessary, because the retraction spring can fit directly into the canine bracket. The PG spring designed by Gjessing is the most efficient current design (Figure 17-31).[17] Closing loops, either in a continuous archwire or with a segmented arch approach, are then used for the second stage of retraction of the incisors (Figure 17-32).

Segmented canine retraction of this type presents two problems. The first is that it is difficult to control the posi-

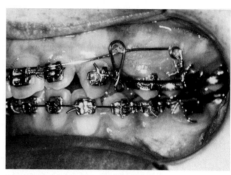

FIGURE 17-31 For canine retraction, the Gjessing retraction spring offers excellent control of forces and moments and probably is the most effective current design of a spring for this purpose.

tion of the canine in all three planes of space as it is retracted. If the canine is pulled distally from an attachment on its buccal surface, the point of attachment is not only some distance occlusal but is also buccal to the center of resistance. This means that without appropriate moments, the tooth will tip distally and rotate mesiobuccally. Both a root-paralleling moment and an antirotation moment must be obtained by placing gable bends in the spring. Control of the vertical position of the canine, particularly after the gable bends in two planes of space have been placed, can be a significant problem.

Second, much more than with en masse retraction using segmented mechanics, segmental retraction of canines does not fail safe. The canine is free to move in three-dimensional space, and there are no stops to prevent excessive movement in the wrong direction if a spring is improperly adjusted or becomes distorted. Loss of vertical control is particularly likely. A missed appointment and a distorted spring can lead to the development of a considerable problem (Figure 17-33), and patients must be monitored carefully.

Maximum Retraction with the 22-Slot Appliance.
The same basic approaches are available with the 22- as with the 18-slot appliance: to increase the amount of incisor retraction, a combination of increased reinforcement

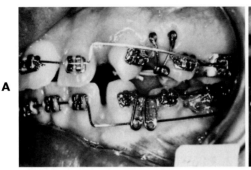
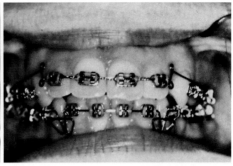

FIGURE 17-32 Canine retraction (**A**) and space closure (**B**) in Ricketts' bioprogressive technique. Instead of stabilizing lingual arches, a base or utility arch from the first molar to the incisors normally is used, with flexible springs that require a root-paralleling gable bend of approximately 60 degrees and an antirotation bend of approximately 20 degrees. After the canines are retracted with segmental closing loops, the four incisors are retracted with continuous arch closing loops, here a contraction utility arch in the upper and a double-delta design in the lower. Neither step in the space closure fails safe.

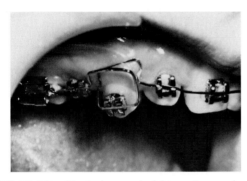

FIGURE 17-33 Vertical control of this canine was lost during retraction with a segmented retraction spring. A box-loop in 16 × 16 wire is being used to regain the correct vertical level (an auxiliary NiTi wire might be used instead in a more modern application). The greatest problem with segmented retraction springs is that they have no fail-safe component, allowing displacements of this type to occur if a spring is distorted and the patient misses scheduled appointments.

of posterior anchorage and decreased strain on that anchorage is needed. All the possible strategies for anchorage control can be used. With a 22-slot appliance in which sliding retraction of canines is the approach to moderate anchorage, the following sequence of steps to increase incisor retraction might be logical:

Reinforcement of Posterior Anchorage with Extraoral Force.
Stabilizing the posterior segments with extraoral force while sliding the canine along an archwire significantly increases posterior anchorage. This approach can be especially helpful in the upper arch, where headgear attached to the molars is easily placed, but the same approach can be used in the lower arch. Wearing two facebows to apply force to upper and lower molar teeth at the same time is difficult but not impossible. Reinforcing the upper arch with headgear, with Class III elastics off the headgear to reinforce anchorage for retraction of the lower canines, is a more typical arrangement.

Application of Extraoral Force Directly Against the Canines to Slide Them Posteriorly.
With this approach, a headgear using four hooks (Figure 17-34) normally is used.[7] The hooks fit over a base archwire, typically 19 × 25 steel, and approximately a 200 gm force is supplied at each point of attachment to slide the canines posteriorly. It is easier to attach extraoral force to the mandibular anterior than posterior region, and this arrangement is tolerated well by patients—much better than two facebows.

Retracting the canines in this way totally avoids strain on posterior anchorage during the first retraction step. The disadvantages are the same as when protruding maxillary incisors are retracted with headgear: this approach requires excellent cooperation by the patient, who should wear the headgear essentially full-time to achieve effective tooth movement. Moreover, friction may cause asymmetric space closure. For cooperative patients, however, this method is quite effective.

The second step, after retraction of the canines, is done with a closing loop as described previously.

Use of Segmented Arch Mechanics for Canine Retraction.
As discussed earlier, use of a segmented arch system to retract the canines independently, followed by retraction of the four incisors, is a practical method for conserving anchorage and equally adaptable to 22- and 18-slot appliances (Figure 17-35). It produces a result approximately equivalent to retracting the canines with headgear, provided that at least a stabilizing lingual arch is used to reinforce posterior anchorage. The problems are also the same as with the 18-slot appliance: the canine can become displaced during its retraction and may become spectacularly malpositioned if something goes wrong, because no fail-safe mechanism is in place.

Segmented Arch Mechanics for Tipping/Uprighting.
Rather than independent retraction of the canines, the recommended procedure in two-step space closure in maximum anchorage cases now is en masse distal tipping

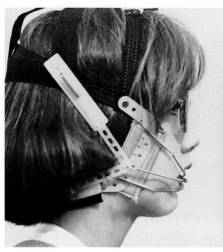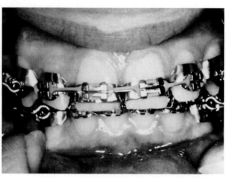

FIGURE 17-34 Four-hook headgear being used for retraction of the canines (in a patient who is also wearing a facebow to the molars). **A,** The hooks extend forward from the headcap and, **B,** attach over the upper and lower archwires mesial to the canines. Bands rather than bonded brackets on anterior teeth, particularly the canines, may be needed if headgear is applied directly to the anterior part of the dental arch.

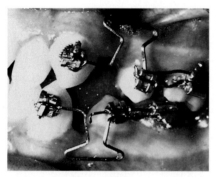

FIGURE 17-35 Retraction of upper and lower canines with T-loops in beta-Ti wire in the segmented arch technique with the 22-slot edgewise appliance. (Courtesy Dr. C.J. Burstone.)

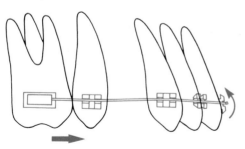

FIGURE 17-36 Torque forces against the incisors create a crown-forward, as well as a root-backward tendency. Preventing the incisor crowns from tipping forward tends to pull the posterior teeth forward, which can be advantageous if it is desired to close space in this way.

of the anterior teeth, followed by uprighting.[18] The segmented arch technique is used but the spring assembly is activated differently from the one needed for space closure in moderate retraction cases. Compared with independent retraction of the canines with loops, the fail-safe characteristics of this approach are much improved (though still not as good as with continuous archwires). Excellent control of anchorage for maximum retraction, without the use of headgear, can be obtained. The segmented arch approach is particularly valuable in treatment of adults (see Chapter 20) but can be used very effectively in adolescents.

Minimum Incisor Retraction

As with any problem requiring anchorage control, the approaches to reducing the amount of incisor retraction involve reinforcement of anchorage (the anterior teeth in this situation) and reduction of strain on that anchorage. An obvious strategy, implemented at the treatment planning stage, is to incorporate as many teeth in the anterior anchor unit as possible. Therefore if extraction of teeth is necessary at all, extracting a second premolar or molar—not a first premolar—is desirable. All other factors being equal, the amount of incisor retraction will be less the further posteriorly in the arch an extraction space is located (see Chapter 8).

A second possibility for reinforcing incisor anchorage is to place active lingual root torque in the incisor section of the archwires, maintaining a more mesial position of the incisor crowns at the expense of somewhat greater retraction of the root apices (Figure 17-36). When the incisors protrude, some degree of forward tipping of these teeth is usually present, so that when the incisors are retracted, they can be allowed to tip lingually at least slightly. Advantage can be taken of this when incisor retraction is desired. Conversely, in patients in whom it is desired to close extraction sites by moving the posterior teeth forward, the incisors are often already upright, and lingual root torque is likely to be desired for both esthetic reasons and control of anchorage. Burstone's segmented arch technique can be used to particular advantage when this strategy for producing differential forward movement of posterior teeth is used.[16]

A third possibility for maximizing forward movement of posterior teeth is to break down the posterior anchorage, moving the posterior teeth forward one tooth at a time. After extraction of a second premolar, for example, it may be desired to stabilize the eight anterior teeth and to bring the first molars forward independently, creating a space between them and the second molars before bringing the second molars anteriorly. This strategy can readily be combined with increased torque of the anterior teeth to minimize retraction.

A final possibility for maximizing protraction of posterior teeth is the use of extraoral force, pulling the teeth forward from a facemask or equivalent device (see Chapter 15). This provides the same opportunities and limitations as any other use of extraoral force for tooth movement. If the patient can be persuaded to wear reverse headgear essentially full-time, excellent tooth movement can be obtained. With less than 12 hours of wear per day, however, the results often are disappointing. Since a reverse headgear inevitably crosses the face, it is difficult to obtain the same level of cooperation as with a conventional posteriorly placed headgear, particularly in adolescents who are the candidates for comprehensive treatment.

As implant/onplant methods to create anchorage are developed, these almost surely will replace extraoral force for tooth movement, and space closure by bringing posterior teeth forward is likely to be one of the first major uses of the new approach. It rarely should be necessary to use involved mechanotherapy to protract posterior teeth. The need for this approach usually arises from an effort to close spaces from congenitally missing teeth, teeth that were lost to decay, or perhaps teeth that should not have been extracted for orthodontic purposes. If the temptation to use first premolars as a routine extraction is avoided, most of the need for minimum retraction mechanotherapy is also avoided.

REFERENCES

1. Stucki N, Ingervall B: The use of the Jasper Jumper for correction of Class II malocclusion in the young permanent dentition, Eur J. Orthod 20:271-281, 1998.
2. Gianelly AA: Japanese Ni-Ti coils used to move molars distally, Am J Orthod Dentofac Orthop 99:564-591, 1991.
3. Hilgers JJ: The pendulum appliance for Class II non-compliance therapy, J Clin Orthod 16:706-714, 1992.
4. Byloff FK, Darendeliler MA: Distal molar movement using the pendulum appliance. Part I, clinical and radiological evaluation, Angle Orthod 67:249-260, 1997.
5. Byloff FK, Darendeliler MA, Clar E, Darendeliler A: Distal molar movement using the pendulum appliance. Part 2, the effects of maxillary molar root uprighting bends, Angle Orthod 64:261-270, 1997.
6. Moffitt AH: Eruption and function of maxillary third molars after extraction of second molars, Angle Orthod 68:147-152, 1998.
7. Hickham JH: Direct edgewise orthodontic approach, J Clin Orthod 8:617, 1974.
8. Kremenak CR, Kinser DD, Harman HA et al: Orthodontic risk factors for temporomandibular disorders (TMD), Am J Orthod Dentofac Orthop 101:13-20, 21-27, 1992.
9. McLaughlin RP, Bennett JC: The extraction-nonextraction dilemma as it relates to TMD, Angle Orthod 65:175-186, 1995.
10. Booth FA: MS Thesis: Optimum forces with orthodontic loops, Houston, 1971, University of Texas Dental Branch.
11. Braun S, Sjursen RC, Legan HL: On the management of extraction sites, Am J Orthod Dentofac Orthop 112:645-655, 1997.
12. Siatkowski RE: Continuous archwire closing loop design, optimization and verification, Parts I and II, Am J Orthod Dentofac Orthop, 112:393-402, 112:484-495, 1997.
13. Burstone CJ, Koenig HA: Creative wire bending—the force system from step and V bends, Am J Orthod Dentofac Orthop 93:59-67, 1988.
14. Ronay F, Kleinert W, Melsen B, Burstone CJ: Force system developed by V bends in an elastic orthodontic wire, Am J Orthod Dentofac Orthop 96:295-301, 1989.
15. Samuels RHA, Rudge SJ, Mair LH: A comparison of the rate of space closure using a nickel-titanium spring and an elastic module, Am J Orthod Dentofac Orthop 103:464-467, 1993.
16. Burstone CJ: The segmented arch approach to space closure, Am J Orthod 82:361, 1982.
17. Eden JD, Waters N: An investigation into the characteristics of the PG canine retraction spring, Am J Orthod Dentofac Orthop 105:49-60, 1994.
18. Burstone C: The segmented arch approach to space closure, Am J Orthod 82:361-378, 1982.

CHAPTER

18

The Third Stage of Comprehensive Treatment: Finishing

Root paralleling at extraction sites

Adjustment of individual tooth positions

Torque of incisors

Correction of vertical incisor relationships

  Excessive overbite

  Anterior open bite

Midline discrepancies

Tooth size discrepancies

Final "settling" of teeth

Removal of bands and bonded attachments

Positioners for finishing

Special finishing procedures to avoid relapse

  Control of unfavorable growth

  Control of soft tissue rebound

By the end of the second stage of treatment, the teeth should be well aligned, extraction spaces should be closed, and the teeth in the buccal segments should be in a normal Class I relationship. In the Begg technique, major root movements of both anterior and posterior teeth still remain to obtain root paralleling at extraction sites and proper axial inclination of tipped incisors. With contemporary edgewise techniques, much less treatment remains to be accomplished at the finishing stage, but minor versions of these same root movements are likely to be required. In addition, most cases require some adjustment of individual tooth positions to get marginal ridges level, obtain precise in-out positions of teeth within the arches, and generally overcome any discrepancies produced by errors in either bracket placement or appliance prescription. In some cases it is necessary to alter the vertical relationship of incisors as a finishing procedure, either correcting moderately excessive overbite or closing a mild anterior open bite.

Although many variations are inevitable to meet the demands of specific cases, it is possible to outline a logical sequence of archwires for continuous arch edgewise technique, and this has been attempted in Box 18-1. The box is based on two concepts: (1) that the most efficient archwires should be used, so as to minimize clinical adjustments and chair time; and (2) that it is necessary to fill the bracket slot in the finishing stage with appropriately flexible wires to take full advantage of the modern appliance. Appropriate use of the recommended finishing archwires and variations to deal with specific situations in finishing are reviewed in some detail later. Similar recommendations and variations in the first two stages of treatment have been provided in the two previous chapters.

ROOT PARALLELING AT EXTRACTION SITES

In the Begg technique, extraction spaces are closed by initially tipping the teeth together, and then uprighting them (Figure 18-1). In the finishing stage, the moments necessary for root uprighting are generated by adding auxiliary springs that fit into the vertical slot of the Begg (ribbon arch) bracket. In most instances, a heavier (20 mil) archwire replaces the 16 mil archwire used as a base arch up to that point, to provide greater stability. Root paralleling is accomplished by placing an uprighting spring in the vertical slot and hooking it beneath the archwire. Since the root-uprighting forces are also crown-separating forces, the crowns must be tied together across the extraction site. The Begg uprighting springs extend only a short distance from the point of insertion into the bracket to the point where they are hooked to the archwire. Therefore it is necessary both to make the uprighting springs from small-diameter wire (usually 14 mil steel) and to increase their length by bending a double helix at the base of the spring.

BOX 18-1

SEQUENCE OF ARCHWIRES, CONTINUOUS ARCH EDGEWISE TECHNIQUE*

18 Slot

Non-extraction
14 or 16 superelastic NiTi (A-NiTi)
16 steel (accentuated/reverse curve)
17 × 25 M-NiTi (if roots displaced)
17 × 25 beta-Ti
17 × 25 steel

Extraction
14 or 16 superelastic NiTi
16 steel (accentuated/reverse curve)
16 × 22 closing loops
17 × 25 beta-Ti (if roots displaced)
17 × 25 steel

22 Slot

Nonextraction
16 A-NiTi or 17.5 twist steel
16 steel (accentuated/reverse curve)
18 steel (accentuated/reverse curve)
21 × 25 M-NiTi
21 × 25 beta-Ti

Extraction
16 A-NiTi or 17.5 twist steel
16 steel (accentuated/reverse curve)
18 steel (accentuated/reverse curve)
19 × 25 steel, A-NiTi coil springs
18 × 22 steel T-loop or 19 × 25 beta-Ti delta-loop
21 × 25 M-NiTi (if roots displaced)
21 × 25 beta-Ti

*For a typical adolescent patient with malocclusion of moderate severity. (Wire sizes in mils.)

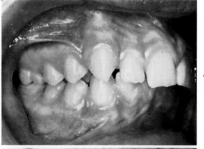
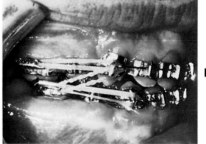
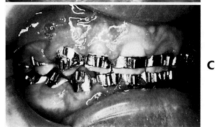
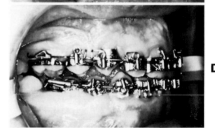
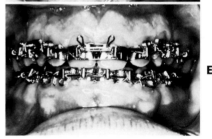

FIGURE 18-1   Stages in Begg technique. **A,** The original Class II, division 1 malocclusion; **B,** space closure during stage 2, using intra-arch elastics plus Class II elastics; **C,** tooth positions at the end of state 2 (note the lingual tipping of incisors and mesiodistal tipping of canines and premolars); **D,** lateral view of the Begg appliance, during stage 3, showing auxiliary root-uprighting springs on second premolars, canines and lateral incisors. These springs extend into the vertical slot of the Begg bracket and hook beneath the archwire adjacent to the tooth. **E,** Anterior view showing a torquing auxiliary to the maxillary central incisors. This auxiliary archwire is "piggy-backed" over the base arch and hooks beneath the base arch posteriorly.

To a considerable extent the original Begg bracket has been replaced by some type of combination bracket (see below) that allows the use of rectangular wire in finishing. With these brackets, however, root paralleling is accomplished with uprighting springs, very much as it was with traditional Begg treatment. The rectangular wire is used primarily for torque (facio-lingual root movement), not the mesio-distal root movement needed for root paralleling at extraction sites.

During space closure with the edgewise appliance, it is almost always a goal of treatment to produce bodily tooth movement during space closure, preventing the crowns from tipping together. If proper moment-to-force ratios have been used, little if any root paralleling will be necessary as a finishing procedure. On the other hand, it is likely that at least a small amount of tipping will occur in some patients and therefore some degree of root paralleling often will be necessary.

Exactly the same approach used in Begg technique can be employed with the edgewise appliance if it includes a

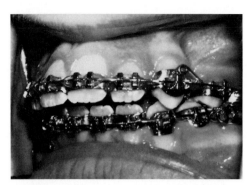

FIGURE 18-2 An auxiliary uprighting spring placed in a vertical slot behind an otherwise standard edgewise bracket, for distal root positioning of the canine tooth. With the introduction of contemporary straight-wire appliances, this use of auxiliary uprighting springs in edgewise technique was almost completely abandoned in favor of preangulated brackets and resilient NiTi or beta-Ti archwires.

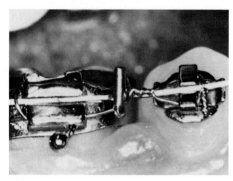

FIGURE 18-3 A rectangular archwire that incorporates active root paralleling moments or torque must be tied back against the molar teeth to prevent space from opening within the arch. If the ligature used to tie back the archwire is cabled forward and also used to tie the second premolar, the tieback is less likely to come loose.

vertical slot behind the edgewise bracket (Figure 18-2). This allows an uprighting spring to be inserted and hooked beneath a base archwire in the same way as in Begg technique. This approach is reasonably effective with narrow edgewise brackets and an undersized round wire (typically 18 mil) in the 22-slot edgewise appliance, but in contemporary edgewise practice, this method has been almost totally abandoned in favor of angulated bracket slots that produce proper root paralleling when a full-dimension edgewise arch is placed as a finishing archwire.

With the 18-slot appliance, the typical finishing archwire is either 17 × 22 or 17 × 25 steel. These wires are flexible enough to engage narrow brackets even if mild tipping has occurred, and the archwire will generate the necessary root paralleling moments. If a greater degree of tipping has occurred, a more flexible full-dimension rectangular archwire is needed. To correct more severe tipping, a beta-titanium (beta-Ti) or even a nickel-titanium (M-NiTi) 17 × 25 wire might be needed initially, with a steel archwire used to obtain final positioning.

With wider 22-slot brackets on the canines and premolars and with the use of sliding rather than loop mechanics, there is usually even less need for root paralleling as a finishing procedure than with narrow brackets and closing loop archwires. If teeth do tip even slightly into the extraction space, however, a full-dimension steel archwire in a 22-slot bracket is much too stiff to produce the needed root-uprighting moment. Even a 19 × 25 steel wire is undesirably stiff. A 21 × 25 beta-Ti wire is the best choice for a finishing archwire under most circumstances, and if significant root paralleling is needed, 21 × 25 NiTi should be used first.

Although superelastic NiTi (A-NiTi) wires perform much better than elastic NiTi (M-NiTi) wires in alignment, this is not true of their performance as rectangular finishing wires. The great advantage of A-NiTi is its very flat load-deflection curve, which gives it a large range. In the finishing stage, however, appropriate stiffness at relatively small deflections, rather than range, is the primary consideration. A-NiTi wires may deliver less force than their M-NiTi counterparts (this will depend on how the manufacturer manipulated the wire—see Chapter 10), and if rectangular A-NiTi is used in the finishing stage, torsional stiffness must be considered in the choice of the wire. M-NiTi usually is the better choice for rectangular nickel-titanium wires.

A root-paralleling moment is a crown-separating moment in edgewise technique just as it is in Begg technique, and this effect is important to remember. Either the teeth must be tied together at the extraction site or the entire archwire must be tied back against the molars (Figure 18-3) to prevent the extraction site from reopening during finishing.

Occasionally, a severely tipped canine tooth will be encountered, and a longer range of action is needed than can be delivered by even the most flexible continuous archwire. In this situation, there are two options: (1) bending a loop into a rectangular archwire to provide the desired flexibility (see Figure 17-33), or (2) using an auxiliary root-uprighting spring (Figure 18-4).

With the 18-slot appliance, the best choice is usually a box loop in 16 × 22 steel wire. The loop is preferred over a very flexible archwire because the malalignment is concentrated at one spot in the arch, and arch form can be distorted by the flexible wire (the same reason that loops are still occasionally indicated for initial alignment). At the same time that the root of the canine tooth is being positioned distally, this loop also can be used to obtain a last bit of space closure.

A similar box loop archwire can be used with the 22-slot appliance, made from 18 × 25 wire (the smallest size that will not twist in a 22-slot bracket), but in this size wire the loop is too stiff for maximum effectiveness. The preferred alternative in 22-slot edgewise is to bypass the tipped canine with a rectangular base arch and use an auxiliary root-uprighting spring tied into the canine bracket (see Figure 18-4).

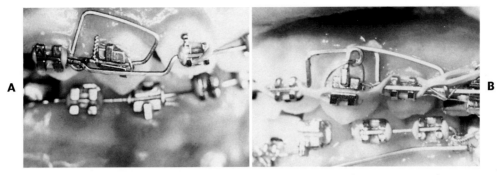

FIGURE 18-4 Auxiliary root springs used with the 22-slot appliance. **A,** An auxiliary root spring in TMA wire, welded to a base arch that bypasses the canine, is tied into the edgewise bracket slot on the canine. **B,** An auxiliary root spring in steel wire, placed in the vertical tube on a Burstone canine bracket and activated by hooking beneath the base arch posteriorly. Note that the base archwire bypasses the tooth being uprighted. (Courtesy Dr. D.J. Burstone.)

ADJUSTMENT OF INDIVIDUAL TOOTH POSITIONS

Root paralleling at extraction sites obviously is not a consideration in non-extraction cases, but the root position of some teeth may require adjustment at the finishing stage, and it is likely that up-down and in-out relationships of some teeth also will need minor change. If the appliance prescription and bracket positioning were perfect, such adjustments would be unnecessary. Given both the variations in individual tooth anatomy and the modest precision of bracket placement, many cases need some adjustment of tooth positions at this stage.

When it becomes apparent that a bracket is poorly positioned, usually it is time-efficient to rebond the bracket rather than place compensating bends in archwires. This is particularly true when the inclination of the tooth is incorrect, so that angulated step bends in wires would be required. After the bracket is rebonded, however, a flexible wire must be placed to bring the tooth to the correct position. Steel finishing wires are too stiff in both the 18 and 22 slot appliances. In the 18 slot appliance, 17×25 beta-Ti usually is satisfactory; in the 22 slot appliance, 21×25 M-NiTi often is the best choice.

Minor in-out and up-down adjustments, typically to obtain perfect canine interdigitation and level out marginal ridge heights, can be obtained simply and easily by placing mild step bends in the finishing archwires. The principle is the same as when brackets are rebonded: these bends should be placed in a flexible full-dimension wire, the next-to-last wire in the typical sequence shown in Box 18-1. Obviously, any step bends placed in the next-to-last wire (17×25 beta-Ti or 21×25 M-NiTi) must be repeated in the final wire that is used for torque adjustments (17×25 steel or 21×25 beta-Ti).

Although the position of a V-bend relative to the adjacent brackets is critical in determining its effect, the position of a step bend is not a critical variable. It makes no

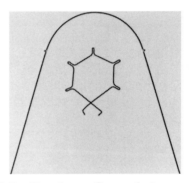

FIGURE 18-5 Torquing auxiliary archwires exert their effect when the auxiliary, originally bent into a tight circle as shown, is forced to assume the form of the base archwire over which it will be placed. This tends to distort the base archwire, which therefore should be relatively heavy—at least 18 mil steel.

difference whether a step bend is in the center of the interbracket span or offset to either side.[1]

TORQUE OF INCISORS

If protruding incisors tipped lingually while they were being retracted, lingual root torque as a finishing procedure may be required. In the Begg technique, the incisors are deliberately tipped back during the second stage of treatment, and lingual root torque is a routine part of the third stage of treatment. Like root paralleling, this is accomplished with an auxiliary appliance that fits over the main or base archwire. The torquing auxiliary is a "piggyback arch" that contacts the labial surface of the incisors near the gingival margin, creating the necessary couple with a moment arm of 4 to 5 mm (see Figure 18-1). Although these piggyback torquing arches come in a number of designs, the basic principle is the same: the auxiliary arch, bent into a tight circle initially, exerts a force against the roots of the teeth as it is partially straightened out to normal arch form (Figure 18-5).

A torquing force to move the roots lingually is also, of course, a force to move the crowns labially (see Figure 17-36). In a typical patient with a Class II malocclusion, anchorage is required to maintain overjet correction while upper incisor roots are torqued lingually. Class II elastics are normally worn during the third stage of Begg treatment to ensure that the maxillary incisor crowns do not become repositioned labially. In addition, the incisors are usually taken to an edge-to-edge relationship during the second stage of Begg treatment, allowing some possibility for the maxillary crowns to move forward during the third stage (see Figure 18-1). The Class II elastics that reinforce the upper arch, however, further add to the tendency to displace the lower arch mesially, and the inclination of the lower incisors will be improved as much by labial tipping as by lingual root torque.

The torquing auxiliaries normally used in Begg technique not only place lingual force against the incisor roots, they tend to alter the form of the arch itself, because the torquing auxiliary wire tends to constrict the base arch posteriorly. A major reason for using a heavier base archwire in the third stage of treatment is to resist this potential distortion of arch form. Better results are achieved with a 20 mil steel base arch during the third stage than with a 16 mil wire, as originally used by Begg.

Precise positioning of individual teeth is difficult to obtain with the Begg appliance. The minimal area of con-

tact between the base archwire and the bracket, though helpful in providing for relatively free tipping and sliding movements, makes it impossible to use the base arch to obtain detailed tooth positioning, and the auxiliaries used for root positioning have no fail-safe component at all. They continue to work until disconnected. Tooth positioners (see following) usually are used with the Begg appliance to detail the occlusal relationships, but a positioner is unable to materially affect root position.

For this reason, modifications of the Begg appliance, so that a rectangular archwire in a rectangular slot can be used for finishing purposes, have been proposed repeatedly. This method requires a combination bracket, incorporating an edgewise bracket slot along with the vertically oriented Begg slot, or a modified edgewise bracket that allows tipping in one direction and that incorporates a vertical slot for uprighting springs. Recent versions of combination brackets are shown in Figures 18-6 and 18-7. With these variations, the first two stages of treatment are carried out largely as in traditional Begg technique. At the finishing stage, root paralleling and torquing are done with Begg-style auxiliary wires, up to a stage of completion approximately equivalent to that at which patients treated with the current edgewise appliances usually enter the finishing stage. Then a rectangular archwire is used in much the same way that it would be in edgewise treatment. With the Tip-Edge combination bracket, however, the rectangular wire fits progressively

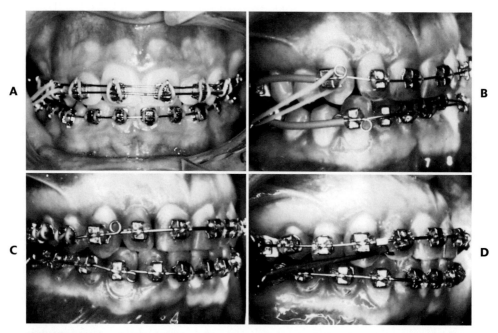

FIGURE 18-6   **A,** The CAT (combination anchorage technique) appliance (also shown in Figure 18-7) uses a combination bracket with both Begg and edgewise slots. A rectangular archwire in the edgewise slot can be used in finishing, either alone as in the lower arch or in conjunction with a wire in the Begg slot, as in the upper arch; **B** to **D,** the Tip-Edge appliance uses a modified edgewise bracket to allow the tipping needed in the initial stages of Begg technique, then employs a rectangular archwire during finishing. (**A,** Courtesy Dr. W.J. Thompson; **B** to **D,** courtesy Dr. P.C. Kesling.)

more tightly as auxiliary springs correct the mesio-distal inclination of tipped teeth, so the action of auxiliary springs is important for torque as well as root paralleling.[2]

In edgewise technique, only moderate additional torque should be necessary during the finishing stage, except in the relatively few maximum anchorage patients in 22-slot edgewise for whom tipping/uprighting was chosen as an anchorage conservation technique (see below). With the 18-slot appliance, a 17 × 25 steel archwire has excellent torsion properties, and active torque with the archwire is entirely feasible. Building torque into the bracket slot initially means that it is unnecessary to place torquing bends in the archwire, making the accomplishment of torque as a finishing procedure relatively straightforward.

With the 22-slot appliance, steel full-dimension rectangular wires are far too stiff for effective torquing, and if incisors have been allowed to tip lingually too much, as can happen in the correction of maxillary incisor protrusion, correcting this merely by placing a rectangular steel archwire is not feasible. Torquing auxiliaries similar to those in the Begg appliance once were commonly used with 22-slot standard edgewise technique, and a number of designs have been offered commercially. These piggyback arches are usually used with round rather than rectangular base archwires.

One of the great virtues of pretorqued brackets is that, even in the 22-slot appliance, tipping of incisors can be largely prevented during retraction and space closure. In addition, full-dimension NiTi or beta-Ti archwires can be

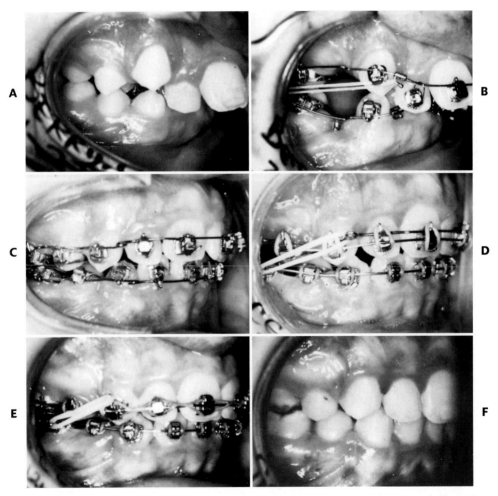

FIGURE 18-7 Stages in treatment with the CAT appliance. **A,** The original Class II crowded malocclusion; **B,** stage 1, using dual-flex archwires. The anterior section is 16 mil NiTi, the posterior section 16 steel. In the initial stage of Begg treatment, the rigidity of steel wire is needed for the anchor bends that control molar position. The dual-flex wires allow the normal posterior anchor bends, without the necessity for loops for alignment anteriorly; **C,** completion of stage 2, with 18 mil steel wires in place (compare with Figure 18-1); **D,** early in stage 3 (finishing), with rectangular NiTi wires in the edgewise slot of both the upper and lower brackets, and an 18 mil steel wire pinned in the Begg slots of the upper brackets for vertical stabilization; **E,** later in finishing, with rectangular NiTi wires alone; **F,** posttreatment occlusion. (Courtesy Dr. W.J. Thompson.)

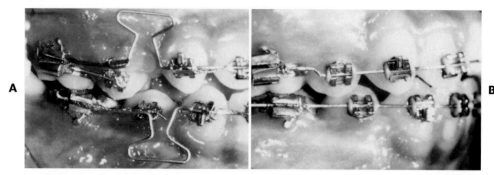

FIGURE 18-8   **A,** Space closure in the segmented arch technique with anterior retraction springs. Note that the posterior segments are stabilized. The retraction springs fit into the auxiliary tubes on the first molars and vertically-oriented auxiliary tubes on the canine brackets. **B,** Rectangular archwires for finishing, later in the same case. (Courtesy Dr. C.J. Burstone.)

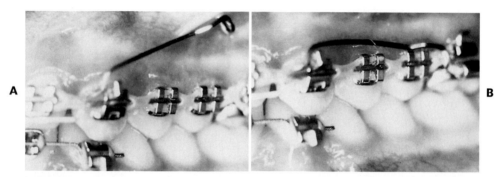

FIGURE 18-9   The Burstone torquing auxiliary (also see Figure 10-41) is particularly useful in Class II, division 2 cases where maxillary central incisors need a large amount of torque. The torquing auxiliary is full-dimension steel wire (21 × 25 or 17 × 25, in 22- or 18-slot brackets respectively) that fits in the brackets only on the central incisors. The base arch (preferably also full-dimension rectangular wire) extends forward from the molars through the lateral incisor brackets, then steps down and rests against the labial surface of the central incisors. When the torquing auxiliary is passive **(A),** its long posterior arms are up in the buccal vestibule. It is activated **(B)** by pulling the arms down and hooking them beneath the base archwire mesial to the first molar. The segment of the base arch that rests against the labial surface of the central incisors prevents the crowns from going forward, and the result is efficient torque of the central incisor roots.

used to torque incisors with 22-slot brackets (provided the brackets have torque built in), further reducing any need for auxiliary arches. For these reasons, torquing auxiliaries for 22-slot edgewise have almost disappeared from contemporary use.

When tipping/uprighting is used with edgewise technique, the segmented arch approach is required, and springs connecting the segments are maintained until the stage of uprighting approaches what would usually be observed at the completion of continuous-arch edgewise space closure (Figure 18-8). At that point, continuous rectangular arches are employed in finishing, as in other edgewise cases discussed in this chapter.

One torquing auxiliary deserves special mention: the Burstone torquing arch (Figure 18-9). It can be particularly helpful in patients with Class II, division 2 malocclusion whose maxillary central incisors are severely tipped lingually and require a long distance of torquing movement,

while the lateral incisors need little if any torque. Because of the long lever arm, this is the most effective torquing auxiliary for use with the edgewise appliance. It is equally effective with the 18- or 22-slot appliance. If all four incisors need considerable torque, a wire spanning from the molar auxiliary tube to the incisors, with a V-bend so that the incisor segment receives the greater moment, is a highly efficient approach.[3]

Two factors determine the amount of torque that will be expressed by any rectangular archwire in a rectangular slot: the inclination of the bracket slot relative to the archwire, and the tightness of the fit between the archwire and the bracket. The variation in torque prescriptions in contemporary edgewise appliances is shown in Table 12-4. These variations largely reflect different determinations of the average contour of the labial and buccal surfaces of the teeth, some differences are also related to the expected fit of archwires. With the 18-slot appliance, it is assumed

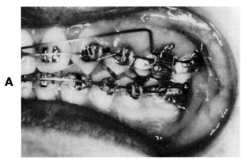
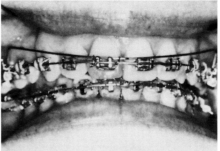

FIGURE 18-10 Use of an auxiliary depressing arch at the finishing stage to correct a mildly excessive overbite. **A,** Lateral view; **B,** anterior view. The auxiliary depressing wire is 17 × 25 beta-Ti. Note that the maxillary base arch (17 × 25 steel) is segmented between the canine and second premolar. If intrusion is desired, the base arch must be segmented.

that the rectangular archwires used for finishing will fit tightly in the bracket slot (i.e., that the finishing archwires will have a minimum dimension of 17 or 18 mil). With the 22-slot appliance, on the other hand, some prescriptions have extra built-in torque to compensate for rectangular finishing archwires that will have more clearance. Torque will not be expressed to the same extent with a 19 × 25 wire in a 22-slot bracket as with a 17 × 25 wire in an 18-slot bracket. The difference amounts to several degrees of difference in incisor inclination. (See Table 12-5 for the "effective torque" of various wire-bracket combinations.) Obviously, when the torque prescription is established, it is important to know what finishing wires are intended.

For full expression of the torque built into brackets in the 22-slot appliance, the best finishing wire usually is 21 × 25 beta-Ti. This wire's torsional stiffness is less than that of 17 × 25 steel (see Figure 10-11 for a comparison of torsional stiffnesses of different types and sizes of wire), but the shorter interbracket distances with 22-slot brackets bring its performance in torsion close to that of the smaller steel wire. Braided rectangular steel wires are available in a variety of stiffnesses, and the stiffest of these in 21 × 25 dimension also can be useful in 22-slot finishing. A solid 21 × 25 steel wire cannot be recommended because of its stiffness and the resulting extremely high forces and short range of action. If a solid steel wire of this size is used (the major reason would be surgical stabilization), it should be preceded by 21 × 25 beta-Ti.

CORRECTION OF VERTICAL INCISOR RELATIONSHIPS

If the first two stages of treatment have been accomplished perfectly, no change in the vertical relationship of incisors will be needed during the finishing stage of treatment. Minor adjustments often are needed, however, and major ones occasionally are required. At this stage, anterior open bite is more likely to be a problem than residual excessive overbite, but either may be encountered.

Excessive Overbite

Before attempting to correct excess overbite at the finishing stage of treatment, it is important to carefully assess why the problem exists, and particularly to observe the vertical relationship between the maxillary lip and maxillary incisor. An excessive curve of Spee in the lower arch still may be the cause of overbite, but by this stage of treatment, the problem is often slight elongation of the maxillary incisors. If so, an auxiliary intrusion arch is the preferred solution.

If a rectangular finishing archwire is already in place, the simplest approach may be to cut this archwire distal to the lateral incisors and install an auxiliary intrusion arch (Figure 18-10). Alternatively, if the patient is still growing and relative rather than absolute intrusion would be satisfactory (see Chapter 17), a light round continuous archwire (16 or 18 mil steel) with an accentuated curve of Spee can be placed and an auxiliary arch added to it. As a general rule, if an auxiliary depressing arch is added to a continuous base archwire, the base archwire should be a relatively small round wire, whereas if the base arch is segmented, the segments should be rectangular wire.

Remember that when an auxiliary intrusion arch is used, a stabilizing transpalatal lingual arch may be needed to maintain control of transverse relationships and prevent excessive distal tipping of the maxillary molars. The greater the desired vertical change in incisor position, the more important it will be to have a stabilizing lingual arch in place, and vice versa. Small corrections during finishing usually do not require placing a lingual arch.

Anterior Open Bite

As with deep bite, it is important to analyze the source of the difficulty if an anterior open bite persists at the finishing stage of treatment. Only rarely is a persistent open bite caused by lack of eruption of the upper incisors, so elongating these teeth usually is undesirable. If the open bite results from excessive eruption of posterior teeth, whether from a poor growth pattern or improper use of interarch elastics, correcting it at the finishing stage can be extremely

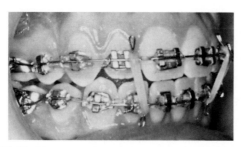

FIGURE 18-11   Anterior vertical elastics used with light archwires to close a mild anterior open bite at the end of the treatment. A 16 mil round wire with a curve of Spee is used in the lower arch, where most of the tooth movement should occur. A full dimension rectangular wire often is preferred in the upper arch. For this patient, two small elastics are being used on the right and left sides. An alternative is to use a single larger elastic in an anterior box configuration.

difficult. High-pull headgear to the upper molars is the best approach if excessive vertical development of the posterior maxilla is the basic problem, and this treatment will have to be continued until growth is nearly complete, usually well into the retention period.

If no severe problems with the pattern of facial growth exist, however, a mild open bite at the finishing stage of treatment usually is due to an excessively level lower arch. This condition is managed best by elongating the lower but not the upper incisors, thereby creating a slight curve of Spee in the lower arch. Because of the stiffness of the rectangular archwires used for finishing, even with 18-slot edgewise, it is futile to use vertical elastics without altering the form of the archwires to provide a curve of Spee in the lower arch. Moreover, it is preferable to replace a heavy rectangular lower archwire with a lighter round wire before using anterior vertical elastics.

The preferred approach is to place a light round wire (16 or 18 mil steel) in the lower arch, with a slight curve of Spee and any vertical steps necessary to correct marginal ridge discrepancies, while retaining a full-dimension rectangular archwire in the upper arch. Posterior marginal ridge discrepancies may also contribute to the open bite and should be eliminated with small vertical steps in the archwires. Light elastic force is then used to augment the action of the archwires, elongating the lower incisors to close the open bite (Figure 18-11). Elongating lower anterior teeth in this way, of course, is no substitute for controlling posterior vertical development. If carried to an extreme, this will produce an esthetically unacceptable relationship even if proper occlusion is achieved.

To summarize: as a general guideline, mildly excessive overbite at the finishing stage usually is treated best by slightly intruding the maxillary incisors, using an auxiliary depressing arch and segmenting the main archwire; but mild open bite at the end of treatment usually is treated best by elongating the lower but not the upper incisors. This is both more esthetic and more stable than elongating the upper incisors.

MIDLINE DISCREPANCIES

A relatively common problem at the finishing stage of treatment is a discrepancy in the midlines of the dental arches. This condition can result either from a preexisting midline discrepancy that was not completely resolved at an earlier stage of treatment or an asymmetric closure of spaces within the arch. Minor midline discrepancies at the finishing stage are no great problem, but it is quite difficult to correct large discrepancies after extraction spaces have been closed and occlusal relationships have been nearly established.

As with any discrepancy at the finishing stage, it is important to establish as clearly as possible exactly where the discrepancy arises. Although coincident dental midlines are an important component of functional occlusion—all other things being equal, a midline discrepancy will be reflected in how the posterior teeth fit together—it is undesirable esthetically to displace the maxillary midline, bringing it around to meet a displaced mandibular midline. A correct maxillary midline is important for good facial esthetics, while a small displacement of the mandibular midline creates no esthetic difficulty.

If a midline discrepancy results from a skeletal asymmetry, it may be impossible to correct it orthodontically, and treatment decisions will have to be made in the light of camouflage vs. surgical correction (see discussion in Chapter 8). Fortunately, midline discrepancies in the finishing stage usually are not this severe and are caused only by lateral displacements of maxillary or mandibular teeth accompanied by a mild Class II or Class III relationship on one side.

In this circumstance, the midline often can be corrected by using asymmetric Class II (or Class III) elastic force. As a general rule, it is more effective to use Class II or Class III elastics bilaterally with heavier force on one side than to place a unilateral elastic. However, if one side is totally corrected while the other is not, the patient usually tolerates a unilateral elastic reasonably well. It is also possible to combine a Class II or Class III elastic on one side with a diagonal elastic anteriorly, to bring the midlines together (Figure 18-12). Coordinated steps in the archwires also can be used to shift the teeth of one arch more than the other.[4]

An important consideration in dealing with midline discrepancies is the possibility of a mandibular shift contributing to the discrepancy. This can arise easily if a slight discrepancy in the transverse position of posterior teeth is present. For instance, a slightly narrow maxillary right posterior segment can lead to a shift of the mandible to the left on final closure, creating the midline discrepancy. The correction in this instance, obviously, must include some force system (usually careful coordination of the maxillary and mandibular archwires, perhaps reinforced by a posterior cross-elastic) to alter the transverse arch relationships. Occasionally, the entire maxillary arch

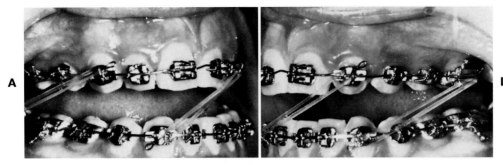

FIGURE 18-12   Midline correction can be approached with any combination of asymmetric posterior and anterior diagonal elastics. **A** and **B**, In this patient, a combination of Class II, Class III, and anterior diagonal elastics are being used, with a rectangular archwire in the lower arch and a round wire in the upper arch, attempting to shift the maxillary arch to the right.

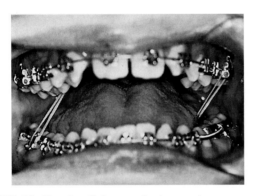

FIGURE 18-13   Parallel cross-elastics, used to correct a mild transverse discrepancy leading to the lateral mandibular shift late in treatment.

is slightly displaced transversely relative to the man-dibular arch so that with the teeth in occlusion, relationships are excellent, but there is a lateral shift to reach that position. Correction again would involve posterior cross-elastics, but in a parallel pattern as shown in Figure 18-13.

If a midline discrepancy is from displacement of mandibular teeth more than maxillary teeth, or vice versa, the difference in stability with rectangular vs. round wires can be used to help in correcting the situation. If the maxillary midline is correct while the mandibular midline deviates slightly toward one side, and a mild Class II relationship still exists on that side, replacing the rectangular mandibular finishing arch with a 16 or 18 mil round wire while retaining a full-dimension rectangular arch in the upper arch can facilitate correction with a unilateral Class II elastic. This approach should be reserved for small discrepancies, and it is important to carefully observe and control any expansion of the lower molar while a Class II elastic is worn against a light archwire. Prolonged use of Class II or Class III elastics during the finishing stage of treatment should be avoided, but a brief period of inter-arch elastic force is often necessary to obtain final positioning of teeth.

TOOTH SIZE DISCREPANCIES

Tooth size discrepancy problems must be taken into account when treatment is planned initially (see Chapter 7), but many of the steps to deal with these problems are taken in the finishing stage of treatment. Reduction of interproximal enamel (stripping) is the usual strategy to compensate for discrepancies caused by excess tooth size. When the problem is tooth size deficiency, it is necessary to leave space between some teeth, which may or may not ultimately be closed by restorations.

One of the advantages of a bonded appliance is that interproximal enamel can be removed at any time. When stripping of enamel is part of the original treatment plan, most of the enamel reduction should be done initially, but final stripping can be deferred until the finishing stage. This procedure allows direct observation of the occlusal relationships before the final tooth size adjustments are made. A topical fluoride treatment always is recommended immediately after stripping is done.

Tooth size deficiency problems often are caused by small maxillary lateral incisors. A small space distal to the lateral incisor can be esthetically and functionally acceptable, but a composite resin build-up of the small lateral incisor usually is the best plan for small incisors (Figure 18-14). It is better to add small amounts of resin on both sides of a small tooth than a large amount on one side. During finishing, segments of coil spring are placed on the finishing archwire to precisely position the small tooth. Precise finishing is easier if the build-up is done during the finishing stage of the orthodontic treatment. This can be accomplished simply by removing the bracket from the small tooth or teeth for a few hours while the restoration is done, then replacing the bracket and arch-wires.[5] Alternatively, the composite build-ups should be done as soon possible after the patient is in retention. This requires an initial retainer to hold the space, and a new retainer immediately after the restoration is completed. The main reason for waiting until after the orthodontic appliance has been removed is to allow any gingival inflammation to resolve itself.

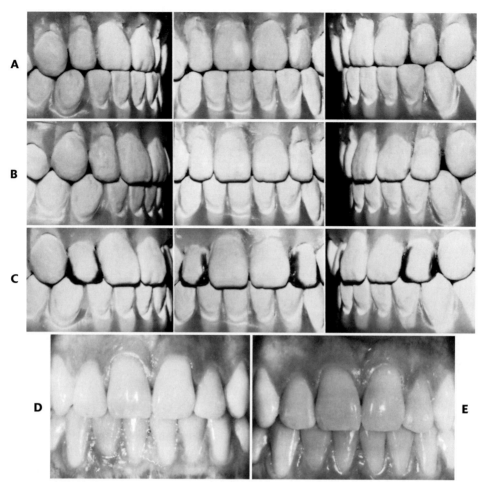

FIGURE 18-14   Small maxillary lateral incisors create tooth-size discrepancy problems that may become apparent only late in treatment. **A,** Setup showing anterior edge-to-edge relationship with the upper incisors in proximal contact; **B,** spaces distal to the lateral incisors with proper overjet/overbite relationship. Leaving a small space distal to the laterals, where it does not show, can be a satisfactory solution for some patients. **C,** Wax-up showing possible addition of composite restorative material to build up the small laterals and allow space closure; **D,** clinical photograph of same patient immediately after; **E,** 12 months after composite build-ups of the laterals. Addition of composite material to bring small lateral incisors to normal size usually is the preferred solution. (From Fields H.W.: *Am J Orthod* 79:176-183, 1981.)

More generalized small deficiencies can be masked by altering incisor position in any of several ways. To a limited extent, torque of the upper incisors can be used to compensate: leaving the incisors slightly more upright makes them take up less room relative to the lower arch and can be used to mask large upper incisors, while slightly excessive torque can partially compensate for small upper incisors. These adjustments require third-order bends in the finishing archwires. It is also possible to compensate by slightly tipping teeth, or by finishing the orthodontic treatment with mildly excessive overbite or overjet, depending on the individual circumstances.[6]

FINAL "SETTLING" OF TEETH

At the conclusion of Class II or Class III correction, particularly if interarch elastics have been used, the teeth tend to rebound back toward their initial position despite the presence of rectangular archwires. In addition, it is not uncommon for a full-dimension rectangular archwire, no matter how carefully made, to hold some teeth slightly out of occlusion.

Because of the rebound after Class II or Class III treatment, it is important to slightly overcorrect the occlusal relationships. In a typical Class II anterior deep bite patient, the teeth should be taken to an end-to-end incisor rela-

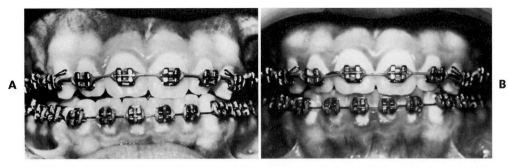

FIGURE 18-15 In finishing, overcorrection of Class II or Class III relationships is necessary to compensate for the rebound that occurs when headgear or elastic force is discontinued. **A,** Occlusion at the time Class II elastics were discontinued; **B,** same patient 8 weeks later, without archwire changes or other treatment.

tionship, with both overjet and overbite totally eliminated, before the headgear or elastic forces are discontinued (Figure 18-15). This provides some latitude for the teeth to rebound or settle into the proper relationship.

No matter what the original malocclusion, a rectangular finishing archwire nearly always requires some first-, second-, or third-order bends to precisely position the teeth. One cannot simply place an ideal rectangular archwire in a straight-wire appliance and assume that the ideal position of each tooth will result. For essentially every patient, variations in tooth morphology and bracket positions will require some adjustments in the final rectangular archwires.

The more precisely the archwire fits the brackets and the more bends that it requires, the more likely that some teeth will be almost but not quite in occlusion. This phenomenon was recognized by the pioneers with the edgewise appliance, who coined the term "arch-bound" to describe it. They found that with precisely fitting wires, it was almost impossible to get every tooth into solid occlusion, although one could come close.

These considerations lead to the formulation of two rules in finishing treatment:

1. Interarch elastics and headgear should be discontinued, and the rebound from their use allowed to express itself, 4 to 8 weeks before the orthodontic appliances are removed.
2. As a final step in treatment, the teeth should be brought into a solid occlusal relationship without heavy archwires present.

The final step of finishing therefore is appropriately called "settling," since its purpose is to bring all teeth into a solid occlusal relationship before the patient is placed in retention. There are three ways to settle the occlusion: (1) by replacing the rectangular archwires at the very end of treatment with light round arches that provide some freedom for movement of the teeth (16 mil in the 18-slot appliance, 16 or 18 mil in the 22-slot appliance) and allowing the teeth to find their own occlusal level; (2) with laced posterior vertical elastics after removing the poste-

rior segments of the archwires; or (3) after the bands and brackets have been removed, with the use of a tooth positioner.

Replacing full-dimension rectangular wires with light round wires at the very end of treatment was the original method for settling, recommended by Tweed in the 1940s and perhaps by other edgewise pioneers earlier. These light final arches must include any first- or second-order bends used in the rectangular finishing arches. It is usually unnecessary for the patient to wear light posterior vertical elastics during this settling, but they can be used if needed (Figure 18-16). These light arches will quickly settle the teeth into final occlusion and should remain in place for only a few weeks at most.

The difficulty with undersized round wires at the end of treatment is that some freedom of movement for settling of posterior teeth is desired, but precise control of anterior teeth is lost as well. It was not until the 1980s that orthodontists realized the advantage of removing only the posterior part of the rectangular finishing wire, leaving the anterior segment (typically canine-to-canine or first premolar-to-first premolar, and using laced elastics to bring the posterior teeth into tight occlusion (Figure 18-17).[7] This method sacrifices a large degree of control of the posterior teeth, and therefore should not be used in patients who had major rotations or posterior crossbite. For the majority of patients who had well-aligned posterior teeth from the beginning, however, this is a remarkably simple and effective way to settle the teeth into their final occlusion. It is the last step in active treatment for the majority of patients at present.

The elastics for this settling are laced around the tubes and brackets as shown in Figure 18-17. A typical arrangement is to use light ¾-inch elastics, with a Class II or Class III direction depending on whether slightly more correction is desired. These elastics should not remain in place for more than 2 weeks, and 1 week usually is enough to accomplish the desired settling. At that point, the fixed appliances should be removed and the retainers placed.

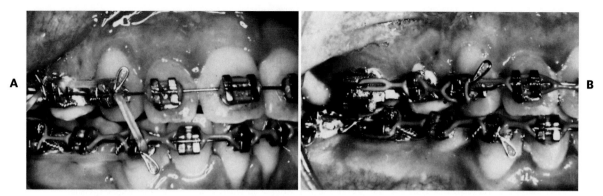

FIGURE 18-16 Use of vertical elastics for settling. **A,** Heavy rectangular archwires have been replaced by 16 mil steel, and ⅛-inch light vertical elastics in a box pattern are being worn to bring the teeth into tight occlusion; **B,** 4 weeks later.

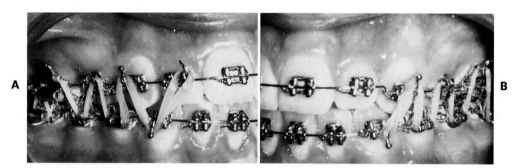

FIGURE 18-17 Use of laced elastics for settling the teeth into final occlusion at the end of treatment. The elastics can be used either with light round archwires, or with rectangular segments in the anterior brackets and no wire at all posteriorly.

REMOVAL OF BANDS AND BONDED ATTACHMENTS

Removal of bands is accomplished by simply breaking the cement attachment and then lifting the band off the tooth—which sounds simpler than it is in some instances. For upper molar and premolar teeth, a band-removing pliers is placed so that first the lingual, then the buccal surface is elevated by the pliers (Figure 18-18). A welded lingual bar is needed on these bands to provide a point of attachment for the pliers if lingual hooks or cleats are not a part of the appliance. For the lower posterior teeth, the sequence of force is just the reverse: the band-removing pliers is applied first on the buccal, then the lingual surface. Maxillary anterior bands are removed from the labial surface with an anterior band-removing pliers, while tightly fitted mandibular anterior bands usually must be slit with a cutting pliers to make it possible to take them off. The difficulty of removing anterior bands is another reason for bonding except in special circumstances.

Bonded brackets must be removed, insofar as possible, without damaging the enamel surface. This is done by creating a fracture within the resin bonding material or between the bracket and the resin, and then removing the residual resin from the enamel surface (Figure 18-19). With metal brackets, applying a cutting pliers to the base of the bracket so that the bracket bends has the disadvantage of destroying the bracket, which otherwise could be reused, but this is the safest method.[8]

Enamel damage from debonding metal brackets is rare, but there have been a number of reports of enamel fractures and removal of chunks of enamel when ceramic brackets are debonded (see Chapter 12 for a more detailed discussion). It also is easy to fracture a ceramic bracket while attempting to remove it, and if that happens, large pieces of the bracket must be ground away with a diamond stone in a handpiece. These problems arise because ceramic brackets have little or no ability to deform—they are either intact or broken. Shearing stresses are applied to the bracket to remove it, and the necessary force can become alarmingly large, even with the special instruments now offered for this purpose (Figure 18-20).

There are three approaches to these debonding problems: (1) grind away the brackets, rather than attempting to break them loose. This is time consuming, and there is the risk of enamel damage from the diamond rotary instruments; (2) modify the interface between the bracket and the bonding resin to increase the chance that when force is

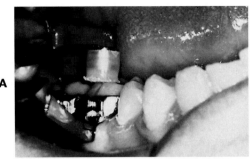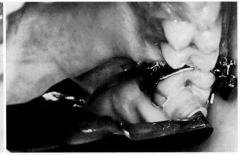

FIGURE 18-18 Removal of molar bands with a band-removing pliers. **A,** Lower posterior bands are removed primarily with pressure from the buccal surface; **B,** upper posterior bands are removed from the lingual surface, using a lingual attachment welded to the band.

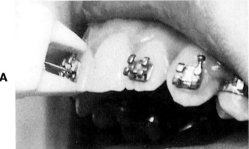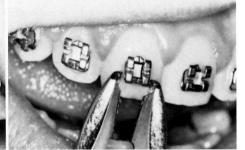

FIGURE 18-19 Removal of bonded brackets. **A,** A special pliers with a wire loop can be used to grasp the one wing of the bracket and apply a shearing force to fracture the bonding resin. This works particularly well with twin brackets. The advantage of this method is that the bracket usually is undamaged; the disadvantage is heavy force that may cause enamel damage; **B,** a cutter can be used to distort the bracket base, which leads to fractures within the bonding resin. The first approach is more compatible with recycling of brackets, but the second is safer.

applied, the failure will occur between the bracket and the bonding material. Chemical bonds between the bonding resin and the bracket can be too good, and most manufacturers now have weakened them or abandoned chemical bonding altogether; (3) use heat to soften the bonding resin, so that the bracket can be removed with lower force.[9] Electrothermal and laser instruments for removing ceramic brackets now are available. There is no doubt that less force is needed when the bracket is heated, and research findings indicate that there is little patient discomfort and minimal risk of pulpal damage. Nevertheless, the ideal solution would be to perfect the second approach so that ceramic brackets can be debonded without heating as readily as metal ones.

Cement left on the teeth after debanding can be removed easily by scaling, but residual bonding resin is more difficult to remove. The best results are obtained with a 12-fluted carbide bur at moderate speeds in a dental handpiece (Figure 18-21).[10] This bur cuts resin readily but has little effect on enamel. Topical fluoride should be applied when the cleanup procedure has been completed, however, since some of the fluoride-rich outer enamel layer may be lost with even the most careful approach.

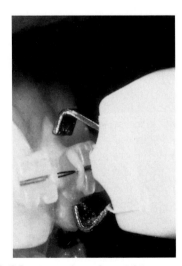

FIGURE 18-20 A number of special instruments have been designed to make removal of ceramic brackets safer and easier. This one creates a torquing force on the bracket. Whatever the special instrument, however, weakening the bond first (with heat or laser) probably is needed for maximum effectiveness.

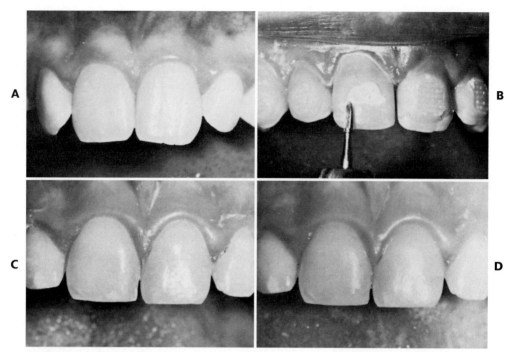

FIGURE 18-21   Removing excess bonding resin is best accomplished with a smooth 12-fluted carbide bur, followed by pumicing. **A,** Close-up view of the virgin surface of upper incisors; **B,** excess resin left on the tooth surface after removal of brackets. Upon debonding, the bond failure usually occurs between the base of the bracket and the resin, leaving excess resin on the tooth. The carbide bur is used with a general wiping motion to remove the resin; **C,** tooth surface after the remainder of the resin has been removed with the bur; **D,** tooth surface after final removal of resin (compare with **A**).

POSITIONERS FOR FINISHING

An alternative to segmental elastics or light round archwires for final settling is a rubber or plastic tooth positioner. A positioner is most effective if it is placed immediately on removal of the fixed orthodontic appliance. Normally, it is fabricated by removing the archwires 4 to 6 weeks before the planned removal of the appliance, taking impressions of the teeth and a registration of occlusal relationships, and then resetting the teeth in the laboratory, incorporating the minor changes in position of each tooth necessary to produce appropriate settling (Figure 18-22). All erupted teeth should be included in the positioner, to prevent supereruption. As part of the laboratory procedure, bands and brackets are trimmed away, and any band space is closed.

This indirect approach allows individual tooth positions to be adjusted with considerable precision, bringing each tooth into the desired final relationship. The positioning device is then fabricated by forming either a hard rubber or soft plastic material around the repositioned and articulated casts, producing a device with the inherent elasticity to move the teeth slightly to their final position (Figure 18-23).

The use of a tooth positioner rather than final settling archwires has two advantages: (1) it allows the fixed appliance to be removed somewhat more quickly than otherwise would have been the case (i.e., some finishing that could have been done with the final archwires can be left to the positioner), and (2) it serves not only to reposition the teeth but also to massage the gingiva, which is almost always at least slightly inflamed and swollen after comprehensive orthodontic treatment. The gingival stimulation provided by a positioner is an excellent way to promote a rapid return to normal gingival contours (Figure 18-24).

The use of positioners for finishing also has disadvantages. First of all, these appliances require a considerable amount of laboratory fabrication time, and therefore are expensive. Second, settling with a positioner tends to increase overbite more than the equivalent settling with light elastics. This is a disadvantage in patients who had a deep overbite initially but can be advantageous if the initial problem was an anterior open bite. Third, a positioner does not maintain the correction of rotated teeth well, which means that minor rotations may recur while a positioner is being worn. Finally, good cooperation is essential.

With modern edgewise appliances, the first advantage is not nearly so compelling as it was previously. It is an error to depend on a positioner to accomplish more than minimal settling of the occlusion. Major movements of teeth simply cannot be accomplished with any degree of

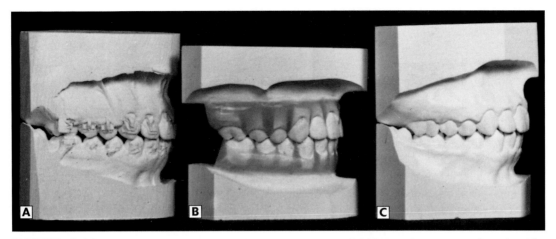

FIGURE 18-22 Use of a positioner for finishing. **A,** Casts 1 month before appliance removal, used to fabricate an immediate positioner; **B,** the positioner setup, with bands and brackets carved off the teeth in the laboratory; **C,** casts 2 weeks after appliance removal and placement of the positioner, showing the teeth settled into their finished relationship.

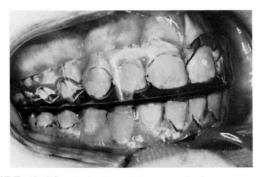

FIGURE 18-23 A tooth positioner made from a transparent plastic material, placed in the patient's mouth. The patient bites into the positioner, which creates forces to slightly displace the teeth and also massages the gingiva. A device of this type is most effective in moving teeth if it is placed immediately after the fixed appliance is removed.

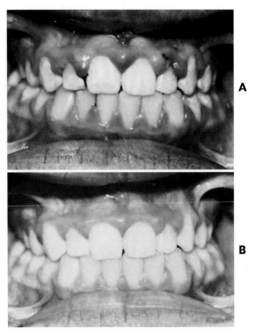

FIGURE 18-24 Gingival improvement with positioner wear. **A,** Swollen maxillary papillae immediately after band removal, just before placement of a positioner; **B,** 2 weeks later. This degree of gingival reaction anteriorly is rarely seen, especially with bonded attachments, but when it occurs, a positioner is one of the best means to resolve it.

certainty. At present, therefore, there are two main indications for use of a positioner: (1) a gingival condition with more than the usual degree of inflammation and swelling at the end of active orthodontics, or (2) an open bite tendency, so that settling by mild depression rather than elongation of posterior teeth is needed. Severe malalignment and rotated teeth, a deep bite tendency, and an uncooperative patient are contraindications for positioner use.

A positioner should be worn by the patient at least 4 hours during the day and during sleep. Since the amount of tooth movement produced by a positioner tends to decline rapidly after a few days of use, an excellent schedule is to remove the orthodontic appliances, clean the teeth and apply a fluoride treatment, and place the positioner immediately, asking the patient to wear it as nearly full time as possible for the first 2 days. After that, it can be worn on the usual night-plus-4 hours schedule.

As a general rule, a tooth positioner in a cooperative patient will produce any changes it is capable of within 3 weeks. Final (posttreatment) records can be taken 2 or 3 weeks after the positioner is placed. Beyond that time, if the positioner is continued, it is serving as a retainer rather than a finishing device (see Chapter 19)—and positioners, as a rule, are not good retainers.

SPECIAL FINISHING PROCEDURES TO AVOID RELAPSE

Relapse after orthodontic treatment has two major causes: (1) continued growth by the patient in an unfavorable pattern, and (2) tissue rebound after the release of orthodontic force.

Control of Unfavorable Growth

Changes resulting from continued growth in a Class II, Class III, deep bite, or open bite pattern contribute to a return of the original malocclusion, and so are relapse in that sense. These changes are not attributed to tooth movement alone, however, but to the pattern of skeletal growth. Controlling this type of relapse requires a continuation of active treatment after the fixed appliances have been removed, rather than specific finishing procedures to prevent relapse. For patients with skeletal problems who have undergone orthodontic treatment, this "active retention" takes one of two forms. One possibility is to continue extraoral force in conjunction with orthodontic retainers (high-pull headgear at night, for instance, in a patient with a Class II open bite growth pattern). The other appropriate option is to use a functional appliance rather than a conventional retainer after the completion of fixed appliance therapy. This important subject is discussed in more detail in Chapter 19.

Control of Soft Tissue Rebound

A major reason for retention is to hold the teeth until soft tissue remodeling can take place. Even with the best remodeling, however, some rebound from the application of orthodontic forces occurs, and indeed the tendency for rebound after interarch elastics are discontinued has already been discussed. There are two ways to deal with this phenomenon: (1) overtreatment, so that any rebound will only bring the teeth back to their proper position, and (2) adjunctive periodontal surgery to reduce rebound from elastic fibers in the gingiva. In some cases, permanent retention is required to maintain the desired relationships, but this need not be planned if either of the two approaches described here would make it unnecessary.

Overtreatment. Since it can be anticipated that teeth will rebound slightly toward their previous position after orthodontic correction, it is logical to position them at the end of treatment in a somewhat overtreated position. Only a small degree of overtreatment is compatible with precise finishing of orthodontic cases as described previously, but it is nevertheless possible to apply this principle during the finishing phase of treatment. Consider three specific situations:

Correction of Class II or Class III Malocclusion. The rebound or settling after Class II or Class III correction has already been discussed. After headgear or elastics have been discontinued, it can be expected that the teeth will rebound 1 to 2 mm (see Figure 18-15), so this degree of overtreatment is required. This rebound is entirely different from re-

lapse tendencies caused by continued growth, which take at least several months to become apparent. The rebound from the forces used for Class II or Class III correction occurs relatively quickly, within 3 to 4 weeks. When elastics are used, therefore, the patient should be taken to a slightly overcorrected position, and elastics discontinued for 3-4 weeks to allow rebound to occur, before appliances are removed.

Particularly when a patient has been wearing Class II elastics, he or she may begin to posture the mandible forward, so that the malocclusion looks more corrected than it really is. For this reason also, it is important to allow a period of time without elastics before ending active treatment, to be sure that the patient really has been corrected and is not just posturing. This is different from rebound, which occurs independently of mandibular posturing, but obviously it is important to detect. Rebound is a 1-2 mm phenomenon; posturing can produce an apparent 4-5 mm relapse. The best plan is to reduce the force on Class II elastics when the apparently correct degree of overcorrection has been achieved but maintain them full-time for 3-4 weeks, then wear them just at night for another appointment period, and finally discontinue them completely for at least 4 weeks before removing the appliances.

Crossbite Correction. Whatever the mechanism used to correct crossbite, it should be overcorrected by at least 1 to 2 mm before the force system is released. If the crossbite is corrected during the first stage of treatment, as should be the case, the overcorrection will gradually be lost during succeeding phases of treatment, but this should improve stability when transverse relationships are established precisely during the finishing phase.

Irregular and Rotated Teeth. Just as with crossbites, irregularities and rotations can be overcorrected during the first phase of treatment, carrying a tooth that has been lingually positioned slightly too far labial, for instance, and vice versa. It is wise to hold the teeth in a slightly overcorrected position for at least a few months, during the end of the first stage of treatment and the second stage. As a general rule, however, it is not wise to build this overcorrection into rectangular finishing archwires.

Similarly, a tooth being rotated into position in the arch can be overrotated. Maintaining an overrotated position can be done by adjusting the wings of single brackets, or by pinching shut one of a pair of twin brackets. Maintaining overcorrected labiolingual positions of incisors is done readily with first-order bends in working archwires. Rotated teeth should be maintained in an overcorrected position as long as possible, but even then, these teeth are often candidates for the periodontal procedures described following.

Adjunctive Periodontal Surgery. A major cause of rebound after orthodontic treatment is the network of elastic supracrestal gingival fibers. As teeth are moved to a new position, these fibers tend to stretch, and they remodel very slowly. If the pull of these elastic fibers could be eliminated, a major cause of relapse of previously irregular and rotated teeth should be eliminated. In fact, if the supracrestal fibers are sectioned and allowed to heal while the teeth are held in the proper position, relapse caused by gingival elasticity is greatly reduced.

Surgery to section the supracrestal elastic fibers is a simple procedure that does not require referral to a periodontist. It can be carried out by either of two approaches. The first method, originally developed by Edwards,[11] is called *circumferential supracrestal fibrotomy* (CSF) (Figure 18-25). After infiltration with a local anesthetic, the procedure consists of inserting the sharp point of a fine blade into the gingival sulcus down to the crest of alveolar bone. Cuts are made interproximally on each side of a rotated

tooth and along the labial and lingual gingival margins unless, as is often the case, the labial or lingual gingiva is quite thin, in which case this part of the circumferential cut is omitted. No periodontal pack is necessary, and there is only minor discomfort after the procedure.

An alternative method is to make an incision in the center of each gingival papilla, sparing the margin but separating the papilla from just below the margin to 1 to 2 mm below the height of the bone buccally and lingually (Figure 18-26).[12] This modification is said to reduce the possibility that height of the gingival attachment will be reduced after

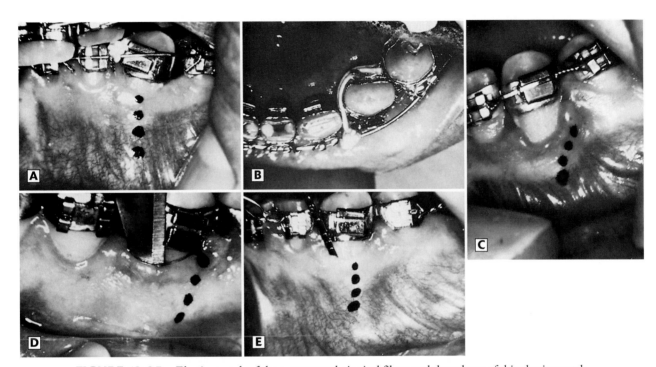

FIGURE 18-25 Elastic stretch of the supracrestal gingival fibers and the release of this elastic stretch by fiber section can be demonstrated by placing tattoo marks in the gingiva. **A**, India ink tattoos placed in the vicinity of a rotated mandibular canine before correction of the rotation; **B**, elastic thread used to rotate the tooth into position; **C**, the tooth rotated to its correct position in the arch. Note the displacement of the gingival tissues, as revealed by the deviation of the tattoo marks. **D**, Circumferential incision around the tooth, penetrating to the crest of the alveolar bone; **E**, after the incision, the gingival tissue returns to its original position. Periodontal probing shows a normal sulcus depth after the incision. (From Edwards JG: *Am J Orthod* 57:35-46, 1970.)

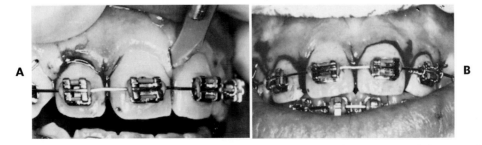

FIGURE 18-26 The "papilla split" procedure is an alternative to the CSF approach for sectioning gingival circumferential fibers to improve post-treatment stability. Vertical cuts are made in the gingival papillae without separating the gingival margin at the papilla tip. **A**, The blade inserted to make the vertical cut; **B**, view at completion of the papilla splits before sutures are placed (see also Figure 21-1). One advantage of this procedure is that it is easier to perform with an orthodontic appliance and archwire in place.

the surgery, and it is indicated for esthetically sensitive areas (i.e., the maxillary incisor region). Nevertheless, there is little if any risk of gingival recession with the original CSF procedure unless cuts are made across thin labial or lingual tissues. From the point of view of improved stability after orthodontic treatment, the surgical procedures appear to be equivalent.

Neither the CSF nor the papilla-dividing procedure should be done until malaligned teeth have been corrected and held in their new position for several months, so this surgery is always done toward the end of the finishing phase of treatment. It is important to hold the teeth in good alignment while gingival healing occurs. This means that either the surgery should be done a few weeks before removal of the orthodontic appliance or, if it is performed at the same time the appliance is removed, a retainer must be inserted almost immediately. It is easier to do the CSF procedure after the orthodontic appliances have been removed, although it can be carried out with appliances in place. An advantage of the papilla-dividing procedure may be that it is easier to perform with the orthodontic appliance still in place. The only problem with placing a retainer immediately after the surgery is that it may be difficult to keep the retainer from contacting soft tissue in a sore area.

Experience has demonstrated that sectioning the gingival fibers is an effective method to control rotational relapse but does not control the tendency for crowded incisors to again become irregular. The primary indication for gingival surgery therefore is a tooth or teeth that were severely rotated. This surgery is not indicated for patients with crowding without rotations.

REFERENCES

1. Burstone CJ, Koenig HA: Creative wire bending—the force system from step and V bends, Am J Orthod Dentofac Orthop 93:59-67, 1988.
2. Parkhouse RC: Rectangular wire and third order torque: a new perspective, Am J Orthod Dentofac Orthop 113:421-430, 1998.
3. Isaacson RJ, Rebellato J: Two-couple orthodontic appliance systems: torquing arches, Sem Orthod 1:31-36, 1995.
4. Gianelly AA: Asymmetric space closure, Am J Orthod Dentofac Orthop 90:335-341, 1986.
5. Kokich V: Esthetics: the ortho-perio-restorative connection, Sem Orthod 2:21-30, 1996.
6. Fields HW: Orthodontic-restorative treatment for relative mandibular anterior excess tooth size problems, Am J Orthod 79:176-183, 1981.
7. Steffen JM, Haltom FT: The five-cent tooth positioner, J Clin Orthod 21:528-529, 1987.
8. Bennett CG, Shen C, Waldron JM: The effects of debonding on the enamel surface, J Clin Orthod 18:330-334, 1984.
9. Bishara SE, Fehr DE: Ceramic brackets: something old, something new, a review, Sem Orthod 3:177-188, 1997.
10. Rouleau BR, Marshall GW, Cooley RD: Enamel surface evaluation after clinical treatment and removal of orthodontic brackets, Am J Orthod 81:423-426, 1982.
11. Edwards JG: A long-term prospective evaluation of the circumferential supracrestal fiberotomy in alleviating orthodontic relapse, Am J Orthod Dentofac Orthop 93:380-387, 1988.
12. Ahrens DG, Shapira Y, Kuftinec MM: An approach to rotational relapse, Am J Orthod 80:83-91, 1981.

At sporting events, no matter how good things look for one team late in the game, the saying is "It's not over till it's over." In orthodontics, although the patient may feel that treatment is complete when the appliances are removed, an important stage lies ahead. Orthodontic control of tooth position and occlusal relationships must be withdrawn gradually, not abruptly, if excellent long-term results are to be obtained. The type of retention should be included in the original treatment plan.

WHY IS RETENTION NECESSARY?

There is extensive literature on retention and post-treatment stability, which has been reviewed recently.[1] Although a number of factors can be cited as influencing long-term results, orthodontic treatment results are potentially unstable, and therefore retention is necessary, for three major reasons: (1) the gingival and periodontal tissues are affected by orthodontic tooth movement and require time for reorganization when the appliances are removed; (2) the teeth may be in an inherently unstable position after the treatment, so that soft tissue pressures constantly produce a relapse tendency; and (3) changes produced by growth may alter the orthodontic treatment result. If the teeth are not in an inherently unstable position, and if there is no further growth, retention still is vitally important until gingival and periodontal reorganization is completed. If the teeth are unstable, as often is the case following significant arch expansion, gradual withdrawal of orthodontic appliances is of no value. The only possibilities are accepting relapse or using permanent retention. Finally, whatever the situation, retention cannot be abandoned until growth is essentially completed.

Reorganization of the Periodontal and Gingival Tissues

Widening of the periodontal ligament space and disruption of the collagen fiber bundles that support each tooth are normal responses to orthodontic treatment (see Chapter 9). In fact, these changes are necessary to allow orthodontic tooth movement to occur. Even if tooth movement stops before the orthodontic appliance is removed, restoration of the normal periodontal architecture will not occur as long as a tooth is strongly splinted to its neighbors, as when it is attached to a rigid orthodontic archwire (so holding the teeth with passive archwires cannot be considered the beginning of retention). Once the teeth can respond individually to the forces of mastication (i.e., once each tooth can be displaced slightly relative to its neighbor as the patient chews), reorganization of the periodontal ligament (PDL) occurs over a 3- to 4-month period,[2] and the slight mobility present at appliance removal disappears.

This PDL reorganization is important for stability because of the periodontal contribution to the equilibrium that normally controls tooth position. To briefly review our current understanding of the pressure equilibrium (see Chapter 5 for a detailed discussion), the teeth normally withstand occlusal forces because of the shock-absorbing properties of the periodontal system. More importantly for orthodontics, small but prolonged imbalances in tongue-lip-cheek pressures or pressures from gingival fibers that otherwise would produce tooth movement are resisted by "active stabilization" due to PDL metabolism. It appears that this stabilization is caused by the same force-generating mechanism that produces eruption. The disruption of the PDL produced by orthodontic tooth movement probably has little effect on the stabilization against occlusal forces, but it reduces or eliminates the active stabilization, which means that immediately after orthodontic appliances are removed, teeth will be unstable in the face of occlusal and soft tissue pressures that can be resisted later. This is the reason that every patient needs retainers for at least a few months.

The gingival fiber networks are also disturbed by orthodontic tooth movement and must remodel to accommodate the new tooth positions. Both collagenous and elastic fibers occur in the gingiva, and the reorganization of both occurs more slowly than that of the PDL itself.[3] Within 4 to 6 months, the collagenous fiber networks within the gingiva have normally completed their reorganization, but the elastic supracrestal fibers remodel extremely slowly and can still exert forces capable of displacing a tooth at one year after removal of an orthodontic appliance. In patients with severe rotations, sectioning the supracrestal fibers around severely malposed or rotated teeth, at or just before the time of appliance removal, is a recommended procedure because it reduces relapse tendencies resulting from this fiber elasticity[4] (see Chapter 18 and Figure 21-1).

This timetable for soft tissue recovery from orthodontic treatment outlines the principles of retention against intra-arch instability. These are:

1. The direction of potential relapse can be identified by comparing the position of the teeth at the conclusion of treatment with their original positions. Teeth will tend to move back in the direction from which they came, primarily because of elastic recoil of gingival fibers but also because of unbalanced tongue-lip forces (Figure 19-1).

2. Teeth require essentially full-time retention after comprehensive orthodontic treatment for the first 3 to 4 months after a fixed orthodontic appliance is removed. To promote reorganization of the PDL, however, the teeth should be free to flex individually during mastication, as the alveolar bone bends in response to heavy occlusal loads during mastication (see Chapter 9). This requirement can be met by a removable appliance worn full-time except during meals or by a fixed retainer that is not too rigid.

3. Because of the slow response of the gingival fibers, retention should be continued for at least 12 months if the teeth were quite irregular initially but can be reduced to part-time after 3 to 4 months. After approximately 12 months, it should be possible to discontinue retention in non-growing patients. More precisely, the teeth should be stable by that time if they ever will be. Some patients who are not growing will require permanent retention to maintain the teeth in what would otherwise be unstable positions because of lip, cheek, and tongue pressures that are too large for active stabilization to balance out. Patients who will continue to grow, however, usually need retention until growth has reduced to the low levels that characterize adult life.

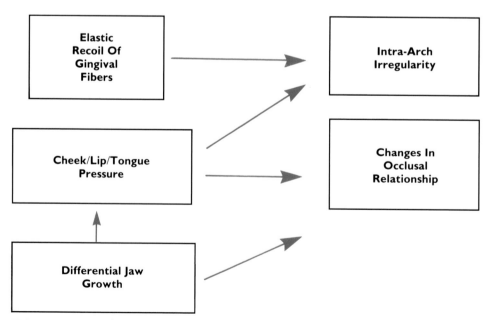

FIGURE 19-1 The major causes of relapse after orthodontic treatment include the elasticity of gingival fibers, cheek/lip/tongue pressures, and jaw growth. Gingival fibers and soft tissue pressures are especially potent in the first few months after treatment ends, before PDL reorganization has been completed.

Occlusal Changes Related to Growth

A continuation of growth is particularly troublesome in patients whose initial malocclusion resulted, largely or in part, from the pattern of skeletal growth. Skeletal problems in all three planes of space tend to recur if growth continues (Figure 19-2). Because transverse growth is completed first, long-term transverse changes are less of a problem clinically than changes from late anteroposterior and vertical growth.

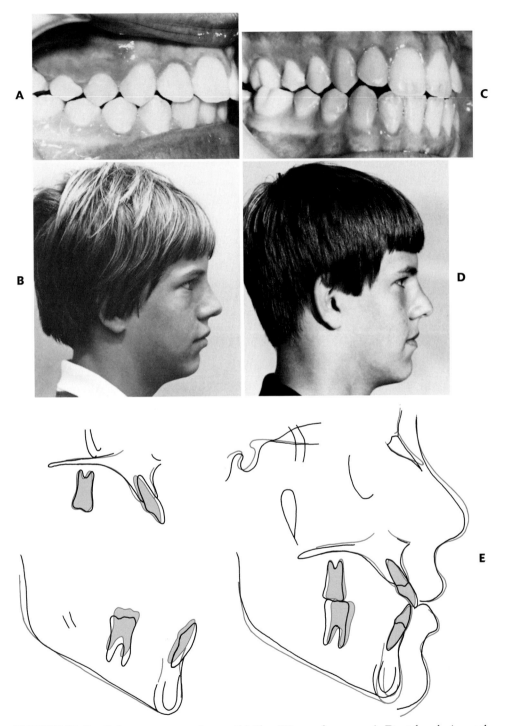

FIGURE 19-2   Relapse accompanying a mild Class III growth pattern: **A,** Dental occlusion at the completion of orthodontic treatment; **B,** profile appearance at the conclusion of active treatment; **C,** occlusal relationships 3 years later; **D,** facial appearance 3 years later; **E,** cephalometric superimpositions showing changes resulting from posttreatment growth (*black*, end of treatment; *red*, 3 years after treatment). Note the mandibular growth, the uprighting of the lower incisors, and the compensatory forward movement of the entire maxillary arch during post-treatment growth.

The tendency for skeletal problems to recur after orthodontic correction results from the fact that most patients continue in their original growth pattern as long as they are growing. Comprehensive orthodontic treatment is usually carried out in the early permanent dentition, and the duration is typically between 18 and 30 months. This means that active orthodontic treatment is likely to conclude at age 14 to 15, while anteroposterior and particularly vertical growth often do not subside even to the adult level until several years later. Long-term studies of adults have shown that very slow growth typically continues throughout adult life, and the same pattern that led to malocclusion in the first place can contribute to a deterioration in occlusal relationships many years after orthodontic treatment is completed.[5] In late adolescence, continued growth in the pattern that caused a Class II, Class III, deep bite, or open bite problem in the first place is a major cause of relapse after orthodontic treatment and requires careful management during retention.[6]

Retention after Class II Correction. Relapse toward a Class II relationship must result from some combination of tooth movement (forward in the upper arch, backward in the lower arch, or both) and differential growth of the maxilla relative to the mandible (Figure 19-3). As might be expected, tooth movement caused by local periodontal and gingival factors can be an important short-term problem, whereas differential jaw growth is a more important long-term problem both because it directly alters jaw position and because it contributes to repositioning of teeth.

Overcorrection of the occlusal relationships as a finishing procedure is an important step in controlling tooth movement that would lead to Class II relapse. Even with good retention, 1 to 2 mm of anteroposterior change caused by adjustments in tooth position is likely to occur after treatment, particularly if Class II elastics were employed. This change occurs relatively quickly after active treatment stops.

In Class II treatment, it is important not to move the lower incisors too far forward, but this can happen easily with Class II elastics. In this situation, lip pressure will tend to upright the protruding incisors, leading relatively quickly (often in only a few months after full-time retainer wear is discontinued) to crowding and return of both overbite and overjet. As a general guideline, if more than 2 mm of forward repositioning of the lower incisors occurred during treatment, permanent retention will be required.

The slower long-term relapse that occurs in some patients who did not have inappropriate tooth movement results primarily from differential jaw growth. The amount of growth remaining after orthodontic treatment will obviously depend on the age, sex, and relative maturity of the patient, but after treatment that involved growth modification, some posttreatment rebound is likely, with more growth of the upper than the lower jaw.

This relapse tendency can be controlled in one of two ways. The first, the traditional fixed appliance approach of

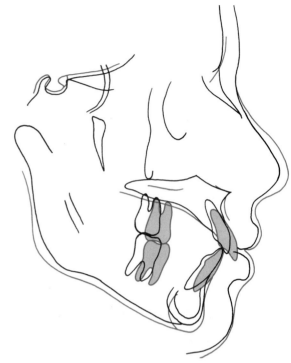

FIGURE 19-3 Cephalometric superimposition demonstrating growth-related relapse in a patient treated to correct Class II malocclusion. *Black*, immediate posttreatment, age 13; *red*, recall, age 17. After treatment, both jaws grew downward and forward, but mandibular growth did not match maxillary growth, and the maxillary dentition moved forward relative to the maxilla.

the 1970s and earlier, is to continue headgear to the upper molars on a reduced basis (at night, for instance) in conjunction with a retainer to hold the teeth in alignment (Figure 19-4). This is quite satisfactory in well-motivated patients who have been wearing headgear during treatment and is compatible with traditional retainers that are worn full-time initially.

The other method is to use a functional appliance of the activator-bionator type to hold both tooth position and the occlusal relationship (Figure 19-5). If the patient does not have excessive overjet, as should be the case at the end of active treatment, the construction bite for the functional appliance is taken without any mandibular advancement—the idea is to prevent a Class II malocclusion from recurring, not to actively treat one that already exists. A potential difficulty is that the functional appliance will be worn only part-time, typically just at night, and daytime retainers of conventional design also will be needed to control tooth position during the first few months. The extra retainer makes sense for a patient with a severe growth problem. For patients with less severe problems, in whom continued growth may or may not cause relapse, it may be more rational to use only conventional maxillary and mandibular retainers initially, and replace them with a functional appliance to be worn at night if relapse is beginning to occur after a few months.

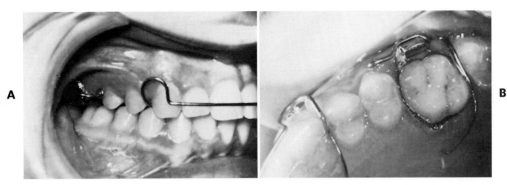

FIGURE 19-4 Retention after Class II correction: bands with headgear tubes remain on the upper first molars so that headgear at night can be continued. This is compatible with a removable maxillary retainer using circumferential clasps that fit under the headgear tubes. **A,** Lateral view; **B,** occlusal view.

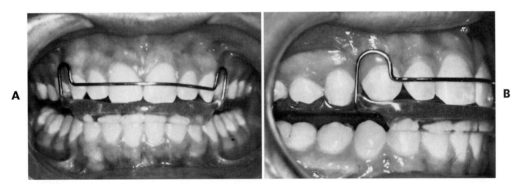

FIGURE 19-5 In patients in whom further growth in the original Class II pattern is expected after active treatment is completed, a functional appliance can be used to maintain occlusal relationships. In a typical Class II deep bite patient, the lower posterior teeth are allowed to erupt slightly, while other teeth are tightly controlled.

This type of retention is often needed for 12 to 24 months or more in a patient who had a severe skeletal problem initially. The guideline is: the more severe the initial Class II problem and the younger the patient at the end of active treatment, the more likely that either headgear or a functional appliance will be needed as a retainer. It is better to prevent relapse from differential growth than to try to correct it later.

Retention after Class III Correction. Retaining a patient after correcting a Class III malocclusion early in the permanent dentition can be frustrating, because relapse from continuing mandibular growth is very likely to occur and such growth is extremely difficult to control. Applying a restraining force to the mandible, as from a chincap, is not nearly as effective in controlling growth in a Class III patient as applying a restraining force to the maxilla is in Class II problems. As we have noted in previous chapters, a chincap tends to rotate the mandible downward, causing growth to be expressed more vertically and less horizontally, and Class III functional appliances have the same effect. If face height is normal or excessive after orthodontic treatment and relapse occurs from mandibular growth, sur-

gical correction after the growth has expressed itself may be the only answer. In mild Class III problems, a functional appliance or a positioner may be enough to maintain the occlusal relationships during posttreatment growth.

Retention after Deep Bite Correction. Correcting excess overbite is an almost routine part of orthodontic treatment, and therefore the majority of patients require control of the vertical overlap of incisors during retention. This is accomplished most readily by using a removable upper retainer made so that the lower incisors will encounter the baseplate of the retainer if they begin to slip vertically behind the upper incisors (Figure 19-6). The procedure, in other words, is to build a potential bite plate into the retainer, which the lower incisors will contact if the bite begins to deepen. The retainer does not separate the posterior teeth.

Because vertical growth continues into the late teens, a maxillary removable retainer with a bite plane often is needed for several years after fixed appliance orthodontics is completed. Bite depth can be maintained by wearing the retainer only at night, after stability in other regards has been achieved.

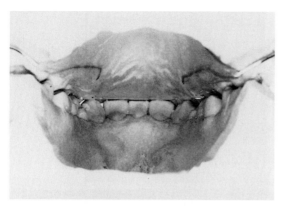

FIGURE 19-6 This view of casts in occlusion, looking from the lingual, shows the biteplate effect of a maxillary retainer. The lower incisors should be just contacting the lingual acrylic of the upper retainer, to prevent deepening of the bite.

Retention after Anterior Open Bite Correction. Relapse into anterior open bite can occur by any combination of depression of the incisors and elongation of the molars. Active habits (of which thumbsucking is the best example) can produce intrusive forces on the incisors, while at the same time leading to an altered posture of the jaw that allows posterior teeth to erupt. If thumbsucking continues after orthodontic treatment, relapse is all but guaranteed. Tongue habits, particularly tongue-thrust swallowing, are often blamed for relapse into open bite, but the evidence to support this contention is not convincing (see discussion in Chapter 5). In patients who do not place some object between the front teeth, return of open bite is almost always the result of elongation of the posterior teeth, particularly the upper molars, without any evidence of intrusion of incisors (Figure 19-7). Controlling eruption of the upper molars therefore is the key to retention in open bite patients.

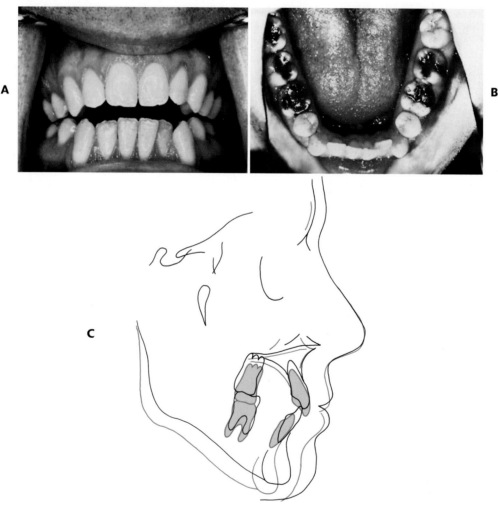

FIGURE 19-7 **A** and **B,** Relapse after comprehensive orthodontic treatment with premolar extraction. Four years after removal of the orthodontic appliances, this 19-year-old has an anterior open bite, 5 mm of overjet with an end-on molar relationship, and severe crowding of the mandibular incisors. Relapse of this type is associated with a downward and backward rotation of the mandible, which is accompanied by excessive eruption of the maxillary posterior teeth. **C,** Cephalometric superimposition showing the pattern of growth associated with this relapse. Note that the increase in both open bite and overjet is related to the downward and backward mandibular rotation, while the incisor crowding is associated with uprighting and lingual repositioning of the incisors as the mandibular rotation thrusts them into the lower lip.

High-pull headgear to the upper molars, in conjunction with a standard removable retainer to maintain tooth position, is one effective way to control open bite relapse (Figure 19-8, *A*). A better tolerated alternative is an appliance with bite blocks between the posterior teeth (an open bite activator or bionator), which stretches the patient's soft tissues to provide a force opposing eruption (Figure 19-8, *B*). Excessive vertical growth and eruption of the posterior teeth often continue until late in the teens or early twenties, making a persistent open bite tendency difficult to control, but this can be accomplished with good patient cooperation over a long enough period.

A patient with a severe open bite problem is particularly likely to benefit from having conventional maxillary and mandibular retainers for daytime wear, and an open bite bionator as a nighttime retainer, from the beginning of the retention period.

Retention of Lower Incisor Alignment. Not only can continued skeletal growth affect occlusal relationships, it has the potential to alter the position of teeth. If the mandible grows forward or rotates downward, the effect is to carry the lower incisors into the lip, which creates a force tipping them distally. For this reason, continued mandibular growth in normal or Class III patients is strongly associated with crowding of the lower incisors (see Figure 19-1). Incisor crowding also accompanies the downward and backward rotation of the mandible seen in skeletal

open bite problems (see Figure 19-7). A retainer in the lower incisor region is needed to prevent crowding from developing, until growth has declined to adult levels.

It often has been suggested that orthodontic retention should be continued, at least on a part-time basis, until the third molars have either erupted into normal occlusion or have been removed. The implication of this guideline, that pressure from the developing third molars causes late incisor crowding, is almost surely incorrect (see Chapter 5). On the other hand, because the eruption of third molars or their extraction usually does not take place until the late teen years, the guideline is not a bad one in its emphasis on prolonged retention in patients who are continuing to grow.

Most adults, including those who had orthodontic treatment and once had perfectly aligned teeth, end up with some crowding of lower incisors. In a group of patients who had first premolar extraction and treatment with the edgewise appliance, only about 30% had perfect alignment 10 years after retainers were removed and nearly 20% had marked crowding.[7] Which individuals would have post-treatment crowding could not be predicted from the characteristics of the original malocclusion or variables associated with treatment. It seems likely that late mandibular growth is the major contributor to this crowding tendency. It makes sense, therefore, to routinely retain lower incisor alignment until mandibular growth has declined to adult levels (i.e., until the late teens in girls and into the early 20s in boys).

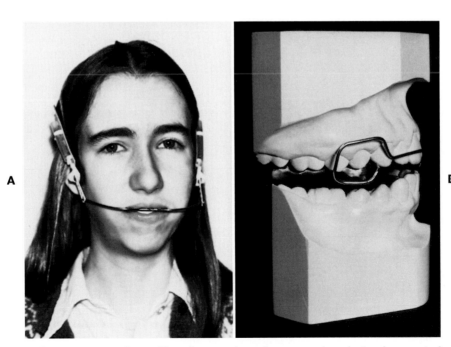

FIGURE 19-8 Controlling the eruption of upper molars during late vertical growth is the key to preventing open-bite relapse. There are two major approaches to accomplishing this: **A,** high-pull headgear, as worn every night by this 16-year-old patient with a long face pattern of growth, to prevent the recurrence of open bite and overjet, and **B,** a functional appliance with bite blocks to impede eruption, continued as a nighttime retainer through the late teens. Although the high-pull headgear can be quite effective in a cooperative patient, the functional appliance is a better choice for most patients, simply because it is easier for the patient to comply.

Timing of Retention: Summary. In summary, retention is needed for all patients who had fixed orthodontic appliances to correct intra-arch irregularities. It should be:

- Essentially full-time for the first 3 to 4 months, except that the retainers not only can but should be removed while eating (unless periodontal bone loss or other special circumstances require permanent splinting)
- Continued on a part-time basis for at least 12 months, to allow time for remodeling of gingival tissues
- If significant growth remains, continued part-time until completion of growth.

For practical purposes, this means that nearly all patients treated in the early permanent dentition will require retention of incisor alignment until the late teens, and in those with skeletal disproportions initially, part-time use of a functional appliance or extraoral force probably will be needed.

REMOVABLE APPLIANCES AS RETAINERS

Removable appliances can serve effectively for retention against intra-arch instability and are also useful as retainers (in the form of modified functional appliances or part-time headgear) in patients with growth problems. If permanent retention is needed, a fixed retainer should be used in most instances, and fixed retainers (see p. 607) are also indicated for intra-arch retention when irregularity in a specific area is likely to be a problem.

Hawley Retainers

By far the most common removable retainer is the Hawley retainer, designed in the 1920s as an active removable appliance. It incorporates clasps on molar teeth and a characteristic outer bow with adjustment loops, spanning from canine to canine (Figure 19-9, *A*). Because it covers the palate, it automatically provides a potential bite plane to control overbite.

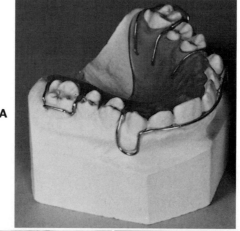

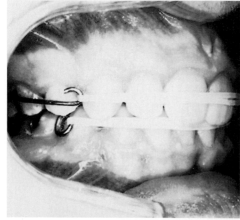

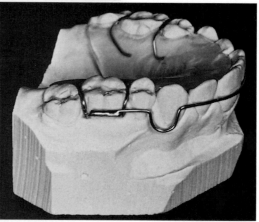

FIGURE 19-9 **A,** A standard maxillary Hawley retainer. Note the canine-to-canine anterior bow, with clasps on the first molars. The anterior bow is the characteristic feature of this retainer design. **B,** Modification of maxillary and mandibular retainers, replacing the Hawley bow with a light elastic across the incisor teeth. This appliance is more esthetic than the standard design but does not give as good control of tooth positions. It is particularly useful when band space must be closed with the retainer, and therefore is rarely used when bonded brackets were employed. **C,** Hawley retainer for premolar extraction patient, with the outer bow soldered to the bridge portion of Adams clasps on the first molars. This design allows the anterior bow to keep the extraction space closed and is usually preferred for extraction cases.

The ability of this retainer to provide some tooth movement was a particular asset with fully banded fixed appliances, since one function of the retainer was to close band spaces between the incisors, and it was sometimes modified to use elastics for this purpose (see Figure 19-9, *B*). With bonded appliances on the anterior teeth or after using a tooth positioner for finishing, there is no longer any need to close spaces with a retainer. However, the outer bow provides excellent control of the incisors even if it is not adjusted to retract them.

When first premolars have been extracted, one function of a retainer is to keep the extraction space closed, which the standard design of the Hawley retainer cannot do. Even worse, the standard Hawley labial bow extends across a first premolar extraction space, tending to wedge it open. A common modification of the Hawley retainer for use in extraction cases is a bow soldered to the buccal section of Adams clasps on the first molars, so that the action of the bow helps hold the extraction site closed (see Figure 19-9, *C*). Alternative designs for extraction cases are to wrap the labial bow around the entire arch, using circumferential clasps on second molars for retention (Figure 19-10); or to bring the labial wire from the baseplate between the lateral incisor and canine and to bend or solder a wire extension distally to control the canines (Figure 19-11). The latter alternative does not provide an active force to keep an extraction space closed, but avoids having the wire cross through the extraction site, and gives positive control of canines that were labially positioned initially (which the loop of the traditional Hawley design may not provide).

The clasp locations for a Hawley retainer must be selected carefully, since clasp wires crossing the occlusal table can disrupt rather than retain the tooth relationships established during treatment. Circumferential clasps on the terminal molar or lingual extension clasps (see Chapter 11) may be preferred over the more effective Adams clasp if the occlusion is tight (see Figure 19-10).

The palatal coverage of a removable plate like the maxillary Hawley retainer makes it possible to incorporate a bite plane lingual to the upper incisors, to control bite depth. For any patient who once had an excessive overbite, light contact of the lower incisors against the baseplate of the retainer is desired.

A Hawley retainer can be made for the upper or lower arch. The lower retainer with the classic Hawley bow is somewhat fragile and may be difficult to insert because of undercuts in the premolar and molar region. If the major reason for lower retention is maintenance of incisor position, a retainer for that region only is a logical alternative, and a wraparound design is preferred.

Removable Wraparound Retainers

A second major type of removable orthodontic retainer is the wraparound or clip-on retainer, which consists of a plastic bar (usually wire-reinforced) along the labial and lingual surfaces of the teeth (Figure 19-12). A full-arch wraparound retainer firmly holds each tooth in position.

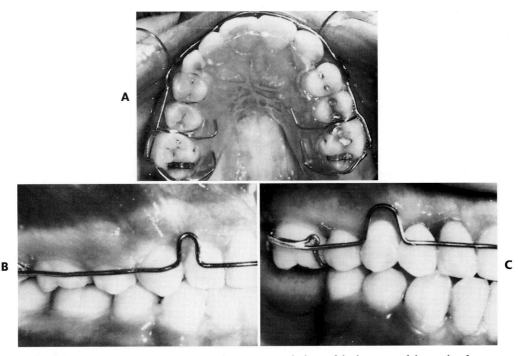

FIGURE 19-10 A wraparound outer bow is particularly useful when one of the goals of retention is to keep extraction spaces closed. **A** and **B,** The bow usually is attached to circumferential clasps on the second molars, but, **C,** also can be soldered to Adams clasps on first molars (note the temporary prosthetic tooth on the retainer in the canine area).

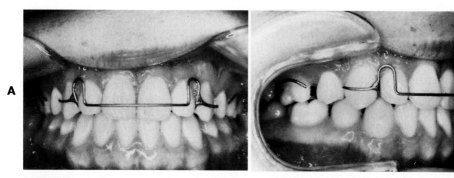

FIGURE 19-11   **A** and **B,** An alternative design for the anterior bow of the retainer, using a distal extension from a short anterior bow to control the maxillary canines. This design is particularly useful when canines were labially positioned initially.

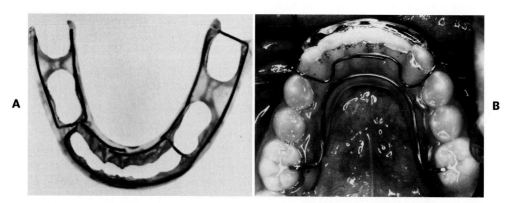

FIGURE 19-12   **A,** A wraparound retainer for the lower arch, out of the mouth, showing the wire reinforcement of the plastic material; **B,** a modified wraparound retainer now often is used in the lower arch, with the wraparound section only used for the anterior segment of the arch.

This is not necessarily an advantage, since one object of a retainer should be to allow each tooth to move individually, stimulating reorganization of the PDL. In addition, a wraparound retainer, though quite esthetic, is often less comfortable than a Hawley retainer and may not be effective in maintaining overbite correction. A full-arch wraparound retainer is indicated primarily when periodontal breakdown requires splinting the teeth together.

A variant of the wraparound retainer, the canine-to-canine clip-on retainer, is widely used in the lower anterior region. This appliance has the great advantage that it can be used to realign irregular incisors, if mild crowding has developed after treatment (see Active Retainers, on p. 610), but it is well tolerated as a retainer alone. An upper canine-to-canine wraparound occasionally is useful in adults with long clinical crowns but rarely is indicated and usually would not be tolerated in younger patients because of occlusal interferences.

In a lower extraction case, usually it is a good idea to extend a canine-to-canine wraparound distally on the lingual only to the central groove of the first molar (see Figure 19-12, *B*). This provides control of the second premolar and the extraction site, but the retainer must be made carefully to avoid lingual undercuts in the premolar and molar region. Posterior extension of the lower retainer, of course, also is indicated when the posterior teeth were irregular before treatment.

Positioners as Retainers.   A tooth positioner also can be used as a removable retainer, either fabricated for this purpose alone, or more commonly, continued as a retainer after serving initially as a finishing device. Positioners are excellent finishing devices and under special circumstances can be used to an advantage as retainers. For routine use, however, a positioner does not make a good retainer. The major problems are:

1. The pattern of wear of a positioner does not match the pattern usually desired for retainers. Because of its bulk, patients often have difficulty wearing a positioner full-time or nearly so. In fact, positioners tend to be worn less than the recommended 4 hours per day after the first few weeks, although they are reasonably well tolerated by most patients during sleep.

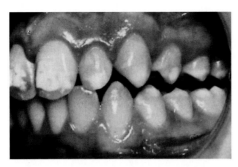

FIGURE 19-13 Separation of the posterior teeth after 3 weeks of intensive positioner wear. This unusual complication results from an incorrect hinge axis in constructing the positioner. A patient wearing a positioner long-term should be observed for problems of this type.

2. Positioners do not retain incisor irregularities and rotations as well as standard retainers. This problem follows directly from the first one: a retainer is needed nearly full-time initially to control intra-arch alignment. Also, overbite tends to increase while a positioner is being worn, and this effect as well probably relates in large part to the fact that it is worn only a small percentage of the time.

A positioner does have one major advantage over a standard removable or wraparound retainer, however—it maintains the occlusal relationships as well as intra-arch tooth positions. For a patient with a tendency toward Class III relapse, a positioner made with the jaws rotated somewhat downward and backward may be useful. Although a positioner with the teeth set in a slightly exaggerated "supernormal" from the original malocclusion can be used for patients with a skeletal Class II or open bite growth pattern, it is less effective in controlling growth than part-time headgear or a functional appliance.

In fabricating a positioner, it is necessary to separate the teeth by 2 to 4 mm. This means that an articulator mounting that records the patient's hinge axis is desirable. As a general guideline, the more the patient deviates from the average normal, and the longer the positioner will be worn, the more important it is to obtain an individualized hinge axis mounting on an adjustable articulator for positioner construction. If a positioner is to be used for only 2 to 4 weeks as a finishing device in a patient who will have some vertical growth during later retention, and if the patient has an approximately normal hinge axis, an individualized articulator mounting may be unnecessary. If a positioner is to be worn for many months as a retainer or if no growth can be anticipated, a precisely correct hinge axis becomes more important.

The usual sign of a positioner made to an incorrect hinge axis is some separation of the posterior teeth when the incisors are in contact (Figure 19-13). Patients wearing a positioner as a retainer should be checked carefully to see that this effect is not occurring.

FIXED RETAINERS

Fixed orthodontic retainers are normally used in situations where intra-arch instability is anticipated and prolonged retention is planned. There are four major indications:

1. Maintenance of lower incisor position during late growth. As has been discussed previously, the major cause of lower incisor crowding in the late teen years, in both patients who have had orthodontic treatment and those who have not, is late growth of the mandible in the normal growth pattern. Especially if the lower incisors have previously been irregular, even a small amount of differential mandibular growth between ages 16 and 20 can cause re-crowding of these teeth. Relapse into crowding is almost always accompanied by lingual tipping of the central and lateral incisors in response to the pattern of growth. An excellent retainer to hold these teeth in alignment is a fixed lingual bar, attached only to the canines (or to canines and first premolars) and resting against the flat lingual surface of the lower incisors above the cingulum (Figure 19-14). This prevents the incisors from moving lingually and is also reasonably effective in maintaining correction of rotations in the incisor segment.

A fixed lingual canine-to-canine retainer can be fabricated with bands on the canines or can be bonded to the lingual surface. A bonded canine-to-canine retainer is preferred for two reasons: (1) unless bands were used during the active treatment, band space can be a problem; and (2) the labial part of a band tends to trap plaque against the cervical part of the labial surface, predisposing this area to decalcification, and is also unsightly.

The fabrication of a bonded canine-to-canine retainer is shown in Figure 19-14. It is attached only to the canines, resting passively against the central and lateral incisors. If the retainer wire is fitted to a cast of the lower arch, a silicone carrier of the type used for indirect bonding of brackets can be made to assist in placing the retainer. An alternative approach is to tie the retainer wire in place with wire ligatures or dental floss around the contacts, to hold it so that it can be bonded.

Fixed canine-to-canine retainers must be made from a wire heavy enough to resist distortion over the rather long span between these teeth. Usually 30 mil steel is used for this purpose (Figure 19-15), with the end of the wire sandblasted to improve retention when it is bonded to the canines.[8]

It is also possible to bond a fixed lingual retainer to one or more of the incisor teeth. The major indication for this variation is a tooth that had been severely rotated. Whatever the type of retainer, however, it is desirable that teeth not be held rigidly during retention. For this reason, if the span of the retainer wire is reduced by bonding an intermediate tooth or teeth, a more flexible wire should be used. A good choice for a fixed retainer with adjacent teeth bonded is a braided steel archwire of 17.5 mil diameter (Figure 19-16).

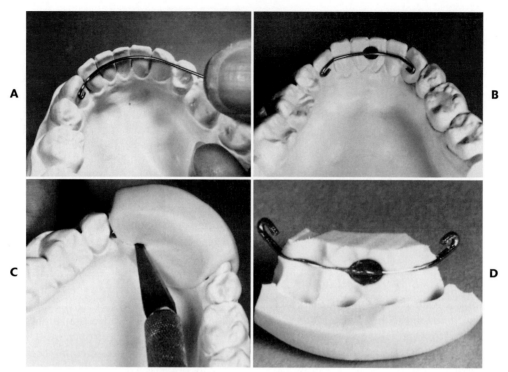

FIGURE 19-14 Steps in the fabrication of a canine-to-canine retainer; **A,** 30 mil steel wire is bent so that it rests against the flat part of the lingual surface of the incisors, with a loop over the cingulum of the canines; **B,** the wire is held in place with candy adhesive; **C,** a silicone carrier material is mixed, placed over the incisors, and trimmed; **D,** wire in place in the carrier, ready to be carried to the mouth for binding. The loop at the ends of the wire now often is replaced with a sandblasted end section (see Figure 19-15, *B*).

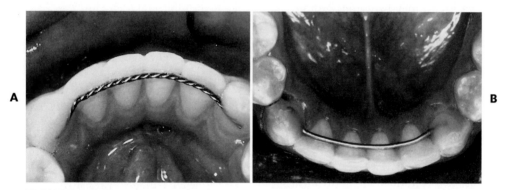

FIGURE 19-15 **A,** A bonded canine-to-canine retainer made from a twist wire, which improves retention of the bonding material. 28 mil wire is recommended if only the canines are to be bonded. If the incisors are bonded, a lighter wire should be used. Heavy twist wire no longer is recommended for canine-to-canine retainers because it has proved not rigid enough. **B,** The preferred canine-to-canine bonded retainer now is made from 30 mil steel wire with sandblasted ends. Roughening the ends of the wire in this way provides excellent retention for the bonding material, without the bulk of wire loops.

2. Diastema maintenance. A second indication for a fixed retainer is a situation where teeth must be permanently or semipermanently bonded together to maintain the closure of a space between them. This is encountered most commonly when a diastema between maxillary central incisors has been closed. Even if a frenectomy has been carried out (see Chapters 7 and 17), there is a tendency for a small space to open up between the upper central incisors. Since this is unsightly, prolonged or permanent retention usually is needed.

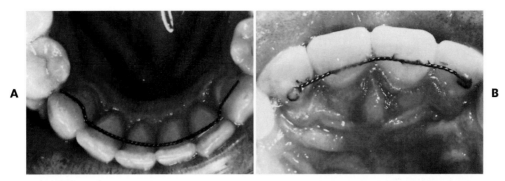

FIGURE 19-16   A fixed lingual retainer bonded to several anterior teeth. If multiple teeth are bonded, a lighter wire, such as the 17.5 mil (3 × 8) twist wire shown here, should be used to prevent splinting the teeth too rigidly. **A,** Mandibular incisor retainer, with the wire lightly bonded to the canines, before the incisors are bonded; **B,** completed maxillary retainer, with all four incisors bonded.

The best retainer for this purpose is a bonded section of flexible wire, as shown in Figure 19-17. The wire should be contoured so that it lies near the cingulum to keep it out of occlusal contact. The object of the retainer is to hold the teeth together while allowing them some ability to move independently during function, hence the importance of a flexible wire.

A removable retainer is not a good choice for prolonged retention of a central diastema. In troublesome cases, the diastema is closed when the retainer is removed but opens up quickly. The tooth movement that accompanies this back-and-forth closure is potentially damaging over a long period.

3. Maintenance of pontic or implant space. A fixed retainer is also the best choice to maintain a space where a bridge pontic or implant eventually will be placed. Using a fixed retainer for a few months reduces mobility of the teeth and often makes it easier to place the fixed bridge that will serve, among other functions, as a permanent orthodontic retainer. If further periodontal therapy is needed after the teeth have been positioned, several months or even years can pass before a bridge is placed, and a fixed retainer is definitely required. Implants should be placed as soon as possible after the orthodontics is completed, so that integration of the implant can occur simultaneously with the initial stages of retention.

The preferred orthodontic retainer for maintaining space for posterior restorations is a heavy intra-coronal wire, bonded in shallow preparations in the future abutment teeth (Figure 19-18). Obviously, the longer the span, the heavier the wire should be. Bringing the wire down out of occlusion decreases the chance that it will be displaced by occlusal forces.

Anterior spaces need a replacement tooth, which can be attached to a removable retainer. This approach guarantees nearly full-time wear and is satisfactory for short periods. Often a better alternative is a fixed retainer in the form of a simple acid-etch bridge, such as a replacement

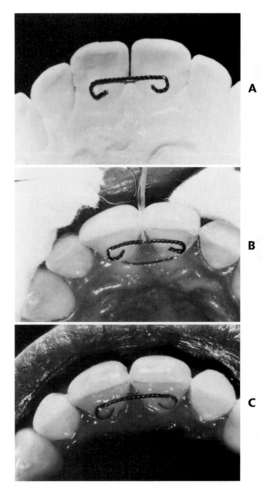

FIGURE 19-17   Bonded lingual retainer for maintenance of a maxillary central diastema. **A,** 17.5 mil twist wire contoured to fit passively on the dental case; **B,** a wire ligature is passed around the necks of the teeth to hold them tightly together while they are bonded. The wire retainer is held in place with dental floss passed around the contact, and composite resin is flowed onto to the cingulum of the teeth, over the wire ends. **C,** The finished retainer. Note that the retainer is up on the cingulum, to avoid occlusal interference with the lower incisors.

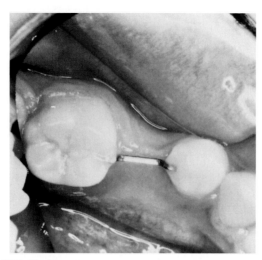

FIGURE 19-18 Fixed retainer to maintain space for a missing second premolar. A shallow preparation has been made in the enamel of the marginal ridges adjacent to the extraction site, and a section of 21 × 25 wire is bonded as a retainer.

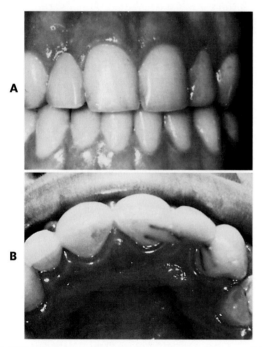

FIGURE 19-19 Bonded bridge using segments of braided orthodontic wire to attach the pontic to the abutment tooth. **A,** Frontal view; **B,** occlusal view in mirror showing the bonded attachment. This type of inexpensive fixed retainer is preferred over a removable retainer with a replacement tooth.

tooth held by twist wires bonded to adjacent teeth (Figure 19-19). If a healing implant is in the area, or if a permanent bridge will be delayed for a long time, a temporary bonded bridge decreases the chance of soft tissue inflammation and provides better stability.

4. Keeping extraction spaces closed in adults (Figure 19-20). A fixed retainer is both more reliable and better tol-

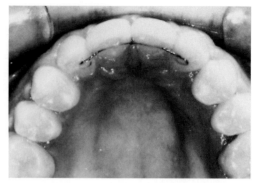

FIGURE 19-20 In the adult with missing maxillary lateral incisors in whom the space was closed and the canines substituted for the laterals, a bonded retainer maintains the space closure. Note the use of 17.5 mil multistrand steel wire bonded to each tooth. A removable retainer worn part-time is less acceptable to the patient and less successful in keeping the space closed than this type of fixed retainer.

erated than a full-time removable retainer, and spaces reopen unless a retainer is worn consistently. It may be better in adults to bond a fixed retainer on the facial surface of posterior teeth when spaces have been closed.

The major objection to any fixed retainer is that it makes interproximal hygiene procedures more difficult. It is possible to floss between teeth that have a fixed retainer in place by using a floss-threading device. With proper flossing, there is no reason that fixed retainers, if needed, cannot be left in place indefinitely.

ACTIVE RETAINERS

"Active retainer" is a contradiction in terms, since a device cannot be actively moving teeth and serving as a retainer at the same time. It does happen, however, that relapse or growth changes after orthodontic treatment will lead to a need for some tooth movement during retention. This usually is accomplished with a removable appliance that continues as a retainer after it has repositioned the teeth, hence the name. A typical Hawley retainer, if used initially to close a small amount of band space, can be considered an active retainer, but the term usually is reserved for two specific situations: realignment of irregular incisors, and functional appliances to manage Class II or Class III relapse tendencies.

Realignment of Irregular Incisors: Spring Retainers

Recrowding of lower incisors is the major indication for an active retainer to correct incisor position. If late crowding has developed, it often is necessary to reduce the interproximal width of lower incisors before realigning them, so that the crowns do not tip labially into an obviously unstable position. The cause of the problem in

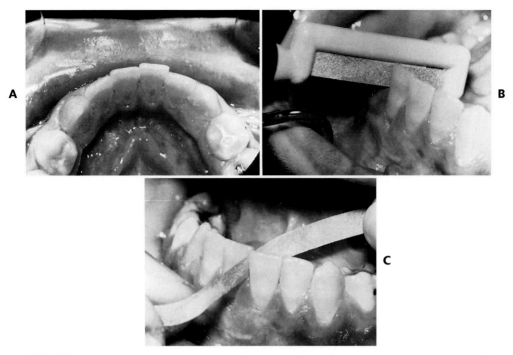

FIGURE 19-21 Stripping of lower incisors to reduce mesiodistal width. **A,** Incisor irregularity before realignment; **B,** interproximal enamel being removed with a relatively coarse steel-backed abrasive strip mounted in a modified electric tooth brush; **C,** enamel surface being polished with a sequence of plastic-backed strips with finer abrasives. Topical fluoride should be applied immediately after stripping procedures.

these cases usually is late mandibular growth, which has uprighted the incisors, and they must be realigned in their more upright position. Not only does stripping of contacts reduce the mesiodistal width of the incisors, decreasing the amount of space required for their alignment, it also flattens the contact areas, increasing the inherent stability of the arch in this region. As with any procedure involving the modification of teeth, however, stripping must be done cautiously and judiciously. It is not indicated as a routine procedure.[9]

Interproximal enamel can be removed with either abrasive strips (Figure 19-21) or thin discs in a handpiece. Obviously, enamel reduction should not be overdone, but if necessary, the width of each lower incisor can be reduced up to 0.5 mm on each side without going through the interproximal enamel. If an additional 2 mm of space can be gained, reducing each incisor 0.25 mm per side, it is usually possible to realign typically crowded incisors.

If the irregularity is modest and if the teeth are to be realigned without moving facially, a canine-to-canine clip-on is usually the active retainer used to realign crowded incisors. The steps in making such an active retainer are: (1) reduce the interproximal width of the incisors and apply topical fluoride to the newly exposed enamel surfaces; (2) prepare a laboratory model, on which the teeth can be reset into alignment; and (3) fabricate a canine-to-canine clip-on appliance (Figure 19-22).

If there is more than a modest degree of relapse, however, placing a fixed appliance for comprehensive retreatment must be considered. With bonded brackets on the lower arch from premolar to premolar, superelastic NiTi wires can be used to bring the incisors back into alignment quite efficiently (Figure 19-23). If the incisors are advanced toward the lip when this is done, a bonded lingual retainer should be placed before the brackets are removed. Permanent retention obviously will be required after the realignment.

Correction of Occlusal Discrepancies: Modified Functional Appliances as Active Retainers

It is possible to describe an activator as consisting of maxillary and mandibular retainers joined by an interocclusal bite block. Although even the simplest activator is more complex than that (see Chapter 15), the description does illustrate the potential of an activator to simultaneously maintain the position of teeth within the arches while altering, at least minimally, the occlusal relationships.

A typical use for an activator as an active retainer would be a male adolescent who had slipped back 2 to 3 mm toward a Class II relationship after early correction. If he still is experiencing some vertical growth (and almost all adolescents fall into this category, even at age 17 or 18), it may

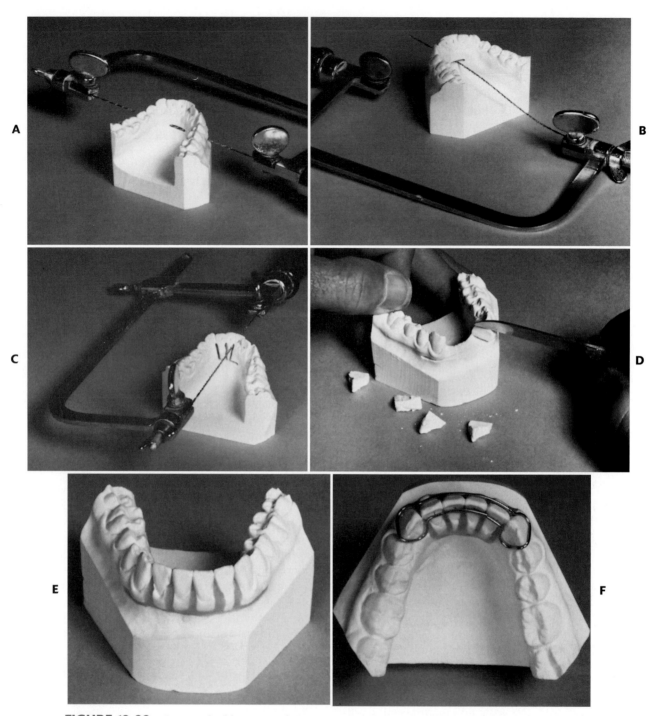

FIGURE 19-22   Steps in the fabrication of a canine-to-canine clip-on appliance to realign lower incisors. **A,** After the teeth have been stripped appropriately, an impression is made for a laboratory cast. A saw-cut is made beneath the teeth through the alveolar process to the distal of the lateral incisors; **B,** the saw blade is then passed from front to back beneath the incisors; **C,** cuts are made up to but not through the contact points; **D,** the incisor teeth are broken off the cast and broken apart at the contact points, creating individual dies, and the cast is trimmed to provide space for resetting the teeth; **E,** the teeth are reset in wax in proper alignment; **F,** 28 mil steel wire is contoured around the labial and lingual surface of the teeth as shown, with the wire overlapping behind the central incisors.   *continued*

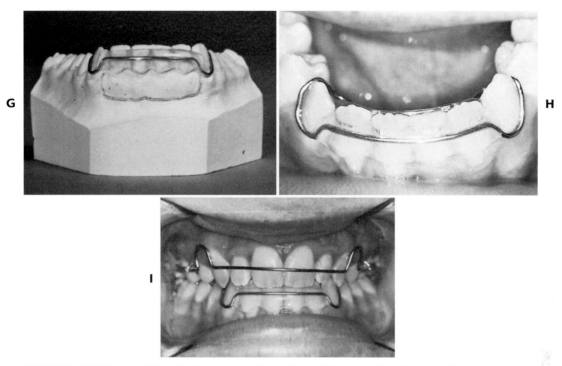

FIGURE 19-22, cont'd   G, A covering of acrylic is added over the wire, completing the retainer; **H,** occlusal view of completed retainer; **I,** facial view, showing the upper and lower retainers for this patient who had premolar extraction for correction of crowded and irregular incisors.

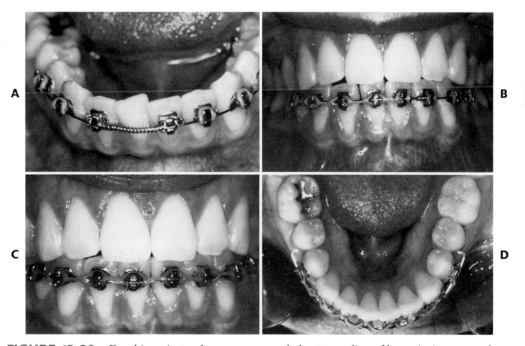

FIGURE 19-23   For this patient, who was concerned about crowding of lower incisors several years after orthodontic treatment, excessive stripping of interproximal enamel would have been required to gain realignment with a clip-on removable appliance. A partial fixed appliance with bonded brackets only on the segment to be realigned is the most practical approach. **A,** Bonded appliance in from first premolar to first premolar, with a coil spring on 16 steel wire to open space for the rotated and crowded right central incisor; **B** and **C,** Alignment of the incisors on rectangular NiTi wire after space is opened; **D,** Re-alignment completed 4 months after treatment began. At this point either a bonded lingual retainer or a new removable retainer, to be worn indefinitely, is required.

be possible to recover the proper occlusal position of the teeth. Differential anteroposterior growth is not necessary to correct a small occlusal discrepancy—tooth movement is adequate—but some vertical growth is required to prevent downward and backward rotation of the mandible. For all practical purposes, this means that a functional appliance as an active retainer can be used in teenagers but is of no value in adults. Stimulating skeletal growth with a device of this type simply does not happen in adults, at least to a clinically useful extent.

The use of an activator as an active retainer differs somewhat from its use to guide skeletal growth during the mixed dentition or when it is used as a pure retainer. In the latter circumstances, the object is to control growth, and tooth movement is largely an undesirable side effect. In contrast, an activator as an active retainer is expected primarily to move teeth—no significant skeletal change is expected. An activator as an active retainer is not indicated if more than 3 mm of occlusal correction is sought, and over this distance, tooth movement as a means of correction is a possibility. The correction is achieved by restraining the eruption of maxillary teeth posteriorly and directing the erupting mandibular teeth anteriorly.

Any of the family of modified activators designed to produce tooth movement is most useful in this active-retention mode, not in early mixed dentition treatment where tooth movement for the most part is undesirable. On the other hand, the more flexible a removable appliance becomes, the less suited it is for the retention part of active retention and the more likely it would be to require replacement with another type of retainer when the occlusal relationship had been reestablished. An activator or bionator with an acrylic framework that contacts most teeth therefore is usually the best compromise when this type of active retention is needed. The appliance is made like any other functional appliance, with a slight advancement of the mandible into the correct occlusal relationship. In contrast to a functional appliance that would be placed as a retainer immediately upon completion of active treatment, some freedom of eruption for posterior teeth normally would be provided.

REFERENCES

1. Blake M, Bibby K: Retention and stability: a review of the literature, Am J Orthod Dentofac Orthop 114:299-306, 1998.
2. Reitan K: Principles of retention and avoidance of post-treatment relapse, Am J Orthod 55:776-790, 1969.
3. Reitan K: Tissue rearrangement during the retention of orthodontically rotated teeth, Angle Orthod 29:105-113, 1959.
4. Edwards JG: A long-term prospective evaluation of the circumferential supracrestal fiberotomy in alleviating orthodontic relapse, Am J Orthod Dentofac Orthop 93:380-387, 1988.
5. Behrents RG: A treatise on the continuum of growth in the aging craniofacial skeleton, Ann Arbor, Mich., 1984, University of Michigan Center for Human Growth and Development.
6. Nanda RS, Nanda SK: Considerations of dentofacial growth in long-term retention and stability: is active rentention needed, Am J Orthod Dentofac Orthop 101:297-302, 1992.
7. Little RM, Wallen TR, Riedel RA: Stability and relapse of mandibular incisor alignment—first premolar extraction cases treated by traditional edgewise orthodontics, Am J Orthod 80:349-365, 1981.
8. Zachrisson BU: Bonding in orthodontics. In Graber TM, Vanarsdall RL (editors): Orthodontics: current principles and techniques, ed 3, St Louis, in press, Mosby.
9. Gilmore CA, Little RM: Mandibular incisor dimensions and crowding, Am J Orthod 86:493-502, 1984.

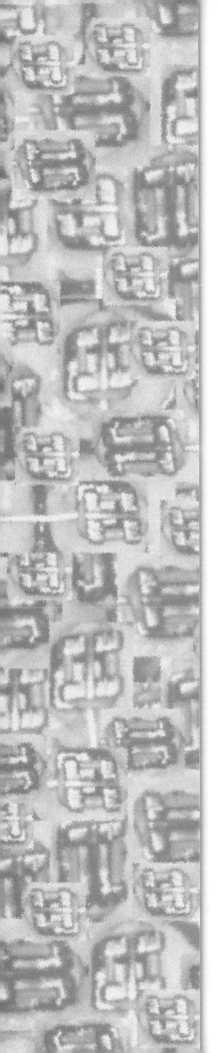

SECTION VIII

TREATMENT FOR ADULTS

Adults who seek orthodontic treatment fall into two quite different groups: (1) younger adults (typically under 35, often in their 20s) who desired but did not receive orthodontic treatment as youths, and now seek it as they become financially independent; and (2) an older group, typically in their 40s or 50s, who have other dental problems and need orthodontics as part of a larger treatment plan. For the first group, the goal is to improve their quality of life. They usually seek comprehensive treatment and the maximum improvement that is possible. They may or may not need coordinated treatment with other dental specialists. The second group seek to maintain what they have, not necessarily to achieve as ideal a result as possible. For them, orthodontic treatment is needed to meet specific goals that would make control of dental disease and restoration of missing teeth easier and more effective, so the orthodontics is an adjunctive procedure to the larger periodontal and restorative goals. Until recently, the younger group have comprised most adult orthodontic patients. Because of the large number of aging "baby boomers" born during the immediate post-World War II era, one can confidently predict that there will be increasing demand for orthodontics from the second group in the early part of the new century.

Adjunctive orthodontic treatment, particularly the simpler procedures, often can and should be carried out within the context of general dental practice, and Chapter 20 is written with that in mind. The discussion in this chapter does not require familiarity with the principles of comprehensive orthodontic treatment, but it does presume an understanding of orthodontic diagnosis and treatment planning. In contrast, the discussion of comprehensive treatment for adults in Chapter 21 builds on the principles discussed in Chapters 16 to 19 and focuses on the aspects of comprehensive treatment for adults that are different from treatment for younger patients. Comprehensive orthodontics for adults tends to be difficult and technically demanding. The absence of growth means that growth modification to treat jaw discrepancies is not possible. The only possibilities are tooth movement for camouflage or orthognathic surgery. Chapter 22, dealing with orthognathic surgery, emphasizes the indications for this type of treatment and the principles that guide the treatment of patients with these complex problems.

CHAPTER

20

Adjunctive Treatment for Adults

THE GOALS OF ADJUNCTIVE TREATMENT

Adjunctive orthodontic treatment is, by definition, tooth movement carried out to facilitate other dental procedures necessary to control disease and restore function. Although malocclusion as classically described is not necessarily an unhealthy condition, some tooth positions are not conducive to long-term oral health. This can be understood best by reference to Amsterdam's concepts of physiologic vs. pathologic occlusion.[1] A physiologic occlusion, although not necessarily an ideal or Class I occlusion, is one that adapts to the stress of function and can be maintained indefinitely, whereas a pathologic occlusion cannot function without contributing to its own destruction. If any of the signs of pathologic occlusion exist, or if restorations needed for other problems would prevent adequate plaque clearance or overstress the support apparatus (e.g., overcontoured anterior crowns to close an unattractive space or a posterior bridge on poorly positioned abutments), then tooth movement should become a part of the overall treatment plan.

Typically, adjunctive orthodontic treatment will involve any or all of several procedures: (1) repositioning teeth that have drifted after extractions or bone loss so that more ideal fixed or removable partial dentures can be fabricated, or so that implants can be placed; (2) forced eruption of badly broken down teeth to expose sound root structure on which to place crowns; (3) alignment of anterior teeth to allow more esthetic restorations or successful splinting, while maintaining good interproximal bone contour and embrasure form; and (4) correction of crossbites if these compromise jaw function (not all do).

Whatever the occlusal status originally, the goals of adjunctive treatment should be to:

- Facilitate restorative treatment by positioning the teeth so that more ideal and conservative techniques (including implants) can be used
- Improve periodontal health by eliminating plaque-harboring areas and improving the alveolar ridge contour adjacent to the teeth
- Establish favorable crown-to-root ratios and position the teeth so that occlusal forces are transmitted along the long axes of the teeth

Adjunctive treatment implies limited orthodontic goals, improving a particular aspect of the occlusion rather than comprehensively altering it. Typically, appliances are required in only a portion of the dental arch and for only a short time. Orthodontic treatment for temporomandibular dysfunction should not be considered adjunctive treatment. Admittedly, the boundary between adjunctive and comprehensive treatment is somewhat indistinct. We consider treatment that requires a complete fixed appliance or that is complex enough to require more than 6 months for completion to be comprehensive, and such treatment is discussed in the next chapter. Treatment with a partial fixed appliance that can be completed in less than 6 months typically is adjunctive. With the distinction made in this way, most of the adjunctive treatment discussed in this chapter can be carried out within the context of general dental practice. Whether one or several practitioners are involved, adjunctive orthodontics must be coordinated carefully with the periodontal and restorative treatment.

PRINCIPLES OF ADJUNCTIVE TREATMENT

Diagnostic and Treatment Planning Considerations

Planning for adjunctive treatment requires two steps: (1) collecting an adequate data base and (2) developing a comprehensive but clearly stated list of the patient's problems, taking care not to focus unduly on any one aspect of a complex situation. The importance of this planning stage in adjunctive orthodontic treatment cannot be overemphasized, since the solution to the specific problems may involve the synthesis of many branches of dentistry.

The steps outlined in Chapter 6 should be followed when developing the problem list. The interview and clinical examination are the same, whatever the type of orthodontic treatment. Diagnostic records for adjunctive orthodontic patients, however, differ in several important ways from those for children. For this adult and dentally compromised population, the records usually should include individual intra-oral radiographs to supplement the panoramic film that often suffices for younger and healthier patients

(Figure 20-1). The panoramic radiograph usually does not give sufficient detail. The guidelines promulgated by the U.S. Public Health Service in 1988 (see Chapter 6) should be followed in determining exactly what radiographs are required in evaluating the patient's oral health status. For adjunctive orthodontics, pre-treatment cephalometric radiographs usually are not required, but it is important to anticipate the impact of various tooth movements on facial esthetics. In some instances, the computer prediction methods used in comprehensive treatment (see Chapter 7) can be quite useful in planning adjunctive treatment.

As for any orthodontic treatment, patients who need adjunctive orthodontics should have dental casts made from impressions that have been fully extended so that not only the crown positions and inclination of the teeth but also the contour of the supporting alveolar bone can be seen clearly. Articulator-mounted cases are more likely to be required if extensive restorative procedures are contemplated or if there are other reasons to suspect pathologic occlusion.

Once all the problems have been identified and categorized, the key treatment planning question is: Can the occlusion be restored within the existing tooth positions, or

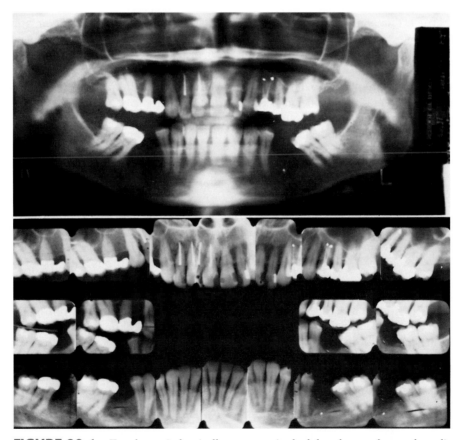

FIGURE 20-1 For the periodontically compromised adults who are the usual candidates for adjunctive orthodontics, periapical radiographs of the areas that will be treated, as well as a panoramic radiograph, usually are needed. Periodontal disease now is the major indication for periapical radiographs. For this patient who is a candidate for adjunctive orthodontic treatment, adequate detail of root morphology, dental disease and periodontal breakdown is obtained only from carefully taken periapical radiographs.

must some teeth be moved to achieve a satisfactory, stable, healthy, and esthetic result? The goal of adjunctive treatment is to provide a physiologic occlusion and facilitate other dental treatment and has little to do with Angle's concept of an ideal tooth relationship.

Possible tooth movements in adjunctive treatment include mesial or distal movement of specific crowns, roots, or both; correction of axial inclination of drifted teeth; correction of the buccolingual position of certain teeth; correction of rotations; and vertical movements of individual teeth. Although intrusion of teeth can be an important part of comprehensive treatment for adults (see Chapter 21), it should be avoided as an adjunctive procedure because of the technical difficulties involved and the possibility of periodontal complications. As a general rule for adjunctive treatment, teeth that are excessively extruded are best treated by reduction of crown height, which has the added advantage of improving the ultimate crown-to-root ratio of the teeth.

Obviously, the time needed for any orthodontic treatment depends on the severity of the problem and the amount of tooth movement desired, but with efficient use of orthodontic appliances, it should be possible to reach the objectives of any adjunctive treatment within six months. As a practical matter, this means that like comprehensive orthodontics, most adjunctive orthodontics requires fixed appliances to get the job done in a reasonable period of time.

Biomechanical Considerations

Characteristics of the Orthodontic Appliance.   In general, control of anchorage requires that anchor teeth not be allowed to tip. This is a major reason that adjunctive tooth movement usually requires a fixed appliance. For adjunctive orthodontic treatment, we recommend the 22-slot edgewise appliance with twin brackets (one-half the width of the crown). The rectangular (edgewise) bracket slot permits control of buccolingual axial inclinations, the relatively wide bracket helps control undesirable rotations and tipping, and the larger slot size allows the use of stabilizing wires that are somewhat stiffer than ordinarily might be used in comprehensive treatment.

Adults traditionally have been somewhat reluctant to wear obvious fixed appliances and often request a removable appliance. However, these appliances are rarely satisfactory for adjunctive (or comprehensive) treatment. Removable appliances make control of root position extremely difficult (see Chapter 10), and it also is difficult to correct rotations at the same time the crown of a tooth is repositioned (Figure 20-2). In addition, removable appliances at best are worn only part of the time. Intermittent forces, though capable of producing tooth movement, are not as efficient as continuous forces, particularly in the presence of occlusal interferences. Discomfort and interference with speech and mastication are far less with a carefully designed and placed fixed appliance than with most removable appliances. In nearly all cases, if the patient is convinced of the importance of treatment, resistance to fixed appliances is minimal.

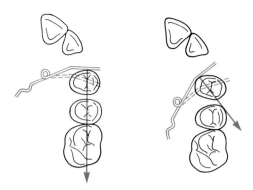

FIGURE 20-2   The direction of tooth movement is always at right angles to the initial contact of a fingerspring on a removable appliance, thus control of tooth position and correction of rotations can be extremely difficult. On the right, applying the spring so that the premolar rotation would improve carries the tooth buccally.

Removable appliances, however, may have an advantage over fixed appliances for some patients with multiple missing teeth. They permit the reaction forces from tooth movement to be spread over adjacent supporting tissues such as the palatal vault and alveolar mucosa as well as the anchor teeth. If many teeth are missing, this approach may be the only way to generate sufficient anchorage.

Modern edgewise brackets of the straight wire type (see Chapter 12) are designed for a specific location on an individual tooth. With the brackets in this position, a rectangular wire bent to ideal arch form, if deflected and fully engaged into the bracket slot, theoretically would produce a force system to move the teeth into an ideal relationship with correct tip, torque, and rotations. For an ideal patient, it would not be necessary to include first-, second-, and third-order bends in the wire, thus the "straight wire" name. If the teeth were severely malposed, of course, a large rectangular wire that would completely fill the bracket slot would be too stiff to use initially, and a series of progressively stiffer archwires would be required to obtain the ideal tooth positions.

Placing the bracket in its ideal position on each tooth implies that every tooth will be repositioned if necessary to achieve ideal occlusion. Since adjunctive treatment is concerned with only limited tooth movements, usually it is neither necessary nor desirable to alter the position of every tooth in the arch. For this reason, in a partial fixed appliance for adjunctive treatment, the brackets are placed in an ideal position only on teeth to be moved, and the remaining teeth to be incorporated in the anchor system are bracketed so that the archwire slots are closely aligned (Figure 20-3). This allows the anchorage segments of the wire to be engaged passively in the brackets with little bending. Passive engagement of wires to anchor teeth produces minimal disturbance of teeth that are in a physiologically satisfactory position. This important point is illustrated in more detail in the sections on specific treatment procedures that follow.

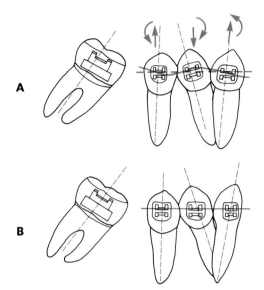

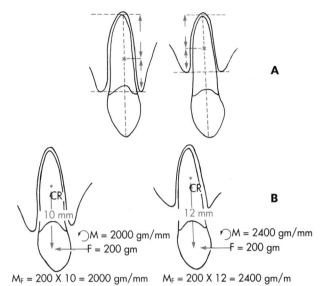

$$M_F = 200 \times 10 = 2000 \text{ gm/mm} \qquad M_F = 200 \times 12 = 2400 \text{ gm/m}$$

FIGURE 20-3 **A,** Brackets placed in the "ideal" position on the anchor teeth. Placement of a straight length of wire will cause uprighting of the anterior teeth as the brackets are brought into alignment. For adjunctive orthodontic treatment, movement of the anchor teeth is often undesirable. **B,** Brackets placed in the position of maximum convenience. Placement of a straight length of wire will maintain the existing bracket and hence tooth alignment. If a rectangular wire is used that closely fits the bracket slot and the brackets are not in the ideal position, the buccolingual position of the teeth can be changed. We recommend the use of fully adjusted "straight wire" brackets and working archwires that are somewhat smaller than the bracket slot, to reduce unwanted buccolingual movement of anchor teeth.

FIGURE 20-4 **A,** The center of resistance of a single rooted tooth lies approximately six-tenths of the distance between the apex of the tooth and the crest of the alveolar bone. Loss of alveolar bone height, as for the tooth on the right, leads to apical relocation of the center of resistance. **B,** The magnitude of the tipping moment produced by a force is equal to the force times the distance from the point of force application to the center of resistance. If the center of resistance moves apically, the tipping moment produced by the force (M_F) increases, and a larger countervailing moment produced by a couple applied to the tooth (M_C) would be necessary to effect bodily movement. This is almost impossible with a removable appliance—for all practical purposes, a fixed appliance is required (see Chapter 10 for more detail).

Effects of Reduced Periodontal Support. Since patients who need adjunctive orthodontic treatment often have periodontal problems, the amount of bone support of each tooth is an important special consideration. When bone has been lost, the periodontal ligament (PDL) area decreases, and the same force against the crown produces greater pressure in the PDL of a periodontally compromised tooth than a normally supported one. The absolute magnitude of force used to move teeth must be reduced when periodontal support has been lost (see Figure 21-13). In addition, the greater the loss of attachment, the smaller the area of supported root and the further apical the center of resistance will become (Figure 20-4).[2] This affects the moments created by forces applied to the crown and the moments needed to control root movement (see Chapter 10). In general terms, tooth movement is quite possible despite bone loss, but lighter forces and relatively larger moments are needed.

Timing and Sequence of Treatment (Figure 20-5)

After the development of a comprehensive treatment plan, the first step is the control of any active dental disease. Before any tooth movement, active caries and pulpal pathology must be eliminated, using extractions, restorative procedures, and pulpal or apical treatment as neces-

sary. Endodontically treated teeth respond normally to orthodontic force, providing all residual chronic inflammation has been eliminated.[3] Prior to orthodontics, teeth should be restored with well-placed amalgams or composite resins. Restorations requiring detailed occlusal anatomy should not be placed until any adjunctive orthodontic treatment has been completed, because the occlusal relationships will inevitably be changed by orthodontic tooth movement, and this could necessitate remaking crowns, bridges or removable partial dentures.

Periodontal disease also must be controlled before any orthodontics begins, because orthodontic tooth movement superimposed on poorly controlled periodontal health can lead to rapid and irreversible breakdown of the periodontal support apparatus.[4] A period of up to 6 months may be needed to allow healing and resolution of inflammation before tooth movement begins. Scaling, curettage (by open flap procedures, if necessary), and gingival grafts should be undertaken as appropriate, before any tooth movement is done. Surgical pocket elimination and osseous surgery should be delayed until completion of the orthodontic phase of treatment, because a significant amount of soft tissue and bone recontouring occurs during orthodontic tooth movement. Clinical studies have shown that orthodontic treatment of adults with both normal and compromised periodontal tissues can be

TREATMENT SEQUENCE: COMPLEX PROBLEMS

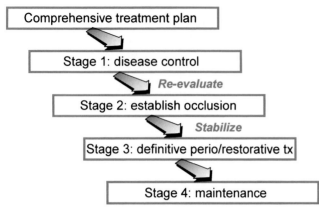

FIGURE 20-5   The sequence of steps in the treatment of patients requiring adjunctive orthodontics. Orthodontics is used to establish occlusion, but only after disease control has been accomplished, and the occlusion should be stabilized before definitive restorative treatment is carried out.

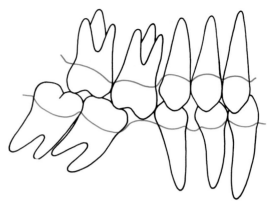

FIGURE 20-6   Loss of a lower molar can lead to tipping and drifting of adjacent teeth, poor interproximal contacts, poor gingival contour, reduced interradicular bone, and supra-eruption of unopposed teeth. Since the bone contour follows the cementoenamel junction, pseudopockets form adjacent to the tipped teeth.

completed without loss of attachment, providing there is good periodontal therapy both initially and during tooth movement.[5,6]

During this preparatory phase, the patient's enthusiasm for treatment and ability to achieve and maintain good overall oral hygiene should be carefully monitored. Repositioning the teeth and attempting to restore the occlusion of patients who are insufficiently motivated to maintain good oral hygiene are doomed to failure. However, if the disease process can be controlled and the patient has demonstrated that he or she is prepared to undergo the necessary treatment, adjunctive orthodontic tooth movement can significantly improve the final restorative and periodontal procedures.

ADJUNCTIVE TREATMENT PROCEDURES

Uprighting Posterior Teeth

Treatment Planning Considerations.   Loss of posterior teeth, usually first permanent molars, is a frequent problem in adults. When a posterior tooth is lost, the adjacent teeth usually tip, drift, and rotate. As the teeth move, the adjacent gingival tissue becomes folded and distorted, forming a plaque-harboring pseudopocket that may be virtually impossible for the patient to clean. The elimination of potentially pathologic conditions associated with tipped molars is probably the most important procedure in adjunctive orthodontics and has the added advantage of simplifying the ultimate restorative procedures (Figure 20-6).

When planning molar uprighting, a number of interrelated questions must be answered. The first is, if the third

molar is present, whether both the second and third molars should be uprighted. For many patients, distal positioning of the third molar would move this tooth into a position where good hygiene could not be maintained, or the uprighted third molar would not be in functional occlusion. In these circumstances, it is more appropriate to extract the third molar and simply upright the remaining second molar tooth. If both molars are to be uprighted, a significant change in technique is required, as described below.

The second question is whether to upright the tipped teeth by distal crown movement (tipping), which would increase the space available for a later pontic, or by mesial root movement, which would reduce or even close the edentulous space (Figure 20-7). This decision will depend on the position of the opposing teeth, the occlusion desired, the anchorage available, and perhaps most importantly, the contour of the bone in the edentulous ridge area. If extensive ridge resorption has already occurred, particularly in the buccolingual dimension (Figure 20-8), mesial movement of a wide molar root into the narrow alveolar ridge will proceed very slowly, and can result in a dehiscence of bone from the mesial, buccal, and lingual root surfaces. Most individuals who need molar uprighting lost their first molars many years previously, and ridge resorption already has occurred. Total space closure for these patients is almost impossible to achieve and maintain. In general, distal crown tipping for uprighting molars is preferred over mesial root movement, but either way, attention must be paid to obtaining a correct axial inclination of the molar. The molar and premolar roots should be parallel or nearly so before a bridge (or implant) is placed.

The third question is whether slight extrusion of a tipped molar is permissible or whether the existing occlusal height must be maintained as the uprighting occurs. Tipping a tooth distally generally extrudes it. This has the merit of reducing the depth of the pseudopocket found on

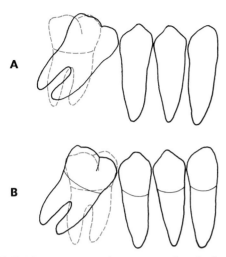

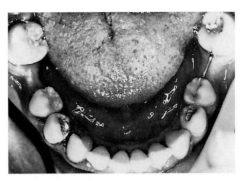

FIGURE 20-7 **A,** Uprighting a tipped molar by distal crown movement leads to increased pontic space, whereas, **B,** uprighting the molar by mesial root movement reduces pontic space and might eliminate the need for a prosthesis—but this can be very difficult, especially if the alveolar bone has resorbed in the area where a first molar was extracted many years previously.

FIGURE 20-8 Loss of the first molar has led to resorption of the alveolar ridge in the edentulous space. The second molars have been uprighted by distal crown tipping since attempts to move the roots mesially would almost certainly have resulted in a dehiscence of bone on the mesiolingual root. Note the teeth on the right side prepared for a stabilizing splint, which has been bonded in place on the left side.

the mesial surface, and since the attached gingiva follows the cementoenamel junction while the mucogingival junction remains stable, it also increases the width of the keratinized tissue in that area. In addition, if the height of the clinical crown is systematically reduced as uprighting proceeds, the ultimate crown-root length ratio will be improved (Figure 20-9). In contrast, maintaining the existing occlusal level as the tooth uprights will require intrusion, which carries with it at least the theoretic possibility of relocating infected crevicular tissue further subgingivally. Moreover, intrusion of molars is technically difficult, requiring precisely directed, gentle and long-acting forces. Unless slight extrusion or crown-height reduction is acceptable, which usually is the case, the patient should be considered to have problems that require comprehensive treatment and treated accordingly.

The final question is whether the premolars should be repositioned as part of the treatment. This decision will depend on the position of these teeth, the existing contacts and the opposing intercuspation, and the restorative plan; but in many cases the answer is yes. It is particularly desirable to close spaces between premolars when uprighting molars, because this will improve both the periodontal prognosis and long-term stability.

Appliances for Molar Uprighting. A partial fixed appliance is preferred to upright tipped molars. Although the design and application may vary slightly, the principles are the same. Each appliance can be separated into an active and a reactive (stabilizing or anchor) unit. To provide appropriate anchorage, all teeth as far forward as the canine in the treatment quadrant should be included. In most cases, the canine on the contralateral side also should be linked to the anchor teeth by the use of a heavy stabilizing lingual arch (Figure 20-10). This is all but mandatory in the man-

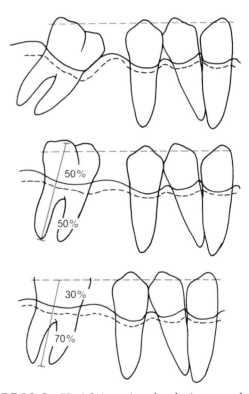

FIGURE 20-9 Uprighting a tipped molar increases the crown height while it reduces the depth of the mesial pocket. Subsequent crown reduction improves the ratio of crown height to supported root length of the molar.

dibular arch and advisable in the maxillary arch, particularly if a premolar also is missing. This canine-to-canine stabilizing arch not only increases the anterior anchorage but also resists buccal displacement of the anchor teeth.

Directly bonded brackets generally are preferred over bands for the premolars and canine teeth in the anchorage unit. The decision as to a band or bonded attachment for the molar(s) depends on the individual circumstance.

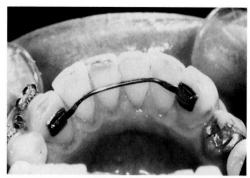

FIGURE 20-10 A bonded canine-to-canine stabilizing lingual arch is needed in most patients who require molar uprighting to increase the anterior anchorage and prevent buccal displacement of the anchor premolars. The wire usually is 30 mil steel. It should be placed up on the cingulum of the incisors for maximum mechanical efficiency and so the patient can maintain good oral hygiene. Retention is improved either by using pre-welded mesh pads on the wire as shown here (available commercially), or by curving the ends of the wire in the area where it will be bonded and roughening the surface (see Figure 19-15).

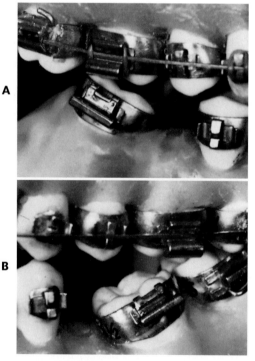

FIGURE 20-11 **A,** If a single molar is to be uprighted, it should carry a wide twin bracket with a convertible cap and gingivally placed auxiliary tube as shown here on the lower second molar. **B,** If two adjacent molars are to be uprighted, the convertible cap on the mesial molar bracket should be removed before cementing the band, and the terminal molar should carry a single tube.

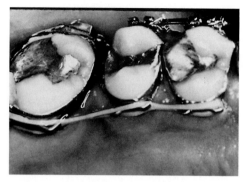

FIGURE 20-12 Lingual buttons or cleats (shown here) permit the use of auxiliary elastics that help in correction of rotations or crossbites. Here, lingual attachments and an elastomeric chain are being used for rotation of the molar. If lingual attachments are needed, they should be welded to a band, not bonded individually.

Bonded attachments for molars are more likely to fail than bonded brackets for premolars or anterior teeth, because of the difficulty in moisture control in the molar region and because occlusal forces against the attachment may be heavy. On the other hand, gingival irritation is greater with bands than bonded attachments. A general guideline is that molar bands are best when the periodontal condition allows, which means for all practical purposes they would be used in younger and healthier patients. The greater the degree of periodontal breakdown around the molar to be uprighted, the more a bonded attachment should be considered. Bonding to metal or porcelain surfaces is less successful than bonding to enamel, so teeth with large restorations on the buccal surface usually are better banded than bonded.

Whether it is banded or bonded, the molar to be uprighted should carry a combination attachment consisting of a wide twin bracket with a convertible cap and a gingivally placed auxiliary tube. This attachment is listed in most orthodontic catalogs as being for first molars but can be adapted easily to second molars. If second and third molars are being uprighted simultaneously, the convertible cap should be removed before the second molar band is cemented or the attachment is bonded, and the third molar should carry a single tube (typically catalogued as being for second molars) (Figure 20-11). If rotations or crossbites are to be corrected, lingual buttons or cleats may be helpful, but if they are used, these lingual attachments should be welded to bands, not bonded individually to the lingual surfaces (Figure 20-12).

Where premolar and canine brackets should be placed depends on the intended tooth movement. If these teeth are to be repositioned, the brackets should be placed in the ideal position at the center of the facial surface of each tooth. However, if the teeth are merely serving as anchor units and no repositioning is planned, then the brackets

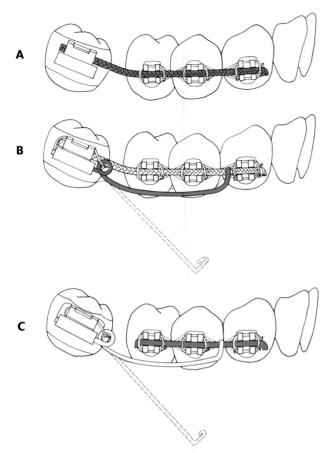

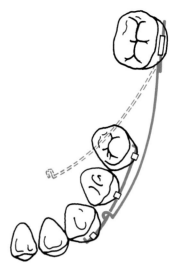

FIGURE 20-14 Because the force is applied to the facial surface of the teeth, a helical uprighting spring tends not only to extrude the molar but also to roll it lingually, while intruding the premolars and flaring them buccally. To counteract this side effect, the uprighting spring should be curved buccolingually so that when it is placed into the molar tube, the hook would lie lingually to the archwire prior to activation (*dotted red*).

FIGURE 20-13 Fixed appliance technique for uprighting a single molar. **A,** Initial bracket alignment is achieved by placing a light flexible wire such as 17 × 25 A-NiTi or 17 × 25 braided stainless steel, from molar to canine; **B,** subsequently, a helical uprighting spring of stiffer wire, 17 × 25 stainless steel is placed in the auxiliary molar tube and activated by engaging the mesial hook over the stabilizing wire. **C,** If the relative alignment of the molar precludes extending the stabilizing segment into the molar bracket, then a rigid stabilizing wire, 19 × 25 stainless steel, is placed in the premolars and canine only (with the brackets bonded so this wire is passive—see Figure 20-3). The mesial arm of the uprighting spring should be adjusted to lie passively in the vestibule before engagement.

should be placed in the position of maximum convenience where minimum wire bending will be required to engage a passive archwire (see Figure 20-4).

Uprighting a Single Molar

Distal Crown Tipping with Occlusal Antagonist. If the molar is only moderately tipped, treatment often can be accomplished with a flexible rectangular wire such as 17 × 25 braided stainless steel or 17 × 25 NiTi. If the anchor teeth require extensive alignment, the best choice is 17 × 25 A-NiTi that delivers approximately 100 gm of force (see Chapter 10 for a more complete description of this modern material). If the anchor teeth are reasonably well aligned, 17 × 25 braided steel wire usually is satisfactory. Providing the wire can be placed in the brackets without

permanent distortion and the occlusal contacts are not too heavy, a single wire may complete the necessary uprighting. From the placement of the initial wire, it is always advisable to relieve occlusal contacts against the molar. Failure to relieve the occlusion prevents the molar from tipping upright, may cause excessive tooth mobility, and greatly increases treatment time.

If the molar is severely tipped, a continuous wire that uprights the molar will also tip the second premolar distally, which is undesirable. It is better therefore to carry out the bulk of the uprighting using a sectional uprighting spring. A stiff rectangular wire (19 × 25 steel) maintains the relationship of the teeth in the anchor segment, and an auxiliary spring is placed in the molar auxiliary tube. The uprighting spring is formed from either 17 × 25 beta-Ti wire without a helical loop, or 17 × 25 steel wire with a loop added to reduce the force level (Figure 20-13). The mesial arm of the helical spring should be adjusted to lie passively in the vestibule and upon activation should hook over the archwire in the stabilizing segment. It is important to position the hook so that it is free to slide distally as the molar uprights. A slight lingual bend placed in the uprighting spring is needed to counteract the forces that tend to tip the anchor teeth buccally and the molar lingually (Figure 20-14).

Because uprighting a tipped molar as described above causes considerable occlusal as well as distal crown movement, this method should be used only when the terminal molar has an occlusal antagonist. Frequent occlusal adjustments are necessary to reduce developing interferences, but even so, the occlusal contacts control the amount of extrusion. The technique will rapidly extrude an unopposed terminal molar.

Uprighting with Minimal Extrusion. If the molar to be uprighted has no occlusal antagonist, if extrusion is undesirable, or if the crown is to be maintained in position while the roots are brought mesially, an alternative uprighting approach should be used. After initial alignment of the anchor teeth with a light flexible wire, a single "T-loop" sectional archwire of 17×25 stainless steel or 19×25 beta-Ti wire is adapted to fit passively into the brackets on the anchor teeth and gabled at the T to exert an uprighting force on the molar (Figure 20-15). When engaged in the molar bracket, this wire will thrust the roots mesially while the crown tips distally.

If the treatment plan calls for maintaining or closing rather than increasing the pontic space, the distal end of the archwire should be pulled distally through the molar tube, opening the T-loop by 1 to 2 mm, and then bent sharply gingivally to maintain this opening. This activation provides a mesial force on the molar that counteracts distal crown tipping while the tooth uprights. The fit of the rectangular wire into the rectangular molar tube controls the position of the tooth in all three planes of space.

Since the extrusive forces generated with this appliance are small, it is ideally suited for patients in whom the opposing tooth has been lost. Severely rotated teeth also may be treated using this appliance, but in this case, the de-

sign of the T-loop is modified so that the end of the archwire is inserted from the posterior aspect of the molar tube (Figure 20-16).

An alternative method is to stabilize the anchor segment as described initially, and use a modified design of the auxiliary uprighting spring with helical loops mesially and distally.[7] Compared with the T-loop, this gives more precise control of the force system against the molar, but less control of its mesiodistal or rotational position.

Final Positioning of Molar and Premolars. Once molar uprighting has been almost accomplished, often it is desirable to increase the available pontic space and close open contacts in the anterior segment. This is done best using a relatively stiff base wire, with a compressed coil spring threaded over the wire to produce the required force system. With 22-slot brackets, the base wire should be 18 mil round or 17×25 rectangular steel wire, which should engage the anchor teeth and the uprighted molar more or less passively. The wire should extend through the molar tube, projecting about 1 mm beyond the distal. An open coil spring over the base wire, when compressed between the molar and distal premolar, should exert a force of approximately 150 gm to move the premolars mesially while continuing to tip the molar distally (Figure 20-17). The coil spring can be either steel or A-NiTi. A steel spring may need to be reactivated by compressing it and adding a split tube spacer over the wire between the coil and the bracket; the very large range of A-NiTi means that adjustments seldom will be necessary.

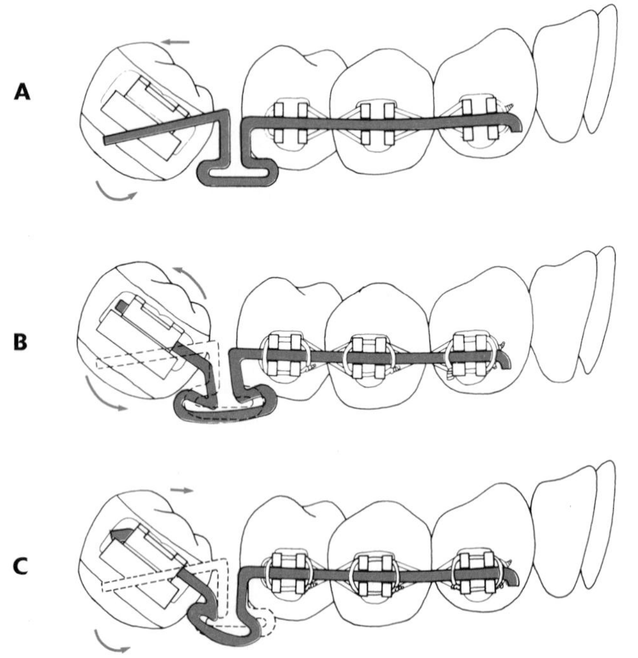

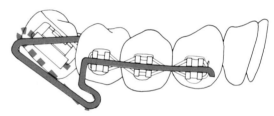

FIGURE 20-16 Modification of a T-loop that may be used to upright a severely tipped or rotated molar. The terminal part of the spring is inserted from the distal opening of the molar bracket.

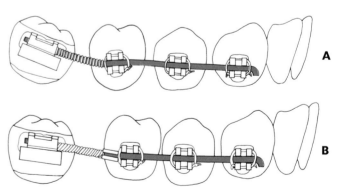

FIGURE 20-17 **A,** Compressed coil spring on a round wire (usually 18 mil steel) may be used to complete molar uprighting while closing remaining spaces in the premolar region. **B,** The coil spring may be reactivated by addition of a splint spacer over the archwire.

FIGURE 20-15 **A,** T-loop spring in 17×25 steel wire, showing the degree of angulation of the wire before inserting it into the molar tube that is necessary to upright a single tipped molar; **B,** T-loop spring active to upright the tooth by distal crown tipping; **C,** pulling the distal of the wire through the molar tube and opening the T-loop generate a mesial force that results in molar uprighting by mesial root movement with space closure.

However, continued use of a compressed coil spring once the premolar spaces are closed may result in anterior displacement of the anchor teeth and incisors. Therefore the occlusion should be checked carefully against the original study casts at each visit and the spring removed when the desired movement has been accomplished. Because of the long range of action of A-NiTi springs, this is particularly important when these springs are used.

The appliances for uprighting a single molar described earlier may be used in the maxilla or the mandible unilaterally (Figure 20-18) or bilaterally (Figure 20-19). However, it must be remembered that during bilateral molar

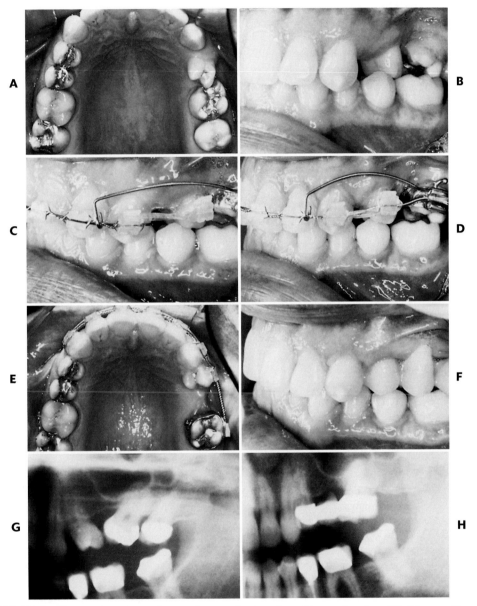

FIGURE 20-18   Unilateral uprighting of a severely tipped maxillary molar. **A** and **B,** The maxillary first molar and second premolar have been lost, with severe tipping and drifting so that molar uprighting and space consolidation are necessary before a pontic can be placed. It is necessary to remove the third molar to reposition the second molar. **C,** For this patient, bonded brackets on the incisors rather than a canine-to-canine lingual arch were used for additional anchorage. Initially, a round wire (16 mil steel) was placed in the incisor brackets and an elastomeric chain was used to bring the first premolar mesially, to provide access for banding the second molar. Then the second molar was banded and an auxiliary spring of 19 × 25 beta-Ti wire was placed to upright the molar. **E,** Once the continuous 16 mil steel wire could be placed, a coil spring was used to move the pre-molar mesially and increase the pontic space, while continuing to upright the molar. Positioning of the teeth was completed with a compressed coil spring on an 18 mil round wire and an elastomeric chain. **F,** The completed bridge in place. **G,** Pre-treatment and **H,** post-treatment radiographs showing improved root inclinations and bone contour. (Courtesy Dr. T. Shaughnessy.)

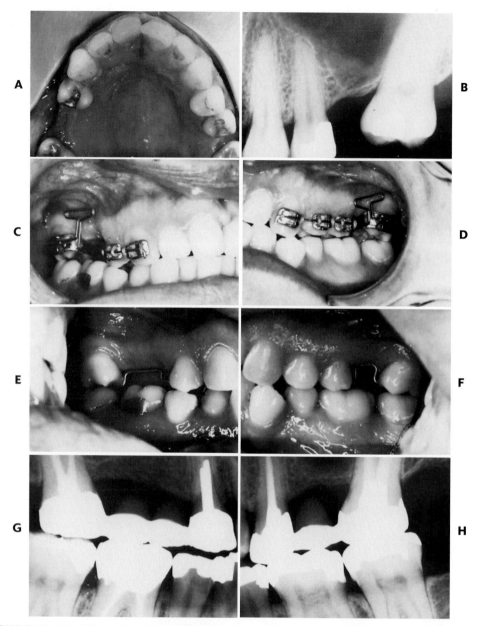

FIGURE 20-19 Bilateral molar uprighting in the maxillary arch. **A,** After the loss of maxillary first molars and one second premolar, the second molars have tipped and rotated mesially; **B,** radiographs show the poor bone contour and degree of tipping. **C** and **D,** T-loop uprighting springs active on the right to bring the root mesially and on the left to tip the crown distally, increasing space for a pontic. **E** and **F,** The uprighted teeth with intracoronal splints in place to stabilize the uprighted teeth until bridge construction; **G** and **H,** Radiographs showing restorative procedures completed. Note the improved root paralleling and alveolar ridge contour.

uprighting, the strain on the anterior anchorage is increased. Very light forces should be used and the anterior occlusion must be monitored carefully. If it appears that the anchor teeth are moving, then it is advisable to deactivate one segment, complete molar uprighting in one quadrant, stabilize those teeth, and then upright the contralateral quadrant.

Uprighting Two Molars in the Same Quadrant. Because the resistance offered when uprighting two molars is considerable, only small amounts of space closure should be attempted. The goal of treatment is to upright the molars with a combination of mesial root movement and distal crown tipping, opening the space slightly. Trying to upright both the second and third molars bilaterally at the same time is not a good idea—significant movement of the anchor teeth is inevitable.

When both the second and third molars are to be uprighted, the third molar should carry a single rectangular tube and the cap should be removed from the convertible bracket on the second molar (see Figure 20-11). Since the second molar is usually more severely tipped than the third

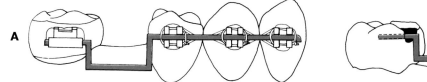
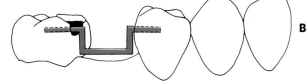

FIGURE 20-20   Stabilization after tooth movement should continue until the prostheses are placed. **A,** An extracoronal splint using 19 × 25 steel wire engaging the brackets passively; **B,** an intracoronal splint when bonded in place with composite resin causes minimal tissue disturbance. The intracoronal splint is preferred, particularly if retention is to be continued for more than a few weeks.

molar, increased flexibility of the wire mesial and distal to the second molar is required. The best approach is to use a modern highly flexible wire initially, and 17 × 25 A-NiTi usually is a good choice. Excessive mobility of the teeth being uprighted can result from either too much force or (more likely if the modern NiTi and beta-Ti wires are used) failure to reduce the occlusal interferences.

The treatment time will vary with the type and extent of the tooth movement required. Uprighting a tooth by distal crown tipping proceeds more rapidly than mesial root movement. Failure to eliminate occlusal interferences will prolong treatment. The simplest cases should be completed in 8 to 10 weeks, but uprighting two molars with mesial root movement could easily take 20 to 24 weeks, and the complexity of doing this puts it at the margin of adjunctive treatment.

Retention.   After molar uprighting, the teeth are in an unstable position until the prosthesis that provides the long-term retention is placed. Long delays in making the final prosthesis should be avoided if possible. As a general guideline, a fixed bridge can and should be placed within 6 weeks after uprighting is completed. Especially if an implant is planned, there may be a considerable delay while the bone graft heals and the implant becomes integrated. For a short time, the orthodontic retainer can be a 19 × 25 steel or 21 × 25 beta-Ti wire designed to fit the brackets passively (Figure 20-20). If retention is needed for more than a few weeks, the preferred approach to intermediate splinting is an intracoronal wire splint (19 × 25 or heavier steel wire), bonded into shallow preparations in the abutment teeth (see Figures 20-8 and 20-19). This type of splint causes little gingival irritation and can be left in place for a considerable period, but it would have to be removed and rebonded to allow bone grafting and implant surgery.

Forced Eruption

Indications.   Teeth with defects in the cervical third of the root or isolated teeth with one or two walled vertical periodontal defects pose a complex dental problem (Figure 20-21). These problems can arise after horizontal or oblique fracture, internal or external resorption, decay, pathologic perforation or periodontal disease. To obtain good access for endodontic and restorative procedures or

to reduce pocket depth, it would be necessary to perform extensive crown lengthening that would produce poor esthetics and adverse changes in the crown-to-root ratio.

Controlled extrusion is an excellent alternative.[8] Extruding the tooth improves endodontic access and can allow isolation under rubber dam when it would not be possible otherwise. Forced eruption also allows crown margins to be placed on sound tooth structure while maintaining a uniform gingival contour that provides improved esthetics. In addition, the alveolar bone height is not compromised, the apparent crown length is maintained, and the bony support of adjacent teeth is not compromised. As the tooth is extruded, the attached gingiva should follow the cementoenamel junction. This returns the width of the attached gingiva to its original level. However, it usually is necessary to perform some limited recontouring of the gingiva, and perhaps of the bone, to produce a contour even with the adjacent teeth and a proper biologic width between bone and depth of sulcus.

Treatment Planning.   Before beginning treatment, it is essential to have good periapical radiographs to examine the vertical extent of the defect, the periodontal support, and the root morphology and position. The ideal morphology is a single tapering root. Flared or divergent roots will result in increasing root proximity with extrusion and the possibility of exposing the root furcation area. In rare instances, hypercementosis or dilaceration of the root may make forced eruption complicated or impossible.

As a general rule, endodontic therapy should be completed before extrusion of the root begins. For some patients, however, the orthodontic movement must be completed before definitive endodontic procedures, because one purpose of extrusion may be to provide better access for endodontic and restorative procedures. In such circumstances, preliminary endodontic treatment to relieve symptoms is done initially, and the tooth is maintained with a temporary root filling or other palliative treatment until it has been moved to a better position.

The distance the tooth should be extruded is determined by three things: (1) the location of the defect (fracture line, root perforation, etc.) that is being treated; (2) space to place the margin of the restoration so that it is

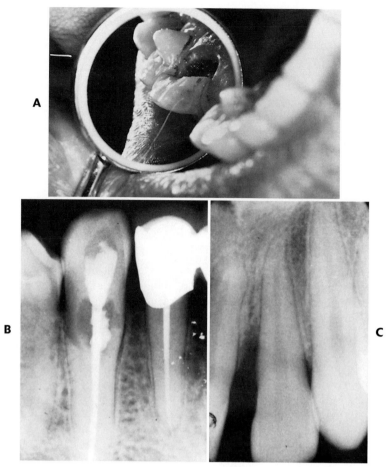

FIGURE 20-21   Situations in which forced eruption of teeth will improve restorative procedures. **A,** Crown fracture at the alveolar crest; **B,** internal root resorption; **C,** isolated vertical periodontal defect.

not at the base of the gingival sulcus (typically, 1 mm is needed); and (3) an allowance for the biological width of the gingival attachment (about 2 mm). Thus if a fracture is at the height of the alveolar crest, the tooth should be extruded about 3 mm; if it is 2 mm below the crest, 5 mm of extrusion ideally would be needed. The crown-to-root ration at the end of treatment should be 1:1 or better. A tooth with a poorer ratio can be maintained only by splinting it to adjacent teeth.

Isolated one or two wall vertical pockets pose a particular esthetic problem if they occur in the anterior region of the mouth. Surgical correction may be contraindicated simply on esthetic grounds. Forced eruption of such teeth, with concomitant crown reduction, can improve the periodontal condition while maintaining excellent esthetics (Figure 20-22).

The length of time required for forced eruption will vary with the age of the patient, the distance the tooth has to be moved, and the viability of the PDL. In general, extrusion can be as rapid as 1 mm per week without damage to the PDL, so 3 to 6 weeks is sufficient for almost any patient. Too much force, and too rapid a rate of movement, runs the risk of tissue damage and ankylosis.

Orthodontic Technique.   Since extrusion is the tooth movement that occurs most readily and intrusion the movement that occurs least readily, ample anchorage is usually available from adjacent teeth. The appliance needs to be quite rigid over the anchor teeth, and flexible where it attaches to the tooth that is being extruded. This contraindicates the use of a continuous flexible archwire, which would produce the desired extrusion but also tip the adjacent teeth toward the tooth being extruded, reducing the space for subsequent restorations and disturbing the interproximal contacts within the arch (Figure 20-23).

Two methods are suggested, one with (Figure 20-24, *A*) and the other without the use of orthodontic brackets (Figure 20-24, *B-D*). It is possible to bond a heavy stabilizing wire, 19 × 25 or 21 × 25 stainless steel, directly to the facial surface of the adjacent teeth.[9] A post and core with temporary crown and pin is placed on the tooth to be extruded, and an elastomeric module or auxiliary NiTi spring is used to extrude the tooth (see Figure 16-22 for the use of NiTi piggyback springs). This appliance is simple, provides excellent control of anchor teeth, and avoids cumbersome orthodontic attachments, but better control can be obtained when orthodontic brackets are used.

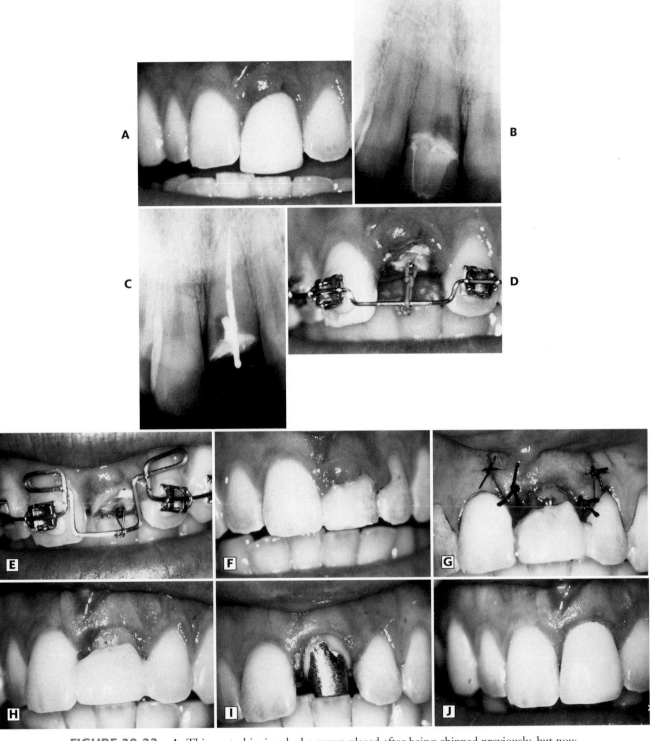

FIGURE 20-22   **A,** This central incisor had a crown placed after being chipped previously, but now showed gingival inflammation and elongation. **B,** A periapical radiograph revealed internal root resorption below the crown margin. The treatment plan was, **C,** endodontic treatment, then elongation of the root so that a new crown margin could be placed on sound root structure. **D,** Initially, an elastomeric tie was used from an archwire segment to an attachment on the post cemented in the root canal; **E,** then loops in a flexible rectangular wire were employed for quicker and more efficient movement. Four mm elongation occurred in as many weeks. **F** to **H,** A gingivally repositioned flap was used to produce the correct gingival contour, then, **I** and **J,** a coping and final ceramic crown were prepared. Extraction of the tooth was avoided and a highly esthetic restoration was possible. (Courtesy Dr. H. Fields.)

The alternative is to bond brackets to the anchor teeth, bond or band the tooth to be extruded, and use a modification of the T-loop appliance described earlier. If the buccal surface of the tooth to be extruded is intact, a bracket should be bonded as far gingivally as possible (Figure 20-25). If the crown is hopelessly destroyed, an orthodontic band with a bracket usually can be placed over the remaining root surface (Figure 20-26). An orthodontic band has the benefit of helping isolation procedures during emergency endodontic treatment. Two or three adjacent teeth should be bonded to serve as the anchor unit. The brackets on these anchor teeth can be

placed somewhat more occlusally than the ideal position. A T-loop archwire is made from 17 × 25 stainless steel or 19 × 25 beta-Ti wire, with the height of the loop being determined by the vestibule depth. The part of the wire engaging the tooth to be extruded should be designed to lie more occlusal than the anchor segment. The wire should fit the anchor segment reasonably passively, unless some additional alignment of this segment is desired, and the T-loop should not impinge on the gingival or facial tissues when engaged. The rectangular wire gives positive three-dimensional control during extrusion.

Whatever appliance is used, the patient must be seen every 1 to 2 weeks to reduce the occlusal surface of the tooth being extruded, control inflammation, and monitor progress. After active tooth movement has been completed, the tooth should be stabilized, either by bending a rectangular wire to fit passively into all the brackets (if they were used), or by tying the pin to the bonded stabilizing wire. Stabilization allows for proper reorganization of the PDL fibers and allows the bone to remodel, discouraging relapse. In general, 3 to 6 weeks of stabilization should be sufficient after extrusion. If periodontal surgery is needed to recontour the alveolar bone and/or reposition the gingiva,

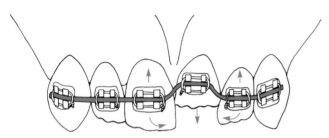

FIGURE 20-23 Although a straight orthodontic wire activated apically will produce an extrusive force on a tooth, it will also cause the teeth on either side to tip toward each other, reducing the space available for the extruding tooth.

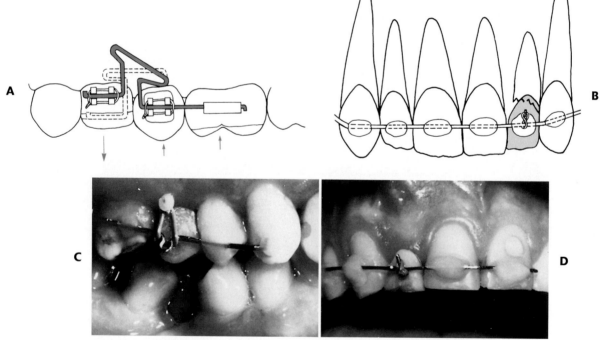

FIGURE 20-24 Possible approaches to extrusion of a single tooth. **A,** With brackets and bands on the teeth, a modified T-loop in 17 × 25 steel or 19 × 25 beta-Ti wire will extrude a tooth while controlling mesio-distal tipping. **B** to **D,** Extrusion also can be done without conventional orthodontic attachments, by bonding a 19 × 25 steel stabilizing wire directly to the facial surface of adjacent teeth. An elastomeric module is stretched between the stabilizing wire and a pin placed directly into the crown of the tooth to be extruded. If a temporary crown can be used for esthetics while the extrusion is being done, as shown in **C** and **D,** it must be progressively cut away to make the tooth movement possible. (**B** to **D,** Courtesy Dr. L. Osterle.)

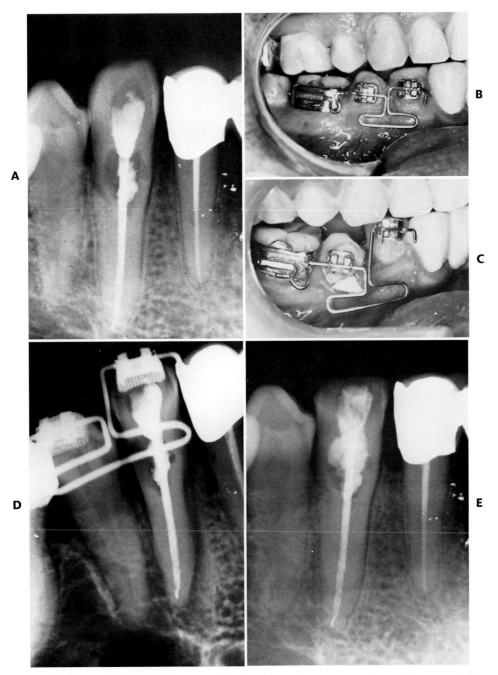

FIGURE 20-25 **A,** Mandibular canine showing internal root resorption and suspected lateral perforation. Access is poor and surgical crown lengthening may jeopardize the periodontal integrity of adjacent teeth. **B,** Segmental T-loop appliance active to extrude the canine. The bracket has been placed as far gingival as possible and the crown must be reduced vertically to permit extrusion. **C,** The canine has been extruded. Note the relationship of the bracket to the gingival margin. **D,** Extrusion has moved the lateral perforation to the alveolar margin, where it is accessible for endodontic treatment. **E,** Two year follow-up showing stable condition. Note the excellent bone height on the adjacent teeth. (From Tuncay OC: *J Prosthet Dent* 46:41-47, 1981.)

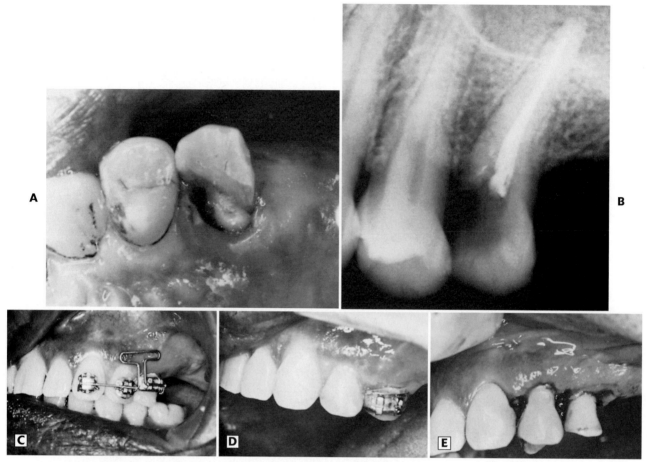

FIGURE 20-26   **A,** Lingual cusp of maxillary second premolar fractured subgingivally at the level of the alveolar crest. **B,** The tooth is treated endodontically to relieve acute symptoms; **C,** an orthodontic band is placed as far gingivally as possible, and a sectional T-loop spring is used to extrude the premolar. **D,** The crown has been reduced occlusally as the tooth is extruded; **E,** excess gingival tissue is removed surgically exposing the fracture margin, and the tooth is now ready for post and core restoration. Note the even gingival contour and comparable functional crown lengths. (From Tuncay OC: *J Prosthet Dent* 46:41-47, 1981.)

this can be done 1 month after completion of the extrusion. As with molar uprighting, it is better to complete the definitive prosthetic treatment without extensive delay.

Alignment of Anterior Teeth

Indications.   The major indications for adjunctive orthodontic treatment to correct malaligned anterior teeth are:

1. To improve access and permit placement of well-adapted and contoured restorations (e.g., when composite resin build-ups to recontour incisors are planned, or when periodontally-compromised incisors must be splinted)
2. To permit placement of crowns and pontics without overcontoured crowns that would produce poor embrasure form
3. To reposition closely approximated roots, to improve the embrasure form and increase the amount of interradicular bone, which in turn increases the chance that periodontal disease can be controlled

4. To position teeth so implants can be placed to support restorations

Rotations, crowding, spacing, tipped teeth, and crossbites all pose problems for restorative and periodontal procedures. Most alignment problems are reflections of crowding or spacing within the dental arch. As such, it is first necessary to assess how much space would be required or created during arch alignment. Moving teeth lingually and correcting rotations of anterior teeth requires additional space within the arch. De-rotating teeth and uprighting tipped teeth usually causes them to occupy less space within the arch, while moving teeth facially increases arch length. Space also may be created by removing interproximal enamel to reduce the mesio-distal width of both anterior and posterior teeth.

Treatment Planning.   Anterior teeth that require alignment should be brought into their proper position before definitive restorative procedures. Progressive interproximal stripping can be used to create space, within the

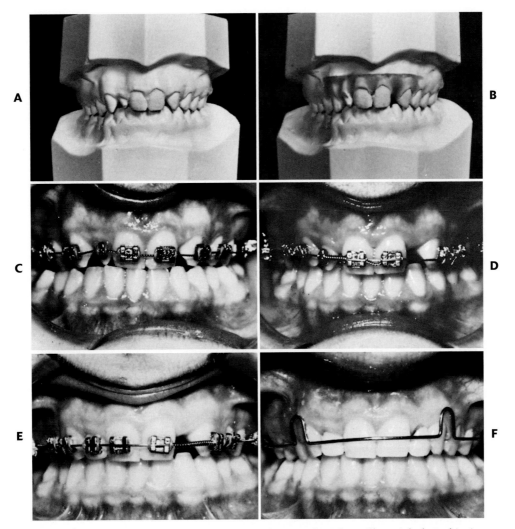

FIGURE 20-27 **A,** Initial models of a patient with a peg-shaped maxillary right lateral incisor, congenital absence of the maxillary left lateral, and one mandibular incisor; **B,** the diagnostic setup suggests retracting both canines, moving the peg-shaped lateral incisor to the right and building it up, and increasing space for the replacement of the left lateral. **C,** A sectioned twin bracket has been bonded on the peg-shaped incisor and a 17.5 mil multistranded wire is used for initial alignment. **D,** Mesial and distal movement of teeth with elastomeric modules or coil spring requires a stiffer wire (usually 18 mil stainless steel) to control tipping. **E,** Note that the peg lateral has been built up with composite resin, and a normal width bracket bonded, as final positioning for replacement for the missing lateral is completed. **F,** A retainer with a replacement lateral incisor can be used for a short time, but long delays in the definitive restorative treatment should be avoided.

limits established by the enamel thickness and the mesio-distal diameter of the crowns at the gingival margin in the maxillary arch. Approximately ½ mm of enamel may be removed from the mesial and distal surface of each maxillary anterior tooth, giving a maximum of 4 mm additional space in the anterior part of the arch. In the mandibular arch, the smaller mesio-distal width of the incisor teeth reduces the amount of interproximal stripping that can be undertaken without producing unacceptable root proximity. For this reason, crowding greater than 3 to 4 mm in the mandibular anterior arch nearly always requires the extraction of a lower incisor.

A "diagnostic setup" is very helpful in planning treatment for alignment problems, particularly if crowding or spacing must be corrected. For this procedure, the study casts are duplicated and the malaligned teeth are carefully cut from the model, crown dimensions are modified if necessary, and the teeth are then waxed back onto the cast in a new position (Figure 20-27). Alternative tooth positions may be tried to determine the optimum for each patient. Once the most satisfactory occlusion has been established, the feasibility of the orthodontic treatment can be evaluated in light of the crown and root movements required, the anchorage available, the periodontal support for each

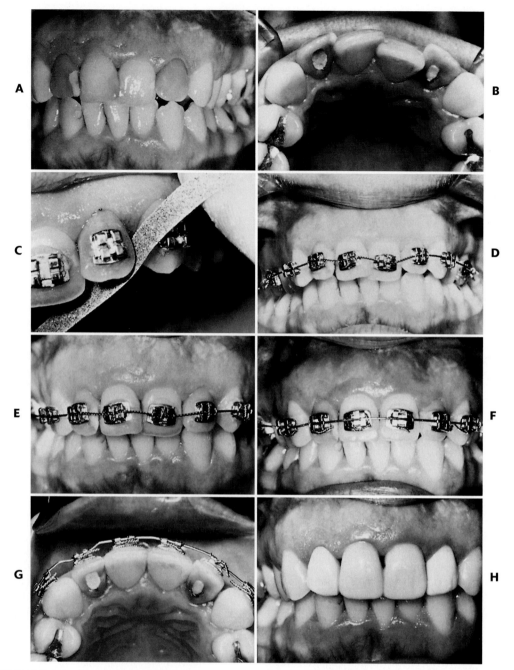

FIGURE 20-28 **A,** Decayed maxillary anterior teeth with discoloration after endodontic treatment; **B,** the occlusal view shows the degree of crowding and rotation; **C,** although the lateral incisor has been treated endodontically, the mesio-distal width of the crown at the gingival margin limits the amount of interproximal stripping possible; **D,** initial alignment is achieved with a highly flexible archwire, 17.5 mil multistranded steel, **E,** which is retied or replaced after 3 to 4 weeks; **F,** final alignment is achieved with a stiffer wire (16 or 18 mil steel). **G,** If anterior crowns are to be placed, minor rotations need not be corrected orthodontically since they can be masked restoratively. This procedure is easier on endodontically treated teeth since there is no danger of accidental pulp exposure during crown preparation. **H,** Temporary crowns in place. Unless the permanent crowns are fused together, retention must be continued to prevent rotational relapse.

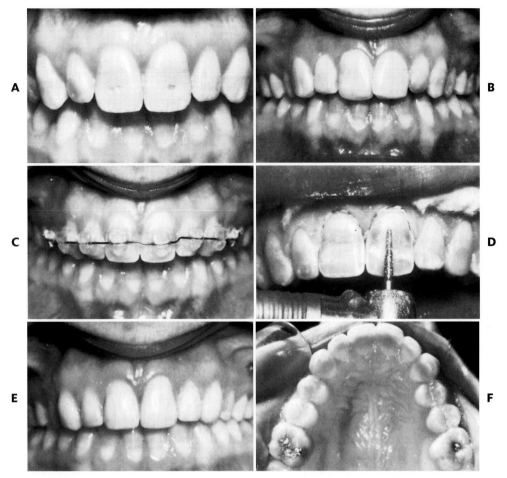

FIGURE 20-29 Adjunctive orthodontic treatment to facilitate treatment of tetracycline staining on rotated incisors. **A,** Marked tetracycline staining; **B,** the color of initial veneers was not satisfactory due to different mesial and distal thickness used to mask the rotations; **C,** a fixed orthodontic appliance was used in conjunction with stripping of mesial and distal surfaces of the incisors to align the teeth; **D,** the realigned teeth are prepared for veneers; **E** and **F,** veneers of uniform thickness produce a significantly better esthetic result. (Restorative work courtesy Dr. H. Heymann.)

tooth, and the possible occlusal interferences. Teeth that can be arranged satisfactorily in a diagnostic setup may not always be as easy to adjust clinically. But if it can't be done on the laboratory bench, there is no reason to attempt it clinically.

While stripping anterior teeth may be an excellent way of gaining a small amount of space, such treatment should be undertaken with caution since it may have an undesirable effect on the esthetics, overbite, overjet, and posterior intercuspation. Treatment of this type should never be undertaken without a diagnostic setup to be sure the teeth will fit satisfactorily. It also is possible to gain space by stripping enamel from posterior teeth.[10] An additional 4 mm can be obtained in this way, but a complete orthodontic appliance is required, and treatment of this type falls into the comprehensive rather than adjunctive category.

Orthodontic Technique

Alignment of Crowded, Rotated and Displaced Incisors. Alignment nearly always requires a fixed appliance (Figures 20-28 and 20-29). The first molars should be bonded or banded to serve as anchorage. This can be augmented if necessary with a rigid lingual arch (see Chapters 9 and 12). Edgewise brackets are bonded on the anterior teeth, usually canine-to-canine, and an initial ideal archwire is placed. This wire must be light and flexible enough to be tied to all the brackets (but not necessarily completely into them) without either becoming permanently distorted or exerting excessive forces on the teeth. A 16 mil A-NiTi archwire is the best choice in most circumstances. If the teeth are only moderately irregular, 17.5 mil braided stainless steel wire also may be suitable (see Chapter 16). Unless the wire is turned gingivally at the distal of the molar tubes, the teeth will flare labially while they align, which is usually undesirable. Crown reduction should be started the day the appliances are placed and continued at subsequent appointments.

If the wire was not seated completely into the brackets initially (this is often possible with A-NiTi wires), it can be tied more tightly at 3- to 4-week intervals. When preliminary alignment has been completed and the wire passively engages the brackets, it may be desirable to place a stiffer round or rectangular wire to complete alignment of the teeth (remember that the use of rectangular wires presupposes the use of modern straight wire brackets). Although round wires can correct rotations and tip teeth into alignment, precise positioning of roots requires the use of a rec-

tangular wire. Rectangular wires should not be used for preliminary alignment, because they may cause undesirable root movement at that stage.

Once the ideal crown and root positions have been achieved, the teeth must be stabilized. Their tendency to relapse after correction of rotation may be reduced by severing the distorted supracrestal gingival fibers (see Chapter 18). A carefully constructed retainer with a closely adapted

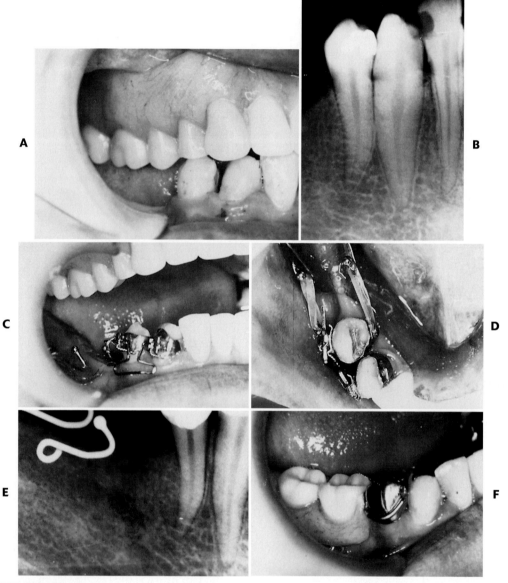

FIGURE 20-30 **A,** Root proximity between the mandibular right premolar and canine poses a prosthetic and periodontal problem. **B,** Radiograph showing the difficulty of restoring the premolar and lack of interradicular bone. The premolar must be moved distally without tipping if damage to the root surfaces of the adjacent teeth is to be avoided. This requires the combination of a translational force and a root-uprighting moment. **C,** A removable appliance was used to augment anchorage, and a T-loop spring was placed between bands on the canine and premolar to provide the moment to move the premolar root distally. **D,** Latex elastics hooked to the removable appliance provided a distal translational force to the premolar. **E,** Radiographs showing the resultant distal bodily movement of the premolar and formation of new interradicular bone. **F,** Partial denture in place with rests on the crown of the premolar. (From Tuncay OC: *J Prosthet Dent* 46:41-47, 1981.)

labial bow must be placed immediately upon removal of the fixed appliance. If a fiber section has been performed, retention should be continued for 6 months. If fibers are not sectioned, then retention should be continued at night for an indefinite period. It is probably advisable to delay any crown construction for 6 to 8 weeks after alignment of incisors to allow bone remodeling to be completed. The retention schedule outlined previously should then be followed unless the crowns are fused together to form a permanent retainer.

Separation of Approximated Teeth. Occasionally two teeth may exhibit close root proximity. The lack of interradicular space at the gingival margin is the critical factor. This not only prevents satisfactory restorative procedures but also predisposes both teeth to rapid progression if periodontal disease develops. If the roots of such teeth must be separated, the necessary tooth movement can be achieved only with a fixed appliance (Figure 20-30), because a force system that applies a moment effective in moving roots must be used (see Chapter 10). The anchorage can be gained from the adjacent teeth or from a removable appliance. Root movement proceeds more slowly than crown tipping, and 8 to 10 weeks should be allowed for such procedures. Periapical radiographs will confirm that adequate root separation has been achieved.

Positioning Teeth for Single Tooth Implants

Treatment Planning. For many patients with missing teeth, either congenitally absent or lost to trauma or dental disease, single tooth implants now provide a preferred method of restoration. This is an especially attractive choice for replacing missing anterior teeth when the adjacent teeth are caries free and one might hesitate to place a full coverage or even resin-bonded bridge. Three critical issues determine the amount of space for an implant: the space needed for the implant itself, the esthetics, and the occlusion.[11]

For satisfactory implant placement, there must be enough room for both the implant and interproximal bone between it and adjacent teeth. The narrowest implants currently available are 4 mm wide at the shoulder or platform. Approximately 1 mm of space is required between the implant and the adjacent tooth to allow for proper healing and to ensure adequate space for the papilla, so 6 mm is the minimum space. Space is needed not only at the crest of the ridge, but also between the roots of the adjacent teeth. The apices of the adjacent teeth must be far enough apart to allow the surgeon to place the implant without damaging the root or apical tissues (Figure 20-31).

When positioning teeth for an implant, the final esthetics must be considered. In general, the contralateral and adjacent teeth will suggest the size of the prosthetic replacement. A lateral incisor is typically about two-thirds the width of the central incisor, and the teeth are bilaterally symmetrical. Establishing a coordinated gingival contour on the teeth adjacent to an anterior implant can also be critical in determining the final esthetics, particularly for those patients with gingival display on smiling.

The occlusion may also influence the size of the replacement crown. If there is any irregularity of the teeth in the opposing arch, as for example the lower incisor crowding so frequently seen in adults, then establishing a Class I canine and molar relationship may result in less than

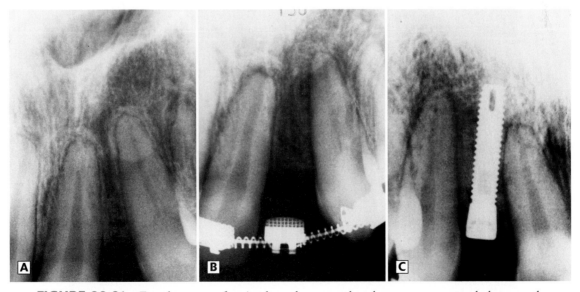

FIGURE 20-31 For placement of an implant, there must be adequate room not only between the crowns of adjacent teeth, but also between the roots. **A,** Although this patient had had orthodontic treatment previously, root proximity at the site of a missing lateral incisor did not allow placement of an implant without further orthodontics to reposition the roots. **B,** A fixed appliance was required to obtain the necessary moments for separation of the roots (note the pontic tied to the orthodontic archwire). **C,** Implant in place after completion of the root separation. (Courtesy Dr. P.M. Thomas.)

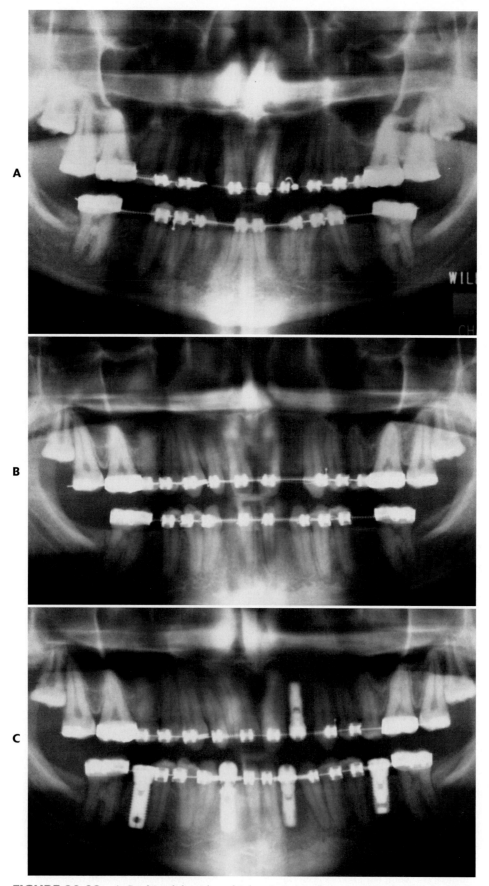

FIGURE 20-32 **A,** In this adult with multiple missing teeth, a complete fixed orthodontic appliance was needed in preparation for placement of implants, so that proper root and crown positions could be obtained; **B,** progress radiograph, showing the improved tooth positions toward the end of orthodontic treatment; **C,** implants in place. (Courtesy Dr. P.M. Thomas.)

ideal space for the implant, unless the patient is left with an increased overjet and/or overbite. Such considerations can turn an apparently simple "adjunctive" case into one requiring far more comprehensive treatment.

Orthodontic Technique. In general, once the plan for regaining the necessary space and any required root positioning has been made, the mechanics are relatively simple, requiring only careful bracket placement and control of anchorage (Figure 20-32). Root movement, which always proceeds more slowly than crown tipping, will determine the duration of treatment. It may take as long as six months to achieve ideal root placement. It is good practice to take progress periapical radiographs to confirm the angulation of the teeth prior to removing the orthodontic appliances.

The timing of implant placement is particularly critical for adolescents and young adults. Implants to support restorations should not be placed until all vertical growth has been completed. For boys this may be as late as their early 20s. Vertical growth in girls is generally complete by age 15-17 years, and implants may be placed correspondingly sooner (Figure 20-33). Once the implant has been placed, no further eruption of this tooth will occur, even though the adjacent teeth continue to erupt in response to increase in the patient's vertical facial height. The implant is analogous to an ankylosed tooth. Even though small differences in the level of the incisal edge might be camouflaged by increasing the crown length, if the adjacent teeth erupt and the implant does not, the gingival contours will become uneven. This can be very unattractive in the anterior maxillary region.

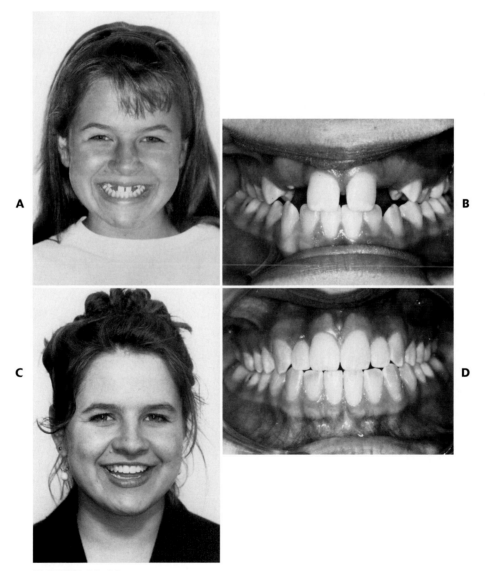

FIGURE 20-33 Replacement of missing maxillary lateral incisors with implants. **A** and **B,** Age 12, prior to orthodontic repositioning of the central incisors and canines in preparation for implants; **C** and **D,** age 17, after implant placement and restorations. Implants usually can be placed at a younger age in girls than boys, but it is important to delay implants until vertical growth is completed. (Courtesy Dr. P.M. Thomas.)

For adults who lose a tooth, placing an implant soon afterward minimizes the loss of alveolar bone in the newly edentulous space. Maintaining primary teeth, even though their roots are partially resorbed, also helps in maintaining alveolar ridge height and width necessary for satisfactory implant placement (see Chapter 21 for a further discussion of implant applications to comprehensive orthodontic treatment).

Anterior Diastema Closure and Space Redistribution.

Loss of posterior teeth, abnormally small teeth, or loss of bone support may all result in drifting and spacing of incisors. Space closure or redistribution will greatly simplify restorative procedures and improve the esthetics. Closure of anterior spaces is usually relatively simple but often requires permanent retention with a bonded lingual retainer, fused crowns or a fixed partial denture. For best esthetics, partial closure of maxillary incisor spacing and redistribution of the space of a central diastema, followed by composite build-ups and/or replacement of missing teeth, often is the treatment of choice.

If the diastema is small or results from adjacent teeth being tipped in opposite directions, a removable appliance with finger springs may be used to close the space by simple tipping. However, if the teeth are bodily displaced or widely separated, a fixed appliance must be used to control both crown and root positions. A wire bent to ideal arch

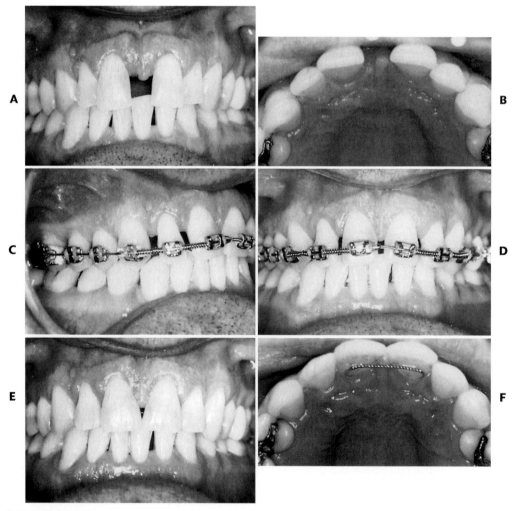

FIGURE 20-34   If spacing of maxillary incisors is related to small teeth and a tooth-size discrepancy, composite build-ups are an excellent solution, but satisfactory esthetics may require redistribution of the space before the restorations are placed, as in this patient. **A** and **B**, Before treatment, age 48; **C** and **D**, redistribution of the space using a fixed appliance with coil springs on a 16 mil steel archwire, immediately before removal of the orthodontic appliance and placement of the restorations (to be done the same day). For this patient, a 17.5 mil multistrand wire was used for initial alignment, before the coil springs were placed; **E** and **F**, completed restorations. Note the bonded retainer of 21.5 mil multistrand wire lingual to the central incisors to prevent partial reopening of the midline space. Surgical revision of the frenum was not performed, partially in deference to the patient's age.

form is used, which may be continuous from molar to molar if several teeth are to be moved, or involve just the anterior segment of the arch if only two or three teeth are to be moved.

Brackets are placed on the teeth to be moved and on appropriate anchor teeth. Initial alignment is carried out using a light wire such as 16 mil A-NiTi or 17.5 mil braided steel. This wire is replaced, 3 to 4 weeks after bracket engagement is achieved, with a 16 or 18 mil round steel wire along which the teeth are repositioned using elastomeric modules or coil springs. Initially the teeth tip, but the stiffness of the wire in the wide brackets counteracts this effect and results in bodily movement. If the spacing is the result of abnormally small teeth in one arch (i.e., a tooth size discrepancy exists), it will be impossible to close all the space while maintaining the posterior intercuspation. In such a case, the teeth must be moved into an ideally separated position and the crowns built up either with composite resins or castings (Figure 20-34). Even if much of the space of a maxillary central diastema was filled with a restorative material, if a diastema has been partially closed there is always a tendency for the space to reopen. Bonding a flexible wire on the lingual of the incisors as a semi-permanent retainer is recommended (note Figure 20-34, *F*).

The restorations are an important part of retention when excess spaces were present in the arch. They should be placed immediately upon removal of the orthodontic appliance. The best plan is to establish the correct position of the teeth, hold them there with the orthodontic appliance for a few weeks at most, and then do the composite build-ups on the same day the orthodontic appliance is removed.

Crossbite Correction

Crossbites may occur in any part of the arch and often cause functional problems such as occlusal interferences, occlusal trauma and improper occlusal loading. Anterior crossbites are an esthetic problem as well. If only one or two teeth are involved, the crossbite usually results from displacement of crowded teeth or ectopic eruption. If a group of teeth are involved, it is more likely that the crossbite is a skeletal problem and will not respond to limited orthodontic treatment. In such a case, if successful restorative or periodontal treatment cannot be done with the teeth in the crossbite position, the patient should be referred for comprehensive orthodontic treatment that may include orthognathic surgery.

If a crossbite is due only to displaced teeth and if the tooth correction requires only tipping movements, then a removable appliance may be used to tip the teeth into a normal position. However, when using a removable appliance, as a tooth rotates labially or buccally into its new position, there is a vertical change in occlusal level (Figure 20-35). Tipping maxillary incisors labially to correct

anterior crossbite nearly always produces an apparent intrusion and a reduction in overbite. This can present a problem during retention, since a positive overbite serves to retain the crossbite correction. A fixed appliance generally is necessary for vertical control in correction of anterior crossbites.

In the posterior segments, crossbites frequently are corrected using "through the bite" elastics from a conveniently placed tooth in the opposing arch. This approach tips the teeth into the correct occlusion but also tends to extrude them (Figure 20-36). Elastics must be used with caution to correct posterior crossbites in adults, because the extrusion can change occlusal relationships throughout the mouth.

If vertical control is critical and/or some degree of bodily movement is required in crossbite correction, an ideal arch system should be used, incorporating the first molars and two or three teeth on either side of the tooth to be moved. Progressively stiffer round wires are placed to align the crown, but the final correction of root position can be achieved only by placing a rectangular wire that will almost fill the bracket slot. The reciprocal force will tend to move the anchor teeth into crossbite. This may be resisted by the use of a transpalatal arch on the molars (Figure 20-37) or the addition of a removable acrylic plate that closely contacts the palatal surface of the adjacent anchor teeth. The rectangular wire can be adjusted to control the tooth in three planes of space.

If a deep overbite exists on the teeth in crossbite, correction will be much easier if a temporary bite plane that frees the occlusion is added. This bite plane should be carefully constructed to contact the occlusal surfaces of all teeth to prevent any supereruption during treatment.

Establishing a good overbite relationship is the key to maintaining crossbite correction. Crown reconstruction can be used to provide positive occlusal indexing, while eliminating any balancing interferences from the lingual cusps of posterior teeth.

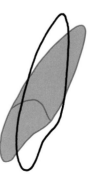

FIGURE 20-35 A labially directed force from a removable appliance will tip the tooth and cause an apparent intrusion of the crown, which reduces the overbite.

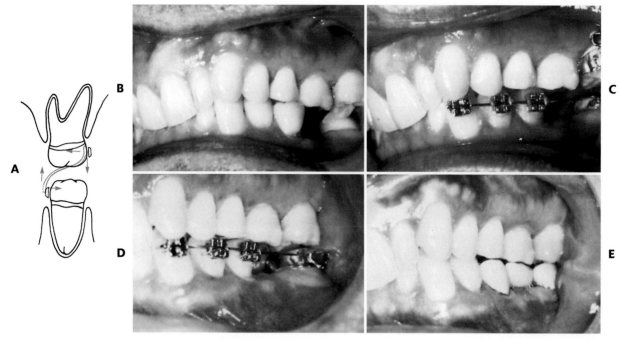

FIGURE 20-36 **A,** "Through the bite" or cross elastics produce both horizontal and vertical forces and will extrude the teeth while moving them buccolingually. If these elastics are used to correct posterior crossbite in adults, care must be taken not to open the bite anteriorly too much. Cross elastics are rarely indicated for an anterior crossbite. **B,** Buccal crossbite of the second molars in a patient at age 50 who had lost the mandibular first molar years previously. The lower second molar had tipped mesially and lingually. **C,** The standard orthodontic appliance for uprighting a lower molar was used, consisting of a band on the mandibular second molar, a bonded canine-to-canine mandibular lingual wire to augment anchorage, and bonded brackets on the facial of the premolars and canine. In addition, a lingual cleat was placed on the lower band, and a band with a facial hook was placed on the maxillary second molar, so that cross elastics could be worn. **D,** The molar uprighting was completed after the crossbite was corrected. **E,** The completed bridge in place. This is classic adjunctive orthodontics. The anterior deep bite and incisor alignment were not problems for this patient and were not corrected.

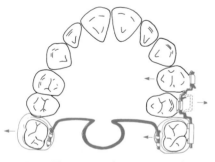

FIGURE 20-37 Tipping and extrusion of a tooth during crossbite correction may be controlled by using a fixed appliance. Anchorage is obtained from adjacent teeth and the contralateral molar if necessary, which can be included via a lingual arch as shown here. A flexible wire engaged in the brackets generates the necessary controlled forces.

REFERENCES

1. Amsterdam M: Periodontal prosthesis: twenty-five years in retrospect. Part II. Occlusion, Compend Contin Ed Dent 5:325-334, 1984.
2. Kusy RP, Tulloch JFC: Analysis of moment-force ratios in the mechanics of tooth movement, Am J Orthod Dentofac Orthop 90:127-131, 1986.
3. Spurrier S, Hall S, Joondeph D et al: A comparison of apical root resorption during treatment in endodontically treated or vital teeth, Am J Orthod Dentofac Orthop 97:130-134, 1990.
4. Wennstrom JL, Stokland BL, Nyman S, Thilander B: Periodontal tissue-response to orthodontic movement of teeth with infrabony pockets, Am J Orthod Dentofac Orthop 103:313-319, 1993.
5. Artun J, Urbue KS: The effect of orthodontic treatment on periodontal bone support in patients with advanced loss of marginal periodontium, Am J Orthod Dentofac Orthop 93:143-148, 1988.

6. Boyd RL, Leggott PJ, Quinn RS et al: Periodontal implications of orthodontic treatment in adults with reduced or normal periodontal tissues versus those of adolescents, Am J Orthod Dentofac Orthop 96:191-199, 1989.

7. Roberts RW, Chacker FM, Burstone CJ: A segmental approach to mandibular molar uprighting, Am J Orthod 81:177-184, 1982.

8. Ziskind D, Schmidt A, Hirschfeld Z: Forced eruption technique: rationale and technique, J Pros Dent 79:246-248, 1998.

9. Osterle LJ, Wood LW: Raising the root: a look at orthodontic extrusion, J Am Dent Assoc 192:193-198, 1991.

10. Sheridan JJ, Ledoux PM: Air-rotor stripping and proximal sealants, J Clin Orthod 23:790-794, 1989.

11. Spear FM, Mathews DM, Kokich VG: Interdisiplinary management of single-tooth implants, Sem Orthod 3:45-72, 1997.

CHAPTER

21

Special Considerations in Comprehensive Treatment of Adults

There are no fundamental differences between treatment for adults and children. The response to orthodontic force may be somewhat slower in an adult than in a child, but tooth movement occurs in a similar way at all ages, and comprehensive treatment for adults can be divided into the same stages discussed in Chapters 16 to 19. Despite this, comprehensive treatment for adults brings with it a set of problems that simply do not exist with younger patients. Special considerations for adults fall into three major categories: (1) different motivations for seeking orthodontic treatment and different psychological reactions to it, (2) heightened susceptibility to periodontal disease, and the possibility that active periodontal disease and the replacement of missing teeth is the reason for seeking treatment in the first place, and (3) a lack of growth, even the small amounts of vertical growth on which orthodontists can rely during treatment in late adolescence. This not only precludes changing jaw relationships without surgery but makes tooth movement more difficult.

Until recent years orthodontic treatment for adults was unusual, but that is no longer the case (Figure 21-1). In 1970, fewer than 5% of all orthodontic patients were age 18 or older. By 1990, 25% fell into that category, and most of the growth in orthodontics in the 1980s was in the adult patient group. In the 1990s, orthodontic practice growth once again was largely in the number of children being treated. Although adults made up about 15% of all orthodontic patients toward the end of the decade, the number of adults receiving comprehensive treatment has remained more or less constant since the 1990 peak.[1] The most recent trend appears to be an increase in the older adult group (age 40 and up), more of whom now are candidates for comprehensive rather than just adjunctive orthodontics.

MOTIVATION FOR ADULT TREATMENT

Psychological Considerations

A major motivation for orthodontic treatment of children and adolescents is the parents' desire for treatment. The typical child accepts orthodontics in about the same way that he accepts going to school, summer camp, and the inevitable junior high school dance—as just another in the series of events that one must endure while growing up. Occasionally, of course, an adolescent actively resists orthodontic treatment, and the result can be unfortunate for all concerned if the treatment becomes the focus of an adolescent rebellion. In most instances, however, children tend not to become emotionally involved in their treatment.

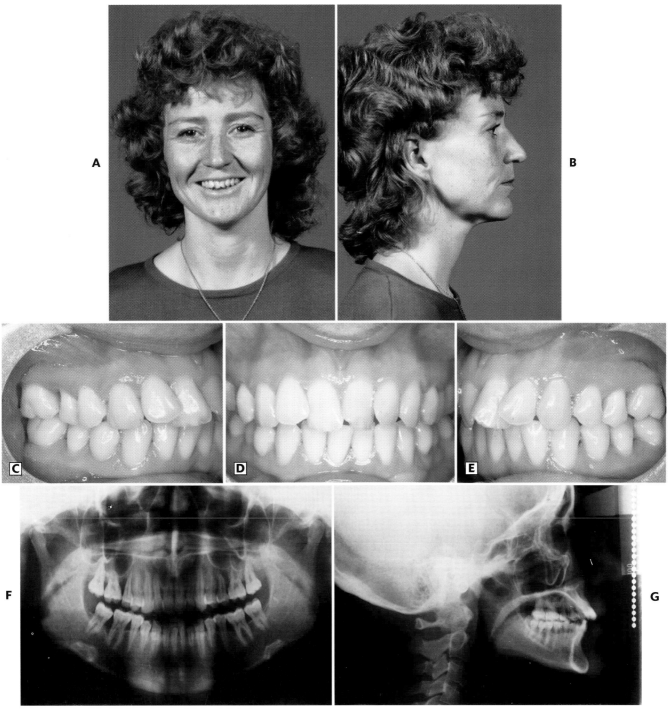

FIGURE 21-1 **A-E,** At age 27, this woman sought orthodontic treatment because her periodontist thought that her periodontal disease perhaps could be controlled better if the alignment of her teeth were improved, and because she had never liked the appearance of her extremely crowded and irregular maxillary incisors. There was a full-cusp Class II molar relationship and minimal overbite. **F,** The panoramic radiograph shows severe bone loss in multiple areas, but active disease was now under control. **G,** The cephalometric radiograph showed a mild skeletal Class II jaw relationship, with moderate maxillary incisor protrusion. The treatment plan called for extraction of maxillary first premolars to allow for alignment of the upper teeth without creating incisor protrusion, plus reduction of interproximal enamel to compensate for the tooth-size discrepancy created by the very large maxillary lateral incisors.

continued

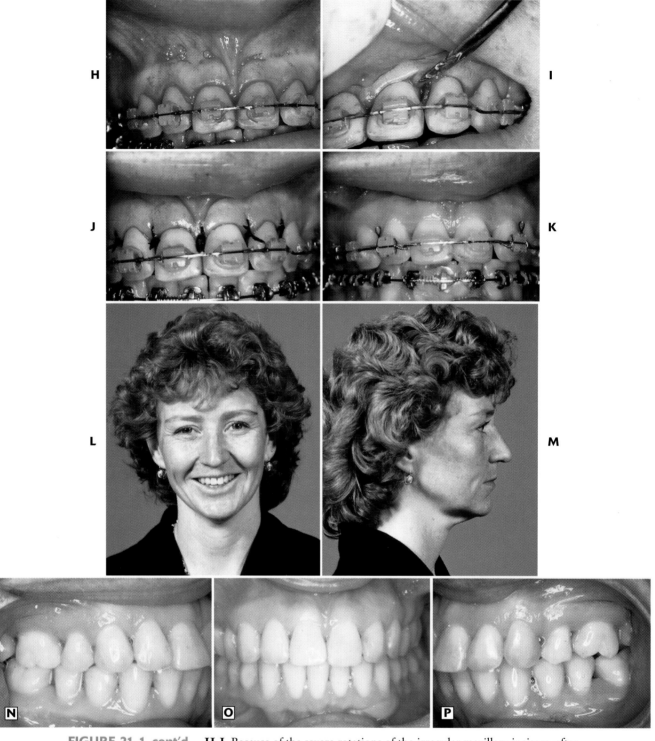

FIGURE 21-1, cont'd   **H-J,** Because of the severe rotations of the irregular maxillary incisors, after alignment was completed but with the orthodontic appliance still in place, repositioning of the maxillary frenum and sectioning of the elastic gingival fibers were carried out; **K,** three weeks later. **L-P,** After 18 months of treatment, both the occlusion and appearance of the teeth were greatly improved. (Periodontal surgery by Dr. R. Williams.)

continued

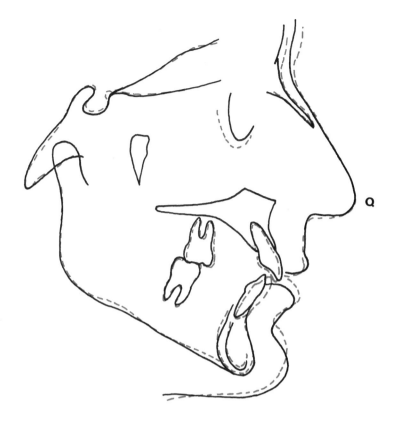

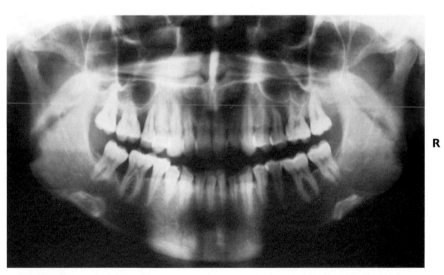

FIGURE 21-1, cont'd **Q,** Cephalometric superimposition shows slight retraction of the maxillary incisors and mild proclination of the mandibular incisors, as was desired in this case. **R,** Panoramic radiograph 1 year after the orthodontic treatment was completed. The periodontal condition remained under good control during and following the orthodontic treatment. (Periodontal surgery by Dr. R. Williams.)

Adults, in contrast, seek comprehensive orthodontic treatment because they themselves want something. That something, however, is not always clearly expressed, and in fact some adults have a remarkably elaborate hidden set of motivations. It is important to explore why the patient wants treatment, and why now as opposed to some other time, to avoid setting up a situation in which the patient's expectations from treatment cannot possibly be met. Sometimes orthodontic treatment is sought as a last-ditch effort to improve personal appearance to deal with a series of complicated social problems. An extreme example might be an individual whose marriage is failing and who thinks that perhaps this would not happen if his or her protruding front teeth were corrected. Orthodontic treatment obviously cannot be relied on to repair personal relationships, save jobs, or overcome a series of financial disasters. If the prospective patient has unrealistic expectations of that sort, it is much better to deal with them sooner rather than later.

Most adult patients, fortunately, understand why they are seeking orthodontic treatment and are realistic about what they can obtain from it. One might expect those who seek treatment to be less secure and less well adjusted than the average adult, but for the most part, those who seek treatment tend to have a more positive self-image than average.[2] It apparently takes a good deal of ego strength to seek orthodontic treatment as an adult, and ego strength rather than weakness characterizes most potential adult patients. A patient who seeks treatment primarily because he or she wants to improve the appearance or function of the teeth (internal motivation) is more likely to respond well psychologically than a patient whose motivation is the urging of others or the expected impact of treatment on others (external motivation). External motivation is often accompanied by an increasing impact of the orthodontic problem on personality (Figure 21-2). Such a patient is likely to have a complex set of unrecognized expectations for treatment, the proverbial hidden agenda.

One way to identify the minority of individuals who may present treatment problems because of their unrealistic expectations is to compare the patient's perception of his or her orthodontic condition with the doctor's evaluation. If the patient thinks that the appearance or function of the teeth is creating a severe problem, while an objective assessment simply does not corroborate that, orthodontic treatment should be approached with caution.

Even highly motivated adults express some concern about the appearance of orthodontic appliances. The demand for an invisible orthodontic appliance comes almost entirely from adults who are concerned about the reaction of others to obvious orthodontic treatment. In an earlier era, this was a major reason for using removable appliances in adults, particularly the Crozat appliance in the United States. However, it is simply impossible to do effective comprehensive treatment with a removable appliance, particularly one that is not worn constantly. In recent years,

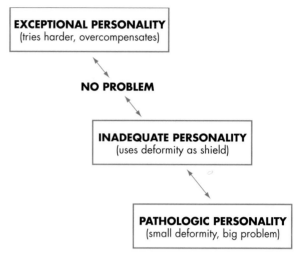

FIGURE 21-2   Dentofacial deformity can affect an individual's life adjustment. Fortunately, most potential adult orthodontic patients fall into the "no problem" category. A few highly successful individuals (who nevertheless may seek treatment) can be thought of as almost overcompensating for their deformity, but they tend to be personable and very pleasant to work with. For some individuals, however, the orthodontic condition can become the focus for a wide-ranging set of social adjustment problems that orthodontics alone will not solve. These patients fall into the "inadequate personality" and "pathologic personality" categories, who are difficult and almost impossible, respectively, to help. An important aspect of orthodontic diagnosis for adults is understanding where a patient fits along this spectrum.

the search for less visible appliances has led to clear or tooth-colored plastic or ceramic brackets (Figure 21-3) and to fixed lingual appliances (see Chapter 12).

At present, it is not possible to produce an invisible or minimally visible appliance that does not compromise the orthodontic treatment. Plastic brackets create problems in controlling root position and closing spaces. Lingual appliances, primarily because of the small interbracket span, also make control of complex tooth movements difficult. Ceramic brackets, though better than anything previously, inevitably make the treatment more difficult because of the problems outlined in Chapter 12. Although there is nothing wrong with using the most esthetic appliance possible for an adult patient, the compromises associated with this approach should be thoroughly discussed in advance. It is unrealistic for a patient to expect that orthodontic treatment can be carried out without other people knowing about it.

The whole issue of the visibility of the orthodontic appliances is much less important, at least in the United States, than many patients fear. Orthodontic treatment for adults is certainly socially acceptable, and one does not become a victim of discrimination because of visible orthodontic appliances. In a sense, the patient's expectations become a self-fulfilling prophecy. If the patient faces others confidently, a visible orthodontic appliance causes no prob-

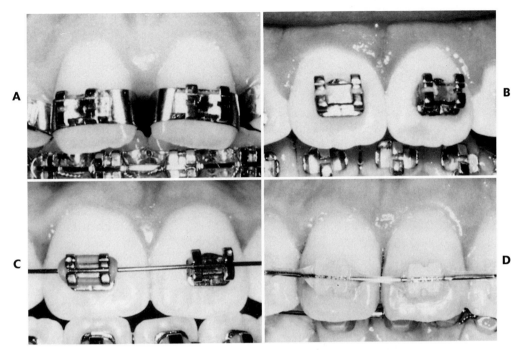

FIGURE 21-3   A sequence of increasingly esthetic brackets for maxillary incisors. **A,** Standard twin brackets on anterior bands; **B,** bonded straightwire brackets, standard size; **C,** bonded straightwire brackets, mini-size; **D,** ceramic brackets. Small bonded metal brackets have less esthetic impact than bands, and ceramic brackets further reduce visibility of the appliance. Lingual appliances (see Figure 12-9) are almost totally invisible. Whether the esthetic improvement from small metal brackets to ceramic brackets to lingual brackets is worth the additional cost, effort, and treatment time is a judgment to be made individually with each patient.

lems. Only if the patient acts ashamed is there likely to be any negative reaction from others.

The question of whether an orthodontic office should have a separate treatment area for adult patients, separated from the adolescents who still constitute the bulk of most orthodontic practices, is related to the same set of negative attitudes. Most comprehensive orthodontic treatment for adolescents is carried out in open treatment areas, not only because the open area is efficient but also because the learning effect from having patients observe what is happening to others is a positive influence in patient adaptation to treatment (Figure 21-4). Should adults be segregated into private rooms, rather than joining the group in the open treatment area? This arrangement is logical only if the adult is vaguely ashamed of being an orthodontic patient. Sometimes, for some adults, treatment in a private area may be preferable, but for most adults, learning from interacting with other patients is extremely beneficial. There are positive advantages in having patients at various stages of treatment compare their experiences, and this is at least as beneficial to adults as to children, perhaps more so.

Despite the fact that adult patients can be treated in the same area as adolescents, they cannot be handled in exactly the same way. The typical adolescent's passive acceptance of what is being done is rarely found in adult pa-

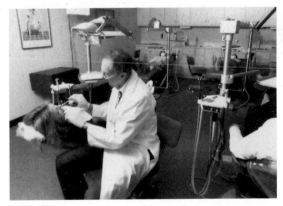

FIGURE 21-4   For most adults, there is a positive advantage in carrying out orthodontic treatment in an open treatment area that allows interaction with other patients, just as there is with adolescents. The interplay between doctor, assistants, and other patients enhances the patient's learning about orthodontic treatment.

tients, who want and expect a considerable degree of explanation of what is happening and why. The fact that an adult can be counted on to be interested in the treatment does not automatically translate into compliance with instructions. Unless adult patients understand why they have been asked to do various things, they may choose not to do them, not in the passive way an adolescent might just shrug it off, but from an active decision not to cooperate. In addition, adults, as a rule, are less tolerant of discomfort and more likely to complain about pain after adjustments and about difficulties in speech, eating, and tissue adaptation. Additional chair time to meet these demands should be anticipated.

These characteristics might make adults sound like less desirable orthodontic patients than adolescents, but this is not necessarily so. Working with individuals who are intensely interested in their own treatment can be a pleasant and stimulating alternative to the less involved adolescents. If the expectations of both the doctor and the patient are realistic, comprehensive treatment for adults can be a rewarding experience for both.

Periodontal and Restorative Needs as Motivating Factors

Although comprehensive orthodontic treatment cannot preclude the possibility of periodontal disease developing later, it can be a useful part of the overall treatment plan for a patient who already has periodontal involvement (Figure 21-5). It may be necessary, for instance, to align teeth and improve occlusal relationships after initial therapy has brought periodontal disease under control, to make definitive periodontal and restorative treatment possible. In a sense, this is adjunctive orthodontic treatment, but even if the major focus of treatment is the periodontal situation, when the orthodontic therapy involves changing the entire occlusal scheme it can be considered comprehensive. Not more than 10% of adult patients have comprehensive orthodontic treatment primarily because of periodontal problems, but periodontal considerations are important for all adults who undergo orthodontic treatment. These are discussed below in some detail.

Temporomandibular Pain/Dysfunction as a Reason for Orthodontic Treatment

Temporomandibular pain and dysfunction (TMD symptoms) rarely are encountered in children seeking orthodontic treatment, but TMD is a significant motivating factor for some adults who consider orthodontic treatment. The relationship between dental occlusion and TMD symptoms is highly controversial, and it is important to view this situation reasonably objectively. Orthodontic treatment can sometimes help patients with TMD problems, but it cannot be relied on to correct them. It is important for patients to understand what may happen to their symptoms during and after orthodontics.

Patients with TMD symptoms can be divided into two large groups: those with internal joint pathology, including displacement or destruction of the intra-articular disk; and those with symptoms primarily of muscle origin, caused by spasm and fatigue of the muscles that position the jaw and head (Figure 21-6, on p. 653). The distinction

in many patients is difficult diagnostically, because muscle spasm and joint pathology can coexist. Nevertheless, the distinction is important when orthodontic treatment is considered. It is unlikely that orthodontic treatment alone will be of significant benefit to the patient who has internal joint problems or other nonmuscular sources of pain. Those who have myofascial pain/dysfunction, on the other hand, may benefit from improved occlusal relationships.

Most of us develop some symptoms of degenerative joint disease as we grow older, and it is not surprising that the jaw joints sometimes show internal degenerative changes (Figure 21-7, on p. 653). Arthritic involvement of the temporomandibular (TM) joints is most likely to be the cause of TMD symptoms in patients who have arthritic changes in other joints of the body. A component of muscle spasm and muscle pain should be suspected in individuals whose only symptoms are in the TM joint area, even if radiographs show moderate arthritic degeneration of the joint.

Displacement of the disk (Figure 21-8, on p. 654) can arise from a number of causes. One possibility is trauma to the joint, so that the ligaments that oppose the action of the lateral pterygoid muscle are stretched or torn. In this circumstance, muscle contraction moves the disk forward as the mandibular condyles translate forward on wide opening, but the ligaments do not restore the disk to its proper position when the jaw is closed. The result is a click upon opening and closing, as the disk pops into place over the condylar head as the patient opens, but is displaced anteriorly on closure.

The click and symptoms associated with it can be corrected if an occlusal splint is used to prevent the patient from closing beyond the point at which displacement occurs. The resulting relief of pain influences patients and dentists to seek either restorative or orthodontic treatment to increase facial vertical dimension. However, orthodontic elongation of all posterior teeth to control disk displacement is not a treatment procedure that should be undertaken lightly. Often the patient whose symptoms have been controlled by a splint can tolerate its reduction or removal, without requiring major occlusal changes. As a general rule, there are better ways of handling disk displacement than orthodontic treatment.

Myofascial pain develops when muscles are overly fatigued and tend to go into spasm. It is all but impossible to overwork the jaw muscles to this extent during normal occlusal function. To produce myofascial pain, the patient must be clenching or grinding the teeth for many hours per day, presumably as a response to stress. Great variations are seen in the way different individuals respond to stress, both in the organ system that feels the strain (those who develop an ulcerated colon rarely have TMD symptoms also) and in the amount of stress that can be tolerated before symptoms appear (tense individuals develop stress-related symptoms before their relaxed colleagues do). For this reason, it is impossible to say that occlusal discrepancies of any given degree will lead to TMD symptoms.[3]

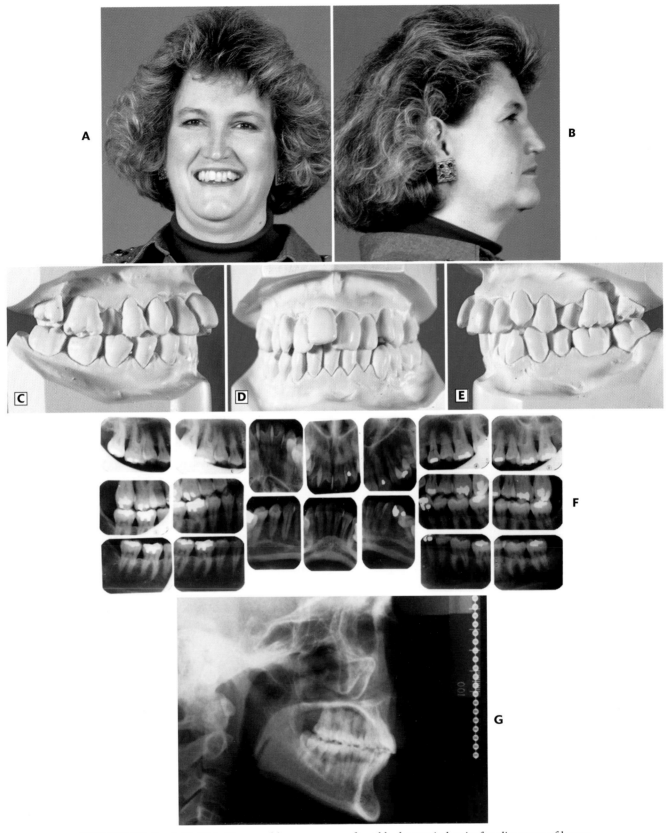

FIGURE 21-5 **A-E,** This 43-year-old woman was referred by her periodontist for alignment of her extremely crowded teeth, so that splinting could be accomplished if required (which was considered quite likely), and to allow better hygiene. **F,** The full series of intra-oral radiographs, indicated for patients with periodontal disease, shows the extent of bone loss; **G,** the initial cephalometric radiograph shows a skeletal Class II tendency with protrusion of maxillary incisors, and reasonable vertical proportions. After initial control of the periodontal condition, the treatment plan called for extraction of maxillary first and mandibular second premolars, with comprehensive orthodontic treatment accompanied by periodontal maintenance appointments at two-month intervals.

continued

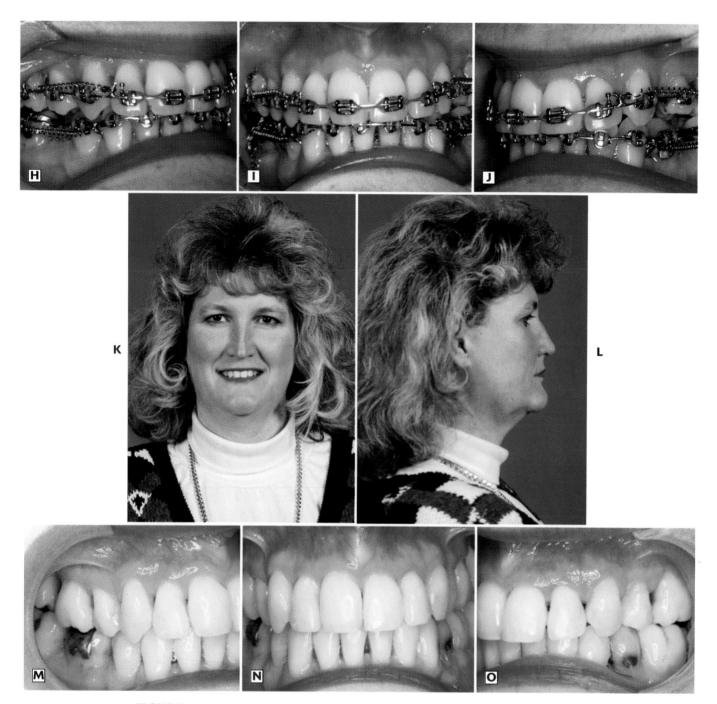

FIGURE 21-5, cont'd   H-J, To keep orthodontic forces as light as possible, space closure was carried out using 150-gm superelastic coil springs; after the spaces were closed, light Class II elastics also were employed for 3 months. **K-O,** After 21 months of orthodontic treatment, both occlusion and alignment were greatly improved, and the patient was pleased with the change in dental and facial appearance.

continued

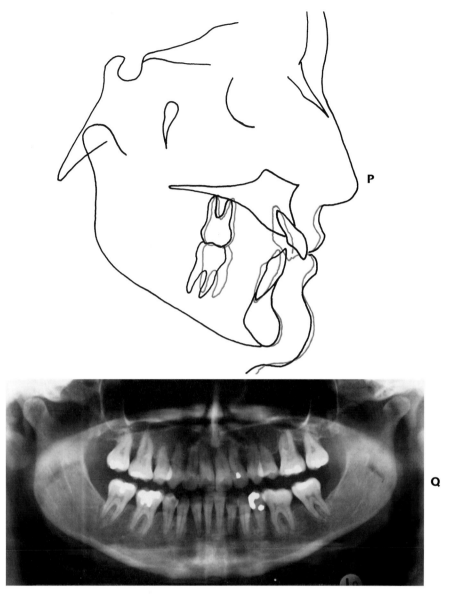

FIGURE 21-5, cont'd P, Cephalometric superimposition shows the changes that occurred, with some retraction of the upper but not the lower incisors. Because of the extreme bone loss, suckdown retainers, which splint the teeth, were used full-time for the first six months, then just at night. **Q,** Panoramic radiograph 1 year after the completion of treatment. Note that the periodontal condition remained stable, but some root resorption did occur during the treatment.

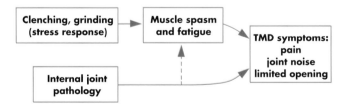

FIGURE 21-6 Temporomandibular dysfunction (TMD) symptoms arise from two major causes: muscle spasm and fatigue, which almost always are related to excessive clenching and grinding in response to stress, and internal joint pathology. As a general guideline, patients with symptoms of muscle spasm and fatigue may be helped by orthodontic treatment, but simpler methods should be attempted first. Orthodontics alone is rarely useful for patients with internal joint pathology.

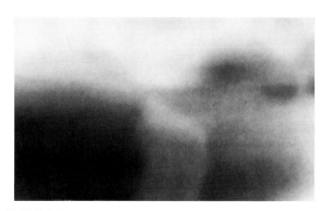

FIGURE 21-7 Radiographic appearance of arthritic degeneration of the mandibular condyle. Note the flattening of the condyle and the lipping posteriorly.

653

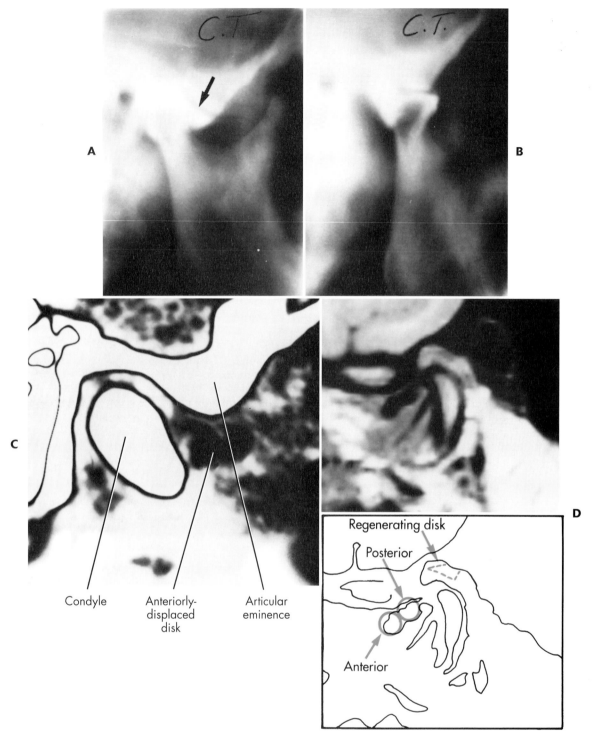

Condyle   Anteriorly-
                displaced
                disk

Articular
eminence

Regenerating disk

Posterior

Anterior

FIGURE 21-8   **A** and **B,** Arthrotomograms showing anterior disk displacement with reduction on opening. In **A,** note the accumulation of dye anteriorly (*arrow*). In **B,** with the patient open, the posterior band of the disk now can be visualized indirectly in the proper position. **C,** Computerized tomographic (CT) view of a displaced mandibular disk, which can be visualized clearly in front of the head of the condyle; **D,** magnetic resonance imaging (MRI) view of displaced disk, with the anterior and posterior bands of the disk indicated on the adjacent sketch. There is evidence on this scan of a regenerating disk, as shown in the dashed area. CT and MRI scans have replaced arthrotomograms for diagnosis of disk displacement, with MRI increasingly preferred because of the absence of ionizing radiation.

It is possible to demonstrate that some types of occlusal discrepancies predispose patients who clench or grind their teeth to the development of TMD symptoms, as well as to construct a rational case for helping control those problems by altering the occlusion. It must be kept in mind, however, that it takes two factors to produce myofascial pain: an occlusal discrepancy *and* a patient who clenches or grinds the teeth. Perhaps the most compelling argument against malocclusion as a primary cause of TMD is the observation that TMD is no more prevalent in patients with extremely severe malocclusion than in the general population.[4] The dictum "let your teeth alone" would solve myofascial pain problems if it could be followed by the patient.

From this perspective, three broad approaches to myofascial pain symptoms can be considered: reducing the amount of stress; reducing the patient's reaction to the stress; or improving the occlusal relationships, thereby making it harder for the patient to hurt himself or herself. Drastic alteration of the occlusion, by either restorative dental procedures or orthodontic treatment, is logical only if the less invasive stress-control and stress-adaptation approaches have failed. In that circumstance, orthodontic treatment to alter the occlusion so that the patient can better tolerate parafunctional activity (which in some instances may involve orthognathic surgery to reposition the jaws) may be worth attempting.[5]

At one time it was thought that TMD was a progressive problem in essentially all patients. Now it is clear that for many individuals, problems gradually resolve over time, with or without treatment. The peak prevalence of TMD symptoms is in the early thirties; after that, there is a considerable decline.[6] This is another reason for caution in attributing the resolution of TMD problems to adult orthodontic treatment.

PERIODONTAL ASPECTS OF ADULT TREATMENT

Periodontal problems are rarely a major concern during orthodontic treatment of children and adolescents, both because periodontal disease usually does not arise at an early age and because tissue resistance is higher in younger patients. For the same reasons, periodontal considerations are increasingly important as patients become older, regardless of whether periodontal problems were a motivating factor for orthodontic treatment.

The prevalence of periodontal disease as a function of age in a large group of potential orthodontic patients with severe malocclusion is shown in Figure 21-9. Note that up to the late thirties, there is nearly a straight-line relationship between periodontal pocketing (defined here as the presence of pockets greater than 5 mm) and age. In contrast, the prevalence of mucogingival problems peaks in the twenties. The odds are that any patient over the age of 35 has some periodontal problems that could affect orthodontic treatment.

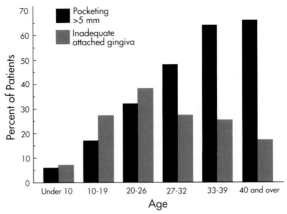

FIGURE 21-9 The prevalence of periodontal pockets greater than 5 mm (*black*) and inadequate attached gingiva (*red*) as a function of age in patients with severe orthodontic problems who were referred to the University of North Carolina Dentofacial Clinic for possible surgical-orthodontic treatment. (Redrawn from Morarity JD, Simpson DM: *J Dent Res* 63, Special Issue A, #1249, 1984.)

There is no contraindication to treating adults who have periodontal disease, as long as the disease has been brought under control. Progression of untreated periodontal breakdown must be anticipated, however, and the periodontal situation must receive major attention in planning and executing orthodontic treatment for all adults.

Periodontal disease is not a continuous and steadily progressive degenerative process. Instead, it is characterized by episodes of acute attack on some but usually not all areas of the mouth, followed by quiescent periods.[7] It is obviously important to identify high-risk patients and high-risk sites. At present, persistent bleeding on probing is the best indicator of active and presumably progressive disease.[8] New diagnostic procedures to evaluate subgingival plaque and crevicular fluids for the presence of indicator bacteria, enzymes, or other chemical mediators show promise and are likely to be clinically useful in the near future.[9] There appear to be at least three risk groups in the population: those with rapid progression (about 10%), those with moderate progression (the great majority, about 80%), and those with no progression despite the presence of gingival inflammation (about 10%).[10]

Minimal Periodontal Involvement

Hygiene Status. Any patient undergoing orthodontic treatment must take extra care to clean the teeth, but this is even more important in adult orthodontics. Bacterial plaque is the main etiologic factor in periodontal breakdown, and plaque-induced gingivitis is the first step in the disease process. Orthodontic appliances simultaneously make maintenance of oral hygiene more difficult and more important. In children and adolescents, even if gingivitis develops in response to the presence of orthodontic appliances, it almost never extends into periodontitis. This cannot be taken for granted in adults, no matter how good their initial periodontal condition.[11]

The difficult area for orthodontic patients to clean is the area of each tooth between the brackets and the gingival margin. Because of the greater length of the clinical crown in adults, however, it is at least easier for adult patients to approach these areas. Hygiene aids such as rubber interdental stimulators and proximal brushes to reach between teeth are often needed. There is some evidence that careful use of modern powered brushes is helpful (but none that one type of powered brush is superior, or that a powered brush is necessary).

Attached Gingiva.   The periodontal evaluation of a potential adult orthodontic patient must include not only the response to periodontal probing but also the level and condition of the attached gingiva. Labial movement of incisors in some patients can be followed by gingival recession and loss of attachment. The risk is greatest when irregular teeth are aligned by expanding the dental arch.

The present concept is that gingival recession occurs secondarily to an alveolar bone dehiscence, if overlying tissues are stressed. The stress can be due to any of several causes. Major possibilities are toothbrush trauma, plaque-induced inflammation, or the stretching and thinning of the gingiva that might be created by labial tooth movement. Once recession begins, it can progress rapidly, especially if there is little or no keratinized attached gingiva and the attachment is only alveolar mucosa.

It was once thought that the width of the gingival attachment determined whether recession occurred. Not all keratinized gingiva is attached. The width of the attached tissue can be observed most readily by inserting a periodontal probe and observing the distance between the point at which the gingival attachment is encountered and the point at which the alveolar mucosa begins (Figure 21-10). Recent animal experiments suggest that the thickness of the gingival attachment, rather than its surface

qualities (keratinized or mucosal), may be the major factor in whether recession occurs.[12] Lower incisors in patients with mandibular prognathism are at particular risk of recession, and thin gingival tissue probably is the reason.

For adult orthodontic patients, it is much better to prevent gingival recession than to try to correct it later. The protective effect of a gingival graft may be due more to the greater gingival thickness than a wider zone of attached tissue. Nevertheless, a gingival graft (Figure 21-11) must be considered in many patients, particularly those for whom arch expansion will be used to align incisors and those who will have surgical mandibular advancement or genioplasty (see Chapter 22).

Moderate Periodontal Involvement

Disease Control.   Before orthodontic treatment is attempted for patients who have preexisting periodontal problems, dental and periodontal disease must be brought under control. Unless a patient can maintain periodontal health after initial therapy, orthodontic treatment is potentially damaging rather than beneficial. A period of observation following preliminary periodontal treatment, to make sure that the patient is adequately controlled and to allow healing after the periodontal therapy, should precede comprehensive orthodontics.

Preliminary periodontal therapy can include all aspects of periodontal treatment except osseous surgery. It is important to remove all calculus and other irritants from periodontal pockets before any tooth movement is attempted, and it is often wise to use surgical flaps to expose these areas to ensure the best possible scaling. Treatment procedures to facilitate the patient's long-term maintenance, like osseous recontouring or repositioned flaps to compensate for areas of gingival recession, are best deferred until the final occlusal relationships have been established.

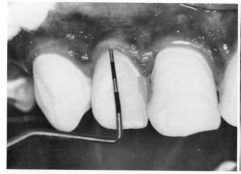 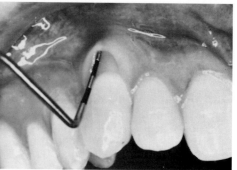

FIGURE 21-10   The amount of attached gingiva is the keratinized tissue between the depth of periodontal probing and the beginning of alveolar mucosa. **A,** In this young and healthy patient, 2 to 3 mm of attached gingiva are apparent; **B,** in this older patient with gingival recession over the canine, the probe penetrates to the mucosal margin, indicating essentially no attached tissue. Note also the thinness of the tissue where recession has occurred over the canine. Before orthodontic treatment, stabilization and thickening of the gingival tissue over a tooth like this, using a gingival graft, would be necessary.

Disease control also requires endodontic treatment of any pulpally involved teeth. There is no contraindication to the orthodontic movement of an endodontically treated tooth, so root canal therapy before orthodontics will cause no problems (Figure 21-12). Attempting to move a pulpally involved tooth, however, is likely to cause a flare-up of the periapical condition.

The general guideline for preliminary restorative treatment is that temporary restorations should be placed to control caries, with the definitive restorative dentistry delayed until after the orthodontic phase of treatment. Temporary restoration, however, should not be taken to mean the use of a cement that will last only a few months.

Short-lived temporaries of this type are incompatible with orthodontic treatment. Composite resin is now the preferred temporary restorative material while orthodontics is being carried out. Cast restorations should be delayed until after the final occlusal relationships have been established by orthodontic treatment.

Periodontal Maintenance.   Because the margins of bands can make periodontal maintenance more difficult, it usually is better to use a fully bonded orthodontic appliance for periodontally involved adults. Steel ligatures or self-ligating brackets also are preferred for periodontally involved patients rather than elastomeric rings to retain orthodontic archwires, because patients with

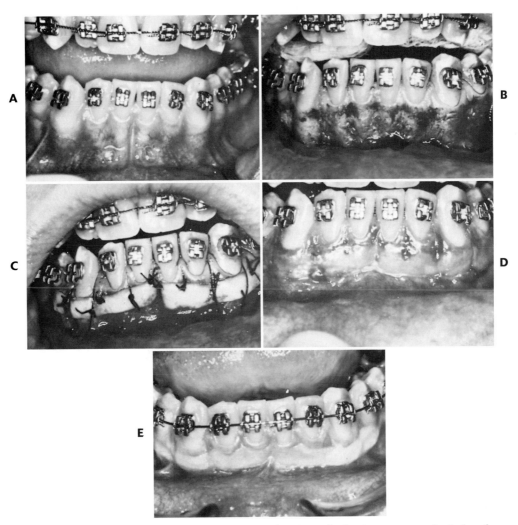

FIGURE 21-11   In adults who will have comprehensive orthodontic treatment, gingival grafting to create adequate quantity and thickness of attached gingiva is important before beginning orthodontic tooth movement. **A,** Lack of attached gingiva and thin gingival tissue in the mandibular anterior region in a patient whose lower incisors must be advanced to align them. Note the alveolar mucosa extending almost to the gingival margin on all anterior teeth; **B,** surgical preparation of a bed for grafting; **C,** grafts sutured in place; **D,** healing 10 days later, showing incorporation of the grafts; **E,** orthodontic alignment nearly completed 5 months later, with the gingival grafts creating both a thicker contour of the gingival tissue and a generous band of attachment. (Courtesy Dr. J. Morarity.)

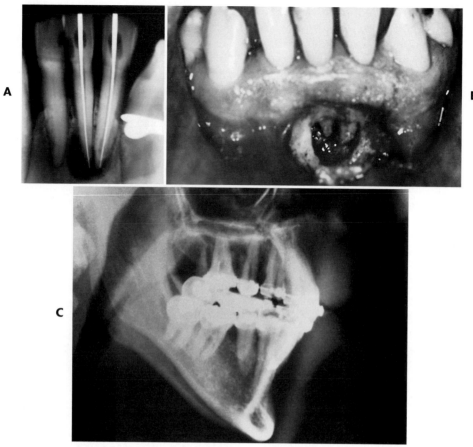

FIGURE 21-12   Any necessary endodontic treatment should precede orthodontic tooth movement. **A,** Periapical lesion around two nonvital mandibular incisors; **B,** apicoectomy and retrograde apical seal in connection with endodontic treatment of these teeth; **C,** cephalometric radiograph during orthodontic treatment. In this patient, the lower incisors were successfully intruded despite the previous endodontic treatment.

elastomeric rings have higher levels of microorganisms in gingival plaque.[13]

During comprehensive orthodontics, a patient with moderate periodontal problems must be on a maintenance schedule, with the frequency of cleaning and scaling depending on the severity of the periodontal disease. Periodontal maintenance therapy at 2- to 4-month intervals is the usual plan. For periodontally involved patients, better hygiene control has been demonstrated with the use of electric toothbrushes,[14] and adjunctive chemical agents (including chlorhexidine if needed) also should be considered.

Severe Periodontal Involvement

The general approach to treatment for patients with severe periodontal involvement is the same as that outlined earlier, but the treatment itself must be modified in two ways: (1) periodontal maintenance should be scheduled at more frequent intervals, with the patient being seen as frequently for periodontal maintenance as for orthodontic appliance adjustments in many instances (i.e., every 4 to 6

weeks); and (2) orthodontic treatment goals and mechanics must be modified to keep orthodontic forces to an absolute minimum, because the reduced area of the periodontal ligament (PDL) after significant bone loss means higher pressure in the PDL from any force (Figure 21-13). Sometimes it is helpful to temporarily retain a tooth that is hopelessly involved periodontally, using it to help support an orthodontic appliance that will contribute to saving other teeth.[15]

Modifications in treatment mechanics are discussed at the end of this chapter.

Orthodontic-Prosthodontic-Implant Interactions

Adults presenting for comprehensive orthodontic treatment often have dental problems that require restorative as well as orthodontic treatment. Such problems include loss of tooth structure from wear and abrasion or trauma, gingival esthetic problems, and missing teeth that require replacement with either conventional prosthodontics or implants.

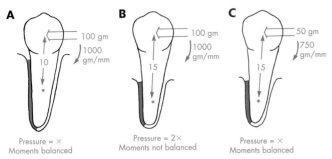

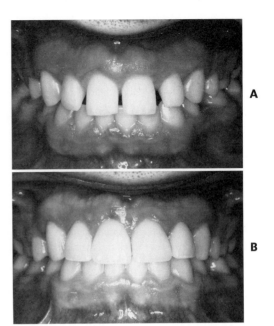

FIGURE 21-13   Bone loss around a tooth that is to be moved affects both the force and the moment needed. **A,** For optimum bodily movement of a premolar whose center of resistance is 10 mm apical to the bracket, a 100 gm force and a 1000 gm-mm moment is needed. **B,** The same force system would be inappropriate for an identical premolar whose bone support had been reduced by periodontal disease so that the PDL area is half as large as it was originally, and so that the center of resistance is now 15 mm apical to the bracket. For such a tooth, the 100 gm force would produce twice the optimum pressure in the PDL, and the moment would not be large enough to prevent tipping. **C,** The correct force system for the periodontally involved tooth would be a 50 gm force and a 15 × 50 = 750 gm-mm moment. Orthodontic movement of periodontally involved teeth can be done only with careful attention to forces (smaller than normal) and moments (larger than normal).

FIGURE 21-14   For this man with very small teeth and concern about a lack of dental prominence, orthodontic treatment was used to create consistent spaces between the maxillary incisors so that porcelain veneers could be placed to bring the teeth to normal size.

Problems Related to Loss of Tooth Structure. The positioning of damaged, worn or abraded teeth during comprehensive orthodontics must be done with the eventual restorative plan in mind. Early consultation with the restorative dentist obviously becomes important. There are three particularly important considerations in deciding where the orthodontist should position teeth that are to be restored: the total amount of space that should be created, the mesio-distal positioning of the tooth within the space, and the bucco-lingual positioning.[16]

When tooth structure has been lost gingivally from the normal contact point, the tooth becomes abnormally narrow, and restoration of the lost crown width as well as height is important. The orthodontic positioning obviously should provide adequate space for the appropriate addition of the restorative material. The ideal position may or may not be in the center of the space mesio-distally—this would depend on whether the most esthetic restoration would be produced by symmetric addition on each side of the tooth, or whether a larger build-up on one side would be better. Similarly, the ideal bucco-lingual position of a worn or damaged tooth would be influenced by how the restoration was planned. If a crown or composite build-ups are planned, the tooth should be in the center of the dental arch. But if a facial veneer is to be used (Figure 21-14), the orthodontist should place the tooth more lingually than otherwise would be the case, to allow for the thickness of the veneer on the facial surface. Finally, better restorations can be done if the orthodontist provides slightly more space than is required, so there is room for the restorative

dentist to finish and polish proximal surfaces. The slight excess space can then be closed with a retainer.

If only a small amount of tooth structure has been lost, as for instance if the incisal edge of one incisor has been fractured, it may be possible to smooth the fractured area and elongate the damaged tooth so that the incisal edges line up. The result, however, will be uneven gingival margins—which means that elongation of a fractured tooth must be done with caution, and with consideration of the extent to which the gingival margins are exposed when the patient smiles. Before acceptably esthetic composite resin build-ups of anterior teeth were available, orthodontic elongation of fractured teeth was a more acceptable treatment approach than it is at present. Now, more than 1-2 mm of elongation rarely is a good plan unless the patient never exposes the gingiva.

Gingival Esthetic Problems. Gingival esthetic problems fall into two categories: those created by excessive and/or uneven display of gingiva and those created by gingival recession after periodontal bone loss.

The importance of maintaining a reasonably even gingival margin in the maxillary incisor area, especially when patients show the gingiva when they smile (as most do), was discussed earlier in the context of whether to elongate a tooth to compensate for a fractured incisal edge. This can be an important consideration when one lateral incisor is missing—substituting a canine on one side almost always results in uneven gingival margins, even if the crown of the substituted canine is recontoured. If several teeth have been worn or fractured, elongating them can create an

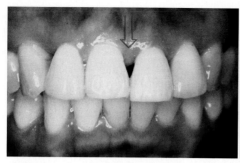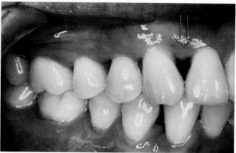

FIGURE 21-15 Bone loss and the associated gingival recession create "black holes" (*arrows*) between the anterior teeth, which can become a major esthetic problem, as they were for this 35-year-old woman. Regeneration of the interdental papillae is impossible, and periodontal surgery to create tissue tends to be unsuccessful. Space closure after reduction of interproximal enamel moves the contact points more gingivally and decreases the interdental space, improving the dental esthetics.

unesthetic "gummy smile" even if the gingival margins are kept at the same level across all the teeth. In that circumstance, it would be better to intrude the incisors to obtain a proper gingival exposure, and then restore the lost crown height. Dental esthetics is not just the teeth—the gingiva play an important role as well.

A particularly distressing problem is created by gingival recession after periodontal bone loss, which creates "black holes" between the maxillary incisor teeth (Figure 21-15). Even if periodontal therapy succeeds in obtaining some regeneration of the lost bony support, there is no way to regenerate the missing soft tissue. One approach to this problem is to remove some interproximal enamel so that the incisors can be brought closer together. This moves the contact points more gingivally, minimizing the open space between the teeth. The more bulbous the crowns were initially, the more successful this approach can be.

Missing Teeth: Space Closure vs. Prosthetic Replacement.

Old Extraction Sites. In adults, closing an old extraction site is likely to be difficult. The problem arises because of resorption and remodeling of alveolar bone. After several years, resorption results in a decrease in the vertical height of the bone, but more importantly, remodeling produces a buccolingual narrowing of the alveolar process as well (see Figure 20-8). When this has happened, closing the extraction space requires a reshaping of the cortical bone that comprises the buccal and lingual plates of the alveolar process. Cortical bone will respond to orthodontic force in most instances, but the response is significantly slower.

An old first molar or second premolar extraction site often poses a particular problem, because mesial drift of the posterior teeth has partially closed it as their crowns tipped mesially. In adjunctive treatment, a mesially tipped second molar usually is uprighted by tipping it distally, and then a bridge is placed (see Chapter 20). If comprehensive treatment is planned, should the space be closed by bringing the

first molar mesially? Mesial root movement is technically much more difficult than distal tipping, but the larger problem is that cortical bone remodeling usually is required to close the space because of atrophy after the old extraction. Such spaces are difficult to close completely and keep closed.[17] The involvement of cortical bone tends to produce a reciprocal space closure, no matter what the apparent anchorage situation is, which means that in the closure of an old extraction site, anterior teeth may be retracted more than anticipated or desired.

If it is desired to move lower molars forward into an old first molar or second premolar extraction site, a temporary implant in the ramus can be used to provide the necessary anchorage and avoid retracting the lower anterior teeth. This technique, pioneered by Roberts,[18] offers a level of control that cannot be obtained in any other way (Figure 21-16). With an appropriate implant, similar treatment could be done in the maxillary arch. Improvements in temporary implants for orthodontic purposes are occurring at a rapid rate.[19] It is likely that implants for orthodontic anchorage will come into widespread use in the near future, especially in orthodontics for adults. Nevertheless, it may be better judgment to open a partially closed old extraction site with simple orthodontic treatment (as described in Chapter 20) and replace the missing tooth with a bridge or implant, rather than plan extensive orthodontics as an alternative. This decision should be considered carefully in consultation between the orthodontist and prosthodontist.

Tooth Loss Due to Periodontal Disease. A space closure problem is also posed by the loss of a tooth to periodontal disease. As a general rule, it is unwise to move a tooth into an area where bone has been destroyed by periodontal disease, because of the risk that normal bone formation will not occur as the tooth moves into the defect. It is better to move teeth away from such an area, in preparation for prosthetic replacement.

However, there is an exception. First molars and incisors are lost in some adolescents and young adults to ju-

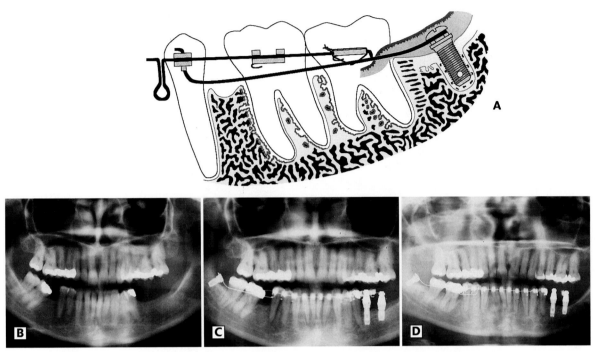

FIGURE 21-16 **A,** Drawing and, **B-D,** panoramic radiographs showing the use of an implant for retromolar anchorage. Note that a wire extending forward from the implant stabilizes the premolar and through it, the anterior teeth, so that they are not pulled posteriorly in reaction to anterior movement of the second and third molars. (From Roberts WE: Dental implant anchorage. In Epker B, Stella JP, Fish LC (editors): *Dentofacial deformities: integrated orthodontic and surgical management,* vol IV, ed 2, St Louis, Mosby, 1999.)

venile periodontitis, which differentially attacks these teeth and is characterized by the presence of a specific microbe, *Actinobacillus actinomycetemcomitans.* Once the disease process has been brought under control, which now typically involves antibiotic therapy, the causative agent seems to disappear.[20] Although bone around the first molars is often totally destroyed, neither the second molar nor the second premolar is significantly affected in most patients (Figure 21-17). Orthodontic closure of the incisor spaces is rarely feasible, but in these adolescent or young adult patients, it often is possible to orthodontically close the first molar extraction sites, bringing the second permanent molar forward into the area where the first molar was lost, without having to resort to implants for additional anchorage (Figure 21-18). The second molar brings its own investing bone with it, and the large bony defect disappears.

This favorable response is attributed to some combination of three factors: the relatively young age of the juvenile periodontitis patients, the fact that the original attack was almost entirely on the first molars, and the disappearance of the specific bacterial flora.[21] In an older patient who has lost a tooth to periodontal disease, it is unlikely that the other teeth have been totally spared or that the bacterial flora have changed, and it would not be good judgment to attempt to close the space.

Comprehensive Orthodontics in Patients Planned for Implants.
If the decision for an individual patient is to re-

place missing teeth rather than close spaces, the second important question is how this is to be done. The success of implants has rapidly made them a preferred way to replace missing teeth. For the orthodontist, the implant vs. bridge decision makes a difference in how the teeth are positioned and in the sequencing of treatment. Major concerns when implants are to be placed are adequate bone in the edentulous area to support the implant, especially when the implant is to replace a congenitally missing tooth, and for single-tooth implants, adequate space between the roots as well as the crowns of the adjacent teeth.

A successful implant requires adequate bone to support it. If there is no tooth to erupt into an area of the dental arch, little or no alveolar bone ever forms. The result is a large defect in the alveolar process that can make implant placement almost impossible. Alveolar bone will form in a 2-4 mm area adjacent to an erupting tooth. For this reason, when an implant is planned as the eventual replacement for a missing maxillary lateral incisor or mandibular second premolar (the most frequent congenitally missing teeth), it is important for a tooth to erupt in the eventual implant area. The primary tooth in the area should be maintained as long as it continues to erupt in concert with growth. Primary teeth, like permanent teeth, bring alveolar bone along with them. If the primary tooth becomes ankylosed or is lost, it then becomes important to try to get the maxillary canine or mandibular first premolar

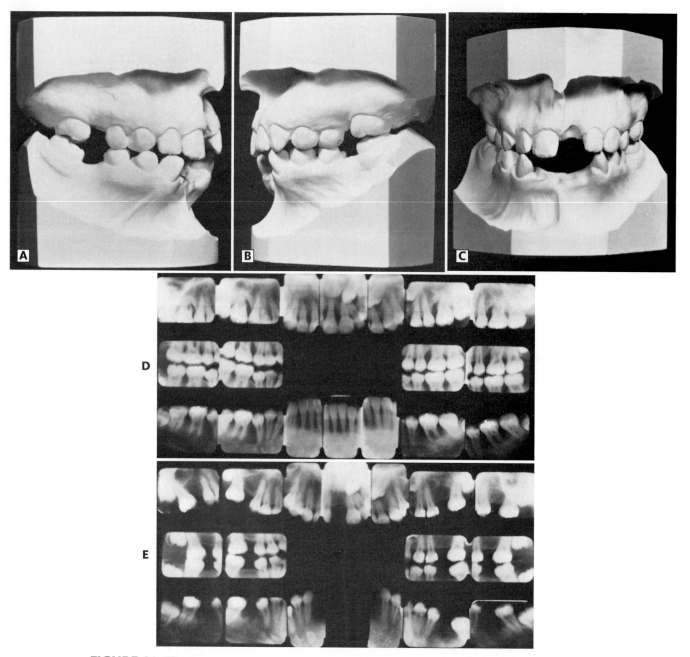

FIGURE 21-17   Pre-treatment records of a girl with juvenile periodontitis. **A** to **C,** Dental casts after the periodontitis had been brought under control, which required extraction of all first molars, the mandibular incisors, and one maxillary incisor. **D,** Periapical radiographs at the time of initial periodontal treatment; **E,** periapical radiographs at the beginning of orthodontic treatment.

to erupt into the edentulous area, with space mesial and distal to it in which bone formation will be stimulated (Figure 21-19). The orthodontic plan would be to open the edentulous space and position the adjacent teeth after the permanent tooth had erupted and to place an implant to support a prosthetic crown after vertical growth is essentially completed.

If an alveolar ridge is created by allowing a permanent tooth to erupt into the area and then opening the space, the orthodontic treatment is likely to be completed at age 14 or 15. Particularly in males, vertical growth is likely to continue into the late teens, so that it is unwise to place the implant for another four or five years after the orthodontic treatment is completed. Implants can be placed sooner in girls, but rarely before age 16 or 17. Fortunately, research shows that an alveolar ridge created by this type of tooth movement does not atrophy nearly as rapidly as it does in the area where a tooth has recently been extracted. The

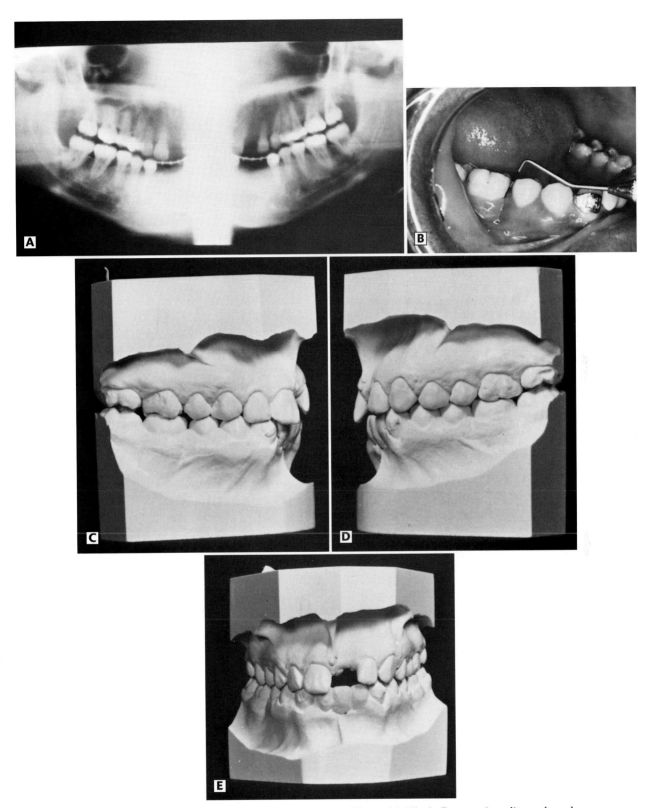

FIGURE 21-18   Orthodontic treatment (patient in Figure 21-17). **A,** Panoramic radiograph at the completion of orthodontic treatment. During treatment, a replacement maxillary central incisor was tied to the archwire. Replacement mandibular incisors were attached to a heavy lingual wire from canine to canine, which is still in place; **B,** at the completion of space closure, pocket depths are normal at the first molar extraction site; **C to E,** dental casts at the completion of orthodontic treatment.

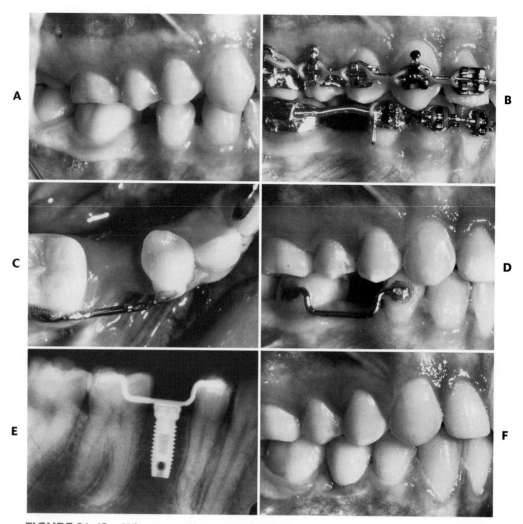

FIGURE 21-19 When a mandibular second premolar is congenitally missing and the primary second molar is lost, it is desirable for the first premolar to erupt distally into the space, to stimulate the formation of alveolar bone in the area so that eventually an implant can be placed. **A,** For this patient the first premolar drifted distally after the second primary molar was lost. **B,** Comprehensive orthodontic treatment repositioned the teeth and created space for an implant, and, **C and D,** a fixed retainer was used to maintain the space until vertical growth was completed in the late teens. **E,** At age 17 an implant was placed, with the space still maintained by the fixed retainer until the implant was integrated and ready for prosthodontic use; and **F,** a restoration was placed on the implant. (Courtesy Dr. V. Kokich.)

ridge created by tooth movement tends to remain satisfactory for implant placement for several years.[22]

Positioning adjacent teeth for a single-tooth implant can be tricky, particularly in the replacement of missing maxillary lateral incisors, because of the small area for implant placement. The orthodontist must provide enough space for placement of a successful implant and must be careful to position the roots of the adjacent teeth so that there is enough room between the roots at the base of the implant (Figure 21-20). Often it is helpful to open slightly more space than will eventually be left for the crown that is placed on the implant, to facilitate the implant surgery, and then to close the extra millimeter or so of space after the implant is in position.

In older patients with long-standing tooth loss, bone grafts in the area of future implants often will be required (Figure 21-21). Usually it is advantageous to go ahead with the placement of grafts in areas that will receive implants, while orthodontic treatment is being carried out in other areas of the mouth. The goal should be to have the patient ready for definitive prosthodontic treatment as soon as possible after the orthodontic appliances are removed, rather than having a considerable delay while both grafts and implants are done. The prosthetic replacements, whether implants or bridges, are an essential part of the orthodontic retention. A rational orthodontic retention plan is much easier to put together after the prosthodontic treatment is completed, than when the prosthodontics

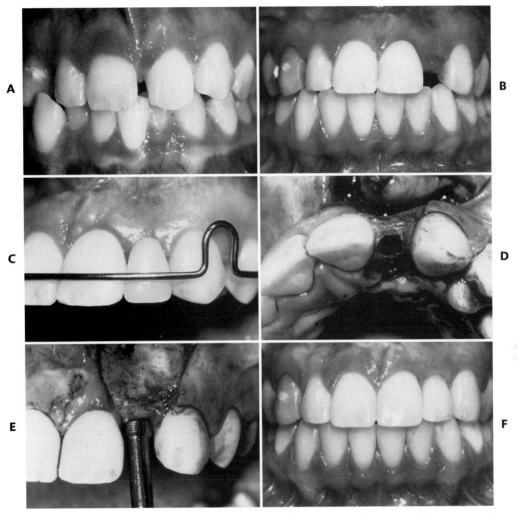

FIGURE 21-20 For replacement of congenitally missing lateral incisors with single-tooth implants, it is particularly important for a permanent tooth to erupt into the lateral incisor area, to stimulate the formation of alveolar bone in that area. **A,** Often this happens spontaneously, as in this patient. **B,** Orthodontic preparation for the implant consists of moving the central incisor mesially and the canine distally, opening the lateral incisor space. **C,** Bone that has formed in such an area does not resorb nearly as rapidly as it would in an extraction site, so the patient can wear a retainer with a temporary replacement tooth for several years after orthodontics is completed. An implant should not be placed until vertical growth is completed, in the late teens. **D,** At that point an implant can be placed, **E,** uncovered after a period for integration, and, **F,** a crown placed as the definitive restoration. (Courtesy Dr. V. Kokich.)

must be coordinated with orthodontic retainers over a period of many months.

After the grafts have matured to the point that implants can be inserted, it may be possible to do the implant surgery too before all orthodontics is finished. Usually, however, orthodontic brackets interfere with placement of the stent that is needed for positioning of the implants at the time of surgery, and it is likely that the orthodontic appliances will be removed before implant surgery in many cases. It is the long delay caused by graft healing and maturation before implants can be placed that is the major problem in orthodontic retention. Almost always, a fixed orthodontic retainer (prefer-

ably bonded on the facial surface to keep it out of the way of the implant surgery) is the best choice to maintain a space in the posterior part of the mandibular arch during implant surgery and incorporation. Supplying a prosthetic replacement tooth as part of the retainer is not important in this area. In the maxillary arch, a prosthetic tooth usually is required for esthetics. Supplying this on an orthodontic retainer can be quite satisfactory, but care must be taken to avoid contact of the retainer base with a healing area after implant surgery. Patients often prefer a temporary resin-bonded bridge, which must be made so that it can be removed for implant surgery and reinserted easily.

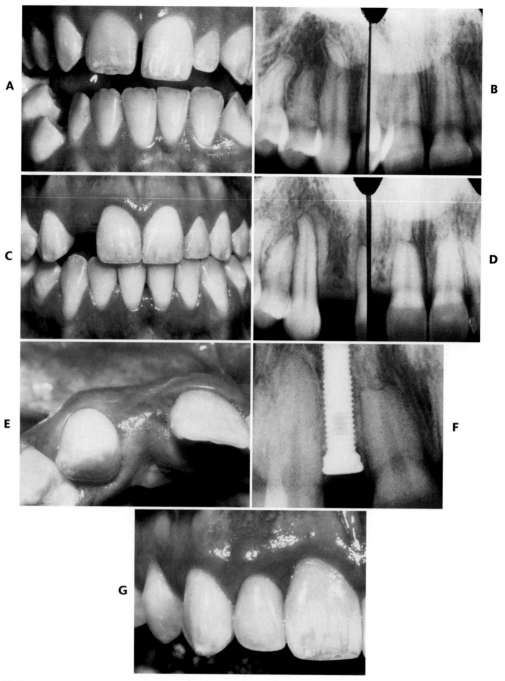

FIGURE 21-21 **A,** For this patient with a missing lateral incisor, **B,** there was almost no space between the roots of the central incisor and canine and, **C and D,** bodily movement was necessary to obtain the space needed for a successful implant (**E and F**) and crown (**G**). Often as much root as crown movement is required in preparation for implants. (Courtesy Dr. V. Kokich.)

A damaged and ankylosed maxillary incisor in a teenager poses a special problem when eventual replacement with an implant is planned. The ankylosed tooth interferes with orthodontic treatment to align the other teeth and can become quite unsightly, but alveolar atrophy will occur if the tooth is extracted before vertical growth is completed and the implant can be placed. In this situation, the alveolar bone can be "banked" by removing the crown of the offending tooth but retaining the root with calcium hydroxide filling the pulp chamber (Figure 21-22). When this is done, the root resorbs over the next 3 to 5 years but bone is retained in the area, and there is a better chance of successful implant placement without a bone graft. Meanwhile, the orthodontic treatment can be completed with a pontic tied to an archwire, and then a temporary resin-bonded bridge until vertical growth is completed and it is safe to place the implant.

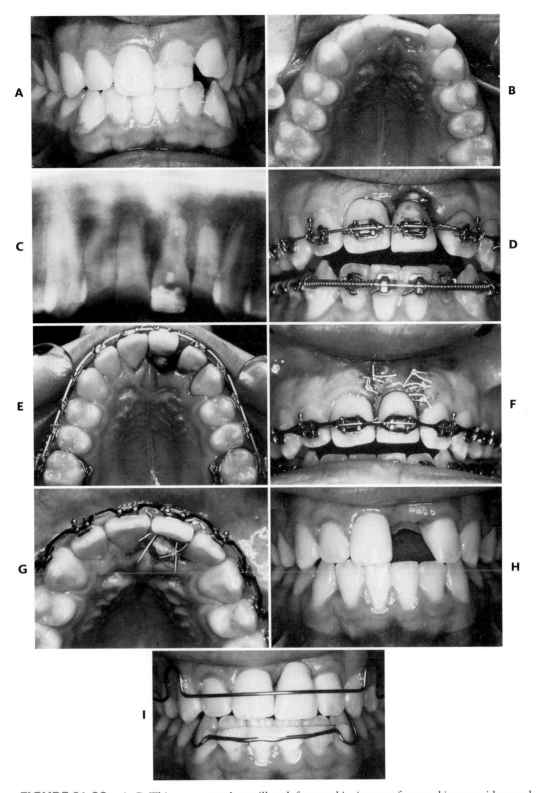

FIGURE 21-22 **A-C,** This young man's maxillary left central incisor was fractured in an accident and became ankylosed, making alignment of the other maxillary incisors and comprehensive orthodontic treatment impossible. **D** and **E,** After initial alignment of the maxillary arch, the crown of the ankylosed central incisor was cut off, the root canal was filled with calcium hydroxide, and the gingiva was sutured over the residual root. A pontic was tied to the archwire, with orthodontic force to close the excess space in the area. **F** and **G,** Three months later, with the excess space closed, gingivoplasty was done in the affected area, and comprehensive orthodontics was completed during the next year. **H** and **I,** At the conclusion of treatment a retainer with a replacement tooth was made, to be worn until an implant could be placed at about age 19, after completion of vertical growth. Resorption of the endodontically-treated root fragment would be expected over the next 2 to 3 years, but resorption of alveolar bone would not occur during that time, so the alveolar bone was effectively "banked" until the time of implant placement.

SPECIAL ASPECTS OF ORTHODONTIC APPLIANCE THERAPY

Both the goals and the stages of comprehensive orthodontic treatment for adults are the same as those in the treatment of adolescents (see Chapters 16 through 18). The orthodontic mechanotherapy, however, often must be modified. Because of the lack of growth, particularly the small amounts of vertical growth that allow some extrusion of the posterior teeth in adolescents without leading to mandibular rotation, intrusion often is required in the leveling of both arches. If the patient has lost some periodontal support, it is especially important to keep forces light. It must be kept in mind that the biologic response is determined by pressure in the PDL, not by force against the tooth (see Figure 21-13). Orthodontic space closure may be contraindicated if teeth have been lost because of periodontal disease, and previous treatment of TMD problems can be a factor in later orthodontic treatment. In adults, an important treatment planning criterion is the extent to which a jaw discrepancy can be camouflaged successfully rather than requiring surgical correction (see Chapters 8 and 22). In the following discussion, it is assumed that an appropriate and feasible treatment plan has been prepared.

Applications of Segmented Arch Technique

The principles of segmented arch treatment have been discussed in Chapter 10, and more specific indications for leveling and space closure are presented in Chapters 16 and 17. The basic idea in segmented arch treatment is to create a stable anchor unit, consisting of several teeth rigidly connected to create the functional equivalent of a single large multi-rooted anchor tooth, and to use this anchorage to provide precisely controlled force against the teeth whose movement is desired. In addition to its use for intrusion, the segmented arch approach also can be helpful in controlling the magnitude of force in space closure. This is even more important in periodontally involved patients than in those with an intact periodontium, because the PDL area over which the force is distributed is smaller (Figure 21-23).

Growth is important in normal orthodontic treatment even for patients who have Class I problems and excellent jaw relationships, because most mechanotherapy has an extrusive component and tends to elongate the teeth. In young patients, the choice between intrusion or extrusion to correct a deep overbite and level an excessive curve of Spee often can be resolved in favor of extrusion, because vertical growth will compensate for it. In adults, the choice often must be intrusion, which can be achieved only by segmented arch mechanics. The practical effect is to make segmented arch treatment more important in adults than it is in younger patients.

Intrusion.   The mechanotherapy needed to produce intrusion in an adult is not different from the methods for younger patients described in some detail in Chapters 10 and 16. In periodontally involved adults, anchorage is likely to be compromised, and careful stabilization of anchor units is especially important. For practical purposes, this is likely to mean greater use of soldered lingual arches for anchorage in adults (see Figure 21-23). Burstone-type depressing arches or (less commonly) Ricketts utility arches, both using a long span from the stabilized posterior segments to the anterior area where intrusion is desired, normally are selected for adults. The use of extremely light force is important, since excessive force will lead to posterior extrusion rather than the desired anterior intrusion. The point at which the intrusion arch attaches to the anterior segment is important, because it influences the extent to which the anterior segment tips buccally or lingually as intrusion occurs (see Chapter 10).

One potential problem with intrusive tooth movement in periodontally involved adults is the prospect that a deepening of periodontal pockets might be produced by this treatment. Ideally, of course, intruding a tooth would lead to a reattachment of the periodontal fibers, but there is no basis for expecting true reattachment in response to orthodontic treatment. What seems to happen instead is the formation of a tight epithelial cuff, so that the position of the gingiva relative to the crown improves clinically, while periodontal probing depths do not increase. Histologic slides from experimental animals show a relative invagination of the epithelium, but with a tight area of contact that cannot be probed (Figure 21-24). It can be argued that this leaves the patient at risk for rapid periodontal breakdown if inflammation is allowed to recur. Certainly intrusion should never be attempted without excellent control of inflammation. On the other hand, if good hygiene is maintained, clinical experience has shown that it is possible to maintain teeth that have been treated in this way, and both dental esthetics and function improve after the intrusion.[23]

The crown-root ratio is a significant factor in the long-term prognosis for a tooth that has suffered periodontal bone loss. Shortening the crown has the virtue of improving the crown-root ratio. The orthodontist should not hesitate to reduce crown height of elongated incisors (especially lower incisors) as an alternative to intrusion, when this would both simplify orthodontic leveling of the arch and improve the periodontal prognosis.

Space Closure

In contrast to leveling of vertical arch discrepancies, continuous arch treatment can be used with adults to correct anteroposterior discrepancies, but segmented arch treatment does have special advantages. The same comments apply to space closure in adults as to adolescents (see Chapter 17), with two exceptions:

1. It is unrealistic to expect an adult to wear a headgear on the nearly continuous basis necessary to produce efficient tooth movement, so direct extra-oral force to slide teeth along an archwire during closure of extraction spaces is impractical. For the same reason, headgear to control anchorage is probably less reliable than it might be in a younger patient and other methods of anchorage control must be sought.

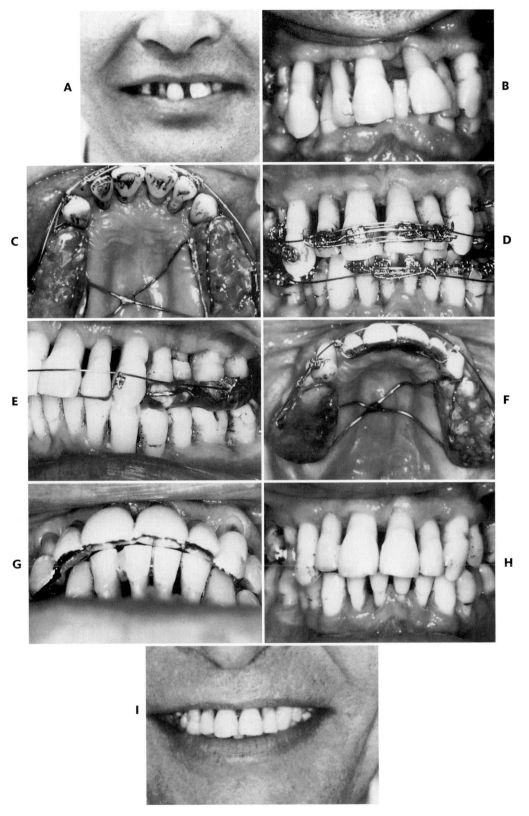

FIGURE 21-23 Orthodontic treatment in a man with advanced periodontal bone loss. **A,** Facial and, **B,** close-up views of the anterior teeth after initial periodontal therapy. **C,** Occlusal view of maxillary arch showing the bonded splint used to supplement posterior anchorage and control extrusion of the posterior teeth while incisors were being intruded. **D,** Burstone auxiliary depressing arches were used in the maxilla and mandible to intrude the incisors, while particular attention was paid to maintaining excellent hygiene. **E,** Occlusal relationships toward the end of orthodontic treatment, with a maxillary splint in place, **F,** continuing to be used for maxillary incisor intrusion. **G,** Incisor teeth were splinted from the lingual at the conclusion of treatment. Permanent retention is required with this degree of periodontal bone loss. **H,** Close-up and, **I,** facial views of the anterior teeth after treatment. (Courtesy Dr. B. Melsen.)

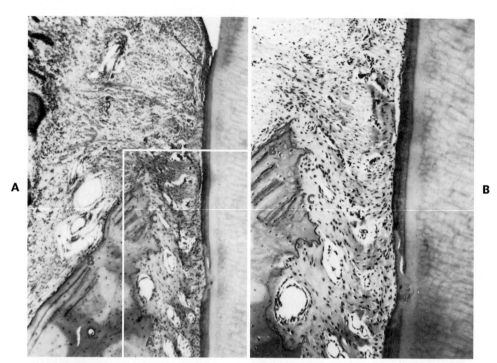

FIGURE 21-24   **A,** Histologic preparation from a dog's lower first premolar that was extruded and slightly tipped buccally for 12 weeks, then intruded for 16 weeks, and finally had 3 days without orthodontic force immediately before sacrifice. Oral hygiene was maintained during the treatment. Tight epithelial cuff is seen where epithelium penetrates apically in consequence of the intrusion (*A*). **B,** Higher magnification view of the alveolar crest area outlined in *A*. Note the formation of new bone (*B*) on the alveolar crest, which occurred during extrusion, and resorption of bone from intrusion only on the PDL side of the alveolar crest (*C*), without loss of alveolar crest height. (Courtesy Dr. B. Melsen.)

The most effective of these is the creation of posterior stabilizing segments with lingual arches and buccal stabilizing wires, the same setup needed for leveling by intrusion. In addition, it may be necessary to use two-step space closure with frictionless mechanics to reduce the strain on anchorage and keep forces as light as possible. Segmental closing loops for retraction of the canines have inherent problems in vertical control of the canines (see Chapters 10 and 17), and therefore if these are used it is particularly important to see the patient on a regular schedule for close supervision. Fortunately, compliance with appointments is less likely to be a problem with adults than with many adolescents.

2. As we have discussed earlier, old extraction sites in adults pose a mechanical and biological challenge in orthodontic treatment. In a young patient, any extraction site is recent and usually can be closed without any particular problems. In an adult, closure of an extraction site many years after the tooth is lost is neither straightforward nor predictable. It may be good judgment not to attempt space closure but rather to plan for prosthetic replacement of the missing tooth.

Finishing and Retention Procedures

Orthodontic finishing with archwires does not differ significantly in adults from the finishing procedures for younger patients, except for those adults who have had a combination of surgical and orthodontic treatment. This circumstance is discussed in Chapter 22. Positioners are rarely indicated as finishing devices for older patients, however, especially those with moderate to severe periodontal bone loss. These patients should be brought to their final orthodontic relationship with archwires and then stabilized with immediately placed retainers before eventual detailing of occlusal relationships by equilibration.

Part of the purpose of a traditional orthodontic retainer is to allow each tooth to move during function, independently of its neighbors, to produce a restoration of the normal periodontal architecture. This clearly does not apply to patients who have had a significant degree of periodontal bone loss and who have mobile teeth. In these patients, splinting of the teeth is necessary both short- and long-term. A suckdown plastic wafer often is the best choice immediately upon removing the orthodontic appliance (Figure 21-25). Other short-term possibilities are an occlusal splint, providing a positive indexing of the teeth and extending buccally and lingually to maintain tooth po-

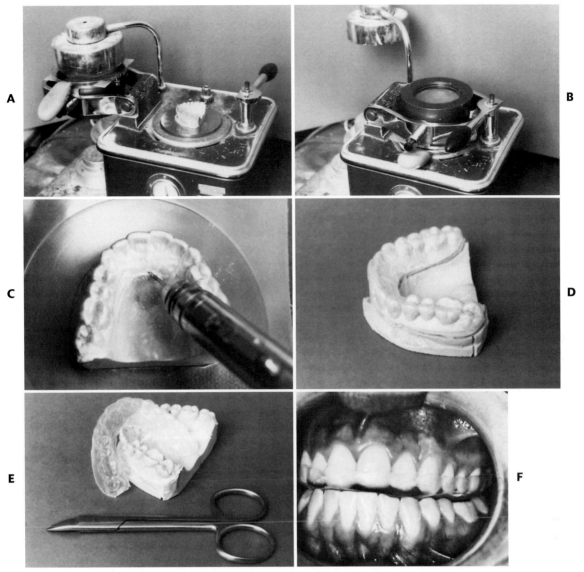

FIGURE 21-25   When orthodontic appliances are removed after treatment of a periodontally-involved adult, a splint-type retainer is needed immediately. These individuals require permanent retention, so the usual orthodontic retention procedures based on gradual withdrawal of the retainer do not apply. Immediately upon appliance removal, the preferred retainer usually is one made from a vacuum-formed thermoplastic material that is tightly formed over the teeth. **A** and **B,** The retention cast on the vacuum-forming machine; **C** and **D,** a bur is used to cut the material away from the palate so that it can be freed from the cast. **E,** Further trimming can be done with scissors. Usually the material extends completely over the teeth and a few millimeters onto the gingiva. Upper and lower retainers are made in exactly the same way; **F,** if desired, and if only one arch needs splint-type retention, a retainer of this type can be modified as shown here by adding soft acrylic to the vacuum-formed base, to form an occlusal splint of the same type often used for initial treatment of patients with TMD problems. Whatever the method immediately after appliances are removed, after a few months a more permanent splint should be made by a restorative dentist.

sition, or a wraparound retainer as illustrated in Chapter 19. Long-term splinting usually involves cast restorations.

Special Treatment Considerations in Patients with Temporomandibular Dysfunction

The extent to which TMD symptoms in many adults diminish and disappear when comprehensive orthodontic treatment begins can be surprising and overly gratifying to those who do not understand the etiologic process of myofascial pain. Orthodontic intervention can appear almost magical in the way that TMD symptoms disappear long before the occlusal relationships have been corrected. The explanation is simple—orthodontic treatment makes the teeth sore, grinding or clenching sensitive teeth as a means of handling stress does not produce the same subconscious gratification as previously, the parafunctional activity stops, and the symptoms vanish. The changing occlusal relationships also contribute to breaking up the habit patterns that contributed to the muscle fatigue and pain. No matter what the type of orthodontic treatment, symptoms are unlikely to be present while movement of a significant number of teeth is occurring, as long as treatment that produces strongly deflective contracts is avoided. Prolonged use of Class II or Class III elastics may not be well tolerated in adults who have had TMD problems and should be avoided (for that matter, prolonged use of elastics should be avoided in most other adult patients as well).

The moment of truth for TMD symptoms comes some time after orthodontic treatment is completed, when the clenching and grinding that originally caused the problem tend to recur. At that point, even if the occlusal relationships have been significantly improved, it may be impossible to keep the patient from moving into extreme jaw positions and engaging in parafunctional activity that produces pain. The use of interocclusal splints in this situation may be the only way to keep symptoms from recurring. In short, the miraculous cure that orthodontic treatment often provides for myofascial pain tends to disappear with the appliance. Those who have had symptoms in the past are always at risk of having them recur.

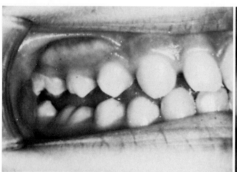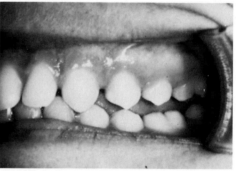

FIGURE 21-26   Occlusal relationships in a 16-year-old girl who had worn a splint covering only the posterior teeth for the previous 8 months. The posterior open bite was created by a combination of intrusion of the posterior teeth and further eruption of the anteriors. Discarding the splint had become impossible.

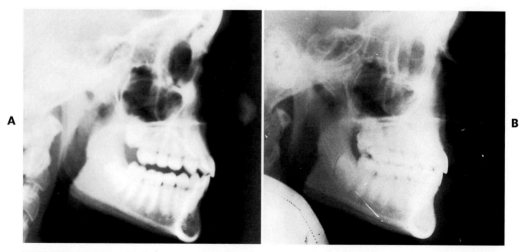

FIGURE 21-27   Cephalometric films for the patient shown in Figure 21-26. **A,** Before and, **B,** after orthodontic treatment to extrude the posterior teeth back into occlusion.

Occasionally, orthodontic treatment is made more complicated by previous splint therapy for TMD problems. If an occlusal splint for TMD symptoms covers the posterior but not the anterior teeth, the anterior teeth that have been taken out of occlusion begin to erupt again and may come back into occlusion even though the posterior teeth are still separated (Figure 21-26). Clinically, it may appear that the posterior teeth are being intruded, but incisor eruption usually is a greater contributor to the development of posterior open bite. In only a few months, the patient may end up in a situation in which discarding the splint has become impossible. The only treatment possibilities are elongation of the posterior teeth, either with crowns or orthodontic extrusion, or intrusion of the anterior teeth.

Orthodontic intervention at this stage is difficult, because TMD symptoms are likely to develop immediately if the splint is removed, and it is not possible to elongate the posterior teeth orthodontically without discarding or cutting down the splint. Placing orthodontic attachments on the posterior teeth and using light vertical elastics to the posterior segments (Figure 21-27) can be used to bring the posterior teeth back into occlusion, if the patient can tolerate this treatment. Some reintrusion of the elongated anterior teeth is likely to occur, but a significant increase in face height is often maintained. Although permanently increasing the vertical dimension to control disk displacement can be accomplished in this way, this treatment plan should be used with extreme caution.

REFERENCES

1. Patient census survey results, Bulletin Am Assn Orthod 15, no. 4, July-Aug. 1997.
2. Phillips C, Broder HL, Bennett ME: Dentofacial disharmony: motivations for seeking treatment, Int J Adult Orthod Orthognath Surg 12:7-15, 1997.
3. Luther F: Orthodontics and the TM joint: where are we now? Part 2: Functional occlusion, malocclusion and TMD, Angle Orthod 68:357-368, 1998.
4. Proffit WR, Phillips C, Dann C IV: Who seeks surgical-orthodontic treatment? Int J Adult Orthod Orthognath Surg 5:153-160, 1990.
5. Rodrigues-Garcia CM, Sakai S, Rugh JD et al: Effects of major Class II occlusal corrections on temporomandibular signs and symptoms, J Orofacial Pain 12:185-192, 1998.
6. Rugh JD, Solberg WK: Oral health status in the United States: temporomandibular disorders, J Dent Educ 49:399-405, 1985.
7. Albander JM: A 6-year study on the pattern of periodontal disease progression, J Clin Periodontol 17:467-471, 1990.
8. Claffey N: Decision making in periodontal therapy: the re-evaluation, J Clin Periodontol 18:384-389, 1991.
9. Armitage GC: Periodontal diseases: diagnosis, Ann Periodontol 1:37-215, 1996.
10. Brown LJ, Brunelle JA, Kingman A: Periodontal status in the United States, 1988-91: prevalence, extent, and demographic variation, J Dent Res 75:672-683, 1996.
11. Boyd RL, Leggott PQ, Quinn RS et al: Periodontal implications of orthodontic treatment in adults with reduced or normal periodontal tissues versus those of adolescents, Am J Orthod Dentofac Orthop 96:191-199, 1989.
12. Wennstrom JL: Mucogingival considerations in orthodontic treatment, Sem Orthod 2:46-54, 1996.
13. Forsberg CM, Brattstrom V, Malmberg E, Nord CE: Ligature wires and elastomeric rings: two methods of ligation, and their association with microbial colonization of *Streptococcus mutans* and lactobacilli, Eur J Orthod 13:416-420, 1991.
14. Timpeneers LM, Wijgearts IA, Gronard NA et al: Effect of electric toothbrushes versus manual toothbrushes on removal of plaque and periodontal status during orthodontic treatment, Am J Orthod Dentofac Orthop 111:492-497, 1997.
15. Matthews DP, Kokich VG: Managing treatment for the orthodontic patient with periodontal problems, Sem Orthod 3:21-38, 1997.
16. Kokich VG, Spear FM: Guidelines for managing the orthodontic-restorative patient, Sem Orthod 3:3-20, 1997.
17. Hom BM, Turley PK: The effects of space closure of the mandibular first molar area in adults, Am J Orthod 85:457-469, 1984.
18. Roberts WE, Nelson CL, Goodacre CJ: Rigid implant anchorage to close a mandibular first molar extraction site, J Clin Orthod 28:693-704, 1994.
19. Costa A, Raffaini M, Melson B: Miniscrews as orthodontic anchorage: a preliminary report, Int J Adult Orthod Orthognath Surg 13:201-209, 1998.
20. Schenkein HA, Van Dyke TE: Early-onset periodontitis: systemic aspects of etiology and pathogenesis, Periodontol 2000 6:7-25, 1994.
21. Folio J, Rame TE, Keyes PH: Orthodontic therapy in patients with juvenile periodontitis: clinical and microbiologic effects, Am J Orthod 87:421-431, 1985.
22. Spear FM, Matthews DM, Kokich VG: Interdisciplinary management of single-tooth implants, Sem Orthod 3:45-72, 1997.
23. Melsen B: Intrusion of incisors in adult patients with marginal bone loss, Am J Orthod Dentofac Orthop 96:232-241, 1989.

CHAPTER

22

Combined Surgical and Orthodontic Treatment

For patients whose orthodontic problems are so severe that neither growth modification nor camouflage offers a solution, surgical realignment of the jaws or repositioning of dentoalveolar segments is the only possible treatment. Surgery is not a substitute for orthodontics in these patients. Instead, it must be properly coordinated with orthodontics and other dental treatment to achieve good overall results. Dramatic progress in recent years has made it possible for combined treatment to correct many severe problems that simply were untreatable only a few years ago.

INDICATIONS FOR SURGERY

Development of Orthognathic Surgery

Surgical treatment for mandibular prognathism began early in the twentieth century. Edward Angle, commenting on a patient who had treatment of this type, described how the result could have been improved if orthodontic appliances and occlusal splints had been used.[1] Although there was gradual progress in techniques for setting back a prominent mandible throughout the first half of this century, Trauner and Obwegeser's introduction of the sagittal split ramus osteotomy in 1959 marked the beginning of the modern era in orthognathic surgery.[2] This technique used an intra-oral approach, which avoided the necessity of a potentially disfiguring skin incision. The sagittal split design also offered a biologically sound method for lengthening or shortening the lower jaw with the same bone cuts, thus allowing treatment of mandibular deficiency or excess (Figure 22-1). During the 1960s, American surgeons began to use and modify techniques for maxillary surgery that had been developed in Europe, and a decade of rapid progress in maxillary surgery culminated in the development by Bell[3] and Epker and Wolford[4] of the LeFort I downfracture technique that allowed repositioning of the maxilla in all three planes of space (Figure 22-2). By the 1980s, progress in oral and maxillofacial surgery made it possible to reposition either or both jaws, to move the chin in all three planes of space, and to reposition dentoalveolar segments surgically as desired. In the 1990s, rigid internal fixation greatly improved patient comfort by making immobilization of the jaws unnecessary, and a better understanding of typical patterns of post-surgical changes made surgical outcomes more stable and predictable. Combined surgical-orthodontic treatment can now be planned for patients with a severe dentofacial problem of any type.

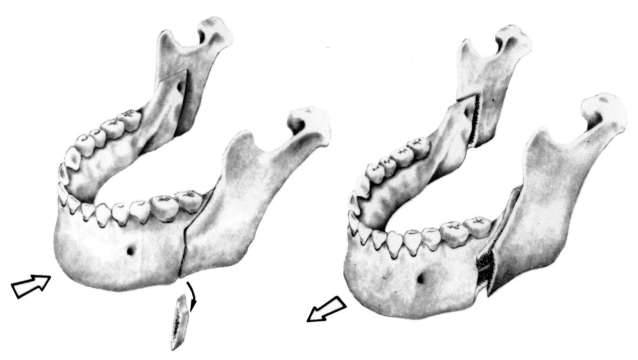

FIGURE 22-1   The sagittal split osteotomy procedure can be used to set back or advance the mandible, as shown on the left and right respectively.

Severity as an Indication for Orthognathic Surgery: The Envelope of Discrepancy

The indication for surgery obviously is a problem too severe for orthodontics alone. It is possible now to be at least semi-quantitative about the limits of orthodontic treatment, in the context of producing normal occlusion. As the diagrams of the "envelope of discrepancy" (Figure 22-3) indicate, the limits vary both by the tooth movement that would be needed (teeth can be moved further in some directions than others) and by the patient's age (the limits for tooth movement change little if any with age, but growth modification is possible only while active growth is occurring). Because growth modification in children enables greater changes than are possible by tooth movement alone in adults, some conditions that could have been treated with orthodontics alone in children (e.g., a centimeter of overjet) become surgical problems in adults. On the other hand, some conditions that initially might look less severe (e.g., 5 mm of reverse overjet), can be seen even at an early age to require surgery.

Keep in mind that the envelope of discrepancy outlines the limits of hard tissue change toward ideal occlusion, *if* other limits due to the major goals of treatment do not apply. In fact, soft tissue limitations not reflected in the envelope of discrepancy often are a major factor in the decision for orthodontic or surgical-orthodontic treatment.[5] Measuring millimeter distances to the ideal condylar position for normal function is problematic, and measuring distances from ideal esthetics is impossible. Diagnostic and treatment planning guidelines for these soft tissue parameters are dis-

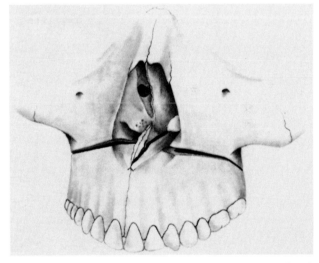

FIGURE 22-2   The location of the osteotomy cuts for the LeFort I downfracture technique. In patients whose mandible is normal in size, the retrognathic appearance results from downward and backward rotation of the chin. Superior repositioning of the maxilla as indicated by the arrow allows the mandible to rotate upward and forward, hinging at the temporomandibular joint, which simultaneously shortens facial height and provides more chin prominence.

cussed in some detail in Chapters 6 to 8. As greater emphasis is placed on soft tissue rather than hard tissue relationships in planning both orthodontic and surgical treatment, more extensive guidelines for clinical examination of facial soft tissues can be anticipated in the near future.[6]

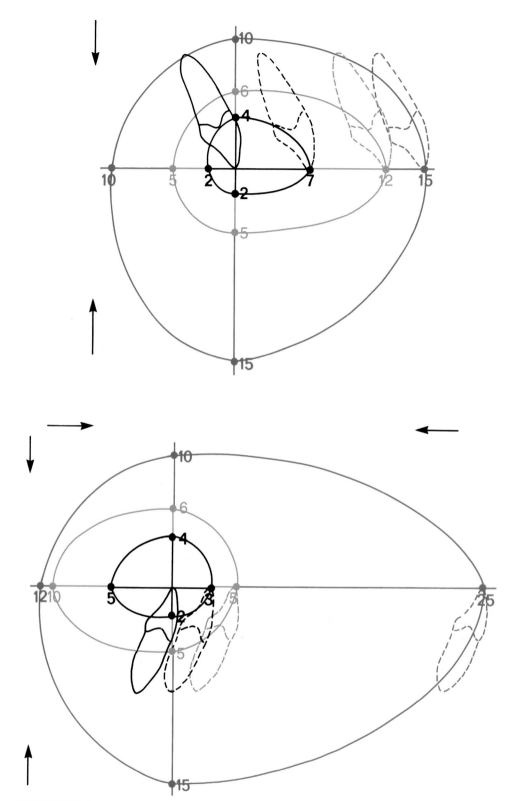

FIGURE 22-3 With the ideal position of the upper and lower incisors shown by the origin of the x and y axes, the envelope of discrepancy shows the amount of change that could be produced by orthodontic tooth movement alone (the inner envelope of each diagram); orthodontic tooth movement combined with growth modification (the middle envelope); and orthognathic surgery (the outer envelope). Note that the possibilities for each treatment are not symmetric with regard to the planes of space. There is more potential to retract than procline teeth and more potential for extrusion than intrusion. Since growth of the maxilla cannot be modified independently of the mandible, the growth modification envelope for the two jaws is the same. Surgery to move the lower jaw back has more potential than surgery to advance it.

Esthetic and Psychosocial Considerations in Orthognathic Surgery

The negative effect on psychic and social well being from dentofacial disfigurement is well documented,[7] and it is clear that this is why most patients seek orthodontic treatment. Those who look different are treated differently, and this becomes a social handicap. Treatment to overcome social discrimination is not "just cosmetic." It is neither vain nor irrational to desire esthetic change that can improve one's total life adjustment.

The motivation to improve facial appearance, not surprisingly, is even stronger for those with the more severe deviations from the norm that might require orthognathic surgery. Although most individuals who are evaluated for orthognathic surgery desire an improvement in function as well as esthetics, several studies have shown that 75%-80% seek esthetic improvement. Data from psychological testing of patients in the University of North Carolina Dentofacial Program, through which orthognathic surgery patients are evaluated and managed, show a high prevalence of psychological distress (15%-37%, depending on the subscale).[8] Those who accept a recommendation for surgical treatment see themselves as less normal than those who decide against treatment, even though cephalometric data for the two groups are similar.[9]

Orthodontic treatment primarily affects the prominence of the teeth and the contours of the lips. Changes in the position of the chin and nose are likely to have a greater impact on facial esthetics than changes limited to the lips, and the effect of orthognathic surgery on the lower face extends the esthetic impact of treatment considerably. If esthetic improvement is a major goal of treatment, it makes sense that changes in the nose, and perhaps other changes in facial soft tissue contours that could be produced by facial plastic surgery should be considered in the treatment planning. The integration of orthognathic and facial plastic surgery is a current, and entirely rational, trend that is well described in Sarver's recent text.[10] Not long ago, treatment planning began with jaw and tooth positions, and then the effect of these changes on the soft tissues was evaluated. A more contemporary approach is to decide how the facial soft tissues should look, and then work backward to determine what would have to be done to the underlying hard tissues to produce the desired soft tissue outcome.

Psychological Reactions to Orthognathic Surgery

On "objective" evaluation, most observers would conclude that both orthodontic treatment alone and orthognathic surgery usually improve facial appearance, but the important consideration is whether patients agree. The best evidence that they do is the high level of satisfaction reported by those who have had treatment. About 90% of patients who undergo orthognathic surgery report satisfaction with the outcome and over 80% (a more revealing number) say

that, knowing the outcome and what the experience was like, they would recommend such treatment to others and would undergo it again.[9]

This does not mean, of course, that there are no negative psychological effects from this type of surgical treatment. First, a few patients have great difficulty in adapting to significant changes in their facial appearance. This is more likely to be a problem in older individuals. If you are 19, your facial appearance has been changing steadily for all your life, and another change is not a great surprise. If you are 49 and suddenly see a different face when you look in the mirror, the effect may be unsettling. Psychological support and counseling, therefore, are particularly important for older patients, and major esthetic changes in older adults may not be desirable. As we have discussed above in Chapters 20 and 21, adults seeking treatment fall into two groups, a younger group who seek to improve their lot in life, and an older group whose goal is primarily to maintain what they have. The older group may need orthognathic surgery to achieve their goal, but for them, often treatment should be planned to limit facial change, not maximize it.

Second, whatever the age of the patient, a period of psychological adjustment following facial surgery must be expected (Figure 22-4). In part, this is related to the use of steroids at surgery to minimize postsurgical swelling and edema. Steroid withdrawal, even after short-term use, causes mood swings and a drop in most indicators of

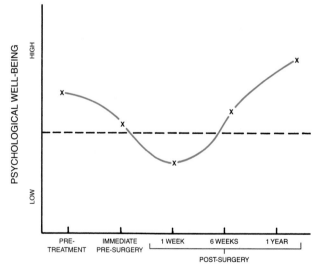

FIGURE 22-4 A generalized representation of the typical psychological response to orthognathic surgery (based on the work of Kiyak).[9] Prior to treatment, patients who seek orthognathic surgery tend to be above the mean on most psychologic parameters. Immediately before surgery, they are not quite so positive, as anxiety and other concerns increase. In the days immediately after surgery, a period of negativism typically occurs (depression, dissatisfaction, etc.). This is related in part to steroid use at surgery and withdrawal afterward, but is not totally explained by this. By six weeks post-surgery, the patients usually are well on the positive side of normal again, and at one year typically rate quite high for satisfaction with treatment and general psychological well-being.

psychological well-being. The adjustment period lasts longer than can be explained by the steroid effects, however. The surgeon learns to put up with complaining patients for the first week or two postsurgery. By the time orthodontic treatment resumes at 3 to 6 weeks postsurgery, the patients are usually—but not always—on the positive side of the psychological scales. Sometimes the orthodontist also has to wait for a patient to make peace with thesurgical experience.

In the short-term, an important influence on the patient's reaction to surgical treatment is how well the actual experience matched what the patient was expecting. Interestingly, orthognathic surgery does not rate high on discomfort/morbidity scales. Mandibular ramus surgery requires about the same pain medication as extraction of impacted wisdom teeth; maxillary surgery is tolerated better than that. From a psychological perspective, it's not so much the amount of pain or discomfort you experienced that determines your reaction, it's how this compares with what you thought would happen. This highlights the importance of carefully preparing patients for their surgical experience.[11]

With current technology, it is possible now to show patients computer simulations of the esthetic impact of surgical treatment. The psychological impact of doing this has been a matter of considerable concern. Current research shows that there is little or no danger of producing unreal-istic esthetic expectations, and on balance, it is better to share the simulations with patients. This is discussed in more detail in the section on interactive treatment planning on p. 696.

For a detailed review of research related to psychological aspects of orthognathic surgery, we recommend the recent review chapter by Phillips.[12]

SURGICAL PROCEDURES AND TREATMENT POSSIBILITIES

To review the changes that can be achieved by contemporary surgical techniques, it is helpful to consider how the jaws can be repositioned in three planes of space.

Correction of Anteroposterior Relationships

Both the maxilla and mandible can be moved forward or backward to correct a jaw discrepancy (Figure 22-5). The mandible can be moved anteriorly or posteriorly in the sagittal plane with relative ease. Extreme advancement may create stability problems associated with neuromuscular adaptation and stretch of the investing soft tissues. The maxilla can be moved forward if bone grafts are interposed posteriorly to help stabilize the new position. Posterior movement of the entire maxilla is not easily achieved because other skeletal components that normally support the

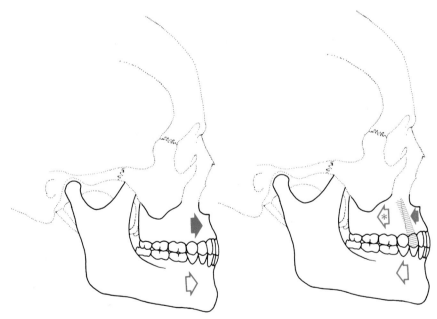

FIGURE 22-5 The maxilla and mandible can be moved anteriorly and posteriorly as indicated by the red arrows in these line drawings. Anterior movements of the mandible greater than 10 to 12 mm create considerable tension in the investing soft tissues and tend to be unstable. Posterior movement of the entire maxilla, though possible, is difficult and usually unnecessary. Instead, posterior movement of protruding incisors up to the width of a premolar is accomplished by removal of a premolar tooth on each side, followed by segmentation of the maxilla. Although the maxilla can be advanced more than it can be retracted, the possibility of relapse or speech alteration from nasopharyngeal incompetence increases with larger movements.

maxilla interfere with moving it back. As Figure 22-5 shows, however, this difficulty is overcome by segmenting the maxilla so that only the anterior portion is retracted.

Maxillary Surgery. The LeFort I downfracture procedure (see Figure 22-2) almost always is used now to reposition the maxilla. If the maxilla is advanced, a graft in the retromolar area or at a step created in the lateral wall usually is required. Various materials, including autogenous and freeze-dried bone and alloplastic substances, can be used. Retraction of the anterior segment is achieved by removal of a premolar, segmentation, and movement of the anterior segment into the space created (see Figure 22-5). Although it is technically possible to move the entire maxilla posteriorly, rarely is this necessary.

Mandibular Advancement. Currently, the bilateral sagittal split osteotomy (BSSO) of the mandibular ramus (see Figure 22-1), performed from an intra-oral approach, is the preferred procedure for most patients who need mandibular advancement. The osteotomy design provides a broad interface of medullary bone for rapid healing. The overlapping of the two segments allows easy rigid internal fixation with screws, and problems with postoperative instability are rare. The early mobilization allowed by this form of rigid internal fixation (RIF) improves jaw mobility in both the short and long term. Although rigid fixation has not eliminated relapse in extensive mandibular advancements, the amount of relapse has been reduced and improved predictability for smaller advances has been reported.

The greatest drawback of the sagittal split is altered sensation post-operatively. Some stretching and retraction of the inferior alveolar nerve are necessary to place the osteotomy cut, and as a result, paresthesia over the distribution of the inferior alveolar nerve almost always is present immediately after surgery. Usually this disappears in 2 to 6 months, but 20% to 25% of patients have some degree of long-term altered sensation.[13]

Mandibular Setback. Reduction of mandibular prognathism can be accomplished by one of two techniques performed in the ramus, each having advantages and disadvantages. The BSSO discussed previously can be used to move the mandible posteriorly as well as anteriorly. It is widely used for setbacks because of excellent control of the condylar segments and because osteosynthesis screws can be employed for fixation.

The transoral vertical oblique ramus osteotomy (TOVRO) is limited to mandibular setback and requires full-thickness overlapping of the segments. This procedure requires less time than the sagittal split osteotomy and is less likely to produce neurosensory changes, but jaw immobilization after surgery is necessary and control of the condylar fragment can be difficult. Especially when both the maxilla and mandible are repositioned in treatment of Class III problems, the advantage of rigid fixation with BSSO outweighs the advantages of TOVRO.

Correction of Vertical Relationships

Problems of excessive and deficient face height, which usually are accompanied by severe anterior open bite and deep bite respectively, were not treated in a reliable manner until the 1970s. At present, as diagrammed in Figure 22-6, the maxilla can be moved up quite successfully but can be positioned downward with less predictability. The mandible can be moved up or down anteriorly but cannot be moved down at the gonial angle with stability.

As a general guideline, this means that long face problems are treated best by superior repositioning of the maxilla. This allows the mandible to rotate around the condyle, thereby reducing the mandibular plane angle and shortening the face. Short face problems, in contrast, are treated most predictably and successfully by mandibular ramus surgery that allows the mandible to move downward only at the chin, increasing the mandibular plane angle by shortening the ramus and opening the gonial angle rather than by rotating at the condyle. When vertical positions of the jaws are changed, it is often necessary to change anteroposterior positions as well.

Maxillary Surgery. The contemporary surgical approach to the skeletal open bite (long face) deformity involves a LeFort I downfracture of the maxilla, with superior repositioning of the maxilla after removal of bone from the lateral walls of the nose, sinus, and nasal septum.

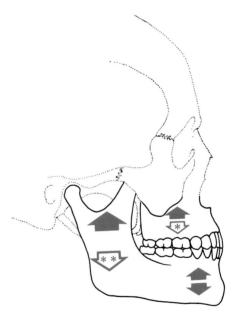

FIGURE 22-6 The surgical movements in the vertical dimension are indicated by the red arrows on this diagram of the skull. The maxilla, mandibular angles, and chin can be moved upward reliably, while downward movement of the maxilla by bone grafting is less predictable (*arrow with single asterisk*). Downward movement of the chin is possible in combination with slight advancement. Lengthening the ramus (*arrow with double asterisks*) stretches the muscular sling and usually results in relapse.

It is important to shorten the nasal septum or free its base so that the septum is not bent when the maxilla is elevated. The inferior turbinate can be partially resected if needed to allow the intrusion, although this procedure rarely is necessary. The overall facial height is shortened as the mandible responds by rotating upward and forward. Neuromuscular adaptation alters both its occlusal and postural positions. Further surgery to correct the anteroposterior position of the mandible may or may not be necessary after this rotation, depending on functional and esthetic concerns (Figure 22-7). Excellent stability of the vertical position of the maxilla is observed post-surgically, but long-term, some continued vertical growth of the maxilla may occur.[14,15]

In contrast, when the maxilla is moved downward to increase face height, it tends to relapse back up post-surgically, so that 20% or more of the vertical change often is lost even when rigid fixation is used.[16] Both the use of more rigid graft materials (like synthetic hydroxylapatite)[17] and simultaneous osteotomy of the mandibular ramus[18] have been reported to improve the stability of downward movement of the maxilla, but this remains one of the more problematic movements (see stability section, on p. 705).

Mandibular Surgery. Patients with a long face, skeletal open bite and anteroposterior mandibular deficiency often have a short mandibular ramus. As Figure 22-6 suggests, surgery to reduce the mandibular plane angle and close the open bite by rotating the mandible down posteriorly and up anteriorly has been found to be highly unstable. Because the fulcrum for rotation is the posterior teeth, this rotation lengthens the ramus and stretches the muscles of the pterygomandibular sling. The instability is attributed primarily to lack of neuromuscular adaptation in these powerful muscles, which can produce relapse to pre-surgical or even worse mandibular positions (Figure 22-8, on p.682). Mandibular ramus surgery in open bite patients should be avoided for this reason, unless it is combined with maxillary intrusion so that lengthening of the ramus does not occur.

Long face patients often have excessive eruption of mandibular anterior teeth, indicated cephalometrically by an abnormally long distance from the incisal edge to the base of the chin. This vertical tooth-chin problem can be corrected by orthodontic intrusion or by anterior segmental surgery to depress the elongated incisor segment. Often, however, the preferred treatment is an inferior border osteotomy of the mandible to reduce the vertical height of the chin at the same time it is augmented horizontally. Many long face patients are treated best with a combination of maxillary intrusion and repositioning of the chin (Figure 22-9, on p. 683).

Patients with a short face (skeletal deep bite) problem are characterized by a long mandibular ramus, square gonial angle and short nose-chin distance. Often the maxillary incisors are tipped lingually in Angle's Class II, division 2

pattern. Despite the deep overbite, excessive eruption of the lower incisors often has not occurred, as demonstrated by a normal distance from the chin to the incisal edge. These patients often have an associated mandibular deficiency, and in many instances could be described as "Class II rotated to Class I" because of the short anterior face height. They are treated best by sagittal split mandibular ramus surgery to rotate the mandible slightly forward and down and the gonial angle area up (Figure 22-10, on p. 684). Orthodontic leveling of the lower arch is required and usually is done after rather than before the surgery (see p. 693 for a discussion of the timing of the orthodontic procedures).

Correction of Transverse Relationships

Transverse problems fall into two categories: those due to symmetrical narrowing or (less frequently) widening of one dental arch and those due to jaw asymmetry.

Expansion and Narrowing of the Dental Arches. It is possible to move the maxillary segments both away from and toward the midline with relative ease and stability (Figure 22-11, on p. 685). The same movements, however, are more difficult to perform in the mandible because of the temporomandibular joint articulation and problems with soft tissue management.

Maxillary Expansion for Lingual Crossbite. Constriction of the maxilla rarely occurs without some coexisting vertical or sagittal problem. Maxillary constriction or expansion can be accomplished easily by segmenting the maxilla in the course of LeFort I downfracture surgery to correct other problems, and this is the usual approach. Expansion is done with parasagittal osteotomies in the lateral floor of the nose or medial floor of the sinus that are connected by a transverse cut anteriorly. A midline extension runs forward between the roots of the central incisors (Figure 22-12, on p. 685). If constriction is desired, bone is removed at the parasagittal osteotomies according to presurgical planning. In expansion, either bone harvested in the downfracture or bank bone is used to fill the void created by lateral movement of the posterior segments.

Orthopedic palatal expansion of the type used in adolescents is not feasible in adults because of the increasing resistance of the midpalatal and lateral maxillary sutures. Surgically-assisted palatal expansion, using bone cuts to reduce the resistance without totally freeing the maxillary segments, followed by rapid expansion of the jackscrew, is another possible treatment approach for adult patients with skeletal maxillary constriction.[19] The implication of this procedure is that the problem affects only the transverse plane of space, and this is when it is most useful (Figure 22-13, on p. 686). Surgically-assisted expansion as the first stage of two-stage surgical treatment, in a patient who would require another operation later to reposition the maxilla in the anteroposterior or vertical planes of space, is not recommended.[20]

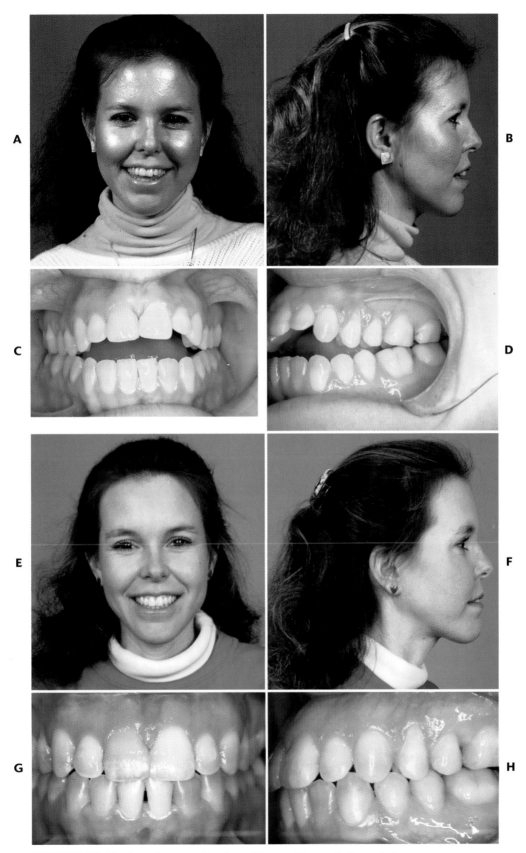

FIGURE 22-7 Superior repositioning of the maxilla usually is needed to correct severe anterior open bite. **A** and **B,** Facial proportions and **C** and **D,** occlusal relationships before treatment. **E** and **F,** facial proportions and **G** and **H,** occlusal relationships after maxillary surgery;

continued

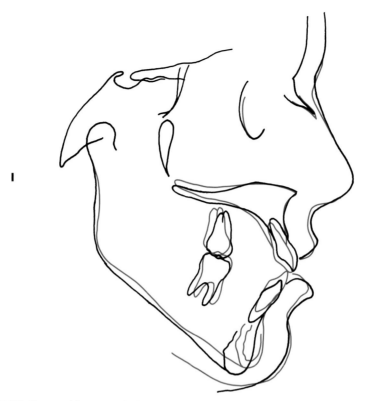

FIGURE 22-7, cont'd **I,** cephalometric superimposition. Note the upward and forward rotation of the mandible, which improved the anteroposterior jaw relationships. When the maxilla is repositioned vertically, both the postural (rest) and occlusal positions of the mandible change.

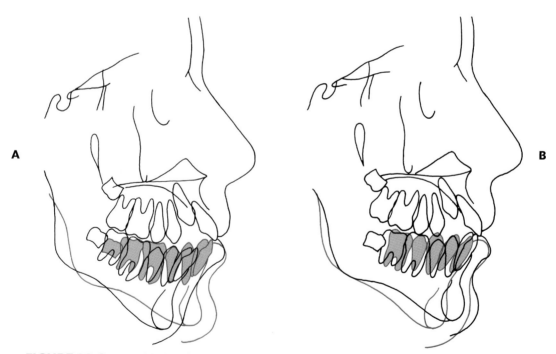

FIGURE 22-8 Mandibular advancement with rotation of the mandible to move the chin upward and decrease the mandibular plane angle is contraindicated because of the high potential for relapse. **A,** Cephalometric superimposition showing the change produced by mandibular ramus osteotomy in a mandibular deficient open bite patient. Note that the chin and mandibular incisors were elevated and advanced, but the mandible rotated around a fulcrum at the molars, and the gonial angle moved down. Lengthening the ramus and stretching the pterygomandibular sling in this way causes instability. **B,** Same patient, superimposition from immediately after surgery to 3 months after surgery. Note the relapse, with return of the anterior open bite caused by rotation of the mandible up posteriorly and down anteriorly.

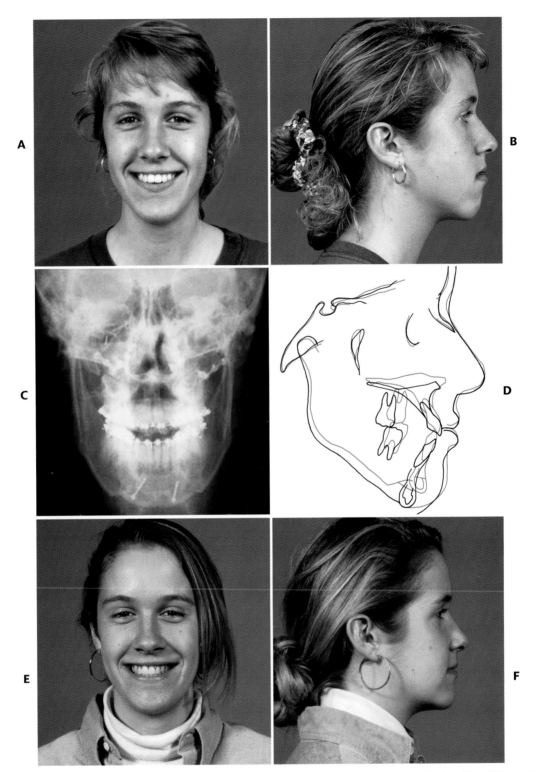

FIGURE 22-9   **A** and **B,** This girl, who had had unsuccessful orthodontic treatment for her Class III open bite malocclusion, was evaluated for surgical-orthodontic treatment at age 17. Note the typical asymmetry observed with excessive mandibular growth, with the chin off to the left. In preparation for surgery, maxillary and mandibular first premolars were extracted, the crowded lower incisors were aligned with minimal retraction, and the protruding maxillary incisors were retracted to produce negative overjet. **C** and **D,** At age 18, the maxilla was moved upward and forward, and a lower border osteotomy with removal of a wedge of bone was used to decrease the vertical height of the chin area and bring the chin to the midline. **E** and **F,** At the completion of treatment 18 months after pre-surgical orthodontics began, there was a significant improvement in facial esthetics. In Class III patients of this type, the combination of maxillary osteotomy and a lower border osteotomy of the chin, avoiding ramus surgery, has advantages of both better stability and better esthetics, particularly in throat form. Note that although the asymmetry of the gonial angles was not corrected, this is not apparent.

683

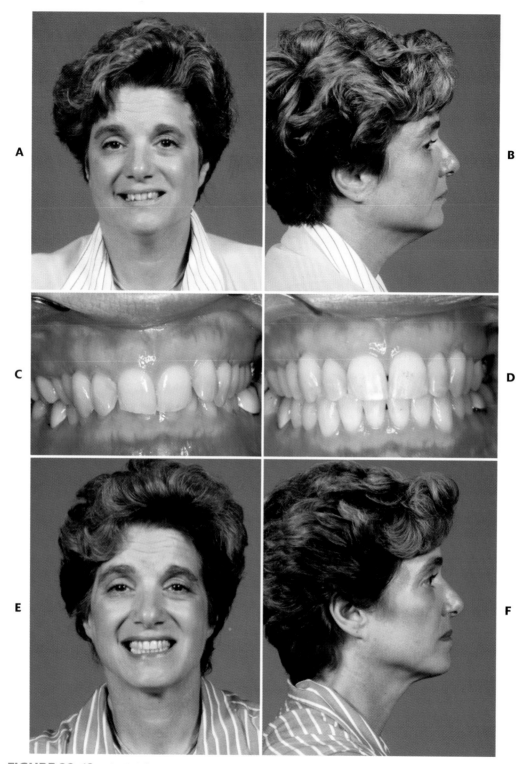

FIGURE 22-10   **A-C,** This 48-year-old woman sought treatment to correct her deep overbite, which was beginning to cause functional problems, and to improve her dental and facial appearance. The treatment plan called for aligning the teeth in both arches without extraction, bringing the upper incisors facially and increasing overjet; surgical mandibular advancement, bringing the mandible forward but rotating the chin downward to increase face height; and post-surgical leveling of the lower arch. **D-F,** In this case, treatment time was 15 months, and both ideal occlusion and improved facial esthetics were obtained. In this age group, mandibular advancement decreases facial wrinkles and tends to make the patient look younger.

continued

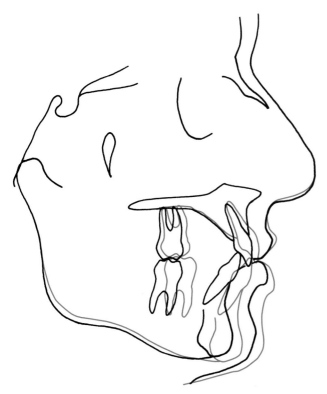

FIGURE 22-10, cont'd **G,** Cephalometric superimposition shows the mandibular rotation, increasing the mandibular plane angle by moving the chin down and the gonial angle up. This is the most stable type of mandibular advancement.

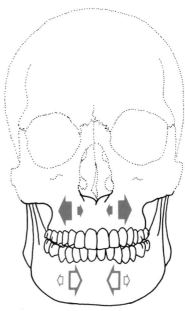

FIGURE 22-11 The surgical movements that are possible in the transverse dimension are shown on this postero-anterior illustration of the skull. The solid red arrows indicate that the maxilla can be expanded laterally or constricted with reasonable stability. The smaller size of the arrows pointing to the midline represents the fact that the amount of constriction possible is somewhat less than the range of expansion. The only transverse movement easily achieved in the mandible is constriction, although limited expansion is possible.

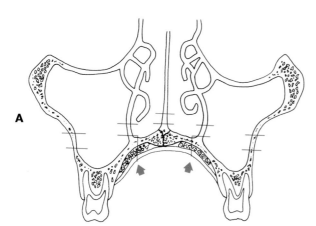

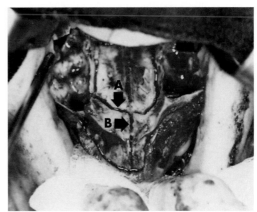

FIGURE 22-12 **A,** The osteotomy cuts necessary to surgically reposition the maxilla using the LeFort I downfracture approach are indicated in red. The arrows point to the vertical cuts that are placed immediately medial or lateral to the nasal wall to allow changes in transverse dimensions. The vertical cuts are placed in this location because there is more loose connective tissue underlying the mucosa in this area than at the mid-palatal suture. This technique allows repositioning with less soft tissue tension than would be experienced if a midline approach were used. **B,** This photograph is the surgeon's view of a downfractured maxilla in which the osteotomy cuts for parasagittal expansion have been completed. The anterior-posterior cuts in the lateral nasal floor are connected by transverse osteotomy (*arrow A*). An extension (*arrow B*) passes between the roots of the central incisors and completes the separation of the maxillary halves.

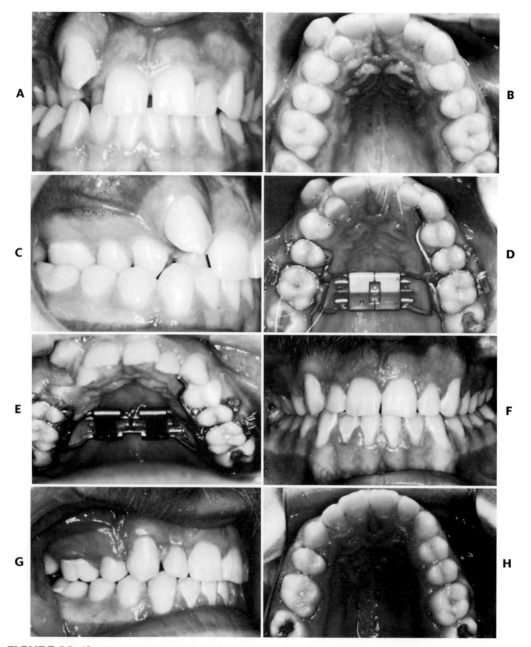

FIGURE 22-13   Surgically-assisted palatal expansion is indicated when an adult has problems only in the tranverse plane of space severe enough to require surgery and may be particularly advantageous when the transverse problem is unilateral, as in this patient. **A** to **C**, Occlusal relationships before treatment in a 17-year-old boy; **D** and **E**, occlusal views before and 1 week after surgery, showing the 4.5 mm of expansion gained following corticotomy of the right maxilla and activation of the jackscrew; **F** to **H**, occlusal relationships at the completion of treatment.

Mandible.   The range of expansion or constriction possible in the mandible is more limited. Movements in the posterior region are limited by the condyle-glenoid fossa relationship. Expansion anteriorly is limited by the need to cover the surgical site with soft tissue. Distraction osteogenesis appears to offer the possibility of augmenting the amount of both bone and soft tissue in the mandibular anterior area.[21] Whether expansion across the mandibular canines would be more stable if produced in this way has not been established. Because pressure against the teeth at the corners of the mouth seems to be the major limiting factor, expansion with distraction osteogenesis may turn out to be no more stable than orthodontic expansion. Constriction by a body ostectomy is possible anteriorly, but removal of teeth is necessary unless adequate interdental spacing exists. Improved techniques and instrumentation have made surgical repositioning of the dentoalveolar process possible, but only to the limit allowed by the underlying bone support.

Asymmetry.   Asymmetry is a surprisingly frequent component of dentofacial deformity. A review of the large data base at the University of North Carolina showed that one-fourth of mandibular deficient patients were asymmetric, and 40% of Class III and long face patients had some degree of asymmetry.[22] The asymmetry primarily involved the chin, but the midface (primarily the nose) also was affected in about one-third of the asymmetric patients. In patients with deficient or excessive mandibular growth, when the chin was off to one side, there was a 90% chance that the deviation was to the left (i.e., more mandibular growth on the right side). Only for the long face patients was there an equal distribution of right-left deviation. Why this occurs is unknown. Although trauma to the mandible can lead to deficient growth on one side and the development of asymmetry, a history of trauma was found in only 14% of the UNC patients with asymmetry. Most normal individuals have slightly more development of the right side of the face—perhaps this tendency is accentuated in those with growth disturbances.

Mandibular asymmetry often leads to a secondary maxillary deformity. More vertical mandibular growth on one side produces compensatory changes in maxillary growth, and a pronounced tilt to the occlusal plane is likely to occur. When the mandible deviates, compensatory changes in the mandibular alveolar process also are likely: the teeth shift back toward the midline as growth continues, and the chin deviates more than the dental midline. For this reason, surgical correction of asymmetry often requires a LeFort I osteotomy to reposition the maxilla, moving it more vertically than transversely, as well as sagittal split osteotomies of the mandibular ramus to advance or shorten one side more than the other (Figure 22-14). A lower border osteotomy of the mandible to reposition the chin transversely and/or vertically also may be indicated. If this procedure is used to bring the chin to the midline, it may be possible to leave the gonial angles slightly asymmetric, which is hardly noticeable, and avoid ramus surgery (see Figure 22-9).

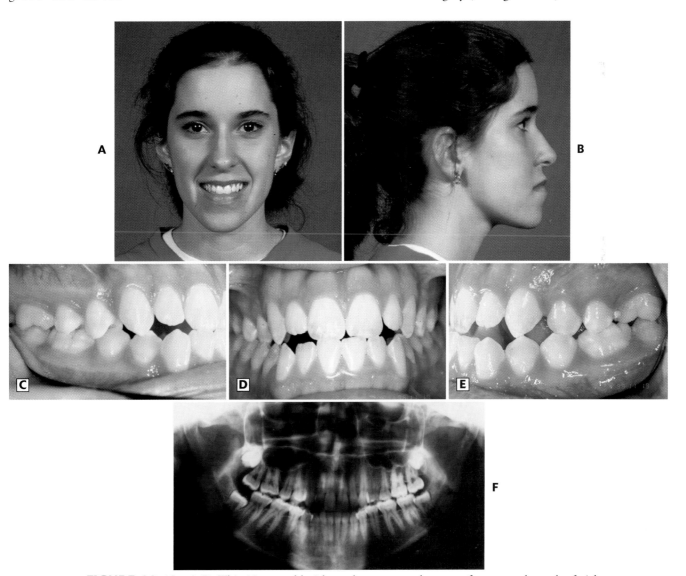

FIGURE 22-14 **A-B,** This 18-year-old girl sought treatment because of concern about the facial appearance created by her prominent and asymmetric chin. **C-E,** A Class III open bite malocclusion was present, with good alignment in both arches but the dental midlines off in the same direction as the chin. **F,** The panoramic radiograph shows a longer condylar neck on the left side of the mandible.

continued

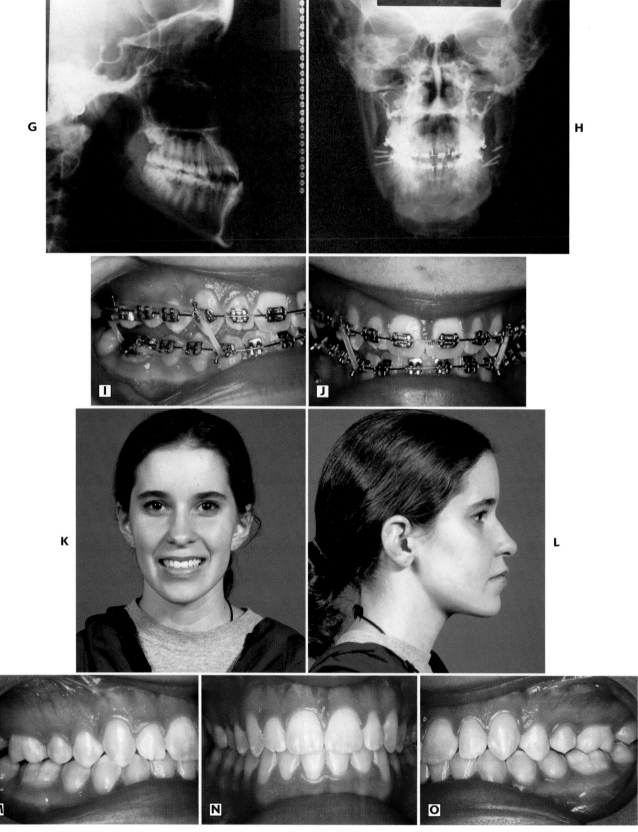

FIGURE 22-14, cont'd **G,** The cephalometric radiograph shows a combination of mandibular prognathism and maxillary deficiency. The plan of treatment was orthodontic alignment and stabilization, then, **H,** LeFort I osteotomy for maxillary advancement combined with BSSO for an asymmetric mandibular setback. **I** and **J,** Postsurgically, orthodontic archwires and light elastics were used to bring the teeth together, leveling the lower arch; **K-O,** Facial and dental appearance after 15 months of treatment;

continued

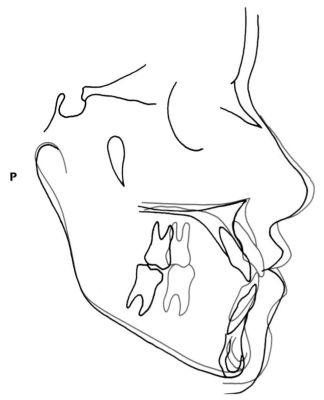

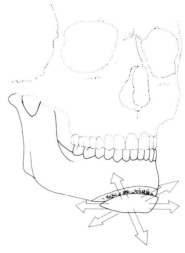

FIGURE 22-15 The chin can be sectioned anterior to the mental foramen and repositioned in all three planes of space. The lingual surface remains attached to muscles in the floor of the mouth, which provide the blood supply. Moving the chin anteriorly, upward, or laterally usually produces highly favorable esthetic results. Moving it back or down may produce a "boxy" appearance.

FIGURE 22-14, cont'd **P,** Cephalometric superimposition showing the changes produced during treatment.

Genioplasty in Orthognathic Treatment

Lack of surrounding anatomic structures gives the surgeon considerable latitude in alteration of chin morphology, and movement of the chin in all three planes of space is possible (Figure 22-15). The chin can be moved in virtually every direction, but esthetic results are unquestionably better and more predictable if the movement increases the soft tissue support rather than diminishes it (Figure 22-16).

Genioplasty Techniques. The chin can be augmented either by using an osteotomy of the lower border of the mandible to reposition the symphysis or by adding an implant material. Addition of a bone graft taken from another area is a possible implant approach but is used rarely because the absence of a vascular pedicle results in loss of viability and significant resorption.

For most patients, the preferred approach to genioplasty is a lower border osteotomy to free a wedge-shaped portion of the symphysis and inferior border that remains pedicled on the genioglossus and geniohyoid muscles. This segment can be advanced to augment chin contour, shifted sideways to correct asymmetry, or downgrafted to increase lower face height. By splitting the segment vertically, the distal aspects of the wedge can be flared or compressed. If narrowing of the anterior portion is needed, bone is removed in that area. When reduction is desired in the distance from the incisal edge to the inferior aspect of the symphysis, a wedge of bone can be removed above the

chin as diagrammed in Figure 22-15 and shown clinically in Figure 22-9.

Silicone implants were commonly placed to augment the chin at one time, but are used infrequently now because of problems with bone resorption under the silicone material and migration of the implant. If an implant must be used, porous hydroxylapatite in block form is a better choice than silicone, but it is difficult to adapt at the time of surgery and is not immune to the problems of resorption and migration.

Less satisfactory results are achieved in the reduction of a prominent symphysis. Degloving the symphysis and cutting away bone produces an undesirable boxy or blunted appearance of the chin. Posterior movement of a pedicled wedge gives results that are better but still less predictable and esthetic than augmentation. If possible, it is better to decrease chin prominence by rotating the body of the mandible downward, which often can be done with a ramus osteotomy while correcting other problems (see Figure 22-10).

Genioplasty as an Adjunct to Non-extraction Orthodontic Treatment. Prominence of the lower incisors relative to the chin traditionally has been treated orthodontically by retracting the incisors to establish proper tooth-chin balance, and indeed this relationship often has been considered a key to orthodontic treatment planning (e.g., as in the Holdaway ratios—see Chapter 6). But when the lower incisors are retracted, the upper incisors also must be retracted. For some patients, this creates the risk of an unesthetic flattening of the lips and can make a large nose appear even more prominent.

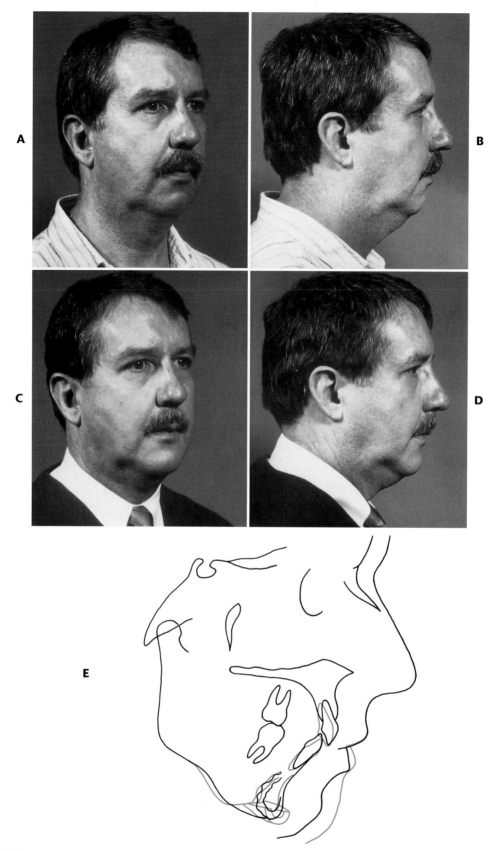

FIGURE 22-16 **A** and **B,** Age 47, prior to orthodontic treatment. His primary concern was impaired facial esthetics, which he related to crowding and protrusion of the upper incisors. The treatment plan was orthodontic treatment to align the incisors without retracting them and advancement genioplasty; **C** and **D,** Age 49, at completion of treatment; **E,** cephalometric superimposition. For this man who wanted improved dental and facial esthetics, orthodontic alignment of teeth solved only part of the problem; the lower border osteotomy to reposition the chin solved the rest. Note the improved throat form and decreased facial wrinkles produced by the genioplasty.

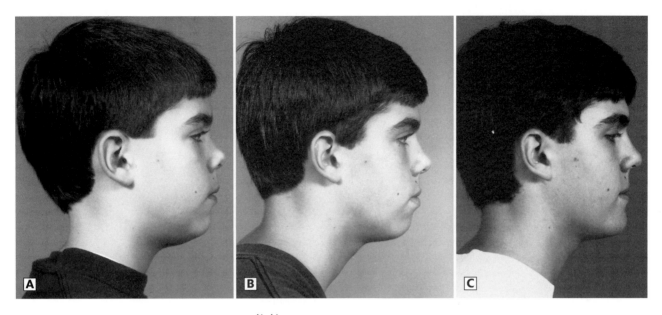

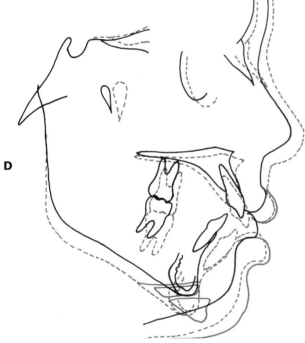

FIGURE 22-17   An attempt at nonextraction treatment for this 14-year-old boy with moderate Class II malocclusion, excessive overjet, and crowded lower incisors (**A**) resulted in unacceptable prominence of the lower incisors and an everted lower lip (**B**). The incisors would not be stable with this degree of protrusion, and facial esthetics are impaired. The traditional orthodontic treatment approach in this situation would be to extract premolars in both arches, retract the protruding lower incisors, and retract the upper incisors to establish ideal overjet, which would produce excellent occlusion and good stability at considerable cost to facial esthetics. An alternative is to improve the balance between lower incisors and chin by advancing the chin, which gives excellent facial esthetics (**C**) and changes lip pressures against the incisors, improving the chance for long-term stability. **D,** Cephalometric superimposition showing the changes from the initial condition (*black*) to corrected occlusion with unacceptable lower incisor protrusion (*dotted red*) to completion of treatment (*red*).

For such patients, a lower border osteotomy to augment the chin provides an alternative to premolar extraction and retraction of prominent lower incisors (Figure 22-17). In theory, advancing the chin decreases lip pressure against the lower incisors and makes them more stable in an advanced position. Although case reports suggest that this may be correct, it has not been established scientifically.

Integration of Orthognathic and Other Facial Surgery

Patients with jaw deformities often also have a nasal deformity, and alterations in the nose can benefit a significant minority of those who seek orthognathic surgery.[10] Rhinoplasty can change the proportions of the nose in a number of ways. It can quite successfully correct the nasal prominence and elevation of the nasal bridge that often accompanies severe Class II malocclusion. Without changes in the nose, retracting protruding maxillary incisors makes the nose even more prominent (Figure 22-18), and even with surgical mandibular advancement, rhinoplasty can greatly augment facial esthetics when a nasal deformity is part of the Class II facial pattern. When jaw asymmetry exists, there is about a 30% chance that the nose also is affected, so it is important to evaluate the nose carefully in asymmetry patients. If the nose deviates in the same direction as the chin, as often is the case, the nasal asymmetry will be accentuated by correcting the jaws and chin. Obviously, it is important to warn the patient that this will occur and to plan rhinoplasty as well as jaw surgery if it is needed.

The timing of rhinoplasty and orthognathic surgery depends on the type and extent of the jaw surgery. It is better for the patient to have both procedures done as part of the same operation, if this is feasible without compromising

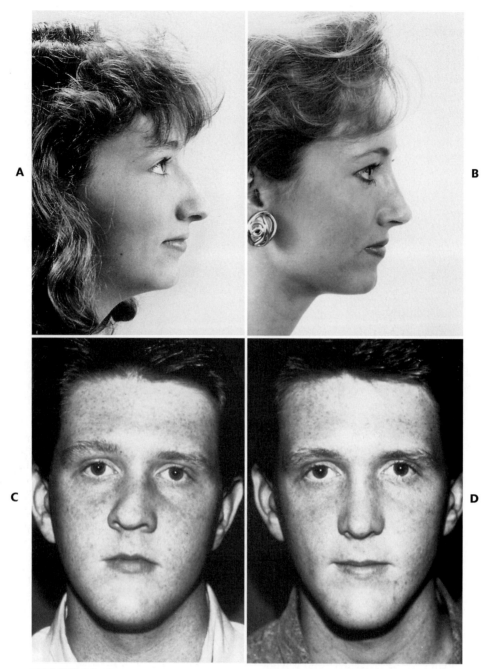

FIGURE 22-18   **A** and **B,** This patient with Class II malocclusion had orthodontic retraction of her protruding maxillary incisors and rhinoplasty to reduce the prominence of her nose and remove its dorsal hump. Retracting upper incisors tends to make the nose more prominent, and changes in the nose may be required for optimal esthetics in conjunction with orthodontic treatment. **C** and **D,** This patient with a nose that deviated to the left and a Class III malocclusion with a mandible that also deviated to the left had both orthognathic surgery and rhinoplasty. Especially if the jaw and nose deviate in the same direction, surgery that straightens the jaw will make the nasal asymmetry more prominent, and it is important for the patient to understand that correction of the nasal deformity also will be needed. (Courtesy Dr. D. Sarver.)

the quality of the result. Simultaneous mandibular advancement and rhinoplasty usually can be accomplished, but it is more difficult to combine maxillary surgery and rhinoplasty, and still more difficult to combine nasal and two-jaw surgery. A second-stage rhinoplasty, typically done 12 to 16 weeks after the jaw surgery, often is the best plan for patients with major asymmetry.

TIMING AND SEQUENCING OF SURGICAL TREATMENT

Early vs. Later Surgery

As noted previously, growth modification is the preferred approach to severe dentofacial problems, whereas surgery is reserved for patients who do not respond to growth modification and whose problems are too severe for camouflage. As a general rule, early jaw surgery has little inhibitory effect on further growth. For this reason, orthognathic surgery should be delayed until growth is essentially completed in patients who have problems of excessive growth, especially mandibular prognathism. For patients with growth deficiencies, surgery can be considered earlier, but rarely before the adolescent growth spurt.

Early Surgery and Growth Excess. Actively growing patients with mandibular prognathism can be expected to outgrow surgical correction and require retreatment

(Figure 22-19), so the timing of this surgery often is a critical consideration. Indirect methods of assessing growth status, such as hand-wrist films to determine bone age, are not accurate enough to use for planning the time of surgery. The best method is serial cephalometric tracings, with surgery delayed until good superimposition documents that the adult deceleration of growth has occurred. Often the correction of excessive mandibular growth must be delayed until the late teens, unless a second later surgical correction can be justified because of psychosocial considerations.

The situation is not so clear cut for patients with the long face (skeletal open bite) pattern that can be characterized as vertical maxillary excess. In a series of patients treated at the University of North Carolina, skeletal stability of the vertically repositioned maxilla was similar in patients above and below the age of 19, but the maxillary posterior teeth tended to erupt after surgery in the younger patients.[14] There appears to be a reasonable chance for stable surgical correction of this problem before growth is totally completed, but the difference in clinical stability between treatment at, for example ages 14 and 18, remains incompletely understood.

Early Surgery and Growth Deficiency. Surgery in infancy and early childhood is required for some congenital problems that involve growth deficiency; craniosynostosis and severe hemifacial microsomia are two examples. The major indication for orthognathic surgery before

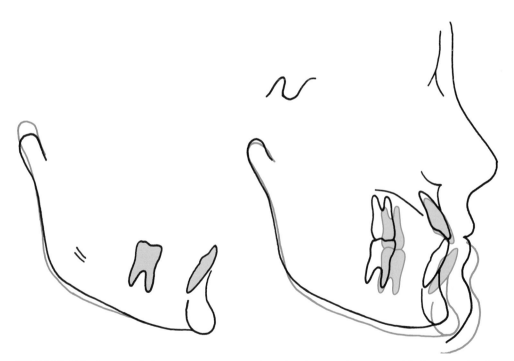

FIGURE 22-19 Cephalometric superimposition showing continued mandibular growth after surgical correction at age 15 (*black tracing*, completion of initial phase of treatment). The red outline, 5 years later, demonstrates the increment of mandibular growth and resulting relapse. Note the eruption of the upper teeth to partially maintain occlusal relationships as the mandible grew.

puberty, however, is a progressive deformity caused by restriction of growth. A common cause is ankylosis of the mandible (unilaterally or occasionally bilaterally) after a condylar injury or severe infection (see Chapters 2 and 4). Surgery to release the ankylosis, followed by functional appliance therapy to guide subsequent growth, is needed in these unusual problems.

A child with a severely progressive deficiency should be distinguished from one with a severe but stable deficiency, such as a child with a small mandible whose facial proportions are not changing appreciably with growth. Although a progressive deficiency is an indication for early surgery, a severe but stable deficiency may not be. In keeping with the general principle that orthognathic surgery has surprisingly little impact on growth, early surgery does not improve the growth prognosis unless it relieves a specific restriction on growth, nor does it produce a subsequent normal growth pattern.

Early Mandibular Advancement. In the 1980s, there was some controversy about the impact of early mandibular advancement on subsequent mandibular growth. It now seems clear that many younger patients have further growth following surgical mandibular advancement. Most of this growth is expressed vertically, however, and results in minimal forward movement at pogonion.[23] In our view, mandibular advancement before the adolescent growth spurt is of questionable utility for patients who do not have extremely severe and progressive deformities. On the other hand, there is no reason to delay mandibular advancement after sexual maturity. Minimal facial growth can be expected in patients with severe deficiency during late adolescence, and relapse from that cause is unlikely. In contrast to mandibular setback, mandibular advancement at age 14 or 15 is quite feasible.

Early Maxillary Advancement. A major reason to consider surgical maxillary advancement at an early age is to help overcome psychosocial problems caused by severe deficiency. Early advancement of a sagittally deficient maxilla or midface remains relatively stable if there is careful attention to detail and if grafts are used to combat relapse, but further forward growth of the maxilla is quite unlikely. In general, maxillary advancement should be delayed until after the adolescent growth spurt unless there are preponderant psychological considerations. In this case, subsequent growth of the mandible is likely to result in reestablishment of the abnormal relationships, and the patient and parents should be cautioned about the possible need for a second stage of surgical treatment later.

Although surgery to reposition the entire maxilla may affect future growth, this is not necessarily the case for the surgical procedures used to correct cleft lip and palate. In cleft patients, bone grafts to alveolar clefts prior to eruption of the permanent canines can eliminate the bony defect, which greatly improves the long-term prognosis for the dentition. A review of cleft palate patients treated with the Oslo protocol (i.e., closure of the lip and hard palate at

3 months, posterior palatal closure at 18 months, and cancellous alveolar bone grafting at 8 to 11 years) showed no interference with the total amount of facial growth.[24] As cleft palate surgery methods continue to improve, the number of cleft palate patients who need maxillary advancement as a final stage of treatment should continue to decrease.

Sequencing Treatment

Surgical and Orthodontic Phases of Treatment. Successful management of combined surgical and orthodontic treatment requires the integration of pre-surgical orthodontic, surgical, and post-surgical orthodontic phases of treatment. In contemporary treatment, dental compensations are removed before surgery and the teeth are properly located in relationship to the individual skeletal components. At this point, heavy archwires are placed and the appliance is used for stability and fixation during surgical reorientation of the bony segments. The contemporary edgewise appliance provides excellent stabilization, better than can be obtained with arch bars or fracture splints. When satisfactory healing has taken place, active orthodontics is reinitiated to refine the occlusion and complete treatment. Although orthognathic surgery can be performed with reasonable precision, it is always desirable to refine the occlusal relationships after jaw discrepancies have been corrected.

Other Dental Treatment. As with any orthodontic patient, dental and periodontal disease must be brought under control before combined surgical-orthodontic treatment is begun. The principles discussed in Chapter 20 are entirely applicable. Three special points should be considered when orthognathic surgery is involved:

1. Incision lines contract somewhat as they heal, and when incisions are placed in the vestibule, this can stress the gingival attachment, leading to stripping or recession of the gingiva. This is most likely to be a problem in the lower anterior area in relation to the incision for a genioplasty (Figure 22-20). Gingival grafting should be completed before genioplasty if the attached gingiva is inadequate.

2. Many young adults being prepared for orthognathic surgery have unerupted or impacted third molars. If the surgeon will use rigid fixation (bone screws) placed in the third molar area, it is desirable to have the teeth removed far enough in advance of the orthognathic procedure to allow good bone healing.

3. If the patient's prime motivation for treatment is temporomandibular dysfunction (TMD), the unpredictable impact of orthognathic surgery must be carefully discussed to avoid unreasonable treatment expectations. TMD symptoms usually improve during active orthodontic treatment, probably because the soreness associated with tooth movement interferes with parafunctional activity, but this im-

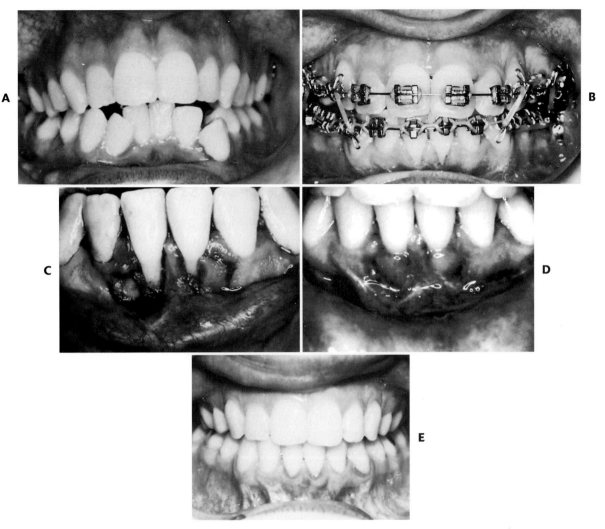

FIGURE 22-20   Mucogingival problems can arise in a patient requiring genioplasty. **A,** Minimal attached gingiva can be seen overlying the lower anterior teeth in this pre-treatment photo. Note the inflammation of the marginal gingiva resulting from inadequate hygiene. **B,** After orthodontic alignment and genioplasty, the stresses placed on the periodontium by orthodontic tooth movement and the contracture of the vestibular incision used in advancement genioplasty have resulted in loss of attachment and dehiscence over the lower central incisors. **C,** Periodontal surgery is indicated to prevent further dehiscence and reestablish gingival attachment over the involved teeth. **D,** Early healing of the laterally positioned flaps as seen at the surgical margins of the central incisors. **E,** Excellent contour and reattachment have been established in this patient. Since early grafting procedures are generally more successful than those to reestablish attachment once dehiscence has occurred, it is better to anticipate problems and plan gingival grafts in questionable areas before initiating treatment.

provement may be transient (see Chapter 21). If surgical-orthodontic treatment can be justified regardless of whether it resolves TMD, there is every reason to proceed with it and hope that the TMD symptoms improve, but the patient should be well aware that they may recur. If joint surgery will be required, usually it is better to defer this until after orthognathic surgery because the joint surgery is more predictable after the new joint positions and occlusal relationships have been established.

As with all adult orthodontic patients, whether or not orthognathic or TM joint surgery is involved, definitive restorative and prosthetic treatment is the last step in the treatment sequence. Initial restorative treatment should stabilize or temporize the existing dentition with restorations that will be serviceable and provide patient comfort during the orthodontic and surgery phases. When the final skeletal and dental relationships have been achieved, it is possible to obtain accurate articulator mountings and complete the final occlusal rehabilitation.

INTEGRATION OF SURGICAL AND ORTHODONTIC TREATMENT

Interactive Treatment Planning

Minimum diagnostic records for potential surgical patients are the same as for any other comprehensive orthodontic treatment. A careful clinical evaluation, with particular attention to facial soft tissue contours and esthetics, is required. To assist in accurate planning, an effort should be made to obtain records with the patient's head normally positioned (i.e., photographs, digital images for computer input, and cephalometric radiographs all should be made in natural head position) (see Chapter 6). It is important for both the orthodontist and the surgeon to be involved in the patient's evaluation from the beginning. Often other consultations are needed initially (especially periodontics and prosthodontics, but occasionally other dental or medical specialists).

It always has been a moral and ethical imperative to allow the patient to make important decisions about what treatment he or she will accept, and now it is a legal obligation as well.[25] Orthodontics and orthognathic surgery are elective procedures. However desirable the doctor may think any treatment approach would be, patients now must be provided enough information to make that decision on their own. Interactive treatment planning, through which the treatment plan is developed as a cooperative effort between the doctor and the patient, therefore is a necessity in the modern world.

Computer Simulation of Alternative Treatment Outcomes: An Important Element in Informed Consent. The objective of treatment simulation is to allow the clinician to visualize and manipulate the dental and skeletal structures so that both the doctor and the patient can compare various treatment alternatives. Since the mid-1990s, computer-generated simulations of profile changes have become the preferred method for doing this. These methods continue to improve rapidly and will be the standard approach in the near future.

Computer simulations are based on algorithms that relate hard tissue changes produced by manipulation of cephalometric tracings, to changes in the soft tissue profile, or vice versa. To accomplish this, the appropriate landmarks from the cephalometric tracing are digitized and entered into a computer. The cephalometric digital model can be the same as that used for other orthodontic purposes, so long as it incorporates enough digitized points to adequately represent the hard and soft tissues relationships. A digital photograph similarly is entered into computer memory. The preferred method now is the output from a 35 mm digital camera; alternatives are a scanned 35 mm photographic slide or the output from a video camera (much less precise because of the smaller image size). Surgical predictions then are produced by moving areas of the digitized cephalometric tracing as they would be at surgery—for instance, the mandible is moved forward and rotated downward, or the maxilla is moved upward and slightly forward—and the computer system produces corresponding changes in the soft tissue image (Figure 22-21).

Although an experienced clinician can judge alternative treatments quite well from cephalometric tracings alone, patients cannot. The major advantage of the computer methods is the greater understanding of treatment options that patients gain from being shown the soft tissue simulations. When these methods were first employed, there was great concern that patients might be led to expect

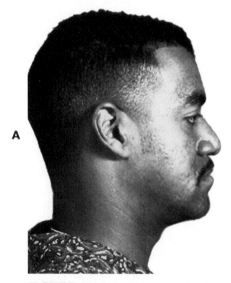 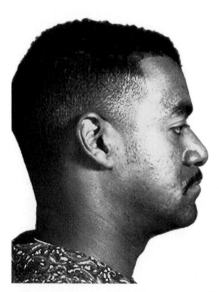

FIGURE 22-21   Computer simulation of maxillary advancement (*right*) to correct Class III malocclusion in a 30-year-old male.

more than the actual treatment could deliver, but patient responses to treatment with and without exposure to computer simulations show that this risk is minimal or non-existent.[26]

Several questions can be asked about this type of simulation and its clinical use:

How Accurate Is It?   The algorithms relating hard to soft tissue changes continue to improve. At present, the prediction of chin position is quite good, the upper lip is reasonably good, and the lower lip is most difficult to predict accurately, especially when vertical changes are involved.[27] The accuracy is good enough to make the simulations quite useful clinically. Similar predictions from a frontal view are just now becoming possible, and it is quite likely that the same pattern will be observed.

What Are the Risks of Showing Computer Simulations to Patients?   A comparison of patients who were and were not shown computer simulations of their possible surgical outcomes showed that seeing the simulations heightened expectations for esthetic improvement, but satisfaction with the treatment outcomes was not different between the two groups (actually slightly higher in those who saw the predictions, but not significantly so).[28] The patients who saw the computer simulations, however, did report more anxiety about the surgical experience and more concern about the possibility of surgical problems, even though both groups saw the same patient education material about this. Apparently the computer simulations made the patients more aware of the surgery as something they really would experience, instead of being a somewhat abstract experience. In this sense also, the simulations perhaps resulted in a more informed consent to treatment.

The Borderline Patient: Camouflage or Surgery?

One of the most difficult decisions facing the orthodontist and surgeon is whether a patient with a borderline skeletal discrepancy can be successfully treated with orthodontics alone. The decision must be made from the very beginning, however, because the tooth movement needed in orthodontic preparation for surgery often is just the opposite of what would be needed for orthodontic treatment alone (see below).

The envelope of discrepancy (see Figure 22-3) should be considered a starting point in making this decision. It gives the limitations of orthodontic treatment in terms of whether the occlusion could be corrected, not whether the deformity could be camouflaged. For a patient whose deformity is within the envelope, the decision must be made in the context of the esthetic impact of the two forms of treatment. This is where the patient's input must be sought and where computer simulations that the patient can understand are particularly valuable (Figure 22-22; also see Figure 22-21). Only the patient can decide whether the esthetic difference between surgical correction of the jaw deformity and orthodontic correction of the malocclusion would be worth it in terms of the additional risk and cost of surgery.

Although the patient can and should decide between the orthodontic and surgical possibilities, it remains true that some conditions can be treated better with orthodontics alone than others, simply because the impact on facial esthetics is likely to be better. Some characteristics that can make the difference between satisfactory camouflage treatment and failure are summarized in Box 22-1. This topic has been addressed in considerable detail by Sarver.[10]

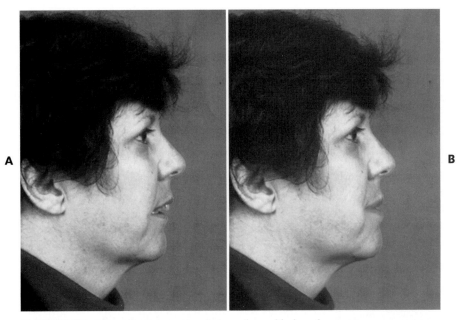

FIGURE 22-22   Computer simulation of mandibular advancement to correct severe Class II malocclusion in a 35-year-old woman. Simulations of this type greatly help patients understand the implications of alternative plans of treatment.

ORTHODONTIC CAMOUFLAGE OF SKELETAL MALOCCLUSION

Acceptable results likely
Average or short facial pattern
Mild anteroposterior jaw discrepancy
Crowding <4-6 mm
Normal soft tissue features (nose, lips, chin)
No transverse skeletal problem

Poor results likely
Long vertical facial pattern
Moderate or severe anteroposterior jaw discrepancy
Crowding >4-6 mm
Exaggerated features
Transverse skeletal component of problem

Pre-surgical Orthodontics

Extraction Patterns. The critical importance of deciding on surgery or camouflage at the beginning of treatment is further illustrated by the difference in extractions needed with the two approaches. In camouflage, extraction spaces are used to produce dental compensations for the jaw discrepancy and the extractions are planned accordingly. For example, with orthodontic treatment alone, a patient with mandibular deficiency and a Class II malocclusion might have upper first premolars removed to allow the retraction of the maxillary anterior teeth. Extraction in the lower arch would be avoided, or if necessary because of leveling or alignment requirements, the second premolars might be chosen to provide needed arch length while avoiding retraction of the lower anterior teeth.

The extraction pattern for this same patient would be quite different if mandibular advancement were planned. Instead of creating dental compensation for the jaw deformity, the orthodontic treatment now would be planned to remove dental compensation, prior to surgical correction of the jaw relationship. Premolar extraction in the lower arch but not in the upper often is needed. Removal of lower first premolars would allow leveling of the arch and correction of the lower anterior proclination often associated with this malocclusion. Often in mandibular deficiency patients the position of the upper incisors relative to the maxilla is normal; if so, retracting them would be undesirable. The upper arch would be treated without extraction, or if some space were needed because of arch length discrepancy, extractions (such as maxillary second premolars) would be planned to avoid compromising the mandibular advancement by over-retraction of the upper anterior teeth.

A similar but reversed situation would be seen in a patient with a skeletal Class III problem. If camouflage were

planned, typical extractions might be lower first premolars alone, or lower first and upper second premolars. As a general rule, Class III problems are less amenable to camouflage than Class II, because retracting the lower incisors may make the chin appear even more prominent, not what is desired in camouflage (Figure 22-23). Surgical preparation of the same patient often would require extraction of upper first premolars so that upper incisors could be retracted, correcting their axial inclination and increasing the reverse overjet. If space were needed in the lower arch, second rather than first premolar extraction would be a logical choice so that the lower incisors were not retracted.

Appliance Systems. In contemporary treatment, the fixed orthodontic appliance is used to stabilize the teeth and basal bone at the time of surgery and during healing. For this reason, the appliance system must permit the use of rectangular archwires for strength and stability. Any of the variations of the edgewise appliance and the combination Begg-edgewise appliance are acceptable. The standard Begg appliance does not provide the control needed, even though a ribbon archwire and special retaining pins can provide some additional rigidity.

Ceramic brackets pose a dilemma in surgical-orthodontic treatment. The appearance of these brackets makes them appealing to esthetically-conscious adults who are also the most likely group of patients to choose surgery, but the brittleness of the ceramic material makes them susceptible to fracture, especially with the manipulation that may occur during the jaw surgery. If ceramic brackets are used, they should be restricted to the maxillary anterior teeth. The surgeon must treat them gently and be prepared to use an alternate stabilization method if they fracture or become dislodged.

Goals of Pre-surgical Treatment. The objective of pre-surgical treatment is to prepare the patient for surgery, placing the teeth relative to their own supporting bone without concern for the dental occlusion at that stage. Since some post-surgical orthodontics will be required in any case, it is inefficient to do tooth movement prior to surgery that could be accomplished more easily and quickly during or after surgery. For example, when a maxillary osteotomy is needed for correction of a vertical or anteroposterior problem, there is no reason to expand the arch transversely during the pre-surgical orthodontics—this can be done as part of the same maxillary surgery. Most patients with deep overbite before treatment need leveling of the lower arch by extrusion of posterior teeth, and this can be done more quickly and easily during the post-surgical orthodontics (see p. 705). On the other hand, it is an error to wait until after surgery to accomplish tooth movement that could lead to relapse. Leveling the lower arch post-surgically by extrusion of posterior teeth can produce undesirable anterior bite opening in patients who were treated for long face, skeletal open bite problems. This means that the treatment sequence for the patient with a

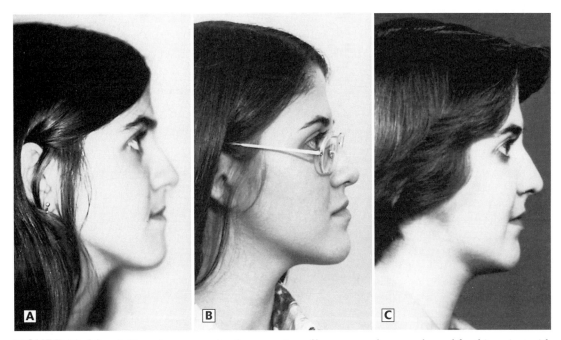

FIGURE 22-23 **A,** Dental compensation by extraction of lower premolars was planned for this patient with average facial height and moderate mandibular prognathism. **B,** Continued mandibular growth and retraction of the lower anterior teeth combined with proclination of the upper teeth has produced reasonable dental occlusion, but overall facial esthetics are compromised by the strong appearance of the chin. At this stage, the patient sought surgical treatment despite her orthodontist's opinion that everything was fine. **C,** Orthognathic surgery has improved the overall facial balance. Treatment was complicated, however, by the dental compensation that had been "built in" to mask the skeletal malocclusion. Patients to be treated with orthodontic camouflage must be carefully selected, since the mechanotherapy and treatment objectives are the opposite of those desired in orthodontic preparation for surgical correction.

long face pattern should be planned so that post-operative tooth movement involves minor settling only.

These guidelines mean that the amount of pre-surgical orthodontics can be quite variable, ranging from only appliance placement in a few patients to 12 months or so of treatment in others with severe crowding or protrusion. The pre-surgical phase should almost never require more than a year, however, unless it is delayed by waiting for growth to be completed. The post-surgical phase of treatment generally requires about 6 months, depending on the amount of detailing needed. Another way to express the goal of pre-surgical orthodontics is that it should prepare the patient so that post-surgical treatment can be completed within 6 months.

Steps in Orthodontic Preparation. The essential steps in pre-surgical orthodontics are to align the arches or arch segments and make them compatible, and to establish the anteroposterior and vertical position of the incisors. Both are necessary so that the teeth will not interfere with placing the jaws in the desired position.

Planning the leveling of the dental arches is particularly important. The guideline is that extrusion generally is done more easily post-surgically, whereas intrusion must be accomplished pre-surgically or handled surgically. Two common problems require special consideration: how to

level an accentuated curve of Spee in the lower arch of a patient with deep overbite, and how to level the upper arch in an open bite patient who has a large vertical discrepancy between anterior and posterior teeth.

Leveling the Mandibular Arch. When an accentuated curve of Spee is present in the lower arch, the decision to level by intrusion of incisors or extrusion of premolars should be based on the desired final face height. If the face is short and the distance from the lower incisal edge of the chin is normal, then leveling by extrusion of posterior teeth is indicated, so the chin will move downward at surgery. If the incisors are elongated and face height is normal or excessive, they must be intruded to prevent problems in controlling face height at surgery (Figure 22-24).

Most short face, deep bite patients can benefit from posterior extrusion. Usually it is advantageous to stage the treatment of short face mandibular deficient patients so that much of the leveling of the lower arch is finished after surgery. Prior to surgery, the teeth are aligned and the anteroposterior position of the incisors is established, but a curve of Spee is left in all the archwires, including the surgical stabilizing wire. This means the surgical splint will be thicker in the premolar region than anteriorly or posteriorly. At surgery, normal overjet and overbite are created, and the space between the premolar teeth is corrected

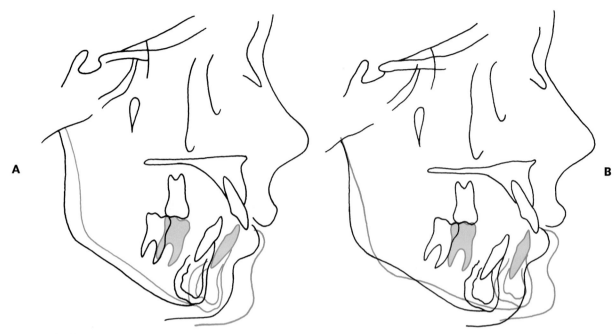

FIGURE 22-24   Effects of orthodontic leveling on the position of the mandible at surgery. **A,** Prediction of correcting mandibular deficiency with no change in the presurgical position of the mandibular incisors (i.e., post-surgical leveling of the lower arch by premolar extrusion). The lower incisors move downward and forward into the proper relationship with the upper incisors, and the chin is projected downward and forward. **B,** Prediction of correcting mandibular deficiency in the same patient after presurgical leveling by intrusion of the lower incisors. The effect is a decrease in face height rather than an increase. If the goal is to maintain or decrease face height when the mandible is advanced, pre-surgical intrusion is required; if the goal is to increase face height, which often is the case in mandibular deficiency patients, pre-surgical intrusion of the lower incisors would be a serious error.

post-surgically by extruding these teeth with flat archwires. This occurs rapidly, typically within the first 8 weeks after orthodontic treatment resumes, because there are no occlusal contacts to oppose the tooth movement. The alternative is to use an auxiliary wire to assist in pre-surgical leveling. An auxiliary leveling wire (see Figure 16-30) can be tied over a continuous reverse curve base archwire to increase its action.

If intrusion is required, a segmented arch approach is indicated in the pre-surgical orthodontics (see Chapters 16 and 21). For the lower arch, surgical leveling rarely is indicated, although a subapical osteotomy to depress the incisor segment is possible. The major disadvantage of this surgical leveling is that all teeth in the segment will be moved the same, although leveling within the incisor segment almost always is required.

Leveling the Maxillary Arch.   In a patient with open bite, severe vertical discrepancies within the maxillary arch are an indication for multiple segment surgery. When this is planned, the upper arch should *not* be leveled conventionally. Leveling should be done only within each segment (Figure 22-25), and the segments are leveled at surgery. If a one-piece osteotomy is planned, pre-surgical orthodontic leveling is required, but extrusion of anterior teeth before surgery must be avoided because even mild orthodontic

relapse could cause a problem with post-surgical bite opening. Segmental leveling at surgery is preferred.

Establishment of Incisor Position and Space Closure.   The anteroposterior position of the incisors determines where the mandible will be placed relative to the maxilla at surgery and therefore is a critical element in planning treatment. This is often the major factor in planning anchorage in the closure of extraction sites.

Incisor positioning before mandibular advancement poses a special problem because different types of postoperative tooth movement can be anticipated depending on which type of fixation is being utilized. With wire osteosynthesis and maxillomandibular fixation during post-surgical healing, the mandible may tend to slip back during the period of approximately 6 weeks that the teeth are tied together. This is caused by the elastic recoil of the soft tissues that were stretched as the mandible was moved forward (Figure 22-26). Thus, while the lower jaw moves back, the teeth are held together in occlusion by the fixation and acrylic splint. The result is a Class II elastic effect with the lower incisors being tipped forward and the upper incisors being retracted. The amount of this movement is related to a combination of tooth mobility from pre-surgical orthodontics, tolerances in the fit of the archwire in the brackets, and the mobility inherent to the intraosseous

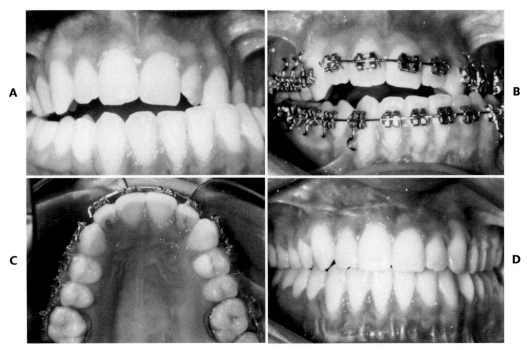

FIGURE 22-25   In preparation for maxillary segmental surgery, often it is better to level and align the teeth only within the planned segments. **A,** Pre-treatment occlusal relationships in a patient with anterior open bite, a narrow maxilla, and posterior crossbite, who was planned for treatment with superior repositioning of the maxilla in three segments. **B** and **C,** Leveling and alignment have been accomplished within the anterior and posterior maxillary segments, and the segments have been stabilized. Note that for this patient, the canines are in the posterior segments. **D,** Post-treatment occlusal relationships.

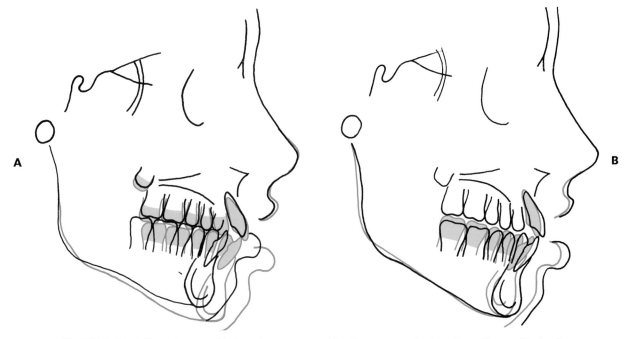

FIGURE 22-26   After mandibular advancement with wire osteosynthesis and maxillomandibular fixation (MMF), the mandible tends to slip posteriorly even though the teeth are wired together (the occlusal relationships are preserved by orthodontic tooth movement). **A,** Superimposition showing changes produced at surgery; **B,** superimposition showing changes during the next 6 months, almost all of which occurred during the 6 weeks of MMF. Note that the mandible has slipped back 2 mm, while the upper incisor has tipped back and the lower incisor has tipped forward, maintaining the occlusal relationships.

wiring technique. These changes stop when bony union occurs at about 6 weeks after surgery. Because the occlusal relationships are maintained, it is not helpful to overcorrect the occlusion at surgery and place the patient in anterior crossbite. Any overcorrection must be done in the pre-surgical positioning of the incisors.

With rigid fixation of the mandibular segments following mandibular advancement, the jaws usually are immobilized for only 2 or 3 days postsurgically, and different patterns of tooth movement are seen. Post-surgical movement of the jaw, when it occurs, is often in an anterior direction rather than in the posterior direction seen in wire fixation cases. Therefore the compensatory tooth movements are in exactly the opposite direction, with the lower incisors tipping posteriorly while the upper incisors flare anteriorly. For this reason, overcorrection of the incisor positions in the pre-surgical orthodontics is less desirable when rigid fixation will be employed.

When several surgical segments are planned for the maxilla, a different consideration arises: the axial inclination of the upper incisors and canines should be established pre-surgically so that rotation of the anterior segment at surgery can be avoided (Figure 22-27). Otherwise, establishing correct torque of the incisors surgically will elevate the canines above the occlusal plane, and proper postoperative repositioning of the canines becomes difficult if not impossible. An extraction site that will be the location of an osteotomy cut should not be completely closed before surgery, but up to one half of the extraction space can be used in the course of adjusting incisor inclination without creating difficulty for the surgeon.

Stabilizing Archwires. As the patient is approaching the end of orthodontic preparation for surgery, it is helpful to take impressions and examine the hand-articulated models for occlusal compatibility. Minor interferences that can be corrected easily with archwire adjustments can significantly limit surgical movement. Second molars should be bonded to increase fixation stability, especially in segmental maxillary surgery. However, they must be positioned carefully to avoid their extrusion, which may induce opening of the bite. This is easy to overlook since they are often out of occlusion preoperatively in patients having a sagittal component to their malocclusion.

When any final orthodontic adjustments have been made, the stabilizing archwires should be placed at least 4 weeks before surgery so that they are passive when the impressions are taken for the surgical splint (usually 1 to 2 weeks before surgery). This ensures that there will be no tooth movement that would result in a poorly fitting splint and potential compromise of the surgical result. The stabilizing wires are full-dimension edgewise wires (i.e., 17×25 steel in the 18-slot appliance, 21×25 TMA or steel in the 22-slot appliance). Filling the bracket slot minimizes tolerance in the appliance system and provides the strength needed to withstand the forces resulting from intermaxillary fixation. Unless the brackets incorporate hooks, brass

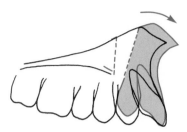

FIGURE 22-27 In segmental maxillary surgery, it is important to establish the correct inclination of the incisors presurgically. Otherwise, it will be necessary to rotate the anterior segment at surgery, which tends to elevate the canine off the occlusal plane and diverge the roots at the osteotomy site.

lugs should be soldered to the archwire as attachments for the fixation wiring (see Figure 22-29). Prefabricated ball-hooks also may be used if welded, soldered, or carefully crimped in place on the archwire. Sliding them over the wire without securing them is undesirable, because they can slip or rotate when they are used to tie the jaws together during surgery. Tight intermaxillary fixation is necessary at least long enough to place rigid fixation.

Patient Management at Surgery

Final Surgical Planning. When the orthodontist considers surgical preparation completed, pre-surgical records should be obtained. These consist of panoramic and lateral cephalometric films, periapical films of interdental osteotomy sites, and dental casts. Casts should be mounted on a semiadjustable articulator if maxillary surgery is planned. To avoid distortion, impressions are best made with the stabilizing archwires removed. The archwires should be passive by the time these final pre-surgical impressions for model surgery and splints are taken.

The final planning requires a repetition of the predictions that were done initially. The difference is that the actual orthodontic movements, rather than predictions of this aspect, are now available. A current cephalometric film is used to simulate surgical movements and evaluate the resulting soft tissue profile. When satisfactory functional and esthetic balance is achieved, the surgical movements are duplicated in the model surgery. For cases involving maxillary surgery, the movements planned with the cephalometric treatment simulation are duplicated and verified on articulator-mounted casts (Figure 22-28) before fabrication of interocclusal surgical splints. It is better for the surgeon to perform this phase, since much insight into the final surgical design can be gained.

Splints and Stabilization. We recommend the routine use of an interocclusal wafer splint made from the casts as repositioned by the model surgery. Since this splint will define the post-surgical result, the orthodontist and surgeon should review the model surgery together. In patients requiring post-operative prosthodontic rehabilitation, the dentist responsible for this phase of treatment should be consulted about the acceptability of abutment and ridge re-

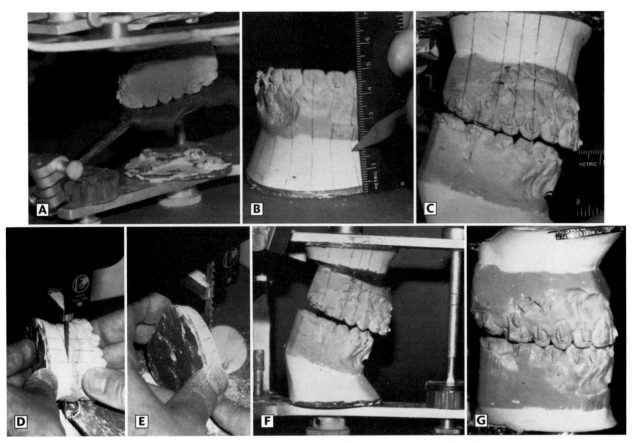

FIGURE 22-28 Steps in model surgery for a patient who will have a total maxillary osteotomy and a mandibular advancement. **A,** The casts are mounted on a semi-adjustable articulator, using a facebow transfer. **B** and **C,** Reference lines are drawn on the mounted casts, and the distance from the mounting rim to each cusp, and from the articulator pin to the central incisor, is recorded so that the magnitude of all movements can be evaluated precisely. **D,** The upper cast is cut away from the mounting ring, using a saw, and, **E,** an additional wedge of mounting material is removed, giving room to reposition the upper cast vertically. **F,** The upper cast is remounted in the desired position, with the measurements checked against the cephalometric prediction for this patient. This is the projected result of the first stage of the surgery, and an intermediate splint is made to this mounting (after the upper cast is stabilized with plaster in its final position). **G,** Then the casts are mounted as they will be after the second stage of the surgery, the mandibular advancement. The second splint is made to this mounting. Note the position of the upper second molars, which were deliberately kept depressed during the orthodontic preparation for surgery so there would be no problems with second molar interferences at surgery.

lationships. Minor changes in model orientation that will facilitate subsequent treatment without compromising the surgery can be made at this time.

Plaster mounting of the models on an articulator avoids the possibility of relationships changing during the laboratory procedures. The splint is made with autopolymerizing acrylic and cured in a pressure pot to prevent distortion. It should be as thin as is consistent with adequate strength. This means that the splint almost never should be more than 2 mm thick at the thinnest point where teeth are separated minimally. When the lower arch has not been leveled presurgically, some teeth can contact through the splint.

The splint should be trimmed on the buccal surfaces to allow good hygiene and permit visual verification of proper seating at the time of surgery. With rigid fixation and early jaw mobilization, the splint should be trimmed so that lateral movements are possible, but a solid occlusal relationship is essential, and the patient should wear the splint until post-surgical orthodontics resumes and the stabilizing archwires are removed. Adding clasps to make the splint removable for cleaning, on balance, is not a good idea. It is a mistake to remove the splint without replacing the stabilizing wires with lighter and more flexible archwires (Figure 22-29).

Surgical Management

Today, the vast majority of dentofacial problems are treated with variations of three surgical procedures: LeFort I maxillary downfracture, bilateral sagittal split ramus osteotomy,

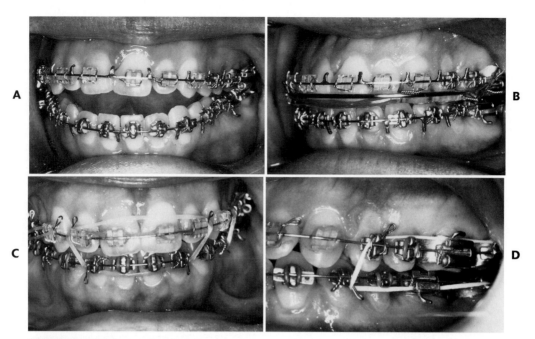

FIGURE 22-29   A, Stabilizing archwires in place prior to surgery (same patient as Figure 22-7). The full-dimension steel wires (17 × 25 in the 18 slot appliance) have soldered lugs for maxillomandibular fixation in the operating room while rigid fixation is being placed. **B,** Four weeks post-surgery, with the splint in place. A 40 mil steel auxiliary wire in the headgear tubes is being used to improve transverse stability, and the patient is functioning into the splint. **C** and **D,** Working archwires and settling elastics after removal of the splint and stabilizing archwires. The light posterior box elastics are worn full-time, including eating, for the first four weeks, and typically are continued full-time except for eating for an additional four weeks. In an open bite patient like this one, an anterior box elastic is worn 12 hours per day for the first 8 weeks. See Figure 22-7 for the result.

and inferior border osteotomy of the mandible to reposition the chin. The few remaining problems can be dealt with using segmental dentoalveolar surgery and mandibular body procedures.

With the trend toward reducing health care costs, hospital stays for modern orthognathic surgery have been reduced considerably. Sagittal split osteotomies of the mandibular ramus often can be performed now on a day-op basis, without overnight hospitalization, and lower border osteotomy of the mandible almost never requires an overnight stay. Maxillary osteotomies typically require overnight hospitalization, and two-jaw surgery almost always requires a 1 to 2 day hospital stay. A well-qualified and experienced nursing team is important in providing the post-surgical care. With early discharge after jaw surgery, telephone access to the nursing team is important. Patients require surprisingly little pain medication, particularly following maxillary surgery. The discomfort associated with prolonged immobilization of the jaws has been reduced by the rigid fixation techniques.

Patients are advised to maintain a soft diet (i.e., milkshakes, potatoes, scrambled eggs, yogurt) for the first week after surgery. Over the next 2 weeks they can progress to foods that require some chewing (soft pasta, meat cut into

pieces), using the degree of discomfort as a guide to their rate of progression. By 6 to 8 weeks after surgery, they should be back on a normal diet. Note that this coincides with the time when orthodontist can allow the patient to eat without the use of elastics (see below).

This progression can be assisted considerably by physical therapy beginning as soon as the initial intracapsular joint edema is resolved—typically about 1 week post-surgically. For the first week after surgery, patients are advised to open and close gently within comfortable limits. Over the next 2 weeks, three 10- to 15-minute sessions of opening and closing exercises as well as lateral movements are indicated. From the third to the eighth week, the range of motion is increased. The goal is to achieve optimum function by 8 weeks. The occlusion and range of motion are carefully monitored at weekly intervals and if problems arise, additional physical therapy may be recommended.

With both rigid and intermaxillary wire fixation techniques, it is important for the orthodontist to see the patient shortly (within 1 week) after surgery to review the patient's occlusal status and to check on the status of the orthodontic appliances. The timing of post-surgical orthodontics depends on the surgeon's estimate of bone healing/stability and on the patient's range of motion.

With rigid fixation, patients who have been placed on a jaw exercise program immediately after surgery often can open satisfactorily 2 to 3 weeks after their operation, allowing for an earlier resumption of active orthodontic treatment. With wire fixation, immobilization for 4 to 6 weeks is required, and active orthodontic treatment is delayed until the patient has achieved a satisfactory range of motion, frequently 3 to 4 weeks after the release of immobilization. With both fixation techniques, when jaw function first resumes the acrylic splint is ligated to one of the arches to key the occlusion, and light elastics are used to guide jaw function.

Post-surgical Orthodontics

Once satisfactory range of motion and stability are achieved, the finishing stage of orthodontics can be started. It is critically important that when the splint is removed, the stabilizing archwires are also removed and replaced by working wires to bring the teeth to their final position. This means that usually the orthodontist, not the surgeon, should remove the splint. Light vertical elastics are needed initially with these working archwires (see Figure 22-29), not so much for tooth movement—the archwires should do that—but to override proprioceptive impulses from the teeth that otherwise would cause the patient to seek a new position of maximum intercuspation. Until the stabilizing archwires are removed, the teeth are held tightly in the pre-surgical position. Removing the splint without allowing the teeth to settle into better interdigitation can result in the patient adopting an undesirable convenience bite, which in turn complicates orthodontic finishing and could stress recent surgery sites.

The type of archwire used for final settling is determined by the amount of movement needed. Minor movement can be achieved rapidly using light round wires (typically 16 mil steel) and posterior box elastics with an anterior vector that supports the sagittal correction. A flexible rectangular wire in the upper arch to maintain torque control of the maxillary incisors (in 18 slot, 17 × 25 TMA; in 22 slot, 21 × 25 M-NiTi or braided steel) often is a good choice, with a round wire in the lower arch. Elastics can be discontinued when a solid occlusion is established. Typically, patients wear the light elastics full-time including eating for the first four weeks, full-time except for eating for another four weeks, and just at night for a third four-week period. Elastics can be discontinued during the final detailing of the occlusion.

Retention after surgical orthodontics is no different than for other adult patients (see Chapters 19 and 21). Definitive periodontal and prosthetic treatment can follow the establishment of the final occlusal relationships.

Post-surgical Stability and Clinical Success

The Hierarchy of Stability and Predictability in Surgical Treatment. The stability of orthognathic surgical procedures has been the subject of numerous studies. Sta-

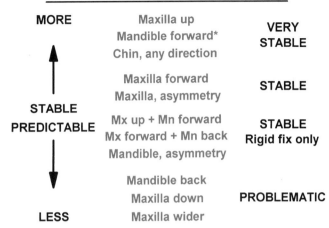

Surgical-Orthodontic Treatment: A Hierarchy of Stability

MORE	Maxilla up / Mandible forward* / Chin, any direction	VERY STABLE
	Maxilla forward / Maxilla, asymmetry	STABLE
STABLE PREDICTABLE	Mx up + Mn forward / Mx forward + Mn back / Mandible, asymmetry	STABLE Rigid fix only
LESS	Mandible back / Maxilla down / Maxilla wider	PROBLEMATIC

* short or normal face height only

FIGURE 22-30 The hierarchy of stability, based on the UNC data base.[29] In this context, very stable means better than a 90% chance of no significant post-surgical change; stable means better than an 80% chance of no change and major relapse quite unlikely; problematic means some degree of relapse likely and major relapse possible.

bility after surgical repositioning of the jaws varies depending on the direction of movement, the type of fixation used, and the surgical technique employed, largely in that order of importance. In a recent review paper, the various jaw movements possible at surgery were ranked in order of stability and predictability (Figure 22-30).[29]

The most stable orthognathic procedure is superior repositioning of the maxilla, closely followed by mandibular advancement in patients whom anterior facial height is maintained or increased. It is important to note that the stability of mandibular advancement is influenced by the pattern of rotation of the mandible as it is advanced. When anterior facial height is decreased by rotating the mandible so that the mandibular plane angle decreases, the gonial angle tends to be pulled downward. This stretches soft tissues in that area, and stability is compromised. For that reason, maxillary surgery is needed when face height is decreased, even if mandibular advancement is necessary at the same time. The combination of moving the maxilla upward and the mandible forward is significantly more stable when rigid internal fixation is used in the mandible.

Forward movement of the maxilla is stable in about 80% of patients. Twenty per cent show modest relapse, but there is almost no tendency for major relapse. In contrast, mandibular setback often is unstable. So is downward movement of the maxilla that creates downward-backward rotation of the mandible. It has been suggested that in mandibular setback, controlling the inclination of the ramus at surgery is a key to stability. For downward movement of the maxilla, interpositional grafting with synthetic hydroxylapatite and simultaneous ramus osteotomy improve stability, but some degree of relapse remains likely. In two jaw Class III surgery, the stability of each jaw appears to be similar to that of isolated maxillary advancement or mandibular setback.

Surgical widening of the maxilla is the least stable of the orthognathic surgical procedures. Widening the maxilla stretches the palatal mucosa, and its elastic rebound is the major cause of the relapse tendency. Strategies to control relapse include overcorrection initially and careful retention afterward, with either a heavy orthodontic archwire or a palatal bar during the completion of orthodontic treatment and then a palate-covering retainer for at least the first post-surgical year. There are no good data to document the effectiveness of these modifications in technique.

If the resistance of the lateral buttresses of the maxilla is reduced by an osteotomy in that area, a jackscrew usually can open the mid-palatal suture, even in adults, by microfracture of interlocking bone spicules at the suture. Although this type of surgically-assisted rapid palatal expansion (SARPE) has been suggested as a more stable alternative to segmental Le Fort I osteotomy, the patterns of movement resulting from the two procedures are different, and differences in stability have not been established. One important difference between Le Fort I segmental oteotomy and SARPE is the pattern of expansion. With a maxillary segmental osteotomy, expansion is typically greater in the posterior maxilla than in the anterior maxilla. With jackscrew expansion, whether orthopedic or surgically assisted, the reverse occurs; there is more expansion anteriorly than posteriorly. This difference in patterns of expansion may contribute to some differences in stability between Le Fort I osteotomy and SARPE.

When a choice exists between SARPE and maxillary segmental osteotomy, an important guideline is that if the patient will require additional maxillary surgery after transverse expansion has been achieved, there is little reason to perform surgery twice. For example, the long-face patient with a narrow maxilla who will require superior repositioning of the maxilla in addition to surgical widening of the palate, can have both procedures performed simultaneously, rather than increasing the risks, cost and morbidity associated with two procedures. It appears that some relapse is inevitable no matter which method of expansion is used, and relapse should be accounted for in the initial treatment planning.

Three principles that influence post-surgical stability can be proposed:

1. Stability is greatest when soft tissues are relaxed during the surgery and least when they are stretched. Moving the maxilla upward relaxes tissues. Moving the mandible forward stretches tissues, but rotating it upward posteriorly and downward anteriorly decreases the amount of stretch. It is not surprising that the least stable mandibular advancements are those that lengthen the ramus and rotate the chin up, while the most stable advance-

ments rotate the mandible in the opposite direction. The least stable orthognathic surgical procedure is widening of the maxilla that stretches the heavy, inelastic palatal mucosa.

2. Neuromuscular adaptation is an essential requirement for stability. Fortunately, most orthognathic procedures lead to good neuromuscular adaptation. When the maxilla is moved upward, the postural position of the mandible alters in concert with the new maxillary movement, and occlusal forces tend to increase rather than decrease.[30] This controls any tendency for the maxilla to immediately relapse downward, and contributes to the excellent stability of this surgical movement. Repositioning of the tongue to maintain airway dimensions, (i.e., a change in tongue posture) occurs as an adaptation to changes produced by mandibular osteotomy. These adaptations of the tongue, and adaptation in lip pressures that also occur post-surgically, contribute to the stability of tooth positions.[31] In contrast, neuromuscular adaptation does not occur when the pterygomandibular sling is stretched during mandibular osteotomy, as when the mandible is rotated to close an open bite. One would expect that if the neuromuscular system reacts to change in the vertical position of the maxilla, adjustment in muscle length should occur when the maxilla is moved downward just as it does when the maxilla is moved upward. Even if the muscles adapt, however, the stretch of other soft tissues apparently can lead to the instability that is observed when the maxilla is moved downward and the mandible is forced to rotate downward and backward.

3. Neuromuscular adaptation affects muscular length, not muscular orientation. If the orientation of a muscle group such as the mandibular elevators is changed, adaptation cannot be expected. This concept is best illustrated by the effect of changing the inclination of the mandibular ramus when the mandible is set back or advanced. Successful mandibular advancement requires keeping the ramus in an upright position rather than letting it incline forward as the mandibular body is brought forward. The same is true, in reverse, when the mandible is set back: a major cause of instability appears to be the tendency at surgery to push the ramus posteriorly when the chin is moved back.

It seems reasonable that by one year post-surgery both physiological adaptation and morphological change resulting from the surgery should be complete (Figure 22-31). Although most patients are quite stable long-term and average changes are small, 5-year follow-up data show a surprising amount of change in the position of skeletal landmarks beyond the first post-surgical year. Long-term condylar resorption is of particular concern. As one would expect, long-term condylar changes are not observed in

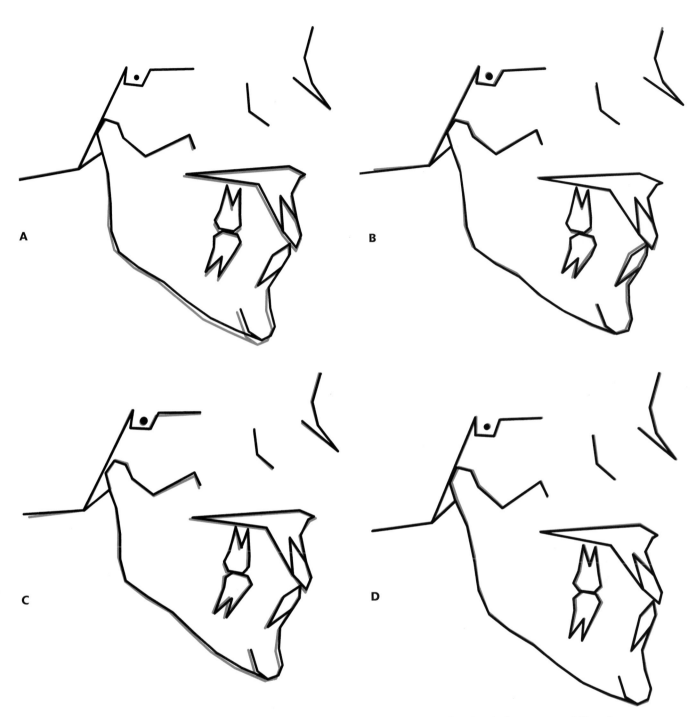

FIGURE 22-31 Computer-generated composite superimpositions showing the long-term stability of **A,** superior repositioning of the maxilla (in long-face patients), **B,** mandibular advancement (short and normal face height only), **C,** two-jaw surgery for Class II problems (superior repositioning of the maxilla plus mandibular advancement), and, **D,** two-jaw surgery for Class III problems (maxillary advancement plus mandibular setback). Note that the mean changes are quite small for each of these treatment procedures, but significant long-term changes do occur in a small number of the patients.

patients who had maxillary surgery only.[15] At 5-year recall, bony changes associated with shortening of the condylar processes (which may not be associated with surgical relapse), were observed in approximately 5% of the relatively large group of patients who underwent mandibular advancement at UNC with or without simultaneous maxillary surgery.[32,33] Surprisingly, although surgical correction of Class III problems is less stable than Class II correction in the short-term post-surgically, it appears to be more stable long-term.[34]

It has not been determined why a few patients are susceptible to long-term changes. It is important to continue to follow well-defined groups of patients who received orthognathic surgery, to improve the quality of the data available, and to resolve questions of long-term stability.

REFERENCES

1. Angle EH: Double resection of the lower maxilla, Dental Cosmos 40:July-Dec, 1898.
2. Trauner R, Obwegeser H: The surgical correction of mandibular prognathism and retrognathia with consideration of genioplasty, Oral Surg Oral Med Oral Pathol 10:671-692, 1957.
3. Bell WH: LeFort I osteotomy for correction of maxillary deformities, J Oral Surg 33:412-426, 1975.
4. Epker BN, Wolford LM: Middle third facial osteotomies: their use in the correction of acquired and developmental dentofacial and craniofacial deformities, J Oral Surg 33:491-514, 1975.
5. Ackerman JL, Proffit WR: Soft tissue limitations in orthodontic treatment, Angle Orthod 67:327-336, 1997.
6. Ackerman JL, Proffit WR, Sarver DM: The emerging soft tissue paradigm in orthodontic diagnosis and treatment planning, Clin Orthod Res 2:49-52, 1999.
7. Eagly AH, Ashmore RD, Makhijani MG, Longo LC: What is beautiful is good, but . . .: a meta-analytic review of research on the physical attractiveness stereotype, Psych Bull 110:109-128, 1991.
8. Phillips C, Bennett ME, Broder HL: Dentofacial disharmony: psychological status of patient seeking a treatment consultation, Angle Orthod 68:547-566, 1998.
9. Kiyak HA, Bell R: Psychologic considerations in surgery and orthodontics. In Proffit WR, White RP, Surgical-orthodontic treatment, St Louis, 1991, Mosby.
10. Sarver DM: Esthetic orthodontics and orthognathic surgery, St Louis, 1997, Mosby.
11. Cunningham SJ, Crean SJ, Hunt NP et al: Preparation, perceptions and problems: a long-term follow-up study of orthognathic surgery, Int J Adult Orthod Orthognath Surg 11:41-47, 1996.
12. Phillips C: Psychologic ramifications of orthognathic surgery. In Fonseca R (editor): Oral & maxillofacial surgery, vol 1, Philadelphia, W.B. Saunders, in press.
13. Cunningham LL Jr, Tiner BD, Clark GM et al: A comparison of questionnaire versus monofilament assessment of neurosensory deficit, J Oral Maxillofac Surg 54:454-459, 1996.
14. Proffit WR, Phillips C, Turvey TA: Stability following superior repositioning of the maxilla by LeFort I osteotomy, Am J Orthod Dentofac Orthop 92:151-161, 1987.
15. Bailey LJ, Phillips C, Proffit WR: Stability following superior repositioning of the maxilla by LeFort I osteotomy: five-year follow-up, Int J Adult Orthod Orthognath Surg 9:163-174, 1994.
16. Proffit WR, Phillips C, Prewitt JW, Turvey TA: Stability after surgical-orthodontic correction of skeletal Class III malocclusion. II. Maxillary advancement, Int J Adult Orthod Orthognath Surg 6:71-80, 1991.
17. Wardrop RW, Wolford LM: Maxillary stability following downgraft and/or advancement procedures with stabilization using rigid fixation and porous block hydroxylapatite implants, J Oral Maxillofac Surg 47:336-342, 1989.
18. Proffit WR, Phillips C, Turvey TA: Stability after surgical-orthodontic correction of skeletal Class III malocclusion. III. Combined maxillary and mandibular procedure, Int J Adult Orthod Orthognath Surg 6:211-225, 1991.
19. Silverstein K, Quinn PD: Surgically-assisted rapid palatal expansion for management of transverse maxillary deficiency, J Oral Maxillofac Surg 55:725-727, 1997.
20. Bailey LJ, White RP, Proffit WR, Turvey TA: Segmental LeFort I osteotomy for management of transverse maxillary deficiency, J Oral Maxillofac Surg 55:728-731, 1997.
21. Weil TS, van Sickels JE, Payne CJ: Distraction osteogenesis for correction of transverse mandibular deficiency: a preliminary report, J Oral Maxillofac Surg 55:953-960, 1997.
22. Severt TR, Proffit WR: The prevalence of facial asymmetry in the dentofacial deformities population at the University of North Carolina, Int J Adult Orthod Orthognath Surg 12:171-176, 1997.
23. Snow MD, Turvey TA, Walker D, Proffit WR: Surgical mandibular advancement in adolescents: postsurgical growth related to stability, Int J Adult Orthod Orthognath Surg 6:143-151, 1991.
24. Roberts HG, Semb G, Hathorn I, Killingback N: Facial growth in patients with unilateral clefts of the lip and palate: a two-center study, Cleft Palate-Craniofacial J 31:372-375, 1996.
25. Ackerman JL, Proffit WR: Communication in orthodontic treatment planning: bioethical and informed consent issues, Angle Orthod 65:253-262, 1995.
26. Sarver DM, Johnston MW, Matukas VJ: Video imaging for planning and counselling in orthognathic surgery, J Oral Maxillofac Surg 46:939-945, 1988.
27. Sinclair P, Kilpelanien P, Phillips C, White R Jr, Rogers L, Sarver D: The accuracy of video imaging in orthognathic surgery, Am J Dentofac Orthop Orthod 107:177-85, 1995.
28. Bell RB, Phillips C, Manente SJ: Patients' expctations following video imaging prior to orthognathic surgery, J Oral Maxillofacial Surg 55 (supplement 3), 88-89, 1997.
29. Proffit WR, Turvey TA, Phillips C: Orthognathic surgery: a hierarchy of stability, Int J Adult Orthod Orthognath Surg 11:191-204, 1996.
30. Proffit WR, Phillips C, Fields HW, Turvey TA: The effect of orthognathic surgery on occlusal force, J Oral Maxillofac Surg 47:457-463, 1989.
31. Proffit WR, Phillips C: Adaptations in lip posture and pressure following orthognathic surgery, Am J Orthod 93:294-304, 1988.

32. Simmons KE, Turvey TA, Phillips C, Proffit WR: Surgical-orthodontic correction of mandibular deficiency: five-year follow-up, Int J Adult Orthod Orthognath Surg 7:67-80, 1992.

33. Miguel JA, Turvey TA, Phillips C, Proffit WR: Long-term stability of two-jaw surgery for treatment of mandibular deficiency and vertical maxillary excess, Int J Adult Orthod Orthognath Surg 10:235-245, 1995.

34. Bailey LJ, Duong HL, Proffit WR: Surgical Class III treatment: long-term stability and patient perceptions of treatment outcome, Int J Adult Orthod Orthognath Surg 13: 35-44, 1998.

INDEX

ISBN 1-5566-4553-8

9 781556 645532

90000

32119